Medical Speech–Language Pathology: A Practitioner's Guide

Medical
Speech–Language
Pathology:
A Practitioner's Guide

Edited by

Alex F. Johnson and Barbara H. Jacobson

Henry Ford Hospital
Detroit, Michigan

1998
THIEME
New York • Stuttgart

Thieme Medical Publishers, Inc.
333 Seventh Avenue
New York, NY 10001

Medical Speech–Language Pathology: A Practitioner's Guide
Alex F. Johnson
Barbara H. Jacobson

Library of Congress Cataloging-in-Publication Data

Medical speech—language pathology : a practitioner's guide / edited by
    Alex F. Johnson and Barbara H. Jacobson.
        p.   cm.
      Includes bibliographical references and index.
      ISBN 0–86577–688–1 (TMP). — ISBN 3–13–110531–3 (GTV)
      1. Speech therapy.   2. Speech disorders.   3. Language disorders.
    I. Johnson, Alex F.   II. Jacobson, Barbara H.
      [DNLM: 1. Speech Disorders.   2. Language Disorders.
    3. Deglutition Disorders.   WL 340.2 M489 1997]
    RC423.M395   1998
    616.85′5—dc21
    DNLM/DLC
    for Library of Congress   97–41324
                                                                        CIP

Important note: Medical knowledge is ever-changing. As new research and clinical experience broaden our knowledge, changes in treatment and drug therapy may be required. The authors and editors of the material herein have consulted sources believed to be reliable in their efforts to provide information that is complete and in accord with the standards accepted at the time of publication. However, in view of the possibility of human error by the authors, editors, or publisher of the work herein, or changes in medical knowledge, neither the authors, editors, publisher, nor any other party who has been involved in the preparation of this work, warrants that the information contained herein is in every respect accurate or complete, and they are not responsible for any errors or omissions or for the results obtained from use of such information. Readers are encouraged to confirm the information contained herein with other sources. For example, readers are advised to check the product information sheet included in the package of each drug they plan to administer to be certain that the information contained in this publication is accurate and that changes have not been made in the recommended dose or in the contraindications for administration. This recommendation is of particular importance in connection with new or infrequently used drugs.

Some of the product names, patents, and registered designs referred to in this book are in fact registered trademarks or proprietary names even though specific reference to this fact is not always made in the text. Therefore, the appearance of a name without designation as proprietary is not to be construed as a representation by the publisher that it is in the public domain.

Printed in the United States of America

5   4   3   2

TNY ISBN 0-86577-688-1
GTV ISBN 3-13-110531-3

This book is dedicated to the members of the Division of Speech–Language Sciences & Disorders, Department of Neurology, Henry Ford Hospital. Our colleagues have served as our best teachers.

Preface

This book is the product of our own experience and commitment to the development and expansion of speech, language, and swallowing services to patients with medical problems. This area of interest within the profession of speech–language pathology is quickly growing. The medical continuum of care in speech–language pathology extends from acute care to rehabilitation to more chronic settings and even to hospice. This growth suggests that the field has discovered that it can contribute to the health and quality of life in patients at virtually every point in their health care delivery system.

Although the medical aspect of our practice is an important part of our heritage, significant developments within the field have worked to expand both knowledge and service. This is reflected not only in the growth in numbers of settings, practitioners, and continuing education opportunities, but is also seen in the establishment of the relatively new publication, *The Journal of Medical Speech–Language Pathology.*

Given the growth of information and interest in medical speech–language pathology, we have attempted to develop a resource book for use by teachers, students, and practitioners. The text is designed to address the breadth of medical speech–language pathology, while giving in-depth attention to some special topics—neuroimaging, pharmacology, language in epilepsy, ethics, psychogenic disorders—which have been underrepresented in most speech–language texts. In addition, the contributors to this text represent a variety of disciplines including speech–language pathology, otolaryngology, neurology, neurosurgery, psychiatry, internal medicine, geriatrics, pharmacology, and radiologic science. As is always the case, the value of the book is increased significantly by the outstanding work of such a diverse group of contributors.

This text is organized into sections, each composed of a variety of chapters by recognized practitioners and scholars within our discipline. Section I provides a brief overview and introduction to the scope and issues involved in service delivery within the field. This section is designed to provide a context for consideration of the subsequent pieces of this comprehensive text. Section II focuses on a range of topics related to the practice of medical speech–language pathology within the context of the health system. In particular, we examine those aspects of patient care that are key points in the continuum of service. In addition, Section II focuses on selected aspects of medical practice that contribute to the care and outcomes in patients with communication disorders. Section III provides substantive discussion of the various aspects of the interplay between neurology and speech–language pathology. In Section IV we consider the relationship of speech–language pathology to otolaryngologic disease and practice. Section V covers basic principles of psychiatry and the interaction between speech–language pathology and psychiatric practice. Section VI examines some of the current issues impacting service delivery in our field—the health reform movement and outcomes assessment.

Review of the list of contributors will reveal the true multidisciplinary nature of medical speech–language pathology and of this text. Many contributors are experts with whom we have had the opportunity to interact on a daily basis. They are professionals whom we hold in high regard and who have positively affected the care of our patients. In addition, over the past several years they have been our friends and our teachers. Other contributors are recognized authorities within the field, whom we have come to know as we have developed this book and its content.

Medical Speech–Language Pathology: A Practitioner's Guide has been designed with multiple purposes. We believe it could serve as a comprehensive text for a course in medical speech–language pathology. It can also function as a support text for traditional courses in dysphagia, aphasia, voice, or motor speech disorders. Finally, and most importantly, this book has been designed to serve as a support text for the clinical practitioner within the discipline.

ALEX F. JOHNSON
BARBARA H. JACOBSON

Acknowledgments

Every person who has authored or edited a book knows the work that is involved. The long tedious process of writing, reading, and editing at times seems never ending. The opportunity to participate in this difficult work with so many wonderful friends and colleagues has been exhilarating. We are, first of all, grateful to all our contributors for their effort in making this book comprehensive and unique.

Next, we thank our editor, Andrea Seils, at Thieme Medical Publishing. Andrea and her staff have been exceptional in offering support and leadership toward the text's completion. We are very grateful to have experienced the benefit of such a strong and committed group of professionals. They have been consistently responsive and sensitive to our needs as authors who were fitting writing in between patients and meetings.

We also thank our colleagues at Henry Ford Health System in Detroit, Michigan. We work with an outstanding group of speech–language pathologists, neurologists, otolaryngologists, and other specialists. Some of them have contributed directly to this text as authors. Others have contributed over the past several years through discussions, lectures, and serving as resources to inform our thinking and our practice. We extend particular gratitude to the clinical and support staff in the Division of Speech–Language Sciences and Disorders. They have served as important contributors, persistent readers, and valued friends. Our secretaries, Carol Mead, Kim Jamerson, and Anita Anderson have also remained friendly despite our mood swings and our pressure to meet deadlines.

We also extend our appreciation to our families. Our spouses (Linda and Gary) and our children (David, Jeffrey, and Cristina) have been very supportive and willing to share their time with us to see the "book" become reality.

Finally, we thank each other!. We have worked together for the past nine years, and this book represents concepts and clinical information that we have developed together. We are grateful for the opportunity to have learned from each other and to have shared ideas, experiences, and patients as our practice has evolved.

A. J.
B. J.

Contents

Contributors

Joan C. Arvedson, Ph.D.
Director
Speech–Language and Hearing Department
Children's Hospital of Buffalo
Buffalo, New York

Michael A. Basha, D.O.
Pulmonary and Critical Care Specialist
Physican Healthcare Network
Port Huron, Michigan

Michael S. Benninger, Ph.D.
Chair
Department of Otolaryngology–
   Head and Neck Surgery
Henry Ford Hospital
Detroit, Michigan

Yue Cao, Ph.D.
Senior Bioscientific Staff
Department of Neurology Research
Henry Ford Hospital
Detroit, Michigan

Carl Coelho, Ph.D.
Assistant Professor
Department of Communication Sciences
University of Connecticut
Storrs, Connecticut

Speech–Language Pathologist
University of Connecticut Health Center
Farmington, Connecticut

Kost Elisevich, M.D., Ph.D.
Senior Staff
Department of Neurosurgery
Henry Ford Hospital
Detroit, Michigan

Susan C. Fagan, Pharm.D.
Associate Professor and Associate Chair
Department of Pharmacy Practice
Wayne State University
Detroit, Michigan

John Fisk
Neuropsychologist
Department of Neuropsychology
Henry Ford Hospital
Detroit, Michigan

Cathy Frank, M.D.
Director
Psychiatric Education
Medical Director
Ambulatory Psychiatry
Department of Psychiatry
Henry Ford Health System
Detroit, Michigan

Carol M. Frattali, Ph.D.
Research Coordinator
Speech–Language Pathology Section
W.G. Magnuson Clinical Center
National Institutes of Health
Bethesda, Maryland

Glendon M. Gardner, M.D.
Senior Staff Otolaryngologist
Department of Otolaryngology–
   Head and Neck Surgery
Henry Ford Hospital
Detroit, Michigan

K. Paige George, M.A., CCC, SLP
Speech–Language Pathologist
Division of Speech–Language
   Sciences and Disorders
Henry Ford Hospital
Detroit, Michigan

Bernice K. Gerdeman, Ph.D.
Voice Pathologist
Institute for Voice Analysis and Rehabilitation
Dayton, Ohio

Leslie E. Glaze, Ph.D.
Director of Clinical Program
Department of Communication Disorders
University of Minnesota
Minneapolis, Minnesota

Keith J. Goulden, M.D., FRCPC
Associate Professor
University of Alberta
    and Glenrose Rehabilitation Hospital
Edmonton, Alberta, Canada

Cindy Grywalski, M.A.
Speech–Language Pathologist
Division of Speech–Language
    Sciences and Disorders
Henry Ford Hospital
Detroit, Michigan

Jackie Hinckley, M.S., CCC-SLP
Head of Aphasia Services
Communicative Disorders Clinic
University of Michigan
Ann Arbor, Michigan

Megan Hodge, Ph.D.
Associate Professor
Department of Speech Pathology
    and Audiology
University of Alberta
Edmonton, Alberta, Canada

Murray B. Hunter, M.D.
Senior Staff Physician
Department of Geriatrics
Henry Ford Center for Seniors
Detroit, Michigan

Barbara H. Jacobson, Ph.D.
Senior Staff Speech–Language Pathologist
Division of Speech–Language
    Sciences and Disorders
Henry Ford Hospital
Detroit, Michigan

Gary Jacobson, Ph.D.
Director
Division of Audiology
Henry Ford Health System
Detroit, Michigan

Alex F. Johnson, Ph.D.
Director
Division of Speech–Language
    Sciences and Disorders
Henry Ford Hospital
Detroit, Michigan

Michael P. Karnell, Ph.D.
Associate Professor
Department of Otolaryngology–
    Head and Neck Surgery
University of Iowa
Iowa City, Iowa

Ann W. Kummer, Ph.D.
Director
Department of Speech Pathology
Children's Hospital Medical Center
Cincinnati, Ohio

Field Service Associate Professor
Clinical Pediatrics
University of Cincinnati Medical Center
Cincinnati, Ohio

Susan Langmore, Ph.D.
Chief
Audiology and Speech Pathology Service
Veteran's Administration Medical Center
Ann Arbor, Michigan

Jeri A. Logemann, Ph.D.
Ralph and Jean Sundin Professor
Department of Communication Sciences
    and Disorders
Northwestern University
Evanston, Illinois

Greg Mahr, M.D.
Division Head
Consultation Liaison Psychiatrist
Henry Ford Hospital
Detroit, Michigan

Janet H. Marsh, M.A.
Speech–Language Pathologist
Children's Hospital Medical Center
Cincinnati, Ohio

Robert M. Miller, Ph.D.
Chief, Audiology and Pathology
Veteran's Administration Medical Center
Puget Sound Health Care System
Seattle, Washington

Nan D. Musson, M.A.
Speech–Language Pathologist
Veteran's Administration Medical Center
Miami, Florida

Daniel Newman, Ph.D.
Director
Hoenselaar A.L.S. Clinic
Department of Neurology
Henry Ford Hospital
Detroit, Michigan

Tami O'Sullivan, Pharm.D.
Clinical Specialist
Internal Medicine
Pharmacy Department
St. Joseph Mercy Hospital
Ann Arbor, Michigan

Thomas R. Palmer, M.D.
Medical Director
Inpatient Geriatric Service
Henry Ford Hospital
Detroit, Michigan

Assistant Professor
Family Medicine
Case Western Reserve University
Cleveland, Ohio

Arlene Pietranton, Ph.D.
Associate Director for Speech–Language Pathology
American Speech–Language–Hearing Association
Rockville, Maryland

Nabih Ramadan, M.D.
Associate Professor of Neurology
Director
Cincinnati Headache Center
Department of Neurology
University of Cincinnati
Cincinnati, Ohio

Danielle N. Ripich, Ph.D.
Professor
Department of Communication Sciences
Associate Dean
College of Arts and Sciences
Case Western Reserve University
Cleveland, Ohio

Brian T. Rogers, M.D.
Chief
Division of Developmental Pediatrics
   and Rehabilitation
Children's Hospital of Buffalo
Buffalo, New York

Rhonna S. Shatz, D.O.
Director
Behavioral Neurology
Department of Neurology
Henry Ford Hospital
Detroit, Michigan

Alice K. Silbergleit, Ph.D.
Senior Staff
Speech–Language Pathologist
Division of Speech–Language
   Sciences and Disorders
Henry Ford Hospital
Detroit, Michigan

Brien Smith, M.D.
Director
Epilepsy Monitoring Unit
Senior Staff Neurologist
Department of Neurology
Henry Ford Hospital
Detroit, Michigan

Joseph C. Stemple, Ph.D.
Director
Institute for Voice Analysis
   and Rehabilitation
Dayton, Ohio

Edythe A. Strand, Ph.D.
Associate Professor
Department of Speech and Hearing Sciences
University of Washington
Seattle, Washington

John D. Tonkovich, Ph.D.
Speech–Language Pathologist
Private Practice
Shelby Township, Michigan

Anne Marie Valachovic, M.A.
Speech Pathologist
Division of Speech–Language
   Sciences and Disorders
Henry Ford Hospital
Detroit, Michigan

Eric M. Vikingstad, B.S.
Student
Department of Neurology
NMR Research
Henry Ford Hospital
Detroit, Michigan

Kathryn M. Yorkston, Ph.D.
Professor
Department of Rehabilitation Medicine
University of Washington
Seattle, Washington

Elaine Ziol, M.H.S.
Research Associate
Department of Communication Sciences
Case Western Reserve University
Cleveland, Ohio

SECTION I

Introduction to Medical Speech–Language Pathology

1

The Scope of Medical Speech–Language Pathology

ALEX F. JOHNSON AND BARBARA H. JACOBSON

CHAPTER OUTLINE

Why Differentiate Medical from Nonmedical Speech–Language Pathology (SLP)?

Medical Speech–Language Pathology: The Continuum of Care

Medical Speech–Language Pathology: Subspecialization

Medical Speech–Language Pathology: Procedures and Competencies

---

The field of speech–language pathology has a rich and long history of service to individuals who suffer from a variety of physical and psychological symptoms and diseases. The study of speech–language sciences and disorders includes attention to:

- The underlying anatomy and physiological processes that are used in thinking about, understanding, formulating, and producing communication.
- The psychological and social mechanisms that nurture communication or destroy it.
- The physical processes that allow sound to be generated, transmitted, and perceived.
- The conditions, both developmental and acquired, that impede the use of communication.
- The environmental inputs and factors that encourage or discourage communication in all its forms.

When such topics are studied from perspectives that emphasize the physical processes, causes, associated signs and symptoms, pathophysiology, and disease processes, then we are using models and tools developed in the medical sciences. Over hundreds of years, those who have studied human medicine and disease have used a common model to expand the understanding of disease and approaches to its treatment. It should be no secret to those in our discipline that our processes and models have evolved from a similar framework, as have those in many other health disciplines (dentistry, optometry, veterinary medicine, psychology, etc.). While those who study medicine have developed and emphasized the use of surgery and pharmaceutical treatments, speech–language pathologists have provided distinctive behavioral and physiological approaches to patient management.

3

WHY DIFFERENTIATE MEDICAL FROM NONMEDICAL SLP?

There are few good reasons for differentiating medical and non-medical speech–language pathology practice. Every clinician practicing in the field needs to know about the care of individuals with a variety of disorders. Regardless of the setting in which he or she practices, the speech–language pathologist must understand the causes and effects of communication disorders. This understanding can only come from an in-depth knowledge of the physical, anatomical, and physiological processes involved in communication and an understanding of the conditions producing the disorders that interrupt it.

It is important to highlight two perspectives regarding the categorization of speech–language pathology into components that are medical and those that are nonmedical. One school proposes that a *distinct* category of professional practice within the field encompasses a body of information and a range of clinical activities that impact a patient's medical status or are impacted by a patient's medical condition. Proponents of this school of thought suggest that this aspect of speech–language pathology practice should be delimited and defined by the term "medical." This approach serves to signal the key feature of the speech–language practice being discussed and also differentiate it from other aspects of the field (i.e., educational, developmental, etc.).

A second perspective suggests that all speech–language pathology is medical. That is, the bases of our understanding of human communication and its disorders are found in an interplay between the physical, biological, and behavioral sciences. This viewpoint emphasizes that, regardless of the setting in which we practice, the types of patients (or clients or students) who we treat, or the nature of our clinical activities, the practice of the profession is based in clinical science and is therefore medical. This group would argue that there is no area of practice that could be considered "nonmedical." While this appears true when one focuses on the understanding of the underlying bases of human communication, it is a less precise description of the service that are delivered in nonhealth care environments. The professional activities of many speech–language pathologists concentrate on the use of language and communication for particular purposes in highly specific settings, such as the school or the workplace. An argument can be made for differentiating this particular set of practices from those directed to more immediate health concerns of the patient.

Our own position represents a compromise between these two perspectives. At the superordinate level, it is easy to recognize the interplay among the behavioral, physical, and life sciences in understanding the nature and treatment of speech, language, and swallowing disorders. At the more direct practice level, the benefit of discussing a "category" of practice within the field helps to align discussion for the important details of clinical diagnosis and treatment for the practitioner. Thus, we recognize the essential contribution of the scientific bases of the discipline, acknowledging that this foundation is shared with other health science professions. At the same time, we argue that there are speech–language patholgists who apply this information in nonmedical settings with persons who may or may not be ill, directed toward expected outcomes that are vocational or educational. Thus, for pragmatic reasons, we feel comfortable in utilizing the term *medical speech–language pathology* to categorize an aspect of speech–language professional practice that is not necessarily specific to a setting. Instead it represents a specific approach to patient care and a specific set of clinical processes and outcomes that are related to the medical, social, and psychological well-being of the patient.

The practice of medical speech–language pathology may be examined from three different viewpoints. These reflect the ways that we can characterize this area of specialization within the larger field of speech–language pathology. These viewpoints also guide how we regard our professional identity and how we plan for the future. Medical speech–language pathology may defined by: (1) *where* it is practiced (the continuum of care); (2) *who* delivers speech–language services (the specialists and subspecialists); and (3) *how* and *what* types of services are performed (procedures and competencies). The contributors in this text reflect these various approaches to medical speech–language pathology in their chapters.

MEDICAL SPEECH–LANGUAGE PATHOLOGY: THE CONTINUUM OF CARE

Medical speech–language pathology can be practiced in a variety of settings including academic facilities (university medical centers), community hospitals, outpatient clinics, subacute hospitals, rehabilitation settings, home care, nursing homes, and hospice. Medical speech–language pathologists can view themselves within the context of these physical environments. The emphasis on

Table 1–1. Dimensions of Speech–Language Pathology Intervention in the Continuum of Care

	Consultative	Rehabilitation	Maintenance
Acute care	X		
Subacute	X	X	
Acute rehabilitation		X	
Subacute rehabilitation		X	
Outpatient clinic		X	
Nursing home		X	X
Home care	X	X	
Hospice	X		X

various skills and knowledge shifts, depending on where services are delivered. For example, clinicians must be attuned to rapid changes in communication and swallowing as well as medical status when they practice in acute care settings. Their focus of management is primarily consultative. In chronic care environments, speech–language pathologists work to strengthen functional communication for patients whose disease processes are relatively stable. Interventions are rehabilitative or monitoring in nature. However, practice in both environments requires a strong base of knowledge in the pathophysiology of communication disorders (e.g., neurologic disease) as well as the effects of other diseases and conditions on patients (e.g., pulmonary disease, drugs). Table 1–1 outlines the various settings where medical speech–language pathology is practiced and its focus.

MEDICAL SPEECH–LANGUAGE PATHOLOGY: SUBSPECIALIZATION

Medical speech–language pathology may also be viewed in terms of areas of specialization. Clinicians often identify themselves by the type of disorders they treat or the kind of patients they see. Some of the areas that have become quite developed within the field include neurogenic communication disorders, voice disorders, swallowing disorders, tracheostomy/ventilator-dependent patients, and a host of pediatric areas. The extent and depth of knowledge necessary for comprehensive diagnosis and treatment in these areas have prompted the need for specialization. This focus by disorder in medical speech–language pathology follows the medical model. Many physicians train in a particular specialty (neurology or otolaryngol-

ogy) and then seek further education in a subspecialty (laryngology or electrophysiology).

Unfortunately, the notion of specialty-based practice assumes that patients present with disorders that are mutually exclusive. Experience tells us that conditions that result in communication and swallowing deficits can affect multiple systems and that along with a specialty focus in a particular disorder group, speech–language pathologists must also acquire a broad base of knowledge in the pathophysiology of communication and swallowing disorders.

The move toward specialty recognition by ASHA can be seen as an indication of the complexity of speech–language pathology practice today. Several Special Interest Divisions (SIDs) within ASHA have begun the process of setting forth standards for speech–language pathologists to obtain specialty recognition. When certain individuals are recognized as having specialized skills and knowledge, referring patients to other clinicians is simplified. In addition, this process can result in a more precise identity for the practitioner within the sphere of health care.

MEDICAL SPEECH–LANGUAGE PATHOLOGY: PROCEDURES AND COMPETENCIES

The practice of medical speech–language pathology may also be defined by a set of tasks, protocols, and competencies. This focus has become more common as diagnosis and treatment rely on technology. Within the last 15 years, practice in voice and swallowing disorders has become dependent on the use of endoscopy and radiographic techniques for definitive diagnosis and treatment planning for dysphonia and dysphagia, respectively.

Because of the potential for risk to patients during various procedures, clearly defined competencies (skill and knowledge based) are required for assurance of safety to patients and for the proper interpretation of results.

This trend for instrumentally based practice is reflected in the development of several practice guidelines by ASHA. In addition, several groups, including the Special Interest Divisions of ASHA, have developed draft competencies for a variety of areas of practice in medical speech–language pathology. Although these competencies are early in their development, it is probable that ASHA and other professional groups will be disseminating information about practice in this area.

As documents that focus on professional competencies are developed, they will specify the information necessary to understand background information from the sciences, psychology, and speech–language pathology; funds of knowledge from the medical field; and skills in service delivery specific to the medical setting. The specific competencies for practice will always be challenged by the emerging technologies and new information that become available to the practitioner, the patient, and the referral source. However, in the current practice environment some areas of clinical knowledge and competence that must be considered include:

- structures and functions related to the processes of language, hearing, speech, swallowing, and respiration
- knowledge of physiology
- physiologic and psychological etiologies of communication disorders and dysphagia

- principles of ethics
- utilization of various computer applications in the measurement, diagnosis, and treatment of communication disorders
- interpersonal communication competencies
- medical terminology and basic medical practices
- knowledge of basic physical signs and symptoms
- basic medical diagnostic tests and their purpose
- medical documentation and confidentiality
- pharmacology related to cognitive processes, language, speech, and behavior
- assistive and augmentative technology
- environmental safety issues
- quality assessment and improvement
- nutrition
- anatomical imaging
- medical and surgical management of communication and swallowing
- knowledge and skill of intrumental assessment and treatment
- speech prosthetics
- skill in communication with providers and patients

These items are, of course, in addition to those skills and funds of knowledge that are generic to speech–language pathology. The core of information about disorders, assessment and diagnosis practices are obviously applicable across situations; however, the SLP practicing in the medical setting must have special knowledge and skills in order to function effectively and efficiently.

2

Issues in Medical Speech–Language Pathology

ALEX F. JOHNSON AND BARBARA H. JACOBSON

CHAPTER OUTLINE

Issues Related to Preparation and Education

Issues in Clinical Practice

Issues in Service Delivery

In addition to being defined by the scope of practice established within the profession (see Chapter 1), medical speech–language pathology has been shaped by a myriad of forces and conditions from within the field and also from outside. In this chapter we have attempted to highlight some of those issues for the reader. We will consider three different categories of professional issues: preparation and education, clinical practice, and service delivery.

ISSUES RELATED TO PREPARATION AND EDUCATION

In the past decade significant attention has been given to the selection, development, education, credentialing, certification, and recognition of speech–language pathologists. The rapid growth of the profession and the dynamic changes in practice content that have occurred have forced consistent attention on the development of methods of establishing and improving competency in practice. Several areas have received considerable attention and are worth noting here.

Undergraduate and Graduate Education

Debate has occurred over the role of undergraduate education in the formation of the professional speech–language pathologist. In recent years far more undergraduate degreed persons are applying to graduate programs, with fewer slots open in graduate programs. This mismatch has resulted in considerable frustration on the part of students and undergraduate programs in speech–language pathology yet has furnished graduate institutions with an excellent choice of strong candidates for graduate study. Is it appropriate for undergraduate programs to produce far more graduates in a specialized major than can expect entrance into graduate school? Is the undergraduate speech–language pathology major in most institutions a general degree that allows for a variety of post-graduate career paths and options? If the response to both questions is "yes," then it is likely to be a satisfactory program of study for individuals who might choose professions other than speech–language pathology if they are unable to gain admission to graduate study. However, if the answer is negative, then some individuals advocate admitting more individuals to graduate study or reconsidering the wisdom of an undergraduate major in speech–language pathology. The debate continues and will receive considerable attention in the next decade. It must be noted that this discussion is further complicated by the shortage of qualified speech–language pathologists in some geographic regions of the United States. Employers in both health and educational settings are arguing for admission of more qualified individuals to graduate school.

Another issue related to preprofessional education in speech–language pathology has been the specific focus on the length of combined graduate and undergraduate education (typically 6+ years), as well as the call from the field for more content in the graduate curriculum on topics related to medical speech–language pathology. Specific concerns have been raised about inclusion of more coursework in topics such as traumatic brain injury, dysphagia, augmentative communication, and ventilator-tracheostomy care. Some have suggested that by moving "basic" information into the undergraduate curriculum, more time during the graduate program could be allotted to the study of specialty information. The call for more "professional" information and practice in the undergraduate program is obviously in conflict with the move, discussed in the previous paragraph, to make the undergraduate degree more generic and less "professional."

Continuing Education

Another area currently debated is the area of professional continuing education. In the past 15 years, considerable attention has been given to the emerging importance of continuing education as a vehicle for transmission of new concepts and practice information to professionals in the field. There has been significant growth in the business of continuing education with hundreds of institutions and private companies offering approved workshops, seminars, teleconferences, and video courses for speech–language pathologists. The "business" of continuing education has become a multimillion dollar activity as organizations compete to provide the best speakers and attract the most registrants. While the trend toward improved continuing education opportunities is both exciting and positive, some concerns have emerged within the field.

Major concerns have been expressed regarding the attempt to mandate continuing education ac-

tivity as a requisite for renewal of the CCC-SLP. The concerns center on the issues of geographic availability of continuing education programs, the cost of enrollment in various courses and workshops, and the wisdom of requiring "recertification" once certification standards are initially met. This is another issue that will be debated over the next several years as the public demand for continued demonstration of competence is felt within all professions.

Professional Doctorate

Within speech–language pathology the area of a professional doctorate has not received considerable attention. However, within the sister profession of audiology, a strong grass-roots movement has resulted in the establishment of a handful of graduate professional programs. Some of the conceptual basis for the development of the professional doctorate in audiology emerged from the call of the prominent medical speech–language pathologist, Arnold Aronson,[1] who argued the need for development of a professional doctoral degree for those working in medical settings.

At the current time, a strong case has not been made either for a speech–language pathology professional doctoral degree or for doctoral entry into the profession. It is likely that the success or failure of the movement within audiology will have an effect on the intensity and popularity with which the issue surfaces within speech–language pathology. Because of the size and diversity of the speech–language pathology profession, major changes regarding certification requirements and entry into the profession will likely occur only after lengthy debate and scrutiny from both within and outside the field.

Distance Learning

Technological advances in the delivery of educational information have afforded many individuals new opportunities for learning. A number of universities have begun to offer coursework via videoconference, teleconference, and the Internet to provide access to individuals who cannot attend classes at the traditional campus.

Of significant importance to the practitioner in medical speech–language pathology is the availability of new learning opportunities for continuing education. Because of the rapid growth in information in this area, the need for rapid access, and the increasing cost of off-site learning opportunities, it is likely that institutions will be willing to invest in appropriate hardware to support on-site efforts. One does not have to stretch one's imagination very far to appreciate the potential for frequent, affordable, on-site learning experiences, as well as case conferencing and video presentations. These types of opportunities have the great potential for improving collaboration among professionals as well as affording strong educational opportunities for practitioners in distant locations.

ISSUES IN CLINICAL PRACTICE

Consultative Practice

In consultative practice, service delivery is characterized by intensive short-term interventions that may or may not include direct treatment with the patient. Chapter 8 contains a more extensive description of this practice modality. In medical speech–language pathology, consultation has evolved primarily in acute care settings as a means of effectively managing the care of patients with communication and swallowing disorders who are hospitalized for a relatively short stay. Instead of following standard evaluation and treatment protocols, practice emphasizes answering the referral question posed by the physician, monitoring communication and swallowing status, patient and family education, and discharge planning. This diversion from the strictly rehabilitative focus maintained in the past can be a difficult adjustment for medical speech–language pathologists. Many practitioners derive a great deal of satisfaction from developing therapeutic relationships with the patients they treat, and those connections may not be possible within the practice of consultation.

The practical implications for the clinician are that he or she must develop strong skills in diagnosis, create education materials that are tailored to patient and family needs, and be aware of community resources for further treatment. In addition, clinicians must develop measures that demonstrate the positive outcomes of consultative practice. These might include patient satisfaction measures, assessments of the success of patient and family education, and referral source satisfaction measures. The process of formalization of the key characteristics of consultative practice will continue in the future.

Specialization and Subspecialization

Specialization within the field of medical speech–language pathology is increasing. As noted in Chapter 1, the sheer volume of information required for providing comprehensive services to various types of patients has grown exponentially. Various subspecialties that are emerging include managing patients with dysphagia, aphasia, voice disorders (including laryngectomy), tracheostomies and ventilator-dependency, and traumatic brain injury. Each of these domains requires that practitioners have competencies (in skills and academic areas) to provide quality care. The move toward specialty recognition acknowledges the change in practice and the depth of knowledge required for particular areas of practice.

However, many practice settings do not have the staffing to allow for an individual specialist in each area. Often, the volume of patients is so small that a subspecialist is not indicated for a particular program. One solution is to "group" areas of practice (e.g., voice and swallowing, neurogenic communication disorders). Another option is to have consultants or contingency speech–language pathologists "on call" for assistance in treating certain patients. Achieving a balance between general and specialty medical speech–language pathology practice will continue to be a challenge. As the parameters for specialty recognition develop within the professional associations, so will new models of delivery that include roles for specialists and generalists.

Technological Developments in Clinical Practice

New technologies that have been applied in speech–language pathology have developed within the past several years. Instrumentation for clinical practice in voice, swallowing, craniofacial anomalies, and other areas involving movement of the speech/swallowing musculature has allowed for new measures and observations of the physiological aspects of speech. Communication aids and tools for the non-oral population also continue to expand options for enhancing interaction and productivity. New computer technologies have also had an effect on practice. General applications for use in business and home are being adapted for clinical settings. In addition, applications are being specifically developed for use by the SLP in clinical and administrative functions. Finally, the Internet is emerging as a source of information and tools for communication among professionals, interaction with resource centers focused on specific topics, and access to new information for incorporation into practice.

The availability and popularity of these technologies will continue to change practice in the field. The major challenge to the clinician in the medical setting will be related to finding funds to purchase and support all the technologies that can assist and expand practice. A second challenge will involve staying abreast of all the technologies and also accessing resources to evaluate rapidly developing systems and programs.

Ethical Issues

Ethical practice refers to the application of standards of service delivery. These standards include avoiding misrepresentation of services, performing only those activities for which one is qualified (i.e., certified, competent), adhering to preferred practice patterns, and providing service in the best interest of the patient, among others.[2] Ethics also may be viewed from the perspective of its formal discipline (see Chapter 10). As the scope of practice expands in medical speech–language pathology, so do the number of situations in which ethical concerns may arise.

The specialty of swallowing has become the most visible area in which ethical issues emerge. The management of swallowing disorders is a high-volume activity for many medical speech–language pathologists. Dysphagia assessment and treatment, along with endoscopy, are service activities that carry the most risk for harm to the patient. Both ethical practice and ethics are important issues in this specialty. The question of competency, in the face of uneven graduation education in dysphagia in the past, continues to be at the forefront of discussion. Decision making in dysphagia practice requires an understanding of the principles of ethics and their application to questions of patient and family decisions regarding type of feeding, withdrawal of feeding, and oral feeding in the presence of aspiration risk. At this writing, most SLPs understand and adhere to ethical standards of practice, but tend to be under-educated in the area of ethics.

Interprofessional Issues

A variety of disciplines and professions interact in medical speech–language pathology practice. Regardless of setting type or clinical specialization area, SLPs come into contact with a myriad of physician specialists and generalists, rehabilitation professionals, nurses, psychologists, audiologists, and others as they go about the business of caring for their patients. As professions attempt to

work together there is sometimes a tendency for individual clinicians engage in conflict over issues of turf, competence, or perceived power. These conflicts increase in frequency (and sometimes intensity) when the practice environment calls for reductions in resource utilization. Some organizations have developed new approaches to delivering services that attempt to avoid the "turf" competition by facilitating team approaches and product line approaches to avoid the traditional departmental structure. These models deserve careful study as vehicles for delivering improved care and quality. However, they do serve as a threat to some aspects of discipline-specific knowledge and skill development. A rush to develop new teams or product lines should not obviate the need for development of specialized skills in meeting the needs of patients with communication or swallowing disorders by the speech–language pathologist.

ISSUES IN SERVICE DELIVERY
Managed Care

The health insurance industry has drastically changed its way of doing business and has caused havoc in the delivery of all health care services, including speech–language pathology. Major effects in all health settings include increased attention to costs and resources used, major attempts to control costs by reducing the length and variety of patient services, an emphasis on prevention over treatment, and measurement of performance from a variety of perspectives and clinical outcomes.

The careful observer of these issues recognizes that the entire process of serving patients via the health care system has changed or is changing. Speech–language pathologists now must understand and appreciate the significance of a variety of new methodologies for funding their programs. These methods, which include capitation arrangements, extend beyond the traditional fee-for-service models. In addition to impacting the financial components of their practice, protocols have been and are being developed that determine who will get service and under what conditions. These factors have moved the speech–language pathologist into the role of needing to work to maintain relationships with referral sources, including insurance companies. The current market also requires that clinicians are continuously able to demonstrate the rationale for their services as well as all costs incurred on behalf of the patient.

Visibility and Marketing

Competition for the health care dollar has been a major issue in the 1990s and will continue to be discussed and debated into the next century. Health care reform may have been postponed in 1996; however, the move toward continuing scrutiny as to who receives payments for services and how much has not abated. Within habilitative and rehabilitative specialties, the competition is obvious. A clear professional identity within the mind of the general public strengthens any specialty's position. The field of speech–language pathology in general has always had only fair recognition within the public at large. Medical speech–language pathologists may have their own difficulties in achieving an identity that is different from providing services in the school setting.

One way to educate consumers regarding our services, certainly within practice settings, is to maintain a high visibility. This visibility promotes marketing efforts. While patients control the health care dollar, in terms of selecting insurance providers, primary care physicians (PCPs) control the referrals. The medical SLP should direct marketing efforts to these two groups. Visibility can be engendered in several ways. The most basic and direct way to create and maintain visibility is through communication about patients (initial reports, occasional progress notes). Answers to referral questions that are prompt and concise provide a service to the referring physician and promote quality care. Many practice settings have newsletters that furnish an opportunity to educate other staff about program activities. Participation in patient and family support groups within facilities allows clinicians to enlarge their presence. These are some activities that can enlarge the scope of marketing efforts in medical speech–language pathology.

Accreditation and Standards

We are in an era in which accreditation governs many of our policies and procedures. If medical speech–language pathology is practiced in a hospital, then JCAHO (Joint Commission on Accreditation of Health Organizations) standards must be followed. If the practice site is a rehabilitation setting, then CARF (Commission on Accreditation of Rehabilitation Facilities) standards guide practice.

In some states, PSB (ASHA's Professional Services Board) accreditation is necessary for Medicaid reimbursement for outpatient treatment.

The process of seeking accreditation can seem bewildering and time consuming. Particularly in small practice settings, resources may not be available for accumulating and collating all the documentation needed to demonstrate compliance with standards. Various accrediting organizations may have similar but slightly different requirements that necessitate duplicative effort. The cost of applying for accreditation and proceeding through a review is not insignificant. Despite these challenges, the benefits of accreditation outweigh the limitations. In developing standards, accrediting agencies have attempted to define practice patterns that assure that quality care is delivered to the consumer. The process of reviewing medical speech-pathology practice to align with externally developed standards provides the opportunity to critically evaluate the status of a program and ensure that it continues to evolve and improve. For example, the PSB standards[3] emphasize several aspects of practice that are crucial to quality service. Standard 3 is devoted to continuous quality improvement that goes beyond the traditional chart audit. By using accreditation standards as guideposts for ongoing program development, medical speech–language pathologists can continue to demonstrate to their consumers (patients, physicians, administrators) that they provide consistent and quality services.

It should be noted that the PSB has recently approved streamlined versions of its accreditation process for programs also accredited by some other recognized bodies such as CARF. This approach represents an attempt to reduce the redundancy of multiple applications and exorbitant staff time, while allowing the program to demonstrate compliance with both sets of standards.

Trends in Inpatient Care

Most practitioners would agree that there is never enough time to complete all the activities required by their job descriptions. In addition to actual patient contact for evaluation and treatment, there are in-person or telephone contacts with referral sources, families, and other medical colleagues, information gathering regarding patient history, discharge planning, preparation time, and documentation. Many clinicians have clear expectations from their supervisors regarding the number of treatment units that they must bill on a daily basis. Balancing these responsibilities is challeng-ing and requires creativity to fulfill them success-fully. Acute care practice can be particularly difficult because of the very short length of stays that have become common for stroke, laryngec-tomy and other head and neck surgeries, and neu-rosurgical procedures. Often, physicians refer patients for assessment just prior to discharge.

Several solutions have been proposed for ac-commodating the restraints caused by too little time and too much to accomplish. Critical path-ways and clinical decision maps have been de-signed as decision and action models for specific diagnoses. They come into operation when the patient is admitted and outline the day-by-day evaluations, decisions, and procedures that move a patient efficiently through the hospital stay. For example, a patient admitted with stroke might re-ceive an MRI, undergo standard laboratory blood work, and have evaluations by internal medicine consult service as needed on day one. On day two, speech–language pathology is consulted as needed, transcranial Doppler tests are completed, and patient and family education regarding stroke begins. These protocols are designed for patients who have *typical* disease courses. Unfortunately, they do not necessarily work well for patients with complicated medical problems (e.g., the patient with a cardiac artery bypass graft who incurs a stroke and then respiratory failure during surgery) or for patients who are admitted to the hospital with multiple problems (e.g., the geriatric nurs-ing home patient with onset of dementia who also has diabetes, possible malnutrition, and hy-pertension). In those cases the speech–language pathologist may be consulted only after medical stabilization has occurred and near to the time of discharge. An obvious presence by the SLP on the hospital wards and floors can often provide the op-portunity for more timely and effective care.

Litigation and Risk Management

By definition, the practice of medical speech–language pathology places the practitioner in a position of risk for litigation. Some high-risk ac-tivities performed by medical SLPs include en-doscopy, use of topical anesthetics (for voice prosthesis placement and endoscopy), videofluo-roscopy, use of latex products, and dysphagia management. Some therapeutic techniques carry the potential for harm to the patient (e.g., glottal effort closure for patients with hypertension). In addition, when SLPs are present for medical or surgical interventions (e.g., BOTOX injections for

spasmodic dysphonia, monitoring laryngeal func-tion during phonosurgery), there is the chance that, should an adverse reaction occur, the SLP will be included in any malpractice suit filed by the patient.

Diagnostic and therapeutic activities performed in the past have been considered relatively "low risk." However, there are several ways in which SLPs may reduce the possibility of litigation. First, SLPs can identify those aspects of their practice that place them at risk. Next, they can develop protocols and competencies for procedures performed at their sites, seek credentialing within their institu-tions for procedures such as endoscopy, and assure that their practice is covered by malpractice insur-ance. Ongoing continuing quality improvement programs that focus on "high-risk, high-volume" activities can assist in maintaining prudent practice standards. For example, monthly sessions to estab-lish reliability in evaluating swallowing function based on videofluoroscopy are helpful in assuring that staff not only have consistent internal stan-dards but also maintain a standard as a group. An emphasis on implementing "best practice" in all areas of medical speech–language pathology and documentation of these activities (through evalua-tion reports, progress notes, staff meeting minutes, and policy and procedure manuals) will enable practitioners to prevent potential adverse effects of their services.

Personnel Issues in Medical Speech–Language Pathology

The development of two areas has potential im-pact for speech–language pathologists, especially those who will be practicing in the future. First, the call for producing "multiskilled" professionals has been proposed as a method for improving effi-ciency in the care of the patient. ASHA has for-mulated a report[4] on this issue basically arguing that SLPs are already providing multiple skills in the service of their patients with speech–language-swallowing-cognitive disorders. The argument is made that increasing the scope of practice to in-clude other rehabilitation activities and goals might not increase efficiency. Instead, quality might be diluted as the result of loss of specialized skills for the very complex functions addressed by SLPs in health settings.

A second area receiving increased attention in recent years is the use of the speech–language pathology assistant as part of the service delivery process. This issue has focused on the develop-ment of standards and recognition for assistants within the structure of ASHA's accreditation programs.[5] The position of the association is that if assistants are functioning in the field, then the public and the professional community should know that they have met certain basic requirements. Some members of the profession argue that the development of a registry or other recognition program will unwittingly promote the use of assistants as a less costly alternative to comprehensive care. At this writing, a number of junior colleges around the country are in the process of developing curricula to comply with the proposed standards for training assistants.

SUMMARY AND CONCLUSIONS

In this chapter we have attempted to highlight some of the professional issues that may be consequential to speech–language pathologists who practice in medical settings. This discussion was not intended to be exhaustive, but to provide a framework and context for consideration of some of the subsequent chapters. Several of the concerns raised in this chapter are discussed in some detail in the chapters by Pietranton and Frattali (Chapters 27 and 28, respectively).

The following suggestions are offered as medical SLPs continue to adapt and grow during this time of change:

1. *Consider continuing education a professional mandate for survival.* The only way for the modern SLP to maintain currency during this highly volatile and variable time is through ongoing acquisition of new information. Medical SLPs should concentrate on information specific to their area of subspecialty to maintain clinical expertise and currency. In addition, attention should be given to reading and attending conferences that address the various social, political, and financial trends impacting the health system.

2. *Know and maintain high standards of practice.* It is essential for practitioners entrusted with the care of their patients' communication and swallowing needs to know the standards of the profession and provide for safe, efficient, and timely care. Resources available include those from a variety of professional associations including ASHA and the various Specialty Interest Divisions; the Standards Council and the Professional Services Board; related professional organizations (Academy of Neurological Communication Disorders and Sciences); and accrediting bodies (CARF and JCAHO). Review of current journals addressing medical speech–language pathology topics can help the professional determine his or her currency and appropriateness in providing quality service that is consistent with the highest standards of practice.

3. *Establish familiarity with other professionals and practitioners.* Medical speech–language pathologists, experts in the communication process, need to have contact and familiarity with various other professionals in the health system who interact in serving patients with communication disorders. The primary physician, specialists, nurses, dietitians, pharmacists, and rehabilitation personnel influence the care of the patient. Thus, as a manager of one aspect of care, the SLP needs to understand the implications and issues of other providers. Establishment of strong positive relationships among the various health care providers serves the interest of the patient.

4. *Consider roles and responsibilities beyond existing models.* Speech–language pathologists are sometimes classified as "rehabilitation" professionals. Although rehabilitation is a key activity in the chain of services provided, much of the expected growth in health care is anticipated in the areas of preventive care, consultation, collaboration in acute and primary care, and so forth. It is important for medical SLPs to participate in these other aspects of the health delivery system.

5. *Professional involvement.* Another way to ensure currency and quality is through ongoing involvement by SLPs in speech–language-hearing associations, related professional organizations, and consumer support organizations. Involvement with such groups provides important vehicles for networking, exchange of information and ideas, and an ongoing source of new resources and data. These inputs to professional practice allow for continuous improvement of the program with attention to those issues that are shaping the current health system environment.

STUDY QUESTIONS

1. What are the key issues affecting medical speech–language pathology practice?

2. What resources do you use (or should you be using) to increase your understanding of key practice issues?

3. How is managed care affecting your practice?

4. What do you see as the primary issues affecting graduate and undergraduate preparation of the medical speech–language pathologist?

5. What continuing education issues and activities are key to your successful practice?

6. What are the actions you can take to improve the currency and appropriateness of your professional practice?

7. List the issues that are affecting service delivery and discuss them from the perspective of the consumer.

8. What resources are available to allow you to gain more information regarding ethical practice that meets professional standards?

SUGGESTED READINGS

1. Aronson A: The clinical Ph.D.: Implications for the survival and liberation of communication disorders as a health care profession. *ASHA* (1987); 29: 35–39.

2. American Speech–Language-Hearing Association: Code of ethics. *ASHA* 1994; 36 (March suppl. 13): 1–2.

3. American Speech–Language-Hearing Association, Professional Services Board: Standards and Accreditation Manual. ASHA, Rockville, MD, 1995.

4. American Speech–Language-Hearing Association: Technical report of the ad hoc committee on multi-skilling. ASHA 1996; 38, 2, 53–61.

5. American Speech–Language-Hearing Association: Guidelines for the training, credentialing, use, and supervision of speech–language pathology assistants. ASHA 1996; 38 (2): 21–34.

SECTION II

General Medical Issues and the Speech–Language Pathologist

3

Dysphagia: Basic Assessment and Management Issues

JERI A. LOGEMANN

CHAPTER OUTLINE

This chapter presents the current status of dysphagia management in acute care hospitals, focusing on the speech–language pathologist's involvement from the time of the initial consultation until the patient is discharged from the acute care hospital. The types of screening and assessment tools utilized by the speech–language pathologist (SLP) are described in the context of cost containment and the integration of treatment into the swallowing diagnostic procedure. We examine the speech–language pathologist's involvement with other professionals in the management of dysphagia in the acute care setting as well as the competencies needed by the speech–language pathologist at each stage of involvement with the dysphagic patient. In addition, protocols are presented for the screening, assessment, and treatment of the oropharyngeal dysphagic patient. Case studies are used to illustrate a number of critical points.

NATURE OF THE DYSPHAGIC POPULATION IN THE ACUTE CARE SETTING

Cost containment is driving every aspect of patient care in the acute care setting, as in most other levels of health care. This translates to a relatively short stay in acute care for most patients with oropharyngeal dysphagia. The population of patients with dysphagia typically seen in acute care are those who have suffered a stroke, head injury, spinal cord injury, those with progressive neurologic disease such as Parkinson's disease, motor neuron disease, multiple sclerosis, Alzheimer's disease, and so on, and those patients receiving treatment for head and neck cancer, systemic diseases such as rheumatoid arthritis and dermatomyositis, and so on.[1–8] Speech–language pathologists in acute care also often see patients on an outpatient basis who are referred for complaints of swallowing difficulty and have no known medical diagnosis. In this type of patient, the speech–language pathologist often serves as a triage officer who assesses the patient's oropharyngeal swallow function as well as speech, voice, and respiratory function and makes the appropriate referrals to a physician for a final diagnosis of the underlying cause of the dysphagia. Our data show that in most cases patients with complaints of oropharyngeal swallowing difficulties usually have had neurologic damage or undiagnosed neurologic disease including brainstem stroke, motor neuron disease, Parkinson's disease, Guillain-Barré, multiple sclerosis, or brainstem tumor.

Numerous clinical anecdotes and experience indicate that the most cost-effective care plan for the patient with a complaint of oropharyngeal dysphagia is a referral to a speech–language pathologist for a modified barium swallow or videofluorographic (VFG) study of oropharyngeal swallow. Following this study, the SLP can make a referral to a particular specialty physician, usually a neurologist, for further diagnostic work-up. Many patients of this sort are referred for videofluorographic studies only after they have already been to see 3 to 5 physicians and have had numerous medical tests at a high cost to the health care system.

CASE ONE

Case One is a 94–year-old woman who was referred by the gastroenterology service because she had a chronic bronchial infection and no known etiology for this problem. She had been treated for the bronchitis for six months by a pulmonologist but no antibiotics were clearing the infection. The pulmonologist, becoming frustrated, referred her to an otolaryngologist for assessment to determine whether there might be some otolaryngologic reason for the bronchitis. The otolaryngologist, after examining her, referred her to gastroenterology for possible reflux disease. The gastroenterologist, after talking with her and her family, thought that dysphagia might be the reason for her bronchitis and referred her to speech–language pathology for swallowing assessment. Informal interview with the patient and observation of her behaviors revealed some degree of thoracic rigidity, a shuffling gait, and a masked facies, all typical of Parkinson's disease. Videofluoroscopic examination (the modified barium swallow) revealed swallowing problems typical of Parkinson's disease including a repeated tongue pumping action making oral transit 10 to 15 seconds per swallow, a delay in triggering the pharyngeal swallow, and residue in the valleculae after the swallow indicating poor tongue base action. This residue was chronically aspirated after the swallow. With the patient's chin down, the aspiration was eliminated. The patient was counseled that her swallowing may be of a neurologic origin, and she was referred to a neurologist familiar with swallowing disorders associated with neurologic disease. She was hospitalized for an in-depth work-up and found to have Parkinson's disease. Throughout her hospitalization, she was fed using the chin down compensatory posture to facilitate her tongue base motion and to improve the clearance of the valleculae and thus reduce or eliminate the aspiration. She was placed on anti-Parkinsonian medications that resulted in improvement of the pharyngeal aspects of her swallowing problem and elimination of the aspiration as viewed by repeat videofluoroscopic study. Her bronchitis cleared up when the aspiration was eliminated.

If this patient had been initially referred to a speech–language pathologist in an acute care setting, those costs for numerous unnecessary referrals would have been saved and the patient would have had an earlier medical diagnosis. Competencies needed by the SLP to serve in this capacity include: knowledge of neurologic disease processes and damage and their characteristic swallowing disorders at various points in recovery or degeneration; skills in conduct and interpretation of VFG studies.

The procedures described and advocated in this chapter are designed to contain costs in the current acute care environment in which rapid decision making is a fact of life and assessment and treatment must be telescoped to have any significant impact on patients' swallowing function while they are often in the acute care setting for only 3 to 5 days.

SCREENING THE INITIAL REFERRAL

The speech–language pathologist's initial contact with a dysphagic patient is often a 10 to 15 minute bedside screening designed to determine whether the patient is exhibiting signs of an oral or a pharyngeal dysphagia or both, since the in-depth assessment procedures for the two dysphagia foci are quite different.[9–10] The screening procedure typically examines the following patient characteristics: (1) general level of alertness; (2) general secretion levels in the mouth, throat, and chest: (3) awareness of secretions, as exhibited by attempts to wipe away drooling, throat clearing, or coughing and attempts to clear chest secretions; (4) vocal quality (i.e., hoarse or gurgly); (5) history of any pneumonias; (6) obvious reduction in oromotor control; (7) history of neurologic insult or other neurologic or structural damage; and (8) medical diagnosis. With these bits of information from an initial screening, the speech–language pathologist may immediately recognize that the patient is at high risk for pharyngeal dysphagia—a disorder in the triggering of the pharyngeal swallow or in any one of the neuromotor aspects that comprise the pharyngeal swallow itself, and that the patient requires an in-depth physiologic assessment to identify the physiologic or anatomic disorder responsible for the patient's dysphagia. Usually this assessment is a modified barium swallow. If the screening locates the patient's dysphagia focus in the oral cavity, then a detailed bedside examination will be completed to identify the nature of the problem and enable the clinician to initiate therapy as well develop a compensatory diet plan for enabling the patient to return to oral intake as quickly as possible. At times, the screening cannot determine the locus of the dysphagia to the SLP's satisfaction and a modified barium swallow is recommended to define the patient's swallow physiology.

CASE TWO

Case Two is a 93–year-old woman with Alzheimer's dementia referred for a videofluoroscopic study of oropharyngeal swallowing because she had begun to refuse to eat and would spit food from her mouth. The preradiographic screening revealed a patient with severe dementia, unable to follow any instructions and only variably alert. The patient refused placement of any food in the mouth when the clinician observed nursing attempting to feed her. If any food did enter her mouth, she immediately spit it out and turned her head away. Observing this behavior, the clinician timed the attempts at food placement and found that each attempt took 2 to 3 minutes and then was unsuccessful as the patient pushed anything that entered her mouth out again. The clinician then talked with the patient's referring physician about the patient's need for non-oral nutrition and also indicated that a radiographic study would be inappropriate. Her clinical opinion was that the patient would not get adequate nutrition or hydration even if her swallowing physiology was normal because of the behavioral and neurologic issues involved in the dementia. After this discussion, the referral for the modified barium swallow was canceled and the patient's family was counseled regarding the need for non-oral nutrition.

CASE THREE

Case Three is a 35-year-old man who suffered a brainstem stroke. The speech–language pathology service received the consultation to screen the patient for dysphagia two days post-stroke. The chart revealed that the stroke was a large medullary lesion, that the patient had indicated complaints of dysphagia, and that the nursing staff had observed coughing at attempts to feed the patient. The diagnosis of brainstem stroke in the presence of patient complaints and observable symptoms is adequate to refer for a modified barium swallow. Brainstem stroke, particularly medullary, almost always involves damage to the timing of pharyngeal triggering, laryngeal elevation, as well as the unilateral pharyngeal wall paresis and sometimes a vocal fold adductor paresis. In this case, the medical diagnosis is enough to immediately refer for a radiographic study because of the extremely high incidence of pharyngeal problems after medullary stroke. Even if the clinician could predict the types of pharyngeal problems that are present, the severity of these problems will vary tremendously from patient to patient, requiring radiographic study to define them and examine the effects of compensatory and other rehabilitation procedures on the swallow. Some of these patients can immediately return to at least partial oral intake using compensatory procedures.

Competencies needed by the SLP to screen for dysphagia include: knowledge of signs and symptoms of dysphagia and medical diagnoses frequently causing dysphagia, and skill in observation of patient behavior and oromotor control.

IN-DEPTH CLINICAL/BEDSIDE EXAMINATION

Once the speech–language pathologist has identified the general locus of the patient's dysphagia (i.e., oral or pharyngeal), the clinician will proceed with an in-depth bedside/clinical assessment.

Review of the Patient's Medical Chart

Prior to entering the patient's room, the clinician should carefully review the patient's medical chart, focusing particularly on the medical diagnosis, any prior or recent medical history of surgical procedures, trauma, neurologic damage, and so on, as well as the patient's current medications. There is a growing body of literature on the nature of swallowing disorders that result from particular medical diagnoses. Therefore, after defining the medical diagnosis, the clinician should immediately consider what physiologic or anatomic swallowing disorders are typical of that diagnosis. Unfortunately, the swallowing function of the vast majority of the patients seen by speech–language pathologists in the acute care setting are not the result of a single diagnosis. Instead, their swallowing ability reflects their medical history including all the neurologic and structural damage they have sustained over the years, chronic medication and other factors influencing the patient's medical status. However, knowing the medical diagnosis and recalling the particular swallowing disorders that are characteristic of that diagnosis can alert the clinician to watch for those possible swallow problems. The presence of a consultation from a neurologist or otolaryngologist should be determined and the results of their assessments noted. History of any respiratory problems should also be identified, including need for mechanical ventilation or tracheostomy tube, the conditions under which these were placed (emergency or planned), and the length of time they were present. In general, any emergency procedure such as emergency tracheostomy or intubation will tend to cause greater scar tissue than a planned procedure. Any history of GI dysfunction should be noted. Prior history of dysphagia from an earlier stroke or head injury, for example, should be highlighted even if the patient or his or her family indicates that the patient returned to oral intake with no apparent difficulty after the prior dysphagia. Very few patients return to entirely normal swallowing after having had a prior dysphagia. Most dysphagic patients become functional swallowers—they exhibit no aspiration, but have a slightly slower swallow with more residue than normal subjects their age and gender. Thus, it should be anticipated that a second injury causing dysphagia will result in more significant swallowing disorders than a single first-time damage. Medical chart review should also reveal the patient's current nutritional status and the presence of any non-oral nutritional support such as a nasogastric tube, a PEG—a percutaneous endoscopic gastrostomy (placed under local anesthetic), a surgical gastrostomy, or a jejunostomy (both surgical procedures requiring general anesthesia). Intravenous feeding, as well as any other nutritional supplements, should also be noted in the patient's chart. The clinician should also be able to identify the patient's general progress, as well as prognosis from this chart review. The presence of any advanced directives should be noted. An advanced directive may be a living will or a medical power of attorney. In either case patients are generally stating their wishes regarding their care at a time of severe illness when no recovery is deemed possible.

BEDSIDE CLINICAL ASSESSMENT

The bedside clinical assessment is designed to define the function of the patient's lips, tongue, velopharyngeal region, pharyngeal walls, and larynx as well as his or her awareness of sensory stimulation.[9] The physiology of some of these structures can be easily assessed at the bedside, while others can only be examined accurately in a radiographic or other instrumental study. The clinical assessment typically begins with an examination of the anatomic structure of the oral cavity including its symmetry and the presence of any scar tissue indicating surgical or traumatic damage. The oral examination should also note the presence and status of any oral secretions, especially the pooling of secretions or excessive, dried secretions. In general, the locus of excess secretions in the oral cavity indicates areas of lesser lingual control or injury.

The clinician's oromotor assessment should then progress to examination of strength, range of motion, and coordination of the lips, tongue, and palate for speech and non-speech tasks, as well as observation of lingual function and lip closure while the patient produces any spontaneous swallows. The clinician will also want to note the frequency of spontaneous swallowing. There is some initial evidence that the frequency of spontaneous swallows is significantly lower in patients who are hospitalized, have dysphagia, and aspirate than in those who do not aspirate. The clinician should define a 5-minute period during which swallows are counted by observing or feeling the laryngeal motion in the patient's neck. Normal saliva swallowing occurs at the rate of approximately 1 to 2 per 5-minute period in awake normal adults. Table 3–1 presents a list of voluntary tasks to be elicited from the patient during the bedside/oromotor assessment. In general, at the bedside, the clinician's goals should be to assess swallow physiology without placing the patient at increased risk of food entering the airway (aspiration). Assessment of chewing and lingual control of material in the mouth can be tested safely at bedside utilizing cloth rather than food. To this end, the clinician can bring into the room four taste stimuli: lemon juice (sour), bitters (bitter), saline solution (salty), sugar water (sweet). In addition, the clinician should bring 4 × 4 in. gauze squares as well as 4 in. squares of satin and burlap. The three types of cloth represent three food consistencies (rough—burlap, smooth—satin, and intermediate texture—gauze). By wrapping each 4 × 4 in. square of cloth around a flexible, disposable straw, the clinician can dip one end of the 4 in. roll into one of the flavors (making it as cold as desired), squeeze out the excess liquid from the cloth, and place the dampened end of the cloth containing the desired texture, flavor, and temperature into the patient's mouth. The clinician can then observe the patient's reaction to the various combinations of stimuli and identify those particular stimuli that result in most normal oromotor activity such as chewing, lateralizing, lifting the tongue tip, and so on. Whatever combination of textures, tastes, and temperatures elicits most normal motor activity is the one that should be introduced in any follow-up radiographic or other instrumental study. In the same way, this cloth can be used to test the patient's chewing ability by placing the damp end of the 4 in. long gauze roll onto the center of the patient's tongue, and asking the patient to lateralize to each side and chew on this roll of cloth. If the patient is unable to control the cloth in the mouth for mastication, and the cloth becomes "stuck" (e.g., two-thirds of the way toward the teeth on one side), the clinician can simply pull the dry end of the gauze from the patient's mouth, replace the damp end in the middle of the tongue, and the patient can return to the task. This eliminates the need to clean the patient's mouth of food that may have gotten stuck, if food were used in this task, and requires that the patient use all the oromotor control needed for chewing. The risk of potentially

losing food in the mouth and having it fall into the pharynx and open airway is eliminated. The task can be made more difficult by using chewing gum once the clinician is sure the patient will not accidentally swallow the gum. This then becomes a therapy exercise as well as an evaluation strategy.

Respiratory Support

Respiratory support should be defined by counting the rate of breaths per minute and observing any obvious stressful or rapid respiration. Patients should be asked to hold their breath for a total of 1 sec, then 3, 5, and 10 sec, and the clinician should observe whether this behavior creates any respiratory distress. Duration of breath-hold should be increased as tolerated by the patient. One important reason for assessing breath-hold ability is to determine whether the patient can tolerate swallow maneuvers or other therapy procedures that increase the duration of the apneic or airway closed period during the swallow. Generally, patients need to be able to hold their breath for at least 5 seconds to use swallow maneuvers comfortably. The patient's coordination of respiration and swallowing should be examined. Most often, normal adults interrupt the exhalatory phase of the respiratory cycle to swallow and return to exhalation after the swallow.[11] This coordination is thought to be a safer coordination than interrupting or returning to inhalation after the swallow, either of which might encourage inhalation of pharyngeal residue after the swallow.

Prolonged Phonation

Prolonged phonation on the vowel /o/ should also be examined in terms of both vocal quality and the respiratory control used. Is the patient able to take an easy inhalation followed by a slow drop of the chest and inward motion of the abdomen to produce a prolonged vowel on sustained phonation of at least 10 seconds?

Gag Reflex

The gag reflex should be tested, not to determine its presence or absence as an indicator of ability or inability to swallow, but to examine the pharyngeal wall motion as part of the motor response for the gag. The pharyngeal wall motion during the gag should be symmetrical. Any asymmetry may indicate a unilateral pharyngeal wall paresis. There is no evidence of a relationship between the

Table 3–1. Voluntary Tasks to be Elicited from the Patient during the Bedside/Oromotor Assessment

Labial

Range of motion
   Lip spread (/i/)
   Lip rounding (/u/)

Asymmetry: Right ____ Left ____

Lip closure at rest

Lip closure on rapid repetitive /pa/

Lip closure during sentence repetition *"Please put the papers by the back door."*

Lingual

Range of motion
   Protrusion
   Elevation of tip (mouth open widely)
   Elevation of back (mouth open widely)
   Point to right side
   Point to left side
   Retraction

Asymmetry: Right ____ Left ____

Rapid repetitive lateralization

Rapid repetitive elevation

Tip alveolar contact on repeated /ta/

Tip alveolar contact during sentence repetition *"Take time to talk to Tom."*

Fine lingual shaping during sentence repetition *"Say something nice to Susan on Sunday"*

Back velar contact on rapid repetitive /ka/

Back velar contact during sentence repetition *"Can you go get the garbage cans?"*

Chewing—ability to lateralize gauze, chew on it, return it to midline, and move it to the other side

Velar Function

Elevation on prolonged /a/

Retraction on prolonged /a/

Symmetry of motion

Oral Sensitivity—Patient awareness of:

Light touch—tongue tip

Light touch—left side
   Lateral margin of tongue
   Posterior tongue
   Anterior faucial arch
   Cheek

Light touch—right side
   Lateral margin of tongue
   Posterior tongue
   Anterior faucial arch
   Cheek

Laryngeal Examination

Vocal quality on prolonged /a/(hoarse, gurgly)

Strength of voluntary cough

Strength of throat clearing

Clarity of /h/ and /a/ during repetitive /ha/

Pitch range (slide up and down scale)

Loudness range (say name soft, conversational, loud)

Respiratory Assessment

Duration of phonation (prolong /o/ as long as you can)

Duration of comfortable breath-hold needed to use swallow maneuvers (1, 3, 5, and 10 sec)

Coordination of respiration and swallowing: Does the patient interrupt inhalation or exhalation to swallow? Does the patient inhale or exhale after the swallow?

presence and normalcy of a gag and the presence and normalcy of a swallow.[12–13] The gag reflex is triggered from surface tactile sensory receptors by a noxious stimulus that does not belong in the posterior oral cavity or pharynx such as vomit or reflux. The motor response of a gag is for the pharynx and larynx to elevate and close/contract to push out any foreign body. In contrast, the swallow is triggered from deeper proprioceptive receptors, as well as surface receptors, and the motor response of a swallow is a coordinated set of muscle contractions designed to carry food from the mouth through the pharynx and into the esophagus, essentially the opposite of a gag motor response. Several studies have shown that the gag reflex can be eliminated by topical anesthetic, while the swallow remains entirely intact. If the deeper proprioceptive receptors are anesthetized, however, then the swallow will be eliminated. Thus, there is no reason to hypothesize that the gag and swallow in any way predict each other, other than to say that if a patient sustains significant neurologic damage, it is quite likely that both the gag and the swallow will be affected because of the extent of damage.

CASE FOUR

Despite the lack of relationship between gag and swallow, both neurologically and physiologically, many physicians learn in their residencies that the gag reflex in some way is predictive of swallow normalcy. Case Four emphasizes this point. This 53-year-old man was referred for a modified barium swallow because he had an asymmetrical uvula and an absent gag reflex. In discussing this test with the patient and taking a brief history prior to the X-ray study, the clinician determined that the patient had no swallowing complaints and no nasality or any other indication of velopharyngeal insufficiency or incompetence for speech. Oral examination did reveal an asymmetrical uvula but good upward–backward motion of the soft palate and visible inward motion of the lateral and posterior pharyngeal walls. Because the patient insisted, the videofluoroscopic study was completed and showed an entirely normal oropharyngeal swallow. In this case, the patient had been referred because the physician thought that an absent gag reflex indicated a swallowing problem and, in combination with an asymmetrical uvula, may indicate neurologic disease. In the report of the radiographic study to the physician, the differences in the gag reflex and swallow were emphasized as was the high incidence of absent gag in normal individuals. The physician indicated that he was extremely grateful for this information.

Laryngeal Function

Laryngeal function should also be assessed by a series of voluntary tasks listed in Table 3–1, with the clinician assessing vocal quality and respiratory support during each task. Increasing loudness and increasing phonation time require coordination between respiratory and phonatory control.

Throughout all the oromotor testing, the clinician will also be examining the patient's general behavioral level, ability to discipline his or her own behavior and focus on the tasks, impulsiveness, and other cognitive and language characteristics that interact with swallow physiology to facilitate the eating situation. Successful eating requires functional swallowing (no aspiration and some manageable residue) *and* behavioral control and language ability. Two patients may exhibit the same swallow physiology, but one with behavioral problems and inability to focus on tasks will generally exhibit longer recovery to oral intake than the patient who is capable of focusing, following directions, and monitoring his or her own performance.

If the patient is taking oral nutrition, the clinician should observe the patient at bedside during a meal to identify the typical postures used, the placement of the food in the mouth, the patient's general awareness of food and reaction to food, and the presence of any behavior that might indicate food entering the airway (aspiration) such as coughing, throat clearing, periods of difficulty breathing, gurgly voice, and so on.[14] An apraxia of swallow should also be noted. Generally, apraxia of swallow is characterized by searching motions in the oral cavity as food is being placed there, or simply no motion in the oral cavity in response to placement of food there.

Once the clinician has collected data on oromotor control, the patient's behavior and language levels, and any symptoms of an oropharyngeal dysphagia, the clinician may wish to attempt some intervention strategies at the bedside. The difficulty, of course, is that if there is a pharyngeal dysphagia, the effects of any treatment strategies, as well as the identification of the actual abnormality in anatomy or physiology causing the patient's symptoms, cannot be accurately identified at the bedside. The clinician may therefore believe that a therapy procedure works because the patient doesn't cough or clear any material from the airway, but food may actually be collecting in the pharyngeal recesses formed by the natural attachment of structures to each other, such as the pyriform sinuses or the valleculae. The patient may appear to be "swallowing" when food is simply resting in these recesses, waiting for a swallow, or may be left in these recesses after an inefficient swallow.

At this point, all the data the clinician has collected from the patient's medical chart and history, as well as direct examination, combine to identify the patient's risk level for a pharyngeal dysphagia and the need for a videofluorographic or modified barium swallow study of the pharyngeal stage of swallowing. As a general guideline, if the patient has any of the behaviors listed in Table 3–2 or the diagnoses listed there, the clinician should recommend a modified barium swallow or other physiologic assessment to directly examine pharyngeal physiology during swallows of various bolus types, as described below. Initial treatment for oral stage problems can be initiated in parallel with conducting the videofluorographic study of the pharyngeal stage of swallowing.

The bedside clinical assessment of oropharyngeal dysphagia is a screening test for the pharyngeal stage of swallowing, but a definitive diagnostic test for the oral stages of swallowing in patients with neurologic lesions in the brainstem or below (i.e., the final common path), and for patients with peripheral structural damage such as surgery or radiotherapy for head and neck cancer, gunshot wounds, or other trauma.[15] For patients with cortical or subcortical neural damage, the effects on oral control may be different for speech and swallowing because these higher neural structures, while involved in both speech and swallowing, are utilized differently for the two functions. Performance on voluntary speech tasks may not reflect performance of the same structures during swallowing.[15]

OTHER BEDSIDE SCREENING TESTS

The clinician may wish to introduce other screening tests at bedside to gain further evidence of the potential of a pharyngeal stage swallowing problem. These include: the blue dye test in tracheostomized patients, cervical auscultation, and the videoendoscopic assessment of pharyngeal swallow known as the Fiberoptic Endoscopic Examination of Swallowing (FEES) by many clinicians. Each of these procedures defines symptoms of swallowing disorders.

Blue Dye Test

The blue dye test involves presenting blue dyed foods to a patient with a tracheostomy and suctioning after each swallow attempt to identify the

Table 3–2. Diagnoses and Patient Behaviors Indicative of Increased Risk for Pharyngeal Stage Disorders and/or Aspiration

Diagnosis at Highest Risk for Pharyngeal Dysphagia	Symptoms Indicating High Risk for Pharyngeal Disorders
Parkinson's disease	Gurgly voice
Motor neuron disease	History of pneumonia
ALS	Difficulty managing secretions
Post polio syndrome	Increased secretions in chest
Brainstem stroke	Coughing or throat clearing during eating
Head and neck cancer patients whether treated with surgery/radiotherapy	Patient report of food "sticking" in throat
Myasthenia gravis	
Guillain-Barré	
Multiple sclerosis (if complaining of swallow problems)	
Dermatomyositis	
Scleroderma	
Oculopharyngeal muscular dystrophy	
Myotonic dystrophy	

presence of any food in the airway below the larynx.[16-17] This test has been found to have both a negative and positive error rate—that is, it misidentifies patients as aspirating who are not and those who are actually aspirating as not aspirating. There is no set protocol for this procedure. Generally clinicians using it prefer to introduce thin liquids, thick liquids, pureed, and mechanical soft foods, all dyed blue, to distinguish the foods from bodily secretions. If the patient loses food out the tracheostomy during or after a swallow or for a period of time after eating, aspiration is indicated and the need for videofluorographic or definitive diagnostic study identified.

Cervical Auscultation

Cervical auscultation involves placing a stethoscope against the patient's neck and listening to the sounds of swallow and respiration.[18-19] The inhalatory and exhalatory phases of the respiratory cycle can generally be identified with auscultation. Also the clinician can define the phase of respiration during which the patient swallows. Unfortunately, the sounds of swallowing have not yet been completely identified, so that the meaning of the sounds heard by the clinician during the swallow is undetermined, nor do we know if clinicians can detect normal from abnormal sounds. In any case, the outcome of auscultation is the identification of a patient's risk for pharyngeal stage dysphagia and its major symptom, aspiration. A definitive diagnostic procedure is needed to identify the exact nature of the dysphagia, plan treatment, and evaluate effects of treatment procedures.

Fiberoptic Endoscopic Examination of Swallowing (FEES)

FEES involves nasal placement of a fiberoptic laryngoscope (generally 3.5 mm diameter) so that the tip of the laryngoscope is positioned posterior to the uvula as seen in Figure 3–1. In this position, the endoscope visualizes the pharynx from above including the valleculae, the airway entrance, and the posterior and lateral pharyngeal walls.[20-22] During the swallow the oral stages are not visible. The bolus becomes visible as it comes over the base of the tongue and into the pharynx. When the pharyngeal swallow triggers and the pharyngeal motor response begins, laryngeal and pharyngeal elevation is partially visualized followed by a period of "white out" when nothing can be seen as the pharynx closes around the endoscopic tube. When the swallow ends and the pharynx relaxes, the pharynx can be visualized again. Any residual food left in the pharynx can be seen. Thus, the swallow itself is not visualized. Instead, FEES examines the pharynx before and after the swallow. FEES can provide information on anatomic changes in the pharynx resulting from surgery or trauma that can be helpful to the clinician trying to understand the patient's altered anatomy. FEES can also be used to supply biofeedback for airway closure maneuvers described later (i.e., supraglottic and super-supraglottic swallow maneuvers).

A rigid endoscope placed transorally can also visualize the pharynx and larynx from above and can be used to provide biofeedback for learning the airway closure maneuvers.

The competencies needed by the SLP in screening and clinical bedside assessment of the dysphagic patient include: (1) knowledge of the range of normal oral anatomy and range, pattern and coordination of lips, tongue, jaw, and palate, and (2) the various screening procedures and their appropriateness for various patients, and skills in: (a) eliciting and evaluating oromotor actions for speech and non-speech tasks in various types of patients, and (b) auditory recognition of normal and abnormal articulation and voice.

MODIFIED BARIUM SWALLOW

The modified barium swallow procedure is a videofluoroscopic evaluation of swallowing that is designed to identify the abnormal anatomy or physiology in the patient's oral and pharyngeal stages of swallowing that are causing the dysphagic symptoms.[10] In addition, the videofluorographic study also assesses the effectiveness of treatment procedures for eliminating the patient's swallowing symptoms and improving the patient's swallowing safety and efficiency. The types of swallows introduced during the videofluorographic study should be selected based on two characteristics: (1) the bolus characteristics that create systematic changes in normal swallowing, including increases in volume and viscosity, as well as (2) the types of stimuli the clinician believes may improve the patient's swallow physiology and thereby eliminate aspiration or significant residue. Since we know that bolus volume and viscosity can cause significant changes in normal swallow physiology, the typical modified barium swallow includes presentation of two to three swallows of 1 ml, 3 ml, 5 ml, 10 ml, and cup drinking of thin liquids, as tolerated.[23-29] Similarly, because bolus viscosity creates significant changes in normal swallow physiology,

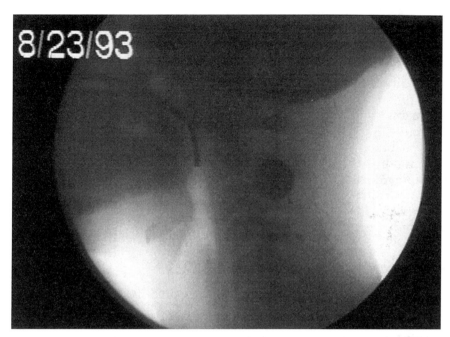

Figure 3–1. Lateral videofluorographic view of the oropharyngeal region showing the placement of the fiberoptic endoscope through the nose and over the soft palate with the tip of the endoscope at the approximate level of the inferior tip of the uvula.

the patient is typically given thin liquids, pudding-type material, and something requiring mastication such as a Lorna Doone cookie. The volume of the pudding is generally restricted to 1 or 3 ml and the amount of cookie presented is usually one-quarter of a Lorna Doone because the volume range of thicker foods is much less than liquids (i.e., 3 to 5 or 6 ml). Generally the thicker the food the smaller the volume per swallow. The cookie is utilized to study mastication. While one might be able to swallow 25 ml of thin liquid, the mechanism is not capable of swallowing 25 ml of pudding; that would require too much distention of the upper esophageal sphincter (UES). Thus, as viscosity increases, the maximum bolus volume per swallow decreases. A given patient may need to have boluses of particular bolus tastes presented such as sour as well as other types of therapy strategies to improve the swallow. Generally, postural techniques are attempted first to eliminate aspiration or large amounts of residue because they are easy for most patients to use and do not require extra muscular work.[30–35] Heightening sensory awareness follows postures and is designed to improve the speed of oral onset and the pharyngeal trigger of the swallow. Swallowing maneuvers and other therapy procedures may be attempted followed by presentation of swallows of thicker foods. In many

cases these strategies can be combined for best effect. For example, if a patient has difficulty in closing the entry of the larynx, the first strategy attempted would be a postural technique (i.e., chin down) that narrows the airway entrance and puts the epiglottis in a more overhanging position to protect the airway. If this posture is not successful and there is any asymmetry in laryngeal function, the patient may be asked to try head rotation to the side of any laryngeal damage, thereby applying extrinsic pressure to the damaged side of the larynx to achieve improved closure. If this posture reduces but does not eliminate aspiration, the two postures may be combined with the head rotated and the chin down, thereby achieving the effects of both. If the patient still continues to aspirate small amounts, the super-supraglottic swallow may be attempted. It is a swallow maneuver to voluntarily close the entrance to the airway. Finally, the two postures and the super-supraglottic swallow may be combined to eliminate the patient's aspiration. Thus, therapy procedures can be assessed separately as well as in combination to identify those procedures that successfully eliminate aspiration or reduce residue and allow the patient to eat. The goal of the radiographic study is not to eliminate oral feeding but instead to find a way in which the patient can eat successfully. Table 3–3 presents all

Table 3–3. Postural Strategies and Their Known Effects on Oropharyngeal Dimensions and Bolus Flow

Disorder for which Posture Appropriate (Symptom of Disorders)	Posture	Effects of Oropharyngeal Dimensions and Bolus Flow
Inefficient oral transit (Reduced posterior lingual propulsion of bolus)	Chin up	Uses gravity to clear oral cavity from bolus
Delay in triggering the pharyngeal swallow (Bolus past ramus of mandible, but pharyngeal swallow is not triggered)	Chin down	Widens valleculae to prevent bolus entering airway; narrows airway entrance, reducing risk of aspiration
Reduced posterior motion of tongue-base (Residue in valleculae)	Chin down	Pushes tongue-base closer to the posterior pharyngeal wall
Reduced closure of laryngeal entrance and vocal folds (Aspiration during the swallow)	Chin down	Puts epiglottis in more protective position; narrows laryngeal entrance
	Head rotated to damaged side	Improves vocal fold closure by applying extrinsic pressure
Unilateral pharyngeal paresis (Residue on one side of pharynx)	Head rotated to damaged side	Eliminates damaged side of pharynx from bolus path
Unilateral oral and pharyngeal weakness on the same side (Residue in mouth and pharynx on same side)	Head tilt to stronger side	Directs bolus down stronger side by gravity
Reduced pharyngeal contraction (Residue spread throughout pharynx)	Lying down on one side	Eliminates effect of gravity on pharyngeal residue
Cricopharyngeal dysfunction (Residue in pyriform sinuses)	Head rotated	Pulls cricoid cartilage away from posterior pharyngeal wall, reducing resting pressure in cricopharyngeal sphincter

the postural strategies and their known effects on the dimensions of the pharynx or the directions of bolus flow. Table 3–4 provides sensory enhancement procedures that generally improve the oral onset of the swallow (i.e., the time from the command to swallow until the oral transit is initiated, and the pharyngeal delay time).[10,36–38] Table 3–5 presents the swallow maneuvers and their known effects on swallow physiology.[10,26,28,39–46]

The outcome of the modified barium swallow should be: (1) the identification of the specific anatomic and/or physiologic dysfunctions in the patient's oropharyngeal swallow; (2) the relationship of the physiology to the patient's symptoms (i.e., the cause(s) of residue or aspiration); (3) the identification of treatment strategies to improve the pharyngeal swallow and the conditions under which the patient can eat safely, if possible; (4) the need for any non-oral supplement or non-oral nutrition if the patient aspirates and the aspiration cannot be stopped by any of the treatment strategies; (5) the type of swallowing therapy needed to further improve the patient's swallow; and (6) the need for and timing of reassessment of the patient's swallow. Because of the relatively short time the

patient spends in acute care, the transfer of this information from the acute care clinician to the clinician in rehabilitation or home health or the skilled nursing facility is critical for the patient's swallowing therapy and recovery to be uninterrupted. The sequence of reevaluation is also critical so that the patient who receives non-oral nutrition in acute care in the first few days or weeks after a stroke, for example, will be evaluated three or four weeks later to determine a continued need for such non-oral nutrition. With the rapid transfer of the patient from acute care to another facility—whether a rehabilitation center, nursing home, or home—the transfer of information from each facility to the next and each clinician to the next is critical for ensuring a smooth continuum of care and optimal recovery for the dysphagic patient.[47] The videofluoroscopic results including all the recommendations and follow-up therapy notes should be transferred with the patient so that the next clinician will be able to provide appropriate care.

Several studies indicate that patients who aspirate during radiographic study are at higher risk for developing pneumonia during the 6 to 12

Table 3–4. Sensory Enhancement Procedures Designed to Improve Oral Onset of the Swallow and Reduce Pharyngeal Delay and Their Method of Presentation (All are helpful in patients with swallow apraxia or reduced sensory input.)

Procedure	Method
Increase bolus volume	Present measured bolus volumes during radiographic study, beginning with 1 ml and increasing to 3, 5, 10 ml as tolerated (if no aspiration). If pharyngeal delay is reduced as volume increased, provide "best" volumes during feeding and therapy.
Increase bolus viscosity	Feed patient those food viscosities that are easiest and safest to swallow.
Change bolus taste	Present liquid with a strong taste such as *"sour" lemonade or salty water.
Increase pressure of spoon on tongue	As spoon is placed in the mouth, press down firmly on the patient's tongue.
Thermal tactile stimulation	Rub a cold size OO mirror up and down 5 times on each anterior faucial arch.
Suck swallow	Ask patient to close his or her mouth and suck in as he or she pumps his or her tongue and jaw up and down.
Chewing	Ask patient to "chew" liquid and paste substances.
Self-feeding	Facilitate the patient's self-feeding. The hand-to-mouth movement may constitute an alerting stimulus to ready the central nervous system to initiate a swallow.

* Do not present if patient is aspirating unless there is radiographic evidence that sour eliminates aspiration. Acidic substances are more irritating to the lungs.

months after the study than patients who are not found to aspirate on videofluoroscopy.[48–50] This is important information to pass along to the patient's physician.

Ideal Equipment for the Modified Barium Swallow

To conduct the modified barium swallow, the clinician needs a video recorder that can be wired directly into the fluoroscopy equipment or attached by cable to the back of the fluoroscopy monitor. The latter arrangement is best since it enables the clinician to use a variety of video recorders. If the video recorder is wired directly into the fluoroscopy, the radiologist or technician can activate the recording at the same time as the fluoroscopy image begins. However, often the video recorder in radiology has a different line rate per inch than standard recorders so that the videotape resulting from the study can only be played in radiology. This makes use of the videotape to educate families, physicians, nurses, and others very difficult. The video recorder, whenever possible, should have a "jog wheel" that enables the clinician to watch the videotape of the radiographic study in slow motion, frame by frame, and forward or backward at any rate. A pause button will not enable the clinician to do the kind of slow motion analysis needed for careful assessment of patient stud-

ies. Both ¾ in. and ½ in. (VHS) tapes are available with a jog wheel feature.

Additional equipment is also helpful, whenever possible. A video counter timer that records numbers on the individual frames or fields of the videotape as it is being recorded enables the clinician to make better notations and measurements of the timing of swallowing events. Another piece of equipment that adds to the ease of the test is a video character generator that allows the clinician to type the patient's name, date, condition of the study, diagnosis, or any other information onto the video screen so that it is visible and recorded at all times on the videotape. This makes finding the patient's study from a tape containing the radiographic studies of 10 or 15 other patients quite easy.

A seating device that enables the patient to be positioned easily into the radiographic equipment is also helpful. A number of chairs are commercially available for this purpose. Table 3–6 lists some of the available chairs and their manufacturers. The chair should allow the clinician (1) to change the patient's posture from true vertical to any degree including true horizontal, (2) to switch from a lateral view to an anterior posterior view without moving the patient from the chair, and (3) to position all types of patients whether they are conscious or not, able to follow directions or not, or have no motor control of their body. One

Table 3–5. Swallow Maneuvers (Voluntary Changes in Selected Motor Aspects of the Oropharyngeal Swallow), Their Purpose, and Instructions

Swallow Maneuvers	Purpose	Problem for which Maneuver Designed	Instructions
Supraglottic swallow	Close vocal folds before and during swallow (Martin et al., 1993)	Reduced or late vocal fold closure	Take a breath, hold your breath, keep holding your breath while you swallow and cough or take a breath, exhale a little, and hold your breath while you swallow and cough.
	Closes vocal folds before and during delay	Delayed pharyngeal swallow	
Super-supraglottic swallow	Tilts arytenoid forward, and pulls false vocal folds in closing airway entrance before and during swallow	Reduced closure of airway entrance	Follow instructions as above, but bear down as you hold your breath.
Effortful swallow	Increases posterior tongue-base movement and pressure generated	Reduced posterior movement of the tongue-base	Swallow hard. Squeeze hard with all your muscles as you swallow.
Mendelsohn maneuver	Laryngeal movement opens the upper esophageal sphincter; prolonging laryngeal elevation prolongs UES opening (Cook et al., 1989; Jacob et al., 1989)	Reduced laryngeal movement	
		Discoordinated swallow	
	Normalizes coordination of pharyngeal swallow events (Lazarus, Logemann, & Gibbons, 1993)		

alternative to a chair is to position the patient on a gurney or cart with a back support narrow enough to fit into the radiologic equipment. In this way, the patient can sit on the gurney with a back support in place. The back support can be shifted from true vertical to various degrees backward until the patient reaches horizontal. This type of back support on a gurney is very helpful for patients with spinal cord injuries, head injuries, or dementia who are sometimes difficult to position. One source for such back support is listed in Table 3–6. The challenge to the clinician is to position patients for the study regardless of their physical or mental limitations.

Competencies needed to complete a modified barium swallow include knowledge of: (1) normal vs. abnormal radiographic anatomy of the head and neck[10,51–52]; (2) the equipment needed for the study; (3) the types and volumes of foods given; (4) the variations in normal swallow based on food characteristics and voluntary control; (5) anatomic and physiologic swallowing disorders; and (6) the range of swallow therapy options that can be introduced into the radiographic study and their rationale and appropriateness for various patients. The skills needed are in: (1) positioning all patient types onto the radiographic equipment; (2) presenting food to the mouth in various ways; (3) interpreting the radiographic study accurately; (4) selecting intervention strategies for the swallow disorder and the patient's diagnosis; (5) evaluating the success of the strategies; and (6) writing a report describing the results and making recommendations.

SWALLOWING THERAPY

Swallowing therapy may be provided to the dysphagic patient in acute care if it is anticipated that the patient's spontaneous recovery will be slow or

Table 3–6. Purchasing Sources for Equipment for Positioning Patients During the Radiographic Procedure

Amigo escort video swallow chair	Durable Medical Equipment Shoppe 1600 Shore Road, Unit H Naperville, IL 60540 (312) 420–7621 or (800) 225–3900
Beach chair w/out seat for back support on standard cart	Northern Speech Services, Inc. 117 North Elm Gaylord, MI 49735 (517) 732–3866
MAMA systems multiple applications and articulations (an infant / child chair)	MAMA Systems, Inc. 4347 Silver Lake Street Oconomowoc, WI 53066 (414) 569–9188
Plywood Sacred Heart chair (plans)	Manager, Radiation Department Sacred Heart Hospital 1545 S. Layton Boulevard Milwaukee, WI 53215 (414) 383–4490
Tumble Form Feeder Seats,™ small, medium, large (Floor Sitter Wedge)	Distributed by: J. A. Preston P.O. Box 89 Jackson, MI 49204 (800) 631–7277
Vess chair	Vess Chair, Inc. 2938 North 61st Street Milwaukee, WI 53210 (414) 932–2203
Video fluoro chair	Rehab Tech, Inc. 6469 Germantown Pike Dayton, OH 45418 (513) 866–4308
Video-fluoroscopic imaging chair (VIC)	Hausted, Inc. 927 Lake Road, P.O. Box 710 Medina, OH 44256–0710 (216) 723–3271; FAX: 725–0505
Video counter timer	Thalner Electronic Lab., Inc. 7235 Jackson Ann Arbor, MI 48103 (313) 761–4506
Dysphagia cup	Jamie H. Stevens MS CCC Inc. 2518 Wheaton Way, Suite 106 Bremerton, WA 98310 (206) 373–7276 FAX: 297–8121

if there is a need to improve specified aspects of swallow physiology.[9,44,53] Swallowing therapy is designed to change the physiology of the patient's swallow and generally includes muscle exercises directed at the specific locus of the patient's physiologic abnormality.

Indirect Therapy

The swallowing therapy may be given *indirectly,* that is, by exercising muscle groups used in swallowing or by practicing specific neuromuscular elements of the swallow without actually using food. In this way, if the patient is aspirating, there will be no increased risk of pneumonia nor will the clinician be placed at any risk. Table 3–7 presents a list of therapy exercises that can be done indirectly and their therapy goal. The directions for each procedure are also given in Table 3–7. In general, patients are instructed to practice these procedures 10 times a day for 5 minutes each if the patient can practice independently. Otherwise, family members can be instructed to work with the patient multiple times per day. The clinician in acute care usually has difficulty reaching the patient even twice a day because of the scheduling of multiple tests and other procedures to be completed during the acute care period. As the patient moves toward the rehabilitation phase or to a subacute unit or skilled nursing facility, there may be more time to provide multiple therapy visits per day to facilitate regular practice.

Table 3–7. Goals and Instructions for Therapy Procedures to be Practiced Indirectly (No Food or Liquid Given) or Directly

Procedure	Goal	Instructions
Range of motion exercises for lips, tongue, or jaw	Increase range of motion	Extend the structure in the desired direction as far as possible, hold for a second in extreme extension, relax.
Adduction exercises	Improve vocal fold movement arytenoid movement	Say "ah" with a hard attack and prolong a clear vocal quality. Repeat "ah-ah-ah" with a hard attack. Cough. Clear your throat, say "ah," and bear down; say "ah" as you lift up on the arms of a chair. Turn your head to the side of the laryngeal damage and say "ah." Listen to the voice quality and maintain the quality as you say "ah" and slowly turn your head to the midline.
Effortful swallow	Improve tongue-base movement improve pressure generation	Swallow saliva "hard" with lots of muscle effort.
Chewing on gauze	Increase tongue control for chewing	Place a 4″ roll of gauze on the patient's tongue so that 2″ of the gauze are in the mouth and 2″ hang out. Ask the patient to move the gauze over to his or her teeth, chew on it, move it across his or her mouth and chew on it. Continue this exercise with gauze until the patient can move the gauze easily. Then move to chewing gum or food.
Bolus control exercises	Improve bolus control by the tongue	Place a lozenge in the patient's mouth. Ask the patient to move the lozenge around and spit it out. When the patient can move the lozenge easily, use a glob of peanut butter, then move to pudding and further liquefy the pudding. The thicker the food, the easier the exercise. Patient can spit out the food without swallowing.
Falsetto	Increase laryngeal range of motion	Slide up the pitch scale as high as possible to the "high, squeaky" level and hold the tone for 2 sec. Then relax.
Thermal tactile stimulation	Improve triggering of the pharyngeal swallow	See **Table 3–4** (use saliva—be sure patient's mouth is damp).
Suck swallow	Improve triggering of the pharyngeal swallow	See **Table 3–4** (use saliva—be sure patient's mouth is damp).
Easy breath-hold (first part of the supraglottic swallow)	Improve vocal fold closure	Take a breath in and hold your breath for 2 sec. Relax.
Effortful breath-hold (first part of the supraglottic swallow)	Improve airway entrance closure (arytenoid and tongue base movement)	Take a breath in, hold your breath and bear down for 2 sec. Relax.

CASE FIVE

A 70-year-old man had undergone a supraglottic laryngectomy a week prior to the radiographic study. This surgical procedure involves removal of all or part of the hyoid bone, part of the base of the tongue surrounding the hyoid bone, the aryepiglottic folds, the false vocal folds, and the topmost portion of the thyroid cartilage. The base of tongue is then sutured to the top of the thyroid cartilage such that the postoperative airway entrance consists of the tongue base and the arytenoid cartilage. The patient was examined radiographically and found to have poor closure of this reconstructed airway entrance; this resulted in food reaching the top surface of the true vocal folds during the swallow. When the patient inhaled after the swallow, the material was aspirated. Attempts at a super-supraglottic swallow designed to improve tongue base and arytenoid motion were not successful in adequately protecting the airway, although improved range of motion was seen. Therefore, the patient was given exercises to improve the airway entrance closure. These included an effortful breath-hold without swallowing. The effortful breath-hold is the critical portion of a super-supraglottic swallow in which the patient holds the breath tightly and bears down; this pulls the tongue base posteriorly and the arytenoid anteriorly as well as closes the true vocal folds. After three weeks of practicing the procedure 10 times a day for 5 minutes per time without food, the patient was returned to X-ray and the effects of the effortful breath-hold were evaluated. Tongue base motion had improved sufficiently as had anterior arytenoid motion to close the airway entrance prior to and during the swallow. The patient was then allowed to begin oral intake using this voluntary airway protection technique. Within three more weeks, the patient was begun on full oral intake.

Direct Therapy

In contrast to indirect therapy, direct therapy is designed to actually change swallow physiology and the procedures are practiced utilizing food or liquid. Generally, direct therapy is not provided if a patient is aspirating. Direct therapy procedures include swallowing maneuvers that are voluntary neuromuscular controls applied to selected aspects of the oropharyngeal swallow. There are four swallow maneuvers: (1) the supraglottic swallow, (2) the super-supraglottic swallow, (3) the effortful swallow, and (4) the Mendelsohn maneuver. These are listed in Table 3–5 along with the neuromuscular aspect of swallow that each maneuver is designed to improve and the instructions given to teach the maneuver. Swallow maneuvers require that the patient be able to follow directions, and are therefore not useful with low-level patients or with infants and young children. These maneuvers also require a level of muscle work and energy that may not be feasible for some patients with extreme fatigue. In general, it is best to introduce the therapy procedures and exercises that are effective and require least effort and are most easily done even by lower level patients.

CASE SIX

Case Six illustrates both the effects of a swallow maneuver and the application of that maneuver during the radiographic or other physiologic assessment. The patient is a 60-year-old woman who suffered a medullary stroke four days before the assessment. As in most medullary strokes, language and cognition were not affected and she was able to follow directions. During the radiographic study, the swallow was characterized by poor laryngeal elevation and unilateral pharyngeal wall paresis as indicated by residue in one side of the pharynx. Both disorders resulted in reduced cricopharyngeal opening. The unilateral pharyngeal wall paresis and the reduced laryngeal elevation resulted in 70% of the bolus remaining in the pharynx with aspiration of most of this material after the swallow when the patient breathed. The first strategy attempted was head rotation to the damaged side of the pharynx that resulted in improved clearance of the bolus, but was not successful enough to clear all the bolus and the patient continued to aspirate. After head rotation, the Mendelsohn maneuver was taught to the patient. This maneuver is designed to increase and prolong laryngeal motion during swallow and thereby improve cricopharyngeal opening. The maneuver resulted in clearing approximately 30% more of the bolus. However, the patient still aspirated the remaining residue after the swallow. Then, head rotation and the Mendelsohn maneuver were combined, resulting in clearance of the vast majority of the bolus with only approximately 20% remaining in the pharynx after the swallow. Aspiration was eliminated. The patient began small amounts of trial oral intake using both head rotation and the Mendelsohn maneuver. The speech–language pathologist continued to follow the patient to assure good use of the Mendelsohn maneuver, and after several days the patient was discharged to her home. She had been in-

Table 3–8. Measures of Swallowing Useful in Defining the Efficacy of Treatment During the Radiographic Study of Oropharyngeal Swallow

Efficacy Measures	Treatment Procedure(s)
Oral transit time	Exercises to improve oral control; tongue range of motion and coordination exercises
Pharyngeal delay time (time from bolus head first reaching mandible to onset of laryngeal elevation assoc. w/swallow)	Therapy to improve triggering of the pharyngeal swallow
	Thermal/tactile stimulation/suck swallow
Duration of velopharyngeal closure	Techniques to improve velopharyngeal closure
Duration of airway closure at entrance (between arytenoid and base of epiglottis or base of tongue)	Super-supraglottic swallow; effortful breath hold adduction exercises
Percent residue in valleculae	Effortful swallow
Percent aspiration	Postures, supraglottic, super-supraglottic, and Mendelsohn maneuver
Duration of cricopharyngeal opening	Mendelsohn maneuver
Coordination of pharyngeal swallow events	Mendelsohn maneuver
Extent of laryngeal elevation*	Falsetto Mendelsohn maneuver
Extent of anterior hyoid motion*	Mendelsohn maneuver
Extent of vertical hyoid motion*	Falsetto Mendelsohn maneuver
Extent of tongue base to pharyngeal wall*	Effortful swallow, tongue-base retraction exercises
Percent residue in valleculae	Effortful swallow, tongue retraction exercises
Percent swallowed into esophagus divided by oropharyngeal transit time	
Oropharyngeal swallow efficiency†	
Oropharyngeal transit time: onset of post. movement of bolus tail till it passes cp region	Any therapy to improve swallow function (compensatory or direct)

* To measure extent of movement, tape a dime at midline under the patient's chin or use a single vertebra as a reference distance to account for magnification.
† Rademaker et al., 1994.

structed to continue this therapy regimen as well as non-oral intake for several more weeks. She was seen for weekly visits by the speech–language pathologist and was reevaluated radiographically at the end of another two weeks. At that time, her swallow showed significant improvement and, using both the Mendelsohn and head rotation, she was able to take all bolus thicknesses and volumes orally and was recommended to begin oral intake. A reassessment at three months post-onset revealed an entirely functional swallow without using either head rotation or the Mendelsohn maneuver. She was then instructed to go ahead and begin full oral intake not using any of the therapeutic strategies.

Throughout the process of evaluation and treatment of the dysphagic patient in acute care, or in any other health care or school setting, it is critical that the clinician is able to understand and explain the rationale for each procedure to the patient's attending physician, other health care professionals, family, as well as the patient. Each procedure in the area of dysphagia management has a strong physiologic rationale that should be communicated to other professionals to validate the procedures used.

PROFESSIONAL INTERACTIONS IN DYSPHAGIA MANAGEMENT

Because of the complexity of some patients' dysphagia, a multidisciplinary team of professionals is often needed. However, in the current cost-contained environment, not every patient needs to see or should see every professional. In most cases the SLP serves as the triage person, suggesting the referrals each patient may need. A successful team depends on communication and mutual respect among all team members. It is not necessary for the team to meet every week. Communication may be effectively maintained by telephone or face-to-face discussions by various team members. Each team member examines the patient from the perspective of their expertise. The patient's attending physician in concert with the patient and family is the ultimate decision maker regarding the patient's care and should be kept well informed regarding the patient's status. Other members of the team include the neurologist, otolaryngologist, gastroenterologist, pulmonologist, pharmacist, radiologist, dietitian, and occupational therapist, as well as the speech–language pathologist. Patients exhibiting oropharyngeal dysphagia with no known medical diagnosis most often are found to have neurologic damage or disease (i.e., Parkinson's disease, motor neuron disease, brainstem stroke, brain tumor, etc.). These patients should be referred to a neurologist on this basis. In many cases the results of the modified barium swallow will point toward the underlying diagnosis because the patient's swallowing pattern is typical of a particular neurologic disease or bolus of damage. These results should be shared with the neurologist to whom the patient is referred.

The dietitian is a critical member of the dysphagia team. Once an optimal diet has been identified that can be swallowed safely and efficiently for a patient, the speech–language pathologist should interact daily with the dietitian to determine whether or not the patient can truly sustain intake to maintain adequate nutrition and hydration on the targeted food types. The dietitian will normally monitor the patient's blood chemistries, calorie intake, and intake of nutrients to ensure that the patient is getting an adequate amount of nutrition as well as an adequate profile of nutrients. If the patient is only able to manage one consistency/viscosity such as pureed food, the dietitian should be determining that the patient is able to get sufficient nutrition in that one single viscosity and that the patient takes an adequate volume without fatiguing. In many cases the patient will need non-oral supplement to get adequate calories and nutrients. Most patients with dysphagia begin oral intake on selected food types while maintaining non-oral nutrition or hydration. Patients should demonstrate adequate oral intake before discontinuing the non-oral nutrition. Generally, oral intake is given first followed by non-

oral nutrition to supplement the oral intake. The particular type of non-oral nutrition is less important then the adequacy of the nutrition received. It is important for the speech–language pathologist to communicate daily with the patient's attending physician to ensure that the physician understands the patient's calorie intake as well as the need for any supplementation. An occupational therapist may be involved with the dysphagic patient if self-feeding is a goal. The patient may need to improve arm and hand control for hand-to-mouth placement of food. The patient may also need assistive devices to improve food placement in the mouth. These are normally supplied by the occupational therapist (OT), and the patient is also trained to use them by the OT.

CHARTING THE PATIENT'S PROGRESS USING OUTCOME AND EFFICACY MEASURES

In today's health care system, each clinician is required to measure the patient's progress at each therapy session. In dysphagia this can be done in two ways: (1) by charting the measured improvement day to day in the patient's target area of dysfunction, and (2) by charting the progress toward oral intake. *Efficacy measures* of treatment present the measured improvement day to day in target functions. For example, the duration of a pharyngeal delay can be measured in seconds during each therapy session, and charted to reflect improvement in triggering over time. If the closure at the airway entrance is being treated, the extent of movement of the arytenoid or base of tongue or front wall of the epiglottis can be measured from one radiographic study to the next. If laryngeal elevation is the target of therapy, the extent of laryngeal elevation observed externally by motion of the thyroid cartilage can be measured in each therapy session with a millimeter ruler on the outside of the patient's neck. Efficacy measures may be temporal, such as the duration of pharyngeal delay, or can include distance measures such as range of motion as in laryngeal elevation. Table 3–7 presents a list of therapy procedures and measures of efficacy of each therapy procedure from session to session.

Outcome measures reflect the broad, ultimate goals for the patient such as safe intake of liquids or return to full oral intake. Each patient should be tracked for these outcomes to define the changes during the patient's acute hospitalization. Unfortunately, with the duration of acute care stays being reduced to a few days, in many cases these ultimate outcome measures may not be observed during the acute care hospitalization unless the patient responds immediately to the treatment procedures introduced in the radiographic study. In that case the patient can be moved quickly to at least partial oral intake. Data show that approximately 25% of patients can increase oral intake after the radiographic study, resulting in a significant cost reduction.

COMMUNICATION WITH PHYSICIANS

Good, constant, knowledgeable communication with the dysphagic patient's attending physician and medical consultants is critical as the speech–language pathologist completes the evaluation and treatment of the patient's swallowing disorders. Communication should be established at the time of the bedside or clinical assessment when the SLP makes a judgment about the need for an in-depth diagnostic study. Communication of the rationale for the diagnostic study is critical. The patient's attending physician must understand that treatment of oropharyngeal dysphagia is directed at the patient's abnormal anatomy or physiology that is creating the dysphagia. Treatment is not directed at symptoms such as aspiration or inefficient eating, but at the physiology causing the symptoms.

The speech–language pathologist should also keep in mind that medical training does not include information on swallowing, either normal or abnormal. The request for an in-depth diagnostic study, such as a radiographic study, should include comments such as: "After reviewing your patient's chart and completing a brief screening, it appears that the patient is at high risk for a pharyngeal dysphagia that may include poor laryngeal elevation, poor airway closure, or poor tongue base action, none of which are visible at a screening. His diagnosis and additional medical problems would put him at risk for abnormalities in any of these areas. Since our treatment is different for each of these disorders, we need an in-depth study to define the specific physiologic abnormalities and evaluate the effects of immediate compensatory treatment that may allow him to begin oral intake right away." Such a discussion by the SLP reflects his or her knowledge base in dysphagia while informing the physician of the goals of dysphagia evaluation—that is, the physiologic understanding of the patient's problem. A radiographic or other diagnostic study should never be requested to define the presence or absence of aspiration. Such a request will often be denied because a clinical observation at bedside may reveal the patient as aspirating or at high risk for aspiration. In the current health care climate with cost containment, most physicians will reject the request for a diagnostic swallowing study if it is designed to simply define presence or absence of aspiration.

Communication with a patient's physician should not only reflect the clinician's knowledge while informing the physician about the assessments that have been completed but should also be timely in relation to patient assessments and treatments. Regular communication about the patient's progress is also critical.

Speech–language pathologists in acute care must work quickly and efficiently to be able to show improvement in efficacy and outcome measures for dysphagic patients. For them to be efficient and effective, clinicians in the acute care setting must gain knowledge about the patient's swallow physiology quickly so that they may target treatment to the exact disorder and move the patient as quickly as possible toward full oral intake.

STUDY QUESTIONS

1. Would you recommend a radiographic procedure for a patient with:
   a. Swallow apraxia
   b. Reduced laryngeal elevation
   Why or why not?

2. What types of treatment strategies might you try for the following patients and why?
   a. Alzheimer's disease with no ability to understand directions
   b. Patient with oral cancer resection
   c. Patient with a supraglottic laryngectomy
   d. Anterior left cortical stroke

3. Your patient has the following problem. Which diagnostic or screening procedures might you use?
   a. Cervical spinal cord injury with tracheostomy
   b. Delay in triggering the pharyngeal swallow
   c. Reduced range of tongue motion

4. Which postures and maneuvers would you combine for each of these patient types and why?
   a. Medullary stroke
   b. Supraglottic laryngectomy
   c. Alzheimer's disease

5. Which postures work best for these problems and why?
   a. Reduced range of vertical tongue motion
   b. Reduced airway closure
   c. Bilateral reduced pharyngeal wall function

REFERENCES

1. Bhutani MS: Dysphagia in myotonic dystrophy. [Letter to the Editor]. *Gastroenterol* 1993; 88:974.

2. Horner MJ, Alberts MJ, Dawson DV, Cook GM: Swallowing in Alzheimer's disease. *Alzheimer Dis Assoc Disorders* 1994; 8:177–189.

3. Lazarus CL, Logemann JA, Pauloski BR, Colangelo LA, Kahrilas PJ, Mittal BB, Pierce M: Swallowing in head and neck cancer patients treated with radiotherapy and adjuvant chemotherapy. *Laryngoscope* 1996; 106:1157–1166.

4. Logemann JA: Management of dysphagia post stroke. In Chapey R (ed): *Language intervention strategies in adult aphasia* (3d ed), pp. 503–512. Williams & Wilkins, Baltimore, 1994.

5. Logemann JA, Pauloski BR, Rakemaker AW, McConnel FMS, Heiser MA, Cardinale S, Shedd D: Speech and swallow function after tonsil/base of tongue resection with primary closure. *J Speech Hearing Res* 1993; 36:918–926.

6. Logemann JA, Rademaker AW, Pauloski BR, Kahrilas PJ, Bacon M, Bowman J, McCracken E: Mechanisms of recovery of swallow after supraglottic laryngectomy. *J Speech Hearing Res* 1994; 37:965–974.

7. Martin RE, Neary MA, Diamant NE: Dysphagia following anterior cervical spine surgery. *Dysphagia* 1997; 12:2–8.

8. Rademaker AW, Logemann JA, Pauloski BR, Bowman J, Lazarus C, Sisson G, Milianti F, Graner D, Cook B, Collins S, Stein D, Beery Q, Johnson J, Baker T: Recovery of postoperative swallowing in patients undergoing partial laryngectomy. *Head Neck* 1993; 15: 325–334.

9. Logemann JA: *Evaluation and treatment of swallowing disorders.* Pro-Ed, Austin, 1983.

10. Logemann JA: *A manual for videofluoroscopic evaluation of swallowing,* 2d ed. Pro-Ed, Austin, 1993.

11. Martin BJW, Logemann JA, Shaker R, Dodds WJ: Coordination between respiration and swallowing: Respiratory phase relationships and temporal integration. *J App Physiol* 1994; 76:714–723.

12. Leder SB: Gag reflex and dysphagia. *Head Neck* 1996; 18: 138–141.

13. Leder SB: Videofluoroscopic evaluation of aspiration with visual examination of the gag reflex and velar movement. *Dysphagia* 1997; 12:21–23.

14. Logemann JA: Factors affecting ability to resume oral nutrition in the oropharyngeal dysphagic individual. *Dysphagia* 1990; 4:202–208.

15. Kennedy G, Pring T, Faucus R: No place for motor-speech acts in the assessment of dysphagia? Intelligibility and swallowing difficulties in stroke and Parkinson's disease patients. *Eur J Disorders Comm* 1993; 28:213–226.

16. Myers AD: Editorial: The blue dye test. *Dysphagia* 1995; 10:174–175.

17. Thompson-Henry A, Braddock B: The modified Evan's blue dye procedure fails to detect aspiration in the tracheostomized patients: Five case reports. *Dysphagia* 1995; 10:172–174.

18. Hamlet S, Penney DG, Formolo J: Stethoscope acoustics and cervical auscultation of swallowing. *Dysphagia* 1994; 9:63–68.

19. Zenner PM, Losinski DS, Mills RH: Using cervical auscultation in the clinical dysphagia examination in long-term care. *Dysphagia* 1995; 10:27–31.

20. Bastian RW: The videoendoscopic swallowing study: An alternative and partner to the videofluoroscopic swallowing study. *Dysphagia* 1993; 8:359–367.

21. Kidder TM, Langmore SE, Martin BJW: Indications and techniques of endoscopy in evaluation of cervical dysphagia: Comparison with radiographic techniques. *Dysphagia* 1994; 9:256–261.

22. Perlman, AL, Van Daele DJ: Simultaneous endoscopic and ultrasound measures of swallowing. *J Med Speech Path* 1993; 4:223–232.

23. Bisch EM, Logemann JA, Rademaker AW, Kahrilas PJ, Lazarus CL: Pharyngeal effects of bolus volume, viscosity and temperature in patients with dysphagia resulting from neurologic impairment and in normal subjects. *J Speech Hearing Res* 1994; 37:1041–1049.

24. Jacob P, Kahrilas P, Logemann JA, Shah V, Ha T: Upper esophageal sphincter opening and modulation during swallowing. *Gastroenterol* 1989; 97:1469–1478.

25. Kahrilas PJ, Logemann JA: Volume accommodations during swallowing. *Dysphagia* 1993; 8:259–265.

26. Kahrilas PJ, Logemann JA, Gibbons P: Food intake by maneuver: An extreme compensation for impaired swallowing. *Dysphagia* 1992; 7:155–159.

27. Kahrilas PJ, Lin S, Logemann, JA, Ergun GA, Facchini F: Deglutitive tongue action: Volume accommodation and bolus propulsion. *Gastroenterol* 1993; 104: 152–162.

28. Lazarus CL, Logemann JA, Gibbons P: Effects of maneuvers on swallowing function in a dysphagia oral cancer patient. *Head Neck* 1993; 15:419–424.

29. Perlman AL, Schultz JG, Van Daele DJ: Effects of age, gender, bolus volume, and bolus viscosity on oropharyngeal pressure during swallowing. *J Appl Physiol* 1993; 75:33–37.

30. Drake W, O'Donoghue S, Bartram C, Lindsay J, Greenwood R: Eating in side-lying facilitates rehabilitation in neurogenic dysphagia. *Brain Injury* 1997; 11: 137–142.

31. Larnert G, Ekberg O: Positioning improves the oral and pharyngeal swallowing function in children with cerebral palsy. *Acta Pædiatrica* 1995; 84:689–692.

32. Logemann JA, Rademaker AW, Pauloski BR, Kahrilas PJ, Bacon M, Bowman J, McCracken E: Mechanisms of recovery of swallow after supraglottic laryngectomy. *J Speech Hearing Res* 1994; 37:965–974.

33. Rasley A, Logemann JA, Kahrilis PJ, Rademaker AW, Pauloski BR, Dodds WJ: Prevention of barium aspiration during fluoroscopic swallowing studies: Value of change in posture. *Am J Gastro* 1993; 160:1005–1009.

34. Shanahan TK, Logemann JA, Rademaker AW, Pauloski BR, Kahrilas PJ: Chin-down posture effect on aspiration in dysphagic patients. *Arch Phys Med Rehabil* 1993; 74:736–739.

35. Welch MW, Logemann JA, Rademaker AW, Kahrilas PJ: Changes in pharyngeal dimensions effected by chin tuck. *Arch Phys Med Rehabil* 1993; 74:178–181.

36. Fujiu M, Toleikis JR, Logemann JA, Larson CR: Glossopharyngeal evoked potentials in normal subjects following mechanical stimulation of the anterior faucial pillar. *Electroencephal Clin Neurophysiol* 1994; 92: 183–195.

37. Logemann JA, Pauloski BR, Colangelo L, Lazarus C, Fujiu M, Kahrilis PJ: Effects of a sour bolus on oropharyngeal swallowing measures in patients with neurogenic dysphagia. *J Speech Hearing Res* 1995; 38:556–563.

38. Rosenbek JC, Rocker EB, Wood JL, Robbins JA: Thermal application reduces the duration of stage transition in dysphagia after stroke. *Dysphagia* 1996; 11: 225–233.

39. Logemann JA: Surgical rehabilitation of adults. In Leahy M (ed): *Disorders of communication: The science of intervention* (2d ed). Whurr, London, 1995.

40. Logemann JA: Therapy for oropharyngeal swallowing disorders. In Perlman A, Schulze-Delrieu (eds): *Deglutition and its disorders: Anatomy, physiology, clinical diagnosis and management*, pp. 449–461. Singular Publishing Group, San Diego, 1997.

41. Logemann JA, Kahrilas PJ: Relearning to swallow post CVA: Application of maneuvers and indirect biofeedback: A case study. *Neurol* 1990; 40:1136–1138.

42. Kahrilas PJ, Logemann JA, Krugler C, Flanagan E: Volitional augmentation of upper esophageal sphincter opening during swallowing. *Am J Phyiol (Gastrointest Liver Physiol)* 1991; 260 (23):G450–456.

43. Lazarus CL: Effects of radiation therapy and voluntary maneuvers on swallowing functioning in head and neck cancer patients. *Clin Comm Disorders* 1993; 3: 11–20.

44. Martin BJW, Schleicher MA, O'Connor A: Management of dysphagia following supraglottic laryngectomy. *Clin Comm Disorders* 1993; 3:27–34.

45. Ohmae Y, Logemann JA, Kaiser P, Hanson DG, Kahrilas PJ: Effects of two breath-holding maneuvers on oropharyngeal swallow. *Ann Otol Rhinol Laryngol* 1996; 105:123–131.

46. Robbins JA, Levine R: Swallowing after lateral medullary syndrome plus. *Clin Comm Disorders* 1993; 3: 44–55.

47. Klor B, Milianti F: Rehabilitation in patients with G-tubes. Presented at the ASHA Convention, Orlando, 1995.

48. Martin BW, Corlew MM, Wood H, Olson D, Gallipol LA, Wingbowl M, Kirmani N: The association of swallowing dysfunction and aspiration pneumonia. *Dysphagia* 1994; 9:1–6.

49. Schmidt J, Holas M, Halvorson C, Redding M: Videofluoroscopic evidence of aspiration predicts pneumonia and death but not dehydration following stroke. *Dysphagia* 1994; 9:7–11.

50. Taniguchi MH, Moyer RS: Assessment of risk factors for pneumonia in dysphagic children. *Devel Med Child Neur* 1994; 36:495–502.

51. Robbins J, Hamilton JW, Lof GL, Kempster GB: Oropharyngeal swallowing in normal adults of different ages. *Gastroenterol* 1992; 103:823–829.

52. Tracy J, Logemann J, Kahrilas P, Jacob P, Kobara M, Krugler C: Preliminary observations on the effects of age on oropharyngeal deglutition. *Dysphagia* 1989; 4:90–94.

53. Ylvisaker M, Logemann, JA: Therapy for feeding and swallowing following head injury. In Ylvisaker M (ed): *Management of head injured patients* (2d ed). Singular Publishing Group, San Diego, in press.

4

Dysphagia in Children

JOAN C. ARVEDSON AND BRIAN T. ROGERS

CHAPTER OUTLINE

Team Approach to Assessment and Management

Aspects of Pediatric Dysphagia That Differ from Adults

Oral-Motor and Feeding Development

Etiologies of Swallowing and Feeding Disorders

Assessment of Pediatric Dysphagia

Management of Pediatric Dysphagia

Swallowing and feeding problems in infants and children are seldom seen as isolated disorders, but are typically observed as part of a broad spectrum of medical and health problems. Issues are usually complex and may involve the neurologic, airway, and gastrointestinal systems, as well as disruptions in caregiver–child interactions, all of which are likely to impact negatively on nutrition. Nutritional status is critical because of the importance of brain development in the first months of life. It is not unusual for children who present initially with physiologically based feeding problems to develop behavioral complications over time. Successful feeding is directly affected by these interrelated factors.

Knowledge of these systems and processes is crucial for accurate diagnosis and effective management of swallowing and feeding disorders in children. Some areas that have an effect on assessment and management of dysphagia differ between children and adults. Professionals need to have a good understanding of anatomic differences, developing systems in infants and young children, interrelationships of physiologic systems and the effect on swallowing and feeding, and the impact on caregiver–child relationships. A description of team concepts will lay the groundwork for a discussion of knowledge needs and the principles for assessment and management of children with dysphagia.

TEAM APPROACH TO ASSESSMENT AND MANAGEMENT

An interdisciplinary team approach is advocated for maximizing the health and development of children with complex medical problems. The expertise of multiple specialists is called for with the realization that certain needs for a specific child may be of higher priority in one time period with other needs becoming a focus at other times. The interrelated concepts integral to interdisciplinary management include a desire to communicate in a collegial way to solve problems, the development of a group philosophy among disciplines for both evaluation and treatment, respect for the expertise of other team members, an organized structure with a well-defined leader, and a shared fund of knowledge that results in creative problem solving and fruitful research.[1]

Interdisciplinary teams may function in outpatient or inpatient settings. Their composition may vary from place to place. Core team members are likely to include a developmental pediatrician or pediatric neurologist, nurse, nutritionist, speech–language pathologist, and occupational therapist. Caregivers are critical members of the team as they must share in information gathering, decision making, and the management plan because they are the primary persons to carry out intervention plans. A social worker and child psychologist have important roles for some children and their families. Other consultant specialties may include gastroenterology, pulmonology, otolaryngology, surgery, and radiology.

The team in a medical setting should be headed by a physician, who usually has a major interest in neurologic or upper GI problems. A speech–language pathologist (SLP) is the primary oral-motor and swallow specialist. An occupational therapist (OT) is the specialist for positioning and sensory issues, as well as self- and assisted feeding. Ideally, patients and families benefit from both SLP and OT expertise on the team. A problem-focused approach allows for streamlined and efficient care so that not all children are seen by all specialists at each clinic visit while team members can consult with each other in person.

Professionals in educational settings should also function in a team mode. The team concept may involve multidisciplinary, interdisciplinary, or transdisciplinary approaches.[2] Needs of individual children may change over time and thus the team functioning may also change in relation to those needs. A physician is not likely to be on site regularly, although a nurse may be available on a regular basis. All educational teams should have a strong link to appropriate professionals in a medical setting. Nonphysician professionals must keep in mind that these medically fragile children are frequently at risk for medical complications (e.g., a child who has cerebral palsy and severe quadriparesis may be at risk for chronic aspiration with oral feeding). Among the critical roles of SLPs in these settings is the awareness of the need for medical referrals and follow-up. This is one area in the practice of speech–language pathology where errors in decision making can be harmful to the patient.

The major goals for all children seen by both medical and educational based feeding and swallowing teams include safe feeding, adequate nutrition, and pleasant mealtimes. The approach emphasizes guidance and support to families, nurses, and aides to ensure adequate nutrition with minimal risk for aspiration consequences. The environment should facilitate caregiver–child interactions for optimal feeding. All persons working in the area of pediatric dysphagia are urged to collect and report efficacy and outcome data.

ASPECTS OF PEDIATRIC DYSPHAGIA THAT DIFFER FROM ADULTS

Anatomic Differences between Infants and Adults

Anatomic differences between infants and adults primarily relate to the size and relationship of the structures involved in swallowing. The infant's small oral cavity and close proximity of tongue, soft palate, and pharynx with the larynx facilitate nasal breathing. This anatomic arrangement enhances airway protection in the first 3 months of life. However, it is not correct to say that infants breathe and swallow simultaneously. A brief cessation of respiration is observed during the pharyngeal phase of swallowing.[3,4] Infants begin to breathe through the mouth in addition to the nose after the first 3 to 4 months. Sucking pads that initially aided in cheek stabilization for sucking disappear as the neck begins to elongate. As growth occurs, more space is available for tongue and soft palate movement. The sloping angle between the nasopharynx and oropharynx gradually changes so that by adulthood it approaches 90°. The larynx descends in the neck from C_4 in infancy to C_6 during childhood and finally to C_7 by adulthood.[5]

Developing System in Pediatric Population

In contrast to adults, swallowing and feeding disorders affect a developing system in the infant or young child. Even a significantly disordered system is likely to show some developmental changes that must be considered in treatment planning. It is likely that the earlier in development disruptions occur, the greater the likelihood that complications can lead to lifelong issues of malnutrition. Assessment of infants and young children is carried out by clinicians who have extensive knowledge regarding normal feeding and swallowing development, as degree and type of deficit are interpreted as differences from "normal" (Table 4–1).

In many ways, the acquisition of feeding skills by children reflects the normal maturation and development of the brain. The gross morphology associated with brain development has been documented for well over a century. A more detailed understanding of the cellular, biochemical, and molecular events associated with brain development has emerged over the past three decades. We will highlight those processes that have been clearly associated with normal and abnormal brain development to emphasize the developmental

"underpinnings" of feeding and swallowing disorders in childhood.

Embryonic Period

The central nervous system (CNS) begins to develop during the third week of gestation. During the embryonic period (4 to 8 weeks gestation), the embryonic disk is transformed into a cylindrical embryo. Initially, part of the ectodermal layer forms the neural plate, an elongated body that expands and rises to become the neural fold and eventually the neural tube. The CNS takes on the appearance of a closed tubular structure with a tail and a head. Lack of closure of the neural tube during this period can result in a variety of anomalies including anencephaly and spina bifida.

After the third week of gestation, the head position of this tubular structure has the distinct outpocketings that eventually form the cerebral hemispheres, brainstem, and cerebellum (Figure

Table 4–1. Oral-Motor and Feeding Skills from Birth to 24 Months

Age (Months)	Progression of Liquid and Food	Oral-Motor and Feeding Skills
0–4	Liquid	Suckle on nipple
4–6	Purees	Suckle → suck
		Suckle off spoon
6–9	Purees	Cup drinking
	Soft chewables	Vertical munching
		Limited lateral tongue movements
		Assist with spoon
		Finger feeding begins
9–12	Ground	Cup drinking independent
	Lumpy purees	Finger feeding
		Grasps spoon with whole hand
12–18	All textures	Lateral tongue action emerges
		↑ independence for feeding
		Straw drinking
		Scoops food, brings to mouth
18–24	More chewable food	Rotary chewing by 24 months
		↓ food intake
24+	Tougher solids	↑ mature chewing for "tougher" solids
		Independent self-feeding
		↑ use of fork
		Cup drinking, open cup and no spilling

Source: Adapted from Arvedson JC, Lefton-Greif, MA: Anatomy, physiology, and development of feeding skills. *Seminars in Speech and Language,* 1994; 17:261–268. Reprinted with permission.

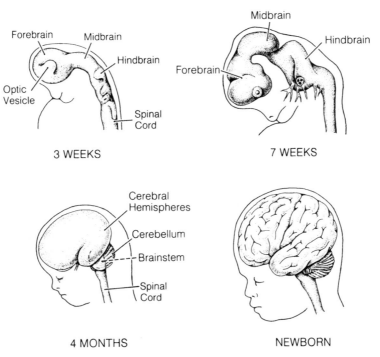

Figure 4–1. Development of the brain during fetal life. A side view illustrates the increasing complexity of the brain over time. The forebrain develops into the cerebral hemispheres, the midbrain into the brainstem, and the hindbrain into the cerebellum. Although all brain structures are formed by 4 months, the brain grows greatly in size and complexity during the final months of prenatal development. *Source:* Batshaw, ML, Perret, YM: *Children with disabilities: A medical primer* (p. 229). Paul H. Brookes, Baltimore. Copyright © 1992. Reprinted with permission.

4–1). These parts of the nervous system begin to bend into their adult shape within the next month. By the end of the embryonic period, the basic structure and form of the CNS are complete.

Cerebral Cortex Developmental Processes

The development of the cerebral cortex is characterized by three major processes including neuronal proliferation (1 to 4 months gestation), neuronal migration (3 to 5 months gestation), and neuronal differentiation (6 months gestation to the third postnatal year). The peak period of neuronal proliferation occurs from the second to fourth month of gestation. Rapidly dividing nerve cells (neuronal and glial stem cell precursors) are located adjacent to the lumen of the neural tube. Cell proliferation in the human forebrain increases exponentially through the first half of gestation (20 weeks) and continues into the second and third postnatal years.[6,7] The regulation of neuronal proliferation in the neocortex is an important deter-

minant of the final number of neurons produced. Disorders that represent the extremes of abnormal cell proliferation include microencephaly (reduced brain size and weight) and megalencephaly (increased brain size and weight). These conditions are commonly associated with multiple congenital anomalies and mental retardation.[8]

Neuronal migration refers to the mass movement of neurons from the ventricular zone that is adjacent to the lumen of the neural tube to various outer layers of the cerebral cortex. The peak period of neuronal migration is between the third and fifth month of gestation. This rapid influx of migrating neurons is associated with the development of cerebral convolutions at 5 months gestation. These cellular events transform the embryonic telencephalic wall into the familiar six-layered structure of the adult cerebral cortex. Early abnormalities of neuronal migration (2 to 4 months gestation) result in severe, usually diffuse anomalies of cortical laminations. Findings may include malposition or absence of large numbers of neurons resulting in a reduction of functional neuronal connections. Schizencephaly (agenesis of part of the cerebral wall), lissencephaly (loss of gyria), and microgyria are examples of early neuronal migrational disorders. Late neuronal migrational disorders result in less severe, often focal defects in the layering of the cerebral cortex (neuronal heterotopias).

The neuronal differentiation and organization period extends from the sixth month of gestation to approximately the third postnatal year. This period is characterized by axonal and dendritic outgrowth, dentritic arborization and spine formation, synapse formation and pruning (synaptogenesis), and expression of neurotransmitters. These processes result in extensive networks of functioning neuronal circuits that are both intrinsic and extrinsic to the cerebral cortex. These neuronal circuits form the functional systems that subserve higher cognitive processes and sensory and motor modalities. The clinical manifestations of disturbances in neuronal differentiation and organization have not been well classified. It is believed that in the absence of other pathologic findings, these disorders may be the primary disturbance in some patients with unclassified mental retardation and seizures.[8]

Myelination

The myelination period begins as early as the fourth month of gestation and continues in some regions of the brain into the third and fourth decades of life. Myelin is a lipoprotein insulation around the axon; it thereby increases the rate and efficiency of electrochemical signaling down the axonal shaft. This myelin membrane is laid down by oligodendroglial cells. Like neurons, these cells originate from primordial cells within the ventricular zone of the embryonic neural plate. The period of cellular proliferation at approximately 20 weeks gestation is a time in which oligodendroglial cells begin to increase rapidly. This proliferation is believed to persist for about 2 years.[6] Myelination stands out as a changing and accessible marker of maturation in the developing infant brain.

Regions of the CNS may differ in the time of onset as well as the rate of myelination.[9,10] Myelination of the human nervous system is characterized by some basic patterns or principles. Proximal pathways myelinate earlier and faster than distal pathways. Sensory tracts myelinate before motor tracts. At telencephalic (cerebral) sites, myelination occurs in projection before associative pathways, central telencephalic sites before poles, and occipital before fronto-temporal poles.[10]

Brain myelination in the fetal and early postnatal periods has been described in great detail by Yakovlev and Lecours.[9] Myelination of the CNS has not been observed prior to the fifth month of gestation. At the end of the fifth month of gestation, the roots of both divisions of the auditory (VIII) cranial nerve are myelinated. Myelination of the roots of the oculomotor (III, IV, and VI) and motor divisions of the trigeminal nerve occurs at about the same time. In addition, at this time, the intramedullary roots of the facial, glossopharyngeal, and hypoglossal nerves show some beginning signs of myelination. These signs of CNS maturation coincide with the appearance of suckling between 18 and 24 postconceptual weeks[11].

The development of the statoacoustic system dominates the early myelination of the central fibers of the brainstem. By five months of gestation, the vestibular and cochlear (statoacoustic) system of fibers in the tegmentum and tectum begins to myelinate and by the ninth month, myelination is completed. Those fiber systems mediating general proprioceptive (muscle sense) and exteroceptive (tactile and pain) somatic experience (e.g., medial lemniscus, outer division of the inferior cerebellar peduncle and brachium conjunctivum) myelinate later and at a slow rate beginning at 6 months gestation and extending to one year postnatally.[9] The reticular formation is a network of much thinner fibers in which longer bundle fibers course through the brainstem. The ventral medial reticular formation around the nucleus ambiguous and the nucleus tractus solitarius in the medulla have been proposed by Miller[12] as sites for the "central pattern generator" responsible for the complex sequence of motor activity involved in swallowing. Both the reticular formation and the tractus solitarius are almost devoid of myelination until term. Myelination continues beyond 2 years of age. This pattern of maturation is associated with well-recognized changes in the timing of the oral and pharyngeal phases of deglutition in the first two years of life.

Cycles of myelination of the specific thalamic projection fibers to respective cortical areas appear to be synchronized with cycles of myelination of descending efferent corticospinal and corticobulbar tracts from these areas. These tracts account for gross and fine motor skills important in efficient oral feeding in children. Myelination of these tracts appears first near term of gestation and undergoes a "burst" of myelination at 8 months postnatally. Feeding skills that coincide with this burst of myelination at 8 months include the development of mature sucking, vertical munching, and mature pincer grasp that is important for self-feeding. By 8 to 9 months postnatally, infants have developed mature sitting balance that is also important in the development of self-feeding skills.

ORAL-MOTOR AND FEEDING DEVELOPMENT

Feeding should be viewed in the context of the major streams of development in childhood. The streams of development include gross motor, fine motor/visuomotor problem solving, language and social-adaptive behavior. Abnormalities of feeding and development are frequently characterized by delays as well as deviancy in skill acquisition. Deviancy is manifested by nonsequential unevenness in the achievement of milestones within one or more streams of development.[13] In deviancy, this nonsequential pattern is intrinsically abnormal for any age.

Oromotor and Primitive Reflexes

Oromotor and primitive reflexes are prominent during the last trimester of gestation and the first 4 to 6 postnatal months. Table 4–2 describes these reflexes, their stimuli, and age of onset and disappearance.

Oromotor Reflexes

The pharyngeal swallow reflex has been observed in delivered fetuses at 12.5 weeks of gestation.[14]

Suckling, the earliest intake pattern, is observed in infants by 18 to 24 weeks. Suckling consists of anteroposterior rhythmic "stripping" movement of the tongue and lips may loosely approximate it.[4] The tongue moves forward for half of the suckle pattern but the backward phase is more pronounced. This pattern persists for the first 4 to 6 postnatal months. Tongue protrusion does not extend beyond the border of the lips.[15] Coordinated suckling and swallowing sufficient for efficient oral feeding can usually be observed by 34 to 35 weeks postmenstrual age (PMA). These events make way for spoon feeding and sucking, which consists of more vertical movement of the tongue rather than the jaw by 6 months of age (transition feeding period).

The gag reflex is elicited by touch over the posterior tongue or pharynx and includes tongue protrusion, head and jaw protrusion, and pharyngeal contractions. The gag reflex is evident by 26 to 27 weeks gestation and is strong by 40 weeks. The gag reflex is independent of swallowing. The absence of a gag reflex does not automatically translate into an inability to swallow safely. Swallow and gag are independently innervated.

The rooting and phasic bite reflexes are useful in initiating nipple feeding in the first few months of life. In an alert, hungry infant the rooting reflex is elicited by light touch to the perioral region followed by turning of the head in the direction of the stimulus. A weak rooting response can first be observed by 28 weeks PMA[16] and dissipates by 3 to 6 months postnatally.

Table 4–2. Development of Oromotor and Primitive Reflexes

Reflex	Stimulus	Age of Onset (Weeks of Gestation)	Age of Disappearance (Postnatal Months)
Pharyngeal swallow	Bolus	12	6–12
Suckling	Nipple in mouth or stroking top of tongue	18–24	6–12
Gag	Touch to posterior tongue or pharynx	26–27	persists
Rooting	Touch corner of mouth	28	3–6
Phasic bite	Pressure on gums	40	9–12
Tonic labyrinthine	Nuchal extension and flexion	30	6
Asymmetric tonic neck reflex (ATNR)	Turn head laterally	25–30	6
Moro	Sudden extension of head	25–30	4–5

The phasic bite reflex is the rhythmic opening and closing of the jaws in response to tactile stimulation of the gums. The reflex is well established by term and persists for the first 9 to 12 postnatal months.

Primitive Reflexes

Primitive reflexes are early automated movement patterns that appear during the late gestational period and are suppressed by higher cortical function before 6 months of age.[17] Primitive reflexes are characteristically prominent and persistent in children with cerebral palsy and neurogenic dysphagia.

Some primitive reflexes are particularly troublesome and interfere with the achievement of optimal positioning and swallowing efficiency. These reflexes are elicited by changes in the position of the head on the trunk. The tonic labyrinthine reflex is elicited by nuchal extension and flexion. Neck extension produces shoulder retraction with secondary flexion of the upper extremities and extension of the lower extremities. Neck flexion results in shoulder protraction and lower extremity flexion.[18] A prominent or obligatory tonic labyrinthine reflex can result in frequent extensor arching of the trunk that may complicate holding or positioning in a chair for feeding. This posture also changes the orientation of the hypopharynx, resulting in a diminished outlet for food to pass into the esophagus.

The asymmetric tonic neck reflex is also known as the "fencer position." Turning the head laterally elicits extension of the upper and lower extremities on the chin side and flexion of the limbs on the occipital side.[18] This reflex is most prominent at about 2 months and rarely is observed past 6 months of age.[19] This reflex when prominent or obligatory results in persistent lateral head turning and an asymmetric trunk posture that may compromise positioning for oral feeding.

The Moro reflex is elicited by sudden extension of the head that results in a rapid symmetrical abduction of the arms and opening of the hands.[18] The Moro reflex is easily elicited in the newborn period and dissipates rapidly by 4 to 5 months of age. When the Moro reflex is strong, minimal extension of the neck can result in an opisthotonic posture. Children with a strong Moro reflex may appear to have frequent "startle" responses to truncal movement, and there may be frequent interruptions of oral feedings.

Oromotor and Gross Motor Development

The normal transitional period from 4 to 6 months represents a time in which primitive reflexes are diminishing while voluntary oral and gross motor skills are rapidly appearing. Munching or vertical jaw movement starts at about 6 months, followed by rotary chewing at 7 months.[20] At this time infants start having lip closure around various feeding devices including the spoon and cup. The efficiency of chewing continues to an adult level of function between 3 and 6 years of age.[21]

The relationship between gross and fine motor development and feeding skills in the first 15 months of life is illustrated in Table 4–3. The first 3 months of life are characterized by increasing truncal balance and midline position of the head and hands. This facilitates midline activities including spoon feeding. The palmar grasp reflex persists until 3 to 4 months of age. This reflex can be elicited by a tactile stimulus to the palm of the infant. This stimulus elicits a quick flexion of all fingers. By 3 to 4 months, infants' hands are predominantly open and are used to reach or bat at objects. By 6 to 7 months, most infants begin to sit independently and are able to reach and grasp objects in a palmar fashion. The use of the forefinger and thumb to pick up objects by 9 to 10 months heralds the appearance of rather efficient finger feeding. More refined hand skills that include grasp and release as well as supination are evident by 12 to 15 months. These hand skills result in more independent feeding skills that include spoon and cup use.

Feeding and Swallowing Development

Suck, swallow, and respiratory patterns are fully functional in the normal term infant. A burst-pause pattern becomes evident during the thirtieth to thirty-third weeks of gestation. This indicates readiness of the infant to attempt oral feeding. Two major prerequisites for successful oral feeding include a strong and rhythmic nonnutritive suck (2 sucks per sec) and a stable airway. Most premature infants can feed by breast or bottle efficiently enough (1 suck per sec) to meet nutritional needs strictly orally between 34 and 37 weeks. It is not unrealistic to find some healthy infants at 32 to 33 weeks of gestation able to meet nutritional needs for adequate weight gain. However, that is not to be routinely expected.

Practices differ across neonatal intensive care units in the United States and Canada regarding

Table 4–3. Gross and Fine Motor Milestones Relevant to Normal Feeding from Birth to 15 Months of Age

Age (months)	Equilibrium and Gross Motor Milestones	Prehension (Fine Motor) Milestones	Feeding Skills
Birth	Prominent primitive reflexes (Moro, tonic labrynthine, and palmar grasp)	Shoulders mildly retracted	Prominent oral reflexes
		Hands frequently closed	Gentle flexor support of head and extremities needed for feedings
	Turn head from side to side in supine position		
	Head lag on pull to sit		
3–4	Primitive reflexes less prominent	Hands open	Oral reflexes (suckle, rooting) less prominent
	Increased midline head position in supine	Midline hand play	Hands frequently placed in mouth
	Head in line with trunk while sitting		Less head and trunk support needed for feeding
			Assisted spoon feedings begin
6–7	Absence of primitive reflexes	Unilateral reach and grasp (palmar-radial)	
	Anterior and lateral propping reactions	Objects to mouth	
			Holds bottle
	Brief independent sitting		
			Reaches for food
			Sits supported in high chair
9–10	Sits steady for 10–15 minutes	Immature pincer grasp	Finger feeding
			Increased independent sitting for feeding
	Stands holding on to person or furniture	Reaches and leans forward, then recovers balance	
12–15	Walks independently		Throws food
		Picks up and releases objects	Holds cup
		Spontaneous supination of hands.	Uses spoon
		Grasps and manipulates long slender objects	

Source: Adapted from Rogers BT: Neurodevelopmental presentation of dysphagia. *Seminars in Speech and Language,* 1996; 17:269–281. Reprinted with permission.

the emphasis placed on breast feeding. Adequate growth is critical in the first months of life. Success of breast or bottle feeding is measured by weight gain and efficiency of the feeding process. Variables that predict outcomes are needed so that parents can take their infants home from the hospital and make feedings pleasant and efficient. If oral feedings are lengthy and stressful for infant and caregiver, there is a high probability that the infant will end up with a diagnosis of Failure to Thrive. Thus, if the best predictions are that the infant can-

not adequately take enough nutrition strictly orally and is likely to require at least a few months to attain full oral feeding status, alternate feeding plans should be made prior to discharge home. The feeding plan may include a combination or oral and non-oral feeds. It is better to have the effective combination worked out in a logical developmental approach rather than a feeding tube placed at some later date after oral feeding has failed.

The concept of a critical period is applicable in consideration of the development of oral-motor and feeding skills, particularly as it relates to chewing in humans[22] and in other animals.[23] The introduction of soft chewable food to human infants is based on developmental status, not strictly chronologic age. Normally developing children are typically ready for soft chewable textures by about 6 to 8 months of age when they are sitting upright, handling thicker textures via spoon, and beginning to reach for objects. The tongue action is altered from suckling to a posterior stripping action of the tongue elicited by solid food that is followed by a swallow.[24] In addition to oral-motor function skills, personality or behavior and environmental factors may complicate feeding. Assessment of children with feeding problems must take into account all the above factors.

Interrelationships of Airway, Neurologic, and Gastrointestinal Systems

The interactions of airway, gastrointestinal, and neurologic systems are complex. Feeding disorders commonly involve these complex interactions. A stable airway for adequate respiration is absolutely essential as a basis for oral feeding. Infants with conditions such as bronchopulmonary dysplasia expend considerable energy for respiration. They may not be able to expend the added energy required for suck/swallow/respiratory sequencing to feed orally and to meet nutritional needs in the first few months of life. These infants are also likely to require increased caloric intake because of the extra respiratory effort. Gastroesophageal reflux is a common complicating factor with a variety of conditions, particularly when there is neurologic impairment.

Impact on Caregiver–Child Interactions

Feeding disorders have an impact on the caregiver–child relationship, and vice versa. Caregivers typically experience stress and frustration whenever there are difficulties related to feeding their infants and children. This stress can be transmitted to a child, which then leads to exacerbation of feeding difficulties. Caregivers are usually very concerned when children do not gain weight appropriately and they put a strong emphasis on the entire feeding process. This stress is likely to lead to forced feeding that makes a bad situation even worse. Mealtimes may become such negative experiences for children that they refuse even more adamantly, and major power struggles can ensue. These negative interactions then affect other areas of caregiver

and child interactions. It is also possible that overall development of oral-motor and feeding skills will be affected negatively.

ETIOLOGIES OF SWALLOWING AND FEEDING DISORDERS

The etiologies of swallowing and feeding disorders in childhood are numerous and vary considerably in their presentation (Table 4–4). The more common disorders that result in dysphagia are presented in a diagnostic framework based on history and physical findings. Great care should be taken in determining the onset and natural history of any feeding problem.

Dysphagia can be conveniently classified into acute and chronic forms. Chronic disorders can either be static or progressive in presentation. In static disorders, chewing and swallowing skills generally remain stable or improve over time. Although feeding efficiency may change during acute illnesses or transition feeding periods, persistent loss of previously acquired oromotor and swallowing skills does not occur with static disorders. Regression or loss of previously mastered feeding skills is seen in progressive disorders and should prompt appropriate medical evaluation.

Neurogenic dysphagia is rarely an isolated finding and usually is associated with more diffuse or global signs of neurologic dysfunction. In static forms of neurogenic dysphagia, children usually have neurologic impairments and dysphagia that are obvious at birth or in the first 3 to 4 months of life. Prognosis is best judged in light of the etiology as well as the severity of the dysphagia and associated neurologic impairments.

Progressive neurologic disorders resulting in dysphagia can present in the neonatal period, infancy, or childhood. Liposomal storage diseases illustrate this variability. Forms of GM_1 and GM_2 gangliosidosis and Krabbe's disease present in the first 2 to 3 months. Infants with metachromatic leukodystrophy have the insidious onset of gait disturbances and dysphagia after their first year of life.

The age of onset is important in the evaluation of any feeding problem. Cardiopulmonary disorders characteristically present in infancy. The proximal and distal airways in infants have smaller diameter than those in adolescents or adults. In addition, the elastic work done by respiratory muscles for a characteristic tidal volume is greater in infants when compared to older children and adults. Conditions including pneumonitis

Table 4–4. Etiologies of Dysphagia in Childhood

Site of Pathology	Acute	Chronic Static	Chronic Progressive
Central nervous system	Hypoxic-ischemic encephalopathy Cerebral infarctions Intracranial hemorrhage Infections 　Meningitis 　Encephalitis 　Poliomyelitis 　Botulism 　Syphilis Acute bilirubin encephalopathy (kernicterus) Metabolic encephalopathies 　Aminoacidopathies 　Disorders of carbohydrate metabolism Neonatal withdrawal syndrome (heroin, barbiturates) Traumatic encephalopathies and brainstem injuries	Arnold Chiari malformation Genetic disorders Familial dysautonomia (Riley-Day) Mobius sequence Congenital anomalies of the brain Cerebral palsy Chronic posticteric encephalopathy	Arnold Chiari malformation Intracranial malignancies 　Tumors 　Leukemia 　Lymphoma Degenerative white and gray matter diseases (examples) 　Lysosomal storage diseases 　(Mucopolysaccharidoses Niemann-Pick, Krabbe's, metachromatic leukodystrophy, Tay-Sachs) 　Peroxisomal disorders (Zellweger's, Leigh syndrome, neuroaxonal dystrophy, adrenoleukodystrophy) 　Purine and Pyrimidine disorders (Lesch-Nyhan) 　Disorders of Metal Metabolism (Wilson's disease, Menkes' disease) 　Hypersensitivity diseases (Cockayne's syndrome) 　Infections (HIV encephalopathy) 　Rett syndrome Spinocerebellar disorders Dystonia musculorum deformans Multiple sclerosis Amyotrophic lateral sclerosis Syringobulbia
Anterior horn cell			Infantile spinal muscular atrophy
Peripheral nervous system	Acute inflammatory polyradiculoneuropathy	Polyneuropathies	Polyneuropathies
Neuromuscular junction	Hypermagnesemia		Myasthenia gravis

Table 4–4. (*continued*)

Site of Pathology	Acute	Chronic	
		Static	Progressive

Muscles	Polymyositis
	Dermatomyositis
		Congenital myopathies
		  Nemaline rod
		  Myotubular
		  Fiber type disproportion
		Myotonic dystrophy
		Congenital muscular
		  dystrophy
		Infantile fascioscapulo
		  humeral dystrophy
			Metabolic myopathies
			  Glycogen storage disease
			  Mitochondrial
			Duchenne's muscular
			  dystrophy

Respiratory tract	Otitis media
	Sinusitis
	Adenotonsillitis and
	  pharyngitis
		Severe chronic lung disease
		  (e.g., bronchopulmonary
		  dysplasia)
		Structural anomalies of
		  upper respiratory tract	

Cardiovascular
  disorders
		Congenital heart disease
		  including cyanotic and
		  congestive heart failure
			Congenital heart disease
			  (may be progressive at
			  times)

Gastrointestinal tract		Gastroesophageal reflux Peptic ulcer	Gastroesophageal reflux and esophagitis Peptic ulcer
Psychological		Disorders of caregiver–child interaction	

Source: Adapted from Rogers B, Campbell J: Pediatric and neurodevelopmental evaluation. In J Arvedson and L Brodsky (Eds.), *Pediatric swallowing and feeding: Assessment and management* (pp. 58–59). Singular Publishing Group, San Diego: 1993. Reprinted with permission.

interstitial edema (congestive heart failure) and fibrosis (bronchopulmonary dysplasia) result in greater airway resistance and work of breathing in infancy. Infants with varying degrees of respiratory distress commonly present with progressive tachypnea or fatigue during oral feeding.[25] Caregivers often report that the infant does well for the first half of oral feeding but then loses interest or refuses the rest of the feeding.

Gastroesophageal disorders are important causes of feeding problems in children. Gastroesophageal reflux (GER) is defined simply as the return of stomach contents into the esophagus and possibly up to the pharynx caused by a dysfunction of the lower esophagus. The presentation may include symptoms such as increased irritability, postural arching, neck hyperextension, and food refusal after a small quantity is taken, but emesis is not necessarily present.[26,27] When emesis does occur regularly, there is a great loss of ingested calories resulting in weight loss and failure to thrive.

The reflux of gastric acid onto the stratified squamous epithelium lining the esophagus can lead to esophagitis. Blood loss from the inflamed tissue may cause nondeficiency anemia, melena, or hematemesis. Esophagitis has been reported in 60 to 80% of infants and children with signs and symptoms of GER.[28,29]

Multiple respiratory complications can result from gastroesophageal reflux. Stridor may be caused by laryngeal dysfunction resulting from a primary laryngeal disorder or inflammation secondary to GER.[30] Other chronic pulmonary disorders including reversible airway disease and recurrent pneumonia have been associated with gastroesophageal reflux.[31]

ASSESSMENT OF PEDIATRIC DYSPHAGIA

A comprehensive assessment of infants and children with feeding and swallowing problems consists of a bedside or clinic assessment that may include the use of some instrumentation. Selected patients may be referred for special studies of swallowing (e.g., videofluoroscopic swallow study

[VFSS]) and other aspects of deglutition. The importance of an accurate diagnosis is once again emphasized as being critical for making realistic prognoses and thus management plans.

Bedside/Clinic Assessment

Criteria for Referral

Major red flags likely to trigger a bedside/clinic feeding assessment include:

- Slow feeding characterized by mealtimes typically longer than 30 to 40 minutes[32]
- New onset of feeding difficulty, or change in feeding patterns that could include
    Increased drooling
    Nasopharyngeal reflux
- Risk for aspiration associated with swallowing and feeding
    Breathing interruptions or apnea during oral feeding
    "Gurgly" vocal quality before and after swallows
    Incoordination of sucking and swallowing in infants
    Oral-motor inefficiencies that delay movement of bolus over back of tongue
    History of recurrent pneumonia and feeding difficulty
- Behavior that can indicate possible gastroesophageal reflux disease (GERD)
    Irritability or behavior problems during mealtimes
    Unexplained food refusal and failure to thrive (FTT)
    Lethargy and decreased arousal during oral feeding
    Emesis not necessarily seen, particularly with neurologic impairment
- Failure to gain weight over 2 to 3 months
- Diagnosis of a disorder associated with dysphagia or FTT
- Delayed development, for example
    No spoon feeding by 9 months
    No chewing of table food by 18 months
    No cup drinking by 24 months

Bedside and Clinic Assessment Protocol

The diagnostic work-up for infants and children with suspected feeding and swallowing disorders includes a detailed health and developmental history, physical examination, and oral-motor and feeding observation. In some instances, findings may lead to instrumental assessments that yield additional specific information necessary for coordinated management recommendations.

There is no single ideal data collection form available at present, although numerous checklists and scales can assist in systematizing observations.[15, 33–42] The Assessment Worksheet presented in Appendix A allows for concise history and feeding observations to be made in primarily a check ($\sqrt{}$) format. A scale is needed to yield standardized observations that can lead to a severity rating to delineate oral and pharyngeal phase components of swallowing, as well as broader aspects of feeding issues. This scale would also allow for data collection across institutions for research purposes.

The interdisciplinary team assessment has been stressed earlier. The focus here is on the oral-motor and feeding assessment. Clinicians are reminded that it can be effective only in conjunction with information from the history and physical examination. The oral-motor and feeding assessment consists of a prefeeding assessment, oral-motor structure and function examination, and feeding observation.[33] However, oral feeding may not be carried out when a child appears at such high risk for aspiration that oral feeding would not be an option at the time (e.g., an infant who has no nonnutritive suck or a child who has a gurgly voice quality when at rest and very limited lip and tongue action).

Prefeeding Assessment

Observations include parent–child interactions, positioning and posture, respiratory status (rate, variability, and effort), responsiveness (level of alertness, affect, and temperament), and ability to self-calm and self-regulate (especially pertinent for infants).[43,44]

Oral-Motor Structure and Function Assessment

This assessment includes examination of oral structures and their function prior to feeding. A cranial nerve examination allows for differentiation of supranuclear and nuclear or peripheral cranial nerve deficits associated with dysphagia (Table 4–5).

Observations for all infants and children include lip and jaw position at rest, status of drooling, tongue at rest and during movement, palatal shape and height, oral reflexes (especially persistent primitive reflexes beyond the age expected for extinction) (Table 4–2), laryngeal function (breathy or gurgly voice quality raise the index of suspicion for aspiration risks), and nonnutritive sucking in infants.

Table 4–5. Clinical Localization of Cranial Nerve Deficits Associated with Dysphagia

Cranial Nerve	Supranuclear	Nuclear or Peripheral
Trigeminal (CN V)	Mandible movements are well preserved but often immature or poorly coordinated	Mandible movements are usually minimal or absent
	Jaw jerk reflex present or exaggerated	Jaw jerk reflex is usually absent
	Tonic bite reflex may be present	Tonic bite reflex is absent
Facial (CN VII)	Paralysis of lower half of face	Paralysis of upper (forehead) and lower half of face
	Paralysis is almost always unilateral	Paralysis can be unilateral or bilateral
Glossopharyngeal (CN IX) and Vagus (CN X)	Muscular palate has normal strength	Weakness of muscular palate
		Asymmetry of muscular palate movement is common
	Normal appearance of palatopharyngeal folds	Flattening of palatopharyngeal folds
	Vocal fold movement preserved	Vocal fold paralysis
Hypoglossal (CN XII)	Tongue movements are dysfunctional but present	Unilateral or bilateral absence of tongue movement
	Tongue protrusion reflex can be exaggerated and prolonged in duration	Tongue fasciculations
		Tongue atrophy

Source: Rogers B, Campbell J: Pediatric neurodevelopmental evaluation. In JC Arvedson, L. Brodsky (Eds.), *Pediatric swallowing and feeding: Assessment and management* (p. 74). Singular Publishing Group, San Diego: 1993. Reprinted with permission.

Feeding Observation

Cranial nerve status related to oral-motor function is also assessed during a feeding observation (Table 4–6). Cranial nerve deficits may be a basis for failure to close lips around a nipple or spoon, failure to form a bolus, lack of tongue elevation, and delay in initiation of a swallow.

Oral Feeders

Children who have been doing oral feeding prior to the feeding assessment are usually observed initially with a familiar feeder. The feeder and the child can be evaluated with a numerical rating to estimate some range of severity (Table 4–7). Bolus formation skills are noted, in relation to lip closure, jaw stabilization, and tongue action. Self-feeding via finger food or spoon is evaluated related to age level expectations, as are chewing and munching skills. Children can be ready for chewable food without necessarily mastering all gradations of pureed textures.[45, 46]

Timing of oral and pharyngeal phases is estimated and the number of swallows per bolus de-termined. Varied textures may be used. The meal starts with textures in the child's repertoire that the caregivers report to be the easiest and then goes on to those textures perceived to be more difficult. New textures may be introduced during the session if pertinent to potential management decisions. The risk for aspiration may be texture related.[47] For example, reduced tongue motility and delayed pharyngeal swallow may result in higher risk for aspiration with thin liquids than thicker liquids and food. Following the typical feeding observation, therapeutic changes can be made in positioning, texture, size of bolus, timing between bolus presentations, and utensils. The therapeutic alterations are designed to answer questions in relation to management decisions. Is the child safe to feed orally? If yes, what are the modifications needed in positioning, textures, and nutrition guidelines? If no, what are the alternatives for non-oral feeding? The alternatives may differ whether the anticipated non-oral feeding status is likely to be long term or short term (no more than 3 to 4 months). A gastrostomy is likely to be needed for long-term non-oral feeding, but a nasogastric tube

Table 4–6. Cranial Nerve (CN) Function during Feeding Assessment

CN	Stimulus	Normal Response	Deficit Response
V	Food on tongue	Mastication initiated	Bolus not formed
VII	Sucking	Lip pursing	Lack of lip seal
	Food on lower lip	Lip closure	Lack of lip movement
	Smile	Retraction of lips	Asymmetry or lack of retraction
IX,X	Food posterior in mouth	Swallow—2 sec	Delayed swallow
		Soft palate elevation	Nasopharyngeal reflux
XII	Food on tongue	Tongue shape, point, and protrude	Tongue lacks thinning, elevation and has excessive thrust, atrophy

Source: Arvedson J: Oral-motor and feeding assessment. In J Arvedson & L Brodsky (Eds.), *Pediatric swallowing and feeding: Assessment and management* (p.271). Singular Publishing Group, San Diego, 1993. Reprinted with permission.

Table 4–7. Assessment of Typical Feeding Session

Feeder	Child
Stroking circumoral area	Hypertonic tongue
Stroking under chin	No tongue grooving
Repeated touching of tongue or teeth with spoon or food	Wide mouth opening (inappropriate)
Up–down movement of mandible	No closure of lips around spoon
Scraping food off upper teeth	No tongue lateralization
Collecting drooled food and reinserting into mouth	Drooling
	Bite reflex
	Coughing
	Gagging or sputtering
	Sucking
	Open mouth swallow
	Regurgitation (emesis)
	Food retained in mouth
	Food aspiration

Note: Score 1 for each action or state. Scores of 4 or less show normal function for weight controls, score of 0 expected if ag-controls used, scores of 5–8 marginal, scores of 9 or more reveal inadequate feeding skills.
Source: Adapted from Gisel, EG, Patrick J: Identification of children with cerebral palsy unable to maintain a normal nutritional stage. *Lancet,* 1988; 1, 283–286.

may be appropriate as a supplement when short-term non-oral feedings are predicted.

First Feeding Assessment in Young Infant Feeders

Infants who have never fed orally prior to the assessment are usually examined when they appear to have cardiorespiratory stability, adequate bowel sounds, and no other obvious contraindications to oral feeding attempts. Infants are observed while feeding for 15 to 20 minutes, the expected time range for a full feed. It is important for the examiner to spend that amount of time. Otherwise the infant who does well for the first 5 minutes but then becomes disorganized or fatigues before completing a feed may be mistakenly cleared for regular feeding. On the other hand, some lethargic infants require several minutes to get them roused sufficiently to attempt a PO feed. Both extremes are not unusual with infants demonstrating neurogenic dysphagia.

Bedside/Clinic Instrumental Tools

Pulse Oximetry

Oximetry is the most widely used method for evaluation of oxygen levels. Oximetry measures oxygen saturation of capillary blood flow through an external sensor. This probe sensor is taped around a toe or finger. The saturation level is expressed as a percentage. Most infants have an oxygen saturation level at least 95%. A saturation level below 90% is an indicator of some degree of hypoxia. Physicians may set acceptable parameters for saturation levels for premature infants and children with other known health problems.

Oximetry is useful to determine baseline oxygen saturation, changes in oxygen saturation in response to work (e.g., feeding), and the effectiveness of oxygen therapy. Oximetry is a non-invasive technique that is easily portable and gives ongoing information regarding oxygen saturation. Oximetry is more reliable than observing facial color changes because desaturation can occur with no observable symptoms. The probe can be left in place for long periods to provide continuous measurement and thus variability in oxygen saturations under different circumstances.

Oximetry has some disadvantages that include factors limiting reliability and accuracy. Movement artifact is a complicating factor[48] with a probe placed on toes or fingers that move a lot during feeding. Oximetry may overestimate oxygen saturation levels of darkly pigmented infants[49] since the values are computed by the degree of infrared light absorption. Accuracy can also be affected by external ambient light sources, infrared heating sources used in certain warmers,[50] and anemia or the amount of fetal hemoglobin still present in an infant's blood.[48] Readings can also vary somewhat by the type of oximeter. The relationship between oximetry values and partial pressures of oxygen (PaO_2) that can be obtained through an arterial blood gas needs to be considered.[51]

Cervical Auscultation

A stethoscope is used to detect changes in upper aerodigestive tract sounds that occur during breathing, swallowing, and bolus passage. These changes in sounds may be helpful information, although findings have not been standardized to qualify auscultation as an instrumental procedure for clinical practice. The acoustic characteristics of different stethoscopes are not well defined. Other limitations include the lack of direct visualization of the swallow mechanism, limited ability to detect aspiration events, and lack of ability to define a reason for inferred aspiration. The potential for accurate inferences of pharyngeal phase physiology during swallowing with a simple stethoscope is intriguing. Advantages include the non-invasiveness, easy availability of equipment, prolonged sampling periods possible, no radiation, and no contrast required. However, data are needed before auscultation can be considered a routine **instrumental** procedure in pediatric swallowing and feeding assessment.

Flexible Endoscopy

Endoscopy can be used for multiple purposes. The improved flexible scopes can be employed with even very low birth weight infants at the bedside. The procedure is usually carried out as nasopharyngoscopy when a scope can be passed through the nose allowing visualization of nasal, pharyngeal, and laryngeal regions. Pediatric otolaryngologists typically carry out this procedure to examine upper airways (laryngoscopy) and lower airways (bronchoscopy). Endoscopy can reveal congenital anomalies, stenosis, compression from vascular rings or masses, and structural airway problems such as laryngotracheal malacia.

Any concerns related to the child's ability to protect the airway during swallowing are also indications for nasopharyngoscopy. Observations precipitating referral could include weak or breathy cry and hoarseness that would raise suspicion for vocal fold paresis or paralysis, gurgly vocal quality that could indicate pooling of secretions at the level of the laryngeal vestibule and possible aspiration, increased rate of respirations during feeding, and any observable indications of increased respiratory effort or incoordination of respirations and sucking and/or swallowing.

Endoscopy for specific examination of swallowing (Fiberoptic Endoscopic Evaluation of swallowing—FEES) is in its infancy for infants and young children.[52] The potential for more accurate inferences of pharyngeal physiology without the use of radiation during swallowing is encouraging. The same problems that occur with adults are magnified in young children (Table 4–8).

Instrumental Assessments of Swallowing and Other Aspects of Deglutition

A variety of instrumental procedures are used in the evaluation of pediatric patients with dysphagia (Table 4–8). The procedures include, but are not limited to, videofluoroscopic modified barium swallow study (VFSS), ultrasound, upper gastrointestinal study (UGI), and scintigraphy. In addition, manometry can help to define UES pressures related to relaxation timing and degree of upper esophageal sphincter (UES) opening, as well as esophageal spasm during food ingestion.[53] Esophageal manometry measures pressures in the upper and lower esophageal sphincters that can aid in assessing the competence of these sphincters. Failure of UES relaxation (cricopharyngeal achalasia) can be documented with manometry.

These procedures examine different swallow and feeding components. Specialized studies can be categorized as procedures that evaluate a specific aspect of swallow function, those that examine factors that may contribute to swallow dysfunction, and others that determine consequences of the dysfunction. Each procedure is carried out for specific purposes and has advantages and disadvantages. All pediatric feeding/swallowing specialists should be familiar with these procedures even when they are not directly involved in carrying them out. They need to understand purposes, processes, and interpretations of findings.

Instrumental procedures are carried out as part of a comprehensive feeding and swallowing evaluation, and are interpreted with other information obtained through case history, nutrition assessment, physical examination, and feeding observation with oral-motor examination. Instrumental procedures are likely to be recommended when information is needed to define the potential ability to feed safely by mouth, identify physiological underpinnings for the impairment in deglutition, and clarify nutrition status. The videofluoroscopic swallow study (VFSS) is the most frequently used instrumental examination in pediatrics that focuses on pharyngeal and upper esophageal physiology. This chapter is not intended to be a procedural manual for VFSS, and thus detailed descriptions are not given. The major issues for clinicians are described briefly.

Videofluoroscopic Swallow Study

The videofluoroscopic swallow study (VFSS) continues to be the procedure of choice for defining pharyngeal physiology and documenting aspiration events before, during, or after swallows.[54] Other terms commonly used to describe the study include "modified barium swallow study," "three phase swallow study," and "oropharyngeal swallow study." Speech–language pathologists and radiologists conduct the study together. SLPs must demonstrate appropriate didactic knowledge and technical skills as approved by the Legislative Council of the American Speech–Language-Hearing Association.[55] In addition, SLPs should have extensive experience with dysphagia in children that includes clinical experience as well as training in interpretation of findings, both for accuracy of interpretation and for relationship to health history and clinic information so that coordinated recommendations are made for optimal management. This study is one piece of a puzzle that must have all the pieces fitting together for the best care of the child. The procedure is described by Logemann (Chapter 3) with focus for adults. Procedures for pediatric patients are similar although some specific cautions exist for infants and young children. Details of procedures with infants and children can be found in other sources (e.g.,[56,57]).

Typically, therapeutic maneuvers are very limited as fluoroscopy time is kept to a minimum while maximum information is obtained to aid in comprehensive decision making. Questions should be defined clearly ahead of time so the study can be focused to address the major concerns. It is important that the infant or child is calm and as responsive as possible to simulate a typical feeding situation. A primary caregiver is frequently an active participant in carrying out the study. Familiar food and comfort items can be brought from home. Barium contrast materials are added to the food and liquid.

Findings are reviewed with caregivers and integrated with information from the history and clinic findings in relation to etiology and prognosis. Clinical competencies for SLPs working in dysphagia are being developed through the Special Interest Division (SID) 13 (Dysphagia), ASHA.

Table 4–8. Instrumental Procedures Used in the Evaluation of Pediatric Patients with Dysphagia

Instrumental Procedure	Components of Swallowing Examined	Advantages	Limitations
Videofluoroscopic Swallow Study (VFSS)	Defines anatomy and physiology of the swallowing mechanism during deglutition Identifies bolus and positioning variables, and feeding strategies or maneuvers that enhance the safety of swallowing Defines "reason" for dysphagia Detects aspiration	Dynamic view of oral preparatory, oral, pharyngeal, and cervical esophageal phases of swallowing Routine procedure in most centers Attempts to simulate "typical" feeding situation	Radiation exposure Samples swallowing performance for brief time period Requires contrast (barium sulfate) Requires patient cooperation
Ultrasound Imaging (US)	Defines oral preparatory and oral phases of deglutition Visualizes temporal relationships between movement patterns of oral and pharyngeal structures	Dynamic and multiple plane views of oral preparatory and oral phases of swallowing Non-invasive, can sample swallows repeatedly and for prolonged time period No contrast required, uses "real" food or liquid Equipment available at major medical centers	Does not detect penetration or aspiration Does not provide definitive structural landmarks Does not define "reason" for dysphagia or aspiration Availability of trained personnel may be limited
Fiberoptic Endoscopic Evaluation of Swallowing (FEES)	Views pharyngeal and laryngeal structures prior to and immediately following swallowing Displays pooling and aspiration of salivary secretions Assesses pharyngeal and laryngeal response (sensation) to direct stimulation Detects velopharyngeal insufficiency and vocal fold abnormalities	Dynamic view of nasal, pharyngeal, and laryngeal structures before and after swallowing No radiation exposure, can sample swallowing repeatedly and for prolonged time periods No contrast required, uses "real" food or liquid Equipment is portable Routine office procedure used by otolaryngologists	Does not view interactions between oral, pharyngeal, and cervical esophageal structures during actual swallow Requires patient cooperation Invasive, may be uncomfortable Potential risk factors include vasovagal reaction, laryngospasm, and nasal hemorrhage
Upper Gastrointestinal Study (UGI)	Defines anatomy and functional integrity of esophagus, stomach, and duodenum Detects esophageal strictures, ulcer disease, vascular rings, extrinsic lesions compressing the esophagus, and foreign bodies in esophagus Detects GI tract obstructions and malformation of the intestines Screens oropharyngeal function Detects gross pharyngeal anomalies and concomitant aspiration	Dynamic view of swallowing mechanism, from oral cavity through duodenum Routine procedure Rapid procedure Without discomfort	Radiation exposure Samples swallowing performance for brief time period Requires contrast medium (barium sulfate) Misses manifestations of oropharyngeal deglutition disorders that appear after bolus passes into esophagus May pose increased risk of aspiration to patients with oropharyngeal dysphagia Fails to simulate a typical meal Not useful to develop a feeding plan

Table 4–8. (*continued*)

Instrumental Procedure	Components of Swallowing Examined	Advantages	Limitations
Radionuclide Imaging Studies	Quantifies esophageal and gastric emptying Quantifies aspiration from saliva or GER	Multiple static images of concentrated regions of tracer residue over prolonged period of time Quantifies aspiration Sensitive to timing of tracer clearance	Does not display swallowing structures Radiation exposure Costly procedure Availability may be limited

Source: Adapted from Lefton-Greif MA, Loughlin, GM: Specialized studies used in the evaluation of the pediatric patient with dysphagia. *Seminars in Speech and Language,* 1996; 17:311–330.

Some clinical competencies will be the same whether the SLP is specializing in dysphagia with children or with adults. SLPs working with infants and young children should demonstrate other competencies that reflect knowledge about how pathologies interact with a developing system. Some form of specialty recognition is likely to be developed in the near future. Professionals with high levels of expertise in the assessment and management of persons with dysphagia will go through some type of examination process to demonstrate knowledge and skills. This specialty recognition will give patients and families the opportunity to seek out the most qualified practitioners.

In summary, the diagnostic workup for children with feeding and swallowing problems must be comprehensive (1) to establish etiology, (2) to describe structures and function in all aspects of feeding and swallowing, (3) to clarify oral, pharyngeal, and esophageal phase physiology and the risk for aspiration with oral feeding, and (4) to delineate nutrition status and risks.

MANAGEMENT OF PEDIATRIC DYSPHAGIA

All intervention strategies have the major goal of adequate nutrition with minimal risk for aspiration. Management of swallowing and feeding problems in infants and children necessitate individualized treatment plans that take into account multiple interactive factors. Management plans must *not* be based on isolated techniques. Medical and surgical interventions may be needed, but they will not be discussed in detail here. Thus management decisions related to nutrition, positioning, oral-motor and swallow function, and behavioral/interaction issues will be discussed in the rest of this chapter.

Nutrition

Optimal nutritional status is essential for all infants and children. The provision of adequate fluid, calories, protein, and micronutrients is a requirement for normal growth and development. Growth velocity as well as calorie and fluid requirements per kilogram of body weight are highest in the first month of life and undergo deceleration during infancy and childhood. Feeding and swallowing problems, if not recognized early, may rapidly result in malnutrition and growth failure in those infants and children with little nutritional reserve.

Normally, a newborn loses weight during the first week of life and then gains about 20 to 30 grams per day for the first 3 months. By 4 to 6 months, the birth weight has doubled and by one year, it is tripled. Between 6 and 12 months, weight gain slows to 10 to 13 grams per day. From 1 to 6 years of age, weight gain averages about 5 to 8 grams per day. Height velocity also decreases from 1.1 cm per day in the first 3 months, to 0.5 cm per day between 6 and 12 months, and 0.2 cm per day from 1 to 6 years.[58] In the first 3 months of life, head circumference increases at a rate of 2 cm per month, 1 cm per month from 3 to 6 months, and from 7 to 12 months, 0.5 cm per month. Head growth averages 1 cm per month between 1 and 3 years of age.[59] In summary, velocity of growth is most rapid immediately after birth and then falls off significantly in the first 2 years of life. From age 2 years until puberty, the rate or velocity continues to decelerate slowly.

The average daily caloric requirement of full-term infants is 80 to 120 Kcal/Kg during the first few months of life and about 100 Kcal/Kg by 1 year. Individual variations can be broad at this age and for many infants intake of this order exceeds caloric needs. After one year, there is a 10 cal/Kg decrease in daily caloric requirement over each succeeding 3-year period. Although nutritional requirements for unit body weight constantly decrease with increasing age (110 Kcal/Kg in infancy; 50 Kcal/Kg at 15 years), the need for calories as well as for proteins, vitamins, and minerals is relatively greater in children than adults.

The need for water is related to caloric consumption, to loss through body tissues, and to the specific gravity of the urine. The infant must consume much larger amounts of water per unit of body weight compared with the adult; however, when calculated per unit caloric intake, the amounts required are almost the same.[60] The daily consumption of fluid by a healthy infant is equivalent to 10 to 15% of body weight compared with 2 to 4% in the adult.

The rate and amount of oral feedings change dramatically in the first year of life.[60] In the first few weeks of life, infants take an average of 2 to 3 oz formula approximately 6 to 8 times per day. Generally by 6 months, infants are taking 7 to 8 ozs, 4 to 5 times daily. At one year of age most infants are taking 8 oz formula 3 times daily. The average duration of oral feedings in the first 2 years of life ranges from 10 to 30 minutes. The duration of oral feedings is a helpful measure of oral feeding efficacy and efficiency. Infants and toddlers who take >30 minutes to feed are considered slow feeders.[32] Prolonged oral feedings may be an indication of oral-motor/swallowing dysfunction or psychosocial problems.

Feeding and swallowing problems that begin in infancy tend to persist and can result in reduced growth in height and weight.[61–63] Dysphagia frequently results in a general decreased intake of all macronutrients rather than specific nutritional restrictions (primary protein-energy malnutrition [PEM]). Serum protein and vitamin concentrations are usually well preserved.[31] Chronic PEM is a relatively common complication in children with quadriplegic cerebral palsy.[64] Longer mealtimes do not compensate for poor nutrition in children with severe cerebral palsy.[37] Wasting associated with severe cerebral palsy can be corrected quickly with nasogastric feeding[65] or gastrostomy tube feedings.[66] Nasogastric feeding tends to be a short-run solution, but is not appropriate for long-term feeding. Energy needs of children with cerebral palsy can be calculated to assist in nutrition guidelines.[67] Further investigations are needed to examine the efficacy of nutritional interventions and to find satisfactory long-term solutions for children with dysphagia.

Posture and Positioning

Functional posture is basic to oral-motor function for feeding and speech. Oral-motor development is a part of a total developmental process and must be considered in that light if appropriate treatment is to be provided.[68] Postural control against gravity is necessary for all other movement to occur. A point of stability and a point of mobility are necessary for producing a movement. The development of balanced stability and mobility occurs as a child learns to use musculature actively against gravity in response to shifts of weight through anterior, posterior, lateral, and diagonal planes of movement. Gradually a sensorimotor feedback system is established that influences all further movement development.

Seating and positioning systems are designed to provide a child with necessary support to have balanced stability and mobility capabilities, but not to restrict potential movement. The majority of infants eventually diagnosed with CP initially demonstrate a low postural tone base or hypotonia.[68] These infants attempt to achieve stability by fixating in proximal parts of the body. They frequently demonstrate significant tongue retraction and head-neck hyperextension. Infants with significant respiratory problems may use head-neck hyperextension to enlarge the pharyngeal area to increase air intake. The abnormal movements involved in fixating then interfere with the development of active antigravity extension and flexion. Children with a variety of CNS disorders commonly present with hypertonia that is accompanied by normal or mildly decreased strength, normal or increased deep tendon reflexes, and strong and persistent primitive reflexes. They are at risk for developing physical deformities, such as flexion contractures. It is not possible to work on the oral-motor system in isolation. Unless improved and functional posture can be attained, any focus on the oral-motor system is likely to be met with lack of progress and frustration on the part of children, their caregivers, and clinicians.

Central Postural Alignment

Proper positioning during mealtime can assist in providing a more stable base of central stability with good body alignment from which more functional oral-motor, oral-pharyngeal, respiratory, and sensorimotor functioning can be produced. Proper central alignment is the first step in positioning adjustments. Central alignment is basic for coordination of the body and mouth for effective oral-motor and feeding activities. Central alignment includes:[69]

1. Neutral head flexion (symmetry, midline, stability), with a balance between flexion and extension
2. Neck elongated
3. Shoulder girdle stable and depressed
4. Trunk elongated
5. Pelvis stable and symmetrical and in neutral position
6. Hips at 90°, with neutral base of abduction and rotation
7. Feet in neutral with slight dorsiflexion and never plantarflexed

Positioning Goals

No single seating or positioning system is effective for any one individual in all situations at all times because of the child's variability throughout a day and also over longer periods of time. Children get tired, excited, and stressed. Overall sensory and motor skills change as children grow. Pediatric physical and occupational therapists who have developed expertise in working with children with motor disabilities can assess children's needs and then work with technicians to devise the best seating system possible. Numerous commercial chairs are available. Some may "fit" a particular child, and other children may need some customization. In general, the more severely involved the child is motorically the greater the need for a customized seating system. The seating system should assist in optimizing tone along with stability for movement patterns. Tone and movement patterns throughout the entire body must be optimal prior to expecting any specific changes to the oral-motor system.

Oral-Motor/Swallow Intervention

Oral-motor therapy has a primary goal of developing coordinated movements of the mouth, respiratory, and phonatory systems for communication as well as for oral feeding.[15] The assessment of eating and drinking skills[40] determines whether a child has the requisite oral-motor skills to benefit from oral-motor therapy. Total oral feeding is not necessarily the goal for all children. Oral feeding may become a by-product in some instances. A systematic developmental approach focuses on heightening sensory awareness, perception, and discrimina-

tion within the mouth. In addition, oral movement is used to explore the world (for details, see Arvedson and Morris and Klein).[70, 15] Food may not even be a regular part of the treatment because the goals of oral-motor development can be met in multiple ways. On the other hand, food may be used to experience smell, taste, texture, and temperature variations.

Oral-motor intervention recommendations must be considered in relation to the potential for meeting nutritional requirements. An estimate of severity of the eating dysfunction strongly influences treatment decisions.[71] Eating efficiency of 27 children with cerebral palsy and moderate eating impairment were studied to determine frequency of aspiration and the effect of 10 and 20 weeks of oral sensorimotor therapy on eating efficiency and measures of growth based on weight and skinfold thickness.[72] The oral-motor function focused on tongue lateralization, lip control, and vigor of chewing in treatment sessions that lasted between 5 and 7 minutes daily before lunch or snack in a school setting. The eating efficiency of the children did not change markedly in response to oral sensorimotor therapy. Children who aspirated had significantly poorer oral-motor skills in spoon feeding, biting, chewing, and swallowing than children who did not aspirate.[72] Aspiration was only on liquid. This finding is consistent with radiographic findings of the prominence of silent, trace aspiration with liquids for larger numbers of children.[47] Gisel and colleagues[46] suggest that eating efficiency is not a good estimator of treatment outcome, but rather a diagnostic indicator of the severity of eating impairment. Clinical implications of the findings are that prolonged mealtimes and oral-motor therapies may be adequate through the childhood years, but oral caloric supplementation is likely to be needed to provide the necessary energy for growth as children get older. Nutritional rehabilitation is needed as soon as eating skills can no longer keep up with growth demands.

Oral-motor treatment for anatomic structure problems is directed at improving the oral function that can affect timing and coordination of the swallow, but often in an indirect way (Table 4–9). Tone and movement patterns are altered similarly to the way whole body tone and movement patterns were altered before one could even think about oral-motor intervention. Given that most children learn motor skills primarily by sensory input, techniques should attempt to normalize the ability to accept and integrate visual, auditory, tactile, vestibular, taste, and temperature information before direct facilitation of new oral feeding patterns in attempted.[70] Outcome measures are needed.

Table 4–9. Oral-Motor Treatment for Anatomic Structure Problems

Structure	Problem	Treatment
Jaw	Thrust	Mouth play with fingers and toys
		Assisted tooth brushing
		Soft object held between teeth
	Clenching	Mouth play to get gradual opening
		Pleasurable stimulation on face
	Retraction	Prone positioning
		Forward pull under jaw
	Instability	Activities to encourage jaw closure
	Tonic bite reflex	Pressure at temporomandibular joints
		Sensory stimulation
		Coated flat spoon to protect teeth
Lips	Retraction	Finger tapping or vibration to cheeks and lips
		Jaw control procedures
	Limited upper lip movement	Varied food textures and temperatures
		Tapping and stroking
		Straw drinking with low tone
Cheeks	Reduced tone and sensory awareness	Stroking and tapping especially at temporomandibular joint
		Varied food textures and temperatures
Tongue	Thrust	Jaw control
		Thickened liquid released at lip
		Food placed at side of gums
		Exercises for lateral tongue movement
		Spoon placed at midtongue downward pressure
	Retraction	Prone position
		Tongue stroking from back to front
		Chin tuck position when upright
		Upward tapping under chin
	Hypotonia	Varied textures and tastes to increase sensory input
		Food or liquid added gradually
	Deviation	Maintenance of head midline
		Stimulation of less active side with finger, toys, toothbrush
	Limited movement	Varied textures, temperatures, tastes
		Vibration
Palate	Nasopharyngeal reflux	Upright or prone position
		Angled bottle used for prone position
		Cheek and tongue function activities
		Thickened liquids (if normal swallow)

Source: Arvedson J: Management of swallowing problems. In J Arvedson & L Brodsky (Eds.), *Pediatric swallowing and feeding: Assessment and management* (p.331). Singular Publishing Group, San Diego, 1993. Reprinted with permission.

Behavioral Intervention

Feeding of infants and children is an interactive process. Typically, at least one caregiver is present for mealtimes. Infants and young children are fed by caregivers. Toddlers and older children are supervised by caregivers for a variety of reasons to include safety, development of more mature feeding skills, and socialization. Behavioral issues may become prominent when a child tries to exert control over the environment, especially in the presence of a caregiver who lacks necessary skills to be supportive and carry out consistency of mealtimes. It is not the purpose of this section to discuss the etiologies of Failure to Thrive, nor to describe the range of treatment approaches. Rather this discussion focuses on basic "food rules" for mealtimes for essentially all children once they reach a transition feeding stage (Table 4–10). Children who are at risk for malnutrition, whose motor skills are severely impaired, and who are at risk for aspiration may need nonoral feedings with limited tastes orally in the context of family mealtimes to meet the basic goals of adequate nutrition, efficient mealtimes, and minimal risk for aspiration. It is to be remembered that not all children can be total oral feeders.

High-quality feeding interactions assist the infant and young child to develop physically and grow. In addition, they are also positively linked to subsequent cognitive and linguistic competence and more secure attachments to major caregivers.[73] Some basic principles apply to all young children at mealtimes. The principles are especially important when behavioral issues are prominent or when weaning children off tube feedings. Toddlers around the age of 2 years typically reject new foods initially but learn to like them with time and repeated neutral exposure.[74] The food rules described by Chatoor and colleagues[75] are applicable to children beyond infancy (Table 4–10). Cultural and ethnic differences must be considered when clinicians make observations and judgments about what is expected of children at certain ages and stages.[76]

The identification of infants, children, and families at risk for Failure to Thrive should occur as early as possible with aggressive nutritional and behavioral intervention to minimize the duration and long term consequences of undernutrition.[77] Behavioral intervention is likely to be most effective with a team approach having a psychologist or other behavioral specialist as a central member. Regimens are described for outpatient treatment[78–80] and for intensive inpatient treatment.[81–86] Speech–language pathologists and other members of the feeding team can assist in carrying out the program and also in reinforcing guidelines with the child and family. In-

Table 4–10. Food Rules for Caregivers Applicable to Children Beyond Infancy

Aspect of Mealtime	"Rules" for Caregivers
Scheduling	Regular mealtimes; only planned snacks added
	Mealtimes no longer than 30 minutes
	Nothing offered between meals, except water if child is thirsty (no bottles or cups of milk or juice)
Environment	Neutral atmosphere (no forcing food or commenting on intake)
	Sheet under chair to catch mess
	No game playing
	Food never given as reward or present
Procedures	Small portions
	Solids first, fluids last
	Self-feeding encouraged as much as possible (e.g., finger feeding, holding spoon)
	Food removed after 10–15 minutes if child plays without eating
	Meal terminated immediately if child throws food in anger
	Wiping mouth and cleaning up only after meal is completed

Source: Arvedson J: Behavioral issues and implications with pediatric feeding disorders. *Sem Speech Lang* 1997; 18:51–70. Reprinted with permission.
Adapted from: Chatoor I, Dickson L, Schaefer S, et al.: A developmental classification of feeding disorders associated with failure to thrive: Diagnosis and treatment. In Drotar D (Ed.), *New directions in failure to thrive: Implications for research and practice.* Plenum Press, New York, 1986.

terested readers should seek out the descriptions by the people who developed them.

Although there are varied approaches, treatment typically begins with the least intrusive intervention. Other treatment components can be added as necessary. The concept of intervention in the least restrictive environment would make outpatient treatment desirable whenever the child and family appear to be suitable candidates. However, inpatient care may be perceived to be necessary for some patients. In this period minimal length of hospitalization, short-term family based intervention is more likely than long-term hospitalization. Types of treatment approaches based on behavioral modification with motivational and skill deficit problems, transactional approach, cognitive behavioral therapy alone or with pharmacologic treatment are reviewed by Arvedson.[43]

SUMMARY

It is not possible in one chapter to cover all the aspects of knowledge and experience that are needed for a clinician to be competent in assessing and managing infants and children with dysphagia. The most important "take home" message is that SLPs must demonstrate high-level skills related to the knowledge base and procedural competencies as well as abilities to work effectively with other medical and nonmedical professionals. They must never assess and treat infants and children with complex feeding and swallowing disorders in isolation. A school-based team needs to have links to a medical team, and both need to make sure the caregivers are actively involved in all steps of diagnosis and treatment. All clinicians in all settings should keep treatment efficacy and efficiency data that can assist in establishing outcome criteria.

STUDY QUESTIONS

1. Give examples of disorders caused by neuronal proliferation, neuronal migration, and neuronal differentiation abnormalities.

2. How does myelination during the first two years of life affect deglutition?

3. How do primitive reflexes affect swallowing and feeding?

4. What factors determine infant readiness for oral feeding?

5. An infant presents with reduced pharyngeal motility during swallowing. Which cranial nerves have been affected?

6. When is aspiration most likely observed during fluoroscopy for children with neurological impairment?

REFERENCES

1. Brodsky L, Arvedson J: Introduction: Rationale for interdisciplinary care. In Arvedson J, Brodsky L (eds.): *Pediatric swallowing and feeding: Assessment and management*, p. 2. Singular Publishing Group, Inc., San Diego, 1993.

2. Lefton-Greif MA, Arvedson J: Pediatric feeding/swallowing teams. *Sem Speech Lang* 1997; 18: 5–12.

3. Bosma JF: Pharyngeal swallow: Basic mechanisms, development, and impairments. *Adv Otolaryngol Head Neck Surg* 1992; 6: 225–275.

4. Bosma JF: Development of feeding. *Clin Nutrition* 1986; 5: 210–218.

5. Wind J: *On the phylogeny and ontogeny of the human larynx*, (p. 105). Wolters-Noordhoff Publishing, Groningen, 1970.

6. Dobbing J, Sands J: Quantitative growth and development of human brain. *Arch Dis Childhood* 1973; 48: 757–767.

7. Dobbing J, Sands J: Timing of neuroblast multiplication in developing human brain. *Nature* 1970; 226: 639–640.

8. Capone GT: Human brain development. In Capute AJ, Accardo PJ (eds.): *Developmental disabilities in infancy and childhood*, pp. 25–75. Paul H. Brookes Publishing Co., Baltimore, 1996.

9. Yakovlev PI, Lecours AR: The myelogenetic cycles of regional maturation of the brain. In Minkowski A (ed.): *Regional development of the brain in early life*, pp. 3–70. Blackwell, Oxford, England, 1967.

10. Kinney HC, Brody BA, Kloman AS, et al.: Sequence of central nervous system myelination in human infancy II. Patterns of myelination in autopsied infants. *J Neuropath Exper Neurol* 1988; 47: 217–234.

11. Moore KL: *The developing human: Clinically orientated embryology*, 4th ed. W.B. Saunders, Philadelphia, 1988.

12. Miller AJ: Deglutition. *Physiol Reviews* 1982; 62: 129–184.

13. Capute AJ, Accardo PJ: A neurodevelopmental perspective on the continuum of developmental disabilities. In Capute AJ, Accardo PJ (eds.): *Developmental disabilities in infancy and childhood*, pp. 25–75. Paul H. Brookes Publishing Co., Baltimore, 1996.

14. Humphrey T: Reflex activity in the oral and facial area of the human fetus. In Bosma JF (ed.): *Second symposium on oral sensation and perception*, pp. 195–233. Charles C. Thomas, Springfield, IL, 1967.

15. Morris SE, Klein MD: *Pre-feeding skills: A comprehensive resource for feeding development.* Therapy Skill Builders, Tucson, AZ, 1987.

16. Saint-Anne Dargassies S: Neurological development of the full term and premature neonate. *Excerpta Medica*, New York, 1977.

17. Capute AJ, Accardo PJ: Cerebral palsy: The spectrum of motor dysfunction. In Capute AJ, Accardo PJ (eds.): *Developmental disabilities in infancy and childhood* (2d ed, Vol. I): Neurodevelopmental Diagnosis and Treatment, pp. 1–22. Paul H. Brookes Publishing Co., Baltimore, 1991.

18. Capute AJ, Accardo PJ, Vining EPG, et al.: Primitive reflex profile. In *Monographs in developmental pediatrics.* University Park Press, Baltimore, 1978.

19. Capute AJ, Palmer FB, Shapiro BK, et al.: Primitive reflex profile: A quantitation of primitive reflexes in infancy. *Developmental Med and Child Neurol* 1984; 25: 375–383.

20. Arvedson JC, Rogers BT, Brodsky L: Anatomy, embryology, and physiology. In Arvedson JC, Brodsky L (eds.): *Pediatric swallowing and feeding: Assessment and management*, pp. 5–51. Singular Publishing Group, Inc., San Diego, 1993.

21. Vitti M, Basmajian JY: Muscles of mastication in small children: An electromyographic analysis. *Am J Orthodontics* 1975; 68: 412–419.

22. Illingworth RS, Lister J: The critical or sensitive period, with special reference to certain feeding problems in infants and children. *J of Pediatrics* 1964; 65: 840–848.

23. Denenberg VH: Effects of differential infantile handling on weight gain and mortality in the rat and mouse. *Science* 1959; 130: 629.

24. Schechter GL: Physiology of the mouth, pharynx, and esophagus. In Bluestone CD, Stool SE, Scheetz, MD (eds.): *Pediatric otolaryngology* (Vol. 2, 2d ed.), pp. 816–822. WG Saunders, Philadelphia, 1990.

25. Harris JP: Heart failure. In Ziai M (ed.): *Bedside pediatrics: Diagnostic evaluation of the child,* pp. 313–319. Little Brown, Boston, 1983.

26. Kinsbourne M: Hiatus hernia with contortions of neck. *Lancet* 1964; 1: 1058.

27. Werlin SL, Dodds WJ, Hogan WJ, et al.: Mechanisms of gastroesophageal reflux in children. *J of Pediatrics* 1980; 97: 244–249.

28. Baer M, Maki M, Nurmonen J, et al.: Esophagitis and findings of long term esophageal pH recording in children with repeated lower respiratory tract symptoms. *J Pediatric Gastroenterol Nutrition* 1986; 5: 187–190.

29. Biller JA, Winter HS, Grand RJ, et al.: Are endoscopic changes predictive of histologic esophagitis in children? *J of Pediatrics* 1983; 103: 215–218.

30. Nielsen DW, Heldt GP, Tooley WH: Stridor and gastroesophageal reflux in infants. *Pediatrics* 1990; 85: 1034–1039.

31. Rossi T: Pediatric gastroenterology. In Arvedson JC, Brodsky L (eds.): *Pediatric swallowing and feeding: Assessment and management,* pp. 123–156. Singular Publishing Group, Inc., San Diego, 1993.

32. Reau NY, Senturia YD, Lebailly SA, et al.: Infant and toddler feeding patterns and problems: Normative data and a new direction. *Developmental Behav Pediatrics* 1996; 17: 149–153.

33. Arvedson J: Oral-motor and feeding assessment. In Arvedson J, Brodsky L (eds.): *Pediatric swallowing and feeding: Assessment and management,* p. 249–291. Singular Publishing Group, Inc., San Diego, 1993.

34. Braun MA, Palmer MM: A pilot study of oral-motor dysfunction in "at-risk" infants. *Phys Occup Therapy Pediatrics* 1986; 5: 13–25.

35. Case-Smith J, Cooper P, Scala, V: Feeding efficiency of premature neonates. *Amer J Occup Therapy* 1989; 43: 245–250.

36. Chatoor I, Menvielle E, Getson P, et al.: *Observational scale for mother–infant–toddler interaction during feeding.* Children's Hospital Medical Center: Washington, D.C., 1989.

37. Gisel EG, Patrick J: Identification of children with cerebral palsy unable to maintain a normal nutritional stage. *Lancet* 1988; 1: 283–286.

38. Herman MJ: Comprehensive assessment of oral-motor dysfunction in failure-to-thrive infants. *Infant-Toddler Intervention* 1991; 1: 109–123.

39. Jelm JM: *Oral-motor/feeding rating scale.* Therapy Skill Builders, Tucson, AZ, 1990.

40. Kenny D, Koheil R, Greenberg J, et al.: Development of a multidisciplinary feeding profile for children who are dependent feeders. *Dysphagia* 1989; 4: 16–28.

41. Lefton-Greif MA: Diagnosis and management of pediatric feeding and swallowing disorders: Role of the speech–language pathologist. In Tuchman DN, Walter RS (eds.): *Disorders of feeding and swallowing in infants and children: Pathophysiology, diagnosis, and treatment,* pp. 97–113. Singular Publishing Group, Inc., San Diego, 1994.

42. Perlin WS, Boner MM: Clinical assessment of feeding and swallowing in infants and children. In Cherney LR (ed.): *Clinical management of dysphagia in adults and children* (2nd ed.), pp. 93–131. Aspen, Gaithersburg, MD, 1994.

43. Arvedson JC: Dysphagia in pediatric patients with neurologic damage. *Sem Neurol* 1996; 16: 371–386.

44. Arvedson JC, Rogers BT: Pediatric swallowing and feeding disorders. *J of Med Speech–Language Pathology* 1993; 1: 203–221.

45. Gisel EG: Effect of food texture on development of chewing in children 6 months to 2 years of age. *Developmental Med Child Neurol* 1991; 33: 69–79.

46. Gisel EG, Lange LJ, Niman CW: Chewing cycles in 4- and 5-year-old Down's syndrome children: A comparison of eating efficacy with normals. *Am J of Occupational Therapy* 1994; 38: 666–670.

47. Arvedson J, Rogers B, Buck G, et al.: Silent aspiration prominent in children with dysphagia. *Inter J Pediatric Otorhinolaryngology* 1994; 28: 173–181.

48. Hay WW: The uses, benefits, and limitations of pulse oximetry in neonatal medicine: Consensus on key issues. *J Perinatology* 1987; 7: 347–349.

49. Emery JR: Skin pigmentation as an influence on the accuracy of pulse oximetry. *J Perinatology* 1987; 7: 329–330.

50. Hay WW: Physiology of oxygenation and its relation to pulse oximetry in neonates. *J Perinatology* 1987; 7: 309–319.

51. Murray JF: *The Normal Lung: The Basis for Diagnosis and Treatment of Pulmonary Disease.* W.B. Saunders Co., Philadelphia, 1986.

52. Willging JP: Endoscopic evaluation of swallowing in children. *International J Ped Otorhinolaryngol* 1995; 32: (Suppl.), S107–S108.

53. Allen ML, Mellow MH, Robinson M: Manometry During Food Ingestion Aids in the Diagnosis of Diffuse Esophageal Spasm. *Am J Gastroenterol* 1992; 87: 568–571.

54. American Speech–Language-Hearing Association: Instrumental diagnostic procedures for swallowing. *Asha* 1992; 34: (Suppl. 7), 25–32.

55. American Speech–Language-Hearing Association: Knowledge and skills needed by speech–language pathologists providing service to dysphagic patients. *Asha* 1990; 32: (Suppl. 2), 7–12.

56. Arvedson J, Christensen S: Instrumental evaluation. In Arvedson J, Brodsky L (eds.): *Pediatric swallowing and feeding: Assessment and management,* pp. 293–326. Singular Publishing Group, Inc., San Diego, 1993.

57. Benson JE, Lefton-Greif MA: Videofluoroscopy of swallowing in pediatric patients: A component of the total feeding evaluation. In Tuchman DN, Walter RS (eds.): *Disorders of feeding and swallowing in infants and children: Pathophysiology, diagnosis, and treatment,* pp. 187–200. Singular Publishing Group, Inc., San Diego, 1994.

58. Foman SJ, Haschke F, Ziegler EE, et al.: Body composition of reference children from birth to age 10 years. *Am J of Clin Nutrition Suppl* 1982; 35: (5 suppl), 1169–1175.

59. Karlberg P, Engstrom F, Lichtenstein H, et al.: The development of children in a Swedish urban community. A prospective longitudinal study III. Physical growth during the first 3 years of life. *Acta Pædiatrica Scandinavica,* 1968; 187 (Suppl): 48–66.

60. Barness LA, Curran JS: The feeding of infants and children. In Behrman RE, Kliegman RM, and Arvin AM (eds.): *Textbook of pediatrics,* pp. 151–163. W.B. Saunders Co., Philadelphia, 1996.

61. Dahl M, Kristiansson B: Early feeding problems in an affluent society. IV. Impact on growth up to two years of age. *Acta Pædiatrica Scandinavia* 1987; 76: 881–888.

62. Eid E: A follow-up study of physical growth following failure to thrive with special reference to a critical period in the first year of life. *Acta Pædiatrica Scandinavia* 1971; 60: 39–48.

63. Ramsay M, Gisel EG, Boutry M: Non-organic failure to thrive: Growth failure secondary to feeding-skills disorder. *Developmental Med Child Neurol* 1993; 35: 285–297.

64. Stallings VA, Charney EB, Davies JC, et al.: Nutrition-related growth failure of children with quadriplegic cerebral palsy. *Develop Med Child Neurol* 1993; 35: 126–138.

65. Patrick J, Boland M, Stoski D, et al.: Rapid correction of wasting in children with cerebral palsy. *Developmental Med Child Neurol* 1986; 28: 734–739.

66. Shapiro BK, Green P, Krick J, et al.: Growth of severely impaired children: Neurologic versus nutritional factors. *Developmental Med Child Neurol* 1986; 28: 729–733.

67. Krick J, Murphy PE, Markham JFB, et al.: A proposed formula for calculating energy needs of children with cerebral palsy. *Developmental Med Child Neurol* 1992; 34: 481–487.

68. Alexander R: Oral-motor treatment for infants and young children with cerebral palsy. *Seminars in Speech and Language* 1987; 8: 87–100.

69. Macie D, Arvedson J: Tone and positioning. In Arvedson JC, Brodsky L (eds.): *Pediatric swallowing and feeding: Assessment and management,* pp. 209–247. Singular Publishing Group, Inc., San Diego, 1993.

70. Arvedson J: Management of swallowing problems. In Arvedson J, Brodsky L (eds.): *Pediatric swallowing and feeding: Assessment and management,* pp. 327–387. Singular Publishing Group, Inc., San Diego, 1993.

71. Gisel EG, Alphonce E: Classification of eating impairments based on eating efficiency in children with cerebral palsy. *Dysphagia* 1995; 10: 268–274.

72. Gisel EG, Applegate-Ferrante T, Benson J, et al.: Positioning infants and children for videofluoroscopic swallowing function studies. *Infants Young Children* 1996; 8: 58–64.

73. Barnard KE, Hammond MA, Booth CL, et al.: Measurement and meaning of parent child interaction. In Morrisson F, Lord C, Keating D (eds.): *Applied developmental psychology.* Academic Press, New York, 1989.

74. Birch LL, Marlin DW: I don't like it; I never tried it: Effects of exposure on two-year-old children's food preferences. *Appetite* 1982; 3: 353–360.

75. Chatoor I, Dickson L, Schaefer S, et al.: A developmental classification of feeding disorders associated with failure to thrive: Diagnosis and treatment. In Drotar D (ed.): *New directions in failure to thrive: Implications for research and practice.* Plenum Press, New York, 1986.

76. Phillips CB, Cooper RM: Cultural dimensions of feeding relationships. *Zero to Three* 1992; 12: 10–13.

77. Tolia, V: Very early onset nonorganic failure to thrive in infants. *J of Ped Gastroenterol Nutrition* 1995; 20: 73–80.

78. Babbitt RL, Hoch TA, Coe DA, et al.: Behavioral assessment and treatment of pediatric feeding disorders. *J Developmental Behav Ped* 1994; 15: 278–291.

79. Hampton, D: Failure to thrive—tackling feeding problems: A community-based approach. *Health Visitor* 1993; 66: 407–408.

80. McCann JB: Children with non-organic failure to thrive. *Arch Dis Childhood* 1994; 70: 234–236.

81. Babbitt RL, Hoch TA, Coe DA: Behavioral feeding disorders. In Tuchman DN, Walter RS (eds.): *Disorders of feeding and swallowing in infants and children: Pathophysiology, diagnosis, and treatment,* pp. 77–95. Singular Publishing Group, Inc., San Diego, 1994.

82. Blackman JA, Nelson CLA: Reinstituting oral feedings in children fed by gastrostomy tube. *Clin Ped* 1985; 24: 434–438.

83. Drotar D, Malone C, Negray J, et al.: Patterns of hospital based care for infants with nonorganic failure-to-thrive. *J Clin Child Psych* 1981; 10: 63–66.

84. Field M: Follow-up developmental status of infants hospitalized for nonorganic failure to thrive. *J Ped Psych* 1984; 9: 241–256.

85. MacPhee M, Mori C, Goldson E: Change in the hospital setting: Adopting a team approach for nonorganic failure-to-thrive. *J Ped Nur* 1994; 9: 218–225.

86. Singer, L: Long-term hospitalization of nonorganic failure-to-thrive infants: Patient characteristics and hospital course. *J Developmental Behav Ped* 1987; 8: 25–31.

Appendix A
Clinic/Bedside Oral-Motor Feeding Assessment Worksheet
Children's Hospital of Buffalo

Name _____ Examiner _____
DOB _____ Referral _____
Eval. _____ Examiner _____
C.A. _____ Med Dx _____

Presenting problem_____
_____ Initial Assessment _____ Follow-up (last seen _____)
_____ Videofluoroscopic swallow study (VFSS) in past (date_____)
_____ Feeding oral only _____ Oral + tube _____ NG-tube _____ G-tube (+/− fundoplication)
_____ Tracheostomy (If yes, speaking valve _____ yes _____ no) _____ O$_2$, _____ Suction needs
_____ Medications _____

Reasons for referral
_____ Risk for aspiration
_____ Difficulty swallowing (coughing/gagging, other _____)
_____ Airway issues _____
_____ GI tract issues _____
_____ Texture difficulties: (_____ liquid, _____puree, _____solid)
_____ Other _____

Position for feeding: _____ held by feeder _____ infant seat _____ high chair or regular chair
_____ wheelchair _____ other _____

Posture for feeding: _____ upright _____ semi-upright _____ supine _____ other _____

Primary feeders: _____ mother _____ other family _____ therapists _____ self (assisted/independent)

Liquid (_____ oz in 24 hours) _____ thin _____ thickened
_____ nipple (_____ breast, _____ bottle) _____ cup (_____ open, _____ spout)
_____ straw _____ other _____

Food textures
_____ puree _____ lumpy puree _____ ground _____ chopped _____ solid
_____ finger food: examples _____

Enjoyment/behavior during mealtimes
_____ Eager to eat and completes meal in <30 minutes
_____ Starts out well, then "shuts down" or gets fussy, mealtimes >30 minutes
_____ Typically not eager to eat, apt to be lethargic, and mealtimes >30 minutes
_____ Fussy with struggle to feed
_____ Other _____

Related interfering patterns
_____ Hypertonicity (If yes, _____ trunk _____ face _____upper extremity _____ lower extremity)
_____ Hypotonicity (If yes, _____ trunk _____ face _____upper extremity _____ lower extremity)
_____Difficulties in acceptance of teeth brushing

FEEDING OBSERVATION

General problems
_____ Extensor thrusting during feeding _____ Asymmetric posture
_____ Nasal flaring during feeding _____ Breathing changes during feeding, ex. _____
_____ Quick withdrawal from food: specify textures _____

Oral-Motor function during feeding

Lips: _____ No problem _____ closed at rest _____ apart at rest
_____ functional seal on nipple _____ active pull on nipple _____ liquid loss (nipple/spoon)
_____ limited upper lip movement on spoon _____ lack of closure for bolus formation
_____ lip retraction _____ lip pursing _____ drooling _____ other _____

Tongue: _____ no problem _____ slow initiation _____ limited movement _____ protrusion/thrust
_____ retraction _____ suckle pattern with spoon or cup _____ no lateral movement/chewing
_____ residue in oral cavity _____ food packed in palate _____ other _____

Mandible: _____ no problem _____ wide excursion _____ poorly graded movement _____ tonic bite
_____ jaw thrust _____ jaw clench _____ no chewing _____ vertical chew
_____ rotary chew _____ bruxism _____ other _____

Pharyngeal Phase Inferences of Swallowing	Thin liquid	Thick liquid	Puree food	Ground food	Chopped chewable food
Delayed trigger of pharyngeal swallow _____					
Swallows per bolus (number) _____					
Gurgly voice **B**efore, **A**fter swallow _____					
Increased respiratory rate or effort _____					
Cough **B**efore, **D**uring, **A**fter swallow _____					
Nasopharyngeal reflux _____					
Gag _____					
Reduced laryngeal elevation					

_____

_____

_____

Performance during observation typical per caregiver __ yes __ no

Problem summary

__ Posture/Seating　　　__ Oral-motor/Swallowing　　　__ Aspiration risk
__ Sensory　　　　　　　__ Self-feeding　　　　　　　 __ GER
__ Behavior　　　　　　　__ Nutrition　　　　　　　　　__ Medical/surgical

PO feeding summary

__ Functional for nutritional needs　　　　　__ Gains/progress in recent weeks/months
__ Inadequate to meet nutritional needs　　　 __ Regression in recent weeks/months

5

Speech–Language Pathology in the Intensive Care Unit

Alice K. Silbergleit and Michael A. Basha

CHAPTER OUTLINE

Normal Respiration

Mechanical Ventilation

Medical Conditions That Require Treatment in an ICU Setting

Tracheostomy

Swallowing Issues

Treating a patient in an intensive care unit (ICU) setting presents a series of unique and complicated issues. The feeling of loss of control that may occur when one is admitted to a hospital may be amplified for the ICU patient. The introduction of multiple tubes, the fear and anxiety associated with a serious medical illness, and the sudden loss of the ability to talk if a tracheostomy tube or mechanical ventilation is required may all contribute to a feeling of helplessness. The continued advances of medical technology have lead to life-saving techniques for individuals with stroke, traumatic brain injury (TBI), spinal cord injury (SCI), pulmonary disease, neurodegenerative disease, trauma, and cardiopulmonary conditions. The ICU patient may be of any age and have any one of a myriad of disorders that affects his or her communication and/or swallowing abilities.

The involvement of speech–language pathologists in the care of ICU patients has increased over the past several years. In the earliest stages of ad-

mission to an ICU, medical stability is the primary concern; speech–language pathologists may be asked to assist at this early stage by identifying a mode of communication or establishing a safe method of nutritional intake for a patient. The current trend of limiting hospital stays to decrease medical costs may be one of the reasons for early consultation among a variety of health care specialists who would previously have delayed consultation until a patient was transferred to a regular medical unit.

The purpose of this chapter is to familiarize the practicing speech–language pathologist with some of the more common terminology and issues specific to the ICU environment. Our discussion includes an explanation of the basic processes of normal respiration and mechanical ventilation as well as common illnesses seen in an ICU setting. Because the role of speech–language pathologists working with tracheostomized patients is becoming more popular, we will present a review of various methods of voicing with tracheostomy tubes and speaking valves. In addition, we will discuss decision-making issues regarding a patient's candidacy for oral feeding and various methods of testing for and treating dysphagia, including some ethical considerations related to feeding severely ill patients. The importance of a team approach to diagnosing and treating ICU patients is emphasized throughout. We hope that this information will help the practicing speech–language pathologist to understand the complexities of working with an ICU patient and thus facilitate effective communication with and swallowing care for individuals in an ICU setting.

NORMAL RESPIRATION

In most cases admission to a medical ICU indicates a problem in respiration. To fully understand such disorders, it is essential for us to have a sound knowledge of the normal respiratory process.

The respiratory system is relatively easy to comprehend when one understands the function of its two major components, the lungs and the respiratory, or ventilatory, pump. The lungs are primarily involved in gas exchange; they are responsible for moving oxygen from the atmosphere into the alveoli and then into the pulmonary capillary blood and for moving carbon dioxide from the pulmonary capillary blood to the alveoli where it can be exhaled into the atmosphere. Hence, the lungs ensure a constant supply of oxygen to the blood, which is then distributed to the cells, tissues, and organs of the body, providing the necessary maintenance of normal biochemical and metabolic function.[1] Likewise, the ability of the lungs to excrete carbon dioxide, the major waste product of metabolism, prevents accumulation of this potentially deadly gas in the body. Diseases that primarily affect the working tissue of the lung (lung parenchyma) (e.g., pneumonia, congestive heart failure, pulmonary hemorrhage) interfere with the gas exchange process and lead to low blood oxygen, called hypoxemia, or occasionally to elevated blood carbon dioxide, or hypercapnia.[2]

The function of the respiratory, or ventilatory, pump of the respiratory system is more complex than that of the lungs and involves those elements that are included in the bellows function of the system. Ventilation is the process of eliminating carbon dioxide from the body through the lungs. The respiratory cycle begins in the brainstem in the respiratory centers of the pons and medulla, with the generation of a nerve impulse and the

transmission of that stimulus to the respiratory muscles, primarily the diaphragm (Figure 5–1). The contraction and flattening of the diaphragm result in the shortening of its muscle fibers as it descends in the thorax. When this occurs, intrapleural pressure becomes more negative as intrathoracic volume increases. This increase in negative intrapleural pressure is transmitted to the alveoli and allows intraalveolar pressure to be lower than atmospheric pressure. The gradient between the atmosphere and alveoli causes air to move into the lungs until alveolar and atmospheric pressures are equal.[3] At end-inspiration, when atmospheric pressure equals intraalveolar pressure, airflow into the lungs ceases and expiration begins. Usually expiration is a passive process dependent on the elastic recoil of the lungs, the presence or absence of airway resistance, and the use of the abdominal and intercostal expiratory muscles. At end-expiration, intrapleural pressure has increased back to -2.0 cm H_2O and the whole process is repeated.[4]

The negative intrapleural pressure at end-expiration is created by the opposing forces of the lungs, which normally want to collapse, and the chest wall, which wants to spring outward. These opposing forces keep the lungs expanded and prevent them from collapsing, create negative intrapleural pressure at end-expiration, and allow a volume of air in the lungs prior to the next inspiration, termed functional residual capacity. Functional residual capacity is the beginning point for a new respiratory cycle. Therefore, the normal respiratory cycle in a spontaneously breathing person depends on opposite pressure and volume changes that allow air to move in and out of the lungs. Tidal volume is the volume of air moving into the lungs depending on their compliance. If the lung is stiff (as in idiopathic pulmonary fibrosis), less volume will move into the lung. Conversely, if its compliance is great (e.g., obstructive lung disease), a greater amount of air will constitute the patient's tidal volume.

MECHANICAL VENTILATION

Patients in an ICU setting are frequently assisted in their respiration by mechanical ventilation. Respiratory failure, whether secondary to hypoxemia, hypercapnia, or both, is the primary reason why critically ill patients eventually require ICU care and mechanical ventilation.[5] The majority of patients seen in an ICU have a fulminate course with a dramatic presentation and the institution of me-

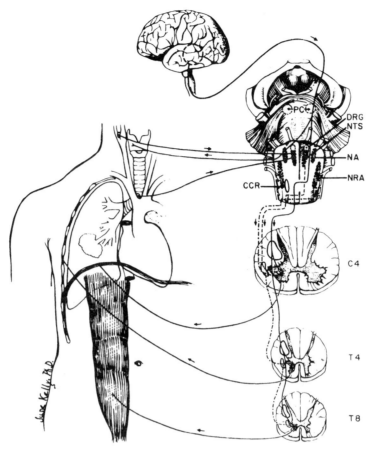

Figure 5–1. Summary of the route of respiration. Reprinted with permission from the American College of Chest Physicians: The diagnosis and management of neuromuscular diseases causing respiratory failure, *Chest* 1991; 99, 6; 1485–1494.

chanical ventilation can be lifesaving once the primary insult is treated or reversed. However, in some cases patients with neuromuscular disease or chest wall abnormalities experience slowly progressive, chronic respiratory failure and are unable to be weaned from the ventilator.

Most adult patients requiring mechanical ventilation in an ICU will be ventilated via positive-pressure, volume-cycled ventilators. This means that gas that is above atmospheric pressure is delivered into the lungs, raising intraalveolar pressure during inspiration. During inspiration from a ventilator, a preset tidal volume is delivered to the patient, and both intrathoracic volume and pressure increase. Therefore, intrathoracic pressure and volume move in the same direction, unlike that of a spontaneously breathing individual. The amount of delivered tidal volume is constant and the pressure is variable, depending on lung compliance and airway resistance.[6] Airway pressure will be high if lung compliance is low (i.e., idio-

pathic pulmonary fibrosis) or airway resistance is high (i.e., tumor, foreign body aspiration, increased pulmonary secretions), or both. At end-inspiration, an exhalation port valve is opened and exhalation is essentially passive, dependent on lung elastic recoil, airway resistance, and the use of expiratory muscles as in a spontaneously breathing patient. The next breath is either triggered by the patient or automatically given to the patient by the ventilator. If the patient is alert or able to initiate a breath, the patient sets the rate of breathing. This mode of mechanical ventilation is referred to as the assist-control (AC) mode and is the preferred mode of early ventilation in patients who develop respiratory failure from a variety of causes. If the patient is unable to set the respiratory rate, the physician can determine the number of minimum breaths per minute. The product of delivered tidal volume and respiratory rate is termed minute volume or minute ventilation; this value varies from patient to patient depending on the underlying disease process.

All ventilator settings are adjusted by a physician, usually a pulmonologist, or respiratory therapist or nurse who follows the orders of a physician. Some patients are uncomfortable with artificial ventilation, which causes them to be anxious and agitated. In those instances, sedation, and in extreme cases, drug-induced paralysis, may be necessary to ensure good patient-ventilator synchrony.

There are other types of noninvasive modes of respiration that may be implemented in less ill patients who may not require conventional ventilation or to forestall more conventional ventilation in patients whose primary disease process can be reversed or controlled. These alternative modes of ventilation deliver positive pressure to the airway via a tight fitting nasal or full facial mask, which are meant to augment the oxygenation and ventilatory processes and reduce the patient's work of breathing.[7] Noninvasive ventilation may also serve as a bridge to more normal spontaneous ventilation as a patient's medical status improves and he or she is ready to be weaned from full mechanical ventilation. Noninvasive airway ventilatory management that is typically seen in an ICU setting may include continuous positive airway pressure (CPAP), pressure support ventilation (PSV), and inspiratory/expiratory positive airway pressure (BiPAP).

Continuous Positive Airway Pressure

CPAP, as its name indicates, is the application of positive pressure to the airways throughout the respiratory cycle (i.e., during both inspiration and expiration). This mode of ventilation can only be used with a spontaneously breathing person. The amount of airway pressure applied is determined by a physician and is usually between 5 to 10 cm H_2O. CPAP may be applied through the ventilator in an intubated patient or via a tight fitting nasal or full face mask in a nonintubated patient. CPAP can be used to assist in weaning a patient from mechanical ventilation or for breath support in patients with frank or impending respiratory failure. CPAP works by splinting open atelectatic alveoli, increasing end-expiratory lung volume, and assisting the inspiratory muscles in reducing the work of breathing.[8]

Pressure Support Ventilation

This method of ventilation, which is patient initiated, has been relatively recently described and used. It is a physician-determined mode that is pressure cycled and flow limited in a spontaneously breathing patient with an intact respiratory center. That is, pressure is applied to the airway only during the inspiratory phase of the respiratory cycle (pressure cycled); and the pressure applied (determined by the physician) ceases once the inspiratory flow drops down below a certain level, [e.g., 5 L/min (flow-limited)]. Exhalation is then passive and no pressure is applied during this part of the respiratory cycle. PSV can be used to entirely support the patient or assist in the weaning of the patient from mechanical ventilation. The more pressure used, the more the patient is assisted and the less the work of breathing for the patient.

Like CPAP, PSV can be used via a mask or through an endotracheal tube in an intubated patient. PSV reduces the work of breathing by unloading the inspiratory muscles. It may be of special value in patients who have increased inspiratory resistance (i.e., central airway mass/tumor, etc.).[9]

Inspiratory/Expiratory Positive Airway Pressure

BiPAP is a technique of noninvasive ventilation in which pressure applied to the airway can be adjusted for both the inspiratory and expiratory phases of the respiratory cycle. Hence, the differential pressures may be used to assist in the ventilation of patients with different disease processes. This modality is used in a spontaneously breathing patient by a tight fitting nasal or full face mask. The pressure applied during inspiration is inspiratory positive airway pressure (IPAP) and during expiration expiratory positive airway pressure (EPAP). IPAP is very similar to PSV and EPAP is similar to positive end-expiratory pressure (PEEP). BiPAP helps to unload the respiratory muscles, reduce the work of breathing, splint open collapsed alveoli, and raise end-expiratory volume. BiPAP is often used in patients who require partial ventilatory support or in those who have impending respiratory failure who might be spared endotracheal intubation if the primary disorder can be quickly reversed.[10]

Mechanical Ventilation Weaning

Although the literature is replete with articles suggesting the best approaches or proper timing for weaning a patient from mechanical ventilation, this process is as much an art as a science.[11] Numerous weaning parameters have been established to aid physicians in the decision-making process, but these parameters do not always predict a successful outcome.[12] As a general rule, the less time a patient is mechanically ventilated and the more quickly reversible the primary insult is, the more accurate these weaning guidelines are for predicting successful weaning. In addition, younger patients and surgical patients tend to wean more quickly from mechanical ventilation than older patients, patients with multiple or complex medical problems, or those with multiple organ dysfunction. A recently described rapid shallow breathing index, which provides a ratio of respiratory frequency divided by tidal volume in liters, seems to predict successful weaning in a number of patients if this ratio is less than 105.[13] Ultimately, many experienced critical care physicians will base the decision to wean on general impressions of patient status. However, as a general principle, weaning usually occurs when the patient assumes a greater work of breathing as his or her clinical condition improves and when gas exchange, as assessed by arterial blood gases, shows stable oxygenation and ventilation.

MEDICAL CONDITIONS THAT REQUIRE TREATMENT IN AN ICU SETTING

This section will review the most common pulmonary and neurologic illnesses that are typically seen in an ICU setting.

Pulmonary Disease

Chronic Obstructive Pulmonary Disease

Chronic obstructive pulmonary disease (COPD) encompasses a group of lung diseases characterized by slow progression and long continuance as well as the presence of expiratory airflow limitation or obstruction. Emphysema and chronic bronchitis are two of the more important diseases that fall under this large category, but chronic bronchial asthma, cystic fibrosis, bronchiectasis, small airway disease, and bronchiolitis all fulfill the broad definition of COPD. About 15 million people in the United States have emphysema and chronic bronchitis, and another 15 million suffer from asthma (total 30+ million, or 11 to 12.5% of the U.S. population).[14] The differences in these diseases are based on histologic, physiologic, radiologic, clinical, and other criteria.

Emphysema

Emphysema is characterized by the permanent destruction and enlargement of the distal air spaces, most commonly caused by cigarette smoking (active or passive).[15] Patients tend to be limited mostly by dyspnea and have significant air trapping and hyperinflation. Because they work so hard to maintain normal or near-normal blood gases, they are often referred to as "pink puffers." They are usually thin and cachectic and rely on pursed lip breathing.

Acute Respiratory Distress Syndrome

Acute respiratory distress syndrome (ARDS, formerly adult respiratory distress syndrome) is a catastrophic disease characterized by significant and acute lung injury leading to respiratory failure usually within 48 hours of the insult. The majority of these patients have profound impairment in gas exchange, are severely hypoxemic, and spend variable amounts of time on a mechanical ventilator. ARDS is most commonly caused by pneumonia, aspiration, polytrauma, multiple transfusions, gram negative sepsis, and pancreatitis. Other organ system involvement and failure occur and the mortality is high (40%).[16]

Cardiopulmonary Illness

Congestive Heart Failure

Congestive heart failure (CHF) is caused by a number of diseases in which impairments in cardiac output allow blood to pool in the pulmonary veins, capillaries, and pulmonary arteries. This pooling of blood leads to lung congestion and gas exchange impairments. Etiologies that can cause CHF include myocardial infarction, valvular heart disease, hypertensive heart disease, cardiomyopathy, and pericardial diseases. The condition can be acute or chronic and almost all patients will suffer with dyspnea, fatigue, exercise intolerance, and lower extremity edema.

Cardiac Failure

Cardiac failure is a nonspecific condition of cardiac or heart dysfunction caused by a variety of diseases. They include hypertensive and ischemic heart disease, pericardial disease, and valvular disease. During cardiac failure, cardiac output is impaired and end-organ perfusion suffers. Patients with cardiac failure may develop stroke, kidney disease, liver failure, and other organ dysfunction. A majority of these patients will also have CHF.

Pulmonary Edema

Pulmonary edema is a condition of excess lung fluid that often leads to respiratory failure because the fluid-filled alveoli are unable to participate in normal gas exchange. CHF and ARDS are causes of pulmonary edema. Important in the evolution of this disease is the type of accumulated lung fluid. Protein-poor edema fluid (as in CHF) is more responsive to diuretic therapy then protein-rich edema fluid (ARDS). Pulmonary edema usually causes dyspnea, fatigue, weakness, exercise intolerance, and peripheral edema.

Neurologic Disease

Amyotrophic Lateral Sclerosis

Amyotrophic lateral sclerosis (ALS) is a degenerative neuromuscular disease that involves the upper motor neurons in the cortex and lower motor neurons in the brainstem and spinal cord.[17] To date, the etiology of ALS is unknown. Viral, toxic, and genetic causes have been speculated.[17] In the United States the ratio of men to women who acquire the nonfamilial form of the illness is 2:1, and the cause of death is usually respiratory failure or pneumonia.[17] Although muscle cramping is commonly the initial symptom of the disease, nearly one quarter of patients present with dysarthria as their initial symptom.[18,19] This illness eventually involves the musculature of speech, swallowing, and respiration. Patients who have made the decision to undergo a tracheotomy and/or mechanical ventilation to assist or prolong their respiratory status may be seen in the ICU. If a patient is anarthric, speech via a tracheostomy tube will not be functional and alternative methods of communication are necessary.

Guillain-Barré Syndrome

Adams and Victor describe this illness as a rapidly progressing ascending inflammatory disease that affects people of all ages and both sexes.[20] The usual clinical presentation is muscle weakness, which can result in total muscle paralysis and death due to respiratory failure within a few days of onset. Facial diplegia occurs in approximately one-half of all cases and arises along with other cranial nerve signs after the arms are affected. The use of plasmaphoresis within two weeks of onset has been known to expedite recovery, including

the length of time patients require mechanical ventilation. The focus of medical treatment is respiratory assistance and careful nursing care as the disease resolves naturally. Recovery is complete in the majority of cases. A flaccid form of dysarthria is seen with this disorder and careful speech assessment and short-term treatment may be necessary as the patient recovers.

Stroke

There are many forms of stroke that require ICU placement for a patient. Stroke may result from an intracranial hemorrhage or a thrombolic or embolic event. Patients who develop brainstem strokes are likely to spend their acute phase of hospitalization in an ICU because respiration may be compromised. As the course of the illness progresses, the patient should be followed closely from a communication and swallowing standpoint.

Traumatic Brain Injury

Patients with acute traumatic brain injury (TBI) may be followed by the speech–language pathologist for basic cognitive stimulation in the ICU. Because intubation and eventual tracheotomy are common occurrences in such situations, thorough diagnostic therapy from a communication and swallowing standpoint is imperative. TBI patients may exhibit rapid changes in neurologic status in a short period of time and thus constant contact with nursing and medical staff are necessary for anticipating the patient's ability to try new methods of communication and feeding, particularly as this relates to voicing and swallowing with a tracheostomy tube.

Spinal Cord Injury

Patients with acute spinal cord injury (SCI) above the level of C_3 will likely have breathing problems and require mechanical ventilation.[21] As the patient stabilizes, communication and swallowing issues will arise. Communication may progress from simple eye blinks for yes/no responses to voicing with a tracheostomy tube as the patient's condition improves. Ongoing monitoring and diagnostic therapy will be necessary to provide the most effective and efficient methods of communication for the patient.

Laryngeal Injury

According to Tucker, the larynx is relatively protected within the neck by the sternocleidomastoid muscles laterally, the cervical vertebrae and other muscles of the neck posteriorly, and the mandible from above.[22] Laryngeal injuries occur from a number of causes ranging from blunt trauma to the larynx, as seen in seat belt or steering wheel injuries in car accidents, to penetrating trauma—bullet or knife wounds. Blunt injury to an older, more calcified larynx may result in arytenoid dislocation or laryngeal fracture of the cartilaginous structures of the larynx whereas the same blow may produce little damage to a young, flexible larynx.

The ICU patient with a laryngeal injury will commonly have a tracheostomy tube. It is important to discuss the full extent of the patient's laryngeal injuries and the surgical repair procedures with the physician to anticipate short- and long-term voicing conditions. Counseling regarding voice use in the early stages of hospitalization is recommended with close monitoring, and voice therapy, with or without the presence of a tracheostomy tube, may be necessary.

TRACHEOSTOMY

During their initial days in an ICU patients may be ventilated via nasal or oral intubation with an endotracheal tube. However, many of these patients will require a tracheotomy to facilitate respiration. Decisions about the proper timing and indications for changing the airway access to a tracheostomy tube seem to be less controversial than in the past, but a variety of opinions still exist. The trend in recent years has been toward earlier insertion of tracheostomy tubes after initial nasal or oral intubation in critically ill patients. For spontaneously breathing patients a tracheostomy tube is placed to improve ventilation. The tracheostomy tube provides direct access to the lower respiratory tract. The patient inhales and exhales directly via the tracheostomy tube, which is usually inserted at or below the second or third tracheal ring, thus bypassing the nose and mouth. A tracheotomy is usually performed in cases when upper respiratory obstruction occurs due to illness, injury, or surgery.[23]

Components of a Tracheostomy Tube

There are three basic parts to a tracheostomy tube: the obturator, the outer cannula, and the inner cannula (Figure 5–2).[23] The obturator is used for insertion of the outer cannula of the tracheostomy tube and is replaced by the inner cannula once the outer cannula is securely in place. The inner cannula remains in place to collect secretions that could po-

tentially obstruct the airway. At times these secretions may be viscous or may collect and dry within the inner cannula. If the inner cannula is not in place and secretions become encrusted within the outer cannula, the potential for airway obstruction exists, which, in extreme cases, may require a total tracheostomy tube change. For this reason it is highly recommended that the inner cannula remain in place and undergo cleaning on a regular basis. Disposable inner cannulas are available that may be replaced without cleaning, and single cannula tracheostomy tubes are also available that are made of a silicone plastic and do not require the use of an inner cannula. The silicone material is intended to reduce the risk of encrustation of secretions.[24]

Types of Tracheostomy Tubes

Tracheostomy tubes may be cuffed (Figure 5–3) or uncuffed (Figure 5–4). The cuff is inflated and deflated via a syringe that inserts into the pilot balloon. When the cuff is inflated, the route of air travel is directly via the trachea to the lower airway, thus bypassing the nose and mouth as shown in Figure 5–5. In most cases, as a patient's medical status improves, the cuff may be deflated or a cuffless tracheostomy tube inserted. In either of these scenarios, air is then able to pass through the upper airway and vocal folds, enabling the patient to voice with a tracheostomy tube as shown in Figure 5–6.

Many manufacturers offer tracheostomy tubes of varying sizes, yet as noted in Table 5–1 tube sizes are usually not comparable between the different manufacturers. For example, a standard no. 6 Shiley tracheostomy tube does not have the same dimensions as a no. 6 tracheostomy tube made by Portex. For this reason, it is important to know the inner and outer cannula dimensions, and not just the given size of the tube, when substituting tubes from one manufacturer to another.

Advantages to Tracheostomy Tube Placement

As with any procedure there are advantages and potential complications to the placement of a tracheostomy tube. In addition to the primary advantage of providing airway access, advantages to the placement of a tracheostomy tube include:[23,25]

1. Ease of access to the lower respiratory tract for suctioning.
2. A decrease in the risk of laryngeal granuloma and subglottic stenosis due to the

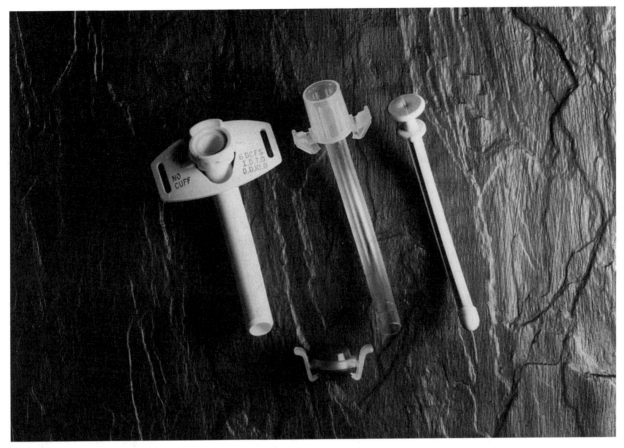

Figure 5–2. Shiley outer cannula, inner cannula, and obturator (left to right). Photo courtesy of Mallinckrodt Medical, Inc.

elimination of constant pressure of an oro-tracheal tube at the level of the vocal folds and subglottis.

3. Improved weaning from mechanical ventilation because (a) the design and placement of a tracheostomy tube lessens the resistance to airflow that is seen in endotracheal tubes and (b) air volume is delivered directly to the lungs thereby reducing the amount of dead space in the airway (areas within the airway that do not participate in gas exchange) and allowing for greater volumes of inspired air available for oxygen exchange.

4. An increase in patient comfort compared with nasal or orotracheal intubation.

5. Improved options for oral communication and swallowing compared with nasal or orotracheal intubation.

6. Improved oral hygiene due to improved access to the oral cavity without the presence of an endotracheal tube.

Complications of Tracheostomy Tube Placement

The following are some complications of tracheostomy tube placement:[23,25–28]

1. Loss of taste and smell due to an absence of airflow through the nose and mouth.

2. An increase in secretions secondary to the presence of the tracheostomy tube as the body reacts to the presence of a foreign object.

3. Tracheal granuloma secondary to abrasion at the stoma site.

4. Tracheomalacia, a softening or degeneration of the elastic and connective tissues of the trachea, may occur when there is any trauma to the tracheal walls that exposes the cartilage and leads to tissue breakdown.

5. Tracheal stenosis occurs when the trachea narrows as part of the healing process after trauma. Stenosis may occur at the stoma site or near the cuff of the tracheostomy tube.

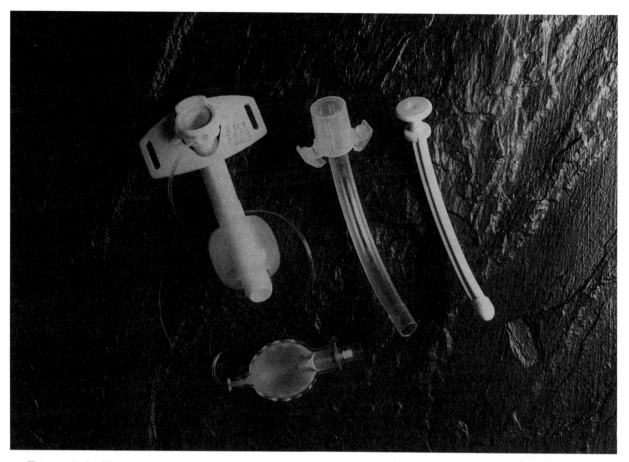

Figure 5–3. Shiley cuffed tracheostomy tube (left). Photo courtesy of Mallinckrodt Medical, Inc.

Tracheal stenosis at the stoma site may result from frequent infections, tube changes, a stoma that is too large and begins to close as part of the healing process, or continuous tugging on the tracheostomy tube from ventilator tubing. Constant pressure on the tracheal mucosa or abrasive movements of the cuff as the tube moves up and down during breathing, swallowing, or changes in body position may contribute to tracheal stenosis at the cuff site.

6. Limitation of laryngeal elevation with a cuffed tracheostomy tube during swallowing, which may lead to aspiration.

7. Tracheoesophageal fistula, a connection between the trachea and the esophagus, may occur from pressure on the anterior esophageal wall from an overinflated tracheostomy tube cuff in conjunction with the presence of a large nasogastric feeding tube. Necrosis of the tracheal and esophageal walls then takes place. Infection and poor nutrition may contribute to this problem.

8. Tracheoinnominate fistula occurs when a tracheostomy tube is inserted too low within the trachea, usually below the third cartilaginous ring. The tube may impinge on the innominate artery, causing eventual erosion, the creation of a fistula and potentially life-threatening hemorrhage. This is a dangerous but rare complication of tracheostomy.

9. Respiratory infection due to changes in bacterial colonization within the airway following tracheotomy. Tracheal wound infections, a severely ill patient, and a reduction in tracheal mucociliary clearance after tracheotomy all contribute to the risk of pneumonia in tracheostomized patients.

Communication with a Tracheostomy Tube

Patient Assessment

Before recommending voicing with a tracheostomy tube, the patient should be assessed to determine whether he or she is a viable candidate for use of

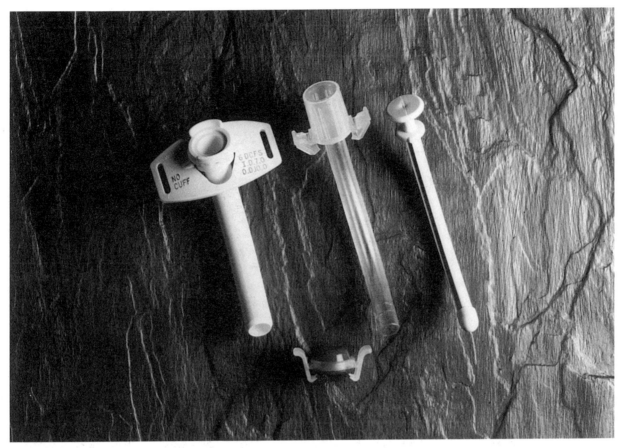

Figure 5–4. Shiley uncuffed tracheostomy tube (left). Photo courtesy of Mallinckrodt Medical, Inc.

this mode of communication. Evaluation includes a review of the patient's medical condition, vocal fold status, oral-motor status, and general communicative/cognitive condition.

Medical History

A thorough review of the patient's medical history will help to anticipate any problems with verbal communication from a linguistic/cognitive, speech, and voice standpoint. In particular, the patient's respiratory and neurologic status should be discussed thoroughly with the patient's physician.

Otolaryngologic Examination

A laryngeal evaluation is important so that any problems with voicing arising from vocal fold paralysis or granulation tissue in the posterior commissure of the glottis may be anticipated. These findings do not preclude the use of a tracheostomy tube for voicing but will prepare the patient for changes in expected vocal quality.

Oral-Motor Status

This evaluation is necessary for determining if a patient will be a candidate for verbal communication. Severely restricted lingual, labial, and buccal movements secondary to neurologic impairment or head and neck surgery may limit the effectiveness of voicing with a tracheostomy tube, making alternative modes of communication necessary. In many cases patients with mild to moderate dysarthria are able to effectively communicate verbally via their tracheostomy tubes.

Voicing Options for Patients with Deflated or Cuffless Tracheostomy Tubes

Several different options are possible for voicing with a tracheostomy tube. In almost all cases the cuff must be deflated or a cuffless tube must be in place. Medical clearance is always necessary when manipulating a tracheostomy tube. When a tracheostomy tube is in place and the cuff is inflated, air is being inhaled and exhaled directly to and from the trachea. Therefore, to redirect the air

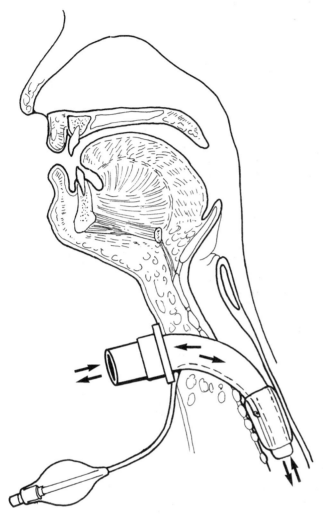

Figure 5–5. Arrows show route of airflow to and from the lower airway with an inflated tracheostomy tube cuff.

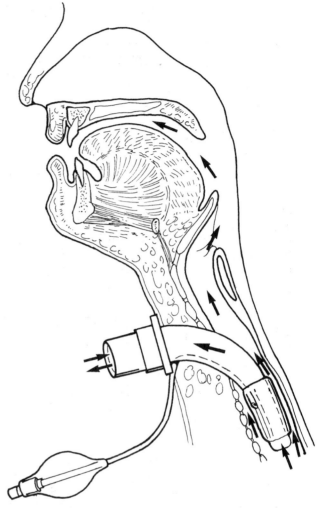

Figure 5–6. Arrows show the route of airflow to the upper airway as well as the lower airway when a tracheostomy tube cuff is deflated.

through the vocal folds, the cuff must be deflated so that air can then travel around the distal end of the tracheostomy tube. The proximal opening of the tube must be occluded so airflow will not escape through the tracheotomy tube to the atmosphere outside, but will be redirected through the vocal folds and out the patient's mouth and nose. There are several ways of doing this:

1. Keep the inner cannula in place while using digital occlusion over the proximal opening of the tracheostomy tube. The patient inhales, the inner cannula is digitally occluded, and the patient voices on exhalation.

2. If the tube is fenestrated, removing the inner cannula will enable air to flow both around the distal end of the outer cannula and up through the fenestration, thus allowing for greater airflow and a stronger voice while

the proximal end of the outer cannula is digitally occluded or capped. Because air will flow through the path of least resistance, it is important to occlude the outer cannula for more efficient use of breath support and a louder voice, otherwise air will flow both out of the tracheostomy tube and the patient's mouth and nose, and a weak, breathy voice will occur that requires much effort on the patient's part to increase volume. If a patient's tracheostomy tube has a fenestrated inner and outer cannula, removal of the inner cannula for voicing in this situation is not necessary.

3. Remove the inner cannula in a cuffless or cuff-deflated nonfenestrated tube and use digital occlusion or capping of the outer cannula for voicing.

Table 5–1. Cross Reference Chart of Tracheostomy Tube Sizes

Adult Tracheostomy Tube CROSS REFERENCE

BIVONA CODE NO.	ID mm	OD mm	APPX French	APPX Jackson	Length mm
850150	5.0	7.3	22	3	60
850160	6.0	8.7	26	4	70
850170	7.0	10.0	30	6	80
850180	8.0	11.0	33	7	88
850190	9.0	12.3	37	8	98
850195	9.5	13.3	40	10	98

SHILEY CODE NO.	ID mm	OD mm	APPX French	APPX Jackson	Length mm
4DCT	5.0	8.5	26	4	67
6DCT	7.0	10.0	30	6	78
8DCT	8.5	12.0	36	8	84
10DCT	9.0	13.0	39	10	84

PORTEX CODE NO.	ID mm	OD mm	APPX French	APPX Jackson	Length mm
503060	5.0	8.5	26	4	67
503070	6.0	9.9	30	6	73
503080	7.0	11.3	34	7	78
503090	8.0	12.6	38	8	84
503100	9.0	14.0	42	10	84

BIVONA CODE NO.	ID mm	OD mm	APPX French	APPX Jackson	Length mm
850150	5.0	7.3	22	3	60
850160	6.0	8.7	26	4	70
850170	7.0	10.0	30	6	80
850180	8.0	11.0	33	7	88
850190	9.0	12.3	37	8	98
850195	9.5	13.3	40	10	98

SHILEY CODE NO.	ID mm	OD mm	APPX French	APPX Jackson	Length mm
5SCT	5.0	7.0	21	3	58
6SCT	6.0	8.3	24.9	4	67
7SCT	7.0	9.6	28.8	6	80
8SCT	8.0	10.9	32.7	7	89
9SCT	9.0	12.1	36.3	8	99
10SCT	10.0	13.3	39.9	10	105

PORTEX CODE NO.	ID mm	OD mm	APPX French	APPX Jackson	Length mm
530060	6.0	8.3	24	4	55
530070	7.0	9.7	30	6	75
530080	8.0	11.0	33	7	82
530090	9.0	12.4	36	8	87
530100	10.0	13.8	40	10	98

BIVONA CODE NO.	ID mm	OD mm	APPX French	APPX Jackson	Length mm
670150	5.0	7.3	22	3	60
670160	6.0	8.7	26	4	70
670170	7.0	10.0	30	6	80
670180	8.0	11.0	33	7	88
670190	9.0	12.3	37	8	98
670195	9.5	13.3	40	10	98

SHILEY CODE NO.	ID mm	OD mm	APPX French	APPX Jackson	Length mm
4FEN	5.0	8.5	26	4	67
6FEN	7.0	10.0	30	6	78
8FEN	8.5	12.0	36	8	84
10FEN	9.0	13.0	39	10	84

PORTEX CODE NO.	ID mm	OD mm	APPX French	APPX Jackson	Length mm
513060	5.0	8.5	26	4	67
513070	6.0	9.9	30	6	73
513080	7.0	11.3	34	7	78
513090	8.0	12.6	38	8	84
513100	9.0	14.0	42	10	84

Uncuffed Tracheostomy Tube CROSS REFERENCE

BIVONA CODE NO.	ID mm	OD mm	APPX French	APPX Jackson	Length mm
60N025	2.5	4.0	12	000	30
60N030	3.0	4.7	14	00	32
60N035	3.5	5.3	16	0/1	34
60N040	4.0	6.0	18	2	36

SHILEY CODE NO.	ID mm	OD mm	APPX French	APPX Jackson	Length mm
OONT	3.1	4.5	14	00	30
ONT	3.4	5.0	15	0	32
INT	3.7	5.5	17	1	34

PORTEX CODE NO.	ID mm	OD mm	APPX French	APPX Jackson	Length mm
553025	2.5	4.5	13	00	30
553030	3.0	5.2	15	0	32
553035	3.5	5.8	16	1	34

BIVONA CODE NO.	ID mm	OD mm	APPX French	APPX Jackson	Length mm
60P025	2.5	4.0	12	000	38
60P030	3.0	4.7	14	00	39
60P035	3.5	5.3	16	0/1	40
60P040	4.0	6.0	18	2	41
60P045	4.5	6.7	20	3-	42
60P050	5.0	7.3	22	3+	44
60P055	5.5	8.0	24	4	46

SHILEY CODE NO.	ID mm	OD mm	APPX French	APPX Jackson	Length mm
OOPT	3.1	4.5	14	00	39
OPT	3.4	5.0	15	0	40
1PT	3.7	5.5	17	1	41
2PT	4.1	6.0	18	2	42
3PT	4.8	7.0	21	3	44
4PT	5.5	8.0	24	4	46

PORTEX CODE NO.	ID mm	OD mm	APPX French	APPX Jackson	Length mm
555025	2.5	4.5	13	00	30
555030	3.0	5.2	15	00	36
555035	3.5	5.8	16	01	40
555040	4.0	6.5	18	02	44
555045	4.5	7.1	19	03	48
555050	5.0	7.7	21	4-	50
555055	5.5	8.3	23	4+	52

BIVONA CODE NO.	ID mm	OD mm	APPX French	APPX Jackson	Length mm
60A150	5.0	7.3	22	3	60
60A160	6.0	8.7	26	4	70
60A170	7.0	10.0	30	6	80
60A180	8.0	11.0	33	7	88
60A190	9.0	12.3	37	8	98
60A195	9.5	13.3	40	10	98

SHILEY CODE NO.	ID mm	OD mm	APPX French	APPX Jackson	Length mm
4CFS	5.0	8.5	26	4	67
6CFS	7.0	10.0	30	6	78
8CFS	8.5	12.0	36	8	84
10CFS	9.0	13.0	39	10	84

PORTEX CODE NO.	ID mm	OD mm	APPX French	APPX Jackson	Length mm
550060	6.0	8.3	24	4	55
550070	7.0	9.7	30	6	75
550080	8.0	11.0	33	7	82
550090	9.0	12.4	36	8	87
560100	10.0	13.8	40	10	98

Source: Courtesy of Bivona Medical Technologies.

4. Use a one-way speaking valve with the inner cannula in place.

If a fenestrated tube is in place and cuff deflation is not an option from a medical standpoint, the inner cannula may be removed for short periods and voicing may occur through the fenestration alone when the outer cannula is digitally occluded. However, if the cuff cannot be deflated, this is probably the result of an excess of oropharyngeal and tracheal secretions. Therefore, thorough suctioning prior to removal of the inner cannula should be done to limit the risk of a patient aspirating secretions that may fall through the fenestration. This method could produce a weaker sounding or strained voice because airflow is limited to travel through the small fenestration and is recommended for vocalization of only a few phrases, for a short time.

One-Way Speaking Valves

Although digital occlusion of a tracheostomy tube is usually effective for voicing under the proper conditions, the patient is at risk for infection if the person occluding the tracheostomy tube is not wearing gloves. Also, digital occlusion may not be an option if the patient or caretaker is unable to occlude the tube because of extremity weakness. A speaking valve eliminates the need for digital occlusion of a tracheostomy tube for voicing or swallowing. Speaking valves continue to allow inhalation via the tracheostomy tube, but exhalation occurs via the nose and mouth as the valve closes and air is then redirected to the upper airway. Many long-term tracheostomized patients become accustomed to airflow through the tracheostomy tube, which bypasses the nose and mouth. When the patient is ready to begin weaning from a tracheostomy tube, a speaking valve may be less anxiety provoking than sudden capping (and redirecting of inhalation and exhalation through the upper airway) of the tracheostomy tube. The valve thus may act as an intermediate step between full breathing from a tracheostomy tube and capping of the tube. According to Frey and Wood, use of the Passy-Muir speaking valve assisted in the weaning process of a group of long-term mechanically ventilated patients and led to independent breathing in 33% of the patients.[29]

All speaking valves must be used with a completely deflated cuff or cuffless tracheostomy tube. In addition, the use of a speaking valve is not recommended with foam cuffed tracheostomy tubes because a foam cuff usually does not completely deflate. If a cuff is inflated while a speaking valve is in place, the patient will not be able to exhale. Air will become trapped beneath the level of the cuff, unable to travel to the upper airway due to the inflated cuff and unable to travel through the outer opening of the tracheostomy tube because of the seal created on exhalation by the valve. Figures 5–7 and 5–8 demonstrate the route of airflow when a speaking valve is attached to a tracheostomy tube when the cuff is deflated and when it is inflated. The amount of pressure required to open a speaking valve varies between valves.[30] The following are common valves currently on the market.

Passy-Muir One-Way Speaking Valve

This valve attaches to the standard 15 mm hub of an inner cannula (Figure 5–9). It is unique from other speaking valves in that it is biased toward the

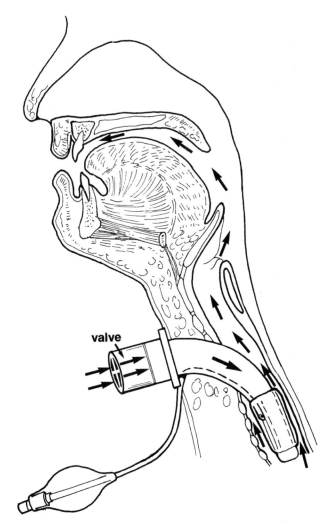

Figure 5–7. Arrows show the route of inhalation through a speaking valve and exhalation via the upper airway with a speaking valve in place and the tracheostomy tube cuff fully deflated.

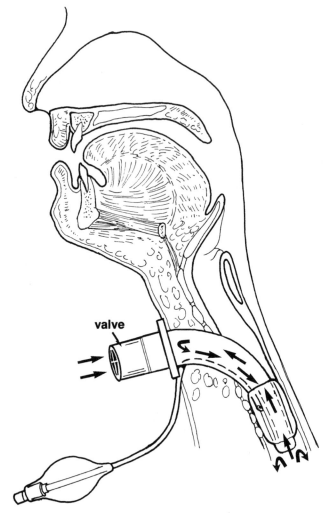

Figure 5–8. Arrows show inhalation through the speaking valve and trapping of air within the trachea during attempts to exhale when a speaking valve is in place and the tracheostomy tube cuff is inflated.

closed position. The valve is continuously closed and only opens when the patient inhales. The valve then begins to close prior to the completion of the inspiratory cycle.[31] The advantage to having the valve resume a closed position prior to the completion of inhalation is that a column of air then becomes trapped within the valve and tracheostomy tube. This column of air acts as a buffer and helps prevent occlusion of the valve by tracheal secretions. An additional advantage to the biased closed position is that it requires less effort for a patient to close than valves that have an open bias.[31] It has been reported that the use of the Passy-Muir speaking valve improves oxygen saturation and assists in patient tolerance of the ventilatory weaning process.[29] This valve is available in several different models as seen in Figure 5–9. The aqua valve is designed specifically for in-line use with ventilators to accommodate the ventilator tubing; it can also be used with nonmechanically ventilated patients with tracheostomy tubes. The clear and purple valves are low profile and are available with an optional attachment to secure the valve to the tracheostomy tube collar so that the valve remains near the patient should it become dislodged (e.g., during a cough).

Hood Speaking Valve

This is a one-way valve designed to adapt to all 15-mm connectors for tracheostomy tubes (Figure 5–10).[32] The valve is also available in a model designed to attach to two sizes of the Hood Stoma Stent, thus eliminating finger occlusion for voicing for patients wearing the stent.

Montgomery Tracheostomy Speaking Valve

This valve fits onto the standard 15-mm hub of an inner cannula (Figure 5–11). It has a unique cough release feature that helps prevent the valve from popping off of the tracheostomy tube during a cough. When coughing occurs, the silicone diaphragm partially dislodges. It is easily tucked back into its housing following the cough.[33] This valve is also available in a model specifically designed for in line use with a ventilator, called the VENTRACH speaking valve (Figure 5–11).

Olympic Speaking Valve

This one-way valve also fits onto the standard 15-mm hub of an inner cannula (Figure 5–12). The valve is held open by a stainless steel spring until the patient exhales, at which time the spring closes the valve, thereby diverting air up through the larynx, allowing the patient to voice. When exhalation is completed, the spring forces the valve back into the open position. The valve is T-shaped and therefore can be used while a patient is receiving oxygen or humidification. In addition, it is not necessary to remove the valve during suctioning because there is a removable cover on the distal end of the tube that can accommodate passing of a suction catheter.[34]

Shiley Phonate Speaking Valve

This valve attaches to the standard 15-mm hub of an inner cannula (Figure 5–13). It is available with or without an oxygen port to allow for supplemental oxygen and/or humidification. It has a flex-

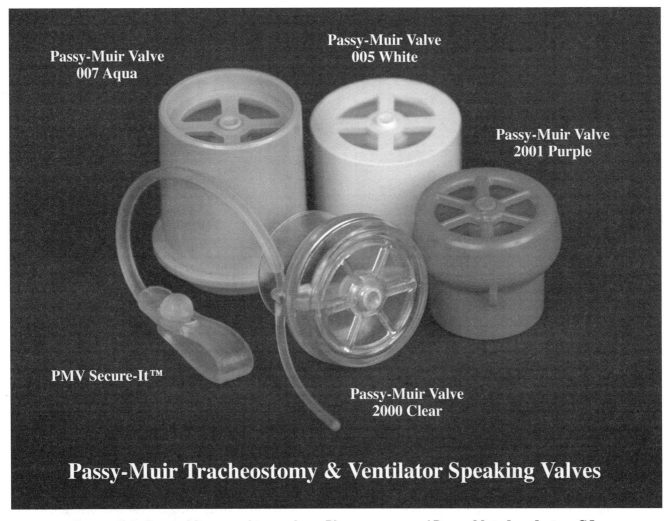

Figure 5–9. Passy-Muir speaking valves. Photo courtesy of Passy-Muir, Inc., Irvine, CA.

ible diaphragm that can be easily pushed back into the housing should it become displaced after a cough or sneeze.[35]

Suggested Protocol for Placement of a Speaking Valve

Preplacement Issues: In some instances the speech–language pathologist may be consulted at the first signs of alertness from a patient. This is particularly true if a patient has had a long hospital course and the medical staff and family members are anxious to communicate with the patient. However, prior to requesting a tracheostomy tube change by the patient's physician and manipulating tracheostomy tube cuffs, it is important to thoroughly assess the patient's potential for communication. Sometimes, using an electrolarynx for a few days may be appropriate while assessing the patient's general cognitive/communicative level

and following medical progress. Once consideration for a speaking valve is made, several pre-placement issues should be addressed. Many of the following suggestions are also applicable to voicing via a cuffless tracheostomy tube without the use of a speaking valve as mentioned earlier.

1. Normal, or near normal, oral motor examination—Although a dysarthric patient may be a candidate for a speaking valve, a patient who is anarthric or has had extensive oral or head and neck surgery and has limited lingual or mandibular movement may not be an effective speaker with a valve. In such instances, the patient may be a more effective communicator via nonverbal methods.

2. Patient is attempting to communicate—A patient may have a normal oral-motor and speech and voice examination, but if he or she is not motivated to verbalize, has diminished cognition, or is too fatigued or ill to speak, the patient may not be an appropriate candidate for a valve. Placement

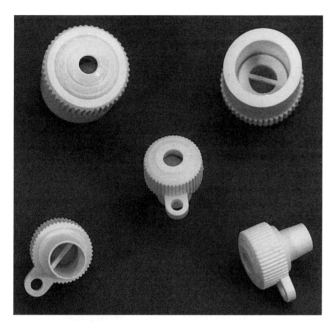

Figure 5–10. Hood speaking valves for tracheostomy tubes (top row); Hood speaking valves that attach to the Hood stoma stents (middle and bottom rows). Photo courtesy of Hood Laboratories, Pembroke, MA.

may then have to be postponed until medical status, cognitive status, or motivation improves.

3. Alertness for most of the day for at least 2 consecutive days—In some cases a valve may be used for short periods for communication of needs or questions to health care providers or family members. However, in general, ongoing communication is best facilitated in a patient who is alert for most of the day and interested in communicating with people within the environment.

4. Tracheostomy tube in place 24 to 48 hours—It is good practice to withhold trials of a valve for 1 to 2 days following initial tracheostomy tube placement to ensure that voicing with the valve will not interfere with the healing process of the tracheotomy.

5. Normal laryngeal examination by physician, or at least identification of laryngeal pathology that may compromise vocal quality—The same reasons previously outlined when considering digital occlusion or capping a tracheostomy tube for voicing apply to the consideration of placement of a speaking valve.

6. Cuff deflation is allowed or cuffless tracheostomy tube is in place—For a patient to use a speaking valve, the cuff of a tracheostomy tube must be fully deflated or a cuffless tube must be in place as previously described.

7. Assessment of viscosity of secretions—If tracheal or oropharyngeal secretions are too thick and thus have the potential to obstruct the airway or interfere with communication, the patient may not be a candidate for a speaking valve until the secretions lessen or become thinner. However, the use of a speaking valve may improve a patient's ability to swallow and thus more effectively clear oropharyngeal secretions. As reported by Eibling and Gross, the use of a Passy-Muir speaking valve assisted in significantly reducing or eliminating aspiration in a group of patients known to have aspiration without the valve in place.[36]

8. Assessment of upper airway—Note any upper airway obstruction that may exist such as tracheal or glottal stenosis or granulation tissue. This information is usually obtained through the case history or the physician's reports after viewing the nasal, oral, tracheal, and bronchial structures, usually via endoscopy. Mason points out that assessment of the upper airway may also be made by the clinician digitally occluding the tracheostomy tube and listening or observing exhaled airflow through the nose and mouth.[37] Condensation on a mirror or movement of a feather placed near the nose or mouth may also confirm upper airway patency. However, any sights or sounds of difficulty breathing, such as an excessively gurgly voice or strained or loud breathing, may indicate problems with upper airway airflow, in which case trials of a valve should be postponed until the problem is investigated further by the patient's physician.

9. If the valve is being used with a ventilator dependent patient, a physician must approve deflation of the cuff and modification of ventilator volumes—To ensure that adequate airflow is reaching the lungs during cuff deflation, an increase in tidal volume is often necessary when a speaking valve is being used with a ventilator dependent patient. This is necessary to accommodate for the new air leakage around a deflated cuff. With the cuff deflated, air will flow up and around the tracheostomy tube as well as into the lungs, and therefore close monitoring of tidal volumes is important. Readjustment of the rate of breathing from the ventilator may also be necessary at times when a speaking valve is in place.

10. Arrange for a respiratory therapist and physician or nurse to be in attendance during initial placement trials—The speech–language pathologist's role in evaluation of and treatment with speaking valves with ventilator dependent patients does not usually include respiratory monitoring. For this reason it is important that a health care expert in the area of ventilators and pulmonology is

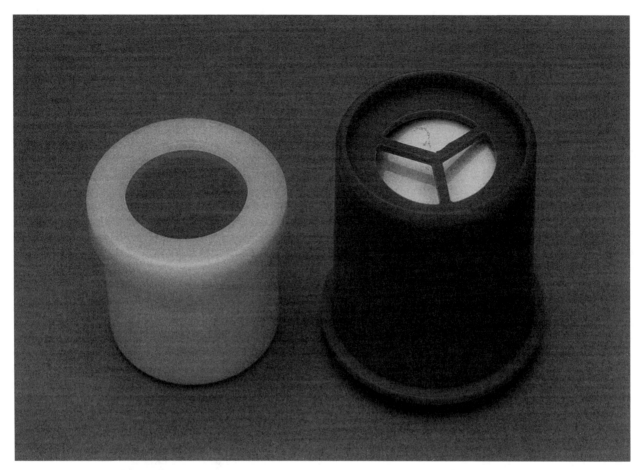

Figure 5–11. Montgomery speaking valve (left) and Montgomery VENTRACH speaking valve (right). Photo courtesy of Boston Medical Products.

present during the initial placement trials. A respiratory therapist alone may then be present for future trials with the speech-pathologist.

Postplacement Issues: The following postplacement issues are based on our clinical experience and as described by Mason and Watkins[31] and Mason.[37]

1. Monitor vital signs—(a) Breathing rate, heart rate, blood pressure, and oxygen saturation levels should all be closely monitored during initial placement of the speaking valve. Problems in these areas may indicate intolerance of the valve, the need to adjust ventilator settings, or patient anxiety as a reaction to the new sensation of upper airway airflow. (b) Skin and nail color should remain similar to preplacement levels. Changes may indicate intolerance to the valve. (c) Measurement of exhaled tidal volume: Once upper airway patency has been established prior to valve placement, measurement of exhalatory tidal volume with the valve in place should also occur. Abnormal exhalatory tidal volume measurements with a

valve in place may indicate a problem with lower, or pulmonary, airway clearance.

2. Be watchful of breath-stacking—If there is an obstruction within the airway, or if the patient has poor pulmonary function, he or she may not be able to fully exhale. If air is not fully exhaled the patient may complain of fullness in the chest, discomfort, or the sensation of actually not being able to inhale. This may present a dangerous situation as the continued building-up or "stacking" of inhaled air may lead to barotrauma.

3. Assess viscosity of secretions—An increase in the amount or thickness of secretions with a valve in place may preclude a patient's candidacy for using a speaking valve until the problem improves.

4. Assess work of breathing—If a patient is observed to attempt to use accessory respiratory muscles to breathe during speaking, airway obstruction should be investigated. In some cases anxiety may cause unnecessary work of breathing and a patient may need relaxation counseling prior to or during use of the valve.

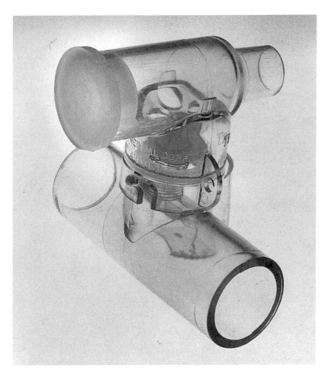

Figure 5–12. Olympic speaking valve. Photo courtesy of Olympic Medical.

5. Assess patient's physical and emotional reaction to valve—For a patient who has not experienced upper airway airflow in weeks or months, the sensation of closure at the level of the larynx may be stressful and anxiety provoking. A patient may report the feeling of not getting enough air to breathe even if adequate ventilation is occurring. Preplacement counseling on the redirection of airflow with a valve in place and reassurance that airway patency has been thoroughly assessed and that adequate breath support is anticipated may assist in acceptance of the valve in a tentative patient. In some cases relaxation techniques, the use of simple anatomy pictures depicting the changes in airflow, and visual imagery techniques may be applied until the patient adjusts to the valve. Another source of anxiety may be the fear that a patient has lost his or her voice after not being able to speak for an extended period. In our clinical experience patients have reported that they "forgot" how to talk after not experiencing voicing for as short a time period as 2 weeks. Again, reassurance and voice therapy will usually lead to increased comfort and effective communication with the valve. Patients are frequently comforted by the sound of their voice, which may lead to early acceptance of a speaking valve.

6. Patient fatigue—Initial placement of the valve should be limited to five minutes with close monitoring of the patient's fatigue level. Gradual increases in the length of time that the valve is used is recommended as the patient adjusts to the valve. A few short speaking times may be scheduled during the day to assist in increasing the patient's comfort and endurance level of voicing with a speaking valve.

7. Education—Educating the patient, caretakers, nursing, and medical staff on the care and use of a speaking valve is imperative. Written instructions posted at the patient's bedside are recommended, with particular emphasis on the necessity of cuff deflation prior to valve placement. The patient and/or caretaker should be trained in cuff manipulation, suctioning, use and care of the valve, and in the case of a ventilator dependent patient, adjusting ventilator settings to accommodate the cuff leak necessary for valve use. Combined training sessions with the respiratory therapist and speech–language pathologist are recommended. If the patient or caretaker is unable to perform the necessary activities for safe use and care of a speaking valve, the patient may not be an appropriate candidate for using a valve, even if he or she is able to communicate well with it in place.

Contraindications to Using a Speaking Valve

As described by Dikeman and Kazandjian,[38] the following situations are contraindications to using a speaking valve.

1. Evidence of airway obstruction. For the patient to fully expel air, a patent airway is necessary.
2. Laryngectomy. A speaking valve is not to be confused with a voice prosthesis such as those used in laryngectomy patients with tracheoesophageal punctures. A laryngectomee is not a candidate for use of a valve since his or her only means of air exchange is directly through the lower airway, thus completely bypassing the upper airway.
3. Cuff inflation or foam cuffed tracheostomy tubes. As previously mentioned, the tracheostomy tube cuff must be completely deflated to use a speaking valve. Foam cuffs do not deflate completely and spontaneously reinflate. Therefore, foam cuffs may actually act as an obstruction in the airway.
4. End-stage pulmonary disease. Patients with end-stage pulmonary disease tend to retain

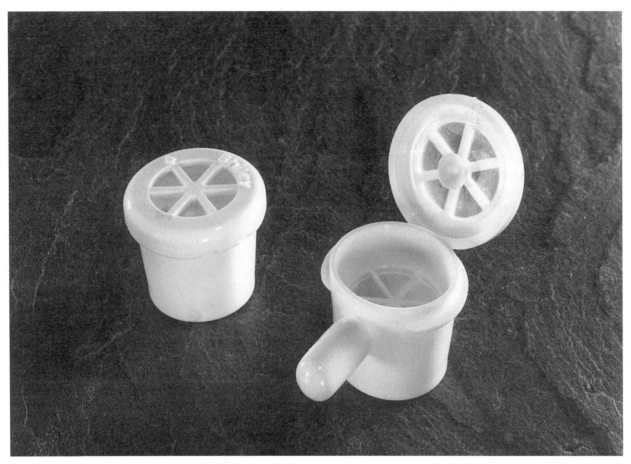

Figure 5–13. Shiley phonate speaking valve with (right) and without (left) oxygen port. Photo courtesy of Mallinckrodt Medical, Inc.

air in their lungs and may therefore have difficulty tolerating cuff deflation.

Voicing Options for Patients with a Tracheostomy and Ventilator Dependency

The decision to insert a tracheostomy tube in a ventilator dependent patient is usually made after some time when it has become clear that the patient will not be able to wean from mechanical ventilation in the foreseeable future. The introduction of a tracheostomy tube will improve a patient's communication options and possibly diminish anxious feelings. It has been reported that the inability to talk is the primary cause of feelings of fear and anxiety or panic in tracheostomized or ventilator dependent patients.[39] In addition, voicing while on mechanical ventilation may be a very important goal to achieve in terminally ill patients who wish to make their medical, financial, or personal needs and desires known to their caretakers, family, and friends. Three basic options are available for voicing in patients who have tracheostomy tubes and are ventilator dependent. These include voicing with a deflated cuff by timing phonation with the respiratory cycles of the ventilator, voicing with a speaking valve that fits in line with the ventilator tubing, such as the Passy-Muir speaking valve, and using a "talking" tracheostomy tube.

Speaking on the Inhalation Phase of the Ventilator Cycle

When a patient is on a ventilator and the cuff of the tracheostomy tube is deflated, the patient may be able to time voicing as the inspiratory cycle begins and a breath is given by the ventilator. During inhalation, air is forced into the lungs, but if a deflated cuff is in place, some of that air will escape around the cuff and travel up through the vocal folds, enabling the patient to phonate. During expiration, recoil of the respiratory system takes place and air is expelled through the ventilator tubing, thus preventing voicing from occurring on exhalation. Hoit et al. studied the timing of voicing of four men and three women who were mechanically ventilated for at least three years.[40] They reported that their subjects initiated speech approximately 0.3 to 0.7 seconds after the onset of inspiratory flow and terminated their utterances 0.7 to 1.1 seconds after the offset of inspiratory flow (or 0.1 to 0.5 seconds after the opening of the expiratory valve). Extemporaneous speaking and reading resulted in earlier speech initiation, later speech termination, and longer speech duration than repetition of sentences and sustained phonation of /a/. They also discovered that in conjunction with voicing during inspiratory flow, their subjects continued to speak during end-inspiratory pause and early expiration.

Since the process of initiating phonation on inhalation is completely contrary to voicing prior to mechanical ventilation, it may be difficult for a patient to adjust to this type of communication. However, most patients are glad to use their own voices for communication and are able to learn how to time speaking with the respiratory cycles provided by the ventilator. Hoit et al. suggest some minor ventilator adjustments and training strategies for optimizing speaking in this manner.[40] These include the following:

1. Lengthening the time of the end-inspiratory pause that patients appear to speak through.
2. Using PEEP to prolong inspiration.
3. Encouraging the patient to continue speaking as far into the expiratory portion of the cycle as possible until voicing fades. This will likely result in linguistically inappropriate silences within an utterance, but the pauses mid-utterance may also serve as a cue to the listener that the patient intends to continue talking.

The Passy-Muir Speaking Valve

As described previously, the Passy-Muir speaking valve is available in a model specifically designed to be used in line with a ventilator. Technically, a ventilator dependent patient may be able to speak on both inhalation and exhalation with the tracheostomy tube cuff deflated and a speaking valve in place. As air is forced into the airway during the inhalation phase of the ventilator, the air that passes around the cuff and through the vocal folds can be used for phonation. During inhalation the

valve opens, allowing air to reach the lungs. It returns to its normally closed position immediately afterward so that exhalation occurs through the mouth and nose. The patient then uses this expiratory air for voicing and speech. It is recommended that patients allow inhalation to occur without using that air to voice and begin voicing on the exhalation phase, as in spontaneous respiration/phonation. In addition, it is important to instruct the patient to completely exhale all the air that has been inspired. The patient should phonate or open his or her mouth during the entire exhalation cycle to ensure full emptying of the lungs before another cycle of inspired air is provided by the ventilator. By adhering to this technique, breath-stacking may be avoided. If the patient appears to be following this technique but reports a sensation of discomfort, fullness, or the inability to inhale, upper airway obstruction should be investigated.[37]

Talking Tracheostomy Tubes

A talking tracheostomy tube is specially designed for patients on mechanical ventilation who are unable to tolerate cuff deflation for voicing. A talking tracheostomy tube has exterior tubing that connects from an outside source of compressed air, such as a wall-mounted oxygen flow unit usually seen at a patient's bedside, to the outer cannula. There is an open port on the connector tube that, when occluded, directs air from the outside oxygen air source through a fenestration that sits above the cuff in the outer cannula of the tracheostomy tube, up through the vocal folds for phonation to take place. When a talking tracheostomy tube is in place, the patient is breathing and phonating from two separate channels. Ventilation takes place as usual but because the cuff is inflated, no connection exists between the lower and upper respiratory airways and phonation is not possible. The outside source of compressed air travels through the extended exterior tubing of the tracheostomy tube, through the fenestration(s) on the outer cannula of the tracheostomy tube, and then up through the vocal folds to enable phonation. Two popular types of talking tracheostomy tubes include the Communitrach I (Figure 5–14) and the Portex Talk Tube (Figure 5–15). The same criteria for candidacy for speaking valves apply to talking tracheostomy tubes except, of course, for the ability to tolerate cuff deflation.

Advantages: The advantage of talking tracheostomy tubes is that they provide voicing for patients who are unable to have the cuff of their tracheostomy

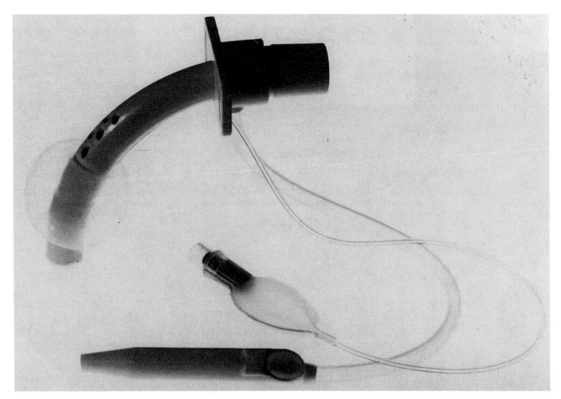

Figure 5–14. Communi-Trach I "Talking" Tracheostomy Tube. Photo courtesy of Spectrum of California.

tubes deflated. Ventilator cycles are not adjusted when talking tracheostomy tubes are in place because breathing and speaking occur from two separate mechanisms. Another advantage is that the patient is able to continually phonate without having to time speaking with the breathing cycle of the ventilator. However, this continuous flow of air leads to complaints of dryness by some patients. It can be alleviated by humidifying the air source, occluding the port on the extended tubing only when speaking occurs, physically turning the exterior air source on and off for speech, or using an environmental control unit (ECU) for patients who are unable to digitally occlude the port. An ECU will allow a patient with upper extremity weakness to activate the air source only during speaking times while the port is permanently occluded, such as when tape is wrapped around the port. The on–off switch to the compressed air source may be activated by, for example, a sip and puff or head activation switch; this is usually best determined by a rehabilitation engineer. Activating the compressed air only when speaking will eliminate the constant flow of air through the pharynx that causes dryness. Another strategy for reducing dryness is to reduce the amount of airflow per minute through the external airflow line. One method of determining op-

timal airflow is to ask the patient to phonate /a/ for an extended period of time while adjusting the airflow rate of the compressed air source until optimal comfort and speaking volume are obtained. It has been recommended by Leder and Traquina that 10 to 15 L/minute of airflow will produce optimum vocal intensity and speech intelligibility with the Communi-Trach I.[41] Kluin et al. reported that 5 L/minute will produce an audible whisper with the Portex "talking" tracheostomy tube while 8 to 10 L/minute will provide normal speaking intensity.[42]

As with any new device, training and counseling are necessary when introducing a talking tracheostomy tube to a patient. Leder and Traquina reported that after insertion of the Communi-Trach I, an average of 5.6 days elapsed before adequate voicing occurred.[41] They reported that this lapse in time was likely due to prolonged intubation leading to reduced vocal fold adduction.

Disadvantages: There are certain disadvantages to talking tracheostomy tubes that clinicians should be aware of when instructing patients and caregivers in their use.

1. The exterior speaking tube or the fenestrations may become occluded with secretions

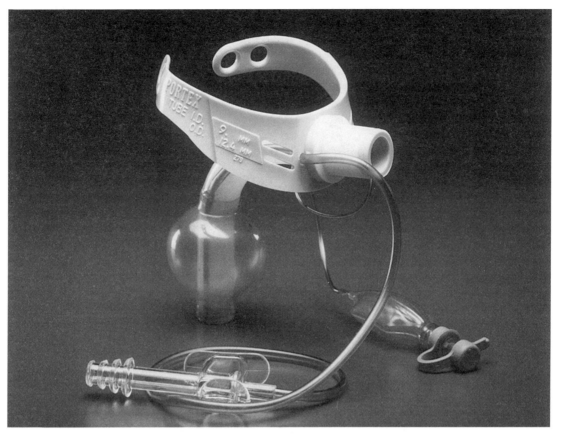

Figure 5–15. Portex "Trach-Talk" Tube. Photo courtesy of Sims Medical Systems.

and frequent suctioning of the speaking tube and oropharynx may be necessary. The Communi-Trach I has eight fenestrations on the superior surface of the outer cannula, which allows for continued airflow should some of the fenestrations become occluded with secretions.

2. The exterior air source must be turned off when the patient is eating. The constant rush of air up through the pharynx will compete with the oral and pharyngeal phases of swallowing as the patient is trying to propel food posteriorly through the oral cavity and inferiorly through the pharynx.

3. The exterior air source must be turned off when the patient is not involved in a conversation or when the patient is sleeping. If the patient's mouth is closed for an extended period of time, the potential exists for the patient to swallow air and subsequent abdominal distension and discomfort may occur.

Suctioning

The authors recommend suctioning a patient orally, pharyngeally, and transtracheally prior to deflating the cuff of a tracheostomy tube for voicing or swallowing purposes. In addition, resuctioning the trachea should take place after the cuff is deflated to remove any secretions that may have collected above the cuff while it was inflated. After secretions are suctioned, the voice is clearer, breathing is easier, and the risk of aspiration of secretions that have collected above the inflated cuff is reduced.

Suctioning should be performed only by a trained individual. This usually includes a respiratory therapist, nurse, or family member. In some cases the speech pathologist is also trained in suctioning technique.

Nonverbal Methods of Communication in an ICU Setting

Nonverbal methods of communication, in general, may range from a simple letter or picture board to a computerized communication system. An ICU patient's initial need for communication may be to request pain medication or suctioning or convey requests concerning medical decisions. For these reasons it is important that the speech–language pathologist establishes a reliable method of communication for the patient. This may include, for example, the use of eye blinks, foot movement, or any other consistently and accurately established muscle movement to indicate a yes/no response. A slightly more advanced method of communication via eye movements is the E-Tran board. This clear acrylic board has strategically placed clusters of letters on its four corners that the patient looks at while the communication partner decodes the message, seated across from the patient, asking for confirmation that he or she has identified the correct letter of the word the patient is spelling. The patient responds and the next letter is chosen.

In most cases, at least initially, nonverbal methods of communication for ICU patients will likely focus on quick and simple strategies that relate to getting basic needs met. The complexity of the system may, of course, increase as the patient's skills and medical status improve.

In summary, key ingredients to successful communication for an ICU patient include a thorough knowledge of the patient's condition, a strong background of voicing options with tracheostomy tubes and speaking valves, patience, counseling, and a team approach.

SWALLOWING ISSUES

Aspiration of oropharyngeal secretions is known to occur in healthy adults as well as critically ill patients. In a study by Huxley et al.,[50] 20 healthy adults and 10 individuals in a coma or stuporous state were studied for aspiration. The results revealed that 45% of the healthy adults aspirated during deep sleep and 70% of the adults with depressed consciousness aspirated. Aspiration was more extensive and occurred more frequently in the latter group. Healthy subjects who did not aspirate awakened frequently during the night or slept poorly, whereas the subjects who did aspirate slept soundly throughout the night. It is suspected that pulmonary infections due to oropharyngeal aspiration are likely related to the frequency, volume, and character of the aspirated material and usually are avoided in healthy individuals because of their ability to more efficiently clear bacteria by pulmonary defense mechanisms.[46,50] Healthy elderly patients may also be at an increased risk for aspiration that may be compounded by the introduction of an illness. Pontoppidan and Beecher[51] found that individuals in their seventies and eighties have reduced laryngeal sensitivity. This finding may contribute to silent aspiration and eventually lead to pneumonia in the elderly.

Aspiration Pneumonia

Treating patients with oropharyngeal aspiration is common practice for speech–language pathologists working in an ICU setting, particularly because most of the patients will likely have several of the risk factors for aspiration pneumonia. These risk factors include acute stroke,[43,44] seizure, alcoholism, tracheostomy tubes, older age, a reduction in mental status, a previous history of pneumonia,[45] and, in general, any state of depressed consciousness.[46] Russin and Adler[47] described three distinct syndromes of aspiration that can lead to pneumonia. These include aspiration of oropharyngeal secretions, inert fluids (i.e., saline or barium solutions), and aspiration of acidic gastric contents. The latter syndrome is considered the most severe because of its rapid progression, which causes irreversible lung damage, and its high mortality rate. Hypoxia is the most characteristic physiologic feature of aspiration of gastric contents[46] and may occur within two hours after aspiration.[47] Sitzmann[48] found that any form of upper enteric feeding such as nasogastric or gastrostomy tubes significantly increased a patient's risk of developing aspiration pneumonia due to a reduction in tone of the lower esophageal sphincter, which may lead to reflux of gastric contents.

Predicting Risk of Aspiration

Many patients in the ICU will be at high risk for aspiration. The ICU patient may be in a stuporous state, have a feeding tube, and be elderly with multiple medical problems. All these factors should be considered prior to initiating the evaluation and should play a role in the planning stages of swallowing treatment. Predicting a patient's likelihood of aspiration during oral feeding may be the first step to take in the intervention process. Several recent studies have attempted to predict aspiration based on clinical presentation.[44,52,53] Horner et al.[44] reported that aspiration occurred equally in left and right hemisphere stroke patients, but more frequently in patients with bilateral stroke. The incidence of aspiration in stroke was further broken down by location of the lesion as studied on computed tomography. The highest percentage of aspiration occurred in patients with combined bilateral cerebral and brainstem strokes (6 of 6, 100%), followed by unilateral cerebral and brainstem stroke (6 of 7, 85.7%), brainstem strokes alone (4 of 6, 66.7%), and cerebral strokes (14 of 33, 42.4%). The most prominent clinical feature of aspirating patients was dysphonia. This included a dry or wet sounding hoarse voice. A diminished or absent gag reflex was equally present in aspirating and nonaspirating patients and therefore was not a prognostically valuable sign for predicting aspiration. The most prominent videofluoroscopic feature of aspirating patients was a delayed swallow response in conjunction with reduced pharyngeal peristalsis. Poor oral motility did not correlate well with aspiration. Interestingly, a single chest X-ray was not predictive of aspirating versus nonaspirating patients. However, the authors concluded that this may have resulted from the NPO status of most of the patients, the degree of aspiration, the acute stage of the patients' illnesses, or the protective nature of the cough reflex.

Linden and Siebens[52] studied clinical signs in 15 patients with pharyngeal dysphagia in an attempt to predict laryngeal penetration on videofluorography. They reported a wet-hoarse voice and impaired pharyngeal gag among 11 patients with laryngeal penetration. Their findings also revealed that laryngeal penetration occurred more frequently with liquids as opposed to semisolids and that a cough was an unpredictable clinical indicator of laryngeal penetration.

Martin et al.[53] reported significantly slower oral transit time during videofluoroscopic swallowing studies in 9 patients with aspiration pneumonia compared to 7 patients with nonaspiration pneumonia. However, most of the patients in the aspiration pneumonia group were neurologically impaired and 1 had undergone head and neck surgery.

A retrospective review of post-stroke patients with and without aspiration during videofluorography was analyzed by Schmidt et al.[49] Their results revealed that the odds of a patient developing pneumonia were 7.6 times greater if he or she aspirated during the videofluoroscopic examination. In addition, patients who aspirated thick or solid consistencies were 5.6 times at greater risk of developing pneumonia than those who did not aspirate or aspirated thin liquids.

In summary, although predicting aspiration based on clinical findings depends on the nature of the illness and the mental and neurologic status of the patient, a voice evaluation should be standard practice and the presence of dysphonia should be an indication to the clinician that the patient is at risk to aspirate. In addition, it is important to remember that the presence of a gag reflex does not reliably indicate that the patient will not aspirate.[54] During videofluorographic examinations for swallowing, treatment strategies should be attempted whenever possible to assess the effectiveness of therapy or the patient's potential to learn a compensatory swallowing technique and avoid aspiration.

Tracheostomy Tubes in Patients with Swallowing Disorders

Adding to the complexities involved in treating an ICU patient for dysphagia is the presence of a tracheostomy tube. The introduction of a tracheostomy tube in any patient presents a series of unique swallowing problems. According to Logemann,[27] an inflated tracheostomy tube cuff creates the possibility of tracheal irritation and the restriction of laryngeal elevation during swallowing. Nash[23] further reports that pressure on the distal esophagus from an inflated cuff may occur when swallowing. Cameron et al.[55] reported an increased incidence of aspiration of oropharyngeal secretions in hospitalized patients with tracheostomy tubes versus orally intubated patients.

As in speech, a patient's swallowing skills are improved when cuff deflation is allowed. Cuff deflation will provide improved laryngeal excursion during the swallow[27] and release the pressure placed on the distal esophagus from a potentially overinflated cuff. In addition, placing a one-way valve, capping, or digitally occluding the outer opening of the tracheostomy tube will assist in creating subglottic pressure through laryngeal closure and the ability to cough and clear the airway should laryngeal penetration or aspiration occur.[56]

Assessing the ICU Patient with Dysphagia

As in all patients with dysphagia, a careful review of the ICU patient's medical condition is manadatory prior to evaluation and treatment. In this population, the speech–language pathologist must ascertain the patient's level of consciousness, length of time the patient was intubated, if and when he or she underwent a tracheotomy, type and size of the tracheostomy tube, presence of cuffed or cuffless tracheostomy tube, anticipated weaning schedule from the ventilator, and cranial nerve status. Because many ICU patients are not able to travel to a videofluorographic swallowing study because of positioning problems in the presence of multiple tubing and equipment, other forms of assessment may need to be initially explored. The following sections will review swallowing assessment techniques that may be performed in the ICU setting.

Blue Dye Testing

In 1973 Cameron et al.[55] described a method of testing for aspiration of oropharyngeal secretions in 61 patients with a tracheostomy tube and 25 patients with oral endotracheal tubes. A 1% solution of Evans blue dye was placed on the patients' tongues every 4 hours for up to 48 hours as routine suctioning took place. The results of the study revealed that 69% of the patients with tracheostomy tubes had evidence of the blue dye marker on suctioning and none of the patients with oral endotracheal tubes exhibited aspiration of oropharyngeal secretions. Since that time, blue dye testing has become a common method of assessing dysphagia in the ICU setting. This method usually takes place when a patient is unable to travel for a videofluorographic swallowing study and the physician is interested in upgrading the patient's nutritional status to oral intake after prolonged tube feeding. Typically this method involves the insertion of blue food dye into a small amount of barium, food, or liquid (usually beginning with 1 cc) and having the patient swallow. In our practice liquid barium is usually used as the initial test medium because aspiration of a small amount of barium places the patient at less risk.[46] Blue is used to differentiate the swallowed material from secretions or gastric contents that may be aspirated. This method is advised for patients with tracheostomy tubes who are either on or off of a ventilator, because suctioning the trachea takes place following the swallow. The patient is usually suctioned immediately after a swallow and periodically during the hour after swallowing. Dikeman and Kazandjian[57] advise suctioning every 15 minutes for one hour after swallowing. Blue dye testing may also be inserted through a feeding tube by a physician or nurse to assess the presence of aspiration of gastric contents.

The obvious limitation to blue dye testing is that if a patient aspirates during swallowing it is impossible to know where along the oropharyngeal tract the difficulty occurred to cause the aspiration. In addition, the absence of blue dye in tracheal secretions during suctioning does not indicate without a doubt that the patient did not aspirate. It is possible that aspiration prior to or between suctioning occurred and the secretions may have traveled too low in the bronchial tree to be completely suctioned. In addition, residual material in the pharynx may remain for an extended period of time, placing the patient at risk to aspirate from pharyngeal residue entering the airway after suctioning has ceased. Although these limitations exist, if a patient's blue dye test is positive, it does provide the clinician with the knowledge that the patient is aspirating and likely is not ready to eat until further testing can be performed such as videoendoscopic or videofluoroscopic evaluations of dysphagia.

If a patient appears to tolerate a small amount of blue dyed liquid, careful monitoring of pulmonary status is strongly suggested as bolus size and texture of consistencies are upgraded. Any signs of difficulty breathing, fever, increase in tracheal secretions, or change in mental status may indicate aspiration and feeding trials should be terminated until further investigation takes place.

Fiberoptic Endoscopic Evaluation of Swallowing (FEES)

As previously mentioned, many ICU patients are unable to undergo a videofluoroscopic swallowing evaluation because of positioning difficulties or the presence of multiple tubes and equipment. In such cases, evaluating a patient's potential to swallow may be assisted by the use of a nasopharyngeal endoscope as discussed by Langmore et al.[58] This technique requires the insertion of a flexible fiberoptic endoscope into the patient's nasopharynx. Viewing the anatomy and physiology while the patient swallows may lead to information regarding aspiration and the patient's ability to clear his or her pharynx. Unfortunately, this type of assessment does not allow full analysis of the oral phase of swallowing and the view of the larynx is obliterated as the patient swallows, precluding analysis of timing of the swallow response and the ability to assess whether aspiration occurred during or after the swallow response. Both factors provide necessary information for planning the appropriate treatment strategies. However, despite these limitations, this technique offers information regarding premature spillage of material, the occurrence of aspiration before a swallow response and insight into the status of pharyngeal peristalsis as noted by any residual material unilaterally or bilaterally in the pharynx after the swallow. These findings, coupled with clinical signs, may be useful in recommending the initiation of swallowing trials with careful clinical monitoring or may provide enough information to recommend withholding swallowing until the patient's medical status improves and a videofluorographic swallowing study can be performed. As with all swallowing evaluation and treatment techniques, formal training is necessary prior to performing FEES. For more complete information regarding endoscopy in the use of swallowing, the reader is referred to Chapter 22.

Auscultation

Cervical auscultation may be useful to determine if a patient is aspirating during swallowing by detecting bubbling sounds during or immediately after swallowing.[59] Typically a stethoscope is placed along various areas of the neck while the patient swallows. The subjective nature of this technique has been made more objective via acoustic analysis of the swallow sounds as reported by Takahashi et al.[59] However, it may be an impractical assessment technique because many facilities may not have the equipment necessary to objectify the data collected. The study may provide general information but should not be a substitute for other methods of swallowing assessment such as videofluorography.

The Use of Videofluorography to Assess Swallowing in Mechanically Ventilated Patients with Tracheostomy Tubes

If a ventilator dependent patient meets the same criteria for candidacy for a videofluorographic swallowing study as would be expected in any patient, that patient should be able to travel to the radiology suite and undergo the examination. These criteria include medical stability, secretion control, adequate oral motor and laryngeal status, and intact cognition so that the patient may follow the instructions provided during the examination and later during swallowing therapy. Ideally, cuff deflation is recommended, coupled with the placement of a one-way speaking valve to facilitate an efficient swallow.[56]

Recently, Siebens et al.[56] described a technique of using the inspiratory phase of the ventilator to clear the larynx and pharynx from aspirated or residual pharyngeal material in mechanically ventilated patients with cuffless or cuff deflated tracheostomy tubes. During videofluoroscopy, aspiration and pharyngeal residue were noted after the patient swallowed. The force of air that was introduced during the inspiratory phase of the ventilator essentially pushed the food up from the trachea and pharynx to then be swallowed by the patient. In their study, this method proved the only way for one of the patients to safely swallow until her respiratory illness improved.

Ethical Issues

Besides the physical aspect of tolerating oral feedings there is usually a complex, psychological advantage given to patients and their families when a patient is able to obtain nutrition orally after prolonged tube feeding. It should be noted that tube feeding does not necessarily preclude a patient's ability to orally eat. In many cases, eating for pleasure occurs in combination with tube feeding for nutritional maintenance. One of the more difficult situations that may arise when treating a patient in an ICU setting is the decision to allow a patient to eat even when obvious signs of aspiration are present. These decisions are not easy to make and, of course, depend on the individual case. For example, a patient with a terminal illness and documented tracheal aspiration may decide to ignore a speech pathologist's recommendation of an NPO status and continue to eat by mouth. In such instances the speech pathologist must consider the quality of life issues involved in the patient's case. Teaching the patient compensatory swallowing strategies to minimize his or her risk of aspiration while eating may be the best route of treatment in some cases. Of course, these decisions are complex and will vary depending on the background training of the speech pathologist, his or her personal philosophical beliefs regarding quality of life issues, the policy of the health care facility, and the decisions expressed by the patient and agreed to by the medical staff. According to Groher,[60] the final decision to feed a patient with known tracheal aspiration ultimately may be more anecdotal than empirical.

SUMMARY

The need for speech–language pathology services is great in the ICU. This chapter has described many voicing, communication, and swallowing options for the tracheostomized and/or ventilator-dependent patient. The ICU setting is a challenging, ever-changing environment. Like most patients in a medical setting, the ICU patient's condition may change on a daily basis and speech–language pathologists must be flexible and ready to alter assessment or treatment strategies on a moment's notice.

Key ingredients to successful management of communication and swallowing include a thorough knowledge of the patient's condition, a strong background in voicing options with tracheostomy tubes and speaking valves, ability to provide appropriate counseling and support, and good team skills. Frequently, speech–langugage pathologists will find themselves working with physicians, nurses, respiratory therapists, psychiatrists or psychologists, and the patient's family, as well as the patient. When possible, we recommend that speech–language pathologists accompany the medical staff on rounds. This opens doors to improved understanding of the patient's medical condition and allows speech–language pathologists to address communication and swallowing needs and to answer questions from other team members in an efficient manner. Clinical experience has shown that this approach allows the speech–language pathologist to intervene, consult, and educate in an effective and efficient manner.

CASE ONE

M. H. is a 29-year-old female who was involved in an auto accident and has been in the ICU for 3 weeks. Her course of recovery was complicated by pneumonia, cardiac arrest, and coma for 10 days. She has now been awake and alert for short periods of time several times throughout the day. She underwent emergent oral endotracheal intubation at the time of hospital admission and a tracheotomy 10 days later. She is on a ventilator. The patient's family is interested in giving the patient ice chips and fluids as she complains of a dry mouth. The medical and nursing staff is hesitant to allow the family to give anything by mouth to the patient as their attempts to do so resulted in immediate coughing by the patient and they are concerned that she is aspirating. The speech pathology service was consulted for cognitive/communicative and swallowing assessment and treatment.

Initial language and cognitive testing with written responses and mouthing words by the patient revealed intact orientation, intact auditory comprehension for simple commands and questions, mild semantic paraphasia in her writing samples, and mild-moderate short-term memory impairment. A right facial droop and mild right lingual weakness were also noted. Prior to evaluating the patient's swallowing skills, the speech pathologist requested an otolaryngologic evaluation to obtain information regarding her vocal fold status. The patient was found to have small bilateral granulomatous tissue formation on the vocal processes and a mild right vocal fold paresis resulting in a mild glottal chink. Her pulmonologist approved cuff deflation trials with a speaking valve to further assess speech, voice, communication/cognition, and swallowing.

The patient's overall medical status improved daily and she tolerated cuff deflation trials well for voicing with a speaking valve in line with the ventilator. During this trial period of voicing and adjusting to the speaking valve, the patient was instructed to practice dry swallows using a modified supraglottic swallow strategy, with the focus on voluntary breath-holding during the swallow. The goal was to begin preparing the patient for swallowing in a modified manner given the knowledge of her vocal fold paresis and incomplete glottal closure. Anticipation for a swallowing evaluation via bedside assessment of blue-dye testing or endoscopic assessment prior to the patient's ability to travel to radiology for a videofluorographic swallowing study was initially planned. However, M. H. was rapidly improving from a medical standpoint and was fully weaned from the ventilator 5 days after speech pathology's initial consultation. She remained tracheostomized with a no. 6 cuffed tracheostomy tube. She was able to travel to the radiology suites for a videofluorographic swallow study with her tracheostomy tube cuff deflated and a Passy-Muir speaking valve in place. Initial liquid trials resulted in penetration of barium into the laryngeal vestibule as a result of impaired timing and coordination of the oropharyngeal swallow. However, with the speaking valve in place, the patient was able to effectively cough and clear the supraglottic area and thus, prevent tracheal aspiration. When M. H. consistently used the modified supraglottic swallow strategy, laryngeal vestibule penetration was avoided on all liquid and solid consistencies. It was recommended that M. H. swallow all consistencies using the modified supraglottic swallow strategy and that she keep the speaking valve on during all eating times to assist subglottic pressure during swallowing and promote an effective cough should tracheal aspiration occur.

CASE TWO

J. M. is a 33-year-old male hospitalized in the ICU for the past 2 weeks with a medical diagnosis of Guillain-Barré syndrome. The speech pathology services were consulted at day 7 of his hospitalization. At that time he was orally intubated and mechanically ventilated. He was almost completely paretic; however, he was observed to have ocular movements. After a short training period of 2 days he was able to consistently move his eyes up and down for a yes and no response. Since J. M. appeared accurate in his yes/no responses, communication via an E-Tran board was attempted. This method of communication was successful, but slow and the patient's family was frustrated by their inability to quickly and accurately understand his needs and thoughts. The patient underwent a tracheotomy after 2 weeks of oral endotracheal intubation. Assessment of the patient's oral-motor movements revealed slow and imprecise lip and tongue motion during isolated tasks; however, J. M. continually tried to communicate by mouthing words. Therefore, a cervical electrolarynx was attempted as a mode of communication and although severely dysarthric, the patient was able to approximate simple single words with enough accuracy and guess work on the part of the listener to make simple needs known. As the patient's medical status improved over the next 2 weeks, cuff deflation and speaking valve trials were approved by the patient's physician. Although J. M. had a weak, breathy voice with an overall moderate-severe flaccid dysarthria, the patient and his family preferred verbal communication over nonverbal methods. Cuff deflation and speaking valve trials occurred twice a day for only 10 minutes at a time because of fatigue by the patient. Gradually the patient's medical condition improved as did his dysarthria. He was able to tolerate longer periods of cuff deflation and voicing with or without a speaking valve. When his cuff was inflated the electrolarynx was used for quick verbal communication needs. J. M. continued to use a speaking valve after he was weaned from the ventilator. He was discharged from the hospital using the speaking valve with a cuffless tracheostomy tube with the goal of decannulation in the near future.

STUDY QUESTIONS

1. You have a 25-year-old TBI patient on your caseload who recently underwent a tracheotomy after 2 weeks of oral endotracheal intubation. He is still on a ventilator, but is expected to be fully weaned from mechanical ventilation within the next 2 to 3 weeks. He has been attempting communication on a regular basis via eye and head movements and facial expressions. His physician has approved cuff deflation trials. Which modes of verbal communication will you attempt with this patient?

2. There is a patient in the ICU who has a tracheostomy tube and is mechanically ventilated. She is intermittently awake for short periods each day. The medical and nursing staff would like you to provide her with a verbal means of communication as soon as possible since it is difficult for them to know what the patient's needs are. Would this patient be a candidate for a speaking valve? Why or why not? If a speaking valve is not an appropriate method of communication at this time, what other types of communication would you currently recommend?

3. One of your patients is very anxious when his speaking valve is in place and reports difficulty breathing while using the valve. Pre and postplacement assessment of vital signs and airway clearance have all turned out to be normal. What are some strategies of improving acceptance of the valve that you could apply with this patient?

4. Your 32-year-old alert, tracheostomized and ventilator dependent patient appears to be aspirating during the initial clinical trials of fluid intake by mouth. What assessment techniques would you pursue? You may assume that cuff deflation during eating has been medically approved.

5. You have a new patient on your caseload who recently had a stroke. He is 89 years old and was orally intubated for 10 days while in a semiconscious state. Following extubation the nursing staff began giving the patient sips of water and noted that he coughs and chokes every time he drinks. What are some of this patient's risk factors for aspiration? What specific clinical signs will you look for that may predict the patient's likelihood of aspiration prior to assessing his swallowing abilities with videofluorography?

REFERENCES

1. Weinberger SE, Schwartzstein RM, Weiss JW: Hypercapnia. N Engl J Med 1989; 321:1223–1231.
2. West JB: Causes of carbon dioxide retention in lung disease. N Engl J Med 1971; 284:1232–1236.
3. Murray JF: The normal lung, 2nd ed. W.B. Sanders, Philadelphia, 1986.
4. Roussos C, Macklem PT: The respiratory muscles. N Engl J Med 1982; 307:786–797.
5. Pingleton SK: Complications of acute respiratory failure. Am Rev Respir Dis 1988; 137:1463–1493.
6. Tobin MJ: Mechanical ventilation. N Engl J Med 1994; 330:1056–1061.
7. Meduri GU, Cook TR, Turner RE et al.: Noninvasive positive pressure ventilation in status asthmaticus. Chest 1996; 110:767–774.
8. Katz JA, Marks JD: Inspiratory work with and without continuous positive airway pressure in patients with acute respiratory failure. Anesthesiology 1985; 63: 598–607.
9. MacIntyre NR: Respiratory function during pressure support ventilation. Chest 1986; 89:677–683.
10. Brochard L, Isabey D, Piquet J et al.: Reversal of acute exacerbations of chronic obstructive lung disease by inspiratory assistance with a face mask. N Engl J Med 1990; 323:1523–1530.
11. Tobin MJ, Yank K: Weaning from mechanical ventilation. Crit Care Clinics 1990; 6:725–747.
12. Sahn SA, Lakshminarayan S: Bedside criteria for discontinuation of mechanical ventilation. Chest 1973; 63:1002–1005.

13. Yang KL, Tobin MJ: A prospective study of indexes predicting the outcome of trials of weaning from mechanical ventilation. *N Engl J Med* 1991; 324: 1445–1450.

14. Feinleb M, Rosenberg HM, Collins JG et al.: Trends in COPD morbidity and mortality in the United States. *Am Rev Respir Dis* 1989; 140:S9–S18.

15. Snider GL, Kleinerman J, Thurlbeck WM et al.: The definition of emphysema: Report of a National Heart, Lung and Blood Institute, Division of Lung Diseases workshop. *Am Rev Respir Dis* 1985; 132:182–185.

16. Ashbaugh DG, Bigelow DB, Petty TL et al.: Acute respiratory distress in adults. *Lancet* 1967; 1:319–323.

17. Mulder DW: The clinical syndrome of amyotrophic lateral sclerosis. *Mayo Clinic Proceedings* 1957; 32:427–436.

18. Mulder DW: Motor neuron disease. In Dyck PJ, Thomas PK, Lambert EH and Bunge R (eds): *Peripheral neuropathy:* Vol. II, p. 1526. W. B. Sanders, Philadelphia, 1984.

19. Rosen AD: Amyotrophic lateral sclerosis. *Arch Neurol* 1978; 35:638–642.

20. Adams RD, Victor M: Diseases of peripheral nerve and muscle. In Adams RD, Victor M: *Principles of neurology,* 3rd ed., p 968. McGraw-Hill, New York, 1985.

21. Rowland LP: Clinical syndromes of the spinal cord. In Kandel ER, Schwartz JH (eds.): *Principles of neural science,* 2nd ed., pp 469–477. Elsevier, New York, 1985.

22. Tucker HM: Laryngeal trauma. In Tucker HM (ed.): *The larynx,* 2nd ed., pp. 199–215. Thieme, New York, 1993.

23. Nash M: Swallowing problems in the tracheostomized patient. *Otolaryngologic Clinics of North America* 1988; 21:701–709.

24. Dikeman KJ, Kazandjian MS: Endotracheal tubes and tracheostomy tubes. In Dikeman KJ, Kazandjian MS: *Communication and swallowing management of tracheostomized and ventilator-dependent adults,* pp 61–96. Singular Publishing Group, San Diego, 1995.

25. Dikeman KJ, Kazandjian MS: Airway management techniques. In Dikeman KJ, Kazandjian MS: *Communication and swallowing management of tracheostomized and ventilator-dependent adults,* pp 35–60. Singular Publishing Group, San Diego, 1995.

26. Heffner JE, Miller KS, Sahn SA: Tracheostomy in the intensive care unit, part 2: Complications. *Chest* 1986; 90(3):430–436.

27. Logemann J: Evaluation of swallowing disorders. In Logemann J: *Evaluation and treatment of swallowing disorders,* pp 87–125. Little-Brown, Boston, 1983.

28. Mason MF: Airway issues. In Mason MF: *Speech pathology for tracheostomized and ventilator dependent patients,* pp 106–125. Voicing, Newport Beach, 1993.

29. Frey JA, Wood S: Weaning from mechanical ventilation augmented by the Passy-Muir speaking valve. Presented at the International Conference of the American Lung Association and the American Thoracic Society, Anaheim, 1991.

30. Fornataro-Clerici L, Zajac DJ: Aerodynamic characteristics of tracheostomy speaking valves. *J Speech and Hearing Res* 1993; 36:529–532.

31. Mason M, Watkins C: Protocol for use of the Passy-Muir tracheostomy speaking valves. *Euro Resp J* 1992; 5, suppl. 15:148s–153s.

32. Hood Speaking Valve Product Information: Hood Laboratories, Pembroke, MA.

33. The Montgomery Speaking Valve: In the Boston Medical Products 1996 Product Catalog, p 18.

34. Olympic Trach-Talk Product Information: Olympic Medical, Seattle.

35. Shiley Phonate Speaking Valve: Product Information Pamphlet, Mallinckrodt Medical, Inc. Irvine, 1994.

36. Eibling DE, Gross RD: Subglottic air pressure: A key component of swallowing efficiency. *Ann Otol Rhinol Laryngol* 1996; 105:253–258.

37. Mason MF: Vocal treatment strategies. In Mason MF: *Speech pathology for tracheostomized and ventilator dependent patients,* pp 336–381. Voicing, Newport Beach, 1993.

38. Dikeman KJ, Kazandjian MS: Oral communication options. In Dikeman KJ, Kazandjian MS: *Communication and swallowing management of tracheostomized and ventilator-dependent adults,* pp 141–195. Singular Publishing Group, San Diego, 1995.

39. Bergbom-Engberg I, Haljamae H: Assessment of patient's experience of discomforts during respiratory therapy. *Crit Care Med* 1989; 17:1068–1072.

40. Hoit JD, Shea SA, Banzett RB: Speech production during mechanical ventilation in tracheostomized individuals. *J Speech and Hearing Res* 1994; 37: 53–63.

41. Leder SB, Traquina DN: Voice intensity of patients using a Communi-Trach I cuffed speaking tracheostomy tube. *Laryngoscope* 1989; 99:744–747.

42. Kluin KJ, Maynard F, Bogdasarian RS: The patient requiring mechanical ventilatory support: Use of the cuffed tracheostomy "talk" tube to establish phonation. *Otol-Head and Neck Surg* 1984; 92: 625–627.

43. Gordon C, Hewer RL, Wade D: Dysphagia in acute stroke. *Br Med J* 1987; 295:411–414.

44. Horner J, Massey EW, Riski JE et al: Aspiration following stroke: Clinical correlates and outcome. *Neurology* 1988; 38:1359–1362.

45. Cogen R, Weinryb J: Aspiration pneumonia in nursing home patients fed via gastrostomy tubes. *Am J Gerentol* 1989; 84:1509–1512.

46. Bartlett JG, Gorbach S: The triple threat of aspiration pneumonia. *Chest* 1975; 68:560–565.

47. Russin SJ, Adler AG: Pulmonary aspiration—The three syndromes. *Postgrad Med* 1989; 85:155–161.

48. Sitzmann JV: Nutritional support of the dysphagic patient: Methods, risks, and complications of therapy. *J Enter Paren Nutr* 1990; 14:60–64.

49. Schmidt J Holas M, Halvorson K et al.: Videofluoroscopic evidence of aspiration predicts pneumonia and death but not dehydration following stroke. *Dysphagia* 1994; 9:7–11.

50. Huxley EJ, Viroslav J, Gray WR, et al: Pharyngeal aspiration in normal adults and patients with depressed consciousness. *Am J Med* 1978; 64:564–568.

51. Pontoppidan H, Beecher HK: Progressive loss of protective reflexes in the airway with the advancement of age. *JAMA* 1960; 174:2209–2213.

52. Linden P, Siebens AA: Dysphagia: Predicting laryngeal penetration. *Arch Phys Med Rehabil* 1983; 64: 281–284.

53. Martin BJ, Corlew MM, Wood H et al: The association of swallowing dysfunction and aspiration pneumonia. *Dysphagia* 1994; 9:1–6.

54. Bleach NR: The gag reflex and aspiration: A retrospective analysis of 120 patients assessed by videofluoroscopy. *Clin Otolaryngol* 1993; 18:303–307.

55. Cameron JL, Reynolds J., Zuidema GD: Aspiration of patients with tracheostomies. *Surg, Gynecol* and *Obst* 1973; 130:68–70.

56. Siebens AA, Tippett DC, Kirby N, et al.: Dysphagic and expiratory air flow. *Dysphagia* 1993; 8:266–269.

57. Dikeman KJ, Kazandjian MS: Program development. In Dikeman KJ, Kazandjian MS: *Communication and swallowing management of tracheostomized and ventilator-dependent adults,* pp 311–334. Singular Publishing Group, San Diego, 1995.

58. Langmore SE, Schatz K, Olson N: Fiberoptic endoscopic evaluation of swallowing safety: A new procedure. *Dysphagia* 1988; 2:216–219.

59. Takahashi K, Groher ME, Michi K: Methodology for detecting swallowing sounds. *Dysphagia* 1994; 9: 54–62.

60. Groher ME: Determination of the risks and benefits of oral feeding. *Dysphagia* 1994; 9:233–235.

Appendix A
Competencies

TRACHEOSTOMY AND MECHANICAL VENTILATION

The reader should be able to perform the following tasks:

1. Discuss a patient's respiratory status with team members and subsequently plan appropriate methods of communication for the patient.
2. Anticipate short and long-term communication needs for an ICU patient, particularly if progression from oral intubation to tracheostomy is expected.
3. Identify situations which preclude the use of a speaking valve.
4. Recommend the appropriate type of speaking valve.
5. Explain to a patient, his or her family and medical staff why a speaking valve must be used with a fully deflated or cuffless tracheostomy tube.
6. Educate a patient regarding the use of a speaking valve and identify signs of patient anxiety related to initial use of a speaking valve.
7. Perform cursory tests of upper airway patency when a speaking valve is in place.
8. Identify signs of breath stacking in a patient using a speaking valve.
9. Identify signs of patient intolerance to a speaking valve.
10. Suggest methods to improve timing of speaking patterns for patients with tracheostomy tubes and cuff deflation who are phonating on the inhalation phase of the ventilatory cycle.
11. Troubleshoot when a patient is unable to voice with a "talking" tracheostomy tube in place.

SWALLOWING

The reader should be able to perform the following tasks:

1. Identify clinical features of a speech and voice assessment which may predict aspiration during a videofluorographic swallowing study.
2. Present the rationale for recommending cuff deflation for swallowing purposes to a patient's physician.
3. Present the rationale for recommending use of a speaking valve, digital occlusion or capping of a deflated tracheostomy tube during swallowing.
4. Discuss the advantages and limitations to alternate methods of assessing dysphagia in an ICU patient who is unable to undergo a videofluorographic swallowing study.
5. Discuss common swallowing problems associated with the presence of a tracheostomy tube.

6. Discuss the importance of suctioning a patient who is undergoing blue-dye testing for dysphagia.
7. Discuss ethical issues regarding swallowing treatment in a patient with known tracheal aspiration with the patient and team members.
8. Plan in-service meetings on communication and swallowing issues for members of the ICU team.

6

Speech–Language Pathology Practice in the Acute Care Setting: A Consultative Approach

ALEX F. JOHNSON, ANNE MARIE VALACHOVIC, AND K. PAIGE GEORGE

CHAPTER OUTLINE

Consultative Approach to Service Delivery in Acute Care

Description of Acute Care Setting

Key Issues in Acute Care Practice

The Process of Consultation

Communicative and Swallowing Monitoring and Intervention

Education in the Acute Care Setting

The acute care environment represents a part of the health care "culture" that provides an exciting and creative opportunity for the speech–language pathologist. Most speech–language pathologists have been prepared extensively for work in various rehabilitation settings while few speech–language pathologists have been specifically educated for practice in the acute care environment. Miller and Groher[1] describe acute care as "a stage in an individual's medical care where symptoms are severe and the duration of the immediate illness is short." It is important for the practicing clinician to appreciate the important differences between this point in the health care continuum and other points of care. In addition, we believe that the role of the speech–language pathologist in acute care is distinguishable from other roles that clinicians may play.

CONSULTATIVE APPROACH TO SERVICE DELIVERY IN ACUTE CARE

A general framework for consideration of key issues in acute care practice is presented in this chapter. Consultation in acute care involves three key professional activities: *evaluation/diagnosis of the communication/swallowing disorder; intensive monitoring of clinical symptoms and intervention; and education/counseling.* These services are referred to as consultative because ideally they are delivered to the patient with consideration of the information needs of the patient, family, and referral source. This emphasis on consultative practice (as opposed to a traditional rehabilitative approach) is called for because of the short length of stay in acute care, the period of rapid change exhibited by most acute patients, and, most important, the need to produce the best outcome in a short time frame. During the acute hospital stay the patient is rarely able to tolerate long periods of treatment that are more typical of rehabilitative care.

In the consultative approach the three aspects of care (diagnosis, monitoring, and education) are delivered in an integrated manner over the patient's stay in the hospital. The consultative model for acute care is presented in Figure 6–1. This simple graphic demonstrates the relatively discrete activities of diagnosis and education, both supported by the careful monitoring of patient change over time.

Implementation of the consultative model for acute care requires a rethinking of the traditional speech–language pathology service delivery system that is currently taught in most graduate programs. Key elements of current training—differential diagnosis, report writing, patient education, clinical supervision, treatment planning, and follow-up—are components of service delivery in acute care. However, the unique arrangement of this environment demands a slightly different emphasis and packaging of patient care. The short-term nature of the patient contact, the demands for quick, accurate, and advanced levels of information and communica-

tion, the day-to-day interaction with many different types of professionals, and the observation and treatment of patients during critical points in illness and recovery dictate adjustments in the standard practice of our discipline.

The role of the acute care speech–language pathologist is to assist the patient and his or her health providers and caregivers to *prepare* for the rehabilitation activities that will follow discharge. This preparation begins with the initial contact with the patient and extends through the acute stay. The activities of preparation for long-term rehabilitation or recovery include:

- Differential diagnosis of the communication and swallowing disturbance
- Assessment of the severity of the problem as the patient progresses (or worsens)
- Aggressive communication with the referring physician, primary care doctor, and other specialists
- Manipulation of the environment to facilitate immediate communication, swallowing, and health needs of the patient
- Education of the family and the patient about the communication disorder including the prognosis and expected follow-up needed
- Intensive monitoring of changes in communication and swallowing function
- Development of a discharge plan and plan for follow-up

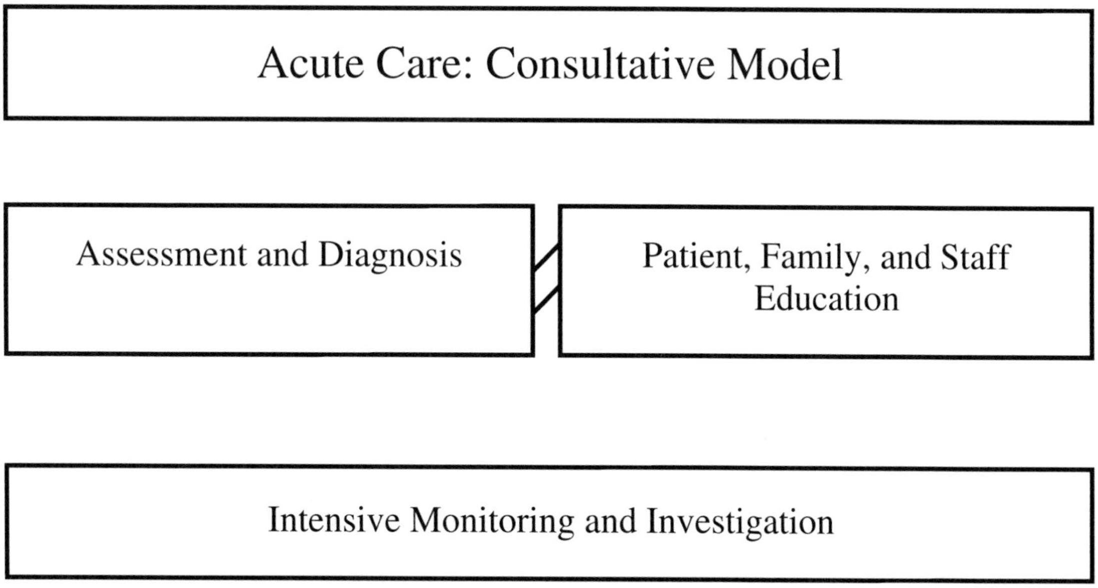

Figure 6–1. The acute care consultative model.

- Provision of short-term treatment to facilitate communication or swallowing in the immediate environment
- Participation in the overall care of the patient

DESCRIPTION OF THE ACUTE CARE SETTING

The modern acute care hospital can be organized in a variety of ways. Acute care services are provided in small community hospitals, large medical centers, or university hospitals. Most acute care facilities include an emergency department through which many patients are admitted, a variety of surgical and medical departments by which physician services are organized, operating rooms, intensive care units, and a range of other services designed to support the primary medical and surgical functions. Some institutions are designed to function in managing the most acutely ill patients. These hospitals tend to be large, technologically advanced, and specialized in the way in which services are delivered. Table 6–1 presents a listing of the major medical departments that could be found in a tertiary care center (one designed for advanced care of acutely ill patients). For a basic review of the major

Table 6–1. Major Medical-Surgical Departments in a Medical Center

Medical departments
  General Internal Medicine
  Cardiology
  Dermatology
  Endocrinology
  Gastroenterology
  Geriatric Medicine
  Pediatric Medicine
  Hematology Oncology
  Infectious Disease
  Nephrology/Urology
  Pulmonary
  Neurology
Surgical departments
  Otolaryngology/Head and Neck Surgery
  Neurosurgery
  Plastic Surgery
  Vascular Surgery
  Trauma Surgery
  Cardiac Surgery
  Thoracic Surgery
  General Surgery

functions of the full range of various medical and surgical specialities, see the texts prepared by Miller and Groher[1] or to Golper.[2]

Common Referral Sources

Speech–language pathologists may interact with any or all of the specialists listed in Table 6–1. However, a few specialties tend to be major referral sources and the speech–language pathologist in the hospital setting should have a keen appreciation for the scope of interest of each of these key specialists as well as an understanding of typical referral concerns and questions. Examples of particular professionals that may provide a high volume of referrals to the speech–language pathologist include neurologists, neurosurgeons, otolaryngologists, pediatricians, internists, geriatricians, psychiatrists, and pulmonary physicians. Because of the rapidly expanding scope of practice of speech–language pathologists, new referral and collaboration relationships are constantly being formed, and so in some institutions the "high volume" list may include many other specialties. Because those specialties mentioned above represent a consistent list of referral sources for acute care speech–language pathology services, it is important for the speech–language pathologist to know their function.

Neurologists

These physicians provide medical diagnosis and care for patients with diseases of the nervous system. In larger centers, neurological services tend to be subspecialized, with providers concentrating in one area of practice. Major subspecialties of neurology that interact frequently with speech–language pathology include: cerebrovascular disease (stroke), epileptology, neuromuscular disease, movement disorders, behavioral neurology, neurooncology, and pediatric neurology. In the acute care practice of speech–language pathology, referrals from any of these subspecialties may be seen. Major diseases and conditions associated with some of these referring subspecialties are listed in Table 6–2.

The neurologist has much to offer the speech–language pathologist in the acute care setting. The detailed neurologic examination, when observed by the astute speech–language pathologist, can reveal important information that may serve to complement the working diagnosis and the ongoing treatment of the communication disorder. Specific types of information that may be obtained in such observation include (1) an understanding of the nonlinguistic aspects of patient's behavior and their effect on communication; (2) appreciation of the role

Table 6–2. Examples of Diseases/Conditions Associated with Some Neurological Subspecialties

Cerebrovascular disease

  Stroke

  Transient ischemic attacks (TIAs)

  Arteriovenous malformation

  Hemorrhage

Epileptology

  Epilepsy

  Pseudoepilepsy

  Ictal/interictal aphasia

Neuromuscular disease

  Amyotrophic lateral sclerosis

  Muscular dystrophy

Movement disorders

  Parkinson's disease

  Progressive supranuclear palsy

Behavioral neurology

  Dementia

  Progressive aphasia

  Nondominant hemisphere involvement

of various neuropharmocologic agents on speech, language, or swallowing; (3) differential diagnosis and localization by the neurologist; and (4) interpretation of various neurological and neurophysiological tests.

The acute care speech–language pathologist has an important role in the care of the patient with neurologic disease and is therefore an important ally to the neurologist. Specific functions provided by the speech–language pathologist include: (1) early assessment of neurogenic speech, language, and swallowing disorders; (2) differential diagnosis of neurogenic communication disorders and determination of their consistency or inconsistency with the presenting neurologic symptoms; (3) objective and sensitive monitoring of patient change in function over the acute care stay; (4) assessment and consultation regarding swallowing function; and (5) prediction and planning for post-acute neurorehabilitation.

Neurosurgeons

Neurosurgeons provide surgical and postoperative care to patients with various neurologic diseases, tumors, malformations, or neurotrauma. Again, in major centers neurosurgeons tend to subspecialize and provide care that is comprehensive and effi-

cient. More common diagnoses referred to speech–language pathologists by neurosurgeons include patients with traumatic brain injury, spinal cord injuries, those who have undergone surgical resection for tumor or intractable epilepsy, and patients with cranial nerve tumors.

In many centers, speech–language pathologists are involved in presurgical evaluations for patients considered at risk for postsurgical development of neurocommunicative or swallowing deficits. In such cases it is essential that sensitive and standardized assessment protocols be used so as to detect the presence of subtle presurgical deficits, as well as document postsurgical effects, recovery, or identify complications that may occur. Postsurgical lack of progress in speech or language, and certainly rapid deterioration at any time in the postsurgical phase, deserve aggressive attention from the patient's physician.

Otolaryngologists

These physicians provide surgical and medical care to patients with diseases of the head and neck. While the close working relationship and types of diagnoses that are of mutual interest are obvious to the general speech–language pathologists, a few words about the special relationship that exists in the acute setting are in order. Otolaryngologists are frequently involved in surgical placement of tracheostomy tubes to assist patients with breathing difficulty. In addition, the assistance of the skilled otolaryngologist is essential in the work-up for patients with suspected vocal fold paralysis. This diagnosis is common in centers where a large number of patients with neurogenic and traumatic disorders are evaluated. Of course, many of these patients are at significant risk for aspiration and the differentiation of their dysphagia/dysphonia is critical to issues of communication and swallowing. In the case of the patient with cancers involving the larynx, jaw, or tongue, collaboration in the communication and swallowing aspects of care is ideal for achieving the best outcomes. In some situations the speech–language pathologist may be called on to collaborate with the otolaryngologist in completing or interpreting videostroboscopy or videoendoscopy for patients in the acute setting. These procedures are described in Chapter 22.

Primary Care Physicians

Pediatricians, geriatricians, internists, and family practitioners are all primary care physicians (PCPs). In the new managed care environment they are considered the gatekeepers to care and they control the patient's access to referral sources, including speech–language pathologists. Increasingly, these groups of physicians are involved in the care of acutely ill patients and their influence in decision making about which patients receive speech–language pathology referrals is being felt. Prior to the strong influence of the managed care movement, these physicians typically turned many of their acutely ill patients over to tertiary specialists who then managed referrals and consultations. It was the specialist who was more knowledgable about the scope of practice in speech–language pathology and therefore made referrals when indicated. Given this new arrangement, it is increasingly important for the speech–language pathologist to learn about the orientation, background, and interests of primary care physicians and then to educate them about the services that can be afforded by skilled speech–language pathologists. It is through ongoing education and effective consultation that these important referral sources may begin to understand what the speech–language pathologist has to offer for patients. PCPs are also influenced toward an appropriate referral decision when a specialty colleague to whom they are referring suggests that the patient might also benefit from evaluation by a speech–language pathologist.

Psychiatry

In the acute care setting, speech–language pathologists come into contact with patients exhibiting a variety of psychiatric disorders (see Chapters 25 and 26). The speech–language pathologists's interaction with psychiatrists and other mental health professionals (psychologists, clinical social workers) usually occurs when both groups are asked to consult on patients exhibiting some behavioral difficulty. Patients with speech, language, or swallowing disorders may also exhibit serious psychological problems that need to be addressed with drugs or other therapies. Likewise, some patients with primary psychological disturbances may exhibit disturbances of communication or swallowing. Because these symptoms can be caused by either physiological or psychological etiologies and can present challenging diagnostic and treatment dilemmas, it is wise for the speech–language pathologist to have a good working relationship with consulting psychiatrists and psychologists.

Pulmonary Medicine

These subspecialists of general internal medicine evaluate and treat patients with diseases of the respiratory system. Pulmonary specialists frequently refer patients from the intensive care setting for communication and swallowing evaluation. Typically, referred patients are seriously compromised at the time of referral and may be dependent on artificial ventilation for oxygen exchange. Speech–language pathologists have much to offer patients in the intensive care setting (see Chapter 5). In addition to the predictable referrals from the intensive care unit, pulmonary physicians may refer patients who are admitted for work-up of suspected functional breathing disorders such as paradoxical vocal fold movement. Jacobson and Silbergleit[3] have presented such a patient who was admitted to the hospital in acute distress.

Other Aspects of Acute Care

In addition to the primary and specialty physician contacts that occur with every patient in the acute care setting might experience, there are many different types of professionals and other services that might be indicated. Examples of some of the services that might be involved in the care of patients with speech, language, and swallowing disorders are listed in Table 6–3. It is important for the speech–language pathologist to understand and

Table 6–3. Hospital-based Professionals and Services Used in Care of Patients with Speech, Language, or Swallowing Disorders

Neurophysiologic procedures
  Electroencepholography (EEG)
  Electromyography (EMG)
  Measures of cerebral blood flow

Radiologic/imaging procedures
  Chest X-ray
  Videoflouroscopy (modified barium swallow; esophogram)
  Magnetic resonance imaging (MRI)
  Computerized axial tomography (CT Scan)

Consultative services (nonphysician)
  Pharmacy
  Physical therapy
  Nursing: Primary nurse
    Nurse clinician
    Nurse practitioner
  Occupational therapy
  Psychology
  Social work
  Discharge planning
  Ethics
  Patient advocate
  Substance abuse
  Dietetics (nutrition)
  Pastoral care

appreciate the unique set of information that each service brings to the data set about the patient. This information is combined with data provided from physician consultation, the patient's history, and the speech–language-swallowing observations to address the referral question. The astute speech–language pathologist uses this *combined* data set to provide a comprehensive interpretation and explanation of the patient's speech–language-swallowing disorder.

KEY ISSUES IN ACUTE CARE SPEECH–LANGUAGE PATHOLOGY PRACTICE

Appreciation and comprehension of these issues are fundamental for effective consultation, assessment, and intervention. This set of issues clarifies the role of speech–language pathology practice in this setting and distinguishes this practice from other points in the continuum of care. In the following discussion, themes that are central to effective practice in the acute setting are presented. These themes include:

- Understanding of a *consultative* model of practice
- Provision of expert level diagnostic services
- Delivery of skilled provision of sensitive, reliable, systematic, and predictive patient *monitoring* over time
- Establishment of multifaceted *educational* services as part of the clinical service program

These overarching themes—consultation, diagnosis, monitoring and education—are emphasized in the remainder of this chapter. Before discussing each topic in detail, we offer some general considerations as the foundation and backdrop to subsequent discussion. These fundamental points serve to justify the need for more specific consideration of consultation, education, and monitoring.

1. *Appreciation for the importance of rapid access to information by all members of the heath care team.* Patients in acute settings change rapidly; sometimes they improve and sometimes their condition deteriorates. In addition to the frequent changes in patient status associated with many diseases of interest to speech–language pathologists, patient stays are decreasing because of improvements in outpatient services and financial pressures on the health system. This decrease in length of stay increases the complexity of scheduling inpatient services, managing communication, carrying out acute rehabilitation activities, and planning for discharge. In many situations patients are now discharged from the hospital so quickly that clinicians are providing discharge information at the time of the initial consultation. Thus, the communication styles called for in the acute care context are brief, direct, and clear written messages. In addition, the message must be delivered within a very brief time after the patient encounter. Table 6–4 highlights a set of communication guidelines that have been used by the Division of Speech–Language Sciences and Disorders at Henry Ford Hospital for inpatient acute care communication.

2. *Knowledge of appropriate observation and treatment methodologies of patients during periods of rapid change in health status.* The approaches to patient care used by the speech–language pathologist in the acute care should be different from those used in the rehabilitation unit or in the long-term care environment. The most effective approach is typically one that integrates consultative activities with differential diagnosis and careful patient monitoring. In the neurological setting, the term *neurocommunicative monitoring* describes the activities used to provide for rapid and sensitive observation over time. This approach is described in some detail later in this chapter. It is presented as an example of monitoring activities provided by the speech–language pathologist that can offer a positive contribution to patient care.

Table 6–4. Sample Acute Care Professional Communication Guidelines

Acute Care Communication Issues and Guidelines

1. Complete all documentation immediately following the patient encounter. This includes chart notes, patient instructions, and counseling with staff or families.

2. For initial consultations, complete the consultation form and place it at the front of the chart and then page the referring physician and review your findings and recommendations.

3. For patients with dysphagia, attempt to communicate on a daily basis with referring physician.

4. Always complete all documentation and place it in the patient's chart by the end of the working day.

5. Document every encounter with your signature, degree, CCC-speech–language pathologist, and your pager number.

6. Return all pages immediately when on the inpatient service.

Source: Henry Ford Hospital, Division of Speech–Language Sciences and Disorders.

Some clinicians may have difficulty embracing a model of care that emphasizes the diagnostic-consultative aspect of clinical function over a rehabilitative-treatment oriented approach. As previously mentioned, shortened patient stays are being implemented in most institutions. It is not unusual for patients to have only one or two visits with a speech–language pathologist prior to being transferred from the acute setting to one that is less intense (rehabilitation, home care, outpatient). For some patients the most appropriate service offered by the speech–language pathologist may be a careful work-up and diagnosis, with adequate plans and recommendations for follow-up. On the other hand, some patients—those that are most sick—may require long hospitalization in a tertiary facility. For these individuals, the speech–language pathologist has the opportunity to follow the patient over many weeks or even months. This allows the speech–language pathologist to provide more long-term rehabilitation while in the acute care phase of recovery.

3. *Communication with a broad audience of other professionals.* The issue of time pressure around professional communication in acute care has been cited as a key characteristic of this practice setting. A second issue of communication relates to the diverse audience of professionals with whom the speech–language pathologist must converse. This factor interacts with the important variable of time to complicate the communication arrangement.

Why is the nature of the audience important or of concern to the speech–language pathologist? Given that one of the major goals of care in the acute setting is to participate in the medical and rehabilitative care of the patient, it is very important that the interaction among care providers be clear, concise, and directed toward patient care. The speech–language pathologist in acute care can affect little change with the patient without the cooperation of other providers. Careful observation, appropriate and accurate diagnosis, and good interaction with the patient, while essential, will not ensure that the patient is positioned properly for eating, has the appropriate level of communication interaction, is using his/her communication device appropriately, has the necessary dietary accommodations, or is receiving appropriate therapies. All these activities and decisions, which might be recommended by a speech–language pathologist, need to be carried out by someone else in the patient's array of care providers. Thus, it is essential that the speech–language pathologist in acute care settings has communication skills that

allow for very specific explanations that provide a clear (and brief) rationale for any recommendation or request; anticipation of the varying information needs of different providers (physician, nurse, OT, psychologist); and the ability to provide background information (justification) for any unusual or unexpected recommendations. It is important to remember also that the speech–language pathologist is as much a receiver as a sender of information. Therefore, good listening skills and the ability to respond critically without confrontation become important. In general, a communication style that is respectful and diplomatic, balanced with directness, and targeted toward a specific professional's interest or concern is desirable.

4. *Dealing with patients and families during times of crisis.* Admission to an acute care situation is never trivial for a patient or the patient's family. In many cases, admissions are non-elective, and both the patient and the family are under considerable stress. It is important for clinicians to remember that they are rarely seeing the "best" communication ability when they evaluate the patient for the first time. Regardless of the etiology of the patient's condition, the psychological state of the patient at the time of evaluation is always an issue. The speech–language pathologist's role is to demonstrate appropriate concern and empathy for the patient and the family, advocate for the patient (especially around issues of communication and/or swallowing, and assist the family in finding resources that might be helpful to the patient. Under very stressful critical care situations, families can exhibit anger, extreme emotionality, withdrawal, and defensiveness. Speech–language pathologists should obtain appropriate information about desirable communication skills in these situations and seek the help of other professionals (social workers, psychologists, pastoral care professionals) when they are not sure how to deal with a difficult patient or family.

Speech–language pathologists should also take care not to overload families or patients with too much information. Constant readjustment of the type and amount of information to be shared should be a goal. In the beginning of the relationship with the family, the clinician should provide clear, concise, and brief explanations. As the relationship continues, it is reasonable to think of expanding information so as to educate the patient about the communication or swallowing disorder, various treatment options, and the patient's communication prognosis.

5. *Providing information that has immediate effect on patient care.* Speech–language patholo-

gists in acute care need to appreciate the pace with which information transfer occurs. Once information is entered into a paper or electronic record, it becomes available for use by anyone with access to the record. This places pressure on the clinician to provide accurate, clear, and essential recommendations. The rapid growth of feeding and swallowing practice in our discipline has highlighted the need for clear communication of results of dysphagia evaluation. Frequently nurses are waiting for these results to feed the patient with the correct consistency or physicians are waiting to determine if a feeding tube is necessary for the patient. Because of the implications of these types of recommendations on cost of care, length of stay, and patient outcome it is essential that information be transmitted as soon as possible. It is equally important that the speech–language pathologist appreciates others' need for information and also understands that once information is provided, follow-up actions will ensue in a timely manner.

6. *Potential for* significant *clinical errors in judgment and/or practice.* The speech–language pathologist in acute care practice has responsibility that affects patient care, satisfaction with treatment, and patient outcome. More than in most other settings, the fast-paced acute care environment affords the opportunity for clinical errors. Some of these errors may cause inconvenience to the patient or caregivers; others can cause serious complications to an illness; and still other bad decisions can be life threatening. A keen knowledge of common clinical pitfalls can serve to prevent clinical errors. A sampling of common errors can be found in Table 6–5.

Speech–language pathologists should *always* be knowledgeable about any potential negative effects that could occur as the result of recommendations or actions on their part. The speech–language pathologist has the responsibility of informing families, physicians, nurses, and other professionals of any potential adverse effects associated with any recommended or completed procedures.

In the unfortunate situation that an adverse effect occurs as the result of a speech–language

Table 6–5. Potential Significant Errors in Speech–Language Pathology Practice

1. Failure to communicate results of high-risk or invasive procedures accurately or in a timely manner.

2. Failure to document detailed recommendations in the chart (especially diet changes or aspiration precautions).

3. Failure to respond to referrals or requests for information from families or physicians in a timely manner, especially when this delay causes interruption of other care or delays discharge from the acute care setting.

4. Performing any procedure without having demonstrated competency.

5. Failure to supervise noncertified personnel when they are completing procedures.

6. Failure to communicate results from language, speech, or swallowing testing that have diagnostic significance and could change the medical plan of care.

7. Failure to observe or report significant changes in patient behavior that may signal an alteration in the medical or psychological status.

8. Performing procedures outside the scope of practice.

9. Performing procedures that are experimental or of questionable benefit without appropriate informed consent.

10. Making diagnostic statements or drawing conclusions that are not substantiated by observation or test data.

11. Failure to make appropriate referrals when indicated.

12. Failure to follow up on recommendations previously made.

13. Failure to explain and document important information to the patient and/or the family.

14. Failure to assure patient confidentiality.

15. Providing services that would be viewed as incomplete or faulty by a group of your peers.

16. Failure to limit opinions and decisions to topics directly related to speech, language, swallowing, cognition disorders and their sequelae.

17. Failure to follow basic procedures for infection control, universal precautions, and safety.

pathology recommendation or procedure, the first issue to be addressed (following appropriate and careful attention to the needs of the patient) should be the reduction of the possibility for the same adverse effect to reoccur. The second issue should involve the careful study of the problem that was presented so that one can learn all that is possible from the situation toward the goal of improved patient care. In medicine, the model for learning from these types of experiences is the "Morbidity and Mortality" Conference. In this educational format, physicians engage in clinical discussion of various unexpected or adverse outcomes that occur in the course of patient care. The intention of these discussions is to learn from the past and prevent similar complications in the future. Speech–language pathologists in hospital settings may wish to model this approach, especially with regard to high-risk areas of practice.

7. *Observing immediate effects of illness, drugs, and surgical management on patient performance, function, and outcome.* One of the most unique learning opportunities for learning afforded to the speech–language pathologist in the acute care setting is the study of the effects that various medical interventions have on the speech, language, cognitive, motor, or swallowing systems. Because these effects can be immediate, sustained, short or long term, it is essential that the clinician come to appreciate the significance of the most common interventions. Many clinicians find it helpful to obtain some of the common manuals used by physicians that present these effects in outline or tabular forms for quick reference. A few of these sources are listed in Table 6–6. Some clinicians develop their own common set of references for quick access as a distillation of these readily available resources. Clinicians working in tertiary care specialty environments such as critical and intensive care units must become familiar with the common medications, treatments, and other procedures that are used by colleagues from their disciplines. This knowledge assists with the speech–language assessment process and also contributes to differentiation of those symptoms and behaviors that are part of the underlying pathophysiology presented by the disease process from those that are iatrogenic (produced by the intervention itself).

8. *Dealing with issues related to patient advocacy and/or ethics.* Another recent development in health care that has affected patient decision making and also involves high-level problem solving and communication among practitioners is the study and practice of ethics. Many institutions have established interdisciplinary teams that in-

Table 6–6. Examples of Common Sources That Summarize Effects of Drugs and Procedures on Cognitive, Communicative, and Motor Systems

The little black book of neurology: A manual for house officers, 2nd ed. J. S. Bonner and J. J. Bonner, Mosby Year Book (1991).

Handbook of symptom oriented neurology, 2nd ed. WH Olson, RA Brumback, V Iyer, G Gascon, Mosby (1994).

Pocket guide to assessment in speech–language pathology, MN Hegde, Singular (1996).

Otolaryngology, 3rd ed. MM Paparella, DA Shumrick, JL Gluckman, WL Meyerhoff (eds.), W. B. Saunders (1991).

Interpretation of diagnostic tests, 6th ed. Wallach and Jacques, Little Brown and Co. (1996).

Current medical diagnosis and therapy, 36th ed. LM Tierney, SJ McPhee, MA Papadakis (Eds.), Appleton and Lange (1997).

Harrison's principles of internal medicine, 13th ed. KJ Isselbacher, E Braunwald, JD Wilson, JB Marin, AS Fauci, DL Kasper (Eds.), McGraw-Hill (1994).

The Merck manual, 16th ed. R Berkow (ed.), Merck Research Laboratories (1992).

clude physicians who have developed expertise in the study of ethical problem solving, members of the clergy, and professionals from behavioral medicine. The recent technological advances that have extended the viability of the patient combined with media attention on these issues have emphasized the role of the patient and the family in decision making about life and death issues as well as the quality of life. Speech–language pathologists tend to be involved in these discussions from a variety of perspectives: Can a patient comprehend a situation and make an informed decision? Will the patient ever be independent in communication or cognitive functioning? What are the implications for a given patient when the decision is made to continue oral feedings when chronic aspiration is documented?

Most speech–language pathologists have not had, as part of their formal training, coursework in medical ethics, death and dying, grief counseling with families, or other topics related to end of life issues. Participation in these discussions with ethics teams can be a valuable learning experience for the clinician interested in learning more about this type of decision making. Most important, however, is the need for speech–language pathologists who are working in tertiary care settings to become familiar with ethical principles, understanding of issues related to death, dying, chronic disability, and interprofessional and family consultation around these topics. When these issues arise in the course of patient care it is important for the speech–language pathologist to inform the patient's primary physician of patient-family concerns, and seek advice from those experienced in management of these issues. These issues are rarely addressed by the speech–language pathologist alone. A review of these issues and their application in medical speech–language pathology are found in Chapter 10.

9. *Understanding the role of the speech-language pathologist in assuring the best outcomes—both rehabilitative and medical.* A final point regarding the role of the speech–language pathologist in acute care is that in addition to providing immediate consultation, diagnosis, and treatment for the patient and the referring physician, the speech–language pathologist has the responsibility to ensure that the more long-term needs of the patient begin to be addressed. Frequently these issues relate to the post-discharge placement of the patient for rehabilitation or nursing care. It is not uncommon for discharge planners or physicians unfamiliar with the complexities of managing communication issues to overlook these needs in planning post-acute care services. Speech–language pathologists have the responsibility of pointing out these needs and recommending suitable referrals or community resources. Every patient should leave the hospital with an appropriate plan for communication treatment (when indicated), and discussion with professionals who will be providing follow-up is an important ingredient to quality care. Speech–language pathologists also have an important role in family education about the patient's communication or swallowing disorder. This can frequently be accomplished in bedside discussions with the patient and the family. For more complex problems, it may be necessary to provide written materials, videos, or other resources designed for patient education. Ideally, patients and families should be given a written plan for follow-up, including scheduling of necessary return appointments, to ensure that the patient is likely to receive those services that will best meet his or her communicative needs.

THE PROCESS OF CONSULTATION

Consultation is an essential component of medical care. It is a highly complex process that is most effective when a model is used to guide the consul-

tation from referral to discharge. The following process is presented as a successful model for guiding consultative activities. A condensed version is provided in checklist format in Appendix A. It may be used as a resource for training fellows or new medical speech–language pathologists to be effective consultants. Consultation is a skill that should be taught formally and perfected through experience, rather than learned in a trial-and-error manner.

Anatomy of an Effective Consultation

Referral Process

The referral of a patient for a speech–language pathology consultation is usually made by a staff or resident physician from the patient's primary service. Typically, referrals are generated directly by the patient's physician, although they may be prompted by a nurse, patient, or family member who reports a concern to the physician. Finally, referrals may be prompted by other consulting services via recommendations.

Once the referral is received, there is a general rule that a response from the consultant is expected within 24 hours. Horwitz et al.[4] found that internist's consultations performed within 24 hours of referral had a significantly increased impact on diagnosis or management than those performed more than 24 hours from initial referral. Therefore, the consultation process is initiated once the referral is received. Before seeing the patient, the speech–language pathologist must be well prepared for the consultation.

Preparation for the Consultation

Once a patient has been referred for consultation, the speech–language pathologist begins with a comprehensive review of the patient's medical chart. The medical chart contains a wealth of information that provides the astute speech–language pathologist with a background of the case and a strong starting point. The following list of medical chart components should be carefully examined and understood by the speech–language pathologist:

- The history and physical form is filled out by a physician from the patient's primary service at the time of admission. It gives the reason for admission, findings of the initial examination, and past medical history.
- Chart notes, or progress notes, are important in understanding the patient's treatment regimen and clinical course since admission.

This section may be integrated so that notes from all disciplines follow one another in chronological order. In some institutions, each discipline has a separate section.

- Review of findings from all tests or procedures, such as CT, MRI, EEG, chest X-rays, pathology reports, and laboratory values.
- Review of the reports from other consultants.
- Medical abbreviations are typically used throughout the medical chart and a speech–language pathologist should be familiar with common ones. Most hospitals produce a book of approved medical abbreviations.

During the chart review, the speech–language pathologist must be aware of signs that indicate significant clinical information. This requires the medical speech–language pathologist to have a working knowledge of pertinent information from related areas of medicine and other disciplines. For example, if the chart indicates that a patient has been intubated for 3 weeks, a voice or swallowing impairment may be suspected; similarly, it is of clinical significance that the patient had progressive mental status changes 6 months prior to admission rather than an acute onset of changes. A history of stroke, pneumonia, or cancer may lead to hypotheses regarding current communication and/or swallowing disorders. Therefore, the consultation process involves application of traditional speech–language pathology skills, as well as the acquisition and practical use of new knowledge from multiple disciplines.

Referral Question

The key to a successful consultation is to accurately identify the referral question(s). According to Lee et al.,[5] "consultants must identify the reasons for which their expertise has been sought." Only when a question has been identified can it be answered. At times, the referring physician may specify the reason for the consultation in verbal communication or in writing on the consultation report. However, in many consultations, no question has been specified. This then becomes a problem-solving endeavor. A thorough medical chart review is critical for identifying the referral question, and if the question does not become clear through chart review alone, a call to the referring physician to clarify the reason for the consultation is indicated.

Physicians most commonly request consultations for the following:[5]

1. Advice regarding diagnosis
2. Advice regarding management
3. Assistance in scheduling or performing a test or procedure

The speech–language pathologist may be consulted for any of these purposes (Table 6–7). Typical referral questions encountered by the medical speech–language pathologist include:

- Is it safe to the patient to eat?
- What type of aphasia does the patient have?
- Is the patient a good rehabilitation candidate?
- Is the presenting behavior consistent with a diagnosis of X disease?

Once the medical chart has been reviewed and the referral question clearly identified, the speech–language pathologist must formulate a plan for the examination.

Plan for the Examination

Based on information from the medical chart review, the speech–language pathologist is able to formulate hypotheses about which communication disorders to expect on examination. A list of differential diagnoses may then be compiled in order of likelihood. As shown in Table 6–8, the differential diagnoses are listed from most to least likely. This facilitates the plan for diagnostic testing because each of the diagnoses must systematically be confirmed or ruled out during the examination.

Formal and informal test measures are selected based on the communication parameters that need to be assessed. In acute care, the main areas to be tested usually include language, cognitive-communication, speech, and swallowing, with perhaps an emphasis in one area based on the

Table 6–7. Main Reasons for Consultation in Acute Care and Examples of How the Speech–Language Pathologist May Fulfill the Purpose of Each Type of Consultation

Reasons for Consultation	Role of Speech–Language Pathologist
Advice on diagnosis	Aphasia classification
	Lesion localization
Advice on management	Feeding status
	Feeding tube placement
Performance of a test	Radiographic assessment of swallowing

Table 6–8. Example of Differential Diagnoses

	Left Hemisphere Lesion	Right Hemisphere Lesion	Brainstem Lesion
Most likely	Aphasia	Cognitive-communication impairment	Dysphagia
	Dysarthria	Dysarthria	Dysarthria
	Apraxia	Dysphagia	Altered level of consciousness
	Dysphagia		
Least likely	Cognitive-communication impairment	Aphasia	Aphasia
	Dementia	Dementia	

referral question. Even if the referral question involves one area, such as swallowing, all parameters are assessed or at least screened. Due to the limited time for testing in the acute setting, brief formal tests are often preferred over more lengthy formal tests that may be more well suited for the outpatient clinical setting. Formal tests may be given in part if they cannot be administered in whole. Informal testing is heavily relied on in acute care due to poor patient tolerance, lack of ability to comply with formal testing, or poor testing conditions.

The organization and sequence of the testing session also must be determined. In general, it is best to first perform the testing needed to answer the referral question. In this manner, the speech–language pathologist has at least obtained the information necessary for addressing the reason for the consultation. Examinations can be limited because of patient fatigue or interruptions for routine medical care or medical tests that temporarily take patients away from their hospital room. Thus, it is important to address the most important issues early in the testing session.

Now that the speech–language pathologist has formulated a list of differential diagnoses and has developed a solid plan for testing, the next step is to examine the patient.

Examination and Diagnostic Testing

In the acute care setting, patients are seen and examined in their hospital room or in the intensive care unit. Examination of the patient involves the administration of formal tests and informal measures according to the plan of action that was developed based on the medical chart review. Even the most experienced and organized speech–language pathologist may not be able to examine the patient according to the original plan because of the unique challenges of the acute care environment. Invariably, modifications in the original plan are necessary as a result of the condition or performance of the patient. A patient may be lethargic due to a neurologic condition or the effects of medication, resulting in a limited assessment and a reliance on behavioral measures; or a patient with severe aphasia may be struggling with formal aphasia tests, requiring the use of informal language measures. These modifications represent an on-line decision-making process that is done throughout the evaluation. It requires skill and experience to determine when such modifications in testing are necessary.

The primary goal of the examination is to obtain sufficient data to answer the referral question—the assessment is not considered complete until this has been accomplished. It is also important to systematically rule out or confirm the presence of each item on the list of differential diagnoses. Finally, the information from the initial assessment provides an important baseline for measuring change.

Documentation: Generation of the Written Consultation Report

The written consultation report is the means by which the consultant's expertise is translated into useable information. Typically, the consultant has less than one page to write a report. This necessitates that the written report be brief, specific, informative, and to the point. Although at times it is difficult to record the necessary information in such a limited fashion, effective consultants are able to relay their findings in a concise manner, with as much content and impact as in a much longer report. The standard information contained in the written consultation report is presented in three sections: the body of the report, impressions, and recommendations. (See Appendix B for examples of written consultation reports.)

Body of the Consultation Report

The first statement of the consultation report usually includes information regarding the patient's age, sex, handedness, date of admission, and reason for hospitalization. This is followed by a statement listing the patient's past medical history. In the next section, the speech–language pathologist consultant provides objective clinical data and key observations obtained during the patient examination. People reading the report benefit from organization by subheadings representing the main areas tested. For example, the subheadings commonly used in reports for patients with neurogenic communication disorders include

- Cognitive-communication
- Language
- Oral-motor examination
- Speech
- Swallowing

Impressions

Following the documentation of objective data, the consultant records diagnoses in the impressions section of the report. Diagnoses are usually given in a list, and it is not uncommon for acutely ill patients to have a list of 3 to 5 diagnosed communication or swallowing disorders. All are listed, whether or not they are related to the referral question. Each diagnosis should be qualified by a severity level (i.e., mild, moderate, severe). It is also beneficial and often appreciated if the suspected etiology of the communication disorder is shared with the referring physician. For example, a phonatory disturbance may be due to prolonged intubation or may have a neurological etiology. If the patient is found to have aphasia or dysarthria, classification according to the traditional profiles should be attempted and stated whenever possible. It is not sufficient to report impressions as "aphasia" or even "receptive aphasia." Referral sources are typically good observers of behavior and know the superficial categories of impairment exhibited by the patient. They seek the expertise of the speech–language pathologist for diagnosing the type of communication or swallowing disorder and interpreting the presenting problem in the context of the patient's physiologic or anatomic distur-

bance. Many neurologists and neurosurgeons are familiar with the Aphasia Classification System proposed by Goodglass and Kaplan[6] or the Mayo Clinic Dysarthria Classification.[7] Using these types of systems may improve communication with physicians and be helpful as they attempt to use the information to localize the lesion or clarify the medical diagnosis.

Recommendations

The last section of the consultation report is the Recommendations section. Based on clinical impressions, the speech–language pathologist provides recommendations to the referring physician regarding patient management. Recommendations should be presented in a concise list and address pertinent issues, including:

- Feeding status: NPO (nothing by mouth) or diet order (e.g., pureed, soft, regular) if it is judged that the patient may safely eat.
- Treatment/management issues: for example, recommendation for modified barium swallowing study; ongoing assessment and treatment of communication/language, swallowing, speech or voice; or augmentative/alternative communication.
- Discharge status: recommendation for continued speech–language follow-up, if indicated, and in what setting (i.e., outpatient clinic, rehabilitation center, home health care, nursing home). In the majority of cases it is not too soon to address this at the time of the initial evaluation.
- Referrals to other services if indicated: the examination may reveal issues that warrant attention from a discipline not already involved in the case. For example, a patient with prolonged dysphonia after extubation may benefit from an examination by otolaryngology. In this case, the recommendation may be written as such: "Recommend otolaryngology consultation to rule out laryngeal pathology."

In all cases, the referring service may be more compliant with recommendations when they are made aware of the reason for the recommendation. All recommendations must be supported by objective information presented in the Consultant's Remarks section of the report. The speech–language pathologist must be prepared to provide the rationale for each recommendation to increase compliance. It is best to recommend tests and treatments that are likely to make a difference in management or outcome[8] and explain the rationale for any recommendations that might be unclear to a particular referral source.

Several factors may influence compliance with recommendations, and these factors should be considered as recommendations are formulated. Compliance may be greatest when recommendations are specific and communicated verbally as well as in writing. Sears and Charlson recommend that consultants limit the total number of initial recommendations; they found that compliance was greatest when fewer than 5 recommendations were provided.[9]

Effective consultants provide a written report with contingency plans and recommendations tailored toward different courses of treatment. They try to anticipate potential problems and provide therapeutic or management options.[10] For example, a speech–language pathologist examined a patient who was admitted with a right hemisphere stroke. After a thorough clinical examination with the patient fully alert, the speech–language pathologist recommended a soft diet, due to the patient's inability to chew solid foods. Review of the medical chart showed that the patient had been exhibiting fluctuating arousal with periods of unresponsiveness over the previous 72-hour period. Therefore, the speech–language pathologist recommended:

1. Soft diet
2. Feed patient only when *fully alert,* NPO when patient is lethargic
3. Dietary consult to monitor nutritional intake
4. Recommend temporary tube feedings to supplement nutrition
5. Speech–language pathologist will follow patient to assess tolerance of diet and manage feeding/swallowing issues

Clearly, these recommendations required the participation of multiple disciplines. The speech–language pathologist spoke personally to the patient's physician, nurse, and family to ensure compliance with these recommendations.

After the consultation report has been written and placed in the medical chart, the effective consultant contacts the referring physician to personally communicate the results and recommendations.

Summary

The written consultation report, supplemented by oral communication when possible, is the primary means for the speech–language pathologist to utilize expertise and influence patient care. When written expertly it can have a positive impact on

the patient's management and clinical outcome. The written consultation report must provide a clear and specific answer to the referral question as well as a clear concise impression of the problem and succinct and direct recommendation.

COMMUNICATIVE AND SWALLOWING MONITORING AND INTERVENTION

As noted earlier, the role of the hospital-based speech–language pathologist differs from that of the outpatient or rehabilitation-based speech pathologist. The acuity of illness in the hospitalized patient requires a different approach to evaluation, management, and therapeutic goal setting. Acutely ill patients can typically have unstable medical and neurologic function that necessitates frequent and serial evaluations to properly chart their clinical course. It also means that intervention goals may change on a day-to-day basis. Goals designed to remediate an impairment one day may not be appropriate the next. Therefore, a primary function of the speech–language pathologist in the acute care setting is careful evaluation and monitoring to assist with initial diagnosis and subsequent care.

Specifically, the acute care speech–language pathologist needs to demonstrate the evolution of speech, language, cognitive, and swallowing abilities during an acute illness. Through serial testing and precise behavioral observation over time, change in these abilities can be demonstrated. Selected tests that provide quantitative measures of communication abilities can be useful indices of change. Precise behavioral descriptions supplement test data and offer a more refined and comprehensive profile of speech, language, cognition, and communication. The information gained provides an objective measure of improvement or deterioration of communication processes as well as signals change in overall medical or neurological condition. The results of communicative and swallowing monitoring activities guide patient and family education and counseling, discharge planning, and judgments regarding prognosis. This section of the chapter reviews the process of monitoring patients with neurogenic communication disorders (neurocommunicative monitoring). This review is offered as an example of the way in which various tools and processes can measure change over time and to intervene appropriately based on these measurements and observations. The process of monitoring is applicable to other patient populations as well, such as those with head and neck cancer or pulmonary dysfunction although different tools would be used to monitor symptom progression.

Neurocommunicative Monitoring Measurement Tools

Depending on the findings from the initial consultation, one or more neurocommunicative monitoring tools may be used in combination to monitor the communication processes of interest (Table 6–9). For example, a patient with aphasia might be tested daily with the Aphasia Diagnostic Profile (ADP)[11] to track the evolution of language behavior. A patient with a traumatic brain injury might be evaluated daily with the Ranchos Los Amigos Scale[12] and the Galveston Orientation and Amnesia Test (GOAT).[13] The choice of test is important because it may be used to predict future recovery levels. Levin[13] found that the period of post-traumatic amnesia as documented serially with the GOAT corresponded to eventual outcome levels. Assessment of outcome was completed on 32 patient 6 months after injury. Subjects with post-traumatic amnesia less than 2 weeks in duration had a "good outcome" as measured on the Glasgow Outcome Scale (see Table 6–10). In addition, monitoring tools must detect subtle change in communication skills while being relatively quick to administer and score. Johnson, George, and Valachovic[29] found the ADP sensitive to subtle change in language performance in the acute setting.

Table 6–9. Neurocommunicative Monitoring Tools for the Acute Setting

Behavioral scales
  Glasgow Coma Scale[14]
  Ranchos Los Amigos Scale[12]

Cognitive measurement tools
  Mini-Mental State Examination (MMSE)[15]
  Galveston Orientation and Attention Test (GOAT)[13]
  Brief Test of Head Injury (BTHI)[16]
  Ross Information Processing Assessment[17]
  Clock Drawing[18] (Freedman, Leach, Kaplan, 1994)
  Rehabilitation Institute of Chicago Evaluation of Communication[19]
  Mini Inventory of Right Brain Injury (MIRBI) (Pimental, Kingsbury[20])

Language monitoring tools
  Frenchay Aphasia Screening Test (FAST)[21]
  Aphasia Diagnostic Profiles (ADP)[11]
  Bedside Evaluation Screening Test (BEST)[22]
  Boston Assessment of Severe Aphasia (BASA)[23]
  Multilingual Aphasia Examination (MAE)[24]
  Boston Naming Test (BNT)[25]

Functional communication measures
  ASHA Functional Communication Measures (FCMS)[26]
  ASHA Functional Assessment of Communication Skills for Adults (FACS)[27]

Table 6–10. Ranchos Los Amigos Scale of Cognitive Levels and Expected Behavior

Level I   Response: Unresponsive to all stimuli.

Level II   Generalized inconsistent, nonpurposeful, nonspecific reactions to stimuli; responds to pain, but response may be delayed

Level III   Localized response. Inconsistent reaction directly related to type of stimulus presented; responds to some commands; may respond to discomfort

Level IV   Confused, agitated, disoriented and unaware of present events. Response with frequent bizarre and inappropriate behavior; attention span is short and ability to process information impaired

Level V   Confused, nonpurposeful random or fragmented inappropriate responses when task complexity exceed non-agitated abilities; patient appears alert and responds response to simple commands; performs previously learned tasks but is unable to learn new ones

Level VI   Confused, behavior is goal-directed; responses are appropriate to the situation with incorrect response because of memory difficulties

Level VII   Automatic, correct routine responses that are robot-like; appropriate, appears oriented to setting, but insight, response judgment, and problems solving are poor

Level VIII   Purposeful, correct responding carryover of new appropriate learning; no required supervision, poor response tolerance for stress, and some abstract reasoning difficulties

Source: Hagen C, Malkmus, D: Intervention strategies for language disorders secondary to head trauma. American Speech–Language-Hearing Association, Atlanta, 1979.

When selecting tools for a particular diagnosis, be aware of several key features that make for a good neurocommunicative monitoring instrument. Neurocommunicative monitoring tools should be:

- **Brief:** The tool needs to be easy to administer and score, ideally taking 30 minutes or less. There is a time pressure to have results available quickly, and patient's testing tolerance may be limited. Lengthier testing instruments with complicated scoring systems would be impractical in the acute setting and might not provide needed information in a timely fashion.
- **Sensitive:** The tool needs to detect subtle change in communication and cognitive skills. The sensitivity of the instrument will depend on the degree of disorder severity. Screening

instruments may indicate a problem, but will not detect subtle change in performance. For a more severely impaired patient, however, a screening instrument might demonstrate small changes. More in-depth diagnostic tools may detect subtle change, but are too lengthy to administer repeatedly. In this case selected subtests might be chosen to monitor progress in the more mildly impaired patient.

- **Quantifiable:** The tool should allow for quantification of the communication process or behavior or interest. Quantification provides an objective index of change and progression of symptoms.
- **Standardized:** Instruments that are standardized provide normative standards of expected performance. This is important in determining whether an observed pattern of behavior is within the normal range for a given population or to what degree the patient's behavior deviates from the norm.

These features are guidelines for choosing a "good" monitoring tool. A number of widely used behavioral scales, language and cognitive tests, and functional assessments meet all or some of these criteria (see Table 6–11). In addition to these measures, clinicians may have developed their own language and cognitive assessment tools to meet their needs. A challenge presented by individualized measurement tools is that typically they do not have normative standards. If individualized tools are used, it is important that some standard testing procedures be employed each session. Varying the testing procedures limits the reliability of the test data.

In addition to data from more formal assessment tools, clinical observations provide another means of monitoring the evolution of speech, language, cognition, and communication.

Clinical Observations

Clinicians make many observations that provide insight into a patient's medical, neurologic, and communication status that extends beyond performance onstandard tests. Changes in these initial observations over time help clinicians to formulate tentative hypotheses about the communication impairment and are later used to signal improvement or decline in function. For the more severely impaired patient, formal testing may be impossible and precise behavioral description may be the only measure of ability. In addition, clinical observations provide information about preserved communication skills not formally tested, the influence of the environment and communication partner on communication abilities, the patient and family's emotional and psychological adjustment, and the patient's rehabilitation potential. The following areas should be considered as the speech–language pathologist interacts with the patient over time.

Table 6–11. Features of Selected Neurocommunicative Monitoring Tools

Instrument	Brief	Sensitive	Quantifiable	Standardized
Glasgow Coma Scale	+		+	+
Ranchos Los Amigos Scale	+		+	+
Mini-Mental State Examination	+		+	+
Galveston Orientation and Attention Test	+	+	+	+
Brief Test of Head Injury	+/−		+	+
Clock Drawing	+		+	+
RIC Evaluation of Right Hemisphere Dysfunction	+/−		+	
Mini Inventory of Right Brain Injury	+/−		+	+
Frenchay Aphasia Screening Test	+	+	+	+
Aphasia Diagnostic Profiles	+/−	+	+	+
Bedside Evaluation Screening Test	+		+	+
Boston Assessment of Severe Aphasia	+/−		+	+
Multi-Lingual Aphasia Test	??		+	+
ASHA FACS	+/−		+	+
ASHA FCMS	+		+	−

Mental Status: The degree of alertness, attention, and orientation must be observed and documented daily. Patients who have decreased alertness or an inability to focus, maintain, and shift their attention will not provide valid and reliable responses on tests of language and cognition. Poor performance, may result from decreased arousal and attention, and not a deficit in higher cognitive or language processing. Formal testing should not continue if a patient cannot maintain an alert state.

General Appearance and Behavior: It is important to note the patient's physical appearance and overall behavior. How does the patient look and behave during the session? What are the patient's mood and affect? Does the patient tend to his/her hygiene and grooming? Is behavior appropriate to the context? Behavioral changes can either be increased or decreased. Both are significant. For example, the abulic patient will show a flat affect, indifferent attitude, and a decreased responsiveness. In contrast the manic patient may be euphoric and impulsive with increased activity.

Medical Status: It is important to determine the patient's medical status. Many acutely ill patients are medically unstable, which can result in fluctuations in language and cognitive function. A review of the medical chart, nurses notes, and daily lab values combined with clinical observation can help clinicians determine the patient's medical status. It is beneficial to note the patient's vital signs including temperature, pulse, respiration, and blood pressure. Fluctuations and irregularity may signal medical instability. There are a wide array of actors that may adversely affect language and cognition. Some of these include cardiovascular dysfunction (i.e., reduced cardiac output, causing a reduction in blood flow to the brain), infection or fever, drug intoxication, metabolic and nutritional imbalance (i.e., hyperthyroidism, dehydration, electrolyte disturbance), neurologic disorders of traumatic, vascular, or infectious origin, and disorders associated with hospitalization (i.e., confusion following anesthesia).[30]

Medical Interventions/Medication: Different tests, medical procedures, and therapies may influence patient performance. Patients may fatigue more readily following a day of tests, or they may have received certain medications that cause drowsiness or confusion. It is important to be aware of the patient's activities and schedule of medications. See Vogel and Carter[31] and Chapter 9 in this text for a review of medications that influence communication.

Medical Devices: It is common for patients in the acute setting to be managed with certain medical devices such as catheters, feeding tubes, intravenous tubes, and oxygen. These devices help clinicians to identify other variables that could influence overall medical and communication functioning.

Motor Function: Observation of posture and motor function has important diagnostic and prognostic indications. Often patients will present with a new physical impairment such as complete or partial paralysis of one side of the body. The functional impact of these limitations should be observed and the compensations a patient implements noted. Abnormal movements such as a tremor or tics may signal the underlying medical diagnosis. Muscle tone, both increased and decreased, should also be observed.

Prosthetics: Many patients will wear glasses, hearing aids, dentures, or another prosthetic. The clinician should note if the patient wears any prosthetic devices and ensure that they are readily available to the patient. A patient might be misdiagnosed if he or she is tested without the aid of his or her glasses or a hearing aid.

Insight and Awareness: Insight and awareness into one's deficits are important prognostic indicators. In the acute setting it is not uncommon for patients to have a lack of awareness about their medical condition and associated deficits. This lack of awareness may be the result of the neurologic insult as in the case of right hemisphere patients or it may be due to a global cognitive decline as seen with demented patients. Patients and family members may show a lack of awareness because the behavioral consequences of an acute illness are so new and foreign. There may also be a degree of denial that serves as a coping mechanism. Initially, both patient and family may be so relieved that the acute event did not result in death that their full awareness of the behavioral consequences is limited. Even with counseling and education, the impact of a stroke or head injury may not be grasped or fully absorbed until after discharge.

Testing and Treatment Tolerance: Another sign of change is testing or treatment tolerance. Patients who fatigue easily may not be candidates for full inpatient rehabilitation and may need a less intensive treatment program following discharge.

Distractibility: Patients with brain injuries commonly suffer from attentional impairments and are easily distracted by competing stimuli. Distractions may be internal such as worries or intrusive thoughts or may be caused by background stimuli, such as bright lights, noises, or other conversations. What is the patient's response to distractions? Can he or she stay on task? What happens when the clinician reduces the distractions by modifying the environment (i.e., turning the television down, drawing the curtain)? The influence of distractions is important to note and may signal improvement when they have less of an impact.

Testing the Limits: At times, strict adherence to standardized testing procedures may not elucidate the underlying cause of failure on a given test item. Clinicians should do what Lezak[32] calls "testing the limits" of the patient. Testing the limits means going beyond the standard test procedures to exploit an individual's full capacities. For example, if a patient is unable to mentally perform arithmetic on an orally administered math test, the cause for failure is unknown. Does the patient not understand the problem? Does the patient's level of attention and concentration interfere? Is the patient unable to hold the numbers in short-term memory long enough to perform the calculation? If the reason for failure is unclear, then the examiner can extend the test by giving the patient a pencil and paper and repeating the failed test items. If the patient can then complete the calculations, attention, concentration, or short-term memory problems may be at the root of the deficit. Testing the limits is done after standard test procedures have been completed, and may yield additional insight about the underlying cause of the deficit.

Response to Cues: Toglia[33] emphasized the importance of investigating a patient's response to cues during an assessment. What effect do cues and the type of cues have on a patient's performance? It is often beneficial to start with the cue of least strength and progress to stronger cues. Toglia describes three levels: (1) error detection and awareness, (2) focusing attention, and (3) strategy use.[33] At the lowest level, feedback cues are given, such as, "How do you think you did?" The examiner is interested in determining the patient's awareness of errors, and whether or not this question may prompt the recognition of an error. At the next level, attention is focused on the error. For example, for a right hemisphere stroke patient with neglect, this level of cue would be, "Did you find all the information on the left?" Finally, at the highest level of cueing, a strategy is provided and the response observed. Patients who are aware of their errors and more responsive to cues show greater rehabilitation potential.

Patient and Family Strategy Use: Often the patient and his or her family members develop compensatory communication strategies without any direct intervention. It is important to observe these strategies and develop related strategies. In addition, note maladaptive strategies or behaviors that impede communication and modify them. For example, talking louder may not necessarily aid comprehension, but shortening instructions will.

Practice: Neurocommunicative monitoring also allows for observations of changed performance with practice. Does the patient recognize items that were difficult on the previous day's testing? Are previously demonstrated strategies spontaneously used by the patient to maximize performance?

Modalities: Which modalities does the patient respond to most/least accurately? Does the patient exhibit greater comprehension in the written or auditory modality? Does the patient write the names of common objects better than he says the names?

As a useful summary, Appendix C presents a form that has been used in patient monitoring over time.

Through observation and interaction with the patient, an experienced clinician can often make a tentative diagnosis of the communication disorder before administering a formal test. Behavioral observations are invaluable as they can be used to demonstrate evolution of communication abilities as well. These observations may capture change in communication more effectively than test data. Objective results from test data combined with behavioral descriptions provide great insight into a patient's speech–language diagnosis, communication strengths and weaknesses, rehabilitation potential, counseling and education needs, and expected level of recovery.

Utilizing Results to Influence Patient Care

As mentioned previously, the information gained through neurocommunicative monitoring is used to influence management of the patient acutely and following discharge. The speech–language pathologist can have a primary impact in several specific ways.

Documenting Improvement or Decline of Function: Neurocommunicative monitoring data provide an objective measure of demonstrating the evolution of speech, language, cognition, and communication. Data are reported comparatively across sessions both quantitatively and through precise behavioral description. The pattern of change will either show improvement, deterioration, or stability. The rate of change can also be demonstrated. Recovery may be rapid or slow. This information has important implications for determining medical and neurological stability and the direction of clinical course.

Determining Functional Communication Abilities: The speech–language pathologist interprets test performance and behavioral observations in functional terms. This is very important as test scores alone do not reflect the impact of the impairment on communicative function.

Establishing Short-Term Goals: The results from neurocommunicative monitoring are used in setting short-term goals. These goals might include (1) more in-depth assessment of a particular deficit area, (2) patient and family education, (3) provision of communication strategies, (4) establishment of an augmentative communication system, and (5) reduction of communication frustration through communication repair strategies. Goals are typically focused at compensation, not remediation of an impairment. The speech–language pathologist provides "surgical strategies" for improving the patient's functional communication skills. These strategies may change on a daily basis given the evolving nature of the impairment. Goals are targeted for hospital staff as well. The nurse and physician benefit from knowing how to optimize communication through strategy use and environmental modifications.

Determining Prognosis: Tracking the rate and pattern of communication change in the acute phase allows for more accurate judgments of prognosis. Determining prognosis in the acute phase can be challenging. If there is no other neurological event, all patients will go through some degree of spontaneous recovery. How much recovery occurs is usually unknown. A number of studies have examined prognosis in aphasic patients.[34–36] Initial severity level is the most significant predictor of later language function. In general, the more severe the initial aphasia, the poorer the eventual outcome. Lengthier hospital stays (thought to be indirectly related to stroke severity) and hemiplegia at discharge have also been shown to be predictive of poorer recovery of language function.[37] The influence of age, education level, gender, and handedness on recovery of language skills has been inconsistent. Many of the variables that influence recovery in patients with aphasia are likely to be similar for patients with right hemisphere cognitive-communication impairments as well.[38] Different variables have been found to influence recovery following head injury. Age has a significant relationship on overall morbidity and mortality following head injury. With increasing age, the percentage of patients with good outcome decreases.[14]

When making statements of prognosis, it is best to be specific. A prognosis of "good" or "fair" does not provide any valuable information, except maybe that some improvement is expected. A statement of prognosis should specify the level and kind of performance and at what point the behavior should be achieved.[38] In addition, it is often helpful to delineate whether a patient will need some type of assistance, such as augmentative communication or compensatory strategies, to achieve maximum function. An example of a well-defined prognosis statement might be: "It is expected that Mr. Jones will communicate well enough to return to work following a one month period of intensive speech–language intervention." In making statements of prognosis it is important to consider the questions that physician and social worker may have in formulating discharge plans. Will the patient's communication skills be adequate for the patient to return home alone? Will they need supervision? Will treatment services be needed to achieve the specified communication level? Knowledge of current literature and ample clinical experience also facilitates accurate assessments of prognosis.

Additional Referrals: Information from neurocommunicative monitoring may also signal the need for additional medical consultation. Careful evaluation and monitoring may reveal symptoms that are inconsistent with the medical diagnosis. For example, more diffuse cognitive deficits observed in patients with a small left hemisphere cortical stroke should prompt further neurological and neuropsychological evaluation. The speech–language pathologist may be the first to notice symptoms of depression and request a psychiatry consultation. A finding of persistent hoarseness following extubation should prompt a referral to otolaryngology to rule out vocal cord injury. Physical and occupational therapy may also be suggested based on the findings from neurocommunicative monitoring. The speech–language pathologists ongoing assessments may be the impetus for these appropriate referrals.

Communicating and Charting Significant Changes

As mentioned earlier, communication is of key importance in the acute setting. It is essential that the speech–language pathologist communicate and chart significant findings shortly after contact with the patient. Findings from test performance and behavioral observations are documented in the medical chart and, when indicated, discussed directly with the nurse and physician. Chart notes should include the findings from repeated assessment and the changes noted since the previous visit. Both objective test scores and precise behavioral descriptions should be reported. In addition, education and counseling performed with the patient and family and any treatment provided should be charted as well. The chart note should end with the updated impressions or diagnoses and recommendations (including discharge recommendations), and a brief plan for the remainder of the patient's hospitalization. It is important that notes be clear and concise and convey significant findings. Progress notes can be written either narratively or following a SOAP (Subjective, Objective, Assessment, and Plan) format. The following outline is useful for the specific information that should be contained. Figure 6–2 provides examples of both formats.

Soap Note Format

Subjective

How the patient reports that he/she feels

Patient complaints

Affect

General mental status: alertness, attention, orientation

Objective/session activities

Test data from language, cognitive, and functional communication assessment tools

Behavioral observations as outlined in the previous section

Behavioral interventions including provision of communication strategies, patient/family education, and counseling

Assessment/impressions

Evaluation of the data and any significant conclusions that can be drawn, including rate and pattern of change in speech, language, cognition, and communication

Prognosis, specifying the specific behavior and time frame

Plan/recommendations

Any new tests or inpatient referrals (i.e., psychiatry, nutrition, occupational therapy)

Strategies for hospital staff to implement to improve functional communication

Short-term goals or interventions, such as patient/family education or direct treatment of communication impairments

Discharge plans, including disposition

Clinical Pathways

Two recent trends have emerged in health care—the need to provide quality services and contain costs. Hospital costs are being contained in part by decreasing the length of acute hospital stays. These shortened stays make the task of acute care speech–language pathologist much more difficult. Within 4 to 5 days, the speech–language pathologist must complete a thorough evaluation to make an accurate diagnosis, monitor the evolution of communicative functions, determine discharge plans and the patient's rehabilitation potential, and counsel and educate the patient and family. In addition, many other disciplines need to intervene with the patient, including the primary care physician, consulting medical services, pharmacy, nursing, social work, physical therapy, and occupational therapy. Clinical pathways have been developed to coordinate scheduling of these services and contain costs while providing high-quality care. Clinical pathways are plans that display goals and outcomes for patients and provide the corresponding ideal timing and sequence of staff actions to meet those goals or outcomes with optimum efficiency.[39,40] Typically, pathways are individualized for an institution based on the makeup of the multidisciplinary team. Pathways are generally diagnosis specific or suited to a particular care setting. Pathways are used to evaluate medical care and clinical practice. Any deviation or departure from the expected pathway (known as a variance) is documented, and the reason for this variance analyzed. This analysis allows for a review of clinical practice, and refinement of the pathway to increase efficiency, timeliness, and appropriateness of care.[41] A speech–language pathology pathway for acute left hemisphere stroke patients is presented in Table 6–12.

Outcome Measurement and Consultative Care

In today's health care climate it is important to demonstrate that services provided had a positive outcome on overall patient care. This section provides a general outline of possible outcomes for the

SOAP NOTE FORMAT

Stroke patient:

S— Patient awake, alert, oriented to person, place, and time. Frustrated by limited verbal communication.

O— Auditory Comprehension: 100% following of 1-step commands;
80% accuracy for object identification; 75% accuracy for short paragraph comprehension
Verbal Expression: Responded to biographical questions with stereotypic utterances and automatic words "Pa"
"Pa" "No." Unable to name or repeat
Writing: Wrote first name only, not last name or address
Reading: 50% accuracy for comprehension of single words and phrases on a short biographical form

Aphasia Diagnostic Profile Severity score = 55

Behavioral Observations: Patient communicated basic needs, such as thirst and feelings of cold with gross gestures.

Educated the patient and his family about aphasia and provided strategies to enhance gestural communication.

A— 1) Moderate-severe Broca's Aphasia—Aphasia Severity score increased by 15 points since yesterday; largely secondary to improvements in auditory comprehension
2) Functional communication limited to the expression of a few basic needs and wants via gestures with minimal assistance.
3) Prognosis: With intensive speech–language therapy, patient's expected to communicate simple ideas via verbal/non-verbal means with familiar communication partners in 1 month.

P— 1) Encourage patient to use gestures and a picture book to answer questions and convey simple ideas.
2) Inpatient Rehabilitation following discharge
3) Will continue inpatient speech–language neurcommunicative monitoring

NARRATIVE FORMAT

ICU patient:

Patient asleep, opens eyes to voice. Does not track objects with eyes. Does not follow verbal commands. No response to yes-no questions. Localizes-to pain. No verbal output. Glasgow Coma Scale score = 9. Ranchos Los Amigos Scale = Level 3; Localized Response. Counseled patient's family on neurological sequelae following a head injury and expected patterns of recovery. Provided literature on CHI and Head Injury Foundation.

Impression:

1) Profound cognitive-cognitive deficits secondary to closed head injury—increased alertness today
2) No functional communication

Recommendations:

1) Will continue family education/counseling
2) Nursing home vs. slow-paced rehabilitation depending upon rate of recovery over next 3–5 days

Figure 6–2. Chart note examples.

acute care setting. The consultative-educational model proposed here will result in different outcomes than a rehabilitative model. For a review of outcome measurement in speech–language pathology, the reader is referred to Chapter 28.

According to Frattali's definitions of outcomes, there are six main categories of outcomes: clinically derived, functional, social, patient-defined, administrative, and financial (see Chapter 28). Some of these outcomes relate directly to the patient, but there are also outcomes for others including the physician and nursing staff who are involved with the speech-langauge pathologist in providing patient care. In addition, there are financial and administrative outcomes as a result of speech–language pathology intervention. Some outcomes specific to the acute care setting are outlined in Table 6–13.

A change in outcome can be objectively demonstrated through a number of published instruments (i.e., handicap scales, ASHA FACS) or accomplished through other outcome assessment methods (i.e., customer satisfaction questionnaires, program evaluations, data registries). The reader is again referred to Chapter 28 for further discussion of methods of outcome assessment.

EDUCATION IN THE ACUTE CARE SETTING

In this chapter a case has been made for emphasizing education in the context of acute care service delivery. To some readers this may come as a surprise, because educational activities are rarely discussed as part of service delivery discussions.

Table 6–12. Acute Care Speech–Language Pathology Left Hemisphere Stroke Pathway

	Day 1	Day 2	Day 3	Day 4
Assessment and evaluation	Review chart Case history Testing/Observation Preliminary Diagnosis(es) Preliminary Recs	Continue further assessment of language (i.e., BDAE, WAB, Token Test, ASHA FACS)	Continue assessment	Continue assessment
Monitoring		Administer Aphasia Diagnostic Profiles (ADP)	ADP	ADP
Treatments	Communication Strategies Augmentative Communication*	Provision of relevant strategies AAC training*	Provision of relevant strategies AAC training*	Provision of relevant strategies AAC training*
Swallowing and nutrition	Complete swallowing evaluation Recommend PO or NPO/type of tube feeding	Observe breakfast Check with nurse if feeder needed	Monitor nutritional status Check diet consistency/change order if needed	Monitor swallowing/feeding status; adjust as appropriate
Pt/family education and counseling	Contact family by phone to introduce self Inform pt/family of speech–language pathologist service Provide literature on aphasia	Continue counseling/education	Continue counseling education Provide literature re: stroke support groups Provide stroke education phone number	Continue counseling/education
Emotional/psycho-social needs	Assess emotional needs Psychiatry referral* Pastoral Care referral*	Monitor psycho-social needs	Monitor psycho-social needs Screen for depression	Monitor psycho-social needs
Referrals/tests	OT/PT* Nutrition* Other medical services* Dynamic Swallowing Study (DSS)*			
Outcomes	Physician/Nursing/PT/Family know speech–language pathologist	Pt/Family/Hospital Staff verbalize speech–language pathologist diagnosis, preliminary tx plan	Demonstration of strategies to facilitate communication Implementation of necessary environmental modifications Pt/family verbalization of community support services	Patient and physician consumer satisfaction Patient eating highest level of diet with greatest independence
Discharge planning	Social work referral*	Determine disposition and rehabilitation potential	Schedule outpatient follow-up*	Instruct pt/family on home program*

* Optional activities, carry out if needed

Table 6–13. Clinical Outcomes Based on Frattali's Definitions

Clinically derived

Patient and family verbalized understanding of speech–language diagnosis

Patient and family identified patient's communication strengths and weaknesses

Patient and family demonstrated strategies (i.e., behavioral techniques or environmental modifications) which enhance communication

Family identified patient safety risks and demonstrated strategies to improve safety

Patient improved on a formal test of speech, language, or cognitive-communication.

Functional outcomes

Communication

Patient demonstrates change on ASHA FACS

Patient demonstrates change on ASHA FCMS

Patient independently communicated basic needs and wants to nursing staff with the aid of augmentative communication or a compensatory strategy

Swallowing

Non-oral to limited oral intake

Limited oral intake to meeting nutritional needs

Limited oral intake to a liquid diet

Liquid diet to a pureed diet

Pureed diet to a mechanical soft diet

Mechanical soft diet to a regular diet

Being fed to feeding self

Social

Patient and family demonstrated effective coping strategies

Patient and family identified support services to meet their emotional and psychosocial needs (i.e., support groups, psychological counseling, stroke hotline)

Patient defined

Increased patient satisfaction

Increased quality of life

Administrative

Patient/family

Verbalized understanding of the treatment plan following the initial intervention session

Verbalized understanding of the discharge plan during last intervention session

Physician/nursing

Increased physician satisfaction

Increased nursing satisfaction

Verbalized understanding of treatment plan

Increased referral source utilization

Increased number of appropriate referrals

Increased timeliness of referral

Implemented communication and swallowing recommendations

Table 6–13. (continued)

Administrative

Discharge planning

Appropriate disposition (home, home with home health, home with OPD, IPD Rehab, Slow-paced Rehab, NH) achieved.

Implemented home program for all home discharges

Schedule outpatient evaluation prior to patient discharge.

Provided diagnosis/disorder specific literature by first patient/family contact

Contacted family/significant other in person or over phone the day of the initial consult.

Completed daily written and verbal communication re: patient progress with physician or nurse

Financial

Decreased length of hospital stay

Increased home vs. nursing home discharges through provision of communication strategies and environmental modifications

Tests/procedures—prevention of unnecessary DSSes/feeding tubes

Prevention of medical complications (i.e., aspiration pneumonia, rehospitalization for fall/safety problems, readmission for dehydration)

However, there are several compelling reasons for including specific educational activities as part of an integrated clinical program. Educational activities to consider fall into three broad categories: (1) patient and family education programming, (2) interdisciplinary education about communication and swallowing disorders, and (3) clinical education and competency development for speech–language pathologists at various professional levels.

Patient and Family Education Programming

Patient and family education is essential in the acute care setting and serves several important functions:

- Provides basic information about the communication or swallowing disorder
- Assists the patient/family in developing an understanding of the expected course of treatment
- Serves as a focus for discussion of patient questions or concerns
- Assists with identification of "information gaps"

Patients and families typically need and want additional information. A common complaint offered by patients and families is that "no one explained what was happening." Tables 6–14 and 6–15 provide some basic considerations regarding the area of communication with patients.

Provides Basic Information

It is easy for the busy professional to forget that a patient may not have an understanding of the communication impairment that is present and seems so obvious and "real" for the clinician. As soon as the professional has a relatively clear picture of the problem, he or she should begin to provide a label and some explanation for the patient. For example, here is a "script" from a conversation between a speech–language pathologist and a patient with a new left hemisphere stroke:

> Mrs. Jones, now that we are through with your testing, I want to tell you a little about what I have learned. First of all, you are having some difficulty talking, as you know. This problem in talking, when it occurs after a stroke, is called *aphasia*. Most people who have aphasia have the most difficulty right after their stroke. Over the next several weeks and months, they usually show improvement in their ability to communicate. No one knows exactly how much you will improve. Over the next few days, while you are here in the hospital, I will be coming in to see you. Together we will see where you might still need some help in talking and begin to plan for your communication needs after you are discharged. Now, do you have any questions?

Obviously, some patients will be interested in additional information, and some will want to hear nothing more. In addition, the comprehension abilities and premorbid educational level of the patient determine the level of complexity that

Table 6–14. Principles of Patient/Family Counseling and Education

Patient education is therapeutic

Educate regarding each of the patient's communication disorders

Encourage and offer a variety of communication methods

Provide written educational material

Use diagrams/pictures to educate

Be positive and encouraging to the patient

Provide prognostic information to assist in preparing for the future

Talk about therapy needs from the beginning

Discuss long-term rehabilitation plans/options

Supply information on community resources (such as stroke clubs)

Table 6–15. Acute Care "Survival Strategies" for Patients and Families

Keep a calendar and clock in the patient's view

Bring pictures and familiar objects into patient's room to elicit conversation and increase memory of past events

Turn off the television and radio before communicating

Establish attention before starting a conversation

Be direct when asking questions

Introduce each new topic of discussion

Avoid quick changes in topic

Speak in shorter sentences with more pauses in conversation

Ask questions periodically to make sure the patient is understanding the conversation

should be used in the presentation. There are several features, however, that should be considered by the clinician in delivering communication or swallowing diagnostic information to the patient for the first time. These features include brevity, clarity, directness, explanation of any clinical terminology, and provision of an opportunity for the patient to respond with comments or questions. This type of simple straightforward discussion provides the patient with a sense of confidence and a preliminary understanding of the direction that will need to be taken.

Subsequent to the first conversation with the patient and/or family, the nature of educational activities becomes individualized to the needs dictated by the situation. Fortunately, the clinician has a variety of resources available to assist with educational goals. Some patients benefit from pamphlets, booklets, or other commercially or clinician produced written materials. In general, patients with communicative disorders need guidance in the use of these materials. Experience teaches that written products can provide a focus for conversations and actually help to structure the content of educational sessions. However, even the most carefully designed materials are rarely used independently by patients or their families in the acute care setting.

Another medium increasingly utilized for patient teaching purposes is video instruction. Many hospitals now have libraries or patient education centers directed at providing basic information about various conditions. The quality of these products varies. Some serve primarily as an advertisement for a dietary product or assistive device, others, usually offered by professional groups or support programs, are more instructional. The clinician should always review materials or videos before recommending that a patient use them.

Assists the Patient/Family to Develop an Understanding of the Expected Course of Treatment

Another dimension of the process of patient education moves beyond the basic instruction that is required for most patients and families as a starting point. This component of instruction deals with the process of speech–language pathology service delivery. Patients must have an understanding of and realistic expectations for what to expect during their acute stay and after discharge. Again, this can be accomplished through a variety of approaches. However, regardless of the method of delivery, no patient should leave the hospital without having learned about his or her problem, necessary follow-up, expected outcomes, community resources for assistance, and the name of a speech–language pathologist to be contacted if follow-up is needed. To the degree possible, the patient should receive written instructions for this type of information, and it should be supplemented with clear verbal explanation and opportunity for questions and conversation. Again, experience teaches that this approach facilitates follow-up and compliance. Specific instructions to the patient without time for the "buy-in" that occurs in conversation rarely produces the same kind of compliance desired.

Serves as a Focus for Discussion of Patient Questions or Concerns

Speech–language pathologists interact with patients around issues of central importance to independent function as a human being. Swallowing, speaking, thinking, communicating, and understanding are all important activities that contribute to one's sense of independence, identity, and satisfaction with life. Interruption in the independent use of these functions is tragic. Speech–language pathologists in the acute care environment, though routinely confronted with serious communication and swallowing disabilities, must fight against becoming desensitized to the profound impact these problems impose on patients and their families. The clinician needs to listen to the concerns, expectations, fears, and confusion of the patient and family members with particular attention to the impact of communication and swallowing problems. Throughout the course of interaction with the patient, the speech–language pathologist should assess the concerns exhibited and try to address them in the context of providing information that might be helpful to allay concerns. For patients with serious language or cognitive disorders, it may be necessary to have frequent conversations with the family separate from the patient to limit confusion. In any case, it is important to include the patient in all discussions about care. When the patient is part of the discussion, the verbal information should be conveyed at the patient's linguistic level. Drawings or other visual aids may serve as useful supplements and assist comprehension. As noted earlier, patients may have significant difficulties adjusting to their new deficit. When these adjustment problems are extreme, it is important for the speech–language pathologist to make appropriate referrals to mental health professionals.

Assists with Identification of "Information Gap"

A final component of patient education addresses the area of information gaps that may be obstacles to progress in treatment. These gaps in knowledge about communication, swallowing, or health service delivery are common. For example, a common confusion exhibited by families (and some health professionals) relates to misunderstanding of the significance of not being able to speak. Those communicating with the patient may not appreciate the level of preserved comprehension and will speak to the patient in a childish or de-

meaning way. The solution for such a problem is in a brief but clear explanation to the family member, perhaps followed by a demonstration of the patient's comprehension level. Some other common "information gaps" are found in Table 6–16.

Preprofessional Education

The acute care environment affords a significant learning environment for students in graduate education programs in speech–language pathology. Students are usually able to see patients in conjunction with an experienced speech–language pathologist. Because of the nature of the inpatient environment in most hospitals, students can be afforded a variety of educational opportunities and challenges. The most unique learning opportunities are related to education about the specific nature of diseases and their effects on human communication and swallowing and the opportunity to learn from other disciplines. In most cases, competency for independent functioning as an speech–language pathologist cannot be attained during a graduate internship lasting 3 to 4 months. It is reasonable, however, to expect students to advance their knowledge about their discipline, to become skilled at bedside speech, language, and swallowing examination, and to develop "basic" skills in documentation and communication in the acute care setting.

Because most graduate programs are not equipped to provide clinical opportunities that prepare students for entry into acute care, it is important for practicum sites to commit to a broad-based educational approach. Ideally, this approach might include such activities as:

- Observation of a variety of patients and clinical activities
- Interaction with physicians and other providers of health care
- Experience in basic assessment of patients in different clinical units within the institution
- Participation in any specialty clinics or multidisciplinary rounds
- Observation of experienced clinicians in service delivery activities
- Participation in Grand Rounds or other educational programs
- Attendance at a staff meeting of the speech–language pathology group
- Observation of patients and their families interacting
- Presentation of cases to more experienced clinical staff

Table 6–16. Common "Information Gaps" for Patients, Families, and Staff in the Acute Care Environment

Information gap: Overestimation of patient's ability

Common statement: "I know he understands what I'm saying."

Results: Information overload to patient, frustration from family when patient does not respond.

Solution: Highlight strengths and weaknesses; teach family to focus on strengths with patient; focus on compensatory strategies to assist with comprehension; teach strategies in context of every contact with the family.

Information gap: Lack of differentiation between language and cognitive disturbances

Common statement: "He seems so confused when he's talking."

Results in: Misinterpretation of patient's behavior, frustration.

Solutions: Clarify differences for family; provide opportunities for family to see patient's strengths and weaknesses, highlighting areas of strength; involve family in daily sessions.

Information gap: Poor understanding of the cause of a comprehension deficit.

Common statement: "You need to talk louder so he can HEAR you."

Results: Patient annoyance or misinterpretation of loud speech as angry speech.

Solutions: Patient/family education concerning specific strengths and weaknesses; provide family with observation tools to observe progress with patient; model appropriate communication style; provide basic reading material for family.

Information gap: Failure to understand NPO status of patient.

Common statement: "They keep refusing to feed my husband. He's going to starve."

Results in: Anger and frustration.

Solution: Explain risks related to oral feeding; explain the alternative method of feeding that is being used. Include family/patient in discussions of results of ongoing swallowing monitoring and evaluation.

Each activity serves many purposes. Students who have engaged in the variety of experiences listed should leave the institution knowing whether or not they wish to pursue medical speech–language pathology or if this area is not a desirable choice for them.

Clinical Fellowship

The ASHA Clinical Fellowship Year (CFY) is a 9-month period of practice under the supervision of an experienced speech–language pathologist. This arrangement is perfect for extended learning opportunities. During this time, speech–language pathologists shape their skills under the tutelage of a mentor; they also have, for the first time in their educational experience, an opportunity for extended practice and the refinement of skills acquired in graduate school. In addition, the extensive clinical focus afforded during the CFY experience allows for the establishment of competence in specific areas. This professional development opportunity is an important step in the establishment of a new career.

Johnson[42] has documented a medical speech–language pathology fellowship program that has been in place for several years at Henry Ford Hospital in Detroit, Michigan. This program, which is a 2-year fellowship, has the following features:

- Completion of ASHA CCC requirements during the first year
- Rotations in neuroscience, otolaryngology, critical care, and pediatrics
- Completion of a 2-month rotation with the inpatient psychiatry service
- Participation in several multidisciplinary clinics
- Completion of a research project
- Establishment of competency in several areas: inpatient consultation, dysphagia, speech production laboratory, tracheostomy/ventilator communication and swallowing, and adult neurogenics

While most programs may not be prepared to commit to a formal fellowship program such as this one, every program that accepts Clinical Fellows should be committed to a vital educational and competency development program for this important group of new professionals.

Teaching Other Professionals

In addition to teaching patients, their families, and new graduates, the speech–language pathologist in the health care setting also has a unique opportunity to influence the knowledge and practice of other providers. Physicians, nurses, dietitians, psychologists, and physical and occupational therapists all need to know more about the best ways of interacting with and managing their patients with communicative and swallowing disorders. Speech–language pathologists should seek every opportunity to provide observation experiences, conduct in-services, participate in multidisciplinary rounds, or present at Grand Rounds. These activities, when delivered effectively, can enhance professional relationships and also improve the service delivery to patients. As professionals from other disciplines become sensitized to the services delivered efficaciously by speech–language pathologists, there is a definite opportunity for increased referrals.

SUMMARY

In this chapter, we have attempted to communicate the science and the art involved in delivering speech–language-swallowing services to patients in the acute care environment. We discussed the role of the clinician in providing effective consultation through skilled diagnoses, effective educational programming, and intensive patient monitoring. We hope this information is useful to individuals preparing for practice in this setting, as well as to experienced colleagues.

STUDY QUESTIONS

1. Discuss the difference between consultative and rehabilitative practice in speech–language pathology.

2. What tools and tests are most useful in acute care practice?

3. Why is it important to be sensitive to the referral question in consultative practice?

4. Who are key referral sources in acute care speech–language pathology?

5. What are some techniques for patient instruction?

6. Discuss the important of the "educational" component in inpatient care.

7. What is "intensive communication and swallowing monitoring?" Why is it crucial to effective service delivery in acute care?

8. Discuss the different methods of evaluation that are useful in acute care service delivery.

9. Review the cases that were presented at the end of the chapter. For each case, answer the following questions:
   a. Who was the referral source and what was his or her question?
   b. How did the findings presented address the referral question?
   c. Was the information presented clear, direct, and organized in an understandable manner?
   d. What would be the expected outcomes if the recommendations were followed?
   e. What would be the expected outcomes if the recommendations were not followed?
   f. Does the follow-up information presented support the original findings? Why? Why not?

10. Evaluate your own information needs regarding practice in the acute care setting. What steps will you need to take to improve your own effectiveness?

REFERENCES

1. Miller, RM, Groher ME: *Medical speech pathology.* Aspen Publisher, Rockville, Md, 1990.
2. Golper, LA: *Sourcebook for medical speech–language pathology.* Singular, San Diego, 1992.
3. Jacobson, BH, Silbergleit, AK: Improvement of functional cough. Paper presented at the Voice Foundation, Philadelphia, 1994.
4. Horwitz R, Henes CG, Horwitz S: Developing strategies for improving the diagnostic and management efficacy of medical consultations. *J Chron Dis* 1983; 36:213–218.
5. Lee T., Pappius E, Goldman L: Impact of Inter-Physician Communication on the Effectiveness of Medical Consultations. *The American J of Medicine.* 1983; 74:106–112.
6. Goodglass H, Kaplan E: *The assessment of aphasia and related disorders,* 2nd ed. Lea and Febiger, Philadelphia, 1983.
7. Duffy J: *Motor speech disorders: Substrates, differential diagnosis, and management.* New York, Mosby, 1995.
8. Rudd P: Contrasts in academic consultation. *Annals of Int Med* 1981; 94:537–538.
9. Sears C, Charlson M: The efficacy of a consultation: Promotion of compliance with recommendations. *Clinical Res* 1981; 29:259 (abstract).
10. Goldman L, Lee T, Rudd P: Ten commandments for effective consultations. *Arch Int Med* 1983; 143: 1753–55.
11. Helm-Estabrooks N: *Aphasia diagnostic profiles.* Riverside Publishing Co., Chicago, 1992.

12. Hagen C, Malkmus D: Intervention strategies for language disorders secondary to head trauma. Paper presented at American Speech–Language-Hearing Association convention, Short Course, Atlanta, 1979.

13. Levin HS, O'Donnell VM, Grossman RG: The Galveston Orientation and Amnesia Test: A practical scale to assess cognition after head injury. *Nerv Mental Dis* 1979; 167:675–684.

14. Teasdale G, Jennett B: Assessment of coma and impaired consciousness: A practical scale. *Lancet* 1974; 40:291–298.

15. Folstein MF, Folstein SE, McHugh PR: "Mini mental state." A practical method for grading the cognitive state of patients for the clinician. *J Psychiatric Res* 1975; 12:189–198.

16. Helm-Estabrooks N, Hotz G: *Brief test of head injury.* Riverside Publishing Co., Chicago, 1991.

17. Ross D: *Ross information processing assessment.* Pro-Ed., Austin, 1986.

18. Freedman M, Leach, L., Kaplan E, et al: *Clock drawing: A neuropsychological analysis.* Oxford University Press, New York, 1994.

19. Burns MS, Halper AS, Mogil SI: *Clinical management of right hemisphere dysfunction.* Aspen, Rockville, MD, 1985.

20. Pimental P, Kingsbury N: *Mini inventory of right brain injury.* Pro-Ed, Austin, TX, 1989.

21. Enderby PM, Wood VA, Wade DT: The Frenchay aphasia screening test: A short, simple test for aphasia appropriate for non-specialists. *Int J Rehabil Med:* 166–170.

22. Fitch-West J, Sands E: *Bedside evaluation and screening test of aphasia.* Aspen Publishers, Rockville, MD, 1987.

23. Helm-Estabrooks N, Ramsberger G, Moran A, Nicholas M: *Boston assessment of severe aphasia.* Riverside Publishing Co., Chicago, 1989.

24. Benton AL, Hamsher K, Sivan AB: *Multilingual aphasia examination.* AJA Associates, Iowa City, IA, 1994.

25. Kaplan E, Goodglass H, Weintraub S: *Boston naming test.* Lea and Febiger, Philadelphia, 1983.

26. American Speech–Language-Hearing Association, *Functional communication measures.* ASHA, Rockville, MD, 1983.

27. Frattali CM, Thompson CK, Holland AL, Wohl CB Ferketic MM: *ASHA functional assessment of communication skills for adults.* ASHA, Rockville, MD; 1995.

28. Jennet B, Bond M: Assessment outcome after severe brain damage: Practical scale. *Lancet* 1975; 1: 480–484.

29. Johnson AF, George KP, Valachovic AM, Acute aphasia: Predicting outcome one and three months post-stroke. Paper presented at the American Speech–Language-Hearing Association Convention. Seattle, 1996.

30. Albert MS: Acute confusional states. In Albert MS and Moss MB (eds.), *Geriatric neuropsychology.* Guilford Press, New York, 1988, 100–114.

31. Vogel D, Carter JE: *The effects of drugs on communication disorders.* Singular Publishing Group, San Diego, 1995.

32. Lezak MD: *Neuropsychological assessment.* Oxford University Press, New York, 1980.

33. Toglia JP: Generalization of treatment: A multicontext approach to cognitive perceptual impairment in adults with brain injury. *Am J Occupational Therapy;* 45:505–516.

34. Basso A: Prognostic factors in aphasia. *Aphasiology* 1992; 6(4):337–348.

35. Pedersen PM, Jorgenssen HS, Nakayama H, Rasschou HO, Olsen TS: Aphasia in acute stroke: Incidence, determinants, and recovery. *Ann Neruol* 1995; 38: 659–666.

36. Kertesz A, McCabe P: Recovery patterns and prognosis in aphasia. *Brain* 1977; 100:1–18.

37. Holland AL, Greenhouse JB, Fromm D, Swindell CS: Predictors of language restitution following stroke: A multivariate analysis. *J Sp Hear Res,* 1989; 32, 232–238.

38. Tompkins CA: *Right hemisphere communication disorders theory and management.* Singular Publishing Group, San Diego, 1995.

39. Pearson SD, Goulart-Fisher D, Lee T: Critical pathways as a strategy for improving care: Problem and potential. *Ann Intern Med* 1995; 123:941–948.

40. Abreu BC, Seale G, Podlesak J, et al: Development of critical paths for post acute brain injury rehabilitation: Lessons learned. *Am J Occup Therapy* 1996; 50(6):417–427.

41. Rossiter D, Thompson AJ: Introduction of integrated care pathways for patients with multiple sclerosis in an inpatient neurorehabilitation setting. *Disability and Rehabilitation* 1995; 17(8):443–448.

42. Johnson AF: Two-year fellowship in medical speech-language pathology. Paper presented at the 1993 Convention of the American Speech-Language-Hearing Association, Anaheim, CA.

Appendix A
Inpatient Consultation
Competency Checklist

Preparation for the Consultation

_____ Medical chart review

_____ Working knowledge of pertinent medical and case history information

_____ Identification of the referral question

Appendix A   Inpatient Consultation Competency Checklist, *continued*

Plan for the examination
_____ List of differential diagnoses in rank order from most likely to least likely
_____ Selection of formal and informal test measures
_____ Organization/sequence of test administration

Examination and diagnostic testing
_____ Administration of formal tests/informal assessment measures
_____ Appropriate modifications in initial plan throughout examination
_____ Sufficient data to answer the referral question

Documentation: Generation of written consultation report
_____ Organization of report with subheadings representing the main areas tested
_____ Accurate diagnostic statement/impressions, including severity levels
_____ Suspected etiology of diagnostic impressions
_____ Classification of aphasia or dysarthria type
_____ Suspected lesion localization of the neurogenic communication disorder
_____ Recommendations appropriate to findings/impressions
_____ Recommendation for referral to other services if indicated
_____ Clear answer to the referral question

Follow-up/management issues
_____ Contact referring physician to report impressions/recommendations
_____ Arrange diagnostic/therapeutic examinations as indicated
       (e.g., videoflouroscopy)
_____ Repeated testing to monitor changes in communication disorders over time
_____ Ongoing patient/family counseling
_____ Treatment of communication disorders
_____ Discharge planning

Appendix B
Examples of Written
Consultation Reports

EXAMPLE 1

REFERRING SERVICE: Neurosurgery
INPATIENT UNIT: Intermediate Intensive Care Unit
DATE OF CONSULTATION: 2/1/97
REASON FOR CONSULTATION: 36-year-old male status post multiple gunshot wounds to the head with left frontoparietal hemorrhage and right frontal contusion. Please evaluate.

CONSULTANT'S REMARKS: The patient is a 36-year-old right-handed male admitted 1/17/97 status post multiple gunshot wounds to the head resulting in a left frontoparietal intracranial hemorrhage and right frontal contusion. Patient is now status post left frontotemporal craniotomy for evacuation of hematoma. Patient was intubated secondary to respiratory failure, extubated 1/31/97. Past medical history unremarkable.

<u>Clinical Examination:</u> Patient laying in bed, fully alert, oriented to person only based on yes/no responses with head nod. Good eye contact with examiner.

<u>Receptive Language:</u> Patient followed axial commands only, unable to follow commands involving extremities. Executed commands with left upper extremity

to imitation only. Reliable yes/no response with head nod to simple questions, unreliable for complex questions. Patient often gestured with left upper extremity to indicate that he did not understand questions/commands.

Expressive Language: Patient mute; no verbal output, no vocalizations, no phonation. Pt attempted to vocalize to command and imitation but was unable to phonate.

Oral Examination: Right facial weakness, tongue deviated to right on protrusion. Decreased left palatal elevation. Absent gag reflex.

Speech Production: No speech production, no phonation.

Swallowing: Excess secretions in oropharynx; patient unable to manage oral secretions. Spontaneous coughing on secretions × 2. Assessment of swallowing with food/liquid was deferred secondary to increased risk of aspiration.

IMPRESSION:
  1. Global aphasia with mutism
  2. Severe oropharyngeal dysphagia
  3. Oral/verbal apraxia (severe)
  4. Probable dysarthria

RECOMMENDATIONS:
  1. NPO/continue tube feedings
  2. Will follow for ongoing assessment and treatment of language/communication, speech and swallowing
  3. Recommend inpatient rehabilitation after discharge—patient is an excellent treatment candidate

Speech–language pathologist intervention during follow-up visits:

- Patient/family education and provision of communication strategies and "survival strategies" in addition to written educational material.

- Implementation of methods to increase vocalizations/verbal output and maximize auditory comprehension via strategies and environmental manipulation.

- Ongoing neurocommunicative monitoring with reclassification of aphasia from global to Broca's aphasia.

- Diagnosis and classification of dysarthria (spastic) once patient began verbalizing.

- Modified barium swallowing study one week after consultation; recommended soft diet.

- Patient discharged to inpatient rehabilitation facility, followed by outpatient therapy.

EXAMPLE 2

REFERRING SERVICE: Cardiothoracic Surgery
INPATIENT UNIT: Cardiac Intensive Care Unit
DATE OF CONSULTATION: 8/8/97
REASON FOR CONSULTATION: 51-year-old male status post coronary artery bypass graft followed by right cerebellar and right posterior parietal infarcts. Intubated for one month. Now awake—please evaluate swallowing and speech.

CONSULTANT'S REMARKS: Patient is a 51-year-old right-handed male admitted 6/28/97 with coronary artery disease. Patient underwent emergent coronary artery bypass graft at that time; now status post stroke × 2, anoxic/metabolic encephalopathy, serratia pneumonia, esophogitis, intubation × 32 days secondary to respiratory failure—extubated yesterday. Past medical history of myocardial infarction one week prior to admission, insulin-dependent diabetes mellitus, hypertension, congestive heart failure, coronary artery disease, chronic renal insufficiency. Patient is current NPO with PEG tube feedings. Referred for evaluation of speech and swallowing.

<u>Cognitive-Communication:</u> Patient sitting up in chair, fully alert. Minimally verbally responsive, provided one-word responses only. No eye contact with examiner. Oriented to name only; disoriented to place ("home"), month, year ("1966"), President. Patient followed simple commands only after multiple repetitions. Patient highly distractible with decreased attention. Limited exam due to decreased attention/responsiveness.

<u>Oral Examination:</u> Left facial weakness. Tongue protruded to left. Decreased right palatal elevation. Positive gag reflex. Nonproductive cough.

<u>Speech/Voice:</u> Harsh/breathy vocal quality. Low volume. Mildly imprecise articulation.

<u>Swallowing:</u> No delay in initiation of swallow. Positive laryngeal elevation. Patient immediately coughed after swallowing 2 cc's of water $\times$ 2. Wet voice after swallowing water.

IMPRESSION:
1. Severe oropharyngeal dysphagia with positive signs of aspiration on clinical exam.
2. Severe aphonia
   #1 and 2 most likely secondary to vocal fold dysfunction (? unilateral paralysis). Etiology: prolonged intubation vs. recurrent laryngeal nerve damage secondary to coronary artery bypass graft.
3. Cognitive-Communication impairment consistent with diffuse cerebral involvement (encephalopathy and ischemia)
4. Probable dysarthria given oromotor weakness

RECOMMENDATIONS:
1. Continue strict NPO status with PEG tube feedings
2. Recommend ENT consultation to rule out laryngeal pathology
3. We will follow patient for ongoing assessment and treatment of voice, swallowing, and cognitive functioning

Speech–language pathologist intervention during follow-up visits:

- Results of ENT consultation—bilateral vocal cord ulcerations. Etiology— prolonged intubation.
- Ongoing assessment of cognitive status and attempts to increase cognitive-communication (orientation, attention, awareness of circumstances).
- Patient/family counseling and education with provision of communication strategies and written information.
- Modified barium swallowing study 2 weeks after initial consultation; recommended soft diet with thickened liquids.
- Patient discharged to inpatient rehabilitation facility.

EXAMPLE 3

REFERRING SERVICE: Internal Medicine
INPATIENT UNIT: General medical floor

DATE OF CONSULTATION: 10/18/97
REASON FOR CONSULTATION: (not filled out by referring physician)

CONSULTANT'S REMARKS: Patient is an 87-year-old right-handed male admitted 10/16/97 status post shortness of breath and cough secondary to right pleural effusion and right mid/lower lobe pneumonia. Patient malnourished/cachectic on admission. Patient lives at home with his daughter. Per daughter, patient with difficulty swallowing >1 month prior to admission. Past medical history significant for prostate surgery. Referred for evaluation of swallowing safety.

Oral Examination: Mild right facial weakness. Tongue deviated mildly to right on protrusion. Left palatal weakness. Absent gag reflex.

Speech Production: Markedly increased rate of speech. Imprecise articulation and decreased speech intelligibility due to rapid speech production. Short rushes of speech. Monopitch/monoloudness. Harsh vocal quality.

Swallowing: Incomplete laryngeal elevation. Delayed initiation of swallow response. Immediate reflexive cough after 3/3 liquid swallows with subsequent wet vocal quality.

Cognitive-Communication: Patient fully alert and oriented. Screening of language and cognitive functions was within normal limits.

IMPRESSION:
1. Severe dysphagia with positive signs of aspiration on clinical examination, unsafe for oral intake.
2. Moderate hypokinetic dysarthria—Etiology most likely Parkinson's disease/basal ganglia lesion

RECOMMENDATIONS:
1. Modified Barium Swallowing Study—We will schedule for tomorrow
2. NPO pending swallowing study
3. Recommend neurology consultation to rule out neurological etiology of dysarthria/dysphagia
4. Will follow for management of speech/swallowing

Speech–language pathologist intervention during follow-up visits:
- Modified barium swallowing study revealed severe dysphagia with repeated aspiration and episodes of silent aspiration. PEG tube was recommended.
- Results of neurology consultation—Parkinson's disease.
- Patient/family counseling and education regarding speech/swallowing disorders. Provided with written material.
- Patient/family provided with low-tech augmentative communication devices/strategies.
- Patient discharged home with home health care.

Although speech and swallowing were not improved due to the speech–language pathologist's intervention (the goal in rehabilitation or outpatient settings), the patient did receive the appropriate care, nutritional services, and awareness of the cause of the speech and swallowing problems as a result of the intervention of the speech–language pathologist. The family became aware of their family history of Parkinson's disease, and they learned about the disease and its consequences. Therefore, the patient and family benefited from the speech–language pathologist consultation.

Appendix C
Checklist for Daily Monitoring of Patients with Communication Swallowing Disorder

Henry Ford Hospital					Patient Name: _____		
Speech–Language Sciences & Disorders					Medical Record No. _____		
Communication and Swallowing Monitoring System							
	Day 1	Day 2	Day 3	Day 4	Day 5		
Mental Status							
Alertness							
Orientation							
Attention							
Comments							
General Appearance/Behav.							
Hygiene							
Grooming							
Physical Appearance							
Mood							
Affect							
Comments							
Medical Status							
Temp.							
Pulse							
Respiration							
Blood Press.							
Condition							
Comments							
Medication Changes							
Comments							
Medical Devices							
Catheters							
Feed. Tubes							
IVs							
Ventilator							
Oxygen							
Glasses							
Hearing Aids							
Dentures							

	Day 1	Day 2	Day 3	Day 4	Day 5		
Motor							
Posture							
Abnormal Movements							
Weakness							
Tone							
Comments							
Insight/Awareness							
Patient							
Family							
Comments							
Testing Observations							
Distractibility							
Emotional Tolerance							
Response to cueing							
Strategy Use							
Practice Effects							
Auditory Modality							
Visual Modality							
Comments							
Motor Speech							
Voice							
Resonance							
Articulation							
Prosody							
Language							
Comprehension							
Production							
Repetition							
Naming							
Fluency							
Pragmatics							
Nonverbal Communication							
Discourse							
Reading							
Writing							
Swallowing							
Oral Feeding							
MBS Results							
Bedside Examination							

7

Issues in Geriatric Medicine

Thomas R. Palmer and Murray B. Hunter

CHAPTER OUTLINE

Issues in Treating the Elderly

Nutritional Needs of the Elderly

Non-Oral Feeding

Pneumonia in the Elderly

Delirium and Dementias

Ethical Issues in Geriatric Practice

Older adults are the most rapidly growing age group among Americans. As of the 1990 U.S. census, 12.5% of the population was 65 and older, and 1.2 % was 85 and older. By 2050, 20.4% of the population is projected to be 65 and over, and 4.8% of the total population age 85 and over[1] (see Figure 7–1). Thus, the "old old" group 85 and older is the most rapidly growing segment of senior adults. This is the group with the most functional and cognitive impairments and the need for professionals to help them will continue to increase.

Geriatrics is the area of medicine that deals with the elderly. Elderly people cannot be treated the same as if they were young adults who happen to be chronologically older. Because of physiological differences, a higher frequency of functional and cognitive impairments, a lack of physiological reserve, a higher frequency of multiple chronic illnesses, a greater number of sensory impairments, and an in-creased chance of being on multiple potentially interacting medications, the elderly must be approached in a specific age-appropriate manner. While these factors make adverse consequences of ill-advised treatments more likely, they also increase the beneficial impact of a well-chosen intervention. For functionally impaired bedridden older adults, for example, the simple act of becoming able to transfer from their bed to a wheelchair makes a tremendous difference in their enjoyment of life.

In this chapter, we will discuss issues that are specific to the management of illness in elderly persons, especially during hospitalization. These include nutritional status, non-oral feeding, pneumonia, dementia and delirium, and ethical considerations. Although this is not meant to be an exhaustive coverage of geriatric medicine, we have highlighted the most frequently occurring conditions and concerns for this group of patients.

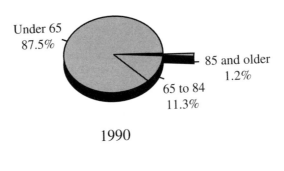

1990

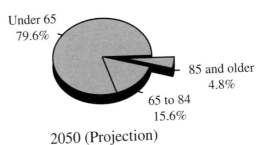

2050 (Projection)

Figure 7–1. Percent distribution of elderly in the United States. *Source:* U.S. Bureau of the Census: *Statistical Abstract of the United States: 1995.* (115th ed.) Washington, DC, 1995

ISSUES IN TREATING THE ELDERLY

The frail elderly are the group most in need of an age-specific, multidisciplinary approach. Frail elderly can be defined as those with a diminished ability to carry out the important practical and social activities of daily living.[2] Many factors can contribute to frailty,[3] and the more factors present, the more dependent a person is likely to be (Table 7–1). Certain problems are more common in the elderly. These include polypharmacy, dementia and delirium, fecal and urinary incontinence, arthritis, visual and hearing deficits, pressure ulcers, malnutrition, osteoporosis, and falls. Because the multiple, complex issues involved in their care are more than an individual professional can deal with alone, these patients benefit from a multidisciplinary team approach to their care.

Functional Status

The most important objective in the care of the elderly is to maximize functional status. For example, there is no value in giving an older person a medicine to help normalize an abnormal laboratory value if in the process they become stiff and unable to walk to the bathroom or if a mild degree of confusion becomes more severe as a result. Assessing functional status is more important than documenting physical findings such as arthritis of the knees or a heart murmur. Functional status is

Table 7–1. Criteria for Frailty

Cerebrovascular accident

Chronic *and* disabling illness

Confusion

Dependence in ADLs

Depression

Falls

Impaired mobility

Incontinence

Malnutrition

Polypharmacy

Pressure sore

Prolonged bedrest

Restraints

Sensory impairment

Socioeconomic/family problems

Source: From Winograd CH, Gerety MB, et al: Screening for frailty: Criteria and predictors of outcomes. *J Am Geriatr Soc* 1991; 39:778–784.

the end result of multiple interacting factors including illnesses, cognitive problems, medicines, nutrition, and social interaction that combine to affect the person's overall wellness.

Functional status is commonly defined by a person's ability to perform the "activities of daily living" (ADLs) and the "instrumental activities of daily living" (IADLs). In the commonly used Katz scale of ADLs, transfers (such as from bed to a wheelchair), dressing, bathing, toileting, continence, and feeding are all evaluated to see whether individuals can do the activity independently, need help, or are totally dependent.[4] To be able to safely live alone without help, a person must be independent in activities of daily living. Likewise, an improvement in the ability to perform ADLs adds to independence and quality of life. The instrumental activities of daily living are using the telephone, traveling, shopping, preparing meals, doing housework, taking medication, and handling money.[5] Assessment of ADLs is also useful in determining how much help a person might need and in monitoring decline or improvement in function over time.

Polypharmacy

Polypharmacy refers to the tendency of many older people to be on numerous medications. Every medicine has potential side effects. For example, nonsteroidal anti-inflammatory drugs such as ibuprofen can cause gastric ulceration (sometimes with bleeding), kidney impairment, edema, liver enzyme elevation, drowsiness, and dizziness—among other side effects. Medicines can also have potential side effects as a result of interactions with other drugs. Ibuprofen can decrease the effect of the diuretic furosemide due to a specific drug interaction. When ibuprofen is taken with the anticoagulant warfarin, the chances of gastrointestinal bleeding are greatly increased over what might be expected from each drug independently. Thus, each additional medicine that a person takes not only can cause side effects by itself, but also from drug–drug interactions. The more medicines a person is taking, the greater the risk of having a single adverse drug reaction. The risk of adverse drug interactions increases exponentially as the number of medicines increases.[6]

Another complication of polypharmacy is the increased risk of noncompliance with taking prescribed medicines. Medication costs may consume a larger proportion of a senior's income, which may be limited. Older persons faced with taking a handful of pills several times a day may more easily decide that they need not take them. Medicare benefits do not presently cover prescribed medicines.

For these reasons, medicines should only be given to older people if they are clearly needed and clearly benefiting the recipient. Over-the-counter medicines must also be considered when reviewing an elderly person's medications. A helpful strategy is to ask the patient or family to place all the medicines being used in a bag and to bring them to appointments or to the hospital. Often, a medicine will emerge that was not previously mentioned. Removing unneeded medicines can result in an improvement in daily functioning or in cognition.

NUTRITIONAL NEEDS OF THE ELDERLY

Dietary Requirements

In general, the nutritional needs of healthy elderly people do not differ much from those of younger healthy adults. The major physiologic changes that occur with aging are a decrease in total body protein, an increase in the proportion of total body fat with a redistribution of fat stores, a reduction in total body water, and a decrease in bone density.[7] Despite the decreased body protein, dietary protein requirements are greater in the elderly than in younger adults.[8] Total energy expenditure is slightly reduced in older women compared to younger women, but about 20% less in older men compared to younger men. The elderly also have a lower resting metabolic rate,[9] which results in less caloric intake being required in the elderly on average. An average calorie requirement for a bed-bound senior to maintain weight is 25 Kcals per kg of body weight. If malnourished, a goal for nutrient intake is 35 Kcals per kg.[10] At least 10% of the calories in the elderly should consist of fat to assure adequate fat-soluble vitamins and essential fatty acids. Usually, this is not a problem since the average American diet consists of 40% fat.[7] Carbohydrates should be of the complex variety, which are less easily digested and add bulk to the stool, and constitute 55 to 60% of calories.[7] Fiber is most easily added in the form of fresh fruits and vegetables, but may also be given as bran supplements, cereals, or psyllium.

Hydration

Drinking fluids is a natural part of life and young adults have no difficulty responding to their thirst sensation by drinking more fluids. The elderly, however, have more problems with dehydration due to various physiological as well as situational causes. Thirst sensation is not as reliable as in younger people and the kidneys do not concentrate urine as well. Often because of problems with incontinence or edema, the elderly purposely may not drink as much as they should. Conditions such as dementia or immobility may prevent adequate fluid intake. Diuretic medicines may contribute to the problem. Hot weather, exercise, or febrile illness may more easily combine with all the above conditions to cause dehydration. Dehydration can often be prevented by educating the elderly person and encouraging fluid intake.

Vitamins

Some vitamins whose lack cause concern in the elderly are B_{12}, C, D, and folate. Vitamin B_{12} deficiency can occur from dietary deficiency, medication interactions, atrophic gastritis, or pernicious anemia and result in anemia, peripheral neuropathy, unsteadiness in walking, and dementia. It is one of the reversible causes of dementia and a part of the laboratory screen for evaluating dementia. Replacement can be given with an intramuscular injection, if poor absorption is the cause, or orally. Vitamin C is a water-soluble vitamin often found to be deficient in the elderly. Deficiency can cause capillary fragility and poor wound healing. Vitamin D is most important in calcium metabolism, and exposure of the skin to sunlight helps convert it to its active form. Deficiency is most common in immobile elderly people in nursing homes or at home with little exposure to sunlight. Replacement is important to optimize calcium absorption and the typical multivitamin contains 400 IU of Vitamin D, which is enough to assure adequate amounts. Folate deficiency also can cause anemia. Absorption of folic acid is decreased by ulcer medicines that lower gastric acidity such as antacids.[11]

Malnutrition

Malnutrition is more common in the elderly, especially the frail elderly. It should be suspected in any thin or frail appearing senior. In its more severe form, it may present as the cachexia seen in end-stage cancer, heart disease, and other illnesses. In cachexia there is severe muscle wasting and atrophy, with prominent bones and a concave abdomen. The goal, however, is to identify malnutrition at an early stage, when intervention may be of most benefit.

Risk Factors

There are many risk factors for malnutrition (see Table 7–2). Alcoholism occurs in the elderly, and appropriate screening questions should be asked in any malnourished person. Persons with even a

Table 7–2. Malnutrition Risk Factors

Alcoholism

Dementia

Depression

Psychosis

Illness causing decreased appetite

Impaired taste, smell, or vision

Polypharmacy

Poor functional status

Poor dentition or edentulous

Poor nutritional knowledge

Limited finances

Living alone and social isolation

Source: From Rauscher C: Malnutrition among the elderly. *Canadian Family Physician* 1993: 39:1395–1403.

mild dementia may forget whether they have eaten and may not prepare an adequate meal. Those with more advanced dementias are usually thin and often have aphasia, agnosia (the failure to recognize sensory stimuli), and apraxia (difficulty with automatic movements)—all have a major effect on eating.[12] A lack of appetite is one of the symptoms used in the diagnosis of major depression and, as it improves, the appetite typically improves. Other mental illness (such as psychosis) commonly affects one's ability to function, thus impairing the ability to prepare or eat food.

Many medical illnesses, both acute and chronic, affect the appetite adversely. In addition, some conditions cause increased nutritional needs, such as wound healing and hyperthyroidism. Impaired sensory input is common in the elderly, and impaired taste, smell, or vision can make it more of a chore to eat than an enjoyment. When teeth are in poor condition or absent and dentures are ill fitting, it may be easier to eat less than to find foods of a texture and nutritional value that can be chewed and ingested well.

As functional status decreases, the risk for malnutrition increases. An inability to shop or prepare meals (IADLs) may result in less food with less variety on the table at mealtime. Difficulty transferring to the table and feeding (ADLs) will also impair nutrition.

Medicines can either independently or via drug–drug interactions adversely affect appetite. Many medicines, including some common antidepressants such as amitryptyline, have anticholinergic side effects that result in dryness of the mouth. Anti-inflammatory medicines for arthritis might cause anorexia from irritation of the stomach or small intestine. Most antibiotics can cause gastric upset. This risk is another reason for older persons to be taking only essential medications.

Knowledge of good nutrition is important for all older people, including the importance of eating foods from the basic food groups. This knowledge may be less available to those from minority groups, especially if they need to follow a special diet for a medical condition incorporating their preferred ethnic foods.[13] Special diets (renal, low salt, low fat, or diabetic) are often tasteless. The need for a certain diet for a medical condition must be balanced against the need for adequate nutrition, especially in the frail elderly. Poor elderly may not have enough money remaining after other expenses to afford an adequate diet. The less human contact a person has, the easier it is for harmful nutritional patterns to continue. Social isolation and living alone are risk factors for malnutrition. Elderly persons may have several risk factors for malnutrition at the same time, and the more factors present, the greater the risk.

Measurement of Nutritional Status

Malnutrition can be suspected by clinical appearance, as mentioned earlier. Certain measurements give more objectivity to the evaluation and can be followed serially in an individual to show improvement or deterioration over time. Body weight is the most basic measurement. A significant weight loss over time is an important indicator of malnutrition (see Table 7–3). Malnutrition can also be suspected in anyone over 65 with a body mass index (BMI) less than 22. BMI is defined as the weight in kilograms divided by the height in meters squared. A desirable BMI is 22 to 27; a BMI over 27 suggests obesity.[13] Triceps skinfold (TSF) measurement is a measure of subcutaneous fat using calipers, but is less reliable in older people because of physical changes with aging such as a redistribution of fat.[14] Mid-arm muscle circumference can be calculated using standardized tables from the mid-arm circumference measurement. A mid-arm muscle circumference falling below the 10th percentile indicates poor nutritional status.[14]

Albumin is a simple protein found in blood that is a good indicator of nutritional status. Like all indicators of malnutrition, it is not perfect and has some limitations. Because of its relatively long half-life it is a reasonable measure of nutritional status during the previous month or so, but not over the previous few days. Conditions such as dehydration

Table 7–3. Important Indicators of Malnutrition

Body Mass Index (BMI) = Wt(Kg)/(Ht(m))2
  <22 = probable malnourished
  22 to 27 = desirable
  >27 = obese

Serum albumin
  Normal 4.0 to 6.5, <3.5 suggestive of protein calorie malnutrition

Total lymphocyte count
  Total white cell count × % lymphocytes in differential
  <1500 is significant

Significant weight loss over time
  >5.0% of body weight in 1 month
  >7.5% of body weight in 3 months
  >10.0% of body weight in 6 months
  >10 pounds of involuntary weight loss in 6 months

Source: From Barrocas A, et al: Nutrition assessment practical approaches. *Clin Geriatric Med* 1995; 11(4):675–713.

may cause it to appear to be higher than it really is. Normal levels are 4.0 to 6.0 gm/dl and levels less than 3.5 gm/dl are suggestive of protein calorie malnutrition. Serum albumin levels less than 2.5 gm/dl have been shown to be helpful prognostic indicators for a limited life expectancy.[15]

Serum albumin levels are also important in certain drug actions. For example, the anticonvulsant phenytoin is a seizure medication that partly binds to albumin in the blood. However, the active portion of phenytoin is the unbound portion. When elderly malnourished patients are given phenytoin, they need a smaller dose because of the lower amount of albumin available to bind the drug, leaving a larger unbound active portion.

Other useful laboratory measures suggesting malnutrition include the total lymphocyte count and hemoglobin. Lymphocytes are a type of white blood cell. Total lymphocyte counts less than 1500 can be caused by malnutrition. Hemoglobin measures the red blood cell concentration. It normally ranges from 12.0 to 16.0 gm/dl in women and from 14.0 to 18.0 gm/dl in men. In malnutrition, the body is not able to make enough red blood cells and a mild anemia with normal sized red blood cells is common. Specific nutritional deficiencies of B_{12} and folate also may cause anemias, but the red cells are usually larger than normal in these cases.

Treatment of Malnutrition

Once a senior is found to be malnourished, or at nutritional risk, solutions vary as much as causes. A simple generic multivitamin taken daily is an inexpensive way to help specific deficiencies such as lack of Vitamin D. Finding ways to help increase food intake with a diet that is tasty but also nutritious is important. Community programs such as Meals on Wheels and congregate nutrition programs are nutritionally helpful; they also provide regular social contact to elders who might otherwise be more isolated. Commercial nutrition supplements can be used for those unable to eat a regular diet and feeding tubes considered for those unable to take adequate food and liquids orally.

NON-ORAL FEEDING

William Beaumont, a physician assigned to Mackinac Island, Michigan, in 1822, treated a French trapper who had suffered a shotgun wound to his abdomen. It healed leaving a direct opening to his stomach. Beaumont did experiments putting various substances, such as meat, into the stomach and observing what happened.[16] In a similar way percutaneous endoscopic gastrostomy (PEG) tubes deliver nutrition via a tube through a hole in the abdominal wall into the stomach. Their placement has become so technically easy that the current protocol might be described as "the patient can't swallow safely or is malnourished; therefore, place a feeding tube." This attitude among health professionals should be discarded and replaced. A more appropriate process should include a thorough discussion of both the risks and benefits of feeding tubes with patients or their decision makers, so they can make an informed decision.

Nutrition not taken by mouth can be divided into two main groups: parenteral and enteral. Parenteral nutrition is given intravenously into either a peripheral vein, or more commonly into a large central vein such as the jugular or subclavian. A central vein allows hypertonic (more concentrated) solutions to be infused. It bypasses the gastrointestinal system. Enteral nutrition refers to nutrition given directly into the gastrointestinal system, allowing more natural absorption of nutrients to occur. It can be given through nasogastric (NG) tubes manually placed, PEG or percutaneous endoscopic jejunostomy (PEJ) tubes placed endoscopically, and gastrostomy or jejunostomy tubes placed surgically or percutaneously with radiologic guidance (Figure 7–2).

Parenteral Nutrition

Parenteral nutrition is indicated in elderly patients needing nutritional supplementation with contraindications to enteral nutrition. The only absolute contraindication to enteral nutrition is mechanical obstruction of the small or large intestine. Relative contraindications include massive small bowel resection and acute pancreatitis.[17] Parenteral nutrition is often used after attempts at enteral nutrition have failed or had complications or after major abdominal surgery. Ideally, it is employed for a short time and discontinued once enteral nutrition can be resumed. Complications include pneumothorax or bleeding during placement of the central line, infection, and venous thrombosis. Confused elderly patients may require restraints or sedation to keep them from pulling out the intravenous line.

Enteral Nutrition

Nasogastric Tubes

Nasogastric tubes are commonly used in hospital and nursing home settings. The standard rigid polyvinyl tube is uncomfortable and can be irritating to the nasal, esophageal, and gastric tissues. Smaller, more flexible tubes made of silicone or polyurethane are more comfortable and thought to be less irritating to the oropharynx, esophagus, and esophageal sphincter.[18]

In addition to discomfort, NG tubes can cause various complications. The tube can be placed inadvertently into the respiratory tract, a potentially lethal problem if nutritional supplements are infused through it. This can be checked by chest X-ray, physical exam, or aspiration of gastric contents to determine pH. Tracheobronchial secretions tend to be alkaline with a pH over 7 while gastric aspirates usually have an acidic pH less than 5.19. Aspiration can occur in patients with NG tubes and gastrointestinal bleeding can result from tube irritation. As with all feeding devices, restraints may be required to keep patients from pulling them out. When restraints are used, there is increased risk for pressure sores, loss of mobility, incontinence, and delirium.

Gastrostomy/Jejunostomy Tubes

Gastrostomy or jejunostomy tubes are preferred for long-term enteral nutrition. With their use, patients no longer have to deal with the nasopharyngeal irritation associated with NG tubes. With intermittent bolus feeding, clothing can cover the tube when the patient is not receiving feedings, allowing fuller freedom to participate in activities without being obvious to others that there is a tube

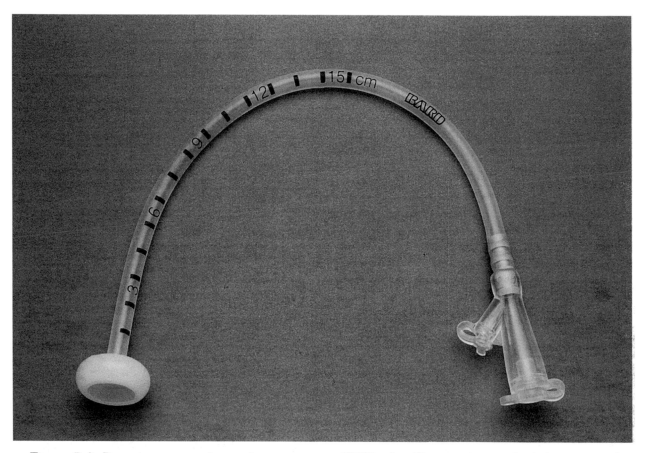

Figure 7–2. Percutaneous endoscopic gastrostomy (PEG) tube. The opening on the left is inserted inside the stomach. The opening on the right is outside the abdomen. Photo courtesy of Bard International Products, Billerica, MA.

present. In those with a tendency to pull tubes out, an abdominal binder can be used to lessen this possibility.

Complications

Gastrostomy tubes have numerous potential complications associated with their use (see Table 7–4). Aspiration can still occur despite precautions such as elevating the head of the bed 30 to 45°.[19] Studies have found rates of aspiration pneumonia to be 23 to 58% in patients with PEG or PEJ tubes.[18] Wound infection or bleeding can occur immediately postoperatively or long after the tube has been inserted. Bleeding might be related to irritation of the gastric or intestinal lining, resulting in ulceration either adjacent to the tube or where the tube tip hits the mucosa. Diarrhea can occur from hyperosmolar formula, rapid bolus feedings, and lactose intolerance. Strategies for alleviating diarrhea include using a more dilute formula, switching to continuous pump feedings, and using a lactose-free formula.[20] Most commercial formulas are lactose free.

Table 7–4. Common Potential Problems with Gastrostomy Tubes

Large residual volume

Wound infection

Aspiration

Bleeding

Diarrhea

Tube obstruction

Tube leakage

Accidental tube removal

Peritube leakage

Hyponatremia or hypernatremia

Restraint use to prevent removal
  Resulting in immobility
  Leading to pressure sores
  Causing agitation

Source: From O'Keefe KP: Complication of percutaneous feeding tubes. *Emer Med Clin NA,* 1994; 12(3): 815–826.

Blocked feeding tubes are a recurrent problem. The blockage may occur from precipitation of medicines given through the tube or from formula solidifying. This is most common with continuous feedings. Periodic flushing as often as every 4 hours with water is the best preventative.[20] Once blockage occurs, irrigation of the tube with cola sometimes unplugs it, but often the only solution is replacing the feeding tube, which may involve another surgical intervention depending on which type of device is present.

Confused patients may pull the tube out, or it may otherwise come out. Once this occurs, the opening quickly closes within hours, again requiring a hospital visit to replace it. Large residual volumes in the stomach are commonly due to gastric atony (a lack of peristaltic waves in the stomach) or other problems. If gastric atony has been identified as the cause, medicines are available that can help. Peritube leakage is more likely to occur with large gastric volumes, but most often results from a chronic infection at the abdominal opening leading to a gradual increase in the size of that opening. Finally, because of the loss of volitional control over intake, fluid imbalance with hyponatremia, hypernatremia, overhydration, and dehydration can occur.

Issues in Decision Making

When a feeding tube is being considered for a patient with a chronic illness, it is important to share all available information with the patient and his or her family. If decision-making capacity is not intact, a surrogate decision maker needs to be involved. The insertion of a feeding tube is such a major decision that, ideally, a meeting should be scheduled so all interested family members can be present. The topic of the meeting should be shared with family and caregivers so that they can be prepared with questions and concerns. It is also wise to have present as many members of the care team as possible to give the perspective of different disciplines and provide the various implications of tube placement.

A number of questions must be answered by the care team and family members to help arrive at the best decision regarding tube placement (see Table 7–5). It is important to know the underlying condition that resulted in feeding tube placement. In addition, the prognosis based on the illness needs to be known. For example, a benign stricture of the esophagus in a functionally active person would have a very different prognosis than dys-

Table 7–5. Feeding Tubes—Questions to Ask

What are the underlying illnesses?

What is the prognosis?

Is the tube needed short or long term?

Is the patient's decision-making capacity intact?

Is there an advance directive or living will?

Did the patient ever express opinions on feeding tubes in the past?

Do the benefits outweigh the risks?

Are there any medical contraindications?

Would a trial of tube feeding be useful?

What are the alternatives?

Is life expectancy 6 months or less? (Hospice appropriate)

phagia in a bedridden, aphasic patient with end-stage Alzheimer's disease. If the need for a tube is expected to be short term—to get over a pneumonia in an otherwise healthy senior, for example—that need would be much clearer than in one with a progressive terminal illness.

If decision-making capacity is intact, patients can decide for themselves, after being given all the information. If they are grossly confused, then family or a guardian will need to make the decision. Advance directives or living wills are very helpful in establishing a cognitively impaired patient's wishes. These documents might be at home or in a safe deposit box and often are not present at the hospital. If they are not available, then the family should be asked about whether the patient ever expressed any opinions about feeding tubes in the past when he or she was cognitively intact.

The benefits as well as the risks of feeding tubes should be discussed by the care team. Sometimes a temporary trial of tube feeding is warranted. Ethically, there is no difference between not starting a feeding tube and discontinuing one when it has been shown to be of no benefit. Despite this, families often have great difficulty in asking for tube feedings to be stopped once they have begun, regardless of whether they are helpful or harmful. Therefore, it is best to have this discussion in the beginning, rather than presenting it as an afterthought.

Finally, it is important to discuss the alternatives to enteral feeding tubes for those with a limited life expectancy. Pureed diets fed in small amounts at a time are usually tolerated, and they can give a great deal of oral satisfaction. The risks of pleasure eating for patients with severe dysphagia should always be presented; however, the patient and family can understand the relative significance of this risk in the context of the patient's overall health. If the underlying disease gives a life expectancy of less than 6 months when the illness follows its usual course, then the hospice approach should also be discussed as an alternative at this time. For many, being unrestrained and able to take small amounts of food orally is preferable to being restrained to be kept from pulling out the tube, drugged to treat the resulting agitation, and developing pressure sores from the resulting immobility during the last days of one's life. These are common and unfortunate results from decisions for feeding tubes in terminally ill seniors.

Eating and feeding are basic to the human condition, and decisions regarding feeding tubes are often difficult for family members. By using a supportive, patient approach the care team can help the decision maker to make a choice based on facts as well as emotion. When prior counseling has taken place, it is easier for the care team to be supportive of whatever choice has been made and then work with the patient to provide the best care given that choice. Ongoing contact with the family is important as changes in status occur. After the initial discussion, patients and families have the information to modify or change their decisions if they so desire.

PNEUMONIA IN THE ELDERLY

The prevention, diagnosis, and management of pneumonia in the geriatric population remains ill understood and controversial despite the proliferation of "pathways," algorithms, and a long tradition of practice and research of this disease. Pneumonia has been seen as the final common lot of the frail elderly, but efforts to reverse or ameliorate this condition have not met with success. The topics that will be covered in this section include: modes of infection, aspiration, diagnostic determinants of pneumonia, community-acquired vs. nosocomial infection, and treatment and prevention issues.

Modes of Infection

The body's response to bacterial invasion ranges from clearance of the offending organisms to overwhelming infection. Bacterial colonization precedes infection. Colonization is the result of inadequate host defense and both immunological and local/ mechanical failures of clearance. A persistent source of bacteria is a predictor of eventual pneumonia. The source may be the nasopharynx in the young, but in the elderly it is almost always located in the oropharynx. Progression of colonization to pneumonia requires additional events and circumstances. Prior respiratory viral infection, a history of smoking, previous antibiotic therapy, malnutrition, and serious illness combine with failure of immune reponse in the elderly to prepare the host for pneumonia. Immobility alone increases the rate of colonization in frail individuals. Excessive pharyngeal secretions, provoked by any kind of enteral feeding device, provide a favorable milieu for bacterial colonization.

Evidence of impaired defense against infection in the elderly includes frequent absence of fever and leukocytosis and diminished cough and expectoration. Tachypnea, tachycardia, and altered cognitive states are the more usual warning signs than fever and elevated white count. In one study, a rise in respiratory rate preceded the clinical diagnosis of pneumonia by 3 to 4 days.[21] Physical signs are often absent in geriatric pneumonias.

Aspiration

Virtually all pneumonia at any age is aspiration pneumonia. This conceptual unity in the understanding of pneumonia has been relatively late in coming. In earlier decades, aspiration pneumonia referred to dramatic instances of large bolus delivery of gastric contents into the respiratory tract as a consequence of alcoholic stupor with vomiting, or with vomiting as a consequence of an illness associated with impaired consciousness from any cause. The offending organisms were thought to be principally Klebsiella and/or anaerobes. The locus of subsequent infection in classic large bolus aspiration pneumonia is the right lower or upper lobe. Large-volume aspiration is actually an uncommon event in seniors. The issue appears to be chronic low-volume aspiration.

Aspiration is the way that colonization of the oropharynx leads to pneumonia. Aspiration is a failure of insulation of the respiratory tract from the gastrointestinal tract. In the elderly, swallowing deficits are most often the result of neurogenic dysfunction. Misdirection of both the food bolus and secretions may occur as a product of impaired consciousness, motor dysfunction (oral and pharyngeal), deficits in sphincter function, ineffectual transport, and slowed esophageal propulsion. The problem is compounded by diminished receipt of sensory impulses and subsequent poor cough to clear the pharynx. Deep sleep favors aspiration, and the use of sedatives constitutes a pneumonia hazard.

Diagnostic Determinants of Pneumonia

Pneumonia is diagnosed during the clinical examination, by X-ray, and through the laboratory. Tubular breathing (breathing characterized by a high "whistling" sound), percussion dullness, and pulmonary rales are the exception in seniors rather than the rule. The chest X-ray radiograph is, however, often far from the gold standard that some clinicians believe it to be. The best X-ray in the evaluation of possible pneumonia is the previous one, ideally obtained at a time of relatively good health and function. Baseline chest film abnormalities abound. One seldom achieves the age of 70 or older without some previous opacity at the costophrenic angles. A proper film may confirm this possibility.

Seniors who get pneumonia have more parapneumonic effusions on the chest film than younger patients. When possible, thoracentesis should be done as an aid in diagnosis, and both chemical and bacteriologic tests performed on the aspirate to ensure precision in diagnosis. The chest tap should be followed by a repeat film with cross table lateral views. Radiologists are most aware of the vagaries of X-ray diagnosis of pneumonia. The now current euphemism of "air space disease" is a consequence of the acknowledged eccentricities in pneumonia diagnosis. The problem is compounded by the frequent presence of coexistent congestive heart failure in seniors with pneumonia. Prior fibrotic disease and other fixed distortions of lung architecture may be present. Diaphragmatic distortion is frequently seen in seniors with infradiaphragmatic difficulties, past or present, and in those with chronic obstructive lung disease. Repeat chest films are seldom of value. It has long been known that clinical changes precede radiological change.

The frequency of bacteremia in pneumonia, particularly in the aged, must be noted. The positive blood culture, if truly caused by the pneumonia, is the clearest guide to antibiotic therapy. What first must be established is the source of the bacteremia. In frail seniors, skin breakdown commonly provokes bacteremia. Urinary tract infection is a more common co-morbidity that may produce positive blood cultures. In any of these three scenarios the antibiotic prescription will likely be the same. What is being treated is the blood culture regardless of the source of the infection.[22]

Sputum culture is rarely of value as a guide to diagnosis or treatment. Gram stains are possibly more valuable, although both are fraught with collection error. As noted above, the white count may be normal and there is likely to be a paucity of immature neutrophils on the differential count. Very high white counts are more often the product of urinary sepsis than of pneumonia.

Influence of Enteral Feeding Devices

The presence of enteral feeding tubes, whether the traditional large or small bore nasogastric tubes or the newer percutaneous endogastric or endojejunal devices, is a risk factor for pneumonia.[20] Endogastric tubes may enhance reflux, particularly under circumstances of high gastric residuals, after PEG tube feeding. No tube prevents aspiration. The jejunostomy route may at least in theory help to prevent pneumonia. Nonetheless these patients also demonstrate increased reflux. Acid gastric contents favor the development of gram-negative bacteria in the oropharynx and trachea, but elevation of the gastric pH by H2 blockers or by alkaline pH feeding tube formulas increases the risk of bacterial overgrowth. If the clinical situation impels gastric mucosal protection, sucralfate, which does not affect pH, is probably the agent of choice. In any case, bleeding from the gut carries a less ominous prognosis than does pneumonia.

The value dilemma in the decision as to whether or not to institute enteral feeding is between meeting the nutritional needs of the patient against the threat of heightening susceptibility to pneumonia. This decision should not be made under circumstances of acute status change. Many patients who fail tests of swallowing may recover this function after acute systemic stress has been alleviated. The enteral tube decision is contextual in nature and should not be made reflexively after a failed swallowing challenge. Delirium, in particular, is always an acute event and its presence is not relevant to the enteral feeding decision.

Community-Acquired and Nosocomial Infection

Pneumonia is often described in terms of the location where it was acquired. "Community-acquired" pneumonia refers to infection that occurs while the patient is not institutionalized and living at home. "Nosocomial" pneumonia is contracted while the patient is hospitalized. The distinction is useful in the original choice of antibiotic therapy prior to receipt of culture data because typically each type of pneumonia tends to be caused by different organisms. But otherwise the distinction may not be important. Both are associated with the aspiration of oropharyngeal microflora and the community in which both are operative is the oropharynx. Institutionally acquired lung infection may be more often associated with gram-negative bacteria. Community pathogens such as chlamydia, H. influenza, mycoplasma, and legionella are seldom seen in seniors admitted for pneumonia. The offending agents in hospital-acquired pneumonia are most commonly staphyloccus or pseudomonas, and initial treatment in this circumstance should cover these pathogens.

Issues in Treatment and Prevention

One does not have to be a historian of biological science to appreciate the fact that recommendations for treatment of pneumonia often change. Even penicillin for pneumoccocus is now somewhat in disrepute. Today, treatment for pneumonia generally begins with a second-generation cephalosporin. Aminogycosides are relatively if not absolutely problematic because of the high incidence of renal impairment in the elderly. Mezlocillin is now active against a variety of gram-negative organisms. Vancomycin is indicated for staphyloccal disease. Clindamycin may be used when anaerobic infection is present. The frequency of antibiotic-associated diarrhea is high with this medication. Imipemen and metranidazole are now commonly employed for refractory infection. Mortality is still high in pneumonia, and treatment failure is seldom due to poor choice of antibiotics but rather to the influence of co-morbidities such as other illness, hypotension, urinary incontinence, alcoholism, and absence of fever.[23]

Preventive maneuvers that are clearly valid include rigorous requirement of hand washing by staff after each patient encounter. Use of H2 blockers should be discouraged. New enteral intubation should never be instituted in the context of current treatment for pneumonia. There is as yet no solid evidence whether feeding tubes already in place should be removed with the supervention of pneumonia. The head of the bed should be elevated in patients with pneumonia and sedatives should not be given. Appropriate antibiotic therapy should be instituted without delay in accordance with the above guidelines. Blood gas determinations should be done in all cases.

Finally, to improve the outcome in pneumonia, careful management of confounding patholo-gies must be vigorously applied. Congestive heart failure must be kept high on the indices of suspicion. Most patients at risk of death from pneumonia will have either cardiac, renal, or cutaneous co-morbidities. Staff who attend geriatric patients with pneumonia must be familiar with atypical presentations, atypical host responses, and the common presence of inadequate tracheopharyngeal function.

DELIRIUM AND DEMENTIAS

As the number of older individuals increases, the number of people with confusional states is also increasing. An understanding of these conditions is important for any health care professional dealing with the elderly. Though cure is usually not available for a dementia, delirium can often be reversed. As with other problems in older people, a measured and considered approach in assessment and treatment will make encounters more rewarding for clinicians and patients and their families.

Delirium is defined as a disturbance of consciousness accompanied by a change in cognition that cannot be accounted for by a preexisting or evolving dementia.[24] Disturbance of consciousness is characterized by an inability to focus on or pay attention to surroundings and a fluctuating level of alertness. For example, you may introduce yourself to the patient and he or she appears to be wide awake and appropriate. Fifteen seconds later, however, this patient might be asleep or rolling the edge of the sheet and not aware of your presence. Delirium has an onset over a relatively short period of time: hours to days. Delirium is often encountered in hospitalized elderly patients. It is important to obtain a history of the patient's baseline functional and cognitive status prior to the illness and hospitalization from a family member or friend. If it was significantly better previously, it is likely that delirium is present. If the presence of delirium is missed, its cause may be overlooked, and the outcome is not likely to be as positive.

Delirium is more common in patients with dementias. For that reason, even if a senior has an established diagnosis of Alzheimer's disease, for example, one should always be aware of the possibility of a concurrent delirium. This awareness allows one to remove any possible contributing factors and help improve the patient's functional or cognitive state.

Possible contributing factors to delirium are numerous and several can be present at one time (see Table 7–6). Illness itself can cause delirium,

Table 7–6. Causes of Delirium

Illness
  Infections
  Metabolic (hypoglycemia, hypoxia, hypercarbia)
  Fluid or electrolyte imbalance
  Hepatic or renal disease
  Thiamine deficiency
  Post ictal

Postsurgical

Change in location

Alteration in sensory cues
  "Sundowner's"

Medicines

Toxins

Withdrawal effects
  Alcohol
  Sedatives, hypnotics, anxiolytics

Source: From DSM-IV Diagnostic and Statistical Manual of Mental Disorders, 4th ed. American Psychiatric Association, Washington, DC, 1994.

and a change in behavior or cognition in a frail elderly person can often be the first sign of an illness. Infections such as pneumonia can present with an onset of confused behavior, but with no fever and cough, in frail, elderly persons. Metabolic causes of delirium such as hypoglycemia, hypoxia, and hypercarbia can be assessed with laboratory tests. Dehydration and hyponatremia or hypernatremia usually result in a decreased level of consciousness. Severe hepatic or renal disease can cause delirium. Thiamine deficiency is common in alcoholics and can cause an acute Wernicke's syndrome, with confusion. Treatment with thiamine is standard in alcoholics to help prevent this. Finally, after a seizure, people commonly have a post ictal state during which drowsiness and confusion are present.

Postsurgical patients can have delirium from the anesthesia, the stress of the illness or surgery itself, or from pain medicines or other medicines given postoperatively. A move to a new location can commonly elicit delirium. This might occur at a new home or during a hospitalization. The confusion is augmented by factors such as a different bathroom location, variation in routine, and new social contacts. When sensory cues are altered (e.g., when it becomes dark and dim), delirium can ensue. Sundowner's syndrome refers to confusion with its onset after nightfall. Typically, patients had no or fewer symptoms of delirium during the day.

One of the most common causes of delirium is adverse effects of medicines. Any psychoactive

drug should be considered a possible cause, including antidepressants, antianxiety medicines, antipsychotics, opioid medications, and lithium (for use in manic-depressive illness). Drugs such as cocaine, marijuana, barbiturates, and alcohol can also cause delirium as a direct effect. Drugs including alcohol, sedatives, hypnotics, and antianxiety medicines can cause delirium as a withdrawal effect: e.g., delirium tremens due to alcohol withdrawal. Any medicine with anticholinergic effects, of which there are many, can cause delirium. Antihistamines that can be obtained over the counter are in this group. Antihypertensives such as propranolol, methyldopa, hydrochlorothiazide, cimetidine (for stomach ulcer), digoxin, and anti-Parkinson's medicines such as levodopa or amantidine are other frequently used medicines with the potential to cause delirium. Any medication taken by an older person with delirium should be considered a possible cause, and as always the case, only medicines that are absolutely necessary should be continued.

The treatment of delirium involves removing the precipitating cause, if at all possible. Subsequent measures are likely to fail unless the cause is identified. The room should be quiet and familiar pictures and objects can help in orientation. A family member or friend can often orient the person to familiar things. If it is dark, turning a light on can often help. In rare instances, medications or restraints may be needed for safety. This should be a last resort because such measures can result in less ultimate benefit to the person.

Dementia

Dementia is characterized by the development of multiple cognitive deficits, including memory impairment. The dementia must be of sufficient severity to cause impairment in occupational or social functioning and must represent a decline from a previous higher level of functioning.[21] The incidence of dementia increases dramatically with age. Dementia is estimated to affect 1% of people from age 50 to 70, and up to 50% of the very elderly.[26]

The diagnosis of dementia starts with the history. Usually this will be collected from the caregiver or family member since it is common for people with dementia to have no insight into their condition. Because the onset is often gradual, families may not be able to state when the problem started without specific probing questions. Inquiries about balancing the checkbook, doing income taxes, paying bills, losing things or getting lost, and forgetting important events are helpful.

For a homemaker, questions about when she last prepared a full meal by herself, when she last did the housework, and if there has been any change in her social functioning are appropriate. Occupational and social history aid in developing the best questions regarding daily functioning that are specific to each person.

Many tests are available for documenting whether there is cognitive impairment. The Folstein Mini Mental State Exam is the most commonly used screening test for dementia[27] (see Table 7–7). It is a highly verbal test and scores have been found to be affected by age, education, and cultural background, but not gender. It has been recommended that it not be used in people with less than an eighth-grade education or in people not fluent in English.[28] A perfect score is 30. Severity ranges for scoring are: no cognitive impairment = 24–30; mild cognitive impairment = 18–23; severe cognitive impairment = 0–17.[25]

Alzheimer's disease is the most common cause of dementia. It is estimated to be present in 76 to 87% of cases of dementia.[29] It is a progressive degenerative neurological disorder that initially most noticeably affects cognition, but in its late stages affects the whole body. Because of its systemic effect, the stage of the disease can be followed by functional status as well as by cognitive status[30] (see Table 7–8). Life expectancy is typically 7 to 10 years after diagnosis. Death most often occurs from pneumonia, urinary tract infection, or infected decubitus ulcers.

Alzheimer's disease is distinguished by a gradual onset and continuing cognitive decline.[21] A sudden onset of symptoms, focal neurologic findings such as hemiparesis or incoordination early in the course of the illness, gait disturbances, or seizures early in the course of the illness make the diagnosis of Alzheimer's disease unlikely.[31]

Vascular dementia is the second most common form of dementia. It can be caused from several types of cerebrovascular lesions. These include multiple infarcts in cortical and subcortical areas, strategic single infarcts in specific areas of the brain, small vessel disease causing lacunar infarcts or white matter lesions, hypoperfusion due to cardiac arrest or other causes, and hemorrhages.[32] DSM-IV criteria include focal neurologic signs and symptoms such as exaggeration of deep tendon reflexes, gait abnormalities, or weakness of an extremity and radiological evidence of lesions, such as multiple strokes on a CT scan. These must be judged as etiologically related to the dementia.[21] The difficulty often lies in determining whether the observed neurological lesions or deficits are responsible for the dementia, or whether Alzheimer's or another condition is also present.

Elderly persons should be screened for "reversible" dementias. These dementias result from hypothyroidism, neurosyphilis, B_{12} or folate deficiency, depression, and normopressure hydrocephalus. Studies have shown that approximately 15% of dementias are caused by "reversible" conditions. However, the few studies that have reported follow-up data have suggested that many of these secondary dementias are not as reversible as commonly believed.[22]

Although there are many causes of dementia, including others not mentioned, the clinical approach to these patients, as well as those with delirium, is similar. To avoid overwhelming patients, one caregiver at a time should interact with them. Any interfering noise such as television or radio should be turned off. An attempt should be made to assess hearing. Ultimately, if important information must be given, it should also be communicated to their family or caregiver. See Chapters 16 and 19 for a more detailed coverage of specific strategies for communicating with patients with dementia.

ETHICAL ISSUES IN GERIATRIC PRACTICE

Ethics are central to geriatric practice. This centrality is not difficult to understand. Decision making in geriatrics must take into account the factors of age itself, life expectancy, frailty, and cognitive impairment. These condition the patient's and the family's sense of the worth of what is left of life. Few practitioners now regard longevity itself as a good. The pivotal issue in geriatrics has, by common consensus, become quality of life.

Quality of Life

Quality of life is difficult to define and even more difficult to measure. No formulaic approach, no algorithm or functional assessment can assign a value to quality of life. The reason is that quality of life is in the arena of subjectivity. The value of the later years, even in the face of frailty, proximity of death, and difficulty with thinking is sometimes underestimated by practitioners. Quality of life is thus an intuitive determination, but as in other intuitive exercises, hidden issues are involved in its valuation. Some of these occult markers are purely social constructs. Is there the balm of love or the perception of love present as an antidote to pain, dysfunction, loss of mobility and loss

Table 7–7. Mini-Mental State Examination

Maximum Score	Score	
		Orientation
5	( )	What is the (year) (season) (date) (day) (month)?
5	( )	Where are we: (state) (county) (town) (hospital) (floor)
		Registration
3	( )	Name 3 objects: 1 second to say each. Then ask the patient all 3 after you have said them. Give 1 point for each correct answer. Then repeat them until he learns all 3. Count trials and record.
		Attention and Calculation
5	( )	Serials 7's. 1 point for each correct. Stop after 5 answers. Alternatively, spell "world" backwards.
		Recall
3	( )	Ask for the 3 objects repeated above. Give 1 point for each correct.
		Language
9	( )	Name a pencil and watch (2 points). Repeat the following "No ifs, ands, or buts" (1 point) Follow a 3–stage command: "Take a paper in your right hand, fold it in half, and put it on the floor" (3 points). Read and obey the following: CLOSE YOUR EYES (1 point). Write a sentence (1 point). Copy design (1 point).
30	( )	**Total score**

ASSESS level of consciousness along a continuum:

| Alert | Drowsy | Stupor | Coma |

Instructions for administration

Orientation

1. Ask for the date. Then ask specifically for parts omitted, e.g. "Can you also tell me what season it is? One point for each correct.

2. Ask in turn "Can you tell me the name of this hospital?" (town, county, etc.). One point for each correct.

Registration

Ask the patient if you may test his memory. Then say the names of 3 unrelated objects, clearly and slowly, about one second for each. After you have said all 3, ask him to repeat them. This first repetition determines his score (0–3) but keep saying them until he can repeat all 3, up to 6 trials. If he does not eventually learn all 3, recall cannot be meaningfully tested.

Attention and Calculation

Ask the patient to begin with 100 and count backwards by 7. Stop after 5 subtractions (93, 86, 79, 72, 65). Score the total number of correct answers. If the patient cannot or will not perform this task, ask him to spell the word "world" backwards. The score is the number of letters in correct order. (e.g., dlrow = 5, dlorw = 3).

Recall

Ask the patient if he can recall the 3 words you previously asked him to remember. Score 0–3.

Language

Naming: Show the patient a wrist watch and ask him what it is. Repeat for pencil. Score 0–2.

Repetition: Ask the patient to repeat the sentence after you. Allow only one trial. Score 0 or 1.

3-stage command: Give the patient a piece of plain blank paper and repeat the command. Score 1 point for each part correctly executed.

Reading: On a blank piece of paper print the sentence "Close your eyes," in letters large enough for the patient to see clearly. Ask him to read it and do what it says. Score 1 point only if he actually closes he eyes.

Writing: Give the patient a blank piece of paper and ask him to write a sentence for you. Do not dictate a sentence; it is to be written spontaneously. It must contain a subject and a verb and be sensible. Correct grammar and punctuation are not necessary.

Copying: On a clean piece of paper, draw intersecting pentagons, each side about 1 in., and ask him to copy it exactly as it is. All 10 angles must be present and 2 must intersect to score 1 point. Tremor and rotation are ignored.

Source: Folstein MF, Folstein SE, McHugh PR: "Mini-Mental State." A practical method for grading the cognitive state of patients for the clinician. J Psychiatr Res 1975; 12:189–198. Repinted with permission.

Table 7–8. Functional Assessment Staging of Alzheimer's Disease (FAST Staging)

FAST Stage	FAST Characteristics
1.	No functional decrement subjectively or objectively
2.	Complains of forgetting location of objects, subjective work difficulties
3.	Decreased functioning in demanding work settings evident to coworkers; difficulty traveling to new locations
4.	Decreased ability to perform complex tasks (e.g., planning dinner party, shopping, personal finances)
5.	Requires assistance selecting attire, may require coaxing to bathe properly
6a.	Difficulty dressing properly
6b.	Requires assistance bathing, fear of bathing
6c.	Difficulty with the mechanics of toileting
6d.	Urinary incontinence
6e.	Fecal incontinence
7a.	Vocabulary limited to 1 to 5 words
7b.	Intelligible vocabulary lost
7c.	Ambulatory ability lost
7d.	Ability to sit lost
7e.	Ability to smile lost
7f.	Ability to hold up head lost; ultimately, stupor or coma

Source: Modified from Reisberg B: Dementia: A systematic approach to identifying reversible causes. *Geriatrics* 1986; 41,4:30–46.

of control of decision making? The most reliable index of quality of life has been found to be, where ascertainable, the patient's own assessment. Quality of life is then what is important to a given individual. Improving or stabilizing quality of life is the principal goal of geriatric practice. An intuitive judgment of reduced quality of life may be presented as a reason for reducing the intensity of therapeutic interventions. Ethics provides constructs for evaluating the various decisions that are made in the care of the elderly.

What Is Ethics?

Ethics is not a determination of good versus evil. Ethics concerns itself with the relative weight of competing goods—the values dilemma.[33] The overreaching good is the primacy of benevolence. The exercise of benevolence is the starting point of ethical action, regardless of the theoretical postulate offered as the structure of ethics. What ethics attempts to resolve is the conflict of goods subsumed under the umbrella of benevolence. Examples abound. Freedom and independence are goods. Protection of the patient is also a good. These may and often do become the poles of an ethical dilemma—when to sacrifice freedom (guardianship, surrogate decision making) in the interests of protection. A good is not to harm. A competing good is to preserve life and health. The value conflict here is to determine what qualities of life may be served by a given intervention when the risk of that intervention cannot be stated a priori with any degree of precision. The work of ethics then becomes the management of uncertainty. The tools of ethics are reason and communication. Ineffective reasoning may sabotage good communication, and faulty communication can undo excellent reasoning. The ethical project is to balance alternatives, each with some merit. If there are no bona fide alternatives, there is no ethical question. The everyday life of the geriatrician is spent navigating through a sea of alternatives—to tube feed or not, to remove a patient from home to an institution or not, to transfer a patient from a therapeutic mode of care to comfort care or not. These are only a few of the value dilemmas in geriatric practice.

Autonomy

In modern medical ethics, autonomy has become the overwhelmingly dominant principle. The primacy of autonomy is a relatively recent development. Autonomy is the individual's right to self-determination.[34] It implies that decisions made are voluntary and intentional and not the result of coercion, duress, or undue influence. For the elderly, particularly the frail elderly, a tradition of reliance on others (learned helplessness) may be established. There may be a history of relying on others for shopping, transportation, physical assistance, money management, and ultimately, for vital decision making.

True autonomy implies sharing information. Careful interaction with the older patient and inclusion of the patient in the work of choice is essential. For such inclusion to be practically applicable, the patient must be deemed capable of an informed choice between alternatives.

Assessment of Decision-Making Ability

The determination of competence is a function of the courts yet physicians are qualified to evaluate a patient's decision-making ability. At the extremes of behavior, there is no difficulty in determining a patient's ability to make decisions in geriatric practice. A patient who can manipulate information, understand the relevance and weight of the choices proposed, and realize the consequences of the alternatives with ease is clearly able to make decisions about medical care. At the other end of the spectrum is the patient who is comatose, unable to communicate, whose thought is disorganized, or who is permanently disoriented. A bedside judgment of impaired decision making ability is, in these circumstances, not difficult to make. The problem is in the vast intermediate zone between these poles of reasoning. Here, consultations with neuropsychiatry are used and there is a resort to formal testing. However, tests of decision-making can be fraught with error. It is certainly possible that an individual may recover this ability after surviving acute illness. In the final analysis, physicians make determinations about decision-making ability in borderline cases. The sensibility of ethics will guide these decisions.

Advanced Directives

The problem of how to proceed in circumstances of lost or impaired decision capacity has been addressed in contemporary practice by recourse to the advanced directive.[35] Advanced directives are considered to encompass the *living will* and *durable power of attorney for health care.*[36] An advanced directive is generally created at a time when the would-be patient is sound in mind and body, and it is a hypothetical instrument. It is intended to govern in circumstances of unspecified future incapacity and cognitive impairment at a future time of crisis. Directives only take effect when the patient is incapable of making or communicating decisions about interventions. One difficulty with advanced directives resides in their hypothetical character. They are determined at a time of detachment yet are to be executed at a time of potential crisis, pain, and fear. However, this may be the best expression of the value of autonomy.

The Living Will

The living will is a statement about specific treatment preferences in the event of terminal illness. It is assumed that the document is drawn up under conditions of competency; however, there are usually no limitations on conditions of revoking a living will.[27] Laws regarding living wills vary from state to state and definitions of terminal illness may vary.

Durable Power of Attorney for Health Care

The durable power of attorney is a document that appoints a health care surrogate in the future event of incompetency. In theory, the surrogate is assumed to behave as a instrument of the incompetent patient's desires. At the time of creation of the durable power of attorney, few would-be patients have discussed the details of decision making with the surrogates. Directions to the surrogate are usually broadly general, such as "I don't want to be on a breathing machine." Surrogates usually wish to create a family consensus before they act in accordance with the terms of the living will.

In geriatric practice, clinicians should understand the principles of ethics and the various legislative statutes and institutional policies that govern decision making. Education and communication with seniors and their families assure sensitivity to autonomy and adherence to standards of ethics. (For more information on ethical principles, see Chapter 10.)

SUMMARY

The assessment and management of seniors require attention to the social, psychological, emotional, and physiological factors that combine to affect their daily functioning and quality of life. A multidisciplinary approach is often the most effective and efficient way of providing the best care. By necessity, each member of the team must be aware of how his or her discipline interfaces with others of the team. Speech–language pathologists supply input on two essential functions: communication and swallowing. The impact of the contribution of the SLP is more significant when there is knowlege of the physician's approach to diagnosis and treatment and a strong foundation in issues in geriatric practice.

CASE ONE

Mrs. Jones was an 87-year-old female admitted to the hospital geriatric service with a history of increasing lethargy and a decreased mental status. Her past history was significant for multiple strokes, vascular dementia, and diabetes of 30 years duration. She had been nonambulatory for 2½ years due to leg weakness from her strokes and lived with her daughter, who cared for her. She had had 6 admissions in the past year including a fractured tibia 7 months previous to this admission. Since that time, she had been confined to bed. She also required total assistance in her other activities of daily living including feeding, dressing, bathing, toileting. She was incontinent of urine and stool. Her most recent admission had been 2 months earlier for pneumonia.

Physical exam was significant for a weight of 53.3 kg (a loss of 22 kg in 6 months). Her height was 160 cm. She had diffuse expiratory crackles bibasilarly. Her extremities were stiff with limited range of motion. She complained of severe pain in both heels and exam revealed a 12 × 3 cm stage 4 decubitis ulcer over her left heel with black eschar and an area of exposed Achilles' tendon. A smaller 4 × 2 cm stage 4 ulcer was on the right heel with exposed bone. She scored 9 of 30 on the Folstein Mini Mental State exam.

Admission laboratory studies were significant for a white cell count of 5300 with 18% lymphocytes (absolute lymphocyte count 954), hemoglobin 9.0 g/dl, glucose 153 mg/dl, ESR 114 mm/hr, and an albumin of 2.3 g/dl. X-rays of her feet showed changes consistent with osteomyelitis of her left heel. Chest X-ray showed a right lower lobe infiltrate consistent with pneumonia. CT scan of the head showed multiple small lacunar infarcts of the brain stem and basal ganglia.

The dietitian recommended she receive 1400 kcal/day, 70 g protein/day, and 1400 cc of fluid/day.

Speech–language pathology was consulted because of difficulty in swallowing. Bedside clinical exam showed pooled secretions in the oral cavity and pharynx. When placed in the full upright position, she drooled. She was able to repeat three word phrases with a soft, strained voice. Naming was delayed but accurate for simple objects. No laryngeal elevation was felt when the patient was asked to swallow, and when 2 cc of water were placed in her mouth, it ran out with no swallow attempts. The impression was dysphagia with flaccid dysarthria and decreased cognition. It was recommended that she have nothing by mouth and that long-term tube feeding with PEG or PEJ tube be considered.

She was treated with intravenous fluids and antibiotics for the infected decubitis ulcer and given transdermal fentanyl and morphine sulfate for the pain. The ulcers were also debrided by a plastic surgeon. Special soft boots were given to relieve pressure and help the heel pain. A conference was scheduled with her family to discuss further care.

Her daughter attended along with her granddaughter. Care team members present were her nurse, social worker, speech–language pathologist, geriatrician, and nurse practitioner, who led the meeting. All took part, with her daughter initially describing how she had been doing over the past years. Mrs. Jones' code status had already been made "do not resuscitate" and she had been consistent in saying to her daughter as well as the care team that she didn't want a feeding tube. The nurse reported that she was more comfortable, but still had some pain when moved. The speech–language pathologist discussed her swallowing problems and high risk of aspiration when fed by mouth. The geriatrician reviewed her medical problems and indicated that no matter what treatments were given, her prognosis was poor. If her illness followed its usual course, she would die within 6 months.

Feeding tubes were discussed, including benefits and risks. The hospice approach of comfort care and focus on maximizing the quality of her remaining life was presented. Her daughter was leaning toward a hospice approach at home, but wanted to discuss it with other family members before making a final decision. The next day she called with her decision for hospice care at home for Mrs. Jones. The intravenous line was removed and antibiotics discontinued. The speech–language pathologist reviewed positions and techniques for pleasure feeding, if desired, to her daughter to minimize risk of aspiration. She was discharged home to hospice care.

At home she took small amounts of food from a spoon, and after 1½ weeks became unable to take anything and was given ice chips and mouth care. The hospice nursing assistant came 3 times weekly as did the nurse to help with her care, make sure she was comfortable, and give support to her daughter. The hospice social worker and spiritual care advisor also made home visits. A small dose of anti-anxiety medicine was added for her comfort, but no adjustment in pain medicine was required. Two and a half weeks after her return home, Mrs. Jones died in her sleep.

STUDY QUESTIONS

1. What other major diagnosis, not mentioned, can be made from the history, physical, and laboratory results of the previous case?

   Answer: Protein calorie malnutrition is the diagnosis. She had a weight loss of 22 kg in 6 months, serum albumin of 2.3 g/dl, and absolute lymphocyte count of 954; all of which support the diagnosis.

2. Mrs. Jones' Folstein Mini Mental State score of 9 is consistent with severe cognitive impairment, and she has a diagnosis of vascular dementia. Should any weight be given to her stating that she doesn't want a feeding tube?

   Answer: If she appears to understand what a feeding tube is and her answers are consistent, then her own statements are important and should be weighed heavily in the ultimate decision.

3. Would Mrs. Jones have lived longer if a feeding tube had been inserted?

Answer: It is probable that she would have lived longer. However, such factors as violation of her autonomy by placing a tube against her will, continued risk of aspiration of oral secretions, possible need for restraint on her wrists to keep her from pulling the tube out with associated risk of developing new pressure sores, as well as other considerations must be balanced with the possible benefits of enteral feeding.

CASE TWO

Ms. Wright was an 80-year-old retired travel agent. She lived independently in a senior apartment building and enjoyed social activities with friends and neighbors. She had a dog, but no living family. Her past medical history was significant for Type II diabetes, a small stroke from which she had recovered with "no problems, but my memory's not as good as it used to be," asthma, and osteoarthritis of her knees. She took six different medicines.

One winter day, with the temperature at a record low of $-20°$, she took her dog outside, slipped on a patch of ice, and was unable to get up. Half an hour later, security personnel in the apartment noticed her dog barking at the entrance. The dog lead them to Ms. Wright, who was awake, but lethargic. She was taken by ambulance to the nearest hospital emergency room.

On physical exam, she could be aroused to speak, but was confused, and fell asleep easily. Her temperature was 90° F. Physical exam was otherwise unremarkable. CT of her head showed several small cerebral lacunar infarcts. She was treated for hypothermia and discharged home after a few days.

Two days later, a visiting nurse saw Ms. Wright in her apartment. She was not taking her medicines, which now totaled ten, correctly. Among them were drugs for anxiety, hypertension, diabetes, asthma, allergies, "heart," and "circulation." Additionally, her nurse learned that the previous night, security personnel had found her wandering in the building hallway, unable to find her apartment. Ms. Wright denied any alcohol use. Her diet appeared adequate, helped by the fact that meals were served in the apartment building's dining room. The nurse did a Folstein Mini Mental State Exam, and Ms. Wright scored 24 of 30. Fingerstick blood glucose was 60 mg/dl.

The visiting nurse called Ms. Wright's physician, who had not cared for her during her hospitalization because she was not on staff there. The physician decided to stop the arthritis, anxiety, allergy, and circulation medicines, as there was no clear need for them. Because her glucose was low, her diabetes pill was also stopped. The nurse arranged to have her other medicines put in a plastic cassette arranged by time of day and day of the week to help Ms. Wright remember if she had taken them or not.

On follow-up visits, Ms. Wright was feeling well and functioning similarly to before her hospitalization. She scored 28 of 30 on a repeat Folstein Mini Mental State Exam. Her dog was given to a friend when she realized the frequent trips outdoors were becoming too much to handle. She was again able to enjoy outings with her friends.

STUDY QUESTIONS

1. What caused Ms. Wright's altered mental state when she arrived at the hospital?

Answer: She had a delirium contributed to by her illness, hypothermia. From her history, she may also have had a very mild underlying dementia, which would make her more susceptible to develop delirium.

2. What was Ms. Wright's problem after her return from the hospital?

Answer: She had delirium with contributions by multiple factors. These would include polypharmacy, adverse effects of individual drugs, and hypoglycemia. Removing unneeded drugs allowed her to return to her baseline cognitive state.

REFERENCES

1. U.S. Bureau of the Census: *Statistical Abstract of the United States: 1995*, 115th ed. Washington, DC, 1995.
2. Brown I, Renwick R, Raphael D: Frailty: Constructing a common meaning, definition, and conceptual framework. *Internat J of Rehab Res* 1965; 18(2):93–102.
3. Winograd CH, Gerety MB, Chung M, et al: Screening for frailty: Criteria and predictors of outcomes. *J Am Geriatr Soc* 1991; 39:778–784.
4. Katz S, Ford AB, Moskowitz RW, et al: Studies of illness in the aged: The index of ADL. *JAMA* 1963; 185:914–919.
5. Lawton MP, Brody EM: Assessment of older people: Self-maintaining and instrumental activities of daily living. *Gerontologist* 1969; 9:179–186.
6. Colley CA, Lucas LM: Polypharmacy: The cure becomes the disease. *J Gen Int Med* 1993; 8:278–283.
7. Chernoff R: Effects of age on nutrient requirements. *Clin Geriatric Med* 1995; 11:641–651.
8. Kerstetter JE, Holthausen BA, Fitz PA: Nutrition and nutritional requirements for the older adult. *Dysphagia* 1993; 8:51–58.

9. Morley JE: Nutrition and the older female: A review. *J Amer Coll of Nutrition* 1993; 12:337–343.

10. Lipschitz DA: Approaches to the nutritional support of the older patient. *Clin Geriatric Med* 1995; 11(4): 715–724.

11. Silver AJ: Malnutrition. In Beck JC, ed., *Geriatrics Review Syllabus: A core curriculum in geriatric medicine* pp. 174–175. American Geriatrics Society, New York, 1991.

12. Cohen D: Dementia, depression, and nutritional status. *Primary Care* 1994; 21(1):107–119.

13. Dwyer J: Nutritional problems of elderly minorities. *Nutrition Rev* 1994; 52:S24–S27.

14. Barrocas A, Belcher D, Champagne C, Jastram C: Nutrition assessment: Practical approaches. *Clin Geriatric Med* 1995; 11(4):675–713.

15. Stuart B et al: *Medical guidelines for determining prognosis in selected non-cancer diseases,* 2d ed. Arlington, VA, National Hospice Organization, 1996.

16. Bald FC: *Michigan in four centuries.* Harper & Brothers, New York, 1954.

17. Rolandelli RH, Ullrich JR: Nutritional support in the frail elderly surgical patient. *Surg Clin of North Amer* 1994; 74(1):79–92.

18. Drickamer MA, Cooney LM: A geriatrician's guide to enteral feeding. *J Amer Geriatr Soc* 1993; 41:672–679.

19. Metheny N: Minimizing respiratory complications of nasoenteric tube feedings: State of the science. *Heart and Lung* 1993; 22(3):213–223.

20. Galindo-Ciocon DJ: Tube feeding: Complications among the elderly. *J Gerontol Nursing* 1993; June: 17–22.

21. McFadden JP, Price RC, Eastwood HD, Briggs RS: Raised respiratory rate in elderly patients: A valuable physical sign. *Br Med J* 1982; 284:626–627.

22. Marrie TJ, Durant H, Yates L: Community-acquired pneumonia requiring hospitalization: Five-year prospective study. *Rev Infect Dis* 1989; 11:586–599.

23. Andrews J, Chandrasekaran P, McSwiggan D: Lower respiratory tract infections in an acute geriatric male ward: A one-year prospective surveillance. *Gerontology* 1984; 30:290–296.

24. American Psychiatric Association: *Diagnostic and statistical manual of mental disorders,* 4th ed. American Psychiatric Association, Washington, D.C., 1994.

25. Arnold SE, Kumar A: Reversible dementias. *Med Clin North Amer;* 1993; 77:215–230.

26. Rossor MN: Management of neurological disorders: Dementia. *J Neurol Neurosurg Psychiatry;* 1994; 57: 1451–1456.

27. Folstein MF, Folstein SE, McHugh PR. "Mini-mental state." A practical method for grading the cognitive state of patients for the clinician. *J Psychiatr Res* 1975; 12:189–198.

28. Tombaugh TN, McIntyre NJ: The mini-mental state examination: A comprehensive review. *J Amer Geriatr Soc* 1992; 40:922–935.

29. Morris JC: Differential diagnosis of Alzheimer's disease. *Clin Geriatric Med* 1994; 10:257–276.

30. Reisberg B: Dementia: A systematic approach to identifying reversible causes. *Geriatrics* 1986; 41:30–46.

31. Stadlan EM: Clinical diagnosis of Alzheimer's disease. In McKhann G, Drachman D, Folstein M, et al., eds., Report of the NINCDS-ADRDA work group under the auspices of Department of Health and Human Services Task Force on Alzheimer's Disease. *Neurol* 1984; 34:940.

32. Roman GC, et al: Vascular dementia: Diagnostic criteria for research studies. Report of the NINDS-AIREN International Workshop. *Neurol* 1993; 43:250–260.

33. Mahowold MB: So many ways to think: An overview of approaches to ethical issues in geriatrics. *Clin Geriatric Med* 1994; 10:403–418.

34. Singer P: *Ethics.* Oxford University Press, Oxford, 1994.

35. Kapp MB: *Legal and ethical aspects of health care for the elderly.* Health Administration Press, Ann Arbor, MI, 1985.

36. McCullough LB, Doukas DJ, Holleman WL, Reilly RB: Advance directives. In Reichel W, ed., *Care of the elderly,* 4th ed. Williams & Wilkins, Baltimore, 1995, pp 597–608.

8

Management of Communicative and Swallowing Disorders in Non-Acute Settings: Home Care, Hospice, Skilled Nursing Facility

JOHN D. TONKOVICH

CHAPTER OUTLINE

Home Care

Hospice Care

Nursing Home

In the past two decades, there has been an increased demand for speech–language pathologists to engage in clinical practice with older adults. This demand has been noted for several reasons, including: (1) declining mortality rates for individuals with strokes;[1] (2) technological advances in prosthetic devices and other devices for providing alternative modes of communication; (3) increased involvement of speech–language pathology interventions for individuals with dysphagia; (4) greater recognition of the role of the speech–language pathologist in medical rehabilitation; and (5) the growing proportion of elderly adults in the general population.

While the demand for speech–language pathology services for older adults has increased, the variety of settings in which services are delivered appears to have increased as well. Acute care hospitals have benefited from financial incentives for discharging medically stable individuals to less costly nonacute settings. This diagosis-related groups (DRG) system authorizes payment of a lump sum to a hospital based on patients' primary and associated diagnoses no matter what the length of the hospital stay.[2] It is to a hospital's advantage, then, to find appropriate discharge sites for patients as soon as possible following acute hospitalization. When individuals need skilled nursing care, discharge to skilled nursing facilities is indicated. Those individuals able to be cared for or who can care for themselves may be discharged to the home. Those with terminal illnesses may be discharged to a hospice setting. Consequently, there has been an increase in the number of speech–language pathologists employed in these nonacute medical settings.

The American Speech–Language-Hearing Association's Omnibus survey,[3] for instance, showed a 200% increase in the number of speech–language pathologists providing home care services from 1990. As the population ages, as forecasters predict, this number is certain to grow.

Although many individuals preparing for careers in speech–language pathology obtain some clinical practicum experiences in acute care hospital and rehabilitation hospital settings, few obtain any practicum experience in the nonacute settings. Further, there is a paucity of literature specifically dealing with the provision of speech–language pathology services in these settings. It is the intent of this chapter, therefore, to provide an overview about services in these other settings, with practical guidelines and suggestions for individuals practicing in these settings.

HOME CARE

Home care represents one of the most rapidly growing segments within the health care delivery system. To qualify for home care, individuals must meet criteria that render them homebound. These criteria might include, but are not limited to: (1) being confined to bed on physician orders; (2) being unable to navigate stairs; (3) ambulating only a few feet or less with limited endurance; (4) using durable medical equipment that is not easily transportable; and/or (5) becoming too fatigued on a trip out of the house for outpatient services to benefit from rehabilitation services. The following criteria, in and of themselves, rarely deem an individual homebound: (1) being elderly; (2) living alone; (3) being unable to communicate; and/or (4) being unable to drive. While homebound status is not revoked when a patient makes occasional visits out of the house for medical appointments, this status becomes jeopardized when an individual ventures out of the home regularly for meals, hair appointments, shopping trips, and other trips of a personal nature. Once an individual is well enough to leave the home on a regular basis, if continued rehabilitation services are necessary, it is appropriate to provide these on an outpatient basis, and home care should be discontinued.

Home care often serves as a bridge between medical/rehabilitation services offered in the acute care hospital setting and the outpatient setting. Often, an individual with communication and/or swallowing problems might complete a course of speech–language treatment provided in the home and not require any additional outpatient services. Sometimes limited resources in the home (particularly for individuals also receiving physical and occupational therapy) require that services be moved to the outpatient setting.

Home care services are provided in a variety of "homes." While the majority of home care services take place in private residences, some home care services are provided to residents of assisted living centers. This venue has been growing in volume, and is expected to grow in the next few decades. Individuals in these settings have their own rooms or apartments, but are offered assistance in the way of housekeeping, meal preparation, medicine administration, and/or nursing support. These settings might be housed within a nursing facility, but, by and large, the individuals in assisted living centers do not require the same level of medical/nursing care as do those in nursing facilities. Some individuals reside in group homes, a small-scale version of an assisted living center. Group homes are typically housed in residential neighborhoods, and a limited number of individuals are cared for by willing caretakers. Home health workers often supply the necessary medical/nursing support for individuals with such needs who reside in group homes. Home care services are generally not provided to the residents of long-term care facilities, skilled nursing centers, or subacute rehabilitation settings. Speech–language pathology service provision in these settings is discussed later in the chapter.

Referrals

Most often, referrals for home care speech–language pathology services are made with a patient's discharge from an acute care hospital setting. Typically, these referrals are to home health agencies, who will assign a team of rehabilitation professionals to the case. A registered nurse usually heads the team and serves as case manager for the home care provided. The nurse typically makes the initial home visit and will gather information about the patient's case history, current problems, and goals and expectations. Following the nurse's visit, speech–language pathologists and other rehabilitation professionals visit the home to assess patient needs and develop a patient-focused treatment plan.

Occasionally, individuals may have a need for home speech–language pathology services, but no apparent needs for services from other home-based health professionals. A referral is made for speech–language pathology services only. In these cases the speech–language pathologist acts as case manager. In this role, in addition to providing direct patient care, the speech–language pathologist is responsible for serving as a liaison between the patient and the physician and takes responsibility for determining if other services might be needed. A person referred for speech–language pathology services for dysphagia, for instance, might actually benefit from having a nurse to monitor temperature and lung sounds and a social worker to provide information about community resources.

The Initial Telephone Contact

Once a referral for speech–language pathology services is received, the case is assigned. Typically a form known as a CPC (continuing patient care) form is given to the speech–language pathologist assigned to the case. The CPC form will contain information about the patient, including name, address, phone, medical diagnoses, dates of hospitalization, medical orders, and plan of treatment, and, in some cases, information about medications, precautions, prior treatments, and unusual circumstances.

When the home care speech–language pathologist receives the referral, it is necessary to contact the patient to arrange for the initial visit. In some cases scheduling of home care visits is done via a central scheduling coordinator; however, in most cases speech–language pathologists call to schedule their own appointments. Because speech–language pathologists may have only cursory information about the patient, the initial contact is important not only for information gathering but also for establishing a positive first impression with the patient and/or significant others. Following an introduction, the speech–language pathologist should gather as much information as possible to help plan for the initial visit. Table 8–1 provides a list of questions that may be appropriate for use during the initial telephone contact.

Answers to these questions may provide a useful springboard for further questions or requests. For instance, if it is determined that the patient has swallowing difficulties and is using thickening agents for liquids, the speech–language pathologist may request that liquids and thickener be made available at the time of the initial evaluation. It is advisable also to contact the previous speech–language pathologist whenever possible prior to the first home visit. This individual can be instrumental in providing the home care clinician with information regarding past interventions; length, duration, and focus of interventions; family and other support systems; patient/family past instructional and current instructional needs; and other pertinent factors.[4] In addition, for dysphagic patients, previous speech–language pathologists can supply useful data regarding videofluoroscopic and/or other swallowing studies, as well as the patient's safety precautions and dietary modifications.

Most individuals have little if any experience with home care, so that when health care professionals phone to set up appointments, patients and/or significant others may need some information about the processes involved in home care rehabilitation. For instance, patients and their significant others often want specific appointment times, and do not understand that speech–language pathologists must coordinate their visit times with other therapists involved in the person's care, as well as other patients on the caseload, and the health care professionals involved in their care. While speech–language pathologists should make every effort to accommodate people and their scheduling preferences (e.g., mornings better than afternoons; patient tires if speech–language treatment is provided immediately after physical therapy), occasionally patients and/or their significant others are not satisfied. In those instances, the speech–language pathologist should offer other options. These options might include having another speech–language pathologist follow the case, scheduling visits early in the morning or early in the evening when daytime visits are problematic, or referring the individual for outpatient rehabilitation services.

The Initial Evaluation Visit

The home care speech–language pathologist is faced with several challenges during the first visit to a patient's home. It is essential that this individual possess or acquire good time management skills. The pace of the initial evaluation visit is rapid, and the speech–language pathologist must attend to a number of requisite details during the visit. In about an hour or so, the home care speech–language pathologist must perform an evaluation to determine the type and severity of communication and/or swallowing disorder, formulate a treatment plan in concert with the patient and his/her significant other(s), instruct the patient and family about evaluation findings and treatment strategies, determine the approximate duration of intervention necessary, envision the patient's communication and/or swallowing status and the end of such intervention, plan for additional services if necessary at the end of the intervention, and, if possible, document all of the above. Unlike acute care, where speech–language pathologists may have opportunities to assess an individual's communication and/or swallowing performance across several sessions or even days, the home care

Table 8–1. Questions for Patients and/or Significant Others During the Initial Telephone Contact for Home Care Visits

How (is s/he/are you) doing with talking?
How (is s/he/are you) doing with swallowing?
How (is s/he/are you) doing with memory?

For those who have suffered cerebrovascular accidents:
    Which side of the body was affected?
    (Is s/he/Are you) left- or right-handed?
    Do(es) (s/he/you) have slurred speech?
    Do(es) (s/he/you) have difficulty putting words together in sentences?
    Do(es) (s/he/you) have difficulty remembering the names of things?
    Can (s/he/you) read and write?

Did (s/he/you) have any speech–language therapy before?
Where was the speech–language therapy provided?
Who was the speech–language pathologist?
What kinds of things were worked on in speech–language therapy?

Can (s/he/you) understand things people say to you?
Can other people understand the things (s/he/you) say(s) to them?

Did (s/he/you) have a swallowing test in the hospital?
What did the swallowing test show?
What (is s/he/are you) currently drinking and eating?
Are any foods, liquids or medicines fed through a tube?

(Does s/he/Do you) have to do anything special when swallowing?
(Does s/he/Do you) have to drink thickened liquids?

(Does s/he/Do you) communicate in other ways than speaking? If so, what are they?

Is there anything else you want to ask me or tell me about (his/her/your) communication and swallowing?

speech–language pathologist must gather all information in one visit.

While standardized test instruments are useful in obtaining diagnostic information during the initial evaluation visit, it is rarely possible for home care speech–language pathologists to administer complete aphasia batteries during this visit. For patients with aphasia, clinicians may find it necessary to administer selected items and/or subtests from standardized tools such as the *Boston Diagnostic Aphasia Examination*[5] or the *Boston Naming Test*.[6] One particularly useful strategy may be to begin by administering the most difficult items of particular subtests. If the patient masters these items, the speech–language pathologist might presuppose that the patient would not have had difficulty with earlier items. Rating scales of communicative function such as the *Communicative Effectiveness Index*,[7] the *Profile of Communicative Appropriateness*,[8] and the *ASHA FACS*[9] may also yield appropriate evaluation information, particularly when significant others are encouraged to participate in the ratings.

For patients with nondominant hemisphere lesions, tools that may be useful during the initial evaluation visit include the *MIRBI—Mini Inventory of Right Brain Injury*[10] and the *RICE-R—RIC Evaluation of Communication Problems in Right Hemisphere Dysfunction—Revised*.[11] Both of these batteries provide quick and broad assessment information about nondominant hemisphere dysfunction. Informal assessment of abilities attributed to the nondominant hemisphere may also be performed. Several tasks for informal assessment of these abilities are provided in Table 8–2.

For patients with dysphagia or suspected dysphagia, a thorough bedside evaluation of swallowing is indicated. As mentioned previously, the home care speech–language pathologist can request that the patient have trial foods available at the time of evaluation. While it may be useful for home speech–language pathologists to bring jars of baby food, applesauce, and thickener to the patient's home, more useful information is often provided when the patient (and/or his/her family) supplies food and/or thickening agents used in the home. By observing the consistently with which a spouse thickens liquids, for instance, the home speech–language pathologist can make recommendations and any necessary modifications.

Table 8–2. Tasks for the Informal Assessment of Nondominant Hemisphere Functions and Impairments

Hemispatial visual neglect

1. Have the patient scan for letters (after Halper).[11] See if more letters are missed in one visual field versus the other.

2. Have the patient produce or copy line drawings of symmetrical objects (e.g., daisy) or drawings that are two-dimensional representations of three-dimensional perspectives (e.g., a house showing two sides and the roof, a bicycle). See if drawings reflect underrepresented or overrepresented detail in one visual field versus the other.

3. Have the person read aloud from the newspaper. Determine if person is missing half of the information relative to midline.

Reasoning/problem solving

1. Have the person identify the missing ingredient or extra ingredient in a list of recipe ingredients read to him/her. Read a list of ingredients aloud and determine whether the person can identify the item (e.g., confectioner's sugar, butter, cocoa, and vanilla = chocolate frosting).

2. Have the person identify potential solutions to hypothetical problems (e.g., the water department will have to turn off your water for a day. What might you have to do to prepare for the water being off?)

3. Ask the person to explain why the punchline of a joke or riddle is humorous.

Organization/relevance/orientation

1. Ask the person to give you directions from his/her home to a landmark in the city or town where you are.

2. Ask the person to provide you with instructions for performing daily living tasks (e.g., changing a flat tire; making biscuits from scratch).

3. Ask the person to tell you about a current news story.

Following a bedside swallowing evaluation, it may be necessary to refer the patient for videofluoroscopy, particularly if aspiration is suspected. The videofluoroscopic swallowing study is ordered by the patient's physician, so it is necessary that the home speech–language pathologist make this recommendation during the initial evaluation visit so that it can be noted in the treatment plan.

When motor speech disorders are apparent in homebound patients, a thorough oral mechanism examination is necessary. Home speech–language pathologists should be particularly aware of any involuntary movements, incoordination, or muscle weakness that would aid in making a specific dysarthria diagnosis. In addition to the oral mechanism examination, evaluation of speech intelligibility might include having patients read a passage (such as *My Grandfather*) aloud, sustain a vowel such as /a/, and perform rapid, alternating movements (oral diadochokinesis). These findings may be used to arrive at a diagnostic classification for the dysarthria. The system proposed by Darley, Aronson and Brown[12] is widely used and provides

practical, descriptive information about the suspected nature of the dysarthria.

When apraxia of speech is suspected, the speech–language pathologist may wish to compare articulatory precision of automatic speech (e.g., counting, saying the days of the week) with that of volitionally produced speech. The speech–language pathologist may also wish to note any articulatory groping and/or struggle, as well as any inconsistencies in articulatory precision, particularly for initial consonant blends and polysyllabic words.

Homebound patients occasionally have memory and/or other cognitive-communication impairments. The *ABCD—Arizona Battery for Evaluating Communication in Dementia*[13] is a useful took for assessing these functions in patients with dementia. Several memory assessment tools are available, and may provide useful information. Home speech–language pathologists may wish to note how patients with memory impairments can benefit from external cueing. A simple way to do this is to use instructions such as these:

I'm going to tell you three words that I want you to remember. Here are the words: suitcase, jam, and baseball. In a few minutes I'm going to ask you to tell me these three words. I'm going to write them down for you. When I ask you to tell me the three words, if you don't remember, I want you to look at this sheet of paper. Then you can just read the words to me. Remember these words: suitcase, jam, and baseball.

This methodology may be modified as necessary to include the date and/or the speech–language pathologist's name. Patients who are able to benefit from having such written aids for memory often benefit from the use of a memory log or journal in aiding recall of important information for daily living.

The evaluation of homebound patients less often requires assessment of patients' voice production, speech fluency, and/or potential for non-oral communication system use. The skillful home speech–language pathologist will develop appropriate tools and/or methods for assessing individuals with these communication needs.

The Evaluation Report and Treatment Plan

At the time of the initial evaluation visit, it is customary for the home speech–language pathologist to write up a summary of evaluation findings and a concomitant treatment plan. Many home health agencies have developed checklist formats to use in summarizing evaluation findings, with opportunities for clinicians to write succinct narratives, as necessary, to clarify any information not available from the checklist alone.

The evaluation summary should in some way address the functional communication limitations of patients. For instance, knowing that an individual can produce automatic sequences without difficulty may be irrelevant information if that individual has severe deficits in comprehension and expression. Home speech–language pathologists may wish to describe the type of daily communication the patient is able to use and the amount of external assistance or guidance needed to perform the communicative function adequately. Table 8–3 gives some examples of functional assessment statements, and contrasts them with statements that are not functionally oriented.

Part of the initial evaluation documentation requires that the home speech–language pathologist, in conjunction with the patient and others (e.g., family member, caregiver), develop a treatment plan. In most instances, the treatment plan must be signed by the patient's physician. This plan should include, as a minimum, the type(s) of speech–language pathology services provided (as indi-

Table 8–3. Some Examples of Assessment Statements with and without Functional Orientation

Functional:	Mr. A. does not consistently use airway protection strategies to promote safe swallowing during mealtimes.
Non-functional:	Mr. A. has moderate to severe oral-pharyngeal dysphagia with laryngeal penetration of thin liquids and pooling in the valleculae.
Functional:	Mr. B. often cannot retrieve specific words he wants to say, but can usually get his message across by providing verbal descriptions of the words he's unable to retrieve.
Nonfunctional:	Mr. B. has a moderate to severe anomic aphasia, typified by an inability to retrieve content words from his lexicon. His output is fluent and circumlocutionary.
Functional:	Mrs. C.'s reading ability is impaired because she does not see words on the left-hand side of the page.
Nonfunctional:	Mrs. C. has an acquired dyslexia resulting from left visuospatial neglect.

cated in Table 8–4), the frequency and duration of proposed treatments, the mutually agreed on goals and/or forecasted outcomes, and the discharge plans. In addition, the treatment plan may include other information such as rehabilitation potential and/or prognosis for improvement, statements identifying when speech–language pathology would be discontinued, and projected functional level of performance at the end of treatment. A sample treatment plan is included in Table 8–5.

Working with Case Managers

While the majority of individuals receiving home speech–language pathology services are funded via the federal Medicare program, an increasing number of patients receiving home-based speech–language pathology services are enrolled in health care plans that are offered by managed care organizations. For these patients, it is usually necessary for the home speech–language pathologist to contact a case manager for a pre-approved number of visits, a process known as *prior authorization*. Case managers provide a link between the health care provider and insurance carrier, and it is important for home speech–language pathologists to maintain positive and successful communicative interactions with these individuals. Most case

Table 8–4. Orders/Treatment Codes
for Speech–Language Pathology
Services Provided in Home Health
Environments

C1 Evaluation

C2 Voice disorders treatment

C3 Speech articulation disorders treatment

C4 Dysphagia treatment

C5 Language disorders treatment

C6 Aural rehabilitation

C7 Reserved[a]

C8 Non-oral communication

C9 Other: (specify under orders)[b]

---

[a]This code is not currently used, but is reserved to
include treatments that might be reflected in expanded scope of practice areas for speech–language pathologists.

[b]This code might be used if physician orders treatment for chewing, arithmetic processes, compensations for visuospatial neglect, and others
not included in the above treatment codes.

managers have little if any direct training in communication and/or swallowing disorders, and when
home speech–language pathologists can furnish
lucid information about specific disorders and
their interventions, this enables case managers to
make sound decisions.

Hecht and Tonkovich[2] suggested the following
guidelines to speech–language pathologists when
working with case managers: (1) develop reasonable goals that are based on the patient's medical
diagnosis and recovery; (2) develop goals that are
realistic relative to the severity of the communication disorder; (3) state goals in terms of functional
outcomes; (4) negotiate with case managers for
patient-specific needs; and (5) invite case managers
and other insurance company representatives to
interdisciplinary team conferences. Each of these
guidelines warrants additional discussion.

Develop Reasonable and Realistic Goals

Home speech–language pathologists should formulate treatment goals while working with patients
and their caregivers. The goals should be based on
the patient's medical diagnosis and presupposed
recovery. Sometimes overzealous speech–language
pathologists wish to restore adult patients with acquired communication disorders to their premorbid skill levels and, consequently, formulate goals
that are not attainable. It would not be reasonable
to expect a patient with a diagnosis of amyotrophic

lateral sclerosis (ALS), for instance, to become able
to produce perfectly articulated speech at the end
of a course of home speech–language therapy. Any
goals of this nature would be considered unrealistic. That the same patient would become able to
utilize an augmentative communication system in
conjunction with speech production to express
daily needs successfully, on the other hand, would
seem a realistic outcome for a course of home
speech–language therapy.

Figure 8–1 illustrates the typical course of recovery from aphasia for individuals following occlusive, hemorrhagic, and traumatic etiologies. It
should be noted that individuals show a more sudden and dramatic recovery relatively soon after the
time of onset following occlusive cerebrovascular
accidents. Those with aphasia attributable to hemorrhagic cerebrovascular accidents, on the other
hand, tend to exhibit slow recovery of function immediately post-onset, but may have a dramatic
peak in recovery several months after the time of
onset. Treatment goals should be reasonable relative to the type of lesion as well. Those experiencing a recovery of function following an occlusive
CVA during the so-called spontaneous recovery
phase would have goals different from an individual who is showing little spontaneous improvement immediately after a hemorrhagic lesion.

In authorizing visits for patients, case managers, many of them with backgrounds in nursing
or social work, will attempt to determine the cost–
benefit ratio of the proposed interventions. That is,
they will attempt to weigh the cost of the speech–
language pathology services with the projected
benefit on communication and/or swallowing to
the patient. Home speech–language pathologists
need to develop skill at formulating attainable
goals that will have some impact on a patient's
ability to communicate and/or eat safely and independently. For a patient with global aphasia,
speech–language treatment provided three times
weekly for six months and solely directed toward
improving yes/no responsiveness to personal information questions may not be reasonable to a
payor. If the treatments are directed toward providing the individual with strategies for non-oral
communication, to include writing, gesture, and
drawing so that the patient has sufficient communication ability to live safely and independently,
the same amount of treatment may be reasonable.

State Goals in Terms of Functional Outcomes

When reviewing treatment plans, case managers
will be more apt to authorize treatments when the
goals are specified in a way that promotes im-

Table 8–5. Sample Speech–Language Pathology Treatment Plan for Home Health Care

Patient: Ned J.	Patient Number: 6400-1	Date of Plan: 02/28/98
Diagnosis: S/P (L) CVA	Onset Date: 01/19/97	Physician: Marlene K, MD

Summary of Major Problems/Severity	Goals
1. Flaccid dysarthria—mild	1. Mr. J. will become independent in his use of strategies that facilitate the production of intelligible conversational utterances (in at least 90% of his attempts).
2. Anomic aphasia—moderate	2. Mr. J. will become independent in his use of strategies that successfully aid him when conversational word retrieval difficulties occur (in at least 90% of his attempts).

REHABILITATION POTENTIAL: ( ) Excellent   (X) Good   ( ) Fair   ( ) Poor

ORDERS/TREATMENT CODES:

(X) C1 Evaluation
( ) C2 Voice Disorders Treatment
(X) C3 Speech Articulation Disorders Treatment
( ) C4 Dysphagia Treatment
(X) C5 Language Disorders Treatment
( ) C6 Aural Rehabilitation
( ) C8 Non-oral Communication
( ) C9 Other

FREQUENCY/DURATION:

2–4X per week for 5–9 weeks, or until goals are met; 45–60 minute sessions.

DISCHARGE PLAN:

(X) Self/Caregiver   ( ) Outpatient   ( ) Rehab Facility
Discharge anticipated in 6 weeks.

HOME PROGRAM PROVIDED AND DEMONSTRATED TO:

(X) Patient   (X) Family/Caretaker   ( ) Other
(X) Patient/Caregiver instructed in Plan of Care, goals, visit frequency

TREATMENT PROVIDED THIS DATE:

Mr. J. was instructed re: evaluation findings. Mr. J. was instructed re: strategies for improving speech intelligibility (e.g., decreasing speech rate, increasing vocal intensity, exaggerating articulatory movements) and re: strategies to use when aphasic word retrieval difficulties occur (e.g., provide verbal descriptions, synonyms, gestures). A written program detailing these strategies was provided and explained to Mr. J. and his wife. Mr. J. agreed with the proposed Plan of Care.

Amy R, MA, CCC-SLP
Speech–Language Pathologist

I have read the above plan and agree.

Marlene K, MD   03/03/98
Physician

---

proved functional use. Home speech–language pathologists should attempt to state goals relative to the impact that they would have on the person's ability to function as independently as possible in daily living activities. Goals should be written to include the kinds of things the patient would be able to do after completing a course of speech–language pathology services. These might include statements such as "to minimize likelihood of aspiration during oral feeding," "to express ideas, thoughts and feelings," "to comprehend sufficiently to meet the demands of daily living needs." These are in contrast to goals such as "to improve auditory comprehension," "to decrease neologistic

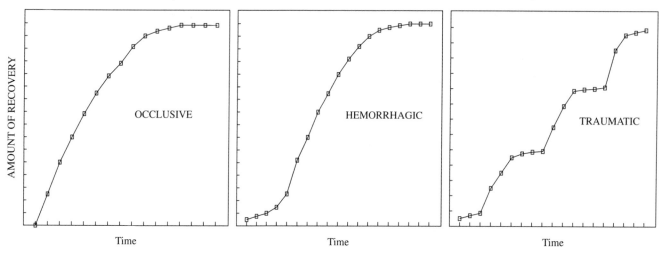

Figure 8–1. The general course of neurologic recovery according to the etiology of the neurologic disorder. The graphs shown here represent the average course of recovery for groups of patients, the recovery of individual patients may differ somewhat from the group averages. These curves are based primarily an clinical experience and anecdotal evidence. There is little objective evidence documenting the course of neurologic recovery following strokes or traumatic brain injuries. *Source:* From Brookshire RH: *An Introduction to neurogenic communication disorders*, 5th ed. Mosby Year Book, St. Louis, 1997. Reprinted with permission.

paraphasia in conversational speech," and "to improve copying of printed words." To determine whether goals are written in terms of functional outcomes, speech–language pathologists should ask themselves, "Does this tell me what the person is going to be doing at the end of treatment?" Examples of appropriate functional outcome type goals are provided in Table 8–6.

Another aspect of goals with a functional-outcome base is that they specify the degree to which the patient performs the behavior independently. The 7-point rating scale used on the *ASHA FACS*[9] utilizes definitions that correspond to the degree to which the patient relies on assistance and/or prompting. Assistance and/or prompting refers to factors that might include repeating, rephrasing, simplifying language, slowing rate of speech, providing help in using assistive/alternative devices, using gestures, writing/drawing pictures, giving additional time for response, asking yes/no questions, and offering a limited choice. These manipulations are provided externally by the patient's conversational partner. The *ASHA FACS* ratings are assigned on the basis of observation of the patient, caregiver's reports, and/or direct testing. A summary of the descriptors associated with these ratings is provided in Table 8–7.

Table 8–6. Some Examples of Goals with Explicit Functional Outcomes

Mrs. W. will take replenishing breaths as needed for appropriate loudness without reminders from her husband in 90% of communication interactions.

Mr. X. will be successful in his use of multiple communication channels (e.g., speaking, gesturing, pointing, drawing, writing) to request information and actions in at least 90% of his communicative interactions with family members.

Mrs. Y. will refer to written cues about airway protection techniques independently to aid her in the use of those techniques for 100% of swallows of food/liquid.

Ms. Z. will refer to her memory notebook independently when she needs assistance in answering questions about recent events.

Negotiate with Case Managers for Patient-Specific Needs

One advantage to working through a case manager is that the speech–language pathologist may request specific items that might otherwise go unfunded. For instance, a particular patient may benefit from an electronic communication device and if the speech–language pathologist has determined that the patient is capable of achieving success using the device, case managers may find the expenditure reasonable and necessary. This would be particularly likely if the speech–language pathologist can demonstrate that the patient would

Table 8–7. Descriptors Associated with Ratings on the ASHA Functional Assessment of Communication Skills[9]

Rating	Descriptor	Definition
7	Can do	Client performs behavior; needs no assistance and/or prompting
6	Can do with minimal assistance	Client performs behavior, rarely needing assistance and/or prompting
5	Can do with minimal to moderate assistance	Client performs behavior, occasionally needing assistance and/or prompting
4	Can do with moderate assistance	Client performs behavior, often needing assistance and/or prompting
3	Can do with moderate to maximal assistance	Client performs behavior, very frequently with assistance and/or prompting
2	Can do with maximal assistance	Client performs behavior only with constant assistance and/or prompting
1	Cannot do	Client cannot perform behavior, even with maximal assistance and/or prompting
0	No basis for rating	Circumstances in which a behavior cannot be observed, directly tested, or available from other sources

be able to live independently and be less reliant on others with this type of communication device.

Some patients immediately post-onset of communication and/or swallowing problems become depressed, and are unable and/or unwilling to participate in speech–language pathology services.[2,15] When this occurs, home speech–language pathologists should suspend speech–language pathology services, particularly if the patient is making little observable progress. Case managers may be amenable to delaying the initiation of speech–language pathology services until a time when the patient can tolerate and benefit from these services.

Invite Case Managers to Interdisciplinary Team Meetings

When interdisciplinary team conferences are held for home care patients, it is often a good idea to invite case managers to participate in the meetings. At these meetings, the case manager has an opportunity to interact with the individuals providing rehabilitation services. Home speech–language pathologists may strengthen their case by discussing ways in which other health care providers can modify their interactions to optimize rehabilitation. For instance, physical therapists often assist patients who have gait disturbances secondary to hemiparesis. These patients may need modifications of instructions to ensure comprehension

(e.g., repeat instructions, write instructions) to enhance what they are able to derive from the physical therapy sessions.

Providing Speech–Language Pathology Services in the Home

Home speech–language pathologists should keep a number of factors in mind when providing services.

1. Remember that you are a guest in the patient's home. Speech–language pathologists should be courteous and ask permission before using the patient's sinks, telephones, and/or other possessions. Use of the phone should be related to brief, professional telephone contacts and never for personal phone calls.

2. Use universal precautions and good infection control techniques. Home speech–language pathologists should practice good infection control techniques. They should carry a bottle of strong, antibacterial liquid soap, and should wash hands vigorously at the beginning and end of each patient treatment session. When tasks require it, speech–language pathologists should wear disposable gloves. At all times, the speech–language pathologist should carry a one-way protective valve for providing cardiopulmonary resuscitation.

3. Be aware of safety issues—yours and those of the patient. Sometimes speech–language pathologists may be asked to provide services to patients who live in settings where there is some real or perceived danger. For instance, patients may be cared for by individuals who physically or verbally abuse them, or who engage in illegal activities such as drug trafficking. The home speech–language pathologist should report suspected safety issues to a designated individual at the home health agency and/or the local protective services agency. If there are circumstances in the patient's home that pose real or perceived danger to the speech–language pathologist, the clinician might insist that these circumstances change prior to returning to the home. For instance, if a number of unfamiliar people enter and leave the patient's home during speech–language therapy visits, the speech–language pathologist, if uncomfortable with this situation, should request that only the patient, significant family member, and clinician be present in the home during scheduled speech–language treatment sessions. Unfortunately, home speech–language pathologists and other rehabilitation professionals are sometimes victims of crime on the job and therefore it is essential to be continuously aware of safety issues.

Not only are there safety issues associated with being in patients' homes, but the nature of the job poses certain other safety concerns. Because most home speech–language pathologists drive their own vehicles to patients' homes, driving issues are an additional consideration. Home speech–language pathologists should ensure that their vehicles are properly and regularly maintained.

4. Maintain skills in cardiopulmonary resuscitation and methods for obtaining vital signs. Know how to access the emergency response system in your area. Home speech–language pathologists are sometimes to the only other person in the patient's home with the patient, and must therefore possess some skills and training in several medical/nursing procedures. At least once every two years, the home speech–language pathologist should demonstrate proficiency in cardiopulmonary resuscitation. Courses are typically offered by the local chapters of the American Red Cross, and require that individuals pass a proficiency exam. In addition, speech–language pathologists should learn how to take blood pressure, pulse, and temperature, even though these skills lie outside the purview of those ordinarily required of speech–language pathologists. In the event patient experiences something extraordinary during a speech–language treatment session, the speech–language pathologist needs to be able to phone a physician or emergency access number and report, at a minimum, the person's vi-

tal signs. An additional skill that might be useful is that of auscultation, listening to the lungs with a stethoscope. This is particularly helpful when working with dysphagic individuals who are at risk for aspiration.

In many parts of the country, the emergency medical response system is accessed by dialing 911. Should something that would require immediate medical attention occur, the home speech–language pathologist should enlist the aid of specially trained emergency medical response system workers. In some rural and remote areas, the emergency medical response system may be accessed through the sheriff's department or some other agency, and the speech–language pathologist should be aware of how to get needed help during a medical emergency.

5. Avoid using materials and procedures that have the potential of misleading the patient. Speech–language pathology interventions should be geared toward providing patients with direct (and preferably functional) therapeutic benefits. Unfortunately, some speech–language pathologists engage in clinical practices that do not afford such benefits.

For example, when patients with dysarthric speech (and a realistic potential for using speech as a communication mode) receive speech–language pathology interventions, the treatment should focus on methodologies with direct impact on the intelligibility of the speech produced. Isokinetic oral motor exercises, often utilized, may or may not have any impact whatsoever, and typically are not the same movements utilized in speech production.[16] When speech–language pathologists focus treatment on such exercises, patients are apt to be misled into thinking that if they practice the exercises, speech intelligibility will improve. It is far more advantageous for the speech–language pathologist to instruct the patient regarding strategies for enhancing speech intelligibility. Such strategies might include increasing vocal intensity, decreasing speech rate, and exaggerating articulatory movements. Patients then practice using the strategies, and the intervention has *direct* impact on the intelligibility of the speech produced, and enhances functional performance.

Information from recent studies have demonstrated, for instance, that some aphasic patients benefit from tasks that may on the surface seem unrelated to the aphasic deficits they present. For instance, individuals with fluent aphasias and poor comprehension have been shown to benefit from exercises requiring visual scanning and visual perception to aid auditory comprehension.[17] When these methods are utilized, speech–language pathologists must have an understanding of the rationale for the approach and there should be some evidence that such approaches are efficacious. Patients and their significant others also need to know why, for instance, you may be working on tasks that seem unrelated to the patient's needs.

6. Provide honest and realistic information about communication and/or swallowing potential to the patient and family members, even when there are serious limitations. Be sensitive to the patient's feelings and needs. Home speech–language pathologists often face difficult and challenging situations, particularly when a patient has a poor prognosis for recovery of oral language or safe swallowing. Information about prognosis should be provided early in the intervention process, and the speech–language pathologist should take care to present the information in a direct, though sensitive manner. A patient with memory difficulties subsequent to anoxic encephalopathy, for instance, will in all likelihood persist in having these difficulties and may always need to rely on a memory notebook or aid, even when speech–language interventions are discontinued. Patients with chronic dysphagia who show laryngeal penetration and aspiration of all food consistencies need to know that they might never eat and drink by mouth again. Patients with chronic global aphasia and their significant others need to understand that alternative communication modalities may be necessary. These are not easy situations for home speech–language pathologists to discuss, nor are they easy for most patients and significant others to hear.

Sometimes patients and their families are unwilling to accept poor prognoses and recommendations made by the speech–language pathologist. For instance, the family of a patient with global aphasia might insist that the patient talk again, even though there is little likelihood of this occurrence and even though the patient might have a reasonably good potential for communicating via some alternate modality. In these situations, home speech–language pathologists may wish to refer the patient to another speech–language pathologist for a second opinion or to another health care professional (e.g., physician, psychologist) for appropriate follow-up. In any event, the wishes of the patient and significant others should always be respected, regardless of whether or not the speech–language pathologist agrees with those wishes. When home speech–language pathologists cannot provide services that match unrealistic goals of patients and/or their significant others, speech–language pathology interventions should be discontinued.

7. Implement intervention strategies that engage others in the patient's home in helping the patient communicate and/or swallow. Whenever patients live with others, the home speech–language pathologist should plan to incorporate these other individuals into the treatment sessions. Just as patients need instruction about strategies for improving communication and/or swallowing, those who live with them require instruction about strategies they can use to help patients. For instance, an aphasic patient may have auditory comprehension difficulties with longer, syntactically complex auditory inputs; those living with the patient might need to be instructed about making requests for action or information short and simple to maximize the likelihood that such requests will be comprehended. Dysphagic patients may require dietary modifications such as nectar-thick liquids to maximize swallowing safety. Others in the home need to be able to thicken liquids to that consistency, and may also need instruction about the dangers associated with aspiration of thin liquids.

Holland[18] describes an aphasia treatment approach called conversational coaching. In this type of treatment approach, the speech–language pathologist prepares a script for a 6 to 8 utterance monologue that is at a level of difficulty just slightly above a patient's current performance level. The speech–language pathologist provides coaching to assist the patient in conveying the information in the monologue and, with the clinician's guidance, the monologue is performed for a family member with no knowledge of the monologue's content. The speech–language pathologist continues to coach the patient regarding strategies (e.g., if you can't say the whole thing, say the one or two most important words). Family members are also coached in the use of strategies that maximize communicative success (e.g., try asking him who he's talking about; ask him if he can draw a picture of it). When feasible, the speech–language pathologist might make a videotape of the interaction and review it with the patient and family members. The procedures are repeated with unfamiliar listeners, and the level of difficulty of scripts is varied, moving from old, known information toward ones involving improbable events or gossip.

Lyon and Sims[19] offered some useful strategies that aid patients with severe aphasic deficits in communicating their messages via drawing. In this approach, aphasic patients are trained to use simple line drawings for conveying information to communicative partners. Speech–language pathologists work with communicative partners, often family members, to help them ask for cues and assistance to improve drawings and maximize communicative success.

In general, methodologies that promote interaction of patients and significant others in the home will likely have the best outcomes for communicative function. For many years, speech–language pathologists have focused intervention efforts primarily on individuals with communication and/or swallowing difficulties and disproportionately on those with whom they must interact and live. The home care setting facilitates involvement of these individuals.

8. Provide meaningful home programs for patients and their communicative partners. In the home setting, speech–language pathologists often think to provide home programs, although sometimes the programs are narrow in scope and focus only on a few movements and/or words (e.g., repeat this word list five times a day). Home programs that provide broad practical guidelines or strategies that can be used throughout the day may afford patients with more efficient home practice opportunities. Table 8–8 offers an example of a home program for word retrieval.

Home programs should not be restricted to patients. Speech–language pathologists should provide the same sorts of broad practical guidelines for others in the home as well. An example of a home program for the conversational partner of a patient with aphasia is provided in Table 8–9.

9. Do not overtreat or undertreat patients. Home speech–language pathologists should take care in providing a sufficient amount of home intervention, but not too much. For instance, sometimes individuals with severe communication and/or swallowing deficits might be discharged too quickly, particularly if they are in an acute phase of recovery and recovering slowly. In these instances, speech–language pathologists should take care to ensure that family members are clear about what they might do to enhance or improve communicative and/or swallowing successes. If speech–language pathology services are about to be discontinued because patients are not able to withstand the rigors of intervention procedures at this point in their recovery,

---

Table 8–8. A Sample Home Program for Word Retrieval

When you have difficulty thinking of the word you are trying to say:

Try to use another word that means the same thing. For instance, say "sofa" if you can't think of "couch."

Try to describe the word. For instance, say "a black and white smelly animal" if you can't think of the word "skunk."

Try to think of the first letter of the word.

Try to think of the first sound of the word.

Try to write the word.

Try to gesture or pantomime the word. For instance, show with your hands how you would play a ukulele, even if you can't think of the word "ukulele."

Try to draw a picture of the word you're trying to say.

Try to say what the word is not. For example, "It's not a tiger, it's not a leopard, it's not a lion. . . ."

Use the first word that comes to mind, even if it's the wrong word. Sometimes the word you think of will be similar to the one you're trying to say, like "caramel" for carousel."

Try to find the item, and show it to someone.

Wait and stop thinking about the word. Sometimes it will come to you on its own.

Table 8–9. A Sample Home Program for the Conversational Partner of a Person with Aphasic Auditory Comprehension Difficulties

To help make sure your spouse/partner understands you better:

Keep your sentences short and simple.

Repeat what you say two or three times.

Use gestures and pointing to supplement what you're saying.

Write down the key words about the topic you're talking about. For instance, if you want to let your partner know that you have to go to the store to get some milk, you might write the words "store" and "milk" when you say them. Point to the printed words and say them again to help your partner understand what you're saying.

When you ask a yes/no question, try asking it a different way and see if your partner responds the same way. For instance, if you ask "Do you want the channel changer?" and he says "no," ask, "Do you want to turn the TV off?" and see if he still says no. Often, people who have difficulty understanding following a stroke say "yes" more often than "no," even when they mean "no." Sometimes they say "no" when they mean "yes." Asking questions several different ways will help you figure out what your partner really wants.

Make sure you have his attention before speaking to him. You might try letting him know you have something to say to him by either calling his name or prefacing your remarks with an alerting sentence like "Here's something for you."

speech–language pathologists should instruct family members about behaviors to watch for—behaviors that might indicate that the person would benefit from speech–language pathology interventions at some point in the future.

At the other end of the continuum are patients who are independently able to communicate most needs, thoughts, feelings, and opinions without assistance from others or who can independently utilize safe swallowing practices. Speech–language pathology interventions for these patients should be discontinued as soon as patients and clinicians agree that they are independent. Similarly, when patients reach a point in recovery where they no longer meet homebound eligibility requirements, they must be discharged to outpatient settings for continued services.

Occasionally patients and their families have a difficult time separating from clinicians once it is time to end home-based speech–language pathology interventions. When this occurs, families should be given the option to pay privately for continued maintenance services—services designed to ensure that patients maintain a particular level of communicative and/or swallowing function. Many home health agencies have divisions for private and extended care, and such maintenance services can be offered through those divisions. Ideally, the patient and family members in these situations should be referred to other community resources that might meet their continuing needs for contact (e.g., community stroke clubs, senior citizen programs).

The home setting provides a unique opportunity for speech–language pathologists to engage the patient and significant others in a natural environment in activities that will enhance communicative effectiveness and/or swallowing safety. The following case is provided to demonstrate how home-based speech–language intervention focuses on maximizing the effectiveness of communicative interactions.

CASE ONE

Mrs. B., age 71, was seen for a speech–language evaluation in her home six weeks after she suffered a left hemisphere CVA. Immediately following the CVA, Mrs. B. was hospitalized at a community acute care hospital and once her medical condition was stabilized, she was transferred to a rehabilitation hospital. During her rehabilitation hospital stay, Mrs. B. received one hour of speech–language therapy five times weekly. Treatment focused on "im-

proving oral motor skills and expressive language skills." The speech–language pathologist at the rehabilitation hospital provided Mrs. B. with a list of 10 oral-motor exercises that she performed during treatment sessions and which she was to practice 10 times each three other times during the day. In addition, treatment sessions included opportunities for Mrs. B. to complete workbook pages from commercially available aphasia workbooks. These workbook pages involved such processes as unscrambling letters to form words, categorization of similar items, and completion of open-ended sentences (e.g., You sleep on a ____). Mrs. B. was discharged to home care, with her husband Mr. B. assuming the role of primary caregiver. Mrs. B. was considered homebound because she could not ambulate without assistance, and home occupational and physical therapy were also ordered.

During the initial home speech–language evaluation, Mrs. B. stated that she wanted to "talk better and say the words that I know." She stated that she was unhappy with her previous therapy because "I hate those exercises and those papers stripped me of my dignity." Selected items from the Boston Diagnostic Aphasia Examination and the Boston Naming Test were administered, and Mrs. B. was determined to have mildly unintelligible speech secondary to a flaccid dysarthria and a moderate anomic aphasia. Mrs. B.'s speech was characterized by consonant imprecision, accompanied by mild breathiness and hypernasality. When provided with items from the Boston Naming Test, Mrs. B. often stated, "I know it but I can't say it." She had no observable self-cueing strategies for word retrieval, but when the clinician provided initial letter cues, Mrs. B. was quick to respond with appropriate words.

Home speech–language therapy was implemented three times weekly for four weeks. Sessions lasted 45 minutes each, on average. Goals were that Mrs. B. would successfully use strategies to facilitate intelligible conversational speech and strategies to aid her when conversational word retrieval difficulties occurred in at least 90% of her attempts.

Mrs. B. and her husband were taught that she should talk slower, talk louder, and open her mouth wider to improve speech intelligibility. Treatment initially focused on having Mrs. B. practice using these strategies in imitation of the clinician's verbal models. Once she became able to imitate sentences consistently, Mrs. B. was observed as she verbally interacted with Mr. B. about conversational topics provided by the clinician. Mr. B. was instructed to tell Mrs. B. when he didn't understand what she was saying, and she in turn was instructed to use strategies to produce the questionable word, phrase, or sentence intelligibly on a subsequent trial.

To remediate Mrs. B.'s conversational word retrieval difficulties, the clinician instructed Mrs. B. and her husband about strategies she might use when word retrieval problems occurred (e.g., provide verbal descriptions; use synonyms; try to gesture or pantomime the word; try to write or draw the word; try to think of the first letter of the word; try to say what the word is not; stop thinking about the word and return to it later). To practice using these strategies, the clinician sat with Mrs. B. and a stack of action photographs clipped from *People* and other contemporary magazines. A file folder was placed upright behind the stack to conceal them from Mr. B.'s view. Mrs. B. was instructed to tell her husband what was occurring in each photograph, with the clinician initially providing cueing regarding strategies Mrs. B. might try. Mr. B. was instructed to ask questions when he was uncertain about something she said, to remind Mrs. B. about strategies she might try, and to guess when he had a reasonable idea about what she was trying to say. During the treatment sessions, the speech–language pathologist provided coaching to the patient and her husband regarding ways of enhancing communicative effectiveness.

Home speech–language therapy sessions were discontinued after four weeks. Mrs. B. had become able to use speech intelligibility strategies independently, and her conversational speech improved from 80% sentence intelligibility to 100% sentence intelligibility. Mrs. B. could then use word retrieval strategies that facilitated retrieval or compensated for retrieval failure in conversational interactions with her husband in as many as 95% of her attempts, up from baseline performance of 67% success. Mrs. B. and her husband were satisfied with the progress she had made and were not interested in additional speech–language therapy.

HOSPICE CARE

In recent years, there has been an increase in the number of terminally ill patients receiving palliative care in hospice programs. Typically, these programs are implemented in patients' homes, or less often, in long-term care settings. The focus of speech–language pathology interventions in these settings is primarily on maintenance goals, with little or no emphasis on restorative goals. In other words, when speech–language pathology interventions are indicated in the hospice setting, they are designed primarily to help the patient maintain an optimal level of communicative and/or swallowing function relative to a declining medical status. The interventions often utilize instruction about compensatory strategies for individuals to use.

Those individuals likely to be referred for services in the hospice setting would include those with progressive degenerative neurological diseases such as amyotrophic lateral sclerosis, Huntington's chorea, Parkinson's disease, and multiple sclerosis; those with degenerative cognitive impairments resulting from acquired immune deficiency syndrome (AIDS) and Alzheimer's disease; and those with terminal metastatic carcinoma. One of the primary objectives of hospice care is to maximize the comfort level of patients and their significant others during the end stages of their illnesses. Therefore, it is incumbent on the speech–language pathologist delivering services in hospice care to develop interventions for patients and their significant others that are directed toward instruction, support, and compensations that promote the maintenance of communication and/or swallowing skills for as long as is feasible.

To date, there has been little demand for speech–language pathology services in the hospice setting, although this area for service delivery can be expected to grow in volume as the proportion of elderly individuals in the population increases drastically during the next few decades. When hospice-based speech–language pathology services are provided, they are typically short-term interventions and usually do not continue until the time a patient expires. It is important for clinicians working in this setting, therefore, to assess needs quickly and develop interventions that might best meet those needs in a relatively short time.

Like the interventions provided in home care, hospice-based services should involve patient input (to the extent possible) as well as input from significant others. Because of the philosophy of hospice care, some patient requests and requests from others pose unique challenges to the speech–language pathologist relative to ethical issues. For instance, a person who has signed an advanced directive statement requesting that no extraordinary measures be used to sustain life may have a severe and irreversible oropharyngeal dysphagia. This individual and others may believe that a PEG tube insertion constitutes an extraordinary measure, and a referral for speech–language pathology services may be initiated. The speech–language pathologist in the hospice setting must instruct the patient and significant others about the risks and probable outcomes associated with eating and drinking as well as those from not eating and not drinking. While the clinician might impart some information about how PEG tubes meet hydration and nutritional needs, and how dysphagic individuals might have minuscule portions of food and drink perorally to supplement the tube feeding, the patient and/or significant others must ultimately decide the course of action. The speech–language pathologist, in this context, serves to instruct the patient and others about the limitations imposed by the dysphagia, and makes referrals to others (e.g., physician, dietitian) if necessary.

Speech–language pathology services delivered in hospice settings need not always have grave consequences such as the scenario just described. Often the speech–language pathologist can offer instruction and advice that enhances the quality of life for the patient and the patient's significant others. This might be something as simple as having patients use some sort of device or system to augment speech production to optimize the successfulness of their interactions with others or keep a memory notebook to aid in the recall of recent events. The value of making final wishes known, participating in life review, and speaking with loved ones cannot be underestimated. The following guidelines for providing speech–language pathology services in a hospice setting may be useful.

1. *Try to anticipate patients' future communicative and/or swallowing needs.* Knowledge about the projected course of illness or disease of patients in hospice care will aid the speech–language pathologist in planning for patients' future needs. For instance, in the case of individuals with degenerative diseases such as amyotrophic lateral sclerosis, speech–language pathologists might anticipate deterioration of communication and swallowing and implement strategies that will aid the patient in the future. Such strategies might include training in the use of some alternate communication system and counseling about non-oral nutrition and hydration, even though the patient is able to use speech and tolerate oral food intake at the time of intervention. As communication and cognitive processes decline in patients in hospice care, caregivers often need advice and instruction about how to anticipate patients' needs for care with them, and the speech–language pathologist might offer suggestions such as those in Table 8–10.

2. *Provide caregivers with suggestions about interacting with patients who are unable to com-*

Table 8–10. Some Suggestions for Anticipating the Physical Needs for Care for Hospice Patients with Declining Communication and Cognitive Skills

Keep the person's room at a comfortable temperature. Provide or remove blankets and/or clothing as necessary.

Make sure the person is fed and hydrated. If oral feedings occur, make sure they are provided often during the day.

If the person is incontinent of bowel/bladder, check the person often and change as necessary.

In the daytime, and during the time when the person is customarily awake, make certain that there is adequate light in the room. Make certain that it is sufficiently darkened in the evenings and when the person is sleeping.

Minimize excessive noise. If the person has a hearing loss and wears a hearing aid, check to see that the hearing aid has working batteries and is inserted properly.

If the person wears glasses, make sure that the lenses are cleaned regularly and that the person is wearing them at appropriate times.

Make sure that the person's clothing is comfortable.

municate and may have severe cognitive limitations. Perhaps one of the most difficult things for significant others of patients in hospice care is to continue to interact with loved ones who have undergone severe cognitive and communicative decline. These individuals need to learn new ways of communicating with terminally ill patients, and the speech–language pathologist can offer suggestions. Some of these suggestions, offered in Table 8–11, include providing passive orientation, offering opportunities for reminiscing and life review, reading aloud, listening to music, and watching television.

3. *Respect the wishes of the patient and significant others, and try to accommodate their needs as best as possible.* By the time terminally ill patients have been referred to hospice care, they have often undergone significant cognitive, communication, and and/or swallowing decline, and patients and significant others have often had time to accept that patients are terminally ill. Speech–language pathologists in the hospice setting therefore must be able to make reasonably rapid decisions about accommodating the requests of patients and their significant others. For instance, sometimes patients who are being fed and hydrated via non-oral means request food or liquid by mouth. While patients might not be able to tolerate entire meals or adequate liquid intake for daily hydration, they

Table 8–11. Some Suggestions for Caregivers for Interacting with Terminally Ill Patients Who May Be Unable to Communicate

Even though the person may be unable to express needs, feelings, and thoughts, do not refrain from talking.

Tell the person what you are doing as you do it. For instance, say, "I'm going to open these blinds to let some more light into the room" as you are adjusting the blinds.

Try to work the day or date into your conversations. For instance, you might say, "It's really hard to believe that it's March 16 because it's 75° out!"

Talk to the person about things that are going on with family members and friends or about current events.

Reminisce about people and events from the person's past. If possible, review old photographs together and talk about them.

Read aloud to the person.

Turn on favorite television programs, even if the person is unable to respond to them. For instance, if a person always liked to watch the game show *Wheel of Fortune* after dinner, turn it on in the evenings.

Play music or sing songs the person likes.

---

might be able to safely tolerate small amounts (i.e., 1/2 teaspoon portions) of thin liquids and purees. Speech–language pathologists may wish to provide instruction regarding other swallowing safety precautions (e.g., chin tucks, multiple swallows) as indicated in these cases.

Sometimes patients with degenerative neurological diseases do not want to use alternate communication systems and insist on talking, even though speech may be severely dysarthric. Speech–language pathologists might wish to implement a system such as an alphabet system for augmenting speech, such as the one described by Yorkston, Beukelman and Bell.[16] With this system, the patient says a word, and if it is not understandable to the listener, the patient points to the first letter of the word as a cue to listeners. Patients who dislike alternate communication systems often find this alphabet system a happy medium that enables them to continue to use speech.

4. *Avoid imposing your preferences and judgments on patients and their significant others.* Sometimes in the hospice setting, patients and caregivers have needs and expectations that do not match those of the speech–language pathologist. The speech–language pathologist needs to be careful to respect the wishes of the patient and caregiver, even if those wishes impede communication

successes or swallowing safety. Patients with severe oral communication impairments who are able to communicate adequately via line drawings may reject drawing as a viable communication option. Patients who are able to tolerate thickened liquids by mouth safely may reject them because they feel that the thickener tastes bad. Speech–language pathologists providing hospice-based speech–language pathology services need to accept these types of situations and when feasible, offer alternate suggestions which match patients' needs with their limitations.

There has been little information about the successfulness and efficacy of speech–language pathology interventions provided in the hospice setting. As the volume of patients treated in this setting continues to grow, more opportunities for speech–language pathologists will be likely. Clinical research efforts regarding hospice-based speech–language pathology interventions are sorely needed.

Speech–language pathology service provided in the hospice setting are unlike those in other settings because their intervention goals are not typically restorative in nature. Often communication and/or swallowing needs of patients and their significant others in the hospice setting define the speech–language pathology intervention strategies. The following case is used to illustrate the concepts we have discussed.

CASE TWO

Mr. Y., age 52, was diagnosed with amyotrophic lateral sclerosis (ALS) four years prior to his speech–language pathology evaluation in hospice care provided in his home. He lived there with his wife, their 22-year-old son and 18-year-old daughter. Mr. Y. was unable to tolerate food and liquids by mouth safely, nor was he able to express basic needs orally because of a severe mixed dysarthria. Mr. Y. was fed and hydrated via a PEG tube. His speech was characterized by severe consonant imprecision, "wet, gurgly" phonation, impaired prosody and slow rate, and on oral diadochokinesis, syllable repetition was slow, and voiced consonants were substituted for unvoiced consonants.

Mr. Y. had had several months of speech–language therapy after the ALS diagnosis was initially made. This treatment had consisted primarily of oral-motor exercises and articulatory drills and had not focused on development of augmentative/alternative communication strategies. Mr. Y. and his family had figured out that he could communicate his needs by pointing to letters on an alphabet board, but as his disease progressed, his precision in doing this accurately was diminishing. He and his family wanted to work on skills that would enable him to communicate more efficiently. In addition, Mr. Y., aware of the risks of aspiration associated with peroral intake, wanted to be able to eat and drink occasionally and stated, "I want to taste it."

Two 45-minute speech–language therapy sessions were conducted weekly for three weeks. Goals were to help Mr. Y. maintain use of his alphabet board for communication purposes and meet his needs regarding the peroral intake of food and liquid. The speech–language pathologist made a few modifications to Mr. Y.'s alphabet board, including the addition of the items "end of word," "end of sentence," "?," and "erase that." Instead of a direct selection approach to the alphabet board (i.e., pointing to each letter individually), Mr. Y. and his family members were instructed in ways of using it with a scanning approach, in which Mr. Y. indicated the row and column of the item he wished to communicate. In addition, he was instructed how to use abbreviated forms (e.g., "2" for "to"/"too"; "B" for "be"/"bee") to maximize communicative efficiency. Mr. Y. and his family preferred the scanning method over direct selection, and the additional modifications to his alphabet board enabled him to communicate most things more effectively and efficiently.

The speech–language pathologist contacted Mr. Y.'s physician regarding peroral food intake, and encouraged the physician to allow Mr. Y. ½ teaspoon portions of thin liquids and pureed consistency foods. Mr. Y. was taught to use a chin tuck and double swallows to help protect the airway during the intake of these "pleasure feedings." Mr. Y. was grateful that he could have these small amounts of food occasionally, and he and his family complied with portion size restrictions and compensatory maneuvers. At the conclusion of speech–language intervention, Mr. Y. was able to maintain use of his alphabet board for communication purposes and enjoy occasional peroral food intake.

NURSING HOME

There has been an increase in the number of speech-pathologists providing services in the long-term care setting, and this number is expected to grow as the proportion of elderly individuals in the population increases. Because it is a lower cost alternative to acute care, there has been growth in recent years in the volume of rehabilitation services offered in long-term care. Specially designated *subacute rehabilitation units* have been developed to meet the needs of individuals with rehabilitation needs following acute illnesses.

Subacute rehabilitation units often serve to bridge the gap between those served by acute rehabilitation programs in freestanding or acute care hospitals and those who cannot tolerate or do not need the intensity of services demanded in acute rehabilitation settings. In acute rehabilitation settings, for instance, patients are expected to be able to participate in at least 3 hours of rehabilitation services daily. Some individuals, because of the acuity and/or severity of their conditions are unable to tolerate 3 hours of daily rehabilitation services, and therefore might be managed more appropriately in a subacute rehabilitation setting until they are able to tolerate this intensity. Some individuals, following an acute episode such as a cerebrovascular accident, may not need 3 hours of daily rehabilitation services. Individuals with Wernicke aphasia, for instance, may not need physical and occupational therapy, but may require speech–language therapy to help them get to a point where they can function independently in their own homes. These individuals might best be served in a subacute rehabilitation program. The intensity of rehabilitation services provided in a subacute setting is presumably greater than the intensity of rehabilitation services provided in other long-term care settings.

Not all long-term care facilities have specially designated subacute rehabilitation units, but most offer speech–language pathology services. There was a dramatic increase in the utilization of speech–language pathology services after the federally enacted Omnibus Budget Reconciliation Act (OBRA) guidelines in 1987. These guidelines mandated that facilities offer services to improve quality of life issues for those they served.

People who reside in long-term care settings are commonly referred to as *residents* and not *patients*. While some have recently acquired conditions, the vast majority of nursing home residents with communication and/or swallowing needs in long-term care settings have chronic conditions, and so the speech–language pathology interventions are necessarily different from those that might be provided in acute rehabilitation settings. The most frequently occurring diagnoses relative to speech–language pathology in long-term care are dysphagia and dementia, and speech–language pathologists in this setting subsequently are likely to be involved in the care of individuals with these diagnoses.

Dysphagia Needs in the Long-Term Care Setting

A relatively large number of nursing home residents are fed and/or hydrated via non-oral means, typically via the use of PEG tubes. The use of non-oral hydration/nutrition is typically ordered by a physician, who may or may not have obtained input about the decision from a speech–language pathologist. Residents may be fed and hydrated via alternate means because they have had recurrent pneumonia or urosepsis secondary to dehydration or because they have severe concomitant dementia and are unable to swallow sufficient amounts to sustain daily nutrition and hydration needs. Some residents may have simply refused to eat because of poor appetite or depression or because they don't like the food. Some residents are discharged from acute care hospitals to long-term care facilities on non-oral feedings because of videofluoroscopic findings following acute episodes (such as a cerebrovascular accident) or exacerbations of progressive illnesses (e.g., Parkinson's disease). It is incumbent on the speech–language pathologist employed in the long-term care setting to assess the very differing swallowing abilities and needs of residents and plan appropriate interventions for them.

When residents are referred for speech–language pathology services because of dysphagia, clinicians should review their medical records and then conduct a bedside swallowing assessment. If the speech–language pathologist cannot make an adequate determination about the resident's swallowing safety and aspiration risks on the basis of this evaluation, it is appropriate to request an order from the resident's physician for a videofluoroscopic swallowing evaluation. Since most nursing homes are not equipped to provide videofluoroscopy, speech–language pathologists in this setting will want to become acquainted with speech–language pathologists in the facility (usually an acute care hospital) where the videofluoroscopies will be conducted.

Following the evaluation of a resident's swallowing abilities (via the bedside swallowing evaluation and/or videofluoroscopic findings), the speech–language pathologist needs to implement an appropriate treatment plan. Residents with severe dysphagia and those who would be unable to sustain daily hydration/nutrition needs perorally will not benefit from further speech–language pathology interventions. Residents who show potential for increasing the amount of oral intake without significant risk of aspiration will be engaged in speech–language pathology intervention programs.

Although it may be appropriate for speech–language pathologists to feed residents with dysphagia for one or two sessions to demonstrate certain swallowing safety precautions, it is important to relinquish this role to a certified nursing assistant, a restorative aide, or to the resident as soon as possible. The speech–language pathologist might observe individuals during mealtimes to ensure that residents are using swallowing safety precautions or that certified nursing assistants are providing adequate portions and/or consistencies of foods, and these services are billable and appropriate. When speech–language pathologists bill insurance carriers for time spent feeding residents with dysphagia, it becomes ethically questionable. Residents should be entitled to have their nutritional needs met without increasing the cost of the meal by the expense associated with a speech–language pathologist. Because nursing home residents are fed at least three times daily seven days a week, it is imperative that the staff responsible for feeding and/or supervision during mealtime is able to manage residents safely. For this reason, speech–language pathologists employed in the nursing home setting may wish to conduct periodic inservice training sessions for those responsible for residents during mealtimes.

Speech–language pathologists in long-term care may often prescribe oral-motor and laryngeal exercises. While these kinds of exercises may not harm individuals with dysphagia, research directed toward substantiating their efficacy is necessary. If speech–language pathologists choose to recommend such exercises to individuals with dysphagia, these individuals should be advised that the exercises may not have any positive effect on swallowing outcomes. Even thermal stimulation, a widely used clinical practice for individuals with a delayed swallowing reflex, has been shown to provide only short-term effects for patients with multiple strokes.[20] A more practical alternative to swallowing exercises is to train the resident with dysphagia and those who may feed the resident or provide supervision during mealtime in compensatory maneuvers that protect the airway. Such maneuvers might include chin tuck, tilting or rotating the head to one side, tongue sweep, and/or the supraglottic swallow technique.[21] Most residents with dysphagia do not benefit from eating in a supine position, so instruction in appropriate posture is often necessary.

The speech–language pathologist should work in close collaboration with the nursing facility's dietitian and dietary staff. These individuals need to know and understand differences between thin liquids and those of nectar, honey, and pudding consistencies. The dietitian can assist in providing calorie counts, particularly when there is a goal of weaning a resident from PEG tube feedings.

There is the potential for abuse and fraud in the long term care setting by speech–language pathologists because of the high incidence of swallowing disorders. Clinicians should therefore take a prudent course of action in these situations without providing more intervention than necessary.

Dementia in the Long-Term Care Setting

A large percentage of nursing home residents have some degree of dementia. Some may have mild symptoms and be relatively independent regarding communication. Others with severe dementia may be unable to communicate even basic needs, and require that caregivers anticipate all their needs. Often, speech–language pathologists are consulted about the communication status of these residents.

The *Arizona Battery for Communication in Dementia*[13] is a useful tool for determining the extent of communication impairment in residents with dementia. Although extensive speech–language pathology interventions are not indicated for individuals with dementia, speech–language pathologists may choose to provide short-term interventions. Because of the nature of the deficits associated with dementia, intervention strategies that are compensatory in nature are indicated. Individuals in early stages of dementing illness can be trained to request repetitions to enhance comprehension and memory.[22] Memory notebooks[23] are often effective with individuals who have more pronounced memory difficulties. It is imperative that nursing home staff members learn how to use the notebooks as well as how to make appropriate entries. For individuals with chronic and severe dementias, nursing home personnel must be trained to anticipate needs for care. Mace and Rabins[24] suggest that in these cases caregivers ensure that residents are warm, fed, wearing comfortable clothing, and toileted. In addition, they offer some suggestions for caregivers about nonverbal ways to interact with persons with severe dementia. These are provided in Table 8–12.

Table 8–12. Some Suggestions for Nonverbal Communicative Interactions with Persons with Severe Dementia

Use body language and facial expressions that convey pleasantness, calmness, and supportiveness.

Express affection in a physical manner, such as smiling, taking the person's hand, and putting an arm around his/her waist.

Maintain eye contact with the person to ensure that the person is attentive. If the person uses body language to signal that he/she is not paying attention, try again later.

Use other signals besides words. You might point to things, or hand the person objects, allowing him/her to get tactile sensations. Use gestures and pantomimes.

Hold hands, hug or sit companionably together to communicate to the severely impaired person that you are concerned and that he/she is protected.

Source: Adapted from Mace N, Robins P: *The 36-hour day: A family guide to caring for persons with Alzheimer's disease, related dementing illnesses, and memory loss in later life,* rev. ed. Johns Hopkins University Press, Baltimore, 1991.

One day in a nursing facility may seem like any other, so it is not uncommon for nursing home residents to become disoriented about time. Many nursing facilities choose to provide ongoing programs of reality orientation,[25] although such programs often do not produce effective outcomes for persons with dementia. There are orientation boards and broadcasts over the intercom about the day, date, and place, which are useful for residents without dementia. While somewhat more controversial, Feil's validation therapy approach encourages caregivers to follow the communicative leads of individuals with dementia.[26] For instance, if a resident believes she is shopping at a department store, the caregiver might ask the resident what she intends to buy and if there are any good sales going on. While validation therapy doesn't aid in orienting residents with dementia, it often has the effect of minimizing the agitation so frequently seen in these individuals and serves to provide a context in which they can continue using communication behavior.

Documentation Issues

In addition to routine evaluation reports, progress notes, and discharge summaries, speech–language pathologists employed in the long-term care setting often have some additional documentation requirements. Typically, any speech–language pathology interventions for communication and/or swallowing disorders need to be entered on a document often referred to as the nursing care plan. This plan includes interventions from all professional disciplines engaged in the care of a resident, and typically notes problems identified, goals established, interventions to be provided, and target dates for completion. The speech–language pathologist should enter any special communication and/or swallowing manipulations for specific residents on the nursing care plan.

Another document that requires input from speech–language pathologists employed in nursing facilities is the Minimum Data Set (MDS) form. This form was developed by the Health Care Financing Administration (HCFA) in 1990 as a national instrument and data base for long-term care resident assessment.[27] Version 2.0 of the MDS form includes identifying and demographic information about residents; information about cognitive, communication/hearing, vision, and mood and behavior patterns; oral/nutritional status; and other assessment information about residents. An associated tool, the Resident Assessment Protocol (RAP), triggers for the staff an identification of problems individual residents may be experiencing. Table 8–13 identifies the information included for each section of Version 2.0 of the MDS form. Input from speech–language pathologists is particularly relevant for the sections and item numbers identified in Table 8–14. While nursing personnel complete the MDS in most facilities, speech–language pathologists may be invited to complete selected portions of the form or provide assessment information to nursing about the form. In 1997 HCFA implemented a mandate requiring nursing facilities to submit the MDS information via computer.

Various other forms may be required depending on the specific nursing facility environment where services are provided. In conjunction with other documentation about speech–language pathology services, clinicians may be required to complete HCFA Forms 700 and 701 for submission of claims for reimbursement.

Treatment Considerations in Long-Term Care

A number of unique features about the long term care setting can be considered in the provision of speech–language pathology services. The following guidelines may be useful to speech–language pathologists providing services in this setting.

1. Offer consultative services regarding communication and swallowing to other nursing facility personnel. Often residents in long-term care are apt to derive more benefits from speech–language pathology services that instruct their caregivers about their communication and swallowing needs. Speech–language pathologists need to work closely with certified nursing assistants who feed residents with dysphagia to ensure that swallowing safety precautions are followed. Well-trained certified nursing assistants can also help long-term care speech–language pathologists identify residents who are having swallowing difficulties. Because there is sometimes a high employee turnover rate for certified nursing assistants, the speech–language pathologist in long-term care will want to be part of new employee orientation for these individuals. Topics to be addressed with newly employed assistants would include information about the risks of aspiration, what NPO status means, positioning, compensatory safety maneuvers (e.g., chin tuck, supraglottic swallow), and how to thicken liquids to appropriate consistencies.

Speech–language pathologists in the long-term care setting will want to work closely with dietitians and dietary staff to ensure that residents with dysphagia are having their daily nutritional and hydration needs met. Some residents, for instance, may be able to tolerate ½ teaspoon portions of thickened liquids safely, but due to limited staffing and residents' dependence on others for

Table 8–13. Outline of the Sections Included in the Minimum Data Set (MDS), Version 2.0[17]

A. Identification and background information

B. Cognitive patterns

C. Communication/hearing patterns

D. Vision patterns

E. Mood and behavior patterns

F. Psychosocial well-being

G. Physical functioning and structural problems.

H. Continence in last 14 days

I. Disease diagnoses

J. Health conditions

K. Oral/nutritional status

L. Oral/dental status

M. Skin condition

N. Activity pursuit patterns

O. Medications

P. Special treatments and procedures

Q. Discharge potential and overall status

R. Assessment information

Table 8-14. Portions of the Minimum Data Set (MDS), Version 2.0 That May Be Particularly Relevant to Speech–Language Pathologists

Section	Items	Descriptions
B. Cognitive patterns	B2. Memory	Compares short- and long-term recall
	B3. Memory/recall ability	Orientation to time, place, person
	B4. Cognitive skills for daily decision-making	Independence in ADL decisions
	B5. Indicators of delirium—periodic disordered thinking/awareness	Distractibility, disorganized speech
C. Communication/ hearing patterns	C1. Hearing	Hearing sensitivity
	C2. Communication devices/techniques	Use of hearing aid, speechreading
	C3. Modes of expression	Speech, writing, sign, communication board
	C4. Making self understood	Expressive communication ability
	C5. Speech clarity	Intelligibility of expressive speech
	C6. Ability to understand others	Auditory comprehension skills
	C7. Change in communication/hearing	Relative to status 90 days ago
D. Visual patterns	D2. Visual limitations/difficulties	Visual neglect; hemianopsia
K. Oral/nutritional status	K1. Oral problems	Chewing problems, swallowing problems
P. Special treatment procedures	P1ba. Therapies: speech–language pathology or audiology services	Number of days and number of minutes of speech–language pathology services provided during the last 14 days
R. Assessment information	R2c. Other signatures	Speech–language pathologist signs and dates MDS form and indicates which section(s) s/he completed

feeding, peroral hydration may be unrealistic. In large facilities, speech–language pathologists might influence dietary departments to consider stocking commercially available prethickened liquids to minimize the likelihood that residents with dysphagia are receiving the requisite liquid consistencies.

Speech–language pathologists will also wish to work collaboratively with nursing facility activity directors and recreation therapy specialists. The activities provided in a facility may serve as appropriate venues for speech–language pathology intervention efforts. For instance, staff may wish to know how to best communicate with aphasic residents with aphasic auditory comprehension deficits during activities, as well as types of activities that may be best suited for these residents. In addition, food and refreshments are served at a number of nursing facility activities, and staff members coordinating these events need to know about the foods dysphagic residents are able to tolerate safely, as well as any additional safety precautions.

Speech–language pathologists should be actively involved in interdisciplinary care conferences in the nursing facility. Because these conferences often involve residents and their families, in addition to staff members from other professions, they provide an opportunity for instruction and education about communication and swallowing disorders and the strategies used in intervention efforts.

2. When possible, pair communicatively and swallowing impaired residents with other residents who are willing to assist them. Lyon[28] and Kagan and Gailey[29] have described programs for enlisting the aid of volunteers to help patients with aphasia communicate. This concept is particularly well suited for use in a nursing facility. Nursing home residents who are more cognitively and linguistically intact, and who show interest in volunteering, may be trained to aid communicatively and/or swallowing impaired residents in implementing intervention strategies outside the context of speech–language pathology treatment sessions. When such pairings are effective, even residents with severe communication impairments are able to participate more fully in daily activities and routines.

3. Help residents and their families reach informed decisions about swallowing issues. A number of nursing home residents with dysphagia become at risk for aspiration and/or dehydration because of degenerative neurological disease or damage, diminished strength and endurance, and/or declining cognitive function. These residents are more safely fed via alternate means. Often the residents and their families reject these alternate feeding options because they do not (or cannot) understand the ramifications of the swallowing problem on daily nutrition and hydration requirements. Speech–language pathologists should provide counseling and instruction about these issues so that residents and their families can make informed decisions about the intake of food. For residents who receive nutrition and hydration via a PEG tube, speech–language pathologists may wish to recommend that physicians amend diet orders to include pleasure feedings of 1/2 teaspoon portions of pureed foods when feasible.

Some residents with dysphagia require thickened liquids and/or pureed foods to minimize the likelihood of aspiration. They frequently reject these dietary modifications because they find the consistencies objectionable. When the speech–language pathologist has provided adequate instruction about why these modifications are necessary and the potential risks of aspiration, and residents continue to reject these foods, residents' wishes should be respected. However, speech–language pathologists, in concert with the administration of the nursing facility, should require that such residents (and/or their legal guardians) sign a written waiver releasing the facility and speech–language pathologist from any complications that may occur as a result of a regular diet and/or thin liquids.

4. Use conversation as the basis of communication interventions when possible. Although speech–language pathology interventions for aphasia often focus on single word inputs and outputs, most adults typically neither speak nor comprehend one word at a time. Kagan and Gailey[29] reinforce the concept that conversation is the basic level of communication interactions and that speech–language pathology interventions should move to the conversational level as quickly as possible. Nursing home residents with auditory comprehension and hearing impairments, for instance, might require conversational interventions that supplement auditory inputs with multimodal presentations. The speech–language pathologist can train others who interact with these residents to gesture, write down key words about a conversation in large print, repeat short bits of information about the conversational topic, and even to draw simple line drawings to facilitate comprehension at a conversational level. These strategies appear to help residents with comprehension impairments function better in the nursing home environment than strategies requiring the resident to point to one object when named from an array of six pictures. Dysarthric residents appear to function better in communication when they learn to apply general intelligibility strategies than ones that focus specifically on articulatory placements, because the strategies can be applied immediately at the conversational level.

5. Help nursing home staff learn to communicate with hearing impaired residents. Most nursing facilities do not have access to audiologists, so it is often incumbent on the speech–language pathologist to serve as a resource for residents with hearing losses. Speech–language pathologists employed in nursing home settings should know, as a minimum, how to change a hearing aid battery, insert a hearing aid, adjust the volume, and troubleshoot common hearing aid problems (e.g., feedback, telephone switch). Caregivers should receive inservice education about hearing losses and hearing aid issues. Sessions might include information about hearing aid care and use as well as how best to communicate with hearing impaired residents. Some hearing impaired residents may benefit from the use of assistive listening devices, particularly when participating in group activities. Speech–language pathologists employed in nursing facilities should establish collegial relationships with audiologists in their communities to assist in meeting the needs of those residents with hearing impairments.

Functional Maintenance Therapy

Nursing home residents with chronic communication and/or swallowing disorders may be eligible for periodic reassessments and interventions to ensure that they are functioning at their highest possible level. The provisions for these functional maintenance programs are authorized in Medicare guidelines that enhance and/or preserve communication and/or swallowing abilities and deter declines in communication and/or swallowing functions obtained from speech–language pathology interventions.

Often individuals may be referred for functional maintenance interventions when there has been a change in status. For instance, someone who was using swallowing safety precautions independently begins to show decreased ability in swallowing. Speech–language pathologists, following an assessment, may recommend a short period (typically two weeks or less) of intervention designed to prevent further declines and maintain the individual's functioning at the highest possible level. Functional maintenance interventions might include providing individuals with new strategies for communication and/or swallowing or reinstruction about previously used strategies. These interventions are not intended to offer remediation for newly acquired impairments or to extend speech–language interventions for someone indefinitely.

Although designed for nursing home residents who are eligible for Medicare benefits, the functional maintenance therapy concept may be appealing to other payors. For instance, residents with needs for functional maintenance therapy might be covered under managed care plans. Speech–language pathologists, in concert with a social worker or case manager from the nursing facility, may be able to negotiate out-of-contract benefits for individuals with chronic conditions who might need a few "tune up" sessions.

CASE THREE

Mrs. E., age 74, was admitted to a long-term care facility from the rehabilitation unit of a hospital. At one month post-onset of a unilateral right hemisphere CVA, she had received 3 weeks of intensive inpatient rehabilitation. Speech–language treatment goals in the hospital focused on "oral motor exercises to strengthen articulatory and swallowing musculature," "dysphagia therapy to maximize safe swallowing behavior," and "higher level language therapy to facilitate judgment and problem solving."

Mrs. E. was seen for a speech–language evaluation following her admission to the long-term care facility. Her speech was mildly unintelligible due to a flaccid dysarthria, and was characterized by breathiness, hypernasality, consonant imprecision, and inhalatory stridor. She was able to verbally express her needs, thoughts, feelings and requests with little difficulty. Mrs. E. had impaired reading and writing skills resulting from a significant left visual field deficit. Attention, memory, orientation, abstract reasoning, judgment, and problem solving were within functional limits, although Mrs. E. was mildly impulsive in her attempts to complete assessment tasks. Mrs. E. reported that she had been having swallowing difficulties, so she was observed during mealtime. Mrs. E.'s diet order was for regular food with thin liquids. A nursing assistant delivered the tray to Mrs. E.'s bedside, and Mrs. E. attempted to eat her meal while in a supine position. She coughed and choked on thin liquids, and had difficulty chewing regular foods. Mrs. E. did not notice food placed on the left side of her tray, and didn't eat it.

The speech–language pathologist contacted Mrs. E.'s physician, who ordered a videofluoroscopic swallowing study. The swallowing study revealed laryngeal penetration of thin liquids without aspiration and pooling in the valleculae for both thin and thick liquids. The residue cleared with double swallows. Laryngeal penetration and aspiration was noted with a barium-coated cookie. On the basis of the videofluoroscopic swallowing study findings, the physician changed Mrs. E.'s diet order to pureed foods with honey-thick liquids.

Speech–language pathology intervention focused on helping Mrs. E. compensate for the left visual field deficit for reading and writing and for other activities she enjoyed. Mrs. E. often participated in the nursing facility's activities and particularly liked to play bingo. Because of the left visual neglect, however, she typically missed numbers on her card. The speech–language pathologist consulted with the facility's activities director to request some modification of Mrs. E.'s bingo cards. The speech–language pathologist recommended that bingo cards be constructed so that all letter and numbers were arrayed in the right visual field. This modification enabled Mrs. E. to participate fully in bingo without difficulty.

For reading and writing activities, Mrs. E. was instructed to take her time, move reading/writing materials slightly to the right, tilt her head a little to the left, while keeping her eyes straight down on the paper to compensate for the visual field deficit. In addition, for reading she was instructed to read aloud, move her finger along word by word as she got through a passage, and remember to go all the way to the left when she approached the end of a line of text. These strategies were written for Mrs. E. in large print and only in the right visual field to maximize the likelihood that she could benefit from referring to them as necessary. During speech–language treatment sessions, Mrs. E. practiced reading articles from newspapers and magazines, initially cued by the clinician to use compensatory strategies. Within two weeks of the introduction of these strategies, Mrs. E. was able to use them independently for reading.

Mrs. E. was instructed to speak slower and louder and open her mouth wider during speech production to maximize speech intelligibility. She independently used these strategies within one week of introduction of intelligibility strategies, and began self-correcting unintelligible productions.

Mrs. E. was instructed about swallowing safety precautions. She was shown that she needed to sit upright during meals, drink liquids of honey consistency, eat pureed foods, and swallow twice after each bite or sip. The speech–language pathologist instructed nursing and dietary staff to make sure that Mrs. E.'s tray contained thickened liquids only and items placed on the right side of the tray. Mrs. E. was observed during mealtimes on three separate occasions, and continued to have difficulty remembering to swallow twice, which resulted in coughing. In addition, she persisted in missing foods on the left hand side of her plate and tray. Trays were being delivered to her with thin liquids and packets of thickener, but Mrs. E. didn't consistently remember that she couldn't have thin liquids.

The speech–language pathologist asked Mrs. E.'s roommate, Mrs. Q., to participate as a helper. Mrs. E. agreed to have Mrs. Q. help her during mealtimes. Mrs. Q. was instructed to remind Mrs. E. about swallowing safety precautions as necessary, particularly about raising the head of her bed prior to eating, to swallow twice if she heard some coughing, and to attend to foods on the left side of the plate and tray. Following three additional sessions conducted during mealtimes, Mrs. E. was using swallowing safety precautions consistently, requiring occasional external verbal cueing from Mrs. Q. Speech–language pathology interventions were discontinued four weeks after initiation because Mrs. E. had achieved treatment goals. Eventually, Mrs. E. and Mrs. Q. began eating lunch and dinner in the nursing facility's dining room, and they asked to be seated at the same table so that Mrs. Q. could help Mrs. E. A follow-up videofluoroscopic swallowing study revealed that Mrs. E. could tolerate thin liquids and solid foods safely, so long as she continued to use double swallows, and her diet order was changed to mechanical soft foods with thin liquids. In time, Mrs. E. also began using regular bingo cards during bingo games and used her visual field compensation strategies independently in this context as well.

SUMMARY

Often individuals with communicative and/or swallowing disorders in non-acute rehabilitation settings receive too little or too much speech–language pathology intervention, and this poses a challenge to speech–language pathologists. Services provided in homes, nursing homes, and hospice offer unique opportunities for speech–language pathologists to meet this challenge and to enlist the aid of others in the environment. Working directly in the patient's environment allows for maximum impact on quality of life and well-being as it relates to communication and swallowing. Services provided in acute care and rehabilitation settings do not have this advantage. When the approach is pragmatic, and when individuals with communication and/or swallowing disorders are given the opportunity to self-monitor and self-cue, communication and/or swallowing abilities can be restored to or maintained at their maximum functional levels.

Acknowledgments

The author wishes to acknowledge Kathleen McAvoy-Black and Gordon H. Krainen for their assistance in the preparation of this manuscript.

STUDY QUESTIONS

1. When are patients with speech–language pathology needs considered homebound?

2. What must the home care speech–language pathologist do during the initial visit?

3. How can home care speech–language pathologists work effectively with case managers?

4. What special skills should home care speech–language pathologists possess?

5. How can family members and significant others become involved in the speech–language pathology interventions of home care patients?

6. How do speech–language pathology interventions provided in the hospice setting differ from those in other settings?

7. How can family members and significant others become involved in the speech–language pathology interventions of hospice patients?

8. How are nursing home residents with dysphagia most effectively managed by speech–language pathologists?

9. Describe ways in which speech–language pathologists in long-term care can serve as consultants to other health care professionals.

10. What is functional maintenance therapy?

REFERENCES

1. Mayo CM, Mayo R: Stroke prevention: A health promotion approach. In Wallace GL, ed: *Adult aphasia rehabilitation.* Butterworth-Heinemann, Boston, 1996, pp 339–354.

2. Hecht JS, Tonkovich JD: Rehabilitation funding. In Wallace GL, ed: *Adult aphasia rehabilitation.* Butterworth-Heinemann, Boston, 1996, pp. 21–38.

3. American Speech–Language-Hearing Association: *Omnibus Survey.* American Speech–Language-Hearing Association, Rockville, MD, 1995.

4. McAvoy-Black K, Tonkovich JD: Issues in the delivery of home-based speech–language pathology services. Short course presented to the American Speech–Language-Hearing Association, Seattle, November, 1996.

5. Goodglass H, Kaplan E: *Boston Diagnostic Aphasia Examination.* Lea and Febiger, Philadelphia, 1983.

6. Kaplan E, Goodglass H, Weintraub S: *The Boston Naming Test.* Lea and Febiger, Philadelphia, 1983.

7. Lomas J, Pichard L, Bester S et al: The communicative effectiveness index: Development and psychometric evaluation of a functional communication measure for adult aphasia. *J Speech Hearing Dis* 1989; 54:113–124.

8. Penn C: The profiling of syntax and pragmatics in aphasia. *Clin Ling Phon* 1988; 2:179–207.

9. American Speech–Language-Hearing Association: Functional assessment of communication skills for adults (ASHA FACS). American Speech–Language-Hearing Association, Rockville, MD, 1995.

10. Pimental PA, Kingsbury NA: *Mini inventory of right brain injury.* Pro-Ed, Austin, TX, 1989.

11. Halper AS, Cherney LR, Burns MS: *Clinical management of right hemisphere dysfunction,* 2nd ed. Aspen Publishers, Gaithersburg, MD, 1996.

12. Darley FL, Aronson AE, Brown JR: *Motor speech disorders.* W. B. Saunders, Philadelphia, 1975.

13. Bayles KA, Tomoeda CK: Arizona Battery for Communication Disorders of Dementia (ABCD). Canyonlands Publishing, Tucson, 1991.

14. Brookshire RH: *An introduction to neurogenic communication disorders,* 4th ed. Mosby Year Book, St. Louis, 1992.

15. Namnum A: Readiness for therapy: Aphasia patient offers insights into rehab process. *ADVANCE for Speech–Language Pathologists and Audiologists* 1995; 5 (26): 11, 38.

16. Yorkston KM, Beukelman DR, Bell KR: *Clinical management of dysarthric speakers.* College-Hill Press, Boston, 1988.

17. Helm-Estabrooks N: Cognitive-Linguistic Task Book. CCICD Publishing Division, Cape Cod, MA, 1995.

18. Holland A: Pragmatic assessment and treatment for aphasia. In Wallace GL, ed: *Adult aphasia rehabilitation.* Butterworth-Heinemann, Boston, 1996, pp 161–174.

19. Lyon JG, Sims E: Drawing: Its use as a communicative aid with aphasic and normal adults. In Prescott TE, ed: *Clinical aphasiology,* Vol 18, pp 11–17. Pro-Ed, Austin, TX, 1989.

20. Rosenbek JC, Robbins J, Fishback B, Levine RL: Effects of thermal application on dysphagia after stroke. *J Speech Hearing Res* 1991; 34: 1257–1268.

21. Logemann JA: Evaluation and treatment of swallowing disorders. College Hill Press, San Diego, 1983.

22. Tonkovich JD: Dementia. In Larson VD, Talbott RE, eds: Grand rounds in communicative disorders. *Comm Dis* 1984; IX (12): 184–188.

23. Bourgeois MS: Communication treatment for adults with dementia. *J Speech Hearing Res* 1991; 34: 831–844.

24. Mace N, Rabins P: *The 36-hour day: A family guide to caring for persons with Alzheimer's disease, related dementing illnesses, and memory loss in later life,* Rev. ed. Johns Hopkins University Press, Baltimore, 1991.

25. Greene JG, Timbury GC, Smith R, et al: Reality orientation with elderly patients in the community: An empirical evaluation. *Age & Ageing* 1983; 12: 38–43.

26. Feil N: *The validation breakthrough: Simple techniques for communicating with people with Alzheimer's type dementia.* Edward Feil Productions, Cleveland, OH, 1993.

27. Morris JN, Murphy K, Nonemaker S: Minimum Data Set 2.0 User's Manual. Briggs Corporation, Des Moines, Iowa, 1995.

28. Lyon JG: Communication use and participation in life for adults with aphasia in natural settings: The scope of the problem. *Amer J Speech–Lang Path* 1992; 1: 7–14.

29. Kagan A, Gailey G: Functional is not enough: Training conversational partners for adults with aphasia. In Holland A, Forbes M, eds: *World perspectives of aphasia.* Singular Press, San Diego, 1993.

9

Drug-Induced Communication and Swallowing Disorders

TAMI O'SULLIVAN AND SUSAN C. FAGAN

CHAPTER OUTLINE

Drug-Induced Dysphonia

Drug-Induced Speech and Language Impairments

Drug-Induced Swallowing Disorders

The use of prescription and over-the-counter medications is increasing, and patients seen by speech–language pathologists are likely to be taking multiple medications for treatment of neurologic and other conditions (see Appendix A). With the use of any drug, a potential exists to cause unwanted effects that can result in serious morbidity or mortality. In 1987, 12,000 deaths and 17,000 hospitalizations were reported to the FDA as a direct consequence of drug therapy. However, these figures are probably gross underestimations due to underreporting; nationally the numbers may be 10 times as high.[1,2] In 1991, it was reported that 3.7% of patients in hospitals experienced a disabling adverse event as the result of drugs.[1] It has also been estimated that up to 11% of hospital admissions are attributable to adverse effects of drugs.[3]

Definition of an Adverse Drug Reaction

An adverse drug reaction (ADR) is "any response to a drug which is noxious and unintended, and which occurs at doses normally used in man for prophylaxis, diagnosis, or therapy of disease, or for the modification of physiologic function."[4] When it is an extension of the expected pharmacologic effect of the drug, it tends to be predictable and dose dependent. However, unexpected, bizarre reactions (idiosyncratic reactions) can also occur that are unrelated to the drug's pharmacologic action.

Health care professionals have an obligation to minimize the risk associated with drugs and to optimize outcomes from drug therapy. Knowledge of drug-induced communication and swallowing disorders will promote prevention, assist in early detection, and ensure prompt action once a reaction has occurred. In this chapter, we will discuss the various adverse effects of drugs that have resulted in communication and swallowing disorders as described in the literature. The classification of these effects into certain categories is at times difficult because authors may use vague descriptions or various labels for a particular communication disorder. For simplification, drug-induced effects consisting of dysarthria, apraxia, and aphasia have been gathered under speech and language effects.

Evaluation of a Patient Experiencing a Drug-Induced Disease

Once an adverse event has occurred, a systematic approach to evaluating the patient will promote proper management and prevention of similar occurrences. First, the clinical status of the patient should be assessed. If the patient is experiencing life-threatening effects, such as those that interfere with airway, breathing, or circulation, then emergency medical attention is imperative. Examples of potentially life-threatening effects include stridor, angioedema, laryngospasm, wheezing, or hypotension. The investigation and action taken in response to other reactions can be prioritized by the degree of compromise the patient is experiencing.

To determine whether the reaction was drug induced, the circumstances surrounding the adverse event must be accurately and thoroughly investigated. Information should be collected directly from the patient if possible and as soon as possible to improve accuracy and reliability of the data. Detailed information is obtained on the complaint, including its location, severity, timing, onset, duration, associated symptoms, modifying factors (what makes it better or worse), and context (under what circumstances does the complaint occur, has it happened before). Determining the patient's current medication history will help in the investigation as well. The clinician must determine what the patient is actually *taking*, including prescription, over-the-counter, and social drugs. The history of dosage changes, initiation of new drugs, and discontinuation of past drugs should also be collected.

Next, previous occurrences of the adverse event should be noted, particularly as they relate to any of the patient's medications. To review adverse effect profiles of drugs, sources such as package inserts (found in drug packaging and in the *Physicians' Desk Reference*), AHFS Drug Information, or *Facts & Comparisons* can be consulted. Direct communication with drug manufacturers is often helpful. They will have reports of postmarketing ADR that are not yet in the package insert and are often able to provide written information on an ADR. Investigation into the primary literature will yield detailed descriptions of drug-induced diseases and is particularly useful for idiosyncratic reactions or reactions from new drugs.

Proving causality between the drug and the adverse event is difficult, and often a clear conclusion is not reached. In general, however, the likelihood that an adverse event is drug induced can be estimated using previously developed criteria (see Table 9–1).[5] Also, comparing the patient's reactions to those discovered in a review of the literature is helpful. The temporal relationship of initiation of the drug or changes in dosage and onset of the event, characteristics of presentation, preexisting risk factors that the patient may possess, the possibility of involvement of drug interactions, alternative causes for the reaction, including symptoms of underlying disease, and other iatrogenic causes can be significant.

A plan of action should be developed and implemented in collaboration with the patient and the patient's primary health care provider based on the acuity and severity of the adverse event and recommendations reported in the literature. This plan should include supportive care and/or direct care for the patient's problem, but could possibly include no treatment at all. The necessity of discontinuing the therapy in question should be addressed. Discontinuing therapy is often the best solution if alternative safe and effective therapy is available. But if the benefits of therapy outweigh the risk of the ADR, therapy may be continued with or without treatment for the ADR. Other drug restrictions should be identified to prevent cross-reactivity with similar drugs.

Implementation of the plan requires informing the patient, the patient's primary health care provider, and the patient's pharmacist of the nature of the reaction and the proposed resolution. Written documentation will support the diagnosis and treatment plan to ensure that information is communicated accurately.

If the reaction has occurred secondary to a new drug or is very unusual or serious, it should be reported to the manufacturer and to the Med Watch program at the Food and Drug Administration (Figure 9–1). Often serious ADR of new drugs are not recognized until they are released for general use due to the low incidence of the event. Reporting the reaction assists the FDA and drug manufacturers in providing information to health care professionals to promote the safe use of medications.

Reporting the ADR in the medical literature is important if it has not been widely described to further improve general knowledge of the adverse effects of the drug and assist other clinicians in their investigation of the topic. Institutional adverse drug reaction forms are also available in most settings, and all ADR should be reported by this mechanism to contribute to internal monitoring of safety of drug therapy.

Table 9–1. Assessment of Likelihood That an Adverse Event Is Drug Induced

	Yes	No	Do Not Know	Score
1. Are there previous conclusive reports on this reaction?	+1	0	0	
2. Did the adverse event appear after the suspected drug was administered?	+2	−1	0	
3. Did the adverse reaction improve when the drug was discontinued or a specific antagonist was administered?	+1	0	0	
4. Did the adverse reaction reappear when the drug was readministered?	+2	−1	0	
5. Are there alternative causes (other than the drug) that could on their own have caused the reaction?	−1	+2	0	
6. Did the reaction reappear when a placebo was given?	−1	+1	0	
7. Was the drug detected in the blood (or other body fluids) in concentrations known to be toxic?	+1	0	0	
8. Was the reaction more severe when the dose was increased, or less severe when it was decreased?	+1	0	0	
9. Did the patient have a similar reaction to the same or similar drugs in any previous exposure?	+1	0	0	
10. Was the adverse event confirmed by any objective evidence?	+1	0	0	
Total score[a]				

[a]Association between drug and reaction: 9—definite, 5–8—probable, 1–4—possible, 0—doubtful.

DRUG-INDUCED DYSPHONIA

Vocal Fold Edema

Inhaled Steroid Preparations

Although few drugs have been associated with changes in voice or dysphonia, inhaled steroid preparations used in the chronic management of lung disease are frequently implicated (Table 9–2). In patients who use inhaled steroids regularly, as many as 50% will report the development of dysphonia.[6–8] The onset of symptoms is highly variable, with some patients developing symptoms immediately on initiation of therapy while the onset in others is delayed up to 112 weeks.[7] Although dysphonia can occur alone, it is often accompanied by other symptoms including oral candidiasis, throat irritation, and cough.

The mechanism of dysphonia associated with inhaled steroids is somewhat controversial. Trauma to the vocal folds from the rapid discharge of propellant from metered dose inhaler preparations may cause voice changes. Dysphonia from the administration of metered dose inhalers without steroid occurs, although at a lower frequency.[9,10] The incidence of dysphonia from other forms of inhaled steroids such as dry powder inhalers seems to be less.[11] However, the use of a spacer device with metered dose inhalers, which eliminates vocal fold trauma from the forceful discharge of the propellant, does not significantly reduce the incidence of dysphonia.[8]

Dysphonia with the use of inhaled steroids could also be caused by local effects of the steroid. It is hypothesized that steroid deposited in the larynx may induce local myopathy of laryngeal muscles that would effect vocal fold function.[7] This would account for the failure of spacers to reduce the incidence of dysphonia since they may actually increase deposition of steroid in the larynx.[12] Also, mouth rinsing after steroid inhaler use has been reported to be protective against dysphonia.[6,13]

Bilateral vocal fold deformities, with and without dysphonia, have been noted in patients receiving inhaled steroids. After discontinuation of the steroid, spontaneous resolution of vocal fold deformity and/or dysphonia occurred in an average of 16 weeks. Recurrence of symptoms was noted in two patients in whom inhaled steroid treatment was reintroduced. Patients who receive more than 1500 mcg/day beclomethasone or equivalent may be at increased risk of developing dysphonia, as well as those who have unusual vocal stress.[6,8] Frequency of dosing does not appear to affect the risk for dysphonia.[6]

MED**W**ATCH

THE FDA MEDICAL PRODUCTS REPORTING PROGRAM

For **VOLUNTARY** reporting
by health professionals of adverse
events and product problems

Page _____ of _____

Form Approved: OMB No. 0910-0291 Expires:12/31/94
See OMB statement on reverse

FDA Use Only

Triage unit
sequence #

PLEASE TYPE OR USE BLACK INK

A. Patient information

1. Patient identifier	2. Age at time of event: or _____ Date of birth:	3. Sex ☐ female ☐ male	4. Weight _____ lbs or _____ kgs

In confidence

B. Adverse event or product problem

1. ☐ **Adverse event**   and/or   ☐ **Product problem** (e.g., defects/malfunctions)

2. **Outcomes attributed to adverse event**
(check all that apply)

☐ death _____ (mo/day/yr)
☐ life-threatening
☐ hospitalization – initial or prolonged

☐ disability
☐ congenital anomaly
☐ required intervention to prevent permanent impairment/damage
☐ other: _____

3. Date of event (mo/day/yr)	4. Date of this report (mo/day/yr)

5. **Describe event or problem**

6. **Relevant tests/laboratory data**, including dates

7. **Other relevant history, including preexisting medical conditions** (e.g., allergies, race, pregnancy, smoking and alcohol use, hepatic/renal dysfunction, etc.)

C. Suspect medication(s)

1. **Name** (give labeled strength & mfr/labeler, if known)

#1

#2

2. **Dose, frequency & route used**	3. **Therapy dates** (if unknown, give duration) from/to (or best estimate)
#1	#1
#2	#2

4. **Diagnosis for use** (indication)

#1

#2

6. **Lot #** (if known)	7. **Exp. date** (if known)
#1	#1
#2	#2

9. **NDC #** (for product problems only)
_____ – _____ – _____

5. **Event abated after use stopped or dose reduced**

#1 ☐ yes ☐ no ☐ doesn't apply
#2 ☐ yes ☐ no ☐ doesn't apply

8. **Event reappeared after reintroduction**

#1 ☐ yes ☐ no ☐ doesn't apply
#2 ☐ yes ☐ no ☐ doesn't apply

10. **Concomitant medical products** and therapy dates (exclude treatment of event)

D. Suspect medical device

1. **Brand name**

2. **Type of device**

3. **Manufacturer name & address**	4. **Operator of device** ☐ health professional ☐ lay user/patient ☐ other:

6.

model # _____

catalog # _____

serial # _____

lot # _____

other #

5. **Expiration date** (mo/day/yr)

7. **If implanted, give date** (mo/day/yr)

8. **If explanted, give date** (mo/day/yr)

9. **Device available for evaluation?**   (Do not send to FDA)

☐ yes   ☐ no   ☐ returned to manufacturer on _____ (mo/day/yr)

10. **Concomitant medical products** and therapy dates (exclude treatment of event)

E. Reporter (see confidentiality section on back)

1. **Name, address & phone #**

2. Health professional? ☐ yes ☐ no	3. Occupation	4. **Also reported to** ☐ manufacturer ☐ user facility ☐ distributor

5. If you do NOT want your identity disclosed to the manufacturer, place an " X " in this box. ☐

FDA

Mail to: MED**W**ATCH
5600 Fishers Lane
Rockville, MD 20852-9787

or FAX to:
1-800-FDA-0178

FDA Form 3500 (6/93)   Submission of a report does not constitute an admission that medical personnel or the product caused or contributed to the event.

Figure 9–1. Med Watch form.

Table 9–2. Drug-Induced Speech and Swallowing Disorders

Agent(s)	Disorder(s)	Proposed Mechanism(s)	References
Alcohol	Dysarthria	Decreased cognition	45
Alendronate	Mechanical dysphagia	Local chemical irritation of the esophagus	84, 85
Anticholinergics	Dysarthria	Reduced activity of acetylcholine	43
Antidepressants	Speech blockage	Unknown	39–41
	Stuttering	Unknown	51–58
Antiepileptics	Dysarthria	Cerebellar damage	46, 47
Antipsychotics	Dysphonia	Tardive dyskinesia	23
	Neurogenic dysphagia	Inhibition of esophageal or pharyngeal/laryngeal motility	89–94, 96–102
		Pharyngeal-laryngeal dystonia	109–113
	Speech arrest	Tardive dyskinesia	115–119
		Acute dystonia	30
	Stuttering	Tardive dyskinesia	32–35
		Imbalance of dopamine, acetylcholine, and norepinephrine	59–61, 65
Benzodiazepines	Neurogenic dysphagia	Inhibition of pharyngeal/laryngeal motility	95
	Dysarthria	Impaired cognition	36–38, 48
	Stuttering	Direct benzodiazepine effect in the brain	67
	Aphasia		48
Botulinum toxin	Neurogenic dysphagia	Impaired laryngeal movement	121–124
Butorphanol	Apraxia	Unknown	44
Chloroquine	Dysphagia	Unknown	128
Cytarabine/methotrexate	Dysphagia	Unknown	133
Digoxin	Dysphagia	Unknown	127
Doxycycline	Mechanical dysphagia	Local chemical irritation of the esophagus	68
Emepronium	Mechanical dysphagia	Local chemical irritation of the esophagus	69–73
		Physical obstruction of esophagus from tablet	88
L-dopa	Dysphagia	Unknown	129
Lithium carbonate	Dysarthria	Neurotoxicity	26–29
Methylphenidate	Stuttering	Increased dopaminergic transmission	66
Metoclopramide	Dysarthria	Antidopaminergic effects	40, 42
Metrizamide (contrast agent)	Stuttering	Immune-mediated or pial vasculature vasospasm	50
	Aphasia		49
Pemoline	Stuttering	Increased dopaminergic transmission	66
Potassium chloride	Mechanical dysphagia	Local chemical irritation of the esophagus	74–80
		Physical obstruction of esophagus from tablet	86
Tetrabenazine	Dysphagia	Unknown	130–132
Theophylline	Stuttering	Unknown	64
Quinidine	Mechanical dysphagia	Local chemical irritation of the esophagus	80–83
		Physical obstruction of esophagus from tablet	87
Steroids, inhaled	Dysphonia	Vocal fold trauma or deformities	6–8, 11–13
Steroids, androgenic	Vocal virilization	Vocal fold inflammation	14–17
Vinca alkaloids	Vocal fold dysfunction	Neurotoxicity	18–21
	Dysphagia	Unknown	134

Androgenic Steroids

Virilization of the voice occurs as an extension of the pharmacologic effect with the use of androgenic steroids, particularly in women (Table 9–1). Danazol is known to cause deepening of the voice, hoarseness, and vocal instability in as many as 38% of patients.[14] It is hypothesized that the mechanism of voice virilization is inflammation of the vocal folds.[15] Increased vocal fold rigidity has been noted and was thought to be due to a local increase in muscle tissue with concomitant decrease in connective tissue.[16] Voice virilization from androgenic steroids usually occurs within the first 3 months of therapy and is often irreversible, even on discontinuation of therapy.[14,15,17]

Vocal Fold Paresis and Paralysis

Vinca Alkaloids

Drug-induced vocal fold paresis and paralysis are unusual but have been reported (Table 9–2). The most frequently implicated agents are the vinca alkaloids—namely, vincristine and vinblastine. These agents are known to be generally neurotoxic, and presenting symptoms usually include constipation, urinary retention, decreased deep tendon reflexes, paresthesia, and distal sensory loss. Vocal fold paralysis rarely occurs, and is thought to be another manifestation of neurotoxicity.[18] It has been hypothesized that the vinca alkaloids may combine with neural proteins, leading to accumulation of neurofilaments and ultimately impairing axoplasmic flow and causing neural degeneration.[19] Vocal fold dysfunction with vincristine and vinblastine is thought to be dose dependent, although it has been reported in a patient receiving low-dose vincristine as well.[18,20] Other risk factors may include underlying neuropathy or autoimmune disease.[20]

The presentation of vinca alkaloid-induced vocal fold paralysis is somewhat variable. Hoarseness, dry cough, sore throat, neck pain, aphonia, and stridor have been reported.[18–20,21] These complaints can be accompanied by symptoms consistent with general neuropathy, such as hypotonia, constipation, and paresthesia.[19,21] On visualization of the vocal folds by direct or indirect laryngoscopy, unilateral and bilateral vocal fold paresis and paralysis have been noted. Onset of symptoms occurs 2 weeks to 7 months after administration of the first dose of vincristine or vinblastine, and resolution of signs and symptoms usually occurs within 6 weeks after drug discontinuation.[18–21]

Thorium Dioxide

Thorium dioxide, an angiographic contrast agent used extensively until 1955, has been reported to cause vocal fold weakness in two patients in whom the dose of thorium dioxide had extravasated into the carotid sheath. In these patients, the onset of symptoms was approximately 30 years. The patients complained of voice hoarseness, local burning sensation, and a feeling of fullness in the neck. Roentgenographic studies of the neck revealed local thorium dioxide deposits and vocal fold paralysis was noted on visualization of the larynx. No information was provided on the ultimate outcomes of the patients.[22]

Neuroleptic Agents

Vocal fold dysfunction has rarely been reported with the use of neuroleptic agents (Table 9–2). Haloperidol and fluphenazine have induced dysphonia in a patient after three years of therapy. It was felt that dysphonia was associated with the development of tardive dyskinesia because it improved with the administration of physostigmine and discontinuation of haloperidol. However, 4 weeks after initiating therapy with fluphenazine, the dysphonia recurred. Again, the patient's symptoms improved with physostigmine and discontinuation of therapy. Subsequent therapy with clozapine was successful.[23]

DRUG-INDUCED SPEECH AND LANGUAGE IMPAIRMENTS

Agents reported to influence speech and language do so by either direct injury to the involved tissues or, more commonly, by altering neurotransmitter function in the central and peripheral nervous systems (Table 9–2). A drug can alter neurotransmitter function by: (1) increasing or decreasing the amount of neurotransmitter in the synapse available for interaction with the receptor, (2) preventing reuptake of the neurotransmitter—allowing it to persist in the synapse longer, (3) blocking the receptor so that the neurotransmitter cannot stimulate the receptor (an antagonist), and (4) stimulating the receptor directly (an agonist). Neurotransmitters affected by pharmacologic agents are acetylcholine, norepinephrine/epinephrine, gamma aminobutyric acid (GABA), serotonin, dopamine, and, most recently, glutamate (see Table 9–3).

Table 9–3. Neurotransmitters and Their Interactions with Common Medications

Neurotransmitter	Actions	Drugs Inhibiting	Drugs Promoting
Acetylcholine	Excitatory; parasympathetic; memory	Anticholinergics; antidepressants; antiarrythmics; antihistamines	Tacrine; pyridostigmine; neostigmine
Norepinephrine/ Epinephrine	Mood; anxiety; alertness; autonomic nervous system	Beta-blockers; alpha-blockers	Epinephrine; stimulants; pseudoephedrine; phenylpropanolamine
GABA	Inhibitory; throughout nervous system		Benzodiazepines; barbiturates; some anticonvulsants
Serotonin	Sleep–wake cycles; emotion; mood; vessel constriction	Cyproheptadine; methysergide	Antidepressants; sumatriptan; ergots
Dopamine	Inhibitory; movement; psychoses; gastrointestinal function	Antipsychotics; metoclopramide	Levodopa; bromocriptine; pergolide; antidepressants
Glutamate	Excitatory; predominant throughout nervous system	Lamotrigine; riluzole ketamine; phencyclidine (PCP)	

Dysarthria

It is quite common for drugs active in the central nervous system to cause changes in speech as part of a symptom complex resulting from adverse cognitive effects of the drug.[24,25] "Slurred speech," dysfluency, and word unintelligibility are used to describe the dysarthria reported to be related to medication usage.[26] More uncommon, however, are the speech disorders occurring as a solitary symptom of the adverse effects of the drug. Dysarthria, aphonia, mutism, and speech blockage have all been associated with administration of drugs, with various degrees of severity and duration.[26]

Lithium Carbonate

Lithium carbonate is used extensively in bipolar disorders and has been associated with both transient and persistent dysarthria when the drug is used alone or in combination with neuroleptic therapy.[26–29] Blood lithium concentrations above 2 mEq/L have been consistently associated with slurred speech, which is usually accompanied by other signs of lithium toxicity such as tremor. However, in some cases the onset of the dysarthria ranges from weeks to years after the initiation of therapy and is not always related to toxic concentrations of lithium in the blood. In all cases withdrawal of lithium was associated with improvement of symp-

toms, but persistent dysarthria, suggested to be due to an irreversible neurotoxicity of the drug, has been reported.[26–28]

Antipsychotic Agents

Neuroleptics may cause speech arrest or inability to articulate words by either of two distinct mechanisms.[30–34] The first occurs early (hours to days after initiation) in treatment and is a result of an acute dystonic reaction. The speech difficulty may be accompanied by oculogyric (eye movement) crisis, choreoathetosis and cervicolingual masticatory crisis and usually responds quickly to discontinuation of the agent and administration of an anticholinergic medication.[30] Young patients receiving phenothiazine or butyrophenone (haloperidol) derivatives by parenteral routes seem to be at particular risk of this adverse effect.[30] The second type of speech disorder associated with neuroleptic administration has been associated with tardive dyskinesia.[32–35] These movement disorders are delayed in onset (usually months) and are thought to be related to the duration of therapy. The symptoms of tardive dyskinesia usually include purposeless movements of the arms, hands, legs and face (akathisia), and the disorder tends to persist and worsen after the discontinuation of the neuroleptic. Increasing the neuroleptic dose may alleviate the symptoms temporarily, but no benefit of anticholinergic medication can be expected. Older patients appear to be at greatest risk of tardive dyskinesia, but all patients on prolonged neuroleptic therapy are at risk.

Benzodiazepines

Benzodiazepines are known to adversely affect speech through their effects on cognition.[36] Reports have been made, however, of speech disturbances occurring in the absence of, or in disproportion to, other cognitive effects of the drug. In one case, a 3-year-old girl was given high-dose intravenous diazepam (37.5 mg over 15 hours) for control of agitation after a surgical procedure.[37] Four hours after the final dose of diazepam, the patient was noticed to be anarthric and subsequently dysarthric, which gradually improved and disappeared at 180 hours after the final diazepam dose. In a case involving the short-acting benzodiazepine midazolam, dysarthria accompanied by hypotension and drowsiness developed in a 67-year-old man, 5 minutes after an intramuscular injection of the drug.[38] The hypotension and dysarthria dissipated after 25 minutes but the drowsiness persisted.

Antidepressants

Speech blockage has been reported to occur with many different antidepressants.[39–41] In the majority of patients, the onset of the symptom is within the first few weeks of therapy and resolution occurs within a few days of reduction in the dose or a discontinuation of the therapy. Although it is thought to be more common in older patients,[40] it has been reported in the young and should be considered in this patient population.[41]

Metoclopramide

Metoclopramide is a dopamine antagonist used for its antiemetic and promotility properties. Extrapyramidal side effects such as acute dystonic reactions are not uncommon, but isolated speech disturbance is quite rare.[40,42] One 25-year-old female patient developed dysarthria after receiving high-dose metoclopramide for 72 hours preoperatively.[42] The dysarthria persisted for 6 weeks after she received her last dose of metoclopramide. In another elderly patient, metoclopramide was associated with a severe dysarthria that developed after 6 weeks of chronic therapy for dyspepsia.[40] The dysarthria was accompanied by a resting tremor and decreased tongue mobility. After discontinuation of the metoclopramide, the neurologic problems dis-

appeared over several weeks. In a second elderly patient, the dysarthria developed after a single intramuscular dose and took 8 weeks to resolve.[40]

Other pharmacological agents associated with speech disorders are anticholinergics,[43] intranasal butorphanol,[44] alcohol,[45] and antiepileptics.[46,47] In most cases, the symptoms resolve quickly on discontinuation of the drug. In the cases of anticholinergics and butorphanol, reversal with an acetylcholinesterase inhibitor (physostigmine)[43] and opiate antagonist (naloxone),[44] respectively, have been used with success. In the case of hydantoins, however, chronic neurotoxicity has been reported after long-term therapy and the implication of permanent cerebellar damage has been suggested.[46]

Aphasia

Benzodiazepines

A jargon aphasia related to clobazam, a benzodiazepine used as an antiepileptic agent, was reported in an 18-year-old man with a history of seizures and migraine with aura.[48] After 3 weeks of therapy, he developed minute-long episodes of sudden onset extended neologisms that gradually improved for the 5 days after the discontinuation of clobazam. The authors proposed an interaction between his partial seizures and the clobazam as the cause of the aphasia. In all cases of benzodiazepine-associated language disorders, onset and duration seem to be related to the pharmacokinetic characteristics of the particular agents and no permanent neurotoxicity appears to exist.

Metrizamide

Aphasia has been reported as complication of metrizamide myelography.[49,50] The authors have characterized the aphasia as motor, expressive, and conduction. Onset of symptoms has ranged from 1 to 18 hours after the administration of the drug. The duration of the aphasia is typically brief—approximately 36 hours. The actual mechanism for the aphasia is unknown, but was theorized to be neurotoxic rather than a phenomenon of seizure.

Drug-Induced Stuttering

Antidepressants

Although it is unusual, drugs have been reported to induce stuttering in patients with and without a previous history of stuttering (Table 9–2).

Antidepressants are most frequently implicated, but the mechanism by which they induce stuttering is not entirely clear. Cases of tricyclic antidepressants causing stuttering were first published in the 1970s and may be underreported. Although there are relatively few cases of antidepressant-induced stuttering published, 4 of 98 patients receiving tricyclic antidepressants in one study required discontinuation of their drug due to stuttering.[51]

Amitriptyline and one of its analogs, dothiepin, were associated with stuttering in two cases when the drugs were utilized in relatively low doses.[52] The onset of symptoms was 3 to 4 days and discontinuation of therapy was indicated in both cases. Spontaneous resolution of symptoms followed in 2 days in the amitriptyline patient and in an unspecified time in the dothiepin patient. Stuttering was accompanied by other symptoms that were labeled as dysarthria by the authors, but later described as a nonspecific involuntary movement that interrupted the patients' speech.[53] The authors hypothesized that stuttering was due to anticholinergic effects of the drugs on the cerebellar connections and striatum.

Desipramine is another tricyclic antidepressant that has been reported to cause stuttering in a patient who had previously tolerated another antidepressant, doxepin.[54] The initial event occurred four months after initiating treatment. However, symptoms recurred within one day of rechallenge with desipramine. The patient's serum desipramine level was reported to be 439 ng/ml, which is slightly higher than the therapeutic range of 150 to 300 ng/ml, but is not in the toxic range of >1000 ng/ml. The patient experienced concomitant jaw myoclonus, and the authors did not speculate as to the mechanism of the reaction.

Newer antidepressants that belong to the class of serotonin reuptake inhibitors have produced stuttering. Fluoxetine has been associated with stuttering in two patients within 3 weeks of initiating therapy.[55,56] One patient had a past medical history of stuttering, but the other did not. In both patients, discontinuation of the drug was necessary. In one patient, resolution of symptoms was noted in 2 weeks.[56] However, the other patient had a much slower resolution of the stuttering and required speech therapy.[55] Proposed mechanisms for this reaction were an abnormality in serotonin function[56] or a type of akathisia (motor restlessness and anxiety) due to inhibition of dopamine activity in the right hemisphere by serotonergic or noradrenergic activity of fluoxetine.[57]

More recently, a newer serotonin reuptake inhibitor, sertraline, has been reported to induce stuttering.[58] The onset of stuttering was within 24 hours of drug administration. After continued therapy for 8 days, the drug was discontinued and resolution of stuttering occurred within 48 hours. The authors offered no other mechanism of stuttering than those already proposed, but did state that the excessive caffeine intake in their patient may have predisposed him to the development of stuttering.

Antipsychotic Agents

Many antipsychotic agents have been associated with drug-induced stuttering. The first reports consisted of two patients who were receiving therapy with fluphenazine or chlorpromazine.[59] Both patients had tolerated antipsychotic therapy before, but experienced stuttering 26 days after restarting therapy or 4 days after a dosage increase. In both patients, treatment with diphenhydramine, benztropine, or trihexyphenidyl was unhelpful, but symptoms abated with decreasing the dosage of the offending agent. Both patients re-experienced stuttering with increased dosage of their neuroleptics. The authors speculated that this reaction could be a type of extrapyramidal symptom, but acute dystonia was ruled out because of the lack of resolution after treatment with anticholinergic agents.

Other clincians have noted improvement in antipsychotic-induced stuttering with administration of propranolol.[60] The two patients in this report were receiving therapy with perphenazine/desipramine combination or chlorpromazine/lithium combination. The patient receiving concomitant antidepressant therapy was reported to have tolerated previous therapy with nortriptyline. In both cases stuttering resolved soon after adminstration of propranolol 10 or 20 mg three times daily. In one patient, stuttering reappeared after discontinuation of propranolol, but again resolved with resumption of therapy. This prompted the authors to propose that antipsychotic-induced stuttering has a similar etiology as akathisia (i.e., imbalance of dopaminergic, cholinergic, and noradrenergic systems in the brain) because it responded to the same treatment as akathisia.

A newer antipsychotic agent, clozapine, has also been known to induce stuttering in a single patient.[61] Stuttering, dystonia, and dysarthria were noted 4 weeks after institution of clozapine therapy. Discontinuation of therapy resulted in resolution of symptoms within 5 days, but symptoms recurred on rechallenge with the drug. In addition, the occurrence of symptoms seemed to be dose dependent. Changes on electroencephalography were demonstrated and the authors hypothesized that the patient's symptoms may have been related to a decrease in seizure threshhold.

Metrizamide

Metrizamide, a radiopaque contrast medium used in positive contrast myelography, was shown to induce stuttering in three patients.[62,63] In all patients, stuttering was accompanied by other symptoms originating in the central nervous system, such as confusion and asterixis (motor disturbance marked by intermittent sustained contractions of groups of muscles). Onset of symptoms was within 12 hours of completion of the imaging study and symptom resolution was highly variable. In one patient, symptoms resolved within 7 days, but the other two patients required 3 to 5 months for symptom resolution. In all three patients, distribution of metrizamide to the central nervous system was confirmed by computed tomography scan. It has been proposed that the presence of dye in the central nervous system may induce an immune response or vasospasm of pial vasculature that could contribute to the development of symptoms.[63] Placing the patient in a supine postition after the procedure may facilitate distribution of the dye to the brain,[62] but a semi-upright postition is not entirely protective.[63]

Other drugs that have been associated with stuttering in individual patients are theophylline,[64] prochlorperazine,[65] methylphenidate and pemoline,[66] and alprazolam.[67] Theophylline induced stuttering in a 4-year-old boy who had a documented theophylline level of 12 mcg/ml, which is within the therpeutic range. His stuttering resolved on discontinuation of the drug, but reappeared on rechallenge. No mechanisms for the reaction were proposed.[64] Prochlorperazine caused stuttering in a 39-year-old female within 3 hours of adminstration of two doses, and was accompanied by tongue and laryngeal spasms. Although the dystonias resolved quickly, the stuttering persisted and required speech therapy for 6 weeks. The authors felt the stuttering was initially part of the acute dystonic reaction, but persisted because of behavioral changes by the patient that caused disruption of the rhythm and coordination of her speech.[65] A 3-year-old girl experienced stuttering 3 to 4 days after separate courses of methylphenidate and pemoline. Stuttering resolved spontaneously after therapy was discontinued. The authors proposed that stuttering may have been resulted from increased dopaminergic neurotransmission that is caused by both drugs.[66] Alprazolam caused stuttering in a 22-year-old

female who had previously tolerated other benzodiazepines. Within 2 hours of drug administration, she began to stutter. It resolved within 2 days of discontinuation of alprazolam, and recurred on a double-blind rechallenge. The authors stated that the onset and duration of stuttering paralleled the pharmacokinetic profile of the drug and therefore felt stuttering was due to a direct action of the drug on the brain, and not anticholinergic side effects.[67]

DRUG-INDUCED SWALLOWING DISORDERS

Dysphagia, defined as difficulty in swallowing, is associated with many neurologic disorders, head and neck cancer, and gastroenterologic diseases. However, many drugs have also been implicated as causes of dysphagia (Table 9–2). Normal swallowing is a complex function, and drugs impair swallowing by inducing a mechanical obstruction (mechanical dysphagia) or affecting neuromuscular control of swallowing (neurogenic dysphagia). Often drug-induced dysphagia resolves spontaneously after discontinuation of the offending agent, but complications including esophageal stricture, ulceration, and bleeding, aspiration pneumonia, weight loss, and even death have been reported. Evaluation of all patients with dysphagia should include consideration of drug-induced causes to promote prompt diagnosis and treatment to prevent the occurrence of complications.

Mechanical Dysphagia

Drugs induce mechanical dysphagia most often indirectly by causing esophageal ulceration or inflammation. Doxycycline,[68] emepronium (not available in the United States),[69–73] potassium chloride,[74–80] quinidine,[80–83] and alendronate[84,85] have been reported to cause dysphagic symptoms by this mechanism. These drugs are chemical irritants to the esophageal mucosa, especially when prolonged contact occurs. Less frequently, the drug preparation itself can induce a mechanical dysphagia by lodging in the esophagus and preventing passage of a bolus. Agents associated with this mechanism of injury are potassium chloride,[86] quinidine,[87] and emepronium.[88] Ingesting small volumes of liquid with orally administered medications,[70–73,81,82,84,85] assuming a recumbent position immediately after taking medication,[68,84,85] recent esophageal injury from a nasogastric tube,[80] and an enlarged left atrium[74,76–79,84] have been identified as risk factors for the development of drug-induced mechanical dysphagia. Onset of dysphagia ranges from immediately after the first dose of a drug to several years after initiation of therapy. Although most reported cases are relatively uncomplicated, esophageal perforation with massive hemorrhage,[78] stricture,[75,77,79,80,83,85] mediastinitis,[76] and death[76,78] have occurred. Management of drug-induced esophageal injury should include discontinuation of therapy and supportive treatment involving limiting oral intake, administration of analgesics when necessary, and appropriate medical or surgical management of complications.

Neurogenic Dysphagia

Drug-induced neurogenic dysphagia occurs when a drug causes weakness of muscles involved in swallowing or incoordination of the swallowing process. Several drugs have been implicated in interruption of the normal swallowing process by a variety of different mechanisms. Drugs that have been reported to decrease esophageal motility include clozapine,[89] digoxin,[90] molindone/benztropine combination,[91] and thiothixene/benztropine combination.[92] Many of these agents possess anticholinergic properties that have the potential to inhibit the activity of striated muscle of the pharynx, upper esophageal sphincter, and upper esophagus. Clinical reports of the effect of these drugs on esophageal motility include increased tone of the upper esophageal sphincter (UES),[91] esophageal muscle incoordination,[90] decreased esophageal peristalsis,[89,91] and marked esophageal dilation.[92] Other drugs—namely, haloperidol/benztropine/amitriptyline combination,[93] clozapine,[94] and nitrazepam[95]—have demonstrated an ability to cause dysphagia through impairment of coordination of the pharyngeal and laryngeal phases of swallowing. Clinically, these effects manifest as delayed cricopharyngeal relaxation until after hypopharyngeal contraction,[95] increased oral and pharyngeal transit times,[93] and decreased pharyngeal peristalsis.[94] Onset of dysphagic symptoms ranged from 2 days to 10 months after the offending agents were started. Some cases were complicated by pneumonia due to aspiration,[93,95] but no other complications were noted. Discontinuation or dosage reduction of the offending agent(s) resulted in resolution of dysphagia in most cases.

Antipsychotic Drugs

Soon after widespread use of antipsychotic agents began in the 1950s and 1960s, several reports of sudden death appeared in the literature. Reserpine,[96] chlorpromazine alone[97,98] and in combination with thioridazine and trihexyphenidyl,[99] prochlorperazine and reserpine,[100] prochlorperazine,[101] and reserpine and an antiepileptic agent[102] were implicated. Onset of symptoms ranged from 3 weeks to 10 years after initiating therapy. Although the patients did not complain of dysphagia, they appeared to suddenly asphyxiate while eating. In several patients, food was found in the airway on autopsy.[97,99,102] This prompted many clinicians to propose that perhaps the antipsychotic agents contributed to aspiration of food by impairing cough or gag reflexes.[103] Later reports of antipsychotic agents inducing dysphagia also proposed the same mechanism.[104–106] However, other investigators found no association between sudden death[107] or swallowing difficulty[108] and the introduction of phenothiazine antipsychotics.

Antipsychotics were more definitively associated with neurogenic dysphagia through the induction of pharyngeal-laryngeal dystonia. Antidopaminergic drugs such as fluphenazine,[109] haloperidol,[110,111] fluspirilene,[112] and metoclopramide alone[113,114] and in combination with prochlorperazine[113] have caused dysphagic symptoms. The onset of symptoms is typically acute and occurs within days of initiating therapy or increasing the dosage. Complaints of dysphagia can be accompanied by difficulty in speaking or breathing,[110,114] or a choking feeling[109] without visible evidence of dystonia. Treatment was delayed in some patients due to a lack of recognition of the cause of the complaints and a single case was complicated by aspiration pneumonia.[111] All patients responded rapidly to treatment with anticholinergic drugs such as benztropine, glycopyrronium and diphenhydramine or drug discontinuation. Recurrence has occurred with rechallenge.

Tardive Dyskinesia

Antipsychotics also have the ability to interfere with swallowing by inducing tardive dyskinesia.[115–119] Patients who develop tardive dyskinesia can have persistent, abnormal tongue movements that prevent normal swallowing.[119] This is clinically different from acute dystonia with respect to the onset of symptoms and response to treatment. Onset is typically years after initiation of antipsychotic therapy. Anticholinergic agents and discontinuation of therapy, which are uniformly beneficial in acute dystonia, have been reported to worsen dysphagia caused by tardive dyskinesia.[115,116,120] However, slow improvement in symptoms after discontinuation of antipsychotic therapy can occur.[116,118,119]

Botulinum toxin

Botulinum toxin produces dysphagia in many patients injected locally for torticollis and in those receiving injections in remote sites as well. The incidence of dysphagia in patients receiving injection of botulinum toxin into cervical muscles ranges from 29 to 57%.[121–123] Although less likely, botulinum toxin injected into the right tibialis muscle has been reported to cause dysphagia.[124] The mechanism by which botulinum toxin causes difficulty swallowing is not entirely clear. The toxin may diffuse into pharyngeal muscle from locally injected sites, or it may be transported through the bloodstream.[122–124] The toxin may also have an increased selectivity for pharyngeal muscle presynaptic terminals.[122,125] Onset of symptoms generally occurs within 3 weeks. Decreased laryngeal muscle movement or slowed or prolonged laryngeal movements have been observed.[126] Symptoms are usually mild and do not require treatment other than discontinuation of injections. Occasionally, restriction to a soft food or liquid diet is necessary.[122] On discontinuation of the injections, symptoms resolve spontaneously within 6 weeks. Although preexisting dysphagia is not a risk factor for the development of botulinum toxin-induced dysphagia, patients with preexisting dysphagia may experience slower resolution of drug-induced symptoms.[123,126]

Other drugs, including digoxin,[127] chloroquine,[128] L-dopa,[129] tetrabenazine,[130–132] cytarabine/methotrexate combination,[133] and vincristine[134] have been reported to induce dysphagia rarely. Because of the low incidence of the reactions, the mechanisms of dysphagia are not well elucidated. However, most patients recovered uneventfully after discontinuation of the offending agent.

SUMMARY

This chapter has approached the topic of drug-induced communication and swallowing disturbances by reviewing the available literature regarding specific pharmacologic agents. The speech–language pathologist in the medical setting is likely to come in contact with patients who are being treated with drugs highlighted in this chapter. In addition, patients may be referred for consultation regarding the acute onset of speech and/or swallowing symptoms that may be drug induced. Familiarity with some basic pharmacologic concepts and knowledge of the interaction between drugs and communication and swallowing disorders will enhance the process of differential diagnosis and appropriate treatment. We hope the information presented in this chapter will also provide some basis for interaction between the pharmacist and the speech–language pathologist.

STUDY QUESTIONS

1. What information should be considered when attempting to determine causality between a drug and a potential drug reaction?

2. What steps can be taken to prevent reexposure of a patient with a documented adverse drug reaction to the inciting agent(s)?

3. Describe the proposed mechanisms for inhaled steroid-induced dysphonia. Which is most likely and what steps can be taken to prevent or treat dysphonia related to inhaled steroid use?

4. What are preventable risk factors for the development of drug-induced mechanical dysphagia?

5. Characterize the documented effects of certain drugs on esophageal motility and pharyngeal/laryngeal coordination.

6. Describe the presentation, time of onset, and treatment of botulinum toxin-induced dysphagia.

7. Differentiate the speech dysfunction that can occur with short- and long-term neuroleptic administration. How does treatment differ?

8. Which drugs induce stuttering most frequently?

REFERENCES

1. Manasse HR: Medication use in an imperfect world: Drug misadventuring as an issue of public policy, Part 1. *Am J Hosp Pharm* 1989; 46:929–944.
2. Manasse HR: Medication use in an imperfect world: Drug misadventuring as an issue of public policy, Part 2. *Am J Hosp Pharm* 1989; 46:1141–1152.
3. Beard K: Adverse reactions as a cause of hospital admissions in the aged. *Drugs Aging* 1992; 2:356–367.
4. *Requirements for adverse drug reaction reporting.* Geneva, Switzerland, World Health Organization, 1975.
5. Naranjo CA, Busto U, Sellers EM, et al: A method for estimating the probability of adverse drug reactions. *Clin Pharmacol Ther* 1981; 30:239–245.
6. Toogood JH, Jennings B, Greenway RW, et al: Candidiasis and dysphonia complicating beclomethasone treatment of asthma. *J All Clin Immun* 1980; 65:145–153.

7. Williams AJ, Baghat MS, Stableforth DE, et al: Dysphonia caused by inhaled steroids: Recognition of a characteristic laryngeal abnormality. *Thorax* 1983; 38: 813–821.

8. Williamson IJ, Matusiewicz SP, Brown PH, et al: Frequency of voice problems and cough in patients using pressurized aerosol inhaled steroid preparations. *Eur J Resp Dis* 1995; 8:590–592.

9. Campbell IA: Inhaled steroids and dysphonia. *Lancet* 1984; 1:744.

10. Skinner C, Williams AJ: Dysphonia caused by inhaled steroids: Recognition of a characteristic laryngeal abnormality. *Thorax* 1984; 39:686.

11. Streeton JA: Inhaled steroids and dysphonia. *Lancet* 1984; 1:963.

12. Anon: Inhaled steroids and dysphonia. *Lancet* 1984; 1: 375–376.

13. Toogood JH, Jennings B, Baskerville J, et al: Dosing regimen of budesonide and occurrence of oropharyngeal complications. *Eur J Resp Dis* 1984; 65:35–44.

14. Newman D, Forbes D: The effects of danazol on vocal parameters—Is an objective prospective study needed? *Med J Australia* 1993; 158:575.

15. Boothroyd CV, Lepre F: Permanent voice change resulting from danazol therapy. *Aust N Z J Obstet Gynaecol* 1990; 30:275–276.

16. Gerritsma EJ, Brocaar MP, Hakkesteegt MM, et al: Virilization of the voice in post-menopausal women due to the anabolic steroid nandrologe decanoate (deca-durabolin); the effects of medication for one year. *Clin Otolaryng* 1994; 19:79–84.

17. Wardle PG, Whitehead MI, Mills RP: Non-reversible and wide ranging voice changes after treatment with danazol. *Br Med J* 1983; 287:946.

18. Whittaker JA, Griffith IP: Recurrent laryngeal nerve paralysis in patients receiving vincristine and vinblastine. *Br J Med* 1977; 1:1251–1252.

19. Delaney P: Vincristine-induced laryngeal nerve paralysis. *Neurology* 1982; 32:1285–1288.

20. Alfredsunder P, Hochman MC, Kaplan BH: Low-dose vincristine-associated bilateral vocal cord paralysis. *NY State J Med* 1992; 92:268–269.

21. Tobias JD, Bozeman PM: Vincristine-induced recurrent laryngeal nerve paralysis in children. *Intensive Care Med* 1991; 17:304–305.

22. DeLuca SA, Rhea JT, Weber AL: Vocal cord paralysis: A latent effect of perivascular thorium dioxide. *Arch Otolaryng* 1984; 110:339–340.

23. Lieberman JA, Reife R: Spastic dysphonia and denervation signs in a young man with tardive dyskinesia. *Br J Psychiatry* 1989; 154:105–109.

24. Fayen M, Goldman MB, Moulthrop MA, Luchins DJ: Differential memory function with dopaminergic versus anticholinergic treatment of drug-induced extrapyramidal symptoms. *Am J Psychiatry* 1988; 145: 483–486.

25. Miller PS, Richardson JS, Jyu CA, Lemay JS, Hisock M, Keegan DL: Association of low serum anticholinergic levels and cognitive impairment in elderly presurgical patients. *Am J Psychiatry* 1988; 145:342–345.

26. Bond WS, Carvalho M, Foulks EF: Persistent dysarthria with apraxia associated with a combination of lithium carbonate and haloperidol. *J Clin Psychiatr* 1982; 43: 256–257.

27. Singh VS: Lithium carbonate/fluphenazine decanoate producing irreversible brain damage. *Lancet* 1982; 2: 278.

28. Lewis DA: Unrecognized chronic neurotoxic reactions. *JAMA* 1983; 250:2029–2030.

29. Solomon K, Vickers R: Dysarthria resulting from lithium carbonate. A case report. *JAMA* 231:280.

30. Marcotte DB: Neuroleptics and neurologic reactions. *S Med J* 1973; 66:321–324.

32. Schmidt WR, Jarcho LW: Persistent dyskinesias following phenothiazine therapy. *Arch Neurol* 1966; 14: 369–377.

33. Faheem AD, Brightwell DR, Burton GC, Struss A: Respiratory dyskinesia and dysarthria from prolonged neuroleptic use: Tardive dyskinesia? *Am J Psych* 1982; 139:517–518.

34. Kane FJ, Taylor TW: An unusual reaction to combined Imipramine-thorazine therapy. *Am J Psych* 1963; 120: 186–187.

35. Angrist B, Gershon S: Behavioral profile of a potent psychotoxic compound. *Psychopharm* 1973; 30: 109–116.

36. Gottschalk LA: Effects of certain benzodiazepine derivatives on disorganization of thought as manifested in speech. *Curr Ther Res* 1977; 21:192–206.

37. Ishikawa T, Hato M, Tauchi A, Wada Y: Dysarthria after large doses of intravenous diazepam. *Jpn J Psychiatr Neurol* 1988; 42: 759–761.

38. Matson AM, Thurlow AC: Hypotension and neurological sequelae following intramuscular midazolam. *Anaesthesia* 1988; 43:896.

39. Schatzberg AF, Cole JO, Blumer DP: Speech blockage: A tricyclic side effect. *Am J Psychiatr* 1978; 135: 600–601.

40. Sandyk R: Speech blockage induced by maprotiline. *Am J Psychiatr* 1986; 143:391–392.

41. Sholomskas AJ: Speech blockage in young patients taking tricyclics. *Am J Psychiatr* 1978; 135:600–601.

42. Walsh TD: Chronic dysarthria and metoclopramide. *Ann Neurol* 1982; 11:545.

43. Duvoisin RC, Katz L: Reversal of central anticholinergic syndrome in man by physostigmine. *JAMA* 1968; 206:1963–1965.

44. Gora-Harper ML, Sunahara JF, Gray MS. Intranasal butorphanol-induced apraxia reversed by naloxone. *Pharmacotherapy* 1995; 15:798–800.

45. Sobell LC, Sobell MB, Colemen RF: Alcohol-induced dysfluency in nonalcoholics. *Folia Phoniat* 1982; 34: 316–323.

46. Riely CG: Chronic hydantoin intoxication: Case report. *NZ Med J* 1972; 76:425–428.

47. Jaster PJ, Abbas D: Erythromycin-carbamazepine interaction. *Neurology* 1986; 36:594–595.

48. Wilson A, Petty R, Perry A, Rose FC: Paroxysmal language disturbance in an epileptic treated with clobazam. *Neurology* 1983; 33:652–654.

49. Sarno JB: Transient expressive (nonfluent) dysphasia after metrizamide myelography. *Am J Neuroradiol* 1985; 6: 945–947.

50. Masdeu JC, Glista GG, Rubino FA, et al: Transient motor aphasia following metrizamide myelography. *Am J Neuroradiol* 1983; 4: 200–202.

51. Garvey MJ, Tollefson GD: Occurrence of myoclonus in patients treated with cyclic antidepressants. *Arch Gen Psychiatry* 1987; 44:269–272.

52. Quader SE: Dysarthria: An unusual side effect of thecyclic antidepressants. *Br Med J* 1977; 2:97.

53. Saunders M: Dysarthria with tricyclic antidepressants. *Br Med J* 1977; 2:317.

54. Masand P: Desipramine-induced oral-pharyngeal disturbances: Stuttering and jaw myoclonus. *J Clin Psychopharm* 1992; 12:444–445.

55. Meghji C: Acquired stuttering. *J Fam Pract* 1994; 39: 325–326.

56. Guthrie S, Grunhaus L: Fluoxetine-induced stuttering. *J Clin Psychiatry* 1990; 51:85.

57. Friedman EH, Guthrie S, Grunhaus L: Fluoxetine and stuttering. *J Clin Psychiatry* 1990; 51:310–311.

58. McCall WV: Sertraline-induced stuttering. *J Clin Psychiatry* 1994; 55:316.

59. Nurnberg HG, Greenwald B: Stuttering: An unusual side effect of phenothiazines. *Am J Psychiatry* 1981; 138:386–387.

60. Adler L, Leong S, Delgado R: Drug-induced stuttering treated with propranolol. *J Clin Psycopharm* 1987; 7:115–116.

61. Thomas P, Lalaux N, Vaiva G, et al: Dose-dependent stuttering and dystonia in a patient taking clozapine. *Am J Psychiatry* 1994; 151:1096.

62. Bertoni JM, Schwartzman RJ, Van Horn G, et al: Asterixis and encephalopathy following metrizamide myelography: Investigations into possible mechanisms and review of the literature. *Ann Neurol* 1981; 9:366–370.

63. Pimental PA, Gorelik PB: Aphasia, apraxia and neurogenic stuttering as complications of metrizamide myelography. *Acta Neurol Scand* 1985; 72:481–488.

64. McCarthy MM: Speech effect of theophylline. *Pediatrics* 1981; 68:749–750.

65. Mahr G, Leith W: Stuttering after a dystonic reaction. *Psychosomatics* 1990; 31:465.

66. Burd L, Kerbeshian J: Stuttering and stimulants. *J Clin Psychopharm* 1991; 11:72–73.

67. Elliott RL, Thomas BJ: A case report of alprazolam-induced stuttering. *J Clin Psychopharm* 1985; 5:159–160.

68. Bokey L, Hugh TB: Oesophageal ulceration associated with doxycycline therapy. *Med J Australia* 1975; 1: 236–237.

69. Higson RH: Oesophagitis as a side effect of empronium. *Br J Med* 1978; 2:201.

70. Hughes R: Drug-induced oesophageal injury. *Br J Med* 1979; 2:132.

71. Cowan RE, Wright JT, Marsh F: Drug-induced oesophageal injury. *Br J Med* 1979; 2:132–133.

72. Tobias R, Cullis S, Kottler RE, et al: Emepronium bromide-induced oesophagitis. *S Afr Med J* 1982; 61: 368–370.

73. Leonard RCF, Adams PC, Parker S, et al: Oesophageal injury associated with emepronium bromide (cetiprin). *Br J Clin Prac* 1984; 38:429–430.

74. Pemberton J: Oesophageal obstruction and ulceration caused by oral potassium therapy. *Br Heart J* 1970; 32:267–268.

75. Chesshyre MH, Braimbridge MV: Dysphagia due to left atrial enlargement after mitral starr valve replacement. *Br Heart J* 1971; 33:799–802.

76. Rosenthal T, Adar R, Militianu J, et al: Esophageal ulceration and oral potassium chloride ingestion. *Chest* 1974; 65:463–465.

77. Howie AD, Strachan RW: Slow release potassium chloride treatment. *Br Med J* 1975; 2:176.

78. McCall AJ: Slow-k ulceration of oesophagus with aneurysmal left atrium. *Br Med J* 1975; 3:230–231.

79. Peters JL: Benign oesophageal stricture following oral potassium chloride therapy. *Br J Surg* 1976; 63: 698–699.

80. Twplick JG, Twplick SK, Ominsky SH, et al: Esophagitis caused by oral medication. *Radiology* 1980; 134: 23–25.

81. Mason SJ, O'Meara TF: Drug-induced esophagitis. *J Clin Gastroenterol* 1981; 3:115–120.

82. Kikendall JW, Friedman AC, Oyewole MA, et al: Pill-induced esophateal injury. *Dig Dis Sci* 1983; 28: 174–182.

83. Wong RKH, Kikendall JW, Dachman AH: Quinaglute-induced esophagitis mimicking an esophageal mass. *Ann Intern Med* 1986; 105:62–63.

84. Maconi G, Porro GB: Multiple ulcerative esophagitis caused by alendronate. *Am J Gastroenterol* 1995; 90: 1889–1890.

85. De Groen PC, Lubbe DF, Hirsch LJ, et al: Esophagitis associated with the use of alendronate. *N Engl J Med* 1996; 335:1016–1021.

86. Ashour M, Salama FD, Morris A, et al: Acute dysphagia induced by bendrofluazide-K. *Practitioner* 1984; 228:524–525.

87. Bohane TD, Perrault J, Fowler RS. Oesophagitis and oesopageal obstruction from T in association with left atrial enlargement: A case report. *Australian Paed J* 1978; 14:191–192.

88. Murray K: Severe dysphagia from emepronium bromide associated with oesophageal diverticulum. *Br J Surg* 1982; 69:439.

89. McCarthy RH, Terkelsen KG: Esophageal dysfunction in two patients after clozapine treatment. *J Clin Psychopharmacol* 1994; 14:281–283.

90. Cordeiro MF, Arnold KG: Digoxin toxicity presenting as dysphagia and dysphonia. *Br Med J* 1991; 302: 1025.

91. Moss HB, Green A: Neuroleptic-associated dysphagia confirmed by esophageal manometry. *Am J Psychiatry* 1982; 139:515–516.

92. Woodring JH, Martin CA, Keefer B: Esophageal atony and dilatation as a side effect of thiothixene and benztropine. *Hosp & Comm Psychiatry* 1993; 44:686–688.

93. Sliwa JA, Lis S: Drug-induced dysphagia. *Arch Phys Med & Rehab* 1993; 74:445–457.

94. Pearlman C: Clozapine, nocturnal sialorrhea, and choking. *J Clin Psychopharmacol* 1994; 14:283.

95. Wyllie E, Wyllie R, Cruse RP, et al: The mechanism of nitrazepam-induced drooling and aspiration. *N Engl J Med* 1986; 314:35–38.

96. Wardell KW: Untoward reactions to tranquilizing drugs. *Am J Psychiatry* 1957; 113:745.

97. Farber IJ: Drug fatalities. *Am J Psychiatry* 1957; 114:371–372.

98. Feldman PE: An unusual death associated with tranquilizer therapy. *Am J Psychiatry* 1957; 113:1032–1033.

99. Hollister LE, Kosek JC: Sudden death during treatment with phenothiazine derivatives. *JAMA* 1965; 192:1035–1038.

100. Plachta A: Asphyxia relatively inherent to tranquilization. *Arch Gen Psych* 1965; 12:152–158.

101. Hollister LE: Unexpected asphyxial death and tranquilizing drugs. *Am J Psychiatry* 1957; 114:366–367.

102. Zlotlow M, Paganini AE: Fatalities in patients receiving chlorpromazine and reserpine during 1956–1957 at Pilgrim State Hospital. *Am J Psychiatry* 1958; 115:154–156.

103. Von Brauchitsch H, May W: Deaths from aspiration and asphyxiation in a mental hospital. *Arch Gen Psych* 1968; 18:129–136.

104. Solan GM: Aspiration pneumonia. *W Virginia Med J* 1976; 72:18.

105. Shamash J, Miall L, Williams F, et al: Dysphagia in the neuroleptic malignant syndrome. *Br J Psychiatry* 1994; 164:849–850.

106. Hughes TAT, Shone G, Lindsay G, et al: Severe dysphagia associated with major tranquilizer treatment. *Postgrad Med J* 1994; 70:581–583.

107. Leestma JE, Koenig KL: Sudden death and phenothiazines. *Arch Gen Psych* 1968; 18:137–148.

108. Hussar AE, Bragg DG: The effect of chlorpromazine on the swallowing function in chronic schizophrenic patients. *Am J Psychiatry* 1969; 126:570–573.

109. Solomon K: Phenothiazine-induced bulbar palsy-like syndrome and sudden death. *Am J Psychiatry* 1977; 134:308–311.

110. Flaherty JA, Lahmeyer HW: Laryngeal-pharyngeal dystonia as a possible cause of asphyxia with haloperidol treatment. *Am J Psychiatry* 1978; 1351414–1415.

111. Cruz FG, Thiagarajan D, Harney JH: Neuroleptic malignant syndrome after haloperidol therapy. *S Med J* 1983; 76:684–686.

112. Stones M, Kennie D, Fulton JD: Dystonic dysphagia associated with fluspirilene. *Br Med J* 1990; 301:668–689.

113. Casteels-Van Daele M, Jaeken J, Van der Schueren P, et al: Dystonic reactions in children caused by metoclopramide. *Arch Dis Childhood* 1970; 45:130–133.

114. Newton-John J. Acute upper airway obstruction due to supraglottic dystonia induced by a neuroleptic. *Br Med J* 1988; 297:964–965.

115. Weiden P, Harrigan M: A clinical guide for diagnosing and managing patients with drug-induced dysphagia. *Hosp & Comm Psychiatry* 1986; 37:396–398.

116. Gregory RP, Smith PT, Rudge P: Tardive dyskinesia presenting as severe dysphagia. *J Neurol, Neurosurg & Psych* 1992; 55:1203–1204.

117. Crane GE, Paulson G: Involuntary movements in a sample of chronic mental patients and their relation to the treatment with neuroleptics. *Int J Neuropsychiatr* 1967; 3:286–291.

118. Crane GE: Tardive dyskinesia in patients treated with major neuroleptics: A review of the literature. *Am J Psychiatry* 1968 (suppl); 124:40–48.

119. Yassa R, Jones BD: Complications of tardive dyskinesia: A review. *Psychosomatics* 1985; 26:305–313.

120. Craig TJ, Richardson MA: Swallowing, tardive dyskinesia, and anticholinergics. *Am J Psychiatry* 1982; 139:1083.

121. Jankovic J, Schwartz K: Botulinum toxin treatment of tremors. *Neurology* 1991; 41:1185–1188.

122. Poewe W, Schelosky L, Kleedorfer B, et al: Treatment of spasmodic torticollis with local injections of botulinum toxin. *J Neurol* 1992; 239:21–25.

123.. Comella CL, Tanner CM, DeFoor-Hill L, et al: Dysphagia after botulinum toxin injections for spasmodic torticollis: Clinical and radiologic findings. *Neurology* 1992; 42:1307–1310.

124. Nix WA, Butler IJ, Roontga S, et al: Persistent unilateral tibialis anterior muscle hypertrophy with complex repetitive discharges and myalgia: Report of two unique cases and response to botulinum toxin. *Neurology* 1992; 42:602–606.

125. Sampaio C, Castro-Caldas A, Nix WA, et al: Botulinum toxin and dysphagia. *Neurology* 1992; 42:2233.

126. Sedory SE, Ludlow CL: The swallowing side effects of botulinum toxin type A injection in spasmodic dysphonia. *Laryngoscope* 1996; 106(1 pt 1):86–92.

127. Kelton JG, Scullin DC: Digitalis toxicity manifested by dysphagia. *JAMA* 1978; 239:613–614.

128. Gustafsson LL, Walker O, Alvan G, et al: Disposition of chloroquine in man after single intravenous and oral doses. *Br J Clin Pharmacol* 1983; 15:471–479.

129. Wodak J, Gilligan BS, Veale JL, et al: Review of 12 months' treatment with L-dopa in Parkinson's disease, with remarks on unusual side effects. *Med J Australia* 1972; 2:1277–1282.

130. Snaith RP, Warren H deB: Treatment of Huntington's chorea with tetrabenazine. *Lancet* 1974; 1:413–414.

131. Critchley EM. Peak-dose dysphonia in Parkinsonism. *Lancet* 1976; 1:544.

132. Huang CY, McLeod JG, Holland RT, et al: Tetrabenazine in the treatment of Huntington's chorea. *Med J Australia* 1976; 1:583–584.

133. Marmont AM, Damasio EE: Neurotoxicity of intrathecal chemotherapy for leukaemia. *Br Med J* 1973; 4:47.

134. Chisholm RC, Curry SB: Vincristine-induced dysphagia. *S Med J* 1978; 71:1364–1365.

Appendix A
Pharmacological Treatment for Neurologic Diseases Commonly Occurring in Patients Seen by Speech–Language Pathologists

Disorder	Pharmacological Treatment
Neurologic disorders	
Ischemic stroke	Aspirin, warfarin, heparin, ticlodipine, tissue plasminogen activator
Brain tumor	Dexamethasone, mannitol
Myasthenia gravis	Pyridostigmine, prednisone
Amyotrophic lateral sclerosis	Riluzole
Multiple sclerosis	Adrenocorticoid hormone (ACTH), methylprednisolone, cyclosporine, interferon, cyclophosphamide, azathioprine
Parkinson's disease	Benztropine, biperiden, trihexyphenidyl, amantadine, levodopa/carbidopa, selegiline, pergolide, bromocriptine
Essential tremor	Propranolol, metoprolol
Laryngeal disorders	
Head and neck cancer	Cyclophosphamide, doxorubicin, cisplatin, fluorouracil, carboplatin, vincristine, bleomycin, hydroxyurea, paclitaxel, mitomycin, methotrexate, interferon alfa-2b
Spasmodic dysphonia	Botulinum toxin
Vocal fold edema	Prednisone

10

Medical Ethics and the Speech–Language Pathologist

EDYTHE A. STRAND, KATHRYN M. YORKSTON, AND ROBERT M. MILLER

CHAPTER OUTLINE

Ethical Theories and Principles of Medical Ethics

Factors Contributing to Ethical Dilemmas and Barriers to Ethical Decision Making in Speech Pathology

Factors Contributing to the Resolution of Ethical Dilemmas

Case Examples of Ethical Dilemmas in Speech Pathology

The field of biomedical ethics has seen a rapid expansion in recent years. Controversial and troubling issues related to health care, such as abortion, euthanasia, a patient's right to choose or refuse treatment, and the distribution of health care, have been the focus of numerous debates and publications. Scholars have used philosophical and theoretical foundations of biomedical ethics as a tool for deliberating many ethical dilemmas in medical practice.[1] Clinicians have looked for a way to systematically approach difficult moral decisions in clinical practice. Numerous recent publications have focused attention on a set of basic moral principles for guiding clinical decisions.[2–10] Beauchamp and Childress[11] note that is through examining moral principles and determining how these principles apply to individual cases that one is guided in the discussion and eventual resolution of these problems.

Principles of biomedical ethics are increasingly being taught in medical school curricula as a means of helping physicians and other health care professionals make critical decisions about patient care. While much of the literature relates to moral and legal issues involved in the physician–patient relationship, basic principles related to biomedical ethics are applicable to the speech–language pathologist and other ancillary medical personnel who work closely with patients over a period of time, especially in the medical setting. Discussion of these principles or information about medical ethics in general is not yet routinely included in the curriculum of many speech pathology programs, yet those students who are choosing to practice in medical settings will be faced with many ethical decisions, either as an individual or as part of a rehabilitation team. This chapter introduces the student or speech–language pathologist to basic definitions of some of the principles of medical ethics and gives examples of how these principles might be relevant in the practice of speech–language pathology. (Because these descriptions are necessarily short, we have included a list of references in the Appendix that may be of interest to speech–language pathologists who work in the medical setting.) A number of cases are used to represent difficult ethical problems. These cases involve moral decisions regarding maintenance and/or quality of life, the right of patients to make decisions about their own treatment, the responsibilities of the clinician to be truthful, loyal, and beneficent to the patient, and the access to assessment and treatment in speech pathology.

ETHICAL THEORIES AND PRINCIPLES OF MEDICAL ETHICS

Beauchamp and Childress[10] suggest an approach to moral reasoning that is based on hierarchical levels that they call "levels of moral justification" (Figure 10–1A). They posit that in the process of moral reasoning, different levels of abstraction may be applied. The lowest level of their hierarchy is judgments and actions. A judgment is a decision or conclusion about a particular action. *Rules* state that certain actions may not be done because they are wrong, or conversely, certain actions should be done because they are right. Principles serve as the foundation for rules. They are more general and fundamental in nature. The top level of the hierarchy is that of *theories,* in which the systematic relationship of principles and rules are considered. Therefore, it is an ethical theory that provides the framework for the principles. The principles then guide morally appropriate actions. Figure 10–1B

provides an example of each level of the hierarchy. At the top, an example of an ethical *theory* is deontology, which states that judgments and acts are either right or wrong, regardless of their consequences. A *principle* derived from this theory is veracity (it is right to tell the truth). This in turn provides the foundation for the *rule,* which is "it is wrong to lie." Finally, the action that exemplifies the principle and rule is a physician who tells a patient that his or her mean life expectancy, due to the physician's diagnosis of ALS, is 2 to 5 years. While it is beyond the scope of this chapter to examine ethical theories in any detail, a basic description of two types of theory are presented to illustrate approaches to moral reasoning and decision making.

Two basic types of ethical theories are most predominant:[9,10] deontological theories (sometimes referred to as formalist theories) and utilitarian theories. In deontology, judgments and actions are either right or wrong. The features of the acts themselves, rather than their consequences, make them right or wrong. Therefore, certain rules (e.g., telling the truth) must always be followed, no matter what the consequences. Those who adhere to deontologist theory believe that what is "right" may be independent of what is "good." Therefore, "right" actions are not determined by whether or not they will produce "good consequences."

Utilitarianism, on the other hand, posits that "the end justifies the means." The rules are based, to some degree, on the consequences of decisions or actions. Beauchamp and Childress[11] describe utilitarianism as referring to a moral theory that posits that utility is the one basic principle in

A

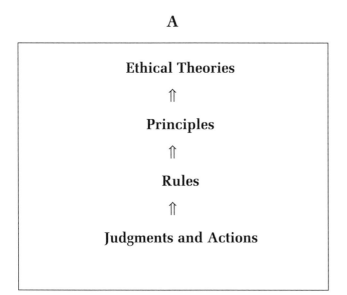

B

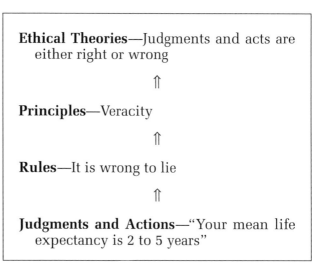

Figure 10–1. Hierarchical levels of moral justification. *Source:* Beauchamp TL, Childress JF: *Principles of biomedical ethics.* New York, New York, Oxford University Press, 1989.

ethics. This principle asserts that we ought always produce the "greatest possible balance of value over disvalue" (p. 26). No action or moral decision is completely wrong in itself, and it is therefore possible for rules to be revised. According to this way of thinking, an action is justified if it results in more good than any other action.

Question: *Can you give an example of how a decision in speech pathology may differ if based on one vs. the other theory?*

Consider a person who comes to you with a hysterical voice problem. If one follows a deontological perspective (an action is either right or wrong), then you must "do what is right" and tell the truth. Therefore, you might tell the patient, "Your voice problem is psychological in origin, and we cannot help you. Instead, we will refer you to a psychiatrist." On the other hand, one who follows a utilitarian perspective would decide the "right" action based in part on the outcome. In this case, the speech pathologist might decide that he or she is likely to get a better outcome for the patient if he or she does not "tell the whole truth." In this case the clinician may say, "Yes, there is something wrong with your voice, and I know exactly what it is. I will show you a few techniques that will make your voice sound better. I am also going to refer you to another doctor, a psychiatrist, who can help this voice problem from coming back." Keep in mind that the outcome was really the same—a referral to the psychiatrist. But, in the second case the clinician made the decision to "not" tell the whole truth, by implying that something was indeed wrong with the patient's laryngeal function.

Although these theories provide a philosophical foundation from which to approach ethical dilemmas, the literature in medical ethics relies heavily on the use of ethical principles as a guide to moral decision making. Authors vary with respect to what principles are most important, how those principles relate to one another, and when one principle takes precedence. Several commonly discussed principles include autonomy, beneficence, nonmaleficence, and justice. In addition, three principles are important to the patient-professional relationship: veracity, confidentiality, and fidelity. A brief discussion of each of these major principles will help illustrate some of the issues involved in ethical dilemmas and how these principles can guide the clinician toward ethical action. We will examine the meaning of each term and then provide an example of how this principle comes into ethical dilemmas in speech pathology.

Autonomy

The principle of autonomy refers to the right of the individual to self-determination.[10] That is, the individual determines his or her own course of action and makes decisions concerning his or her own fate. If a person is autonomous, he or she is free to choose a self-formulated plan of action. He or she is free of control or influence by people or institutions and by personal limitations (such as lack of information or understanding that would prevent making a meaningful decision). Therefore, a person who is in some way influenced or controlled by others because of some diminished competency (i.e., dementia) is considered to have diminished autonomy. A person's autonomy, then, refers to his or her self-contained ability to make personal decisions. In contrast, a person with little or no autonomy is dependent on others, whether or not they are capable of deliberating or acting on their own. In recent years, those involved in the practice of clinical medicine have shifted away from a paternalistic attitude of making decisions for patients, and toward respecting the autonomy of patients to make decisions for themselves.

Question: *What if the patient or family is making the wrong decision? Do they still have the right to autonomy?*

Consider the example of a 42-year-old woman who has a very severe verbal apraxia subsequent to an embolic ischemia (stroke) as a result of surgery. She has a very mild aphasia, and no cognitive deficits. She is educated, self-sufficient in activities of daily living, and well informed about the options open to her. The speech–language pathologist has recommended a high-tech augmentative communication system to maximize her communication efficiency. She refuses, however, because the system "draws attention to her disability." Even though the speech–language pathologist may believe it is in her best interest to use the augmentative system, the apraxic speaker has the right to autonomy—to decide not to invest the time, money, and effort to use a system that is unacceptable to her lifestyle.

Speech–language pathologists often provide assessment and treatment to patients who already experience diminished autonomy, not because it is imposed on them by government or the health care system, but because of diminished competence. As we will see in one of the following cases, the degree to which such reduced competency (e.g., in the early stages of progressive dementia accompanying Parkinson's disease) impacts our respect for patient autonomy presents real ethical dilemmas.

Respect for autonomy, a term also used to describe this principle,[3] is based on the notion of individual liberty. Beauchamp and Childress[11] point out that respect for autonomy also involves recognizing a person's right to make decisions, have opinions, and take actions. But they also posit that respect for autonomy involves recognizing that person's capabilities. (In the above case, the apraxic speaker had the cognitive capability to make a decision regarding augmentative communication.) Further, respect for autonomy involves doing whatever is necessary or possible to enable the person to act autonomously.

Respect for autonomy is one of the most common principles involved in moral dilemmas that face speech–language pathologists who work with patients with degenerative neurologic disease, as well as other disorders that are encountered in the medical setting. While respect for autonomy is one of the fundamental obligations in medical management, it is dependent in part on the maintenance of the patient's ability to communicate. Facilitating communicative efficiency and/or providing some means of augmentative communication may allow the patient to retain personal autonomy and the ability to make personal choices about medical care. However, even when communication is maintained and facilitated, the principle of patient autonomy still presents difficult moral dilemmas. This is especially true when one considers the sometimes contrasting principle of beneficence.

Beneficence and Nonmaleficence

Autonomy and beneficence have been said to be the conflict at the roots of bioethics.[1] In medical practice, the principle of beneficence refers to furthering the optimal health interests of the patient.[3] Beneficence, in its simplest form implies being kind and merciful. Beneficence refers to "doing good," and includes any action that will result in benefiting another. Beneficence implies that positive steps are taken to prevent harm, re-move from harm, as well as contribute to another's welfare.

Beauchamp and Childress[11] note that beneficence goes beyond being kind. They point out the importance of the obligation to balance the potential good against the potential harm that might result from an action or decision. They note that one cannot usually perform actions that are beneficial or that prevent harm without also creating risks. Therefore, the balance of potential good versus potential harm is an important aspect of this principle.

Question: *I have heard the word "paternalism." How does that term fit in?*

Until recently, beneficence often took precedence over autonomy. The doctor, or health care professional, "knew best" and the beneficent decision was made for the patient. This has been known as "paternalism." In fact, paternalism is sometimes considered to occur whenever beneficence outweighs autonomy.

In clinical practice, it is common for autonomy to come in conflict with beneficence. For example, a patient with a progressive swallowing problem may be advised that a percutaneous endoscopic gastrostomy (PEG) is the most appropriate intervention at a particular time and is necessary for adequate nutrition and hydration. The speech pathologist employs the principle of *beneficence* in the recommendation. The patient may be unwilling to accept the recommendation and choose to continue oral nutrition. In this case, autonomy takes precedence over beneficence.

While the principal of beneficence includes acts to prevent harm or remove from harmful conditions, the principle of nonmaleficence refers to the noninfliction of harm on others. These two principles are not easily separable. Beauchamp and Childress,[11] however, consider nonmaleficence to be distinct from beneficence because of the conviction that our obligations to *not* injure someone are distinct from and more stringent than our responsibilities *to* benefit others. Nonmaleficence encompasses both intentional harm, as well as the risk of harm, and the line between them is not always clear. Using the example of the dysphagia patient described previously, we see that the principles of autonomy may conflict with the principle of beneficence, but also that nonmaleficence comes into play because of the risk of harm.

That is, deciding to continue oral feeding risks maleficence because of the risk of aspiration, dehydration, and malnutrition.

Justice

The formulation of a single unifying theory of justice has been an elusive problem.[11] Different theories of justice described in the literature attempt to simplify and give order to diverse rules and judgments. These theories have been used to determine how health care services should be distributed. For example, egalitarian theories emphasize equal access to goods (or health care). Libertarian theories stress invoking fair procedures over outcome. Utilitarian theories emphasize a variety of different criteria to maximize the public good. That is, there are trade-offs in balancing private and public benefit. Important questions concerning the right to equal access to health care, the right to a particular minimum of care, and how to establish priorities when allocating health care resources all involve the principle of justice. How one comes to answers in any particular situation will depend on the theoretical perspective taken.

Question: Can you give me an example of how the principle of justice comes into play in the field of speech pathology?

One example relates to the number of treatment sessions allowed for patients in the rehabilitation setting. Certain reimbursement systems are based on the principle of equal access to treatment, regardless of outcome (libertarian). That is, a given diagnosis allows a specified number of treatment sessions. This allowed number is the same for all patients with that diagnosis. Conversely, those who make decisions from a utilitarian perspective would say the number of sessions should be based on a variety of individualized factors (e.g., severity, prognosis) that relate to the potential outcome.

The principle of justice is often explained in terms of "fairness." In medical ethics, the discussion of justice often focuses on the distribution of services under a particular moral vision. The emphasis is on the comparative treatment of individuals given limited resources. The speech–language pathologist, while not usually in the front lines of establishing systems of health care delivery, does struggle with problems related to patient access to assessment and treatment. We are faced with

determining how much treatment is appropriate, the minimal treatment one can recommend given the financial resources available, and who to treat and not treat given limited resources. Speech–language pathologists in the medical setting have experienced situations of increasingly shorter stays on rehabilitation units and authorization for increasingly fewer number of outpatient treatment visits. And the dilemmas do not stop at the medical setting. Consider the public school therapist who has responsibility for providing treatment to a child who has returned to school on discharge from the hospital following a closed head injury. Cognitive, linguistic, and motor speech disorders are present, yet prognosis for improvement is excellent. The principles of beneficence and nonmaleficence would dictate that the therapist see the child daily on an individual basis. Given a large caseload, however, that would mean denying, or severely curtailing, services to others. This moral dilemma illustrates that ethical decisions are not easily made.

Veracity, Confidentiality, and Fidelity

The principles of veracity, confidentiality, and fidelity are discussed together because they are all important to the patient-health care professional relationship. They also often overlap in practice as well as in principle, and together sometimes come in conflict with the necessity to be beneficent and obey the law. All three principles are often discussed as "obligations" to the patient by the health care professional.

Beauchamp and Childress[11] offer three arguments for the obligation of veracity. First, they posit that veracity is partially obligated because of the respect that is due to others. Second, the necessity to tell the truth comes from the obligation of fidelity, or keeping promises. When health care professionals are in a caregiving relationship with the patient, they "promise" to be truthful and not deceive. Finally, the obligation for veracity stems from the necessary relationship of trust between the health care professional and the patient. The patient expects the professional to be honest, and the professional expects the patient to be truthful and open about concerns, attitudes, and information regarding his or her health and mental status. In addition to being truthful and open, however, there is the expectation that information about the patient's health care status will remain confidential.

The principle of confidentiality involves widespread rules and practices. These have historically been considered of grave importance. In general, this principle implies that the professional may not reveal the confidences entrusted to him or her in the course of medical attention. This principle has been stated in a variety of codes, including the Hippocratic oath and the AMA principles of medical ethics. In practice, confidentiality is often difficult to implement, given the number of people who have access to a patient's chart because they may be directly involved in the delivery of some health care service. Charts typically do not note what information patients desire to keep confidential and what they have given permission to disclose. The speech–language pathologist, for example, may often have much information about a patient's medical history and health care status. The principle implies that we adhere to rules of confidentiality and not disclose information we have access to. That, in fact, is essential to preserving fidelity.

The term fidelity implies the obligation of keeping promises, or agreements inherent in the relationship with a patient. These promises include being beneficent, not doing harm, telling the truth, and maintaining confidentiality. However, the necessity to preserve fidelity (by telling the truth and maintaining confidentiality) sometimes comes in conflict with the duty to obey the laws of country and be beneficent to all persons.

Question: *Can you give me an example of fidelity?*

One speech–language pathologist had been working with a 12-year-old head injured girl for some time. The girl, who had come to trust the speech–language pathologist, confided to her that her father was abusing her. She implored her not to tell anyone. The speech–language pathologist knows that it is her obligation to inform the county social service department. What is the "ethical" course of action here? In this case, the speech–language pathologist decided to have several talks with the girl, until she was able to convince her that it was important to tell someone.

FACTORS CONTRIBUTING TO ETHICAL DILEMMAS AND BARRIERS TO ETHICAL DECISION MAKING IN SPEECH–LANGUAGE PATHOLOGY

The two major areas of functional impairment encountered by speech–language pathologists in a medical setting are communication deficits and swallowing disorders. Inherent in these overlapping populations are factors that potentially contribute to the development of an ethical dilemma, as well as barriers to the resolution of those dilemmas. For example, communication deficits, whether related to cognition, language, or motor speech, may prevent the patient from being able to express wishes and feelings. Patients with acute dysphagia may be experiencing an immediate and insidious threat to their life. Issues of dependency and feeding tubes have a direct impact on a patient's perceived quality of life. Swallowing impairment often connotes negative ideas such as aspiration, choking, gagging, strangulation, drooling, dehydration, and cachexia, all of which evoke emotional reactions. When communication and swallowing impairment coexist, as they often do, the case is ripe for the development of an ethical dilemma.

Ethical dilemmas may arise for any number of reasons, as may barriers to the resolution of those dilemmas. Some factors, however, if recognized, may be controlled to prevent an ethical dilemma from developing or obviate the barriers to ethical decision making. These barriers may include: failure to accede to the principles of medical ethics; developing strict and limiting policies or laws that affect patient care; team communication failures; and acting self-defensively because of a "fear of blame."

Failure to understand or accede to the principles of medical ethics may occur for many reasons. Perhaps the most frequently encountered problem concerns the failure to accept the wishes of a patient who invokes autonomy. For example, a patient who is unable to express his or her wishes regarding alternative forms of nutritional management may have previously declared to the family that they would never accept a feeding tube to sustain their life. A clinician who recognizes a high aspiration risk would be forced to grapple with the seeming conflict between the principles of beneficence and autonomy. The issues revolving around each of these principles must be openly discussed and weighed before determining a clinical course of action. Failure to identify how the two principles are in conflict can be a barrier to the process of decision making and result in dire consequences.

Strict and limiting policies or laws have been encountered that have either contributed to the development of an ethical dilemma or provided a barrier to its resolution. For example, a patient was transferred into a skilled nursing facility (SNF) with a policy that prevented any form of "syringe feeding." After admission, this patient was discovered to be rapidly losing weight and needing IVs to maintain hydration. The patient had been nutritionally maintained with syringe feeding at home, by the family, for two years prior to this SNF admission. There had been no instance of acute airway compromise and no evidence of insidious pulmonary decline related to aspiration. An experienced speech–language pathologist diagnosed an oral stage dysphagia and demonstrated on repeat clinical examinations and during a video fluoroscopic swallow study that the patient showed no evidence of aspiration when formula was placed in the mouth via syringe. Although in general syringe feeding should be discouraged, and utilized only with stringent guidelines and criteria, the unyielding policy of this SNF precipitated an ethical dilemma that escalated to involve the issues of feeding tube placement, surgical risk, and the loss of pleasure derived from eating. A more carefully worded policy could have prevented this dilemma.

Some states have laws that limit a clinician's authority to post patient care instructions at bedside. Such laws prevent a speech–language pathologist from affixing feeding recommendations to direct caregivers in safe swallowing techniques. Although this may be a well-intended law that protects the patient's right to confidentiality, it places some patients in jeopardy. These laws may be enforced even when the patient and family desire to have the information posted. Here, again, is potential for conflict between "best clinical practice standards" and a benevolent principle designed to prevent disclosure of privileged information. The strictly stated policy in this case both precipitated an ethical dilemma and acted as a barrier to solving that dilemma.

Team communication failures also serve as barriers to the processes of ethical decision making. These may occur because the medium most often used for communication is the medical chart. The patient's chart is an artificial mode of communication and is not conducive to complex decision making. In particular, it doesn't facilitate the health care team's ability to come to consensus on important issues, because it is a serial log of communication where consensus cannot easily be developed. Such a method of communication does not then facilitate ethical decisions.

Consider, for example, the case of a terminally ill patient who is suffering from unremitting pain and does not want to participate in medical procedures that are performed for purposes of diagnosis and assessment. All consultants involved with the case should be made aware of the patient's wishes, and intervention decisions should be driven by the

desire to provide comfort and compassion. Unfortunately, the medical chart, a medical/legal document, frequently fails to communicate to all involved health professionals this essential information. Commonly, such patients are transported to radiology for nonessential X-rays or are visited by laboratory technicians to draw blood for analysis. Face-to-face team meetings can facilitate communication for the purpose of coordinating care that is truly in the patient's best interest. Clarity and access to information are essential elements in preventing ethical dilemmas.

Acting self-defensively because of fear of liability or blame has the potential not only to precipitate an ethical dilemma, but to compromise patient care. A speech–language pathologist's decision to recommend a feeding tube in an acutely ill patient may be based on the clinician's subjective fear that the patient might develop complications as a result of oral feedings. Instead of using more objective measures, good clinical judgment, and considering all relevant factors in the individual case, a clinical decision can be unduly influenced by the clinician's anxiety, perhaps based on a previous unfortunate experience. Recommendations regarding nutritional management have the inherent potential of resulting in a medical complication. They are rarely easy decisions, but they are determinations that must be based on the facts of the individual case and in consultation with the primary care team. By allowing fear and anxiety to guide recommendations, the clinician will experience an unresolved conflict between the desire to adhere to the principle of beneficence and avoid maleficence.

FACTORS CONTRIBUTING TO THE RESOLUTION OF ETHICAL DILEMMAS

Despite the best efforts, ethical dilemmas are inevitable in the context of a health care environment. The extreme complexity of modern medical care, technology, and the expanse of human relationships and emotions provide the ingredients for precipitating ethical dilemmas. When such conflicts arise, one should consider a number of techniques that can facilitate their resolution. For example, conflicts should be clearly defined, articulated, and broken down into component parts; available options should be listed and objectively evaluated; and dialogue between all stakeholders should be encouraged whenever possible. Avoiding emotional attachment to a point of view—a major barrier to the resolution of a dilemma—

should be avoided. The following case was presented at a recent regional nurses' conference on ethics to illustrate the facilitating techniques and potential barriers for the resolution of ethical dilemmas.

JR is a 65-year-old patient with an atypical form of basal ganglia disease, similar to Parkinson's disease. The patient's functional limitations include anarthria and severe oral-pharyngeal dysphagia. He is unable to use either his upper or lower extremities in a functional manner, making him totally dependent for all self-care and mobility. He is an avid sports fan and movie buff. Insofar as can be determined, JR had no significant cognitive deficits that limit his ability to make informed choices regarding his health care. He has no clinical signs of depression or other mental illness. His neurologic disease has been slowly progressive over the last 15 years, but his only medical complications in the past have been related to two bouts of urinary tract infection. He has been cared for at his home by a series of health aids. He is unmarried and has no immediate family. He is currently hospitalized for "aspiration pneumonia."

During his hospitalization, nursing notes describe, and the speech–language pathologist confirms, frequent episodes of aspiration during attempts to feed. Radiographic swallowing studies have demonstrated aspiration on all food and liquid consistencies. All compensatory strategies have failed to ameliorate the problem with aspiration. Recommendations from the speech–language pathologist are to keep the patient NPO until safe swallowing can be demonstrated. The attending physician has reported that there is no expectation that the patient's neurologic disease will improve, nor is there any expectation that his dysphagia will resolve.

The dilemma is this: (1) The patient has made it very clear, through previous written documents and in present communication, that he will not accept a feeding tube under any circumstances. He acknowledges that swallowing is unsafe and may lead to his imminent death, but he is unwilling to accept any alternatives to oral feeding; (2) the nursing staff refuses to feed the patient on the grounds that it is tantamount to assisted suicide. The patient is choking on every attempt to ingest food or liquid despite their best efforts. He has required the Heimlich maneuver more than once.

When this case was initially presented at the nursing conference, the audience divided themselves into two camps. Some argued in favor of patient autonomy at all cost, while others declared that nonmaleficence was the primary consideration. During the ensuing discussion it became evident that opinions were strongly divided and emotional attachments developed to different points of view. The presenter halted the discussion and focused the group's attention on the clinical facts of the case, including the patient's functional assets and limitations. A list of potential treatment options was developed and evaluated in a dispassionate manner. Interestingly, a nurse who had withheld any opinion regarding the dilemma offered a potential solution that would allow the patient to continue taking nourishment by mouth while eliminating the concern of caregivers over aspiration and airway compromise. This solution, a total laryngectomy, was the procedure that had been offered to and accepted by JR. In fact, as a result of this surgical procedure, JR was able to be discharged to his home with what he perceived to be a significantly improved quality of life.

CASE EXAMPLES OF ETHICAL DILEMMAS IN SPEECH–LANGUAGE PATHOLOGY

So far in this chapter we have focused on what the principles and theories of medical ethics are and how to avoid some of the barriers to resolution of ethical dilemmas. Emphasis was given to describing what contributes to the dilemma. Now, we'll make an abrupt turn in content and style in an effort to more adequately reflect how ethical dilemmas are dealt with in a medical setting.

Clinical ethics is a term used to describe the discipline that provides a structured approach to identifying, analyzing, and resolving ethical issues in clinical medicine.[7] This approach to examining moral principles is a process, not a construct. It is the process by which principles of medical ethics can be applied to specific situations and cases. To illustrate this process of communication and decision making, we will present four real-life cases where an ethical dilemma occurred. Following each case is a discussion by a small group of practicing speech–language pathologists. These discussions demonstrate the process of applying the principles of medical ethics to difficult situations in which speech–language pathologists often find themselves. The discussions are similar to what might occur in a patient staffing, a rehabilitation team meeting, or perhaps a discharge planning meeting. They point out the principles of medical ethics as they are applied to real cases, and strategies for approaching difficult clinical problems.* This type of forum is an important teaching mechanism for students in the medical professions, yet somewhat neglected in the field of speech–language pathology.

Questions the clinicians asked themselves to guide the discussion included: What are the facts of this case? What other information do we need? What principles of medical ethics are important in this situation? How do the principles of autonomy, beneficence, and nonmaleficence come into conflict? How do the facts of this case help us resolve the conflict? Is there anything the team could or should have done to prevent this situation in the first place? Are there barriers to ethical decision making that the clinician or team should be aware of as they approach ethical dilemmas? What are the important issues relevant to our responsibility in this case? What are our options for action?

Question: Is there any order in which these questions should be asked?

These questions are often structured so that one always begins by reviewing the facts of the case. From the facts, one can list issues that pertain to the principles of medical ethics discussed earlier in this chapter. For example, in the following case, listing the facts leads one to determine that the main issues involved are the questions regarding the patient's cognitive competency, his request for no feeding tube, and the current risks to his well-being. This leads to a discussion of the principles of autonomy, beneficence, and maleficence. The principle of autonomy alone would lead to the decision to let him continue as he has, living alone and eating. The principle of beneficence (doing good and preventing harm) would dictate that any steps necessary be taken to prevent probably frequent aspiration. Some would even argue that allowing this patient oral nutrition so greatly risks his well-being that maleficence is at issue. The discussion is therefore guided by the questions, but the questions do not necessarily lead to one "right" answer.

---

* These cases might be presented in classrooms, proseminars, staff development meetings, and so on to allow students and clinicians an opportunity to utilize principles of medical ethics as they think through solutions to these situations.

The discussion following each case is not scripted, nor was there any attempt to direct it. Each asterisk represents a turn by one of the three speech–language pathologists involved in the discussion. Although no specific directions were given to guide the discussion, there is an approach to the process of discussion that the three speech–language pathologists followed, and it may be helpful when approaching a similar discussion in your workplace. First, make sure there is not a lack of communication or failure to get the people together who are involved in the case. Everyone should have all the facts and the answers to any questions they have. Second, make sure that possible barriers to the resolution of dilemmas, discussed earlier in this chapter, are not impeding the discussion. Then examine the principles involved in the case and how they might come into conflict. Finally, list alternative courses of action.

In the discussion after each case, it will be clear that these are indeed ethical "dilemmas" because the principles do not fall into a "hierarchy" in terms of their importance. Clinical decisions will often be made only after weighing the consequences of possible solutions. In Case One, for example, patient autonomy might be preserved while reducing the risk for maleficence if a full-time caregiver would be available to assist feeding and minimize risks. An alternative decision might be that, in this case, beneficence and maleficence outweigh patient autonomy.

CASE ONE

RL is a 76-year-old man with advanced Parkinson's disease. He has a moderately severe dysarthria and a history of aspiration pneumonia and weight loss. On admission to the hospital, he denied episodes of choking or other difficulty with swallowing. He lives alone, and has a part-time assistant. Prior to admission, he signed an Advance Directive not to have a stomach tube placed at any stage in his disease. The primary physician feels that he is competent enough to make this decision. The speech–language pathologist, concerned about the recent precipitous weight loss, along with the history of aspiration pneumonia, completed a bedside swallow evaluation. She found that the patient had a great deal of difficulty swallowing both thin liquids and some solid food. Further, the patient appeared confused, and had difficulty following directions. This information was presented at rounds.

Excerpts from the Discussion of Case One

The participants begin by making sure they have all the facts they need.

- In reviewing the facts of this case, we see we have an example of a degenerative disease that we know is often accompanied by cognitive changes. In this case we also see a clear risk of aspiration. One of the things we don't know is when this advanced directive was signed. Do we know that this is still his wish?

- This also brings up another question that I have. What is the physician using as a measure of the patient's competence? Is she basing it on current information or on her relationship with the patient 10 years ago? I would want to know a little more about the patient's competency.

- I'd also like to know a little more about the family and how they feel about the patient's decision and his competency to make this decision today. Do they feel his advanced directives are in fact still current and correspond to his wishes? If so, then there are not a lot of options available at this point.

- This case reflects an interesting problem that advanced directives always gives you. We can sit down in our healthy state and write advanced directives, not knowing what tomorrow may bring. When a life-threatening situation actually arises, predetermined directives may well undergo new scrutiny by the patient.

- Another problem this case illustrates is the role of knowledge or understanding of intervention strategies and the possible connotations often accompanying some techniques. Sometimes, the connotations may be quite different than the reality (e.g., that a feeding tube is only used as a life-prolonging measure). So the patient may make a decision based on the connotation of the feeding tube, rather than the reality.

- Also, when the ultimate decision gets closer and closer, something that has been unthinkable becomes more and more attractive.

- The decision about a feeding tube may also have been made prior to the advent of a PEG, with is an entirely different procedure than an open gastrostomy or NG (nasogastric) tube. If this was done over 10 years ago, we would have been talking about a whole different kind of procedure and a different set of potential conflicts.

Now the discussion shifts to examination of the principles involved:

- A lot of what this case presents, too, is the obvious conflict between respect for the patient's autonomy and consideration of the clinician's recommendations that are made in the spirit of "do no harm" and do what is in the best interest of the patient. On the surface, there is not really an ethical dilemma here. The speech–language pathologist, in spite of finding aspiration and swallowing difficulties, could decide to respect the patient's autonomy and his right to make these decisions. In that case, the clinician would simply make certain management suggestions to minimize the risk without ever deciding that it was inappropriate for the patient to eat at all.

- But that leads to the flip side of autonomy that brings into play the principle of beneficence and doing good for the patient. These principles come into conflict here, because if therapists would indeed only respect patient autonomy, allowing the patient to make this decision, they run the risk of not upholding the principle of beneficence. In fact, they risk maleficence, or doing harm to the patient.

- In this case, it's obvious that the major conflict with respect to coming to an ethical decision relates to the typical conflict between patient autonomy and the principle of beneficence. This case also points out that there is no black-and-white answer, and we need to know more before an ethical decision can be made.

- In this case it is also possible that some of the barriers to ethical decision making would arise: emotionality, for example, is probable. One person could get very strongly fixed on one side of advocating for the patient's right for autonomy, whereas a speech–language pathologist might become emotionally involved in the aspect of taking every measure possible so the patient does not aspirate at all (perhaps because of fear of blame). A lot of that can be alleviated by very clear communication. The speech–language pathologist may say, yes, we recognize the risk for aspiration here, but we must take other considerations into account before deciding on a course.

- Communication would be a critical factor in this case. As the scenario reads I could interpret it to mean that all the communication has been done via the medical chart. First there is the advanced directive at some previous date signed in the medical chart. There is the physician's note in the medical chart that the patient is cognitively competent. All these issues could be communicated without any face-to-face communication with all the stakeholders in this matter. Perhaps one way to begin to solve the ethical dilemma is to bring all the players together for an on-line discussion.

CASE TWO

PH is a 43-year-old woman with a recent onset of ALS. Her first symptoms were hypernasality and slurring of speech. She had recently been forced to quit her retail job due to decreasing intelligibility. She was married and had an 11-year-old daughter. With multiple visits to the clinic, it became apparent that speech was becoming more labored and more difficult to understand; she was losing weight and her respiratory status was declining rapidly. Although walking was becoming more difficult, she refused to use a wheelchair. In fact, on one clinic visit she arrived an hour late, in a tearful and exhausted state, having just walked a quarter of a mile from the parking lot. When questioned she indicated that she had not told the parking attendant of her problem and had not asked for parking for the disabled, or a wheelchair and assistance, because she "thought she could make it." When she arrived she was so fatigued that she could not participate in the clinic visit. Her husband declined to attend any clinic visit. She indicated, "He thinks I'm faking it, and if I were stronger I'd be fighting it." Although she declined information about augmentative communication systems or alternative feeding procedures, she indicated she wished to live as long as possible because her daughter "needed her so much." When questioned about these decisions, she indicated that if her husband viewed her as having a disability, "He'd put me in a nursing home."

Excerpts from the Discussion of Case Two

• First, let's review the facts as we know them. She is a young woman with a diagnosis that is terminal. There are some social issues with respect to the family dynamics and their reactions to the disease, as well as the woman's own need to remain independent and her reluctance to ask for help.

• Yet there are contradictory statements here. She states that she wants to be around for her daughter, but she is unwilling to adopt the technology that would compensate for her limitations. It is an inconsistency that is causing a problem for her.

• It causes a problem for us too. There is an ethical dilemma here. One of the ways of helping her at this time is helping her communicate the facts about her illness with her husband. We perceive it as helpful to her to explain to her husband the nature of the disease, what the prognosis is, and what he should anticipate in terms of providing physical and emotional support for her. Conversely, she has a tremendous fear that communicating those facts will have extremely negative consequences for her. So, what do we do? How do we resolve that?

Now that a major dilemma has been identified, the clinicians turn to a discussion of the principles.

• At first glance, it seems clear that we did our job, conveyed information honestly to the patient and gave her advice that we felt would be beneficial to her. It is her choice as to what information she wants shared with her family.

• Yes, but to some degree we struggle a bit by wanting to respect her autonomy to choose not to confide in her husband, but also wanting to "do good" or be beneficent by providing the family with information that should be helpful to her in the long run. The more they know, the easier it will be for them to predict her needs, plan for support systems that will improve her quality of life, as well as provide emotional support.

• This case brings up not only the issues of patient autonomy and our wanting to be beneficent, but also the principles of confidentiality and fidelity. While veracity was maintained in that the clinicians were very honest about the nature of the disease, the course of the disease, and the ultimate outcome of the disease, important ethical decisions are raised with respect to whether or not it is up to the clinicians to speak to the husband to provide some of this information when we know it is the patient's wish that this information not be given to him.

• Following the principle of fidelity, we are guided to the decision that we remain loyal to the patient, that we maintain her wish for confidentiality, and that we also remain available and supportive as new problems arise during the course of the disease.

Now the discussion shifts to barriers:

- Let's talk about what barriers to ethical decisions might be seen in this case. We've avoided some barriers here in that we have no specific policies that state we must always talk to the families or that the families are brought in on every decision, because then this case would definitely have to be an exception to that policy.

- The issue of abandonment could arise in this case as a barrier to ethical decisions. I think there is a potential barrier to making ethical decisions because the health care providers might find themselves resentful of the fact that the patient is reluctant to follow their suggestions. For example, her disinclination to use the wheelchair for long distances; her refusing information about alternative feeding mechanisms, and so on may give the team the impression that she doesn't really want help. There is a danger of the team adopting the attitude, "If you don't do what I say, how can I continue to help you?"

- Yes, I agree. If a health care provider or a health care team really feels their best recommendations are not being followed, there is the risk of the patient's being abandoned.

- So, in this case the clinician is faced with the dilemma of weighing beneficence with patient autonomy as well as being faced with the problem of maintaining a good relationship with the patient with respect to confidentiality and fidelity.

- It also raises the question of what do you, as a health care professional, do when the patient gives you mixed messages, and they appear to have two different divergent and conflicting goals, each of which would result in a very different course of actions. What is your responsibility then?

- Perhaps one responsibility is to help the patient see how those divergent desires or goals are in conflict and how they impact the clinical management of their disease.

- Yes, in this case we see a patient going in a direction that is inconsistent with her own stated goals. She wants to live as long as possible because her daughter "needs her," yet she is refusing information on alternative feeding and refused augmentative communi-

cation that would help facilitate communication with her daughter now, and allow communication to continue for a longer period of time.

- Right, And when we recognize that, we need to maintain our fidelity to the patient by helping her recognize that conflict so *she* can resolve it. That is different than imposing the team's opinion on her.

- Is there an issue of the patient having fidelity to the health care worker? For example, is there some sense of a responsibility on the part of the patient to do what is suggested to take care of him or herself?

- I don't see that the patient has any obligation to maintain fidelity. The obligation is only on the health care professional's side. The patient has the right to go contrary to all the medical opinions they want. It is also important to note that the clinician should not, in that case, abandon the patient with regard to the rest of his or her health care.

CASE THREE

NL was a 52-year-old woman two months post diagnosis of ALS when she was referred to the outpatient clinic. She had just retired from a job she enjoyed that required extensive public speaking. She was accompanied to the first clinic visit by her sister who had just lost her husband to cancer. Although NL's first symptoms were entirely bulbar, she was only mildly dysarthric and denied swallowing difficulty. Both NL and her sister indicated that they knew the natural course of ALS but that they intended "not to give in to the disease." NL returned to clinic every two months. By the third visit, speech, swallowing and respiratory status had all declined. She was also showing increasing evidence of lability. During the second and third clinic visits, the PEG was discussed. It was explained that the procedure would facilitate nutrition and hydration, as well as conserve her energy. She was told she could eat when she wished, and use the tube to provide needed additional calories and liquid. Also, the timing of the PEG placement was discussed, including the need to carefully monitor respiratory status because poor pulmonary function may prevent PEG placement. Each time the PEG was mentioned she said, "Not now, maybe later, I'm not ready." At the fourth visit (8 months post-diagnosis) vital capacity had declined to just over one liter and NL was counseled that a decision about PEG needed to be made soon. Her sister became upset that the team had "waited too long" to ask NL to make a decision, and that this wait put NL at some risk. In an hourlong tearful meeting, in which NL used a portable typewriting system, NL told the team that she felt "railroaded into a fast decision."

Excerpts from the Discussion of Case Three

First, the clinicians try to examine why this problem occurred.

- One of the facts integral to this case is that to put in a PEG, patients need to have at least one liter of air in terms of vital capacity or the procedure itself puts them at too great a risk. So, this patient, although she had had the information explained to her prior to this visit, had probably been in a state of denial, and for that reason kept putting off making the decision to the point at which the decision was now critical.
- The other fact that is important is that as a health care management team we have no crystal ball to determine the slope of the progression of this disorder. So we are using our clinical judgments and guesses about when things need to happen to inform the patient. We are constantly balancing the potential risk of giving the patient too much information too soon or all at one time versus the risk of waiting too long to give information that the patient may need time to digest and accept.
- One of the questions that comes up in this particular case is whether or not there is anything the team could or should have done to prevent this situation. It is more complicated than just a lack of communication or miscommunication. The principle of beneficence comes into play here. Given that the patient was not open to discussing the PEG, should the team have "pushed" the discussion even though the patient did not want to hear it? Would that have been an instance of "going good" for the patient?
- Maybe there is another barrier that comes up here as we are talking about this. This barrier is summarized with the word "connotation." Feeding tubes have a connotation of "life support" about them. The whole idea of sustaining life artificially is fixed in some people's minds. It puts the decision for a medical procedure such as a feeding tube on a whole different level. It becomes a more emotional than objective decision about nutrition, hydration, and quality of life.
- One way, then, for a medical team or a clinician to try to solve the conflict between patient autonomy and beneficence is to explain to the patient that a feeding tube is always *his or her* decision. There is nothing that is being taken away from him or her with respect to his or her ability to decide what it is he or she wants and does not want. As a medical team, we are only asking that patients listen and get the information we have to give them. Maybe that is as far as we can go in "doing good" for the patient.
- This is a great case to point out that perhaps we should have dispassionately presented the facts early, emphasizing that no decision is required at this time and emphasizing that it is just our role to "provide education" about possible interventions: this is what a feeding tube is; this is what it can do for you; this is how it can improve your quality of life; these are other ways it will impact your life; and here are some of the issues around the timing of it.
- I really like your analysis that the decision was too big for this patient to make in one step. If we had broken the decision down into two steps—making a decision about considering a tube at some time in the distant future and then, if there was a decision to have the tube, deciding on the timing and accepting the referral to the gastroenterologist—then perhaps she would have more easily heard what we had to say. Breaking it into steps allows the patient to maintain control but not have the steps be so big it is such a huge decision.
- I might even go further than that and add another step first. Rather than present the patient with the question "Do you ever want a feeding tube?," simply tell the patient "We have information about feeding tubes. You may decide you never want one. That is OK. Today it is our job to tell you about what is available, how they work, and what they can do for you, if you should ever want to consider it."
- The other thing we learned from this case, regarding patient autonomy, is to remind the patient that he or she can change his or her mind about any decision at any time. Nothing he or she decides at any time is irrevocable.
- In this case, though, part of the important information is that patients can change their

minds only up to the point where respiratory capacity is at that critical level. Then they run the risk of the decision's being out of their hands.

Finally, the discussion summarizes some of the principles related to the "patient–health care provider" relationship.

- It would have been really easy in this case for us to violate some issues of fidelity. We were having some fingers pointed at us by the patient and her sister. "This is your fault. You waited too long to tell her about this, and now you are trying to railroad her into a decision." It is not uncommon for health professionals to want to pull away at this point. We have to deal with that and be able to accept blame, whether justified or not, and maintain fidelity to both the patient and significant others.

- Yes, the risk of abandonment is real here. The patient is going into the most difficult progression of the disease. She needs the team's support.

CASE FOUR

TW is a 30-year-old single woman with a diagnosis of Huntington's disease who was referred to the clinic for evaluation of swallowing difficulty by her family physician. The only information we had when we met her, other than her diagnosis, was the clinic nurse's note that she weighed 94 pounds and was 5'8" tall. Explanation of her low body weight was clear when we met the patient. She exhibited severe chorea and was essentially in constant motion. The dietitian estimated that her calorie intake was approximately 1900 calories, but that her calorie needs were between 4000 and 5000 per day. Her swallow was characterized by lack of coordination, mild to moderate risk of aspiration, and difficulty in transport of the food to her mouth. She indicated that eating was a time-consuming activity that she did not particularly enjoy. When alternative means of feeding were discussed, she firmly refused. When risks to health of malnutrition, dehydration, and aspiration were presented, she indicated that she "didn't have much to live for anyway." When the patient left the clinic, a clinician who was just beginning her fellowship year told her supervisor, "She's risking her own death through malnutrition or aspiration. Are we just going to let her do that? Isn't that condoning her suicide? That doesn't seem right. What should I do?" The supervisor motioned the clinician into her office and said, "Let's talk."

- Let's start with a review of the facts in this case. That's a major problem here. There is a lot we don't know in this case. We don't know the degree of dementia. We don't know to what degree this woman presents conflicting wishes with respect to wanting to live. We don't know what the family situation is regarding support. The first dilemma here is whether we can get all the information we need to facilitate decision making regarding this patient's care.

- We do know that she has calorie needs more than she can meet by her oral intake alone, given the degree of motor difficulty she has and that she is already spending an inordinate amount of time per day trying to feed herself. Second, she has a risk of aspiration because of her incoordination and poor swallowing function. Finally, we have the fact that she is adamantly refusing a tube. Here again, we probably have the connotation of a feeding tube (prolonging life) coming into play. We have an obligation at least to educate the patient about what a feeding tube offers in terms of quality of life versus prolonging life. I think a lot of times we see a patient shake their head "no" when the subject is brought up. After we explain what it is, how it is used, and what our experience with patients has been, then they often go, "Oh, this is different than what I thought."

- It was clear that she was viewing the decision about a PEG as a decision about shortening her life. She was not interested in the quality of life issues related to being relieved of the burden of eating.

Now the discussion turns to a poignant issue related to autonomy.

- In a way, this case brings up the most emotional and perhaps difficult ethical decision of all: the patient's right to choose to continue living. What is the role of the speech–language pathologist in contributing to that decision? Do we have any role?

- The reason I remember this patient so vividly and remember what she said to us was that she was a very attractive young woman who was moving constantly, and this gave a very unusual appearance because of the movement. Someone asked her about her decision. As she was moving, she turned to them and said, "Would you want to live like this?" It just stopped the whole conversation.

- This case really emphasizes how, as clinicians, we can't completely divorce our own feelings about the worth of life, our own self-image, and what we would be willing to live and cope with. It also illustrates how we might transfer our own personal feelings to the patient when we help him or her cope with some very difficult personal decisions. One of the questions I have here is why did she come to the clinic, given that we are a speech and swallowing clinic? I see from the chart that she was referred by her family physician. What was she really hoping to get from the visit? It is important to make sure we ask why the patient chose to make the appointment, even if it was due to a physician referral. There would also be a tendency here, on the basis for the facts as presented, for abandonment, by the clinic, throwing up our hands as a unit, saying we have nothing to offer; there's nothing we can do.

- Or, saying if you don't want what we have to offer, namely a PEG, don't come back, because that is what is best.

- I hope what we did was to provide her with some management suggestions to minimize her risk of aspirating; educate her with regard to what her calorie needs were and perhaps provide her with appropriate consultation with other people who might be able to provide her with adaptive aids for self-feeding. Then it would have been important to let her know that we would be there for her as consultants whenever she had questions or issues regarding feeding, swallowing, or communication, making it clear we were available and willing to help; thereby promoting patient autonomy while still being beneficent.

- Could we have broken down the decisions regarding a PEG in this case, as would have been helpful with the last patient?

- I don't think so in this case. Unlike the last patient, this woman came in with a clear desire to end her life. Short of actually doing something to end it immediately, she came in with the notion of making every decision that would hasten that end.

- I remember the patient talking about how she wasn't married, would never be married or have children, and how no one depended on her. "Why do you insist I keep on living?" is what she said to us.

- We do come across patients, on a fairly regular basis, who are making that decision. Or at least who have a desire not to live with a degenerative disease any longer. Including this issue in a chapter such as this points out that our role as a clinician involves more than just assessment and treatment of communication and swallowing disorders. When these issues come up, we have to remember that there is no right answer. We don't really have a role other than to keep in mind that the patient has a right to autonomy, and that our job is to provide information, be supportive, and do as much good for the patient as possible.

Now the discussion turns to our role as educators. How do we help students and CFY clinicians learn to deal with ethical dilemmas?

- This brings us to the final aspect of this case: the distraught clinician beginning her CFY and being unsure how to deal with intervention in this case. How does a young clinician acquire skills in these difficult situations? As an academic institution, how do we teach students to approach a problem from an ethical perspective? How do we provide training for clinical decisions that involve ethical dilemmas?

- It's important to remember that clinicians who are well skilled and have no reservations about their fundamental clinical knowledge are still struggling with issues related to ethical management. How do we expect a student or beginning clinician who is still learning to do a physical exam or choose the appropriate test to give, to do this? How do we put him or her in a position where he or she can productively learn about issues that are less tangible and more tied to principle rather than accepted practice?

- It may be that the supervisor needs to guide the student in steps. One way to do that may be by going through the questions we've used to guide our discussion. That is, what are the facts; what principles are presented in this case; what principles come into conflict; what barriers are there to coming to ethical decisions, and so on.

- Right off the bat we have to recognize that the student or CFY clinician has little experience here and is therefore ill equipped to deal with this. It is likely they will react on a whole different level than those of us who have been in these situations numerous times. The student may first and foremost be absolutely overwhelmed by the devastation they see caused by the disease itself and its consequences related to speech and swallowing. I think they are going to be less equipped to see the big picture and how all of this relates to, in this case, the woman's mortality. I think they will at first react at a very emotional level, and will not be able to rationally look at the facts of the case.

• One important aspect to remember when considering how to train clinicians with respect to clinical decision making involving ethical dilemmas is that one needs to develop a "fund of knowledge" on which to draw. One does that by honing observation skills and learning how to clearly interpret what you see. How does an experienced clinician, who has only recently been introduced to the principles of medical ethics, or a beginning clinician practicing in the medical setting for the first time begin to establish an experience base from which to learn?

• There is no short cut to experience. Every case that a beginning clinician has is a learning experience. It's important to keep in mind that each case is a new learning experience and that we shouldn't generalize too fast. There is a general tendency to take what we learned from the last case and apply it to the current case. Sometimes, even though there may be similarities that are apparent at first, there may be very different sets of circumstances that will require very different approaches to the ethical dilemmas they present.

• It is a very important process to evaluate the cases according to the principles of medical ethics, so that you begin to establish a fund of experience in this area. Issues related to ethical dilemmas and techniques for resolving barriers pose particular challenges, because there are no textbooks that tell you the right answers. There are no checklists or guide-lines for dealing with those clinical problems that involve ethical questions. That is why developing a fund of experience is so important. Clinicians have to learn from each case by talking about them honestly. If they give you problems, discuss them, talk about what worked and what didn't and why.

• Wisdom comes from a lot of experience, including failures as well as successes.

• Yes, it is important that we don't avoid the very uncomfortable process of critically evaluating how we have handled each patient. And it's important to lay the blame on ourselves if blame is appropriate. That is, to say: "I didn't handle this case in the best possible way. How can I apply this experience in the future with other cases? Because that is how we learn."

REFERENCES

1. Engelhardt HT: *The foundations of bioethics.* Oxford University Press, New York, 1986.
2. Ahronheim JC, Moreno J, Zuckerman C: *Ethics in clinical practice.* Little, Brown, Boston, 1994.
3. English DC: *Bioethics: A clinical guide for medical students.* Norton Medical Books, New York, 1994.
4. Dunn PM, Gallagher TH, Hodges MO, et al: Medical ethics: An annotated bibliography. *Ann of Int Med,* 1994; 121:627–632.
5. Pellegrino D: The metamorphosis of medical ethics: A 30-year retrospective. *JAMA* 1993; 269:1158–1162.
6. Gillon R: Medical ethics: Four principles plus attention to scope. *Brit Med J* 1994; 309: 184–188.
7. Jonsen AR, Siegler M, Winslade WJ: *Clinical ethics: A practical approach to ethical decisions in clinical medicine.* McGraw-Hill, New York, 1992.
8. Elliott C, Elliott B: From the patient's point of view: Medical ethics and the moral imagination. *J Med Ethics* 1991; 17:173–178.
9. Harron F, Burnside J, Beauchamp T: *Health and human values: A guide to making your own decisions.* Yale University Press, New Haven, 1983.
10. Beauchamp, TL, Childress JF: *Principles of biomedical ethics.* Oxford University Press, New York, 1983.
11. Beauchamp TL, Childress JF: *Principles of biomedical ethics.* Oxford University Press, New York, 1989.

Appendix A: Selected Resources for the SLP

Bach, J. R., & Barnett, V. (1994). Ethical considerations in the management of individuals with severe neuromuscular disorders. *American Journal of Physical Medicine & Rehabilitation,* 73, 134–140.

Banja, J. D., & Bilsky, G. S. (1993). Discussing cardiopulmonary resuscitation with elderly rehabilitation patients. *American Journal of Physical Medicine & Rehabilitation,* 72, 168–171.

Callahan, D. (1993). Allocating health care resources. *American Journal of Physical Medicine & Rehabilitation, 72*, 101–105.

Dougherty, C. J. (1994). Quality-adjusted life years and the ethical values of health care. *American Journal of Physical Medicine & Rehabilitation, 73*, 61–65.

Haas, J. (1993). Ethical considerations of goal setting for patient care in rehabilitation medicine. *American Journal of Physical Medicine & Rehabilitation, 72*, 228–232.

Jennings, B. (1993). Healing the self: The moral meaning of relationships in rehabilitation. *American Journal of Physical Medicine & Rehabilitation, 72*, 401–404.

Kottke, F. J. (1982). Philosophic considerations of quality of life for the disabled. *Archives of Physical Medicine & Rehabilitation, 63*, 60–62.

Meier, R. H., & Purtilo, R. B. (1994). Ethical issues and the patient-provider relationship. American Journal of Physical Medicine & Rehabilitation, 73, 365–366.

Pearlman, R. A., & Jonsen, A. (1985). The use of quality-of-life considerations in medical decision making. *Journal of the American Geriatrics Society, 33*, 344–352.

Purtilo, R. B. (1986). Ethical issues in the treatment of chronic ventilator-dependent patients. *Archives of Physical Medicine & Rehabilitation, 67*, 718–721.

Purtilo, R. B., & Meier, R. H. (1993). Team challenges: Regulatory constraints and patient empowerment. *American Journal of Physical Medicine & Rehabilitation, 72*, 327–330.

Sivak, E. D., Gipson, W. T., & Hanson, M. R. (1982). Long-term management of respiratory failure in amyotrophic lateral sclerosis. *Annals of Neurology, 12*, 18–23.

Strax, T. E. (1994). Ethical issues of treating patients with aids in a rehabilitation setting. *American Journal of Physical Medicine & Rehabilitation, 73*, 293–295.

Venesy, B. A. (1994). A clinician's guide to decision making capacity & ethically sound medical decisions. *American Journal of Physical Medicine & Rehabilitation, 73*, 219–226.

SECTION III

Neurogenic Communication Disorders and the Speech–Language Pathologist

11

Neurologic Disorders: An Orientation and Overview

DANIEL NEWMAN AND NABIH RAMADAN

CHAPTER OUTLINE

Anatomical Substrates

The Neurological Exam

Neurological Tests

Neurological Diseases and Their Management

Of the various disciplines within medicine, an understanding of neurology is arguably the most important for the speech–language pathologist (SLP). Not only does the nervous system provide for the control of the structures that produce and modify sound into speech, but language itself is organized and constructed solely within the brain.

This chapter will attempt to provide a framework for understanding the neurological approach to problems encountered by the SLP. An anatomical approach to the patient's problem is traditional for neurologists, and although this is sometimes maligned as an effete exercise, it is an efficient method of limiting a potentially huge differential diagnosis. In reality, most of us think in this way all the time.

An example: Your grandmother calls you up and, knowing that you are a SLP, tells you that her neighbor has begun to "talk funny." You think a moment; this could mean anything. You wonder, has the usual content of conversation changed or become inappropriately jocular or puerile? Is the person now speaking in jargon or neologisms? Has

the speech become softer and monotonal? Is it more hoarse or slurred? Whether you know it or not, as you attempt to figure out what Grandma means by "talk funny," you are beginning to try to localize the lesion. Your first question is likely to be, "Is she saying funny things or are the words slurred or mushy?" The answer to this question immediately tells you whether Grandma has noted the onset of a dysarthria, an aphasia, or a disorder of thought.

ANATOMICAL SUBSTRATES

The Motor Unit

Thinking of the neurological aspects of speech as being organized hierarchically is useful. The tissues that actually produce sound and modify speech are either largely muscle (e.g., the tongue) or soft tissues that change their shape through the action of attached or adjacent muscle. These skeletal muscles are innervated by lower motor neurons (LMN), which have their cell bodies in the caudal part of the brainstem, specifically the pons and medulla. The apparatus that functionally connects the lower motor neuron with the muscle is the neuromuscular junction (NMJ). The lower motor neuron, the NMJ, and the muscle are considered the motor unit. Damage or dysfunction of the motor unit will lead to variants of dysarthria that are inevitably flaccid.

Motor Control

The Corticospinal Tract

The motor unit is under the control of a number of descending pathways that originate in the cerebrum and brainstem. They are known collectively as the upper motor neurons (UMN), although, in practice, the corticospinal (projecting to spinal LMNs) and corticobulbar (projecting to the lower cranial nerve LMNs) tracts alone are often given this designation. Because the corticospinal tract descends through the pyramid in the medulla, it is also referred to as the pyramidal tract. The corticobulbar tracts provide the voluntary control over the cranial nerves that produce speech.

A lesion of the corticospinal tract leads to weakness and a loss or reduction of contralateral voluntary movements. In comparison, unilateral lesions of the corticobulbar tract have less of an effect on speech because most lower cranial nerves have fairly prominent bilateral innervation. A notable exception is the innervation of the lower part of the face that receives primarily contralateral (corticobulbar) input. If the corticobulbar tracts are lesioned bilaterally, the dysarthria produced is spastic.

The Basal Ganglia

Other descending pathways (e.g., the rubrospinal and reticulospinal) are primarily concerned with posture and tone of the upper and lower extremities, and their roles in the production of speech are less well understood. Finally, substantial areas of the brain (e.g., the basal ganglia and cerebellum) are involved with motor control but do so by way of complex feedback loops involving cortical and subcortical structures.

Perhaps the best way to think of the interplay of the pyramidal and extra pyramidal motor systems is to consider them as "voluntary" and "involuntary" systems respectively.

Consider a person standing ready to catch a thrown baseball; the ball is thrown to the right of the person. When the person reaches to the right to catch it, only the abduction and extension of the arm and the opening of the fingers are "volun-

tary." The unconscious extension of the left arm and the requisite changes of the trunk musculature are "involuntary." These changes have been largely planned and executed by the basal ganglia using real-time sensory information to maintain balance and utilizing prelearned motor programs to support the rest of the body in a stable posture while catching the ball. The cerebellum primarily smoothes and corrects the voluntary actions of the agonist and antagonist muscles involved in the movements of the right arm as it is directed to and acquires the target.

THE NEUROLOGICAL EXAM

The neurological examination is a structured approach to the patient; its goal is to collect sufficient information to localize the lesion. The examination is usually made up of observations of mental status, cranial nerves, motor function, sensory function, reflexes, gait and station, and coordination.

Mental Status

The mental status examination is usually the first neurological function tested, even if it is done informally. This is covered in greater detail in Chapter 12.

The Cranial Nerves

Olfactory Nerve (CN I): The first-order neurons involved in perception of odors are contained in the olfactory nerves. The patient is asked whether he or she is able to perceive odors through one nostril while the other is occluded. Generally small vials containing volatile agents (e.g., oil of wintergreen or camphor) are used. The absence of the ability to detect odors is termed anosmia.

Optic Nerve (CN II): While the rods and cones in the retina are the sense organs that convert light to electrical impulses, the fibers of the optic nerve are the first-order neurons of sight. The fibers of the optic nerve begin in the retina, exit the globe, and travel posteriorly to the optic chiasm where a partial decussation occurs. The fibers continue and end primarily in the lateral geniculate nucleus of the thalamus. A small percentage of optic nerve fibers end in the midbrain as afferents of the pupillary light reflex. CN II is tested by checking visual acuity with an eye chart as well as the visual fields. In the clinic, visual fields are usually tested by asking the patient to count or detect the movement of fingers or small objects in the visual fields. This is done with the contralateral eye covered and with the patient fixating on the examiner's eye. The examination of the optic nerve also includes a funduscopic examination with an ophthalmoscope.

Occulomotor, Trochlear, Abducens Nerves, (CNS III, IV, VI): Cranial nerves III, IV, and VI provide the lower motor neuron control of eye movements. In addition, the third nerve innervates the levator of the eyelid, the constrictor muscle of the pupil, and the ciliary muscle that controls accommodation. They are tested clinically by having the patient visually follow an object to the cardinal positions of gaze.

Trigeminal Nerve (CN V): The fifth cranial nerve has both motor and sensory components. The motor component of the trigeminal nerve provides for jaw movement. Unilateral lesions are usually well tolerated, but severe bilateral lesions leave the mouth open and unable to be closed.

The sensory portion of the trigeminal nerve supplies sensation to the face as well as the buccal and nasal mucosa. The cells arise largely in the gasserian ganglion and, like all sensory nerves, send processes distal to innervate the periphery and centrally to nuclei within the brainstem. The fibers that course peripherally do so within the three divisions of the trigeminal nerve—the ophthalmic, maxillary, and mandibular branches. The centrally destined processes of the trigeminal sensory neurons enter the lateral pons and course rostrally or caudally in the brainstem depending on the type of sensory information they carry. Those concerned with pain and temperature descend into the medulla and upper cervical spinal cord as the descending trigeminal tract. Those carrying tactile and proprioceptive information ascend to the main sensory nucleus. The motor fibers of CN V leave the pons and innervate the muscles of mastication (the temporalis, masseter, and pterygoids) via the mandibular branch.

Of particular interest to the SLP are the maxillary and mandibular branches. The maxillary branch carries sensation from the maxilla, maxillary teeth, the mucous membranes of the upper mouth, the anterior palate, nose and nasopharynx, the inferior portion of the internal auditory meatus, and the mid face. The mandibular branch conducts sensory information from the skin of the cheek, the lower teeth and jaw, and the mucosal linings of the uvula, posterior hard palate, and nasopharynx. The mandibular branch contains the proprioceptive and other sensory information from the skin on the mandible, ipsilateral side of the tongue, and the buccal surface of the cheek. The ophthalmic division can be tested with the corneal and nasal tickle reflexes. A wisp of cotton gently stroked across the junction of the sclera-cornea should elicit bilateral blinking. Similarly, a wisp of cotton introduced very gently into one of the patient's nostrils should result in the wrinkling of the nose. In both tests, the two sides are compared. The bulk of the masseter and temporalis muscles is tested by palpation of the muscles while the patient clenches his or her teeth. Once bulk has been ascertained, the strength of these muscles is tested by attempting to open the patient's jaw with downward pressure on the chin. The pterygoids provide for lateral movement of the jaw. The jaw will deviate to the side of the weak pterygoid and will be more easily pushed in that direction. Inside the mouth, weakness of the tensor veli palatini may manifest as tilting of the uvula to the weak side. The jaw jerk reflex tests afferent and efferent function of the mandibular division of CN V.

Facial Nerve (CN VII): As another nerve with both motor and sensory components, the facial nerve provides LMN innervation for the muscles of facial expression and the stapedius muscle. The sensory component allows for the innervation of some of the salivary glands and taste for the anterior two-thirds of the tongue.

The facial muscles are tested first by inspection of the face for symmetry and then by examining individual muscles for strength. Patients with weak facial muscles generally have fewer facial lines and wrinkles. The face looks inordinately placid. With unilateral weakness, the palpebral fissure will be wider on the weak side. When the orbicularis oculi are contracted maximally, the patient should be able to "bury" the origins of the eyelashes. Additionally, a good deal of resistance to forced eye opening should be apparent. The nasolabial folds should be roughly symmetrical; the weak side will appear flattened. With unilateral weakness the corner of the mouth will be seen to sag. When smiling, the corners of the mouth should elevate. With bifacial weakness, the smile looks more like a snarl and whistling or drinking through a straw become difficult or impossible. When facial muscle weakness is due to lower motor neuron loss as in amyotrophic lateral sclerosis (ALS), fasciculations may be seen.

A key clinical point with respect to facial weakness is the distribution of the deficit. Lower motor neuron weakness, as in Bell's palsy, generally involves all ipsilateral muscles. In a typical upper motor neuron lesion, such as a stroke, the muscles below the eyes are generally much weaker than those of the forehead and of eye closure.

Acoustic Nerve (CN VIII): Cranial nerve VIII provides innervation for the cochlea and the end organs of the vestibular apparatus. Thus, hearing and the ability to sense vertical, horizontal, and rotatory accelerations are provided by this nerve.

Hearing may be tested at the bedside by having a patient listen for the ticking of a watch or recognize whispered words. A tuning fork is used to test whether air conduction is greater than bone conduction, as is normal. Vestibular function may be glimpsed by observing the eyes for movements in primary gaze or during pursuit movements. Detailed vestibular function testing is beyond the scope of this chapter.

Glossopharyngeal Nerve (CN IX): This nerve supplies somatic sensation to the middle ear and the sense of taste to the posterior third of the tongue. The stylopharyngeus is the sole muscle innervated by this nerve. This muscle raises and dilates the pharynx.

Testing of the glossopharyngeal nerve is accomplished by testing the gag reflex. A cotton-tipped applicator or tongue blade that gently touches the posterior wall of the pharynx should elicit elevation and constriction of the pharyngeal musculature, as well as retraction of the tongue. While the afferent arc of this reflex is carried through the glossopharyngeal nerve, the efferent function is conducted through the vagus. Some people, however, do not gag, so this should be considered unequivocally abnormal only if the gag is lost unilaterally.

Vagus Nerve (CN X): The vagus nerve is a long and complex structure. It provides motor and sensory innervation to the palate, pharynx, and larynx. Additionally, it contains visceral sensory information from and parasympathetic innervation to thoracic and abdominal viscera. Some of the taste receptors on the posterior tongue and pharynx are vagally innervated as well. The thoracic and abdominal aspects of vagus function not relevant to speech will not be covered further in this chapter.

Functionally, the vagus nerve is extremely important for both swallowing and phonation, innervating most of the muscles involved with speech and swallowing except for the stylopharyngeus (IX) and tensor veli palatini (V). For the SLP, the three relevant branches of the vagus are the pharyngeal, the superior laryngeal, and the recurrent laryngeal. After these segments have branched, the vagus nerve is concerned primarily with the viscera of the thorax and the abdomen.

Shortly after exiting the skull, CN X breaks into branches. The pharyngeal branch descends to the inferior pharyngeal constrictor where it mingles with the glossopharyngeal and external branch of the superior laryngeal nerve as the pharyngeal plexus. From this plexus, efferent fibers innervate all of the muscles of the palate and the pharynx, except those noted above.

The superior laryngeal nerve, the second important branch of CN X, divides into internal and external branches. The external laryngeal nerve supplies the inferior pharyngeal constrictor and the cricothyroid muscle. The cricothyroid muscle controls pitch by lengthening the vocal cords. The internal laryngeal nerve is a pure sensory nerve that receives mucosal sensory information from the pharynx down to the level of the epiglottis, the aryepiglottic folds, and the arytenoid cartilages. It also contains proprioceptive information from the muscle spindles of the vocal apparatus.

The third relevant branch of the vagus is the recurrent laryngeal nerve. Both the left and right recurrent branches are so named because after descending to the level of the branching great vessels in the mediastinum, they double back on themselves and ascend to the larynx. The right recurrent laryngeal loops under the right subclavian artery and the left loops beneath the arch of the aorta. Both recurrent laryngeal nerves innervate all intrinsic muscles of the larynx except for the cricothyroid.

Several functions of the vagus nerve are easily tested during the neurological exam. Inspection of the palate will reveal it to look lower and less archiform on the unilaterally weak side. When saying /a/, there will be deviation to the normal side. The gag reflex will be reduced or abolished on the affected side. Unless palatal weakness is bilateral, hypernasality or nasal regurgitation of liquids during swallowing is not noticeable. In bilateral weakness of the palate, speech becomes hypernasal and there is nasal regurgitation of liquids during deglutition.

Normally the vocal folds are abducted during inspiration and adducted during phonation and coughing. With unilateral abductor weakness, the voice may be hoarse but there will not usually be dyspnea. With bilateral abductor weakness, there is often severe dyspnea and inspiratory stridor.

The voice may be hoarse but because both vocal folds can still be adducted, speech will not be severely affected. In a complete unilateral LMN lesion, the vocal fold will lie motionless in mid-abduction. The voice will be low pitched and hoarse, but phonation may not be much affected as the normal cord may be able to cross the midline. With bilateral LMN weakness, there is inspiratory stridor, dyspnea, and loss of phonation.

Accessory Nerve (CN XI): The eleventh nerve is derived from anterior horn cells from the upper four or five cervical segments. Its fibers enter the skull through the foramen magnum, travel briefly with the vagus nerve, and ultimately innervate the sternocleidomastoid (SCM) and the upper part of the trapezius (TPZ) muscles. (The lower part of the TPZ is innervated by the third and fourth cervical roots through the cervical plexus.) The SCM is tested by asking the patient to turn the head away from the muscle as it is being palpated.

If the TPZ is weak, the shoulder will appear depressed in repose, and will wing somewhat. This will be accentuated with the arm abducted. Also, because the supraspinatus and deltoid can only abduct the arm to approximately horizontal, to elevate the arm above this point, the TPZ is needed. The muscle strength of the upper part of the TPZ is tested by having the patient shrug the shoulders.

Hypoglossal Nerve (CN XII): The hypoglossal nerve is a mixed nerve that innervates the tongue. The nucleus lies in the medulla beneath the floor of the fourth ventricle. It innervates all muscles the tongue except the palatoglossus, which is innervated by the vagus. The sensory portion of the hypoglossal nerve is concerned chiefly with tactile information and is therefore important for chewing, swallowing, and articulation.

Tongue motor function is tested by having the patient protrude the tongue. Unilateral lesions of the twelfth nerve lead to unilateral wasting, deviation of the tongue toward the weak side, and fasciculation. Strength may be tested by asking the patient to push the tongue against the inside of the cheek, lateral to the mouth while the examiner resists the pressure. With practice, the examiner should develop an appreciation of what is within the normal range. With UMN lesions, tongue movements are slower and weaker, particularly with lateral extension. In severe bilateral UMN lesions, as in ALS, the tongue may have relatively good bulk but be essentially plegic with attempted voli-

tional movement. When the patient gags or yawns, however, greater degrees of tongue movement may become apparent. This disassociation between volitional movement and reflex movement indicates that although substantial loss of the corticobulbar tracts may have occurred, the intrinsic bulbar reflex pathways are still relatively intact.

Motor Examination

The goal of the motor examination is an assessment of the function of the motor unit and the various direct and indirect motor pathways. For the ambulatory patient this begins with an inspection of the posture of the limbs and a visual assessment of the bulk of the musculature. For example, fixed postures across joints (contractures) may be indicative of long-standing lesions of the upper motor neuron. The presence of hammer toes generally indicates long-standing LMN loss of the extensors of the toes leading to unopposed toe flexion. In essence, one's resting posture is a unfailing indicator of the combined descending forces acting through the motor unit.

After the inspection and palpation of the limbs and muscles at rest, the tone of muscles is tested by passively stretching them. Spasticity, the characteristic "clasp-knife" tone seen in corticospinal tract lesions or the "rigidity" seen in Parkinson's disease may be appreciated. Acute cerebellar lesions manifest as hypotonia. It is useful to observe the outstretched arms with the hands supinated while the patient closes the eyes. A "pronator drift" (the drift of the hand to pronation) indicates a subtle corticospinal tract lesion. An upward or outward drift of the arm may be an indication of a sensory system lesion, demonstrating that with the eyes closed, the brain no longer "knows" where the limb is in space.

After the bulk and tone are assessed, the strength and speed of individual muscles are tested. Numerous grading scales are used but one of the most common is the Medical Research Council system in which muscle strength is graded on a 0 to 5 scale, listed below.

Medical Research Council Muscle Strength Scale[1]

0	No contraction
1	Flicker or trace of contraction
2	Active movement, with gravity eliminated
3	Active movement against gravity
4	Active movement against gravity and resistance
5	Normal power

Sensory Examination

Sensory information ascends from the periphery through the spinal cord and brainstem to the thalamus in a number of tracts that differ in the type of information encoded. Thalamocortical fibers relay the information to relevant cortex. In a patient without sensory complaints, this part of the exam is often limited to the detection of light touch (with a wisp of cotton) and pinprick on the face and the distal aspects of the hands and feet. Additionally, vibration sense and position sense are tested in the fingers and toes. In a patient with sensory complaints, the examination would be more detailed with an attempt made to determine the distribution, nature, and degree of anesthesia.

If the lesion involves the sensory cortex or the thalamocortical radiations, a different type of sensory defect is produced. Although the ability to detect the "primary" sensations of light touch, pinprick, and vibration may not be impaired, the ability to perform certain other sensory tasks will be. "Two point touch" can be tested with the two points of a compass, for example. The patient is asked if the examiner has touched the skin with one or two points. Normally, one can detect two distinct points separated by several mm on the finger tips. Below this distance, the two points are experienced as one. On the back or trunk, several cm or more are needed to make this distinction. The ability to detect letters or numbers written on the palm or finger tips is referred to as "graphesthesia." Finally, the ability to recognize objects placed in the hands by virtue of their shape and texture is called "stereognosis." These abilities are also impaired in cortical (and some subcortical) sensory lesions.

Reflexes

The examination of reflexes provides important objective information about the integrity of the nervous system in two ways. First, most reflexes are mediated by mono- or oligosynaptic pathways that have afferent arcs outside the CNS, enter the CNS, and efferent arcs that mediate a motor function in the periphery. Thus, the integrity of the nervous system in a "horizontal" sense can be assessed with the tap of a tendon.

For example, tapping on the triceps tendon at the elbow produces an afferent volley in the radial nerve that ultimately enters the spinal cord through the C7 dorsal root. The large sensory nerve fibers mediating the reflex synapse directly on lower motor neurons also in the C7 spinal cord segment. These are induced to fire and an efferent volley goes down some of the LMN destined to innervate the triceps producing the triceps contraction. If the peripheral nerve, the dorsal or ventral root, or the spinal cord segment itself are damaged, the reflex may be abolished or reduced.

The second kind of information that reflexes provide is in a vertical sense. The briskness of a reflex is determined by the descending corticospinal tract tone. An UMN lesion will produce hyperreflexia below the level of the lesion. Therefore, a mid-thoracic spinal cord lesion would produce hyperreflexia in the legs but the reflexes in the arms and cranial innervated structures would remain normal. Similarly, a unilateral corticospinal tract lesion at the level of the frontal lobe would be expected to produce hyperreflexia in all contralateral muscles that receive its projections. This is the most common scenario following a cerebral infarct producing contralateral hemiparesis.

Gait and Station

The assessment of gait and station is an essential part of the neurological examination that may provide an enormous amount of information about many different areas of the nervous system. Standing upright is possible only with adequate proprioceptive information concerning the location of the body and limbs in space, muscular power to maintain the erect posture, and vestibular and visual input to centers involved in "righting reflexes." Locomotion involves voluntary sequential firing of flexors and extensors of the legs but also abundant "unconscious" input to the arms, legs, and trunk muscles. A detailed discussion of the physiology of gait is beyond the scope of this chapter, but some examples of the insight provided by an examination of the gait are useful.

Hemiparetic gait: The involved leg is slow and weaker, particularly in movements involving flexion of the hip and dorsiflexion of the foot. Because of this, the patient circumducts the leg in an attempt to avoid premature striking of the toe. There is decreased arm swing on the involved side, and the arm may be held flexed and abducted.

Sensory ataxic gait (an ataxic gait due to polyneuropathy or spinal cord disease): Without having a precise knowledge of the position of the feet and limbs, the patient needs a widened stance. The individual movements of the legs are exaggerated in force and degree. The visual system may provide a partial compensation for these deficits;

that is, watching the ground may help compensate for the loss of proprioceptive information. Consequently, under these circumstances, the gait will worsen in low light situations or when the eyes are closed. A similar gait is seen in disease affecting the portions of the cerebellum that normally coordinate the gait.

Parkinsonian gait: The gait in parkinsonism is fairly stereotypic. The patient stands somewhat stooped with the head forward and the arms slightly flexed. The steps are shortened and perhaps shuffling. There is decreased arm swing and the patient may "festinate," that is, involuntarily speed up and begin to shuffle forward (propulsion) or backward (retropulsion). In severe parkinsonism, these abnormalities, as well as the loss of "righting reflexes" may make independent ambulation impossible.

Myopathic gait: If there is sufficient weakness of the hip flexors and other muscles of the pelvic girdle, the patient will manifest a waddling gait. Normally, when one is walking, the gluteal muscles on the weight-bearing leg elevate the contralateral hemi-pelvis slightly to allow the free forward swing of the nonweight-bearing leg. If these muscles are weak, when the patient walks, the pelvis tilts downward on the side of the free swinging leg, producing a waddling from side to side. This same abnormality occurs in neurogenic weakness if it prominently affects the hip girdle muscles, particularly the gluteus medius.

Coordination

Tests of coordination primarily test the cerebellum. Acute cerebellar hemispheric lesions produce a constellation of signs ipsilateral to the lesion: hypotonia, ataxia, tremor, and a slight amount of weakness. These signs often improve over time. Two common tests of cerebellar function are the "finger–nose–finger" test (in which the patient alternately touches the examiner's finger, their own nose, the examiner's finger, etc.), and the "heel–shin" test (in which the patient carefully slides his or her heel along the contralateral tibia from knee to ankle). The cerebellum is vital for the motor control of coordinated movement. With cerebellar lesions, there is decomposition of the planned movement. In the "heel–shin" test, for example, one might see jerky movements that represent abnormalities in the degree, duration, and timing of the contraction of the quadriceps (as the

heel slides distally), and the relaxation of the hamstrings and ileopsoas muscles.

NEUROLOGICAL TESTS

Electrophysiological Tests

Electroencephalography (EEG) and electromyography (EMG) are both diagnostic testing modalities based on the fact that nerve cells and muscle are electrically active tissues. They maintain measurable voltages (potentials) across their membranes at rest and generate changes in these potentials as a means of integrating and communicating information to and from other cells. EEG and EMG exploit these properties for diagnostic purposes.

Electroencephalography

An electroencephalogram (EEG) is a record of the electrical activity of the brain as recorded by electrodes positioned on the scalp. The electrodes are placed in a standardized format that uses common anatomic landmarks as points of reference. The recorded activity directly reflects the activity of the cortex below, specifically the postsynaptic potentials of the large vertically oriented pyramidal cells (Figure 11–1). Indirectly though, structural or functional abnormalities of the underlying white matter or of the thalamo-cortical projections may produce characteristic changes as well.

The EEG is principally used to classify and prognosticate seizure disorders. For example, some EEG patterns are pathognemonic of a given epileptic syndrome and therefore predictive of effective treatment with one or another class of anticonvulsants. Certain EEG patterns are suggestive of heritable, though benign and self-limited seizure disorders. In others, the pattern suggests a severe disorder of brain function and portends a dismal future for the patient.

Generally, a localized "spike and wave," "spikes," or other paroxysmal activities can be suggestive of a seizure focus. The electroencephalographer looks for either the maximal amplitude of the spike discharge or phase reversal of the spike between adjacent electrodes to localize the focus on the underlying brain (Figure 11–2b).

Other major uses of the EEG are in the functional evaluation of normal and abnormal states of consciousness. Many patients experience "spells," whose nature may be unclear under the best of circumstances. An EEG may help confirm or exclude the possibility that the spell is epileptic in origin. Certain factors improve the diagnostic yield of

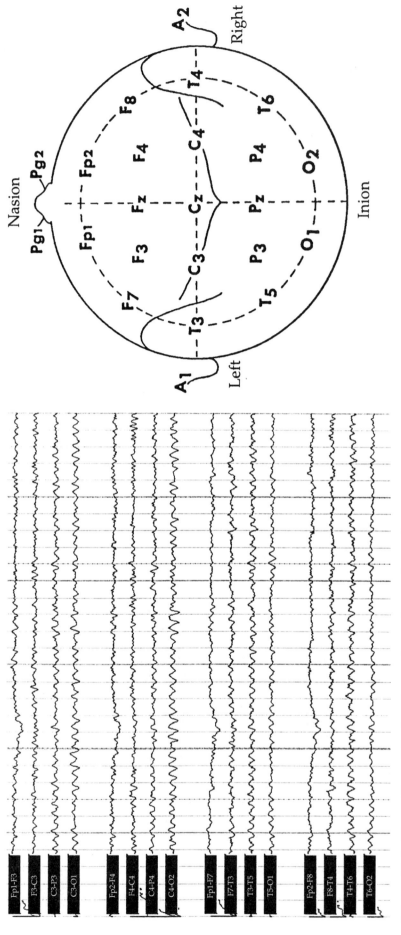

Figure 11–1. The outline of the head, seen from above, shows the standardized placement of electrodes according to the International 10-20 system. The EEG record indicates a normal 16-channel EEG recorded in an anterior to posterior bipolar montage.

EEG such as 24-hour sleep deprivation, sleep, hyperventilation, and photic stimulation. In epileptic patients studied repeatedly over time, at least 90% will ultimately demonstrate epileptiform EEG activity.[2]

The EEG is very sensitive but nonspecific in the evaluation of metabolic encephalopathy. Generally, as encephalopathy deepens, there is desynchronization and slowing of the alpha rhythm and the appearance of slower wave forms in the theta and delta ranges. With continued worsening these slower wave forms predominate (Figure 11–2a).

Other uses of EEG in the inpatient setting include its function as one of the criteria of brain death (i.e., the irreversible cessation of brain function). In this circumstance, a "flat" or isoelectric record is obtained.[3] EEG is also one of the modalities used in surgical monitoring of cerebral function—for example, during carotid endarterectomy.[4] Finally, the EEG is sometimes called on to help localize a functional problem in the brain when imaging studies are either not available or have been negative. In many areas of the United States, the MRI has largely supplanted this function.

Electromyography and Nerve Conduction Studies

Conventionally, an electromyogram (EMG) is a test constructed of two parts: the nerve conduction studies (NCS) and the needle exam (NE), which is, strictly speaking, the electromyogram. Nerve conduction studies are capable of assessing peripheral motor and sensory nerve function, as well as that of the neuromuscular junction.

While peripheral nerves are found in a wide variety of diameters, only the large myelinated (and hence rapidly conducting) fibers are measured using most conventional techniques. Essentially, the smaller fibers generate such small signals that without special techniques, they are lost in the "noise."

To understand the NCS changes seen in pathological conditions, it is useful to imagine a plastic-covered telephone wire as a model for a myelinated nerve fiber. The central copper wire is analogous to the axon. It carries the information encoded in the electrical current; if it is severed, the call is lost. The plastic coating, analogous to the myelin sheath synthesized by the Schwann cell, provides for isolation and insulation of the line. If the plastic sheath is damaged, there can be cross talk or "shorts" between wires. Additionally, in myelinated nerve fibers (but not phone lines), the relationship between the normal sheath and the axon it envelops is vital for normal conduction. If the myelin sheath is damaged, conduction in the axon may slow or cease altogether, something known as "conduction block."

NCS are generally performed by percutaneously stimulating an accessible portion of peripheral nerve and simultaneously recording from a proximal or distal portion of the nerve or a muscle innervated by the nerve. In the case of sensory nerves, the recording is made with applied disk or ring electrodes directly above the nerve. When recording from motor nerves, disk electrodes are placed directly over the muscle innervated by the nerve. The resulting evoked response is actually generated by the muscle itself. Because of these differences, while sensory nerve action potentials are in the microvolt range, motor-evoked responses, representing the depolarization of many grams of electrically excitable muscle tissue, are in millivolt range. The data obtained using these techniques include conduction velocity, terminal or distal latencies, and measurements of the sensory and motor-evoked response amplitudes.

Disorders of peripheral nerve generate a fairly limited number of abnormalities of these measures despite the limitless number of insults or diseases that can affect them. Figure 11–3 illustrates the characteristic abnormalities seen in common disease states.

Axonal Neuropathy

In an axonal neuropathy, as individual axons are lost, the number of individual elements participating in the conduction are decreased and the resulting amplitude is diminished. Although Figure 11–3b illustrates a motor fiber with its connection to the muscle, the situation is exactly analogous with a sensory conduction. Because axonal disease does not involve the Schwann cell (i.e., the myelin sheath), the distal latency and conduction velocity are relatively spared. The results are summarized in Table 11–1.

Demyelinating Neuropathy

As can be seen from Figure 11–3, in an acquired multifocal demyelinating neuropathy (e.g., Guillain-Barré syndrome), with proximal stimulation, individual motor unit action potentials (MUP) may be delayed. This has several consequences. First, the terminal latency can be delayed, and the resulting conduction velocity will be slowed. Second, as the individual motor unit action potentials are delayed, the resulting compound motor unit action

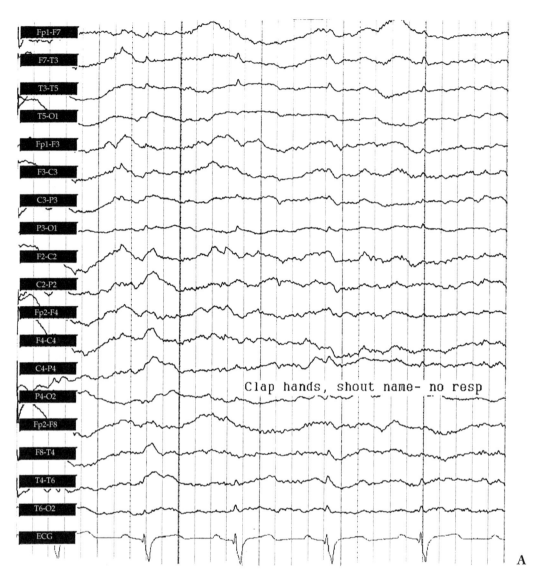

Figure 11–2. (A) EEG in severe diffuse encepalpathy. The bottom line is ECG. Note that the record is characterized by slow irregular activity that is unresponsive to loud clapping and calling the patient's voice. Note also that some of the sharper wave forms are actually ECG artifact.

potential (CMAP) is less synchronous with respect to time. As the individual motor unit action potentials are temporally dispersed, their positive and negative phases begin to cancel electrically. This results in a CMAP that is of lower amplitude and potentially spread out with respect to time or "temporally dispersed."

If a sufficient portion of the myelin sheath has been damaged by the process causing the demyelinating neuropathy, "conduction block" of that axon may take place. In essence, while still

alive and functioning in many ways, the individual motor fiber may cease to participate in voluntary contraction of the muscle. This manifests clinically as weakness.

Focal Neuropathy

The NCS are very useful for detecting focal neuropathies, and the carpal tunnel syndrome (CTS) is a common and prototypical example. Carpal tunnel syndrome represents the clinical manifesta-

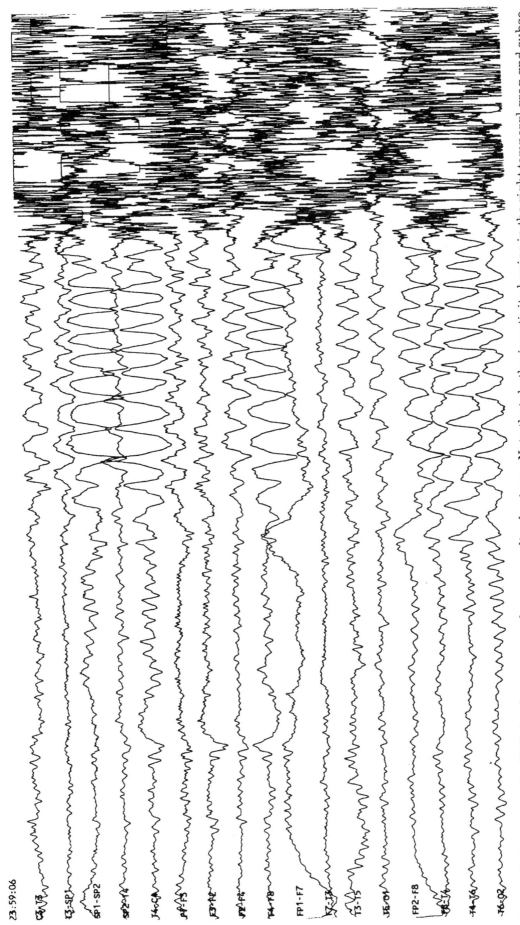

23:59:06

C3-V3
T3-SP1
SP1-SP2
SP2-T4
T4-C4
A1-F3
F3-F2
FZ-F4
T4-F8
FP1-F7
X-T3
T3-T5
T5-O1
FP2-F8
OE-T4
T4-T6
T6-O2

Figure 11-2 (*continued*). **(B)** A focal onset secondary generalized seizure. Note that rhythmic activity begins in the right temporal area and subsequently spreads to involve the whole brain. The dark sharp lines on the right side of the record are motor/muscle artifact caused by the onset of tonic-clonic activity in the muscles of the head and face.

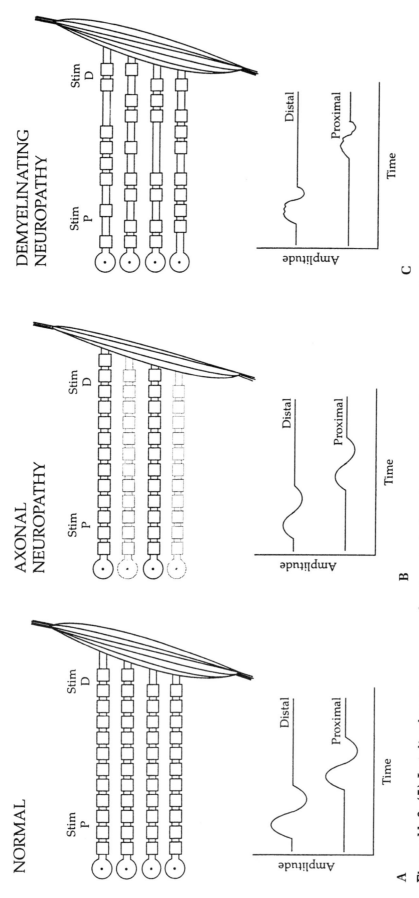

Figure 11–3. (A) A stylized motor nerve conduction study. The four myelinated nerves are stimulated distally and proximally to yield the two traces shown below. The "compound motor unit action potential" or CMAP is the summed electrical potential of the four individual motor unit action potentials. The amplitude and latencies of the responses are usually recorded. **(B)** In axonal neuropathies, or in any axon loss lesion, the loss of axons leads to a loss of muscle bulk and hence a loss of the summed individual action potentials. Note that the latencies and therefore the calculated conduction velocity are relatively spared. **(C)** In demyelinating neuropathies the random multifocal loss of internodes of myelin leads to the unpredictable slowing in individual nerve fibers. The third fiber from the top has lost too many internodes to conduct and fails to activate its muscle fibers. The resulting waveforms are therefore delayed, "dispersed," or notched because of the temporal dissynchronization of the individual motor unit action potentials, and of lower amplitude because of the complete loss of conduction of one of the nerve fibers.

Table 11–1. Nerve Conduction Findings in Peripheral Neuropathy

Type of Neuropathy	Terminal Latency	Conduction Velocity	Amplitude
Axonal	Nl or slightly dec.	Nl or slightly dec.	Reduced
Demyelinating	Increased	Decreased	Nl or slightly dec.

tions of median nerve compression as it passes through a bony tunnel of wrist bones with nine flexor tendons. The roof of this tunnel is an unyielding sheet of connective tissue. If for any reason the space needed by the nerve is compromised (e.g., by edematous swelling of the contents of the tunnel during pregnancy), the myelin sheaths of the median nerve axons may become sufficiently distorted to cause conduction slowing, conduction block, or, when extreme, axonal loss. These three features are seen in median neuropathies at the wrist (CTS) and essentially all other focal neuropathies as severity progresses.

Tests of Neuromuscular Transmission

In the previous figures illustrating the effects of demyelination and conduction block on the measured aspects of motor nerve conduction, the neuromuscular junction was omitted for simplicity. Several disorders of neuromuscular transmission are of great clinical relevance to the neurologist and SLP. The most common and prototypical disorder of neuromuscular transmission is myasthenia gravis (MG). MG is characterized by fatiguable weakness of striated muscle caused by dysfunction at the neuromuscular junction. It may present as and be confined to the extraocular muscles causing ptosis and diplopia. In more severe cases it involves all axial and appendicular muscles including those of swallowing, speaking, and breathing. Myasthenic involvement of swallowing and respiratory function is considered a life-threatening illness.

Several tests of neuromuscular transmission are used to diagnose MG or measure the effect of therapy. Repetitive nerve stimulation (RNS), known as the Jolly test, and single fiber EMG (SFEMG) are the most common. Before describing these tests, it will be worthwhile for us to have a brief overview of the physiology of neuromuscular transmission.

When a motor nerve is stimulated, a wave of depolarization proceeds toward the nerve terminal. Close to the terminal, the motor axon branches into many small nerve endings, each of which ends in close apposition to a single muscle fiber. When the wave of depolarization proceeds to the end of each nerve terminal, the resulting voltage change induces an influx of calcium from the extracellular space. The rise in calcium concentration at the nerve terminal causes the release of many membrane-bound packets of the neurotransmitter acetylcholine (ACh) into the synaptic cleft. The ACh quickly diffuses across the cleft and binds to postsynaptic ACh receptors (AChR) on the muscle fiber. When a molecule of ACh binds to the AChR, a conformational change occurs in the receptor that causes a small depolarization of the muscle membrane to take place. There are many AChR on the muscle membrane, and if enough are stimulated, the small depolarizations of the muscle membrane summate and cause the muscle fiber to reach "threshold." At threshold, a muscle fiber action potential takes place. As the muscle fiber depolarizes along its whole length, it begins to contract and generate force, a process known as "excitation-contraction coupling."

MG is an autoimmune disease characterized by the production of autoantibodies to the postsynaptic AChR. When the antibody binds to the receptor, it causes its premature destruction. Thus, in MG there is a paucity of functionally useful AChR.

One other fact must be appreciated to understand the physiology of fatiguable weakness in MG. When the nerve terminal depolarizes and the waiting packets of ACh are released into the synaptic cleft, there is a normal diminution of the number of packets released with each successive stimulation. If the first stimulation induced the release of, say, 100 packets, by the fourth stimulation perhaps 50 would be released. Under normal circumstances 50 would be more than enough to produce a muscle action potential, but in MG, if a large percentage of AChR have been destroyed or are nonfunctional because of antibody attack, the 50 packets of ACh may be inadequate to cause the depolarization of the muscle fiber. The failure to depolarize is manifested clinically as weakness.

In the technique of RNS, stimulating electrodes are placed on a motor nerve and recording electrodes on a muscle supplied by the motor nerve. Four to 10 shocks at 2 to 3 Hz (aptly named repetitive stimulation) are given and the amplitude of the evoked motor responses are measured at the first and fourth stimulation. Amplitude decrements of greater than 10% are considered pathological and suggestive of a defect in neuromuscular transmission (Figure 11–4).

SFEMG is a more sensitive and more complex test used to detect defects of neuromuscular transmission.[5] In SFEMG, a specialized needle electrode with an extremely small pickup area (25 uM[2]) is introduced into the muscle. The patient is asked to barely activate the muscle while the needle is maneuvered until two spike potentials firing "simultaneously" are identified. With normal neuromuscular transmission, the variation in time with consecutive discharges between the firing of the first potential and the second is extremely small, on the order of 20 to 45 microseconds (Figure 11–5). The measurement of this variability is called "jitter." In MG the reduced reliability of neuromuscular transmission leads to an increased variability or jitter in the firing of a given muscle fiber action potential with respect to a second fiber from the same motor unit. Sometimes, the firing of the second fiber fails altogether, an event termed "blocking." SFEMG is abnormal in greater than 95% of patients with generalized MG.[6]

The Role of the Needle Exam in EMG

The needle exam (NE) is an essential part of the EMG, providing vital information on the function of the motor unit. If there is weakness from a disorder of the motor unit, the needle exam should be able to detect it. Even in weakness due to disorders of the upper motor neuron, abnormalities of diagnostic significance are often apparent (e.g., changes in motor unit firing patterns or frequencies).

In the NE a small needle electrode is inserted into the muscle of interest. The tip of the needle acts as a recording electrode from within the muscle and the activity is displayed on a video monitor. EMG machines assign sounds to the wave forms based on their morphologies.

The question asked of the electromyographer determines which muscles will be sampled. Laryngeal EMG, both percutaneously and endoscopically performed, is becoming more common in the United States. Figure 11–6 illustrates characteristic findings during the needle exam.

Another method of directly obtaining information regarding the electrical activity of muscle during the EMG is by recording the surface activity of muscles (SEMG). In SEMG, the active recording electrode is placed over the belly of the muscle and the reference electrode is placed along a tendinous insertion. SEMG is insensitive to whether a muscle is denervated or whether the muscle has myopathic or neurogenic features, but it is able to provide other kinds of useful information.

SEMG is used in a number of clinical and research situations. It is particularly useful in "Central EMG"—studying the patterns and timing of muscle activation in movement disorders or other disorders of central motor control. SEMG can also be used to provide auditory or visual signals for biofeedback.

Transcranial Doppler Ultrasonography

Transcranial Doppler ultrasonography (TCD) was first introduced for use in clinical practice in 1982.[9] The technique is based on the Doppler principle—the sound frequency difference between an ultrasound signal transmitted onto a moving target and the reflected signal from that target is proportional to its speed. In clinical medicine, using some assumptions and approximations, the Doppler principle can be used to assess the velocity of blood flowing in the major arteries of the brain (Figure 11–7).

The measurement of blood flow velocity (BFV) allows us to determine whether the diameter of the artery is normal, increased (dilated), or reduced (constricted). This information is important in searching for stenosis (constriction) of the arteries that could lead to, or cause, strokes. Also, temporal changes in BFVs in patients with subarachnoid hemorrhage (SAH—blood in the subarachnoid space) and head trauma may warn us of impending and potentially lethal arterial vasospasm (severe constriction of the arteries as a response to the presence of blood around them). Early recognition of vasospasm could direct the treating physician to the appropriate intervention aimed at stopping serious sequelae such as ischemic stroke (neuronal injury from poor tissue oxygenation) or death. Furthermore, TCD is used to detect abnormalities in brain blood vessels (e.g., aneurysms or arteriovenous malformations [AVM]). Brain aneurysms or AVMs manifest as headache or seizures and tend to bleed, resulting in severe neurological deficits or death. Finally, TCD is a complementary test to the neurological examination in assessing brain death. Brain death is defined as the absence of brainstem functions. Patients who are brain dead are unable to sustain vital functions (e.g., breathing) independently. Early determination of brain death, by clinical examination and TCD, hastens the decision to withdraw life support measures; it is an important step in planning organ donation.

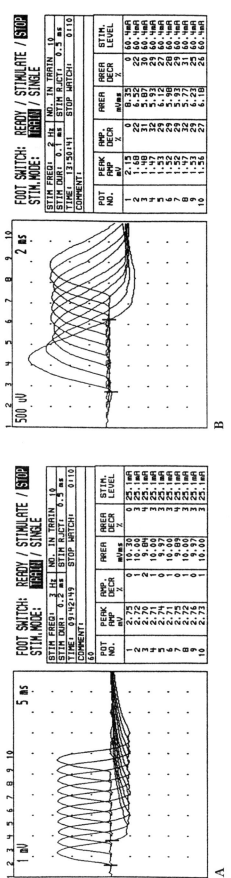

Figure 11–4. (A) A normal repetitive nerve conduction, or Jolly test. The CMAPs were recorded from the hypothenar muscle while the ulnar nerve was stimulated at 3 Hz. Note that each waveform differed in amplitude or area by less than 4%. **(B)** This Jolly test was performed on a patient with myasthenia gravis (at 2 Hz in this case). Note that with repetitive stimulation there is a marked reduction of amplitude, most prominent from the first to the second potential and reaching a nadir with the fourth stimulation. See the text for an explanation of this phenomenon.

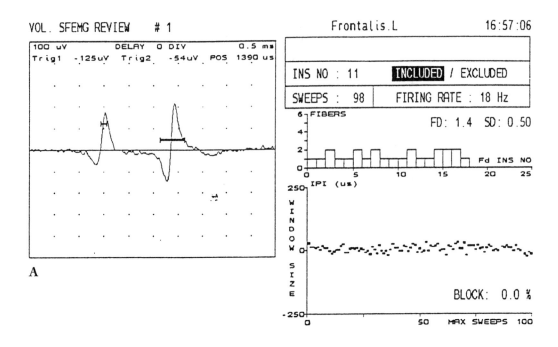

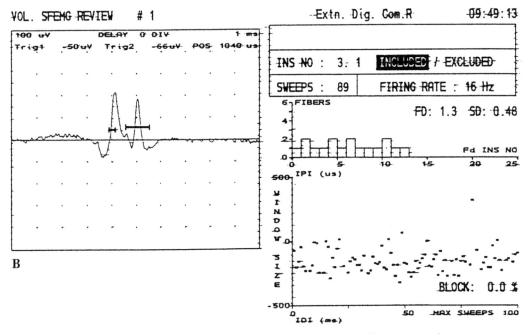

Figure 11–5. (A) Normal SFEMG from the frontalis muscle. The two spikes represent the potentials from two individual muscle fibers of the same motor unit. The bold horizontal lines crossing the potentials above the baseline represent "triggers" (voltage thresholds for the computer program to recognize) for the display of the potential and the calculation of when the second spike fires relative to the first. From the IPI (interpotential interval) seen in the graph in the lower right, a calculation is made of the "jitter," or variability between the firing of the first and second muscle fibers. Most of this variabililty results from neuromuscular transmission. In this case the jitter was 11 microseconds, (normal <45 μsec). **(B)** This abnormal SFEMG from a patient with MG demonstrated jitter of 99 μsec.

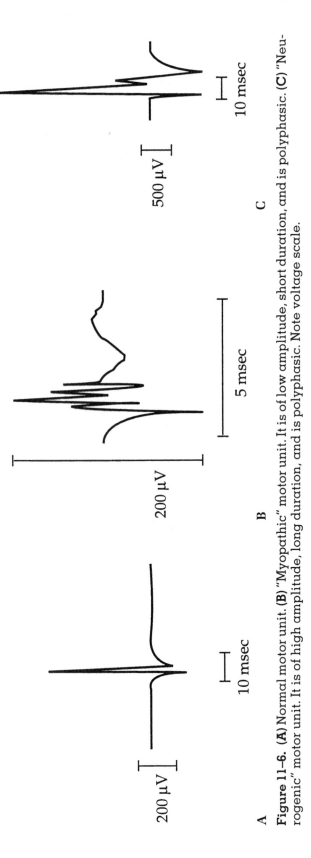

Figure 11-6. (A) Normal motor unit. **(B)** "Myopathic" motor unit. It is of low amplitude, short duration, and is polyphasic. **(C)** "Neurogenic" motor unit. It is of high amplitude, long duration, and is polyphasic. Note voltage scale.

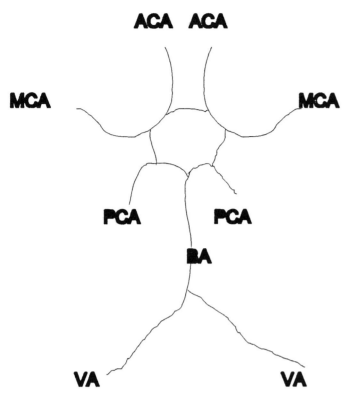

Figure 11–7. Diagrammatic representation of the circle of Willis showing the arteries that are studied by TCD. MCA = middle cerebral artery; ACA = anterior cerebral artery; PCA = posterior cerebral artery; BA = basilar artery; VA = vertebral artery.

Also, early recognition of brain death is aimed at reducing the emotional burden on the family and avoiding unnecessary hospital costs.

An expert panel of the American Academy of Neurology[10] determined that the above applications are definite indications for the use of TCD in clinical medicine. Other potential indications currently under research include:

1. *Detection of cerebral embolism:* Emboli are particles or debris that form in the bloodstream and travel in the blood vessels to points where they can't move any further. At these locations, they generally block blood flow and, hence, the delivery of important nutrients and oxygen to tissues (e.g., brain tissue). This results in ischemic strokes. Emboli produce a characteristic "chirping" sound of at least 15 dB as they travel past the recording TCD probe.
2. *Evaluation of the dizzy patient:* Dizziness may be due to many reasons including medications, fluid imbalance, narrowing of the VA or BA (Figure 11–7), and so on. TCD detects VA or BA stenosis and can therefore

guide us in the evaluation and treatment of patients with dizziness.

Imaging Studies

The field of neuro-imaging has substantially expanded in the last 25 years with the advent of computerized axial tomography (CT scan) in the early 1970s and magnetic resonance imaging (MRI) in the early 1980s. In addition, cerebral angiography remains a cornerstone in the evaluation of patients with cerebrovascular disease.

CT Scan

This technique is an X-ray computerized method used to identify abnormal structures based on (1) tissue electron density differences and contrasts; (2) displacement of normal structures; and (3) enhancement properties. Generally, structures that do not attenuate the X-ray signal are hypodense or black on CT. An example would be water or cerebrospinal fluid. On the other hand, tissues that maximally attenuate the X-ray beam are hyperdense or white on CT; a good example of a hyperdense tissue is bone. The density of brain tissue and spinal cord lies between these two extremes; they appear gray on CT images. Conditions that increase the water content of brain tissue (e.g., ischemic stroke or cerebral edema) render the CT image hypodense (dark). Alternatively, stagnant blood has a higher density than that of brain tissue or spinal cord; it appears white on CT. Table 11–2 lists the density characteristics of normal brain tissue and some commonly seen abnormalities. Occasionally, the contents of an abnormal brain or spinal cord lesion have the same density (isodense) as that of the surrounding tissue. Thus, the CT image is not able to give us the contrast needed

Table 11–2. Normal and Abnormal CT Scans

CT Image	Example
Normal	Minor head injury; pseudotumor
High density	Cerebral hemorrhage; calcium-containing lesions (e.g., tuberous sclerosis)
Mixed density	Malignant brain tumors
Isodensity	Isodense subdural hematoma; benign tumors; low grade glioma
Low density	Cerebral infarct; cysts; lipid-containing lesions; MS plaque

to identify that lesion, unless additional information is obtained. In such instances, a close attention to disruption of the normal nervous system anatomy and the topographical relationship of different brain or spinal cord structures, and/or unusual enhancement following the administration of a contrast agent (usually an iodine-based compound that appears white on CT) may delineate the sought-for abnormality.

CT scanning is an important tool in the diagnostic evaluation of many neurological conditions (Table 11–3). Most patients with one of these conditions/diseases are better evaluated with MRI than with CT for reasons described below; demonstration of fresh blood (<24 hours) and fractures may be the exceptions. CT scanning is more commonly used and more readily available than MRI because it is cheaper and quicker to perform.

Magnetic Resonance

The technique of MRI depends on the mobile hydrogen concentration in tissues. Also, magnetic resonance can visualize blood vessels and fluid flow (spinal fluid or blood), and analyze tissue chemistry (magnetic resonance spectroscopy). The MR signal is a function of deflected mobile hydrogen atoms, relaxation times referred to as T_1 and T_2 (tissue magnetization times), MR pulse sequences (e.g., T_1-weighted and T_2-weighted images), imaging protocol, and the MRI system used. On T_1-weighted images, cerebrospinal fluid is hypo-intense and white matter is hyper-intense relative to gray matter. This translates into an image where CSF is black, gray matter is dark gray, and white matter is light gray. In contrast, T_2-weighted images show a white CSF signal and a gray matter signal that is lighter (more hyper-intense) than that of white matter. Generally, abnormalities that increase mobile tissue water darken the T_1- and lighten the T_2-weighted image (e.g., ischemic stroke). On the other hand, subacute and chronic hemorrhage appears white (hyper-intense) on both pulse sequences.

Contrast material is used with MRI to provide tissue contrast enhancement. The most commonly used MRI contrast agent is gadopentetate dimeglumine (gadolinium or Gd-DTPA); it shortens T_1 and T_2.

MRI is more sensitive than CT in detecting most brain and spinal cord abnormalities. It provides a better delineation of normal and abnormal tissues and is particularly suitable in evaluating the brain stem where CT scanning has a relatively limited value.

The indications for MRI are listed in Table 11–3. MRI is certainly more advantageous than CT in identifying MS plaques, lesions in the brain stem, early ischemic strokes (infarcts), acoustic neuromas (tumors of the eighth cranial nerve), pituitary tumors, and spinal cord cavities. MRI is very helpful in determining the age of a cerebral hemorrhage. Vascular malformations, aneurysms, and arterial occlusion are well delineated on MRI. Also, MR angiography (MRA) is a noninvasive technique that allows the visualization of arteries and veins without injecting a dye in the vessels. On MRA, arterial stenosis or occlusion, AVMs, aneurysms, and venous thrombosis are very well seen. Finally, intravenous Gd-DTPA is more sensitive than CT contrast in identifying small metastatic tumors.

Table 11–3. Indications for CT or MRI Scan in the Neurological Work-Up

Condition/Disease	Examples
Cerebrovascular disease	Ischemic stroke; cerebral hemorrhage
Infections	Toxoplasmosis; brain abscess
Neoplastic disease (tumors)	
Primary benign brain tumors	Meningioma
Primary malignant brain tumors	Glioblastoma multiforme
Metastatic brain tumors	Melanoma
Spinal cord tumors	Schwannoma; metastatic breast cancer
Demyelinating disease	Multiple sclerosis
Head trauma	Contusion; fractures
Congenital malformations	Chiari; cerebral cysts

Angiography

This technique was introduced in clinical medicine over 50 years ago and remains very valuable in the evaluation of patients with neurological complaints. Cerebral and spinal angiography are performed under local anesthesia; spinal angiography is rarely performed. The procedure involves the percutaneous (across the skin) introduction of a catheter in the arterial tree (most commonly the femoral artery) and, guided by X-ray images, the injection of a dye at the desired site. The radio-opaque dye highlights the injected vessel and hence permits the detection of abnormalities in the cerebral arterial or venous system. This invasive radiological procedure carries a small risk of complications that include stroke, infection or blood clot formation at the site of the cannulation (introduction of the catheter), or even death from a severe allergic reaction (anaphylaxis) to the dye.

Cerebral angiography is the mainstay of diagnosis of stenotic disease of the major cerebral arteries. It is also indicated in the evaluation of patients with suspected venous sinus thrombosis, although MR venography is gaining ground over conventional angiography in the diagnosis of this condition. Angiography is also used in the diagnosis of AVMs, aneurysms, and inflammation of the blood vessels (vasculitis). Cerebral arteriography is superior to MRA in detecting intracranial arterial stenosis and small cerebral aneurysms. Arterial vasospasm can be appreciated on TCD (see above) but is best delineated on angiography.

NEUROLOGICAL DISEASES AND THEIR MANAGEMENT

A thorough review of neurological disease and its management is beyond the scope of this chapter. The following topics are meant to introduce the non-neurologist to the common and major categories of neurological disease. For more specific information, the reader is referred to comprehensive texts in the area.[7,8]

Cerebrovascular Diseases

Stroke is the third most common cause of death and the leading cause of disability in the United States.[11,12] The annual incidence of stroke in the United States is 500,000, and one-third of these patients die. Stroke is subdivided into ischemic and hemorrhagic (SAH, ICH—intracerebral hemorrhage). Patients with SAH or ICH are more likely to be severely disabled or die from stroke than those afflicted by cerebral infarction. There is some evidence that the incidence of cerebral infarction is declining partly because of better control of hypertension, but the incidences of ICH and SAH are unchanged.

Cerebral Ischemia

Cerebral ischemia is the most common cause of stroke; 75 to 85% of all strokes are ischemic. Cerebral ischemia could be permanent (i.e., cerebral infarction), or transient (i.e., transient ischemic attack [TIA]). The case fatality of cerebral infarction is less than 10% in subjects under 65 years old and approximately 20% in older individuals.

Risk factors for cerebral infarction are divided into nonmodifiable (age, male gender, black race, family history of cerebral infarction, previous stroke, high blood fibrinogen levels) and modifiable ones (atrial fibrillation, hypertension, myocardial infarction, diabetes mellitus, prior TIA, cigarette smoking, *excessive* alcohol consumption). Oral contraceptive pills, high blood lipids, obesity, and a sedentary life style were risk factors for cerebral infarction in some studies but not in others.[11]

Despite major advances in the investigative studies for cerebral infarction, over 40% of ischemic strokes are of unknown etiology (cause). The most commonly identifiable causes of cerebral infarction are (1) atherosclerosis (hardening) of the large arteries supplying the brain; (2) embolism from the heart; and (3) disease of the small cerebral arteries (lacunar disease). *Atherosclerosis* results in cerebral infarction when a thrombus (a complex lesion that forms on the vessel wall, consisting that consists of fatty debris and blood products such as platelets and red blood cells) dislodges from one site of the diseased artery (usually at sites where shear force is maximal such as the bifurcation of the common carotid artery into the internal and external carotid arteries) and blocks the distal portion of that vessel, preventing nutrients and oxygen from being delivered to the brain tissue. Less commonly, a clot does not dislodge, but the reduction in the large artery diameter at the site of the thrombus is severe enough to hamper flow beyond the point of constriction; this mechanism is known as hemodynamic stroke. *Cerebral cardioembolism* refers to ischemic strokes caused by emboli that break off from a heart chamber (e.g., left atrium) or valve. These emboli travel in the cerebral blood vessel to a point where they can't move any further and block the delivery of blood flow at that site. *Lacunar disease* is a condition where the small vessels that penetrate into the brain substance are constricted and/or occluded; lacunar disease is caused mostly by hypertension.

Uncommon causes of cerebral infarction include blood clotting abnormalities (e.g., coagulation or platelet disorders), increased blood viscosity, sickle cell disease, migraine, dissection (tear) of the cerebral arteries, use of illicit (cocaine) or licit (oral contraceptives, phenylpropanolamine [found in cough medicines]) substances, and so on. (See Tables 1, 4, 7, 8, and 9 in Reference 13).

Cerebral infarcts and TIAs manifest similarly with one exception; by conventional definition,[14] TIAs last less than 24 hours. It is important to note, however, that true TIAs (transient symptoms and signs without any evidence of brain damage) are 2 to 15 minutes in duration; symptoms that last more than 60 minutes are unlikely to reverse.[15] The onset of symptoms with cerebral ischemia is usually abrupt. The neurological deficits are reflections of dysfunctional or nonfunctional brain tissue supplied by the occluded artery (Table 11–4). The MCA territory is the most common site for cerebral infarcts. Cerebral ischemia is more likely to occur in the anterior (MCA, ACA) than the posterior (PCA, VA, BA) cerebral territories.

Acute Management

Optimal blood pressure control (not high but also, and equally important, not too low), control of fluid and/or electrolyte imbalance, adequate oxygenation, and maintenance of euglycemia (normal blood sugar) are some general measures used in caring for the patient with acute ischemic stroke. Patients with significant aphasia, drowsiness, obtundation, and/or brainstem stroke are best kept NPO until it is determined that they are safely able to eat. This precautionary measure is intended to avoid aspiration pneumonia, a common morbidity in patients with acute stroke. Urinary tract infections are best avoided by using condom catheters in men and intermittent catheterization in women, instead of indwelling catheters. Frequent turning in bed helps prevent pressure ulcers. Venodyne boots should be worn and subcutaneous heparin should be administered (unless intravenous heparin is used) to avoid deep venous thrombosis and pulmonary embolism. Stool softeners are also recommended.

Ischemic stroke is a neurological emergency. Every effort is exerted to evaluate and treat the patient early to avoid irreversible brain damage. Over the last eight years, a major public aware-

Table 11–4. Clinical Manifestations of Cerebral Infarction

Arterial Territory	Common Symptoms and Signs
MCA	Contralateral weakness and/or sensory loss (face and arm more than leg); aphasia (dominant MCA); neglect; apraxia (nondominant MCA)
ACA	Abulia; contralateral leg weakness and/or sensory loss; urinary incontinence; transcortical motor aphasia (dominant ACA); initial mutism
PCA	Contralateral hemifield loss; visual perceptual problems
VA	Lower cranial nerve dysfunction (hoarseness, double vision, facial paralysis, swallowing difficulty, etc.); dizziness; vertigo; unsteadiness; hiccups; nausea; vomiting
BA	Locked-in-syndrome (paralysis form neck down); stupor; coma; oculomotor abnormalities (diplopia, ptosis); abnormal motor movements (chorea, hemiballismus)

ness campaign was launched to emphasize the seriousness of cerebral ischemia and stress the need for stroke victims to seek medical attention very early. These measures allowed the evaluation of the role of thrombolytics (agents that lyse or dissolve blood clots) in the acute treatment of cerebral infarction. The efforts were fruitful as rt-PA (recombinant tissue plasminogen activator) was demonstrated to be an effective treatment in cerebral ischemia.[16] rt-PA was recently approved by the U.S. Food and Drug Administration as the first proven treatment for ischemic stroke. The role of many other drugs in stroke therapy is currently under investigation.

The patient with acute ischemic stroke is best managed in a special care unit (e.g., stroke unit) where continuous neurological and cardiovascular monitoring is performed by skilled medical personnel. The value of close monitoring is in the early recognition and aggressive management of some of the potentially devastating sequelae of stroke such as cerebral edema or significant hemorrhagic conversion (development of blood in the area of cerebral ischemia).

Medical Prevention

Patients with acute cerebral infarction are prone to ischemic stroke recurrence, particularly in the first month after the initial event and especially in patients with cerebral cardioembolism. In this high-risk group, anticoagulant therapy (heparin) is sometimes indicated. Other preventive medical measures include long-term use of oral anticoagulant (e.g., warfarin) or antiplatelets agents such as aspirin, ticlopidine, clopidogrel (not yet available for use), and dipyridamole.

In addition to the above medical therapies, patients with ischemic stroke are educated to minimize stroke risk factors (i.e., stop smoking, comply with anti-hypertensive and/or blood sugar medications, exercise, avoid excess alcohol use, etc.) (Table 11–5).

Surgical Management

Patients with ischemic stroke or TIA in the territory of a severely narrowed (70 to 99%) internal carotid artery are best managed by carotid endarterectomy (CEA) in addition to the medical therapy described above, provided the surgical risk is low.[17] Also, it is suggested that men with asymptomatic stenosis of the internal carotid artery should undergo CEA.[18] Carotid endarterectomy is a vascular surgery aimed at dissecting out the plaque (lesion composed of fat and blood products) from the diseased carotid artery. Surgical therapy in the posterior circulation is not standard care. Transluminal angioplasty (introduction of a balloon catheter in the artery and expanding the stenosis) is a promising experimental intervention.

Massive cerebral infarction and edema can result in hydrocephalus (increased size of the cerebral ventricles from blockage of CSF flow). Patients with hydrocephalus sometimes require the insertion of shunts into the ventricles to drain CSF. Also, a large infarct can cause brain herniation (displacement of the brain through rigid structures) requiring lobectomy (removal of the cerebral lobe where the infarct occurs) or hemispherectomy (removal of the diseased hemisphere) in rare instances. Finally, cerebellar ischemic strokes may be devastating unless a cerebellectomy is performed and the infarcted cerebellar hemisphere surgically removed.

Intracerebral Hemorrhage

Intracerebral hemorrhage accounts for 5 to 10% of all strokes in the United States and 20 to 30% in Japan.[12] The mortality rate of ICH declined dramatically from 90% in 1945–1974 to less than 50% in the 1980s.[19] Most ICH-related deaths occur in the first week of the event, a reflection of devastating complications such as brain herniation or massive edema. The major predictors of mortality after ICH are (1) hemorrhage size, (2) low Glasgow Coma Scale (a scale that assesses the patient's neurological status), and (3) presence of intraventricular hemorrhage.[12] Less than 50% of patients with ICH are functionally independent at one year following the hemorrhage. Similar to ischemic strokes, long-term complications following ICH include pneumonia, urinary tract infections, seizures, and deep vein thrombosis with potential pulmonary embolism.

Intracerebral hemorrhage is classified as traumatic or nontraumatic. Over 50% of nontraumatic ICH is related to hypertension. Less common causes are listed in Table 11–6. Cerebral amyloid angiopathy is an age-related abnormality in the cerebral blood vessels pathologically characterized by the deposition of amyloid material (an abnormal protein) in the walls of the arteries. The use of illicit drugs, particularly cocaine, led to a sharp rise in the incidence of ICH in the young. Sympa-

Table 11–5. Medical Management of Ischemic Stroke

General Measures	Acute Treatment	Medical Prevention	Risk Factor Control
Adequate oxygenation	rt-PA	Antiplatelet agents	Blood pressure
Blood pressure control	Aggressive treatment of cerebral edema (e.g., mannitol)	Anticoagulants	Diabetes
Control of blood sugar			Exercise
NPO until judged safe			Weight loss
Frequent turning in bed			Lipids
Optimize hemodynamics			Cigarette smoking
Continual monitoring			Excess alcohol

Table 11–6. Non-hypertensive Causes of Nontraumatic ICH

Cause	Example
Blood vessels abnormality	Amyloid angiopathy; AVM; aneurysms; moyamoya disease
Blood abnormality	Leukemia; clotting factor deficiency; platelet dysfunction
Medications	Anticoagulants; thrombolytics; sympathomimetics (e.g., diet pills)
Illicit drugs	Cocaine; amphetamines (speed); heroin and opiates
Brain tumors	Melanoma; choriocarcinoma; lung and renal cancer; glioblastoma

Table 11–7. Clinical Manifestations of ICH by Location

Location	Symptoms and Signs
Putamen	Abrupt hemiplegia and hemisensory loss; homonymous hemianopsia; impaired consciousness; paralysis of conjugate gaze
Thalamus	Hemisensory loss; forced downward gaze; unreactive small pupils; short-term memory loss; convergence paralysis
Hemisphere	Variable depending on the lobe involved and the side
Cerebellum	Unsteadiness; dysequilibrium; vertigo; nausea and vomiting; limb incoordination
Pons	Rapid development of coma; quadriplegia; abnormal breathing; horizontal gaze paralysis; ocular bobbing

thomimetics include over-the-counter drugs used for cough and weight loss; they are rarely implicated in ICH. Finally, any brain tumor can result in ICH, although metastatic lesions more commonly bleed than primary neoplasm (e.g., glioblastoma).

The neurological symptoms and signs of ICH depend on its location (Table 11–7). The majority of hypertension-related ICHs occur in the deep brain structures. In decreasing frequency, the putamen, thalamus, cerebral hemispheres, and cerebellum are the most common locations of ICH. Nonhypertensive ICH is seen in the hemisphere.

General measures of acute ICH management are similar to those used in patients with ischemic stroke (Table 11–4). Particular attention is paid to lower blood pressure since many patients are hypertensive and the pressure is often extremely elevated. Additional treatment strategies include (1) early endotracheal intubation of patients with depressed level of consciousness and those with large brain stem ICH; (2) aggressive treatment of cerebral edema (e.g., mannitol); and (3) early recognition and treatment of the syndrome of inappropriate anti-diuretic hormone (SIADH) secretion. Correction of coagulation abnormalities, when appropriate, prevents further bleeding.

The role of surgical therapy in patients with ICH is controversial.[20] Cerebellar hemorrhages larger than 3 cm in maximal diameter are the exception; patients with this type of ICH are best managed by surgical evacuation of the hematoma (blood clot). Other potential candidates for surgi-

cal intervention are (1) younger patients, noncomatose, generally healthy prior the ICH, whose hemorrhage volume is less than 50 ml; (2) patients with lobar hemorrhage, particularly in the nondominant hemisphere, whose symptoms and signs are progressing; and (3) patients who require the surgery for diagnosis (e.g., suspected tumor with unknown primary).[21]

Subarachnoid Hemorrhage

Ruptured saccular aneurysms and SAH account for 6 to 10% of all strokes and up to 25% of stroke mortality.[22] Aneurysmal SAH occurs mostly in the fifth or sixth decade; it is more common in women than men, blacks more than whites. Over 40% of patients with SAH either die or are severely disabled one year following the hemorrhage. Determinants of morbidity and mortality include age, neurological status at presentation, presence of hydrocephalus and/or intraventricular hemorrhage, thickness of the SAH layer on initial CT scan, aneurysmal location, and medical and surgical complications.[12,22]

The majority of nontraumatic cases of SAH are related to the rupture of berry aneurysms (saccular). Berry aneurysms typically form near the circle of Willis (Figure 11–7); most form in the anterior circulation (anterior communicating, anterior cerebral, middle cerebral, internal carotid arteries). They are believed to develop from degenerative changes in the wall of the blood vessel secondary to hemodynamic stress.[22,24] Risk factors for the development of berry aneurysms include hypertension, smoking, alcohol use, and systemic diseases affecting connective tissues such as polycystic kidney disease, Marfan's syndrome, sickle-cell disease, fibromuscular dysplasia, pseudoxanthoma elasticum, and coarctation of the aorta. Other types of aneurysms (mycotic or infectious; atherosclerotic), vasculitis, coagulation disorders, and licit or illicit drugs are other rare causes of SAH.

Aneurysms can expand and cause signs and symptoms related to local compression of neighboring structures. These manifestations include headache, facial pain, double vision, oculomotor nerve paralysis, weakness, and visual field defects.

Approximately 20% of aneurysmal SAHs are preceded by warning signs such as headache, dizziness, visual or ocular symptoms, nausea, or transient sensorimotor deficits.[22] These are believed to be the result of minor hemorrhage. When they occur, warning signs precede SAH by up to three months in 92% of the cases.

The characteristic presentation of aneurysmal rupture is explosive headache, altered consciousness, neck stiffness, and photophobia (light sensitivity). Other symptoms that may develop include diplopia, sensorimotor deficits, aphasia, vertigo, and unsteadiness of gait. Approximately 25% of patients develop seizures shortly after the aneurysmal rupture. Hunt and Hess developed a grading scale that proved important in determining the surgical risk and prognosis of patients with SAH[25] (Table 11–8); patients with grade I or II have a good prognosis whereas those with grade IV or V do not fare well.

All patients with suspected SAH should undergo an emergency head CT. If the CT is negative and the suspicion of SAH is still high, a lumbar puncture (LP) is indicated. The yield of CT in the diagnosis of SAH is 95% in the first day, 90% in the second day, and 50% a week after the aneurysmal rupture.[12,24] A spinal tap may not demonstrate hemorrhage in the first 6 to 12 hours after SAH; it is 100% accurate between 12 hours and two weeks.

Once the clinical diagnosis of SAH is confirmed radiologically or by LP, cerebral angiography should be performed to look for one or several aneurysms. An initially negative angiogram should be repeated in 2 to 3 weeks to safely determine that an aneurysm is not present.

The general medical management of SAH is similar to ICH and ischemic stroke.[22,24] Particular attention should be paid to keeping the room quiet

Table 11–8. Hunt and Hess Classification

Category	Criteria
Grade I	Asymptomatic or minimal headache and slight neck rigidity
Grade II	Moderate to severe headache, neck rigidity, neurological deficit limited to cranial nerve paralysis
Grade III	Drowsiness, confusion, mild neurological deficits
Grade IV	Stupor, moderate to severe hemiparesis, early decerebrate rigidity, vegetative disturbances
Grade V	Deep coma, decerebrate rigidity, moribund appearance

Source: From North American Symptomatic Carotid Endarterectomy Trial Collaborators: Beneficial effect of carotid endarterectomy in symptomatic patients with high grade carotid stenosis. *N Engl J Med* 1991; 325:445–453.

to avoid agitation and having the head elevated so that venous drainage is optimally maintained. Corticosteroids and anti-epileptic drugs are used to prevent cerebral edema and seizures, respectively. Nimodipine is a standard medical therapy used to avoid the complications of vasospasm; "triple-H" therapy (hypervolemia, hypertension, hemodilution) is also employed routinely.

Surgical therapy of aneurysmal SAH consists of ligation of the aneurysm, within 48 hours of the onset of hemorrhage in patients with grades I-III and 10 to 14 days later in those with grades IV and V.[22,24] Balloon occlusion or placement of detachable coils are recent promising therapies of inoperable or partially obliterated aneurysms. Transluminal angioplasty is occasionally used to treat vasospasm.

Neuromuscular Diseases

Diseases of muscle can be roughly divided into those due to inherited defects (the muscular dystrophies) and those that are acquired. This distinction is admittedly arbitrary as some myopathies may occur as hereditary disorders in some families and sporadically in others (e.g., inclusion body myositis).

The Muscular Dystrophies (MD)

Duchenne's, muscular dystrophy (DMD) is the most common muscular dystrophy in this country. As an X-linked recessive disorder, it occurs essentially only in boys. Mutations in the gene for dystrophin are associated with an absence or near absence of this protein in the muscle. Dystrophin is a membrane-associated structural protein; in its absence muscle fibers are rendered too physically frail to withstand the normal wear and tear of contraction. The incidence is approximately 1 per 3500 male births.[26] In a minority of cases, the disease appears to represent a new mutation. Affected boys are normal at birth but begin to manifest subtle signs of weakness when they begin to stand and walk. Although patients do acquire walking, most are wheelchair bound by 12 years. The disease is inexorably progressive and death usually occurs from respiratory failure or pneumonia. The facial and bulbar muscles are usually spared until very late.

Treatment consists of corticosteroids, which reduce the rate at which muscle function is lost,[27] and the physical bracing of weakened limbs to allow the patient to remain mobile as long as possible.

Oculopharyngeal MD is a late onset autosomal dominant disorder that is extremely rare below the age of 45. In the United States it is primarily seen in families of French Canadian descent.[28] The muscle biopsy is often characteristic. The disease usually manifests with ptosis and later, dysphagia. Oculopharyngeal MD is progressive and currently without definitive treatment. The dysphagia may be treated with cricopharyngeal myotomy. If this does not provide sufficient relief, gastrostomy should be performed.

Myotonic dystrophy (MyoD) is the most common form of MD in the adult and is the form most likely to involve the muscles of swallowing and speaking. It is a multisystem disease that involves other tissues such as the lens of the eye, endocrine tissues, as well as smooth and cardiac muscle. The disease is caused by an expansion of an unstable region of the gene for myotonin protein kinase.[29] Clinically, the small muscles of the hands and forearm are often the first to become weak and wasted. Facial and pharyngeal muscles are invariably involved with ptosis, facial, masseter, and sternocleidomastoid wasting and weakness giving the face a characteristic look. Pharyngeal and laryngeal weakness produce a weak hypernasal voice. There is currently no treatment for MyoD other than supportive care. Because many patients develop cardiac arrhythmia or heart failure, routine cardiac follow-up is very important.

Inflammatory Myopathies

Polymyositis (PM), dermatomyositis (DM), and inclusion body myositis (IBM) are inflammatory myopathies. They are a group of disorders characterized histologically by the presence of inflammation within muscle.[30] PM is an autoimmune disorder caused by the invasion and destruction of muscle cells by mononuclear cells. DM is an immune-mediated vasculitis affecting the small blood vessels of muscle and skin. The pathophysiology of IBM is less certain. Clinically these disorders are most commonly characterized by the subacute onset of weakness of skeletal muscle. While most have a predilection for proximal muscles, IBM commonly causes distal weakness as well. Characteristic skin and nail changes are seen in DM. Dysphagia occurs in all inflammatory myopathies but is more common in DM and IBM. DM is the only inflammatory myopathy that occurs to any extent in children. Treatment of PM and DM consists of immunosuppression with steroids and other agents. Most patients can be controlled with these measures. IBM is notoriously difficult to treat, though some improvement may be seen with corticosteroids and IVIG for a time. The disease is essentially progressive and ultimately quite disabling.

Disorders of Neuromuscular Transmission

Myasthenia Gravis

Myasthenia gravis (MG) is an autoimmune disorder that produces fatiguable weakness of skeletal muscle. It is caused by the production of autoantibodies to the postsynaptic acetylcholine receptor (AChR) on the muscle membrane.[31] These antibodies cause premature destruction of the AChR and lead to failure of neuromuscular transmission. This is manifest by decrement of the compound muscle action potential (CMAP) during repetitive stimulation at low rates (see above).

MG is relatively rare with a prevalence of perhaps 5 per 100,000. It has a peak incidence in woman in their twenties and thirties and in men in their sixties and seventies. There is an increased incidence of thymoma in patients with MG. In some patients the disease remains confined to the extraocular muscles. In others it is generalized, involving all skeletal muscle including bulbar and respiratory muscles. Myasthenic crisis is a sudden severe decline in strength usually accompanied by respiratory failure and severe bulbar weakness. It is a life-threatening emergency requiring intubation and mechanical ventilation.

The mainstay of treatment for mild MG is anticholinesterase inhibitors such as pyridostigmine. By delaying the destruction of ACh at the NMJ, an improvement of neuromuscular transmission is achieved. More severe cases are treated by immunosuppression with corticosteroids, steroid sparing agents such as azathioprine, or other immunosuppressant drugs like cyclosporin. For patients in crisis, plasma exchange is used to rapidly remove the offending autoantibodies. Thymectomy, even in patients without thymoma, results in an increased probability of remission in MG and is usually recommended for patients with generalized disease. The reason for this is unclear.

Lambert-Eaton Myasthenic Syndrome (LEMS)

LEMS is an another autoimmune disorder of neuromuscular transmission due to antibodies to the voltage sensitive calcium channel in the motor nerve terminal. Antibody-mediated loss or inactivity of these channels leads to a reduction in the calcium influx that accompanies depolarization of the nerve terminal and hence a reduction in the amount of ACh released The failure of neuromuscular transmission by this mechanism leads to proximal weakness with relative sparing of the cranial innervated muscles. Another feature of the disease is autonomic failure manifested by xerostomia, decreased sweating, impotence, and orthostatic hypotension. Men outnumber woman by about 5:1[32] and in about two-thirds of patients a malignancy is present, usually a small cell carcinoma of the lung. The remaining patients have LEMS on an autoimmune basis. The findings on electrophysiological testing are distinct from that in MG. As with MG there is decrement of the CMAP at low rates. At high rates (30–50 Hz), or immediately following maximal volitional activity, there is a profound incrementing response of the CMAP, often over 200%. Because this is an antibody-mediated disease, treatment consists of corticosteroids and steroid sparing agents.[33] In neoplastic LEMS, tumor regression following chemotherapy and/or radiation reduces the severity of disease and may result in remission.[34]

Botulism

Botulism is a paralytic condition caused by the ingestion of botulinum toxin from food contaminated by Clostridium botulinum.[35] The first signs are usually xerostomia (dry mouth), abdominal cramps, and diarrhea. Generalized weakness occurs, most prominently in bulbar and ocular muscles. Diagnosis is based on the physical examination and electrophysiological abnormalities similar to those described in LEMS. Treatment is with parenterally administered antitoxin as well as supportive care.

Disorders of Nerve

The disorders of peripheral nerve most likely to be encountered by the SLP are few but important because of their combined incidence and severity.

Guillain-Barré Syndrome (GBS)

Every year at large hospitals, numerous patients are admitted with Guillain-Barré syndrome. The annual incidence is about 1 to 2 per 100,000 per year. Characteristically, the syndrome develops 1 to 3 weeks following a viral upper respiratory or gastrointestinal syndrome. The onset is often heralded by paresthesia or pain in the lower extremities. In days to weeks, an ascending progressive paralysis develops that may be complete. Severe cases develop bulbar and respiratory muscle weakness requiring mechanical ventilation and tube feeding. The dysarthria seen in this condition is flaccid.

The diagnosis of GBS is made by clinical examination, CSF exam (which demonstrates high CSF protein and few or no white blood cells), and findings consistent with multifocal demyelination on the NCS. (For a review of all aspects of this syndrome, see reference 36.)

Treatment is with either plasma exchange[37] or intravenous immune globulin.[38] Most patients recover completely or nearly so. However, a minority are left with significant residual weakness and a few percent die in the acute phase, usually from cardiac arrest.

Amyotrophic Lateral Sclerosis (ALS)

ALS is an idiopathic degenerative disease of upper and lower motor neurons that is inevitably fatal. The annual incidence is about 2 per 100,000 and the median age of onset is in the mid-fifties in most populations studied. The disease is more common in men. The mean survival from symptom onset is less than three years in most studies with death usually coming from respiratory failure or pneumonia. (For a historic review, see reference 39.) Most cases (at least 90%) occur on a spontaneous basis but a minority are inherited, almost always in an autosomal dominant manner. Approximately 20% of the familial cases in the United States result from missense mutations in the gene for Cu/Zn superoxide dismutase (SOD1). This enzyme functions intracellularly as a dismutase—that is, it neutralizes an extremely reactive and potentially damaging form of oxygen that is ubiquitously produced in an intermediate reaction. It has become clear that the damage of motor neurons and their subsequent death are not solely due to the SOD1 being less efficient as a dismutase. Recent studies suggest that the mutant enzyme acquires new and toxic functions, a phenomenon known as "toxic gain of effect."[40] The pathophysiology of this disease is currently an area of active research.

Although the classic form of the disease is characterized clinically by symptoms and signs of both upper and lower motor neuron loss, individual patients are seen whose dysfunction seems to be due to either primarily UMN or primarily LMN dysfunction. Over time, however, most patients develop clear evidence of both UMN and LMN signs.

Approximately one-third of patients experience symptomatic onset of the disease in the lower extremities or upper extremities and about one-quarter have onset in bulbar muscles. In occasional patients, the onset is heralded by generalized weakness, respiratory failure, or fasciculation. Regardless of the site of onset, most patients ultimately experience weakness referable to bulbar musculature and are referred to the SLP.

It has been the experience of one of the authors that patients with bulbar onset disease, especially those characterized by primarily UMN features, are the group that seems to take the longest time to be referred to the neurologist. In adult patients with the insidious onset of spastic or spastic/flaccid dysarthria, ALS should always be included in the differential diagnosis.

Recently, the U.S. Food and Drug Administration approved the drug riluzole for the treatment of ALS. In two studies riluzole seemed to impart a modest survival advantage compared to placebo.[41,42] Unfortunately, no statistically significant reduction in the rate of functional progression was seen.

The management of dysphagia and dysarthria are the main challenges for the SLP confronted with an ALS patient. With respect to dysphagia, a fluoroscopic swallowing study provides anatomical information that may help determine safe swallowing strategies. If aspiration is demonstrated or if bulbar function is becoming so impaired that nutritional status is beginning to suffer, percutaneous gastrostomy is offered. It is recognized that ALS patients with poor respiratory function are at higher risk for morbidity and mortality following the procedure. One group has used a FVC (forced vital capacity) greater than 1 liter and pCO2 less than 45 mm Hg as criteria for percutaneous endoscopic gastrostomy and had a 24-hour mortality of 3.6%.[43] There is some evidence that nutritional support provided by gastrostomy prolongs life.[44]

Movement Disorders

Hypokinetic Movement Disorder

Parkinson's Disease: Parkinson's disease (PD) is a degenerative disorder of the basal ganglia; specifically, the pigmented cells of the substantia nigra, the locus ceruleus, and the dorsal motor nucleus of the vagus are depleted. The disease affects approximately 1% of people over the age of 65 throughout the world. The disease is rarely familial and essentially all cases are sporadic. Even in identical twins there is poor concordance for the disease. Environmental exposures may modify risk. For example, the disease is more common in men and nonsmokers.[45] Lifelong occupational exposure to metals, particularly copper or manganese, seems to be a risk factor.[46] Clinically, the disease is characterized by bradykinesia or akinesia, rigidity, tremor, and a loss of postural reflexes. Patients have a characteristically inexpressive or "masked" face and they blink less. When sitting, there are fewer small adjustments of posture than usual; when standing up from a chair the patient does not use the arms to push up. There may be a resting ("pill rolling") tremor of the hands. When walking, the patient is stooped, the arms flexed, the gait short-stepped, and ultimately characterized by shuffling. The loss of postural reflexes leads to falls. Given this constellation of motor signs, it is not surprising that the dysarthria of PD is hypokinetic, monotonous, and monopitched.

Rational treatment of PD is directed at reducing the pathological effects of the loss of the dopaminergic nigrostriatal pathway. The administration of drugs containing L-dopa, a precursor of the neurotransmitter dopamine, as well as dopaminergic agonists themselves (e.g., bromocriptine, pergolide, lisuride) form the mainstay of treatment. Centrally acting anti-cholinergic drugs such as trihexyphenidyl are used as well, particularly in patients with prominent tremor.

In patients with advanced disease, speech becomes progressively less understandable and the dysphagia may progress to the point where enteral feeding becomes necessary. Speech and swallowing symptoms generally are not improved by the various drug treatments.

Hyperkinetic Movement Disorders

Huntington's Disease: Huntington's disease (HD), also known as Huntington's chorea, is an autosomal dominant neurodegenerative disease characterized by dementia and a choreoathetoid movement disorder. It is progressive and fatal. The disease is now known to be due to an expansion of a region on chromosome 4. The gene product, a protein named "huntingtin," has been identified but its function is not currently known. HD occurs in people of northern European descent with an incidence of about 5 per 100,000. The usual age of onset is in the thirties and forties, but cases are seen occasionally in the teens or after the age of 70. The disease is usually not difficult to diagnose because of family history. Patients at risk for the disease can be most reliably detected by genetic analysis for the mutation. Because there is no treatment for the disease, genetic testing under these circumstances should be performed only at specialized centers with genetic counselors familiar with the medical and ethical issues.

The disorder often begins with psychiatric manifestations such as subtle changes in personality; sometimes frank psychosis develops. Depression is common. At some point, the movement disorder begins. At first patients may seem merely fidgety, but ultimately a choreoathetoid movement disorder becomes obvious. Speech in HD is characterized by a hyperkinetic dysarthria with variable rate and loudness and imprecise consonants. Symptomatic treatment of chorea is usually accomplished with haloperidol.

Essential and Familial Tremor: One of the more common hyperkinetic movement disorders is tremor; this may occur as an autosomal dominantly inherited form or it may appear sporadically, in which case it is known as essential tremor. It has an estimated incidence of over 400 per 100,000.[47] The disorder may begin in childhood but is more prevalent as a population ages. The action tremor (present when using the limb, not at rest or when supported) usually begins in the arms or as a side-to-side movement of the head. Over time, it worsens and may become quite disabling. In some patients, the cranial innervated muscles are involved and there is a wavering property to the voice. Many patients have themselves noted that the tremor abates after one or two drinks of alcohol.

Treatment is with beta blockers such as propranolol or with the anticonvulsant primidone.

Multiple Sclerosis (MS)

MS is a relatively common demyelinating disease of the CNS. The pathological process causes relapsing/remitting multifocal demyelination in the brain, spinal cord, and optic nerves. The axons are relatively spared. The disease has a number of intriguing features. In most countries or continents studied, there is a gradient of incidence that is lowest toward the equator and rises with latitudes above or below the equator. In African Americans in the United States, at all latitudes the incidence is lower than whites.[48] The same is true in Japan. In studies of migrants, the risk of the disease seems to be largely acquired by the age of 15. There is a higher incidence of MS in first-degree relatives of patients with the disease, especially identical twins. Fraternal twins have an incidence of nontwin siblings.[49]

While the lesions in MS certainly represent immune mediated demyelination (there is evidence of antibodies directed at components of myelin and active plaques are infiltrated with certain subtypes of lymphocytes), there is no autoantibody in the classical sense.

Clinically, the disease may present with or be characterized by many different manifestations. One way to think of the possible symptoms and signs is to recall that all motor, sensory, and visual information is carried by myelinated pathways. Hence, unilateral visual loss, sensory loss or paresthesias, varying combinations of motor weakness and spasticity can be seen. Spinal lesions may lead to complete or incomplete transverse myelitis.

While most patients have a relapsing remitting course, over time there is a tendency for the disorder to become chronic and progressive in many patients.

Because of the multifocal nature of demyelination in MS, many different types of speech disorder can be seen. In some patients speech is normal, in others it is primarily ataxic, in still others it is spastic/ataxic.[50,51]

Treatment involves modulation of the immune system as well as symptomatic aid. High-dose oral or parenteral glucocorticoids have been shown to reduce the period of the exacerbation, but they do not change the ultimate course of the disease. Other immunosuppressants such as azathioprine and cyclophosphamide may slow the course of decline in chronic progressive MS but not without potentially dangerous side effects—in particular, lymphoreticular malignancies. More recently, interferon beta has been shown to reduce the demyelinating activity as seen on MRI.[52] Whether this will have long-term clinical benefits is unclear at this time.

Symptomatic treatment of spasticity may be accomplished with baclofen or the new antispasticity agent tizanidine. The spasticity of the bladder may be treated with oxybutynin or propantheline. Fatigue is sometimes effectively treated with amantadine.

Epilepsy

A seizure is a symptom of brain dysfunction characterized by disorderly electrical discharges of nerve cells. The abnormal discharge (1) may occur in a silent area of the brain causing no clinical symptoms; (2) could be limited to an island of neurons resulting in focal symptoms and signs; or (3) could spread to many areas of the brain leading to multiple symptoms and signs, and sometimes loss of consciousness. Recurrent unprovoked seizures are known as epilepsy.

It is estimated that the prevalence of epilepsy is 6 per 1000—which translates into more than 1.5 million Americans;[53] blacks may be more prone than whites. Also, more than 200,000 epileptics have more than one seizure per month, and approximately one-fourth of patients have recurrent seizures despite treatment.[54] Risk factors for epilepsy include mental retardation/cerebral palsy, repeated and focal febrile seizures, family history of epilepsy, central nervous system infections, moderate and severe head injury, cerebrovascular disease, brain tumors, Alzheimer's disease, excessive alcohol use and drug abuse (e.g., heroin), and a history of asthma.[54]

The majority of epilepsies are idiopathic (unknown cause).[55] Definite causes of seizures are multiple (Table 11–9). Idiopathic epilepsy is more common in children and adolescents than in adults; symptomatic epilepsy is more prevalent in adults.

Seizures are either generalized or partial (focal, local); partial seizures are further subclassified into simple partial, complex partial (indicating an impaired level, but not loss, of consciousness), and partial evolving to generalized tonic-clonic (GTC) convulsions.[56]

Generalized seizures are characterized by initial involvement of both hemispheres with impaired level of consciousness, bilateral motor symptoms, and widespread and bilateral neuronal discharges on electroencephalography. Grand mal and petit mal are the two main forms of generalized seizures. With grand mal, patients loose consciousness abruptly, there is tonic contraction of muscles (stridor or cry if the respiratory muscles are affected), and they fall to the ground. Soon after, convulsive movements occur for a variable period of time and are followed by a muscle relaxation phase where the unconscious patients breath

Table 11–9. Causes of Seizures

Cause	Example
Trauma	Contusion; penetrating injury; hemorrhage
Cerebrovascular disease	SAH; ICH; subdural hematoma; ischemic stroke; cerebral venous thrombosis
Infections	Meningitis; encephalitis; cerebral abscess
Neoplastic disease	Primary tumors; metastatic disease
Metabolic	Hypo- and hypernatremia; hypo- and hyperglycemia; hypoxia; hypo- and hypercalcemia; kidney and liver failure
Drugs and toxins	Alcohol intoxication and withdrawal; withdrawal of anti-epileptics; environmental toxins (e.g., lead)
Inherited diseases	Phenylketonuria; tuberous sclerosis; urea cycle disorders
Others	Sleep deprivation; fever in children

deeply. Tongue biting, urinary and/or fecal incontinence, frothing at the mouth, and grunting occur during the GTC phase. Occasionally, patients develop a vague and ill-described feeling before they lose consciousness. When epileptic patients are awakened after a seizure, they usually feel sore and may have headache. Grand mal seizures can occur in childhood or in adult life. They do not recur as frequently as petit mal seizures.

Petit mal or absence seizures are characterized by a brief (few seconds) interruption of consciousness, a blank stare, and sometimes uprolling of the eyes. Absence seizures can be isolated or could be accompanied by clonic, tonic, atonic activities, or by automatisms such as lip smacking, cloth fumbling, and so on. Typical absence seizures occur in 4- to 12-year-old children. Simple partial seizures take the form of motor (any portion of the body may be involved in repetitive motor activities), somatosensory (manifest as numbness or tingling), special sensory (visual, auditory, gustatory, or olfactory hallucinations; vertigo, floating sensations), autonomic (pallor, perspiration, pupillary dilatation, etc.), or psychic seizures with cognitive impairment (aphasia, déjà vu, fear, anger, etc.).

Sometimes, partial seizures affect multiple body areas sequentially (Jacksonian march). Complex partial seizures can evolve from simple partial or can be associated with an initial impairment of the level of consciousness.

Rare types include myoclonic (single or multiple sudden and brief shock-like contractions of the face, trunk, or extremity); clonic (similar to GTC without the tonic component); tonic (GTC without clonic component); and atonic seizures (sudden loss of muscle tone).

Status epilepticus (SE) is an epileptic seizure that is "frequently repeated or so prolonged as to create a fixed and lasting condition."[56] Unless attended to emergently, patients with SE are at a high risk of significant morbidity or death.

One of the most important elements in the management of patients with suspected epilepsy is to first establish the diagnosis. Many conditions can mimic seizures, including syncope (brief loss of consciousness), hyperventilation, sleep disorders, migraine, or psychiatric dissociative states. Once the diagnosis of epilepsy is made with confidence, a cause for the seizures is explored (Table 11–9).

Avoidance of the offending mechanism (e.g., alcohol abstinence) is the treatment of choice for nonrecurrent seizures. The therapy of epilepsy is guided by the its type, medication cost, and patient preference. Monotherapy (a single agent) is the recommended strategy. If an anti-epileptic drug (AED) is not effective or causes significant side effects, it is preferable to change the AED rather than add another one. Commonly used AEDs, their indications, and side effects are listed in Table 11–10. New AEDs (e.g., gabapentin) are undergoing intense testing to evaluate their usefulness as primary or adjunctive therapy for epilepsy.

Routine blood testing (complete blood count, electrolytes, liver and kidney function tests) is performed before initiating AED therapy. When appropriate, these tests are repeated and serum blood levels of AEDs are obtained during the course of therapy.

Some patients with epilepsy fail multiple drug regimens. These patients are candidates for referral to specialized epilepsy centers that evaluate epileptics for possible surgical intervention. Localized resection of the area generating the seizures is an effective and long-term treatment in some patients with temporal lobe epilepsy.[57] Large resections (e.g., hemispherectomies) are occasionally performed to control intractable seizures in infants and small children.

The management of SE requires an emergent approach; the longer it takes to control SE, the worse the prognosis. The essential "ABCs" are: protect the airway, draw blood (AED levels, glucose, sodium, calcium, gases, urea nitrogen, drug screen), assess and stabilize cardiac function. Rapid administration of AEDs in the first few minutes is essential. A benzodiazepine (lorazepam or diazepam) is given intermittently to stop the seizures while the AED is infusing in the vein. Sometimes patients are put into pharmacological coma (e.g., pentobarbital) to stop the continuous electrical brain discharges that are causing SE.

SUMMARY

A basic understanding of functional neuroanatomy provides a useful and rational approach to the diagnosis and treatment of neurogenic communication and swallowing disorders. In general, diseases of the motor unit lead to flaccid dysarthria and disorders of the basal ganglia and cerebellum affect the quality of movement. Degenerative, vascular, inflammatory, and neoplastic disorders of the cerebrum ultimately impact on the motor unit via central mechanisms of control. While it is beyond the scope of this chapter to provide exhaustive coverage of all neurological disease, we have presented the fundamental ap-

Table 11–10. Commonly Used Anti-Epileptic Drugs

Medication	Indications	Common Side Effects
Phenytoin	First drug of choice for partial epilepsy	Gum hypertrophy; increased body hair; nausea; drowsiness
Phenobarbital	Alternative therapy for partial epilepsy	Sedation; cognitive impairment; sexual dysfunction
Carbamazepine	First drug of choice for partial epilepsy	Gastrointestinal distress
Valproate	Drug of choice for primary generalized epilepsy	Weight gain; hair loss; nausea; tremor

proach used by neurologists in their assessment of patients with symptoms of neurological origin. This information complements the practice of speech–language pathology.

STUDY QUESTIONS

1. What are the elements of the motor unit?

2. Which tract provides the principle means of voluntary control over the cranial nerve nuclei involved in speech and swallowing?

3. Which branch of the vagus nerve is most important for controlling vocal pitch?

4. The EEG is useful in the diagnosis and prognosis of epilepsy—true or false?

5. The EMG should be abnormal in a disorder of the motor unit—true or false?

6. What are the various advantages and disadvantages of clinical imaging studies?

7. What are the most common causes of stroke?

8. How do ICH and SAH differ (other than by site)?

9. Lambert-Eaton myasthenic syndrome (LEMS) and botulism are disorders of the NMJ that largely spare the bulbar muscles—true or false?

10. Describe the various types of epilepsy.

REFERENCES

1. *Aids to the examination of the peripheral nervous system.* Medical Research Council. Memorandum No. 45, Her Majesty's Stationery Office, London, 1946.

2. Marsan CA, Zivin LS: Factors related to the occurrence of typical paroxysmal abnormalities in the EEG records of epileptic patients. *Epilepsia* 1970; 11:361.

3. Silverman D, Saunders MG, Schwab RS, Masland RL: Cerebral death and the electroencephalogram. Report of the Ad Hoc Committee of the American Electroencephalographic Society on EEG Criteria for Determination of Cerebral Death. *JAMA* 1969; 209:1505–1510.

4. Sundt TM, Sharbrough FW, Piepgras DG, et al: Correlation of cerebral blood flow and electroencephalographic changes during carotid endarterectomy: With results of surgery and hemodynamics of cerebral ischemia. *Mayo Clin Proc* 1981; 56:533–543.

5. Stalberg E, Ekstedt J, Broman A: Neuromuscular transmission in myasthenia gravis studied with single fiber electromyography. *J Neurol Neurosurg Psychiatry* 1974; 37:540–547.

6. Konishi T, Nishitani H, Matsubara F, Ohta M: Myasthenia gravis: Relation between jitter in single-fiber EMG and antibody to acetylcholine receptor. *Neurology* 1981; 31:386–392.

7. Adams RD, Victor M, Ropper AH: *Principles of neurology,* 6th ed. McGraw-Hill, New York, 1997.

8. Bradley WG, Daroff RB, Marsden CD, Fenichel GM: *Neurology in clinical practice. The neurological disorders.* 2nd ed. Butterworth-Heinemann; Boston, 1996.

9. Aaslid R, Markwalder TM, Nornes H: Noninvasive transcranial doppler ultrasound recording of flow velocity in basal cerebral arteries. *J Neurosurg* 1982; 57:769–774.

10. Therapeutic and Technology Assessment Subcommittee of the American Academy of Neurology: Assessment of transcranial doppler. *Neurology* 1990; 40: 680–681.

11. Bowler JV, Hachinski V: Epidemiology of cerebral infarct. In Gorelick PB, ed., *Atlas of cerebrovascular disease.* Philadelphia, Churchill Livingston, 1996; 1.1–1.22.

12. Davis PH, Torner JC: Epidemiology of subarachnoid hemorrhage and intraparenchymal hemorrhage. In Gorelick PB, ed., *Atlas of cerebrovascular disease.* Philadelphia, Churchill Livingston, 1996;2.1–2.15.

13. Ramadan NM, Mitsias P: Nonatherosclerotic stroke. In Gorelick PB, ed., *Atlas of cerebrovascular disease.* Philadelphia, Churchill Livingston, 1996;7.1–7.16.

14. Special Report from the National Institute of Neurological Disorders and Stroke (Whisnant JP, chairman). Classification of cerebrovascular diseases. *Stroke* 1990; 21:637–676.

15. Levy DE: How transient are transient ischemic attacks? *Neurology* 1988;38:674–677.

16. The National Institute of Neurological Disorders and Stroke rt-PA Study Group. Tissue plasminogen activator for acute ischemic stroke. *N Engl J Med* 1995; 333: 1581–1587.

17. North American Symptomatic Carotid Endarterectomy Trial Collaborators: Beneficial effect of carotid endarterectomy in symptomatic patients with high grade carotid stenosis. *N Engl J Med* 1991; 325:445–453.

18. Executive Committee for the Asymptomatic Carotid Atherosclerosis Study: Endarterectomy for asymptomatic carotid stenosis. *JAMA* 1995; 273:1421–1428.

19. Broderick JP, Phillips SJ, Whisnant JP et al: Incidence rate of stroke in the eighties: The end of the decline in stroke. *Stroke* 1989; 20:577–582.

20. Minematsu K, Yamaguchi T: Management of intracerebral hemorrhage. In Fisher M, ed., *Stroke therapy.* Boston, Butterworth-Heinemann, 1995; 351–372.

21. Kelly MA: Management of intracerebral hemorrhage. In Gorelick PB, ed., *Atlas of cerebrovascular disease.* Philadelphia, Churchill Livingston, 1996; 20.1–20.10.

22. Weaver JP: Subarachnoid hemorrhage. In Fisher M, ed., *Stroke therapy.* Boston, Butterworth-Heinemann, 1995; 399–435.

23. Curtin JC, Kelly MA: Subarachnoid hemorrhage. In Gorelick PB, ed., *Atlas of cerebrovascular disease.* Philadelphia, Churchill Livingston, 1996; 5.1–5.8.

24. Schievink WI: Intracranial aneurysms. *N Engl J Med* 1997; 336:28–40.

25. Hunt WE, Hess RM: Surgical risk as related to time of intervention in the repair of intracranial aneurysms. *J Neurosurg* 1968; 28:14–20.

26. Emery, AEH: Population frequencies of inherited neuromuscular diseases—A world survey. *Neuromusc Disord* 1991; 1:19–29

27. Mendell JR, Moxley RT, Griggs RC, Brooke MH, Fenichel GM, Miller JP, Kinger W, Signore L, Pandya S, Florence J: Randomized double-blind six month trial of prednisone in Duchenne's muscular dystrophy: *N Eng J Med* 1989; 320:1592–1597.

28. Tome FMS, Fardeau M: Nuclear inclusions in oculopharyngeal dysstrophy. *Acta Neuropathol* 1980; 49: 85–87.

29. Fischbeck KH: The mechanism of myotonic dystrophy. *Ann Neurol* 1994; 35:255.

30. Dalakas MC: Polymyositis, dermatomyositis, and inclusion body myositis. *N Eng J Med* 1991; 325:1487–1498.

31. Drachman DB: Myasthenia gravis. *N Eng J Med* 1994; 330:1797.

32. Elmqvist D, Lambert EH: Detailed analysis of neuromuscular transmission in a patient with the myasthenic syndrome sometimes associated with bronchogenic carcinoma. *Mayo Clin Proc* 1968; 43:689–713.

33. Newsome-Davis J, Murray NMF: Plasma exchange and immunosupressive drug treatment in the Lambert-Eaton myasthenic syndrome. *Neurology* 1984; 34:480–485.

34. Chalk, CH, Murray NMF, Newsom-Davis JH, Oneill JH, Spiro SG: Response of the Lambert-Eaton myasthenic syndrome to treatment of associated small cell carcinoma. *Neurology* 1990; 40:1552–1556.

35. Swift T, Rivner M: Infectious diseases of nerve. In Vinken PJ, Bruyn GW, and Klawans HL, eds., *Handbook of clinical neurology.* Amsterdam, Elsevier Publishing, 1987; 179–194.

36. Ropper AH, Wijdicks EFM, Truax BT: Guillain-Barré syndrome. F.A. Davis, Philadelphia, 1991.

37. McKhann GM, Griffen JW, Cornblath DR, et al: Plasmapheresis and Guillain-Barré syndrome: Analysis of prognostic factors and the effect of plasmapheresis. *Ann Neurol* 1988; 23:347.

38. van der Meche FGA, Schmitz PIM and the Dutch Guillain-Barré Study Group: A randomized trial comparing intravenous immune globulin and plasma exchange in Guillain-Barré syndrome. *N Eng J Med* 1992; 326:1123.

39. Williams DB, Windebank AJ: Motor neuron disease (amyotrophic lateral sclerosis). *Mayo Clin Proc* 1991; 66:54.

40. Gurney ME, Pu H, Chiu AY, Dal Canto MC, Polchow CY, Alexander DD, et al: Motor neuron degeneration in mice that express a human Cu,Zn superoxide dismutase mutation. *Science* 1994; 264:1772–1775.

41. Bensimon G, Lacomblez L, Meininger V: A controlled trial of riluzole in amyotrophic lateral sclerosis. ALS/Riluzole study group. *NEJM* 1994; 330: 985–991.

42. Lacomblez L, Bensimon G, Leigh P, Guillet P, Meininger V: Dose-ranging study of riluzole in amyotrophic lateral sclerosis. ALS/Riluzole study group II. *Lancet* 1996; 347:1425–1431.

43. Mathus-Vliegen LM, Louwerse LS, Merkus MP, Tytgat GN, Vianney de Jong JM: Percutaneous endoscopic gastrostomy in patients with amyotrophic lateral sclerosis and impaired pulmonary function. *Gastrointest Endosc* 1994; 40:463–469.

44. Mazzini L, Corra T, Zaccala M, Mora G, Del Piano M, Galante M: Percutaneous endoscopic gastrostomy and enteral nutrition in amyotrophic lateral sclerosis. *J Neurol* 1995; 242:695–698.

45. Morens DM, Grandinetti A, Reed D, White LR, Ross GW: Cigarette smoking and protection from Parkinson's disease: False association or etiologic clue? *Neurology* 1995; 45:1041–1051.

46. Gorell JM, Johnson DD, Rybicki BA, Peterson EL, Kortsha GX, Brown GG, Richardson RJ: Occupational exposures to metals as risk factors for Parkinson's disease. *Neurology* 1997; 48:650–658.

47. Haerer AF, Anderson DW, Schoenberg BS: Prevalence of essential tremor. *Arch Neurol* 1982; 39:750.

48. Kurtzke JF, Beebe GW, Norman JE Jr: Epidemiology of multiple sclerosis in U.S. veterans: I. Race, sex and geographic distribution. *Neurology* 1979; 29:1228.

49. Ebers GC, Bulman DE, Sadovnick AD: A population-based study of multiple sclerosis in twins. *N Eng J Med* 1986; 315:1638.

50. Darley FL, Aronson AE, Goldstein NP: Dysarthia in multiple sclerosis. *J Speech Hear Res* 1972; 15: 229–245.

51. Beukelman DR, Kraft GH, Freal J: Expressive communication disorders in persons with multiple sclerosis: A survey. *Arch Phys Med Rehabil* 1985; 66:675.

52. Arnason BGW: Interferon beta in multiple sclerosis. *Neurology* 1993; 43:641.

53. Hauser WA, Kurland LT: The epidemiology of epilepsy in Rochester, Minnesota, 1936–1967. *Epilepsia* 1975; 16:1–66.

54. Hauser WA, Hesdorffer DC: Epidemiology of epilepsy. In Anderson DW, ed., *Neuroepidemiology: A tribute to Bruce Schoenberg.* Boca Raton, CRC Press, 1991; 97–119.

55. Annegers JF: The epidemiology of epilepsy. In Wyllie E, ed., *The treatment of epilepsy: Principles and practice.* Philadelphia, Lea and Febiger, 1993; 157–164.

56. Commission on Classification and Terminology of the International League Against Epilepsy: Proposal for revised clinical and electrographic classification of epileptic seizures. *Epilepsia* 1981; 22:489–501.

57. Goodman RR: Surgical treatment of epilepsy. In Chokroverty S, ed., *Management of Epilepsy.* Boston, Butterworth-Heinemann, 1996; 309–328.

12

Behavioral Neurology

RHONNA S. SHATZ

CHAPTER OUTLINE

The Three Axes of Behavior

The Vertical Axis

Lateral Axis

Horizontal Axis

Speech and language are two segments of the behavioral repertoire of the brain. In total, these brain behaviors are termed cognition: arousal, attention, affect, memory, executive functions, visuospatial function, gnosis, and praxis. Although the fields of neurology and psychiatry share evaluation and treatment of these functions, their assessments are based on different assumptions. In neurology, behaviors have a known association with different structures and regions of the brain; they are anatomically based. A step-by-step testing of behavior yields a region-by-region assessment of cognitively relevant brainstem and cortex. By the end of a behavioral screen, a neuroanatomic syndrome is defined and etiologies of disorders affecting those regions can be determined. In psychiatry, behaviors, although believed to be anatomically based, have less well-defined relationships to brain structure. The variety and variability of behavior in psychiatric disease are greater and more difficult to relate to disruption of specific anatomic regions of the brain. Behavioral neurology isolates and tests each element of cognition and then clusters and sorts behaviors to find an anatomic pattern common and predictable to disease or dysfunction. The behav-

ioral neurology exam begins in an orderly fashion by assessing behavior and collating findings into an anatomic pattern. The following sections detail the neuropsychological and anatomic underpinnings of aspects of behavior and provide descriptions of bedside tests (See Appendix A).

THE THREE AXES OF BEHAVIOR

Despite the complexity of behavior, we can conceptualize the neuroanatomy of behavior in three axes: the vertical axis, the horizontal axis, and the lateral axis (Figure 12–1).

Vertical Axis

The vertical axis is the most basic axis of behavioral function. The vertical axis runs vertically in the midline from the brainstem through the hemispheres to the cortex. It is assessed first, because its integrity is integral to the functioning of all the other axes. Any time one of its components is disrupted, the functioning of the other axes is affected and interpretation of the behaviors tested in those

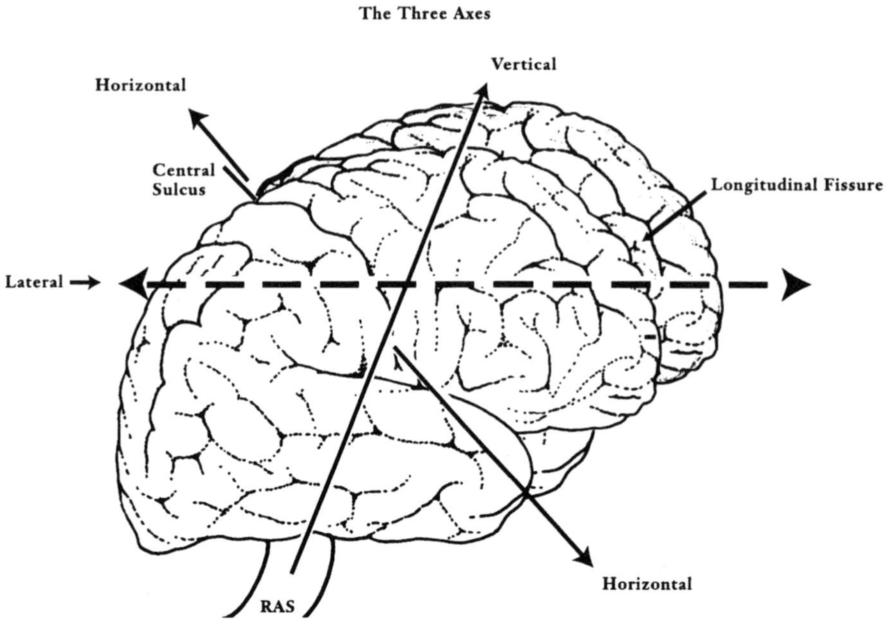

The Three Axes

Vertical

Horizontal

Central
Sulcus

Longitudinal Fissure

Lateral →

Horizontal

RAS

Figure 12–1. The three axes of behavior.

must take into account basic defaults in attention, control of attention, or level of consciousness. Like a fence post, the vertical axis literally keeps an individual upright; it is responsible for the postures and behaviors of alertness and alerting. In hierarchical order, the behaviors of the axis are arousal, attention, memory, affect, and executive functions. The anatomic area underlying the behavior is the reticular activating system with its limbic and cortical connections.[2] The principal neurotransmitter of the system is acetylcholine, though dopamine, serotonin, noradrenalin, and excitatory monoamines contribute.

Arousal

Anatomy of the Reticular Activating System

The anatomical basis of the vertical axis is the reticular activating system (RAS). The reticular activating system is an alarm system. If an alarm is to function in awakening, its signal must be anatomically widespread. The reticular activating system, therefore, stretches through the brain as a core of gray matter from the brainstem, the midline thalamic nuclei, and the white matter to the cortical regions termed the association areas[3] (Figure 12–2). The association areas are the great conferencing regions of the hemispheres. Information from like areas of the region converge to be compared and analyzed in this space, and then processed or associated with other areas of the brain. One association area exists for each of the three subdivisions of

behavioral function: prefrontal in the inferior frontal lobe for the convergence of motor functions; posterior in the inferior parietal lobule, the melting POT of sensory information from the pareital, occipital, and temporal lobes; and the parahippocampal region, where memory and emotion from the vertical axis are processed. Neurons in the system are few, but reticular; the interconnectivity and reach of the system are achieved by the branching of a few neurons through multiples of dendritic extension. The cholinergic projections from the basal forebrain excite extensive portions of the sensory cortex relevant to behavior and are significant in the pathology of Alzheimer's disease.[4] Almost all areas of the cortex project back to the reticular nucleus of the thalamus. Feedback from the cortex to the thalamus is excitatory, but projections from the brainstem to the same thalamic nuclei are inhibitory. The reticular nucleus, therefore, is an intermediary between cortical excitatory and brainstem inhibitory influences and can mediate or gate attention to voluntary or reflexive stimuli of interest.[5]

Lesions of the RAS

The reticular connectivity of the system causes all parts to function as a whole in affecting consciousness. A lesion in any system structure leads to loss of signal to the whole brain and, like the loss of voltage in a wire to a lamp, the whole brain dims. Clinically, reticular organization of the sys-

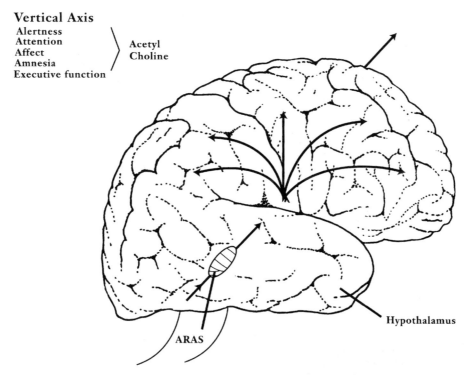

Vertical Axis
Alertness
Attention
Affect
Amnesia
Executive function

Acetyl
Choline

Hypothalamus

ARAS

Figure 12–2. The vertical axis and the reticular activating system.

tem means that a diminished level of consciousness could result from a single lesion of the brainstem, midline thalamus, or association area, or bilateral white matter reticular tracts, or all the components of the system at once.[6–11] Single lesions of the system generally result from tumors or vascular disease. Lesions affecting bilateral white matter tracts or all the components of the RAS are usually due to metabolic derangements of the rest of the body: hyper- or hypoglycemia, sepsis, hypoxia, uremia, hepatic failure, drugs, or intoxication. The disorder of consciousness that results from the latter is therefore often called metabolic encephalopathy.

To illustrate the function of the reticular activating system, observe the Johnson and Johnson string doll (Figure 12–3). The yellow cord connecting the doll's head, torso, and legs is the core of gray of the RAS. Like the RAS it runs vertically from head to toe. If the cord is pulled taut, the parts of the doll are aligned upright; the doll has the posture and appearance of wakefulness. If the cord is slack, its hold on the body and the brain is loosened and the doll falls down; it now has the posture and appearance of sleep or a disturbed level of consciousness (Figure 12–4). A rightly connected RAS is necessary for the appearance of alertness; and loosening of the cord leads to the disorders of consciousness.

Testing Level of Consciousness

Clinically, the first test of behavior is the level of consciousness. The classification of consciousness, as well as all other behaviors, takes into account the notion that all output is dependent on input. Brain functions are organized into circuits of incoming or internally generated sensory cues and outgoing thoughts or actions. To classify the level of consciousness, there is a hierarchy of stimuli and actions (Table 12–1).

Hierarchy of Sensory Inputs: With decreasing levels of consciousness, the intensity of stimulus needed to arouse and activate the RAS declines. In a state of full alertness, the cortex is operational and perceives and interprets sensory information at the most complex level; therefore, just the presence of someone in the room will usually elicit a response, or the uttering of a person's name will stimulate a verbal answer, the turning of the eyes and body to the speaker, a gesture of hello or welcome. When a person is less than fully alert, it implies the cortex is faulty; sensory information is perceived incompletely or distorted. Responses may be more stereotyped and reflexive. Different inputs are needed to stimulate the system than those involving language. Because the RAS is an alarm system, the inputs to it are also stimuli that

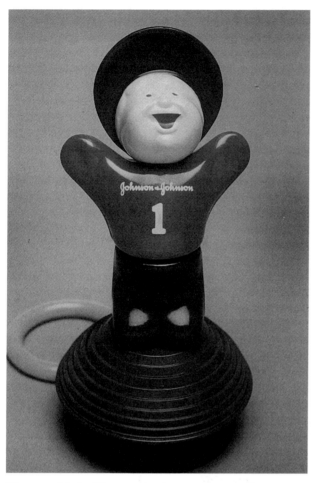

Figure 12–3. The reticular activating system: awake, alert.

convey warnings of danger. To a human being, danger is signaled by sudden movements or flashes of light, sudden or loud sounds, or pain. Therefore, there must be tracts to the RAS from the auditory, visual, tactile, and pain pathways. When cortical dysfunction impairs voluntary attention, a point of access to the RAS can frequently be obtained by forcing attention with a loud sound, a shout or a clap, shaking the body, or inflicting

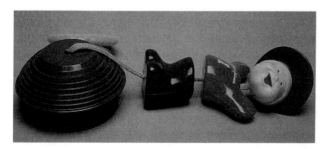

Figure 12–4. The reticular activating system: comatose.

pain. Pain is processed at two levels: fine discriminative, well-localized pain, usually describable as sharp that is carried by the spinothalamic tract and diffuse, poorly localizable, aching pain, that is carried by the spinoreticular tract.[12] Spinothalamic projections are somatotopically organized in the thalamus and somatosensory cortex. A pinprick can be localized to the finger because the tract from the receptor to the cortex maintains its somatotopic fidelity (an almost one-to-one relationship between receptor and cortex) and is consciously recognized. Spinoreticular pain is diffuse because of the convergence of many pain receptors onto portions of the tract; there is little anatomic organization to the tract and virtually no correspondence of receptor location to projection in the thalamus. Its fibers project to the periaqueductal gray matter and midline laminar thalamic nuclei of the RAS. Because of these connections, pain in this tract serves arousal, emotive, or affective purposes. It only requires brain area from receptor to upper brainstem to be functional. Pain from sternal rub, supraorbital pressure, and knuckle crushing is less well localizable and results in a response that may be nonspecifically aversive, such as a flailing of the arm, startle response, or a fragment of a reflexive avoidance response called decerebrate or decorticate posturing.

Hierarchy of Motor Inputs: In a fully alert and responsive individual, a painful stimulus can reach the cortex and elicit both a reflexive withdrawal, such as the quick movement of the hand away from a flame, and volitional aversive activity, such as hand shaking or treating the hand with analgesics and ice. The volitional activities require integrated cortical inputs and corticospinal tract outputs. The reflexive activity can be processed by lower motor pathways: rubrospinal, vestibulospinal, and intraspinal tracts. The rubrospinal tract originates in the midbrain's red nucleus and coordinates gross arm and forearm flexion and lower extremity step activity. In lower animals, this system replaces the corticospinal system for movement. When the brain is dysfunctional above the midbrain, but doesn't include the red nucleus, an aversive stimulus can activate the remaining rubrospinal pathway to cause flexion of the upper extremities and extension of the lower extremities, called *decorticate posturing*. It is decorticate because it is the motor activity of efferent tracts below the cortex. Lesions below the midbrain but above the vestibular nuclei in the pontomedullary junction allow aversive stimuli to cause decerebrate posturing: extension of the arms and legs. This posturing results from

Table 12-1. Testing Level of Consciousness

Level of Consciousness	Stimulus	Movement Observed
Alert: appears awake	Walk into the room; address patient by name	Spontaneous, purposeful, complex
Lethargic: appears sleepy; remains awake once aroused	Shout name; shake head and body	Less spontaneous, purposeful
Obtunded: sleepy; remains awake only as long as stimulus is present	Pain inflicted superficially by pin or deeply by supra-orbital nerve pressure, sternal rub, knuckle crush	Brief unsustained movement; fragmented, aversive, may respond reflexively with decorticate or decerebrate posturing.
Comatose: asleep	Unarousable	Unresponsive

vestibulospinal pathways. Vestibulospinal tracts are responsible for upright posture of the trunk. The function of this tract is illustrated by the position of the body that a figure skater makes after immediately stopping a spin; head, neck, and trunk are extended, arms are extended and abducted from the body, and the legs are rigidly extended at the knee. This position allows maximal stability of the trunk when vestibular stimulation signals that there has been a disruption in the position of the head and trunk. It is decerebrate because the cerebrum is not necessary for this brainstem pathway to cause movement. Intraspinal pathways coordinate simple withdrawal of upper and lower extremities to pain or tactile stimuli. These movements, as well as deep tendon reflex responses, are still possible in a comatose individual with no cerebral function. In the coma evaluation, the task is to determine the highest level of functioning of the nervous system. If function is localized below the vestibular system—in other words, there is no arousal to any stimuli or movement is limited to spinal reflexes—a person is considered brain dead.

The orderly evaluation of consciousness by stimulus, as pain or other sensory input, and response, as voluntary or reflexive movement, allows a survey of the midline RAS from peripheral receptor (pain, auditory, tactile) to cortex and then from cortex to periphery via corticospinal, rubrospinal, vestibulospinal, and intraspinal pathways. It is the first assessment of the anatomy of behavior.

Attention

After establishing a sufficient level of wakefulness, the next task is to determine if a person can focus the energy of wakefulness to a specific task. As in assessing the level of consciousness, this function involves a sensory or input limb and a motor or output limb; attention entails both the ability to detect and orient to stimuli and the ability to direct thinking or activities.[13,14] Attention consists of both conscious and voluntary processes and unconscious and involuntary processes. The failure to detect or orient to stimuli is termed stimulus neglect or hemi-inattention. These processes involve vertical axis input, but also additional processing in the right hemisphere, and therefore are discussed in the lateral axis. Concentration is the term used for the voluntary, purposeful, conscious act of directing thoughts or actions to one or more specific stimuli or tasks. Clinically, three aspects of concentration are assessed in the vertical axis: span of attention, divided concentration, and vigilance.

Span of Attention

Span of attention refers to the amount of information that can be concentrated on simultaneously. This information can be in the form of numbers (digit span), words (immediate memory), or figures and objects (immediate visual memory). Any lesion of the caudate nuclei,[15] or the association areas of the inferior frontal lobe, parahippocampal region, or inferior parietal lobule can impair concentration span. Concentration can vary for different types of information based on lesion localizations; left-sided lesions located in the structures above affect spans for words and digits and right-sided lesions affect spans for figures, objects, and spatial tasks.[16]

Disorders of Span of Attention: Amnestic Korsakoff's syndrome patients and depressed patients do not have diminished digit spans, but effort in performing the task may be poor in depressed patients. In Alzheimer's disease, digit spans of 7 forward and 5 backward remain until late in the disease; if digit span is diminished in the disease, it may be due to an overlying metabolic encephalopathy, usually an infection such as a urinary tract infection or pneumonia.[17] Diminution of attention span is a cardinal sign of delirium and metabolic encephalopathy.

Testing: All tests of span of concentration involve the immediate reproduction of information that is divided into equivalent, discrete units. Typically, digit span, verbal span, and spatial span are assessed.

In digit span, the most common test of attention, random sequences of numbers are repeated forward or backward. Portions of the Wechsler Memory Scale and Wechsler Adult Intelligence Scale (WAIS) include the digit span task, normal for age and education.[18] Digit span decreases with age, but until age 70 remains at 7 forward and 5 backward. Education below grade 8 decreases the upper value of digit span. The ability to attend to only 7 pieces of information at one time governs everyday life. Think of the following sequence of numbers:

8747172

This random appearing set of numbers may be familiar in this form:

874-7172

Telephone numbers are 7 digits long, average sentence length is 7 words, perhaps even the division of weeks into 7 days implies that the brain conceives of time in finite 7-unit sequences.

The clustering in phone numbers illustrates another principle of brain function. Though our maximal attention at any one time is 7 units long, it is still easier to bunch information into smaller units of 1 to 2. When telephone numbers are given with a pause in between a cluster of 3 and a cluster of 4 instead of 7 units, the number is now in 2 units, each unit on either side of the hyphen. During bedside exams of digit span testing, care must be taken to avoid reciting numbers in clusters; otherwise, instead of testing a span of 7 digits, testing would be a span of 2 units.

Verbal span is usually tested as part of "immediate memory." Patients repeat random 3- to 5-word sequences after the examiner. Repetition of sentences of increasing word length, a part of the Boston Diagnostic Aphasia Examination,[19] is a form of verbal span testing; failure to repeat sentences with greater numbers of words may indicate a disorder of concentration and not language.

A visual analogue of the verbal subtests, the spatial span subtest of the WAIS-R NI, involves replication of the order of tapping over a series of 10 cubes randomly attached to a board. Norms do not exist for this test. In situations where language or speech is impaired or patients are not native English speakers, patients can be asked to duplicate the tapping sequence of random patterns of colored squares in forward or reverse order.

Divided Attention

Divided attention allows for the simultaneous performance of two or more tasks, the proverbial ability to do "2 things at once." The performance of either task alone is relatively well preserved, but a decrement in performance of one task occurs when a second task is added.[13] Impairment of divided attention is greater when tasks are very similar (e.g. two verbal tasks, as compared to one that is verbal and one that is motor) or when performance of the tasks depends on the same brain areas. Most commonly, this function of cognition is associated with the top of the vertical axis as part of the frontal lobe executive functions. It is impaired with lesions of the frontal lobe, the corpus callosum,[19] especially in the frontal area,[20] "diffuse" brain damage, such as in head injury,[21] and perhaps has a greater association with lesions in the right hemisphere.[16] Disorders of divided attention can be inferred from history: Patients may complain that they cannot listen to music and simultaneously read, write, or draw. At work, a teacher may complain that he or she cannot lecture, write on the board, and be conscious of student activity all at once. Formal measurement tools are not available.

Vigilance

Vigilance is the ability to sustain attention on a discrete set of stimuli while ignoring other distracting external stimuli (e.g., noise in the next room) or internal stimuli (e.g., thoughts of the weekend during work). When vigilance is disrupted, the disorder is called distractibility. Like divided attention, this function is part of the executive functions of the frontal lobe; lesions in the dorsolateral frontal lobe, especially on the right,[101] corpus callosum,[19] and medial pathways cause distractibility. A distractible patient will answer questions posed by someone in another conversation, fail to respond to a stimulus after a long waiting period, or have a decline in performance of a task sustained over time. For two similar tasks, performance on one will be greater if the patient has more interest in that task. Performance is very sensitive to the complexity of the task. Impairments of vigilance are seen as part of idiopathic attention deficit disorder.

Vigilance can be tested by asking a patient to indicate by tapping the table whenever the letter "A" is heard as the examiner repeats a list of letters at a rate of one per second:[22]

L T P E A O A I C T D A L A A

A N I A B F S A M R Z E O A D

P A K L A U C J T O E A B A A

Z Y F M U S A H E V A A R A T

The stimulus "A" appears with greater than random frequency. Errors are virtually never made on this test by normals. More than two omissions (failing to identify an "A") are indicative of inattention. Two errors of commission (indicating by tapping that the letter "A" was heard when it wasn't said) are indicative of impulsivity. Perseveration and periods of continued tapping regardless of which target stimulus is given are abnormal even if they occur only once.

The assessment of attention, therefore is a measure of how well a patient may be able to focus and sustain focus for the subtests of cognition to come. It is important to establish integrity or impairment of the attention system before administering tasks in other axes (e.g., language in the lateral axis) so that poor performance on a task can be correctly attributed to a language disorder and not an attention disorder. Though attention deficits exist as idiopathic disorders, they often co-exist with deficits in arousal and contribute to the behavioral aberrations of delirium or metabolic encephalopathy.

Memory

How is memory related to alertness or alerting? A record of past experience can serve as a cue for interpreting the present. Consider a caveman hunting for mastodon. The first time the hunter approaches the animal head on, he is mauled and perhaps goes hungry because the hunt cannot be completed. With memory, the unpleasant record of prior experience rouses thinking about different hunting techniques so that injury and starvation can be avoided. This function of cognition aids in survival. It not only helps save the body, it preserves the soul. Memory provides records of who one is and what one has done. Memory disorders lead to behaviors that endanger patients. A coffeepot left boiling on a stove burner eventually could cause a house fire. Lack of knowledge about past experience leads to faulty judgment in making financial decisions. Identity is lost in amnestic disorders. Amnestics cannot recollect memories about their likes and dislikes or who is family. They cannot form relations or relationships; they live for the moment in a "perpetual present."

Types of Memory

Memory can be conceived of as a continuous record of an organism's experience. Though the molecular and cellular processes underlying memory are ancient and identical across species from insects to humans, it is functionally diverse to embody the whole of human experience.[23] Memory is not a unitary phenomenon.[24] Like a library, it contains stacks, organized logically and chronologically. Shelves contain yearbooks; references to an individual's experience over time, called long-term memory, are arranged so that the most recent year is the most recent book on the shelf. Long-term data related to sensory experiences—material specific memory—are shelved according to Brodmann's number in the appropriate sensory cortex. Less permanent information can be displayed on computer terminal screens for minutes, short-term memory, hours, middle-term memory, or in files that can be retrieved days later with the option for printouts to long-term memory, called anesthesia resistant memory. Data can be stored in the form of words like books in the left hemisphere, verbal memory, or in the form of images like videotapes in the right hemisphere, visuospatial memory. Information can be collated, unedited in the form of eidetic or photographic memory, or it can be filtered and consciously associated with other sensory, motor, and emotional funds of information like in a computer search as cognitive memory using the limbic-cortical circuit. Files that become associated arbitrarily due to frequent use are linked as habit memory; they require no cognitive or conscious association and are therefore controlled by subcortical, subconscious striatal circuitry. They are the foundations for more complex, purposeful behaviors, but because they are subconscious, they aren't remembered. That is why events from infancy and early childhood are not recalled. In addition to the content of memory, its location must be committed to a map; spatial memory mediated by the hippocampus permits memories to have location in space as well as time.

Anatomy of Memory: Material Specific

If memory is not one phenomenon, the anatomy and physiology of it must not be unitary. Memory is the sum of a cascade of processes beginning with a sensory stimulus.[25] Sensory information reaches the cortex and is processed in areas of the brain specific for each stimulus: occipital cortex for vision, temporal cortex for audition, parietal cortex for touch, insular cortex for taste, and inferior frontal cortex for smell.

The sensory cortex is arranged for serial and parallel processing of the stimuli it receives. (See the discussion on the horizontal axis for concepts related to the sensory cortex). Highly processed sensory stimuli from the sensory cortex are transmitted to the limbic structures: the amygdala and hippocampus in the medial temporal lobe. Each structure contributes equally to the formation of new learning termed recognition memory. Recognition memory is the ability to consciously recognize what has been sensed before. The amnesia that results from lesions to the amygdala and hippocampus is graded in severity depending on the extent of damage to the two structures. Each structure substitutes for the other in recognition memory, but if both are lesioned bilaterally, amnesia is anterograde, affecting learning for all new information presented since the time of the lesion, global, affecting all sensory information, and severe, not improving with semantic or phonemic cues.

Amygdala: Sensory Associative Memory: In addition to recognition memory, the amygdala is specialized for sensory associative memory.[26] The result of associative memory is the ability to link the sight of a flower to its smell, or the pain of a fire to the smell of its smoke. If the amygdala is bilaterally injured, memories still form of the smell or taste or touch of an object, but the sight of an object would not conjure up the other sensory memories of the object, such as smell, taste, or feel. Hippocampal lesions would only partially affect sensory associative recall; performance on sensory association tasks remains about 90% accurate. A clinical manifestation of amygdala dysfunction exists as the Klüver-Bucy syndrome.[27] First described in monkeys, the syndrome consists of constant, seemingly purposeless manipulation, tasting, and smelling of objects. Without sensory association functions of the amygdala, when monkeys feel an object, they cannot conjure up how it tastes, so they lick it, and once licked, they cannot associate that with its smell, so they sniff it. Therefore the object is handled with each sense in isolation.

Amygdala: Emotional Association: In Klüver-Bucy syndrome, monkeys also display inappropri-

ate reactions to objects; they don't avoid objects previously associated with pain or gravitate to those associated with reward. Even in the case of the caveman, it is obvious that avoidance of mauling was not simply a rational decision, but an emotional one. Emotions influence learning; they help provide the filter or "significance" to the indiscriminate jumble of incoming sensory information. Not all incoming sensory stimuli is recorded permanently. Part of the decision about which information should be inscribed permanently is based on the strength of the emotional association attached to the stimulus.[28] The amygdala helps in the selective attention and inscription of emotionally charged events by coordinating sensory associations with data from the hypothalamus regarding emotional state. Anatomically, this is accomplished by reciprocal amygdala connections first to the hypothalamus and then to the S3 sensory cortex. The release of endorphins from amygdala nerve terminals in the S3 cortex is associated with strengthening of the memory trace.

Amygdala and the Role of Reward: The link of the amygdala to the hypothalamus also explains enhanced learning in the presence of a reward.[28] Monkeys learn to identify neutral objects faster if the neutral object is associated with a food reward. Associative learning could still occur, though, even in the absence of a reward; it would just proceed more slowly and require a greater number of trials. Complaints of poor memory and effortful memory in depressed patients could be related to lack of endorphin-enhanced associative learning.

Hippocampus and Spatial Memory: Just as the amygdala specializes in certain memory tasks, so does the hippocampus. Whereas the amygdala receives sensory input related to the identity of an object, the hippocampus receives inputs related to the spatial location of an object, termed spatial memory.[29] Spatial memory is formed by a pathway from the visual cortex to the hippocampus that carries information related to object location.[30] Lesions of the hippocampus impair the ability to determine where an object is located, where it was seen, or how one traveled to see it.

Amnesia does not only occur with lesions of the limbic system's amygdala and hippocampus. Projections from the limbic system to dorsomedial thalamus, mamillary bodies, and prefrontal cortex cause amnesia as well.

Anatomy of Memory: Chronologic

Memory not only has sensory and spatial attributes, but also contains the variable of time.[23] "Immediate memory," the immediate repetition of information, is more precisely a measure of attention or concentration than memory. After immediate memory, chronological divisions of memory occur for short-term recall, medium-term recall, anesthesia resistant recall, and long-term recall. Acquisition of memory into long-term stores must follow this chronological sequence. Long-term memory is permanently stored information or an engram, which is the result of a physical change in molecules and cellular connections that is very resistant to disruption and persists for years.

The cAMP System: The chemical system that parallels the clinical sequential development of long-term memory is the cyclic AMP (cAMP) system. This system creates energy for protein synthesis. Early events in the cAMP system are responsible for short-term and medium-term memory and later events for long-term memory. Each phase is under the influence of its own discrete set of genes and therefore the expression of these memory phases is dependent on gene-directed protein synthesis. The purpose of protein synthesis is to form, strengthen, or increase the number of synapses between cellular arrays that are the physical connections that underlie memory associations. The characteristics of molecular activity parallel clinical features of memory. Short- and medium-term memory genes are easily activated and as a consequence these forms of memory are easily acquired. Long-term memory is less easily acquired; as any student knows, the best recall for exams occurs after repeated studying with breaks in between. Cramming, or massed practice without breaks allows acquisition of memory for several hours, reaching the status of anesthesia resistant memory, but these memories are not resistant to forgetting. Facts are generally lost the next day.

The gene underlying long-term memory encodes a protein known as CREB: cAMP responsive element-binding protein. Activator and repressor forms of the protein exist. Activator forms enhance long-term memory acquisition or repress long-term memory acquisition. During studying, both forms seem to be equally active; during rest, however, repressor activity falls more rapidly than activator activity and so there is relatively more activation of CREB during rest. Rest is necessary after a drill because time is needed for activator proteins to increase to the critical functional levels that ultimately produce the proteins associated with the formation of long-term memory. In long-term memory cellular arrays become "crystallized" intelligence from many protein-based synapses.

Memory and Development

Why should long-term memory acquisition be effortful and require repeated exposure to the information? Early in life, this memory is actually less effortful; children easily acquire facts in almost a photographic or eidetic manner. Sometimes this eidetic memory persists into adulthood and these individuals can memorize and repeat entire phone books or each word of *War and Peace*. This memory, however, is not functional. A collection of facts does not make meaningful memory. Mnemonists who recite tables, facts, or contrived mathematical formulas cannot combine the facts and associate them with times or people. Their minds are like the movie room where all the takes of each scene run in order, unedited so that the significance and power of the whole story are lost. After childhood, when there is an initial eidetic acquisition of a basic foundation of factual knowledge, memories are subject to filters that help sort out what information is significant to remember. The first test of significance is whether the information occurs repeatedly. Therefore, the cAMP system evolved to encode into permanent memory only the information that repeats enough to stimulate activator proteins. The second test looks for connections with intense emotions. Therefore, there are connections between the amygdala and the sensory cortex. Finally, coordinated memories are more efficient than a collection of unrelated facts about an object. The amygdala coordinates sensory data regarding objects and people and the hippocampus provides spatial information.

Clinical Disorders of Memory

Amnesias can result from lesions in diverse sites of the brain and can vary in their behavioral expression (Table 12–2).

Clinical correlates to the anatomy of memory occur. Rubenstein-Taybi syndrome causes loss of the ability to form long-term memory due to the absence of a CREB binding protein.[31] In Alzheimer's disease (AD), degeneration of the basal forebrain system and association areas (S3) that mediate the formation of memory at first causes a short-term

Table 12–2. Memory Disorders

Disorder	Anatomy	Type of Memory Loss
Anoxia (cardiac or pulmonary arrest, carbon monoxide)	Diffuse; Hippocampus bilateral	Global anterograde; recognition better than recall; Mild retrograde
Herpes simplex encephalitis	Hippocampus, bilateral	Global anterograde, defective spatial memory, retrograde amnesia, significant
Posterior cerebral artery infarctions	Hippocampus, bilateral, fornix, mammillary bodies	Global anteograde, rapid rate of forgetting
Paramedian artery infarction	Dorsomedial thalamic nuclei	Global anterograde, severe; normal forgetting; encoding by superficial features
Traumatic brain injury	Frontal and temporal poles	Global anterograde and retrograde amnesia, severe
Temporal lobectomy and temporal lobe epilepsy	Left or right inferomedial temporal lobe and varying degrees of hippocampus and amygdala	Material specific (verbal or visuospatial); severity proportional to amount of hippocampus removed; if preserved side is sclerotic, can be severe; global anterograde
Chronic alcoholism	Third ventricular degeneration; Dorsomedial thalamic nuclei	Greater visuospatial than verbal long term deficits; mild to moderate in severity
Wernicke-Korsakoff (thiamine deficiency; idiopathic or acquired in alcoholism or poor nutrition)	Periventricular damage; Dorsomedial thalamic nuclei mammillary bodies	Temporally graded retrograde amnesia; Global anterograde
Anterior communicating artery aneurysms	Basal forebrain; septal nuclei; nucleus accumbens, substantia innominata	Retrograde and anterograde; confabulation; material specific depending on side of aneurysm; may not know that they know; (defect in declarative memory) severity varies by individual and recovery can occur; benefit from cueing
Alzheimer's disease (early)	Neurofibrillary tangles sequentia involving the hippocampus, amygdala, temporal, parietal, and frontal association areas; a disconnection syndrome of association areas from frontal attentional systems	Memory loss earliest predictor of Alzheimer's disease; Abnormal acquisition or material not helped by semantic cueing; Abnormal delayed recall
Normal aging (typical)		Acquisition of material declines linearly across decades; learning acquisition enhanced by semantic encoding; declarative memory or free recall impaired, but semantically cueable; delayed recall preserved

memory loss and then a chronologic loss of long-term memory, akin to removing yearbooks off the shelf, one by one.[31,33] Initially, patients with Alzheimer's fail to make new memories or learn new information, so they repeat questions or stories. The loss of short- and medium-term recall leads to recollections about remaining frames of reference, past memories. As past memories face and frames of references reach further into the past, mistakes in interpreting the present occur; patients will look at their spouses and believe that they are their parents. Young children will be misinterpreted as siblings. Patients won't recognize their own homes and continuously ask to go home, referring to their childhood homes. In individuals destined to have Alzheimer's, there may be metabolic abnormalities in the regions associated with Alzheimer's disease decades before symptoms or cognitive signs occur.[34–36] In these individuals, a continuum of cognitive function can be defined from normal, to mildly impaired to demented and each point may have markers in isolated but predictive memory tasks, neuroradiological findings, and distribution of neuropathology.[37,38]

In typical aging, attention span, long-term memory, syntax, semantics, comprehension, and processing of simple perceptions remain stable. Executive functions, acquisition and retrieval of memory (cueing and recognition memory better than free recall), naming, fluency, complex perceptions, and problem solving are mildly decreased.[39] There is dependence on associating new semantic features; for example, a rote list of words: "bat," "watermelon," and "beach" would be more easily remembered if categorized as things related to summer. In Alzheimer's, the memory deficit is different; it involves poor delayed recall as well as poor acquisition, and lack of benefit from cueing or semantically encoding information. The concentration of pathology of Alzheimer's in the hippocampus, amygdala, medial temporal lobe, and neocortex correlates with the qualitative and quantitative memory changes of Alzheimer's. In normal aging, although the neurofibrillary tangles (NFT) and senile plaques (SP) occur, they are concentrated in hippocampus and amygdala, and not found in the neocortex or in the numbers seen with AD.

Testing

The aim of bedside memory testing is characterization of memory disorders into deficits over time: short-term versus long-term loss; material specific deficits: verbal versus visuospatial; and severity: effect of phonemic and semantic cueing on re-trieval. The testing yields anatomical information on limbic-cortical system, left versus right hemisphere, and evidence for partial versus total involvement of memory substations respectively.

A patient is given a sheet of paper with 3 words randomly paired with 3 meaningless pictures, asked to copy the information, and remember it for later recall.[40] To prevent rehearsal as soon as the patient completes the writing and drawing, another demanding task is given. After several delays of 5 to 60 minutes, the patient can be asked to recall the information—write the words and reproduce the drawings of the figures. If free recall, unaided reproduction of the stimuli cannot be done, cues as to the category of the words can be given. If recall still fails after semantic cueing, phonemic cueing, using the first sound of the target words, can be given. Finally, if neither cue stimulates remembering, a recognition trial is performed: for each of the 3 words, 3 choices are provided. Alternatively, a second sheet of paper with 10 choices, including the 3 target words and figures is shown, and the patient is asked to identify which stimuli he or she saw before.

Variations of this testing include oral administration of 3 words and oral recognition tasks after cueing plus co-administration of a complex drawing for immediate and delayed reproduction. If cueing and recognition tasks fail to cue memory either for verbal or visuospatial material, the patient is said to have an amnestic syndrome. This is typical for disorders involving bilateral limbic circuits, as in Alzheimer's disease. Failure to recall only verbal or visuospatial information may point to a focal lesion of one hemisphere, such as in stroke, tumor, or malformation. Memory disorders aided by cueing are more typical of subcortical dementias, such as those seen with Parkinson's disease, multiple sclerosis, multiple infarcts, spinocerebellar degenerations, or in normal aging.[41] The most common memory disorders seen clinically are anterograde; they affect new learning, but leave past memories intact. Retrograde memory disorders (loss of information chronologically backward from the time of the lesion) occur commonly in moderate to severe head injuries, anterior communicating artery aneurysms, and Wernicke-Korsakoff syndrome.[42] In Wernicke-Korsakoff, the retrograde amnesia can be persistent, but in head injury, the extent of loss shrinks from months to years over time to involve minutes to days before the insult.[43] Testing can be done by first interviewing a family member or close friend regarding 5 to 8 significant past events encompassing the period of retrograde amnesia plus 2 or 3 extra years. The informant's memory of the events must be detailed. From this battery of information, the examiner constructs open-ended questions. The patient is asked to recall the events first unaided, then cued, such as by holiday: "Christmas 1994."

Affect

Why are feelings alerting? Emotions are motivating; when we feel, we are moved. The root word for emotion, "motus," to move out, implies movement. Movement can be in the form of facial expression, gesture, readiness for action, thought, or as discussed above, a hormone and chemical cascade to consolidate memory. The subjective experience and outward expression of emotion is under the control of the limbic system, striatum, and right frontal lobes.[44] Observations of patient mood states, facial expression, gesture, emotional intonation, and prosody help in localizing disorders.

Flat Facies

Depression: A masked, fixed, and staring expression characterizes "flat" facies. Depression is the most commonly associated affective disorder with a flat facies. Psychomotor retardation describes the accompanying lack of spontaneous movement and thought that a depressed affect causes. A bedside measure of depression is self-report; ask a patient if he or she feels depressed. Vegetative signs, poor sleep, poor appetite, and low energy are characteristic of primary depressions, but the depression of degenerative diseases may not include these signs or the signs may occur because of cognitive decline.[45] Degenerative disease not associated with obvious signs of cognitive decline is sometimes heralded by a first-time depression at age 50 or more, which is uncharacteristic of the idiopathic primary affective disorders. Tearfulness, especially if repetitive more than five times during the interview and if brief, and stereotyped, may present a pseudobulbar affect rather than an expression of depression.[46] Depression can affect performance on other cognitive tests. Typically, in primary depression, effort is poor; speeded tasks, such as performance measures of the WAIS-R, linearly decline with the severity of depression; and answers of "I don't know" occur in response to examiner's questions. The cognitive deficit of early Alzheimer's disease, complicated by depression yields a patient who is struggling for answers to questions, confabulates, or answers questions incorrectly, and cognitive performance doesn't improve when the

depression is treated and resolved. Inventories of depression, such as the Beck Inventory Screen for Depression, can identify the presence of depression in a patient who may also have cognitive complaints. To differentiate the depression of dementia from the dementia of depression, the serotonin reuptake inhibitor antidepressants (SSRIs) (Prozac, Zoloft, Paxil, and Effexor) can be given for 3 to 6 months and then cognitive function retested and compared to the initial results. If mood improved and cognition didn't, dementia can be inferred. Post-stroke depression is physiologic and not related to the burden of the somatic disability from the stroke. Loss of interest, rather than sadness, is more characteristic of post-stroke depression. In the acute stroke period, depression is associated with anterior lesions of the left hemisphere.[47] Parietooccipital strokes of the right hemisphere acutely cause depression;[48] cerebral blood flow studies reveal inverse relationships of blood flow and degree of depression. Improved mood increases blood flow. Acute depression may subside spontaneously; if it is still present after 3 months, treatment with SSRIs are preferable to tricyclic antidepressants (TCAs) to avoid the anticholinergic effects on memory from the tricyclics.[49] Depression persisting one year after stroke is likely to be intransigent; combined SSRIs and TCAs or electroconvulsive shock therapy (ECT) and sympathomimetics (Ritalin) may be needed.[46,50]

Flat Facies without Depression: Facies can be flat without depression. In these disorders, patients deny depression. Right frontal lobe injury leads to an expressive aprosodia, which causes an expressionless face and voice, and lack of gesturing.[51] Subjectively, the patient may report mood changes, but they are not revealed on the face. In Parkinson's disease and other extrapyramidal disorders, hypophonia, a whispered voice, and bradykinesia and bradyphrenia (slow movements and responses) adjoin the expressionless face. Abulia consists of flat facies with an accompanying disorder of extreme apathy and lack of motivation and initiative. In abulia, motivation is so impaired that a person who is asked "Will you please pass the salt?" may only answer "Yes." and not pass the shaker. This is typical of frontal dementias of the non-Alzheimer's type,[52] head injury,[53] or tumors of the frontal lobe, such as butterfly gliomas.[16]

Pseudobulbar Affect

In contrast to a stable low level of expression, the patient with pseudobulbar affect experiences sudden, exaggerated, or inappropriate laughing or crying whose intensity is not matched to internal mood state. The episodes are triggered by trivial stimuli, such as the mention of a sad book. Movements are stereotyped and brief, lasting from 30 seconds to 1 to 2 minutes. Patients are often embarrassed by the outbursts, which may reoccur continuously throughout the day and can lead to social withdrawal and depression. Pathologic crying is more characteristic of bilateral lesions of the corticobulbar tracts of the hemispheres, whereas pathologic laughing is more common with bilateral lesions of the corticobulbar tracts in the brainstem near their terminus in the facial nuclei.[46] Multi-infarct dementia or subcortical lacunar states differently affect the white matter of the frontal lobes because the greatest volume of white matter occurs in this area and therefore pseudobulbar affect involves more inappropriate crying than laughing. The cerebellar degenerations, the olivopontocerebellar atrophies, affect brainstem white matter predominantly and therefore create more pathological laughing. In addition to counseling and educating the patient and family regarding the mechanisms behind the behaviors, low doses of Elavil (amitriptyline) from 25 to 50 mg may help diminish the frequency of the episodes.[54]

Testing

Classification of abnormal affects requires observation of facial expression, amount and appropriateness of gesturing and spontaneous movement, direct questioning regarding mood state, listening for monoprosody and hypophonia, and reports from family members regarding the patient's ability to both understand and express feelings to others. For aprosodia, patients can be tested on the comprehension, expression, and imitation of emotion in sentences in a manner similar to the simple survey of language in these domains. An emotionally neutral sentence, such as "I went to the movies" is used as the universal stimulus in three tasks:[55]

1. *Imitation:* The examiner varies the intonation pattern in the sentence to indicate anger, happiness, or sadness. The patient is asked to repeat the sentence exactly as the examiner says it.
2. *Comprehension:* The examiner again varies the intonation pattern in the sentence to indicate anger, happiness, or sadness. The patient is asked to label the emotion evoked

by the recitation of the sentence as happy, angry, or sad.
3. *Expression:* The examiner asks the patient to recite the sentence to indicate happiness, sadness, or anger.

Aprosodia is classified as motor if imitation and expression are faulty, sensory if imitation and comprehension are faulty, and finally, as global if imitation, comprehension, and expression are all impaired.

Executive Functions

The executive functions, or frontal lobe functions, are the behaviors associated with the combined circuitry of the top of the vertical axis with the anterior or motor portion of the horizontal axis. The frontal lobes help in execution of action; to act with motive is motor in nature. A lack of initiative leads to no action or the condition of abulia mentioned above. Once initiative is established, the frontal lobes help with the channeling of arousal, attention, emotion, and recollections to:

1. *Focus:* narrow the scope of activity
2. *Sustain:* maintain the activity for the appropriate amount of time
3. *Shift:* change activities when appropriate

If these functions fail, a person is said to be tangential, distractible, or perseverative, respectively. These areas not only focus on what to do, but when; they add an element of timing. In the English language, the importance of *speed* to intelligence is reflected in the words used to describe intellect. A smart person is "quick," "quick-witted," "adroit," or "nimble." A stupid person is "slow," "retarded," "cloddish," or "lame-brained." Speed and action are combined to form aptitude. Timing also requires impulse control. The patient with Pick's disease who spontaneously grabs a partner and dances and sings in the office exhibits a lack of impulse control known as *disinhibition.* The frontal lobes are inhibitors of actions that otherwise might occur reflexively in response to environmental cues.[56] An extreme disinhibition of exploring behavior occurs in frontal degenerations called *utilization behavior.*[52] These patients pick up any object in their field of vision and purposelessly manipulate them. In Alzheimer's disease, a patient may pick at clothing or strings on the floor to such a continuous degree that relatives have formed large fiber balls from the threads.

Testing

The measurement of executive function is initially achieved by monitoring behavior during the clinical interview. Lack of initiative is suggested by family comments that a person is "withdrawn," "lazy," or "just sits there" and confirmed by the observation that the patient doesn't initiate comments and answers only when asked. When distractible, family members report that patients do not finish tasks, thoughts, or maintain conversations. During the examination, a patient may respond to questions being asked of someone in the next bed, cease a task when other activities occur in the room, and ramble in conversation. Perseveration of thought appears as the repeated mention of a story or concern or a perseveration of action in the repetitive arranging or rearranging of clothes or objects.[57] During the examination, perseverative patients respond with an action that was required of an earlier task. For example, a person who earlier was asked to count the fingers seen in peripheral vision will continue to count the examiner's fingers when asked to just follow the finger for testing of extraocular movements. A feeling of impatience with a patient may arise from slowness of response or movement: bradyphrenia or bradykinesia. Disinhibited patients eat with their hands, grab food off of others' plates, solicit sexually in public, or make "blunt," "opinionated," or "outspoken" comments. During the interview, questions may be answered almost before the query is finished. This manifestation of disinhibition, called automaticity, may cause a person to answer with an unintended response, for example, "Yes" instead of "No."

Tests of executive function are divided into whether impersistence occurs with movements or with thoughts. Movements of the eyelids, extraocular muscles, tongue, and upper extremities are rated on the following criteria.[13,58]

1. *Speed:* The capacity to blink, perform saccades, move tongue in and out or side to side, and tap rapidly with hands palm side down for 5 seconds.
2. *Persistence:* The capacity to sustain a steady rate of movement for 20 seconds.

Perseveration is measured with rapid alternating or sequential movements. Once weakness and ataxia are ruled out, the following bedside tests can be performed:[13,59]

1. *Rapid pronation and supination:* One at a time, each hand alternately pronates and supinates over a flat surface, 15 alternations in 10 seconds. Note how many alternations are accomplished in the 10 seconds and whether performance is slow or clumsy.
2. *Alternating hand positions:* The right hand is placed palm down on a flat surface with fingers clenched, while the left hand lies next to it with fingers open. The patient is asked to shift rapidly between clenching and unclenching the fingers of each hand so that one hand is flat while the other is clenched for 20 shifts in 10 seconds. Note how many shifts are accomplished and if performance is slow, clumsy, or if clenching positions are simultaneous instead of alternating.
3. *Tandem reciprocal movements:* This procedure is from Luria's Neuropsychological Investigation.[60] By demonstration and not by explicit verbal instruction, the examiner indicates that the patient is to hold up two fingers when the examiner holds up one finger and the patient is to hold up one finger when the examiner holds up two. A response set is established by holding up the same number of fingers for several trials and then suddenly shifting to a different number of fingers to see if the patient shifts response accordingly. Administer 11 trials, shifting after every second response: one finger, one finger, two fingers, two fingers, one finger, etc., and then administering a second block of 16 trials in which each block shifts after the third response. When errors are made, quickly correct, "No, you should have held up two fingers" and then continue. One or both hands may be tested. The number of correct responses in 27 trials is recorded separately for each hand. Two types of errors are noted: slavist imitation of the examiner's movement and failing to shift to a new response when the examiner shifts to a different number of fingers. In normals, only one or two errors are expected.

For measuring speed, persistence, and shifting abilities in thinking, the following tasks can be performed:[40]

1. *Writing the alphabet:* The patient is asked to write the alphabet as fast as possible. The time to perform the task is recorded. Ability to complete the task is a measure of persistence and the time to complete it.
2. *Shifting figures:* The patient is asked to copy the following designs that vary by periodicity or shape:

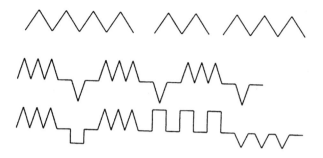

The ability to make the correct shifts in copying the designs is a measure of the ability to shift; a failure to change designs indicates perseveration.

Although these tests are specifically designed to measure executive functions, if disorders of these functions are present, patients may make errors on subsequent tests that are due to perseveration. For example, on a test for finger gnosis, the person may respond with a number instead of the name of the finger, which would represent a perseverative response from an earlier test of counting fingers for visual field determination.

Delirium

Phenomenology of Delirium

Diffuse dysfunction of the vertical axis causes a predictable set of behaviors known as delirium.[3,61] To illustrate these behaviors, consider the story of *A Nightmare in My Closet* by Marcel Mercer.[62] It is night. The boy misinterprets the shadows behind his closet door—an illusion. He exhibits mild paranoia; he is afraid to look back at his closet as he walks to his bed. The paranoia escalates to a paranoid delusion; he believes something. A MONSTER, is after him. The delusion is still environmentally dependent; it appears in the area of a blowing curtain.

He switches on the light, and the monster still remains. No longer environmentally dependent, this figment of his imagination is a hallucination. The appearance of the monster fosters agitation, anger, and aggression. He attempts to shoot it. Moods spontaneously normalize and he calms, inviting the monster to sleep with him. The lights are again switched off. As he once again looks back at the closet, another monster appears. One can expect renewed hostile encounters with the monster and sleeplessness, a cycling or fluctuation in perception.

Delirium occurs as a result of a defect in arousal, a function at the basis of the vertical axis and basic for all other aspects of cognition (Table 12–3). As a result of a diminished level of consciousness, therefore, a diffuse disturbance in vertical axis function appears.

The persistence of the need to go home in delirium and the attending disorders of perception are best illustrated by the story *Harold and the Purple Crayon,* by Crockett and Johnson.[63] Harold is an insomniac. He is sent to his bedroom, but cannot sleep. His attention waxes, he takes his crayon and is drawn to images on the wall. He's delirious. He draws himself out of his room; his mind wanders. As he outlines the train tracks, he loses perspective. Perceptions are altered.

Increasingly, his drawings loom large, become out of hand, and his image of self diminishes. Objects take on frightening proportions. He believes that he's fallen into a hole and cannot get back home. Simple persecutory delusions have developed. The pictures become real and he addresses the birds and flowers. He hallucinates. A lucid interval appears, a sign of fluctuation. For a moment he realizes that "This is only a picture" and crosses out the drawing.

As delirium improves, he regains perspective: "I am back to my usual size." His sense of self returns as he draws himself in the mirror.

Lessening of fear occurs as he realizes that he is "back home" in his own room. But delirium heightens again as he picks up his purple crayon to draw more pictures.

Management of Delirium

This story contains all the elements of the behaviors of delirium. Like Harold, the problem of delirium is most likely to occur at night, a phenomenon known as sundowning.[45,64] Maintaining strong lighting, orienting patients with familiar objects, food, treats, or activities such as prayer and diminishing distracters such as TV and noisy grandchildren help to lessen anxiety and fear. Avoiding activities at this time, such as bathing, dressing, or going to sleep prevents the triggering of anger. Establishing sleep hygiene helps the patient to understand that the bed is for sleeping. Wandering may appear for many reasons and it is important to ask the patient where he or she is going and why. Sometimes a patient is looking for the bathroom and is too disoriented to find it. Sometimes a patient is bored, like Harold. In many cases, a reason cannot be ascertained, and it is best to safeguard against leaving the house or falling down the stairs by installing baffle locks, locks in unusual locations, such as at the top of the main exit doors, and

Table 12–3. The Cognitive Disorder of Delirium

Arousal	Fluctuates: sleepiness and periods of perfect alertness alternate. Alteration in sleep-wake cycles: daytime sleeping and nighttime wakefulness
Attention	Distractibility: unable to complete thoughts, tasks, movements.
Memory	Short-term memory: impaired Confabulation: defects in recall filled in with any available information
Affect	Fear, paranoia: may not be directed at an identifiable source. Aggression: usually in response to hallucinations or delusions. Apathy, Abulia: more common in the elderly.
Executive functions	Distractibility Perseveration: leads to difficulty in distracting patients away from delusions and hallucinations. Bradykinesia, bradyphrenia
All other axes	All axes are dependent on the vertical axis, and when it is disrupted, so are the others.
Horizontal	Motor: restless or inert; poor sequencing abilities for movements. Sensory: distortions in vision, touch, and hearing in the form of hallucinations, delusions, and illusions.
Lateral	Language: anomia, extended jargon (fragments of sentences or meaningless combinations of sentences); not aphasia. Visuospatial: disorientation to place; wanting to "go home," even if at home.

on doors to stairways or unsafe rooms. The Alzheimer's and Related Disorders Association Safe Return Program catalogues information on patient appearance, caregivers, and home so that local police stations can return wandering patients safely to their homes. Regular physical activity, such as walking, can lessen the need to wander and improve sleep. Agitation or simple oppositional behavior such as shouting "NO" to a request to change clothes is not amenable to medication. It's best to move on to a different activity and return to the original one later.

Other Delusional Behaviors

On the other hand, hallucinations and delusions do require treatment with antipsychotics.[65] In Alzheimer's disease, the most common delusions are simple persecutory: Things and people are "after" patients. When lost items can't be found, the delusions take the form of fear that someone is burglarizing the house or specific people may be accused of stealing. In the Othello syndrome, delusional jealousy takes the form of accusations that the spouse is unfaithful. Although only 30% of Alzheimer's patients exhibit these delusions in the mid-stages of their disease, and even though they are temporary, lasting 6 months to a year, they are the most disturbing behavior to families besides incontinence.[66] Their appearance often hastens placement of the patient in a nursing home. The early appearance of delusions and paranoia before pronounced deficits in memory and other areas of cognition in patients without a prior history of psychiatric disease may herald Lewy body dementia or frontal dementia of the non-Alzheimer's type.[67] Acute, episodic confusion without alteration in level of consciousness and Parkinson's-like features to the motor exam also suggest Lewy body dementia in a patient with isolated delusions. Parkinson's-like side effects occur from antipsychotic treatment and therefore the lowest possible doses and the least likely antipsychotics to cause these side effects are chosen. Traditionally, Haldol is prescribed, 0.5 mg twice daily or every hour to a maximum of 5 mg until the aberrant behavior lessens. Two newer antipsychotics, Risperdal and Clozaril, cause less Parkinson's side effects, but can cause insomnia and require monitoring for blood dyscrasias, respectively. Used judiciously, these medications may be the best choice for controlling hallucinations and agitation without compromising abilities to perform or participate in other activities. Delusions in the Capgras' syndrome cause patients to believe that there is an exact duplicate for a person or a place, and the one before them is an imposter.[68] They usually insist on being taken to the "real" place or person. Although described in Alzheimer's disease,[69] it is associated with vascular lesions, endocrine disorders, inflammatory disorders, head injury, and tumors, especially of the right frontal-parietal region.[70] Multiple imposters appear in the Fregoli syndrome.[71] In epilepsy, a person can appear to take on the physical appearance of others (intermetamorphosis) or form an exact double (heutoscopy).[72] In mania, delusions of grandiosity, that someone is or can be the president, a king or queen, or a millionaire, can be combined with de Clermbault syndrome, a delusion that one is secretly loved by another. Infestations of bugs crawling from the walls, on the floors, or under the skin occurs in delusions of infestation. Alcohol withdrawal, sedative drug withdrawal or intoxication, infections, and other metabolic disturbances cause these latter delusions. One particular class of drugs is most likely to create the disorder: the anticholinergics. Antihistamines, antipsychotics, antidepressants, and many other medications have anticholinergic properties and are more likely to cause delusions in patients who are already cognitively compromised. Acetylcholine, the neurotransmitter most associated with the vertical axis,[5] is necessary for the functioning of the entire vertical axis and disorders in which the chemical is diminished, such as Alzheimer's disease[73,74] or with the use of anticholinergics, not only delusions of infestations, but delirium is likely to occur.

LATERAL AXIS

The lateral axis, found anatomically along the longitudinal fissure, separates the two hemispheres of the cerebrum into left and right halves: "left brain" and "right brain." Left brain functions are language related or cognitive, analytical, and specialized for internal functions; right brain functions are visuospatial, gestalt, and specialized for external functions (Figure 12–5). The left brain dissects information and sequences it (temporal processing); the right brain integrates information and assembles it (spatial processing).[40] All the functions of the right brain can be codified as functions for dealing with the outside world and other people whereas the left brain processes information for our inner world, ourselves.

The left brain digests and interprets information; it "cuts nature up and organizes (it) into concepts."[75] Language clarifies mental tasks because the task can be broken down into verbal steps. Language can be thought of as a tool of analysis; words provide detail, fine tune a thought, and supply nuance. The thinking that involves language is of a different kind; it is the reasoned thinking of problem solving, telling stories, and planning strategies. It is rational, directed, logical, and propositional. It involves deductive thinking—solving problems by using a given set of rules, as in working out an arithmetic problem. The formal properties of language, syntax, and semantics are themselves results of temporal sequencing or deduction. Syntax is word order and sequencing. Semantics, the process of fitting a word to an idea, is the result of deductive reasoning through a semantic network (Figure 12–6). The left hemisphere is verbal, temporal, analytical, propositional, and deductive.

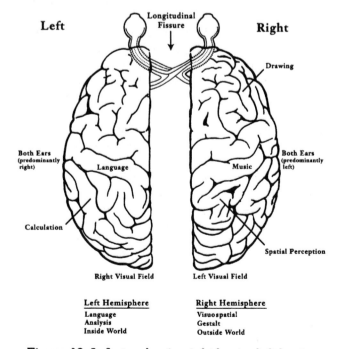

Figure 12–5. Lateral axis: right brain–left brain.

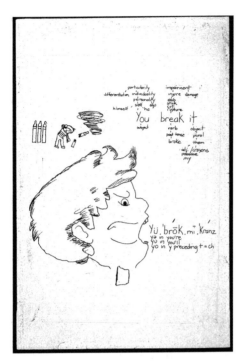

Figure 12–6. Thought, language, and speech: the semantic network and grammar.

Right brain thinking, on the other hand, is akin to the thinking beyond words of artists; composers "hear" the music they want to write, artists "see" their painting before the brush is on the canvas, and our language to explain our emotions in response to a beautiful painting or unpleasant incident is "hard to explain, beautiful beyond words." It is the hemisphere of emotion: communication of feeling, not rational thought. The comprehension and expression of emotion through changes in voice inflection, gestures, and facial expression (prosody) is mediated by the right hemisphere.[51] The musicality of voice that communicates emotion to others is closely related to the right hemisphere function of musical and nonlinguistic sound pattern recognition and production.[76,77] Aprosodia and amusia may both result from deficiencies in right hemisphere processing of pitch, harmony, timbre, and intensity that are components of voices, musical instruments, or tunes.[78,79] The left hemisphere, on the other hand, analyzes sounds for words and the temporally dependent characteristics of rhythm and melody recognition found in speech, lyrics, and environmental sounds.[80,81] A person with a right hemisphere lesion can't sing, but because the left hemisphere knows the words and rhythm, he can rap. The perception of faces is vital because humans interact with other humans and must recog-

nize and differentiate them. The right hemisphere is specialized for face recognition,[82] perhaps because the representation of faces is mainly based on a gestalt, an overall structure, that is not decomposed into individual parts.[83] Alexia, the disturbance of visual recognition of words, is mediated by the left hemisphere, because words must be decomposed into parts. Reading by the right hemisphere can be demonstrated, but it is executed by whole word recognition and has a high association with nouns and image ability—"visualness."[84,85] The visualness and gestalt functions of the right hemisphere are also reflected in its contribution to drawing and construction. Drawings of right parietal lesioned patients are disorganized into parts whereas simplification or lack of detail occurs in left hemispheric lesioned patients.[86–88] The right hemisphere contributes to storytelling and comprehension. The ability to determine plots, morals, and the contextual reference of words combined into paragraphs and stories are functions of thinking that involve relating individual parts to the whole.[89,90] The left hemisphere, in contrast, tells stories point by point, line by line. Inherent in right brain functioning is the role of space.[91] It is the predominant receptor and executor of left space, intrapersonal and extrapersonal, and a contributor with the left hemisphere to right space. The neglected space in right hemisphere lesions can be either real or imagined,[92] and independent for vision,[93] tactile stimuli,[94] eye and limb movements.[14] The disassociation of neglect or spatial disorientation across different sensory or motor functions suggests that spatial processing is a supramodal function. Right hemisphere contributions to movement are in directing aim or providing feedback about accuracy of spatial coordinates. The right hemisphere is spatial, paralinguistic, gestalt, and emotional.

Left Brain: Language, Analysis, and Internal Functions

Although the whole left hemisphere is specialized for language-related activities, it is subdivided by the horizontal axis into anterior motor and posterior sensory fields. Like any other function of the brain, language can be conceptualized as sensory, requiring input processes, and motor, requiring output processes. Instead of classifying language disorders by eponyms and lists of characteristics, the aphasias can be predicted by associating symptoms with the anatomy. For language, the motor and sensory fields are created by division of the left hemisphere into quarters by the central sulcus and sylvian fissure.

Anatomy of Language: Sensory Limb

Language processes follow a neuroanatomic sequence. The sensory or input limb begins with sound perception at the peripheral receptor, the cochlea. From the auditory nerve, sound is processed subcortically in way stations until it reaches the superior temporal gyrus or Heschl's gyrus, located in the sensory portion of the left hemisphere posterior to the line of the sylvian fissure and central sulcus. After elementary sound processing in the form of frequency and rate information, speech sounds are associated with meaning: semantic processing. In semantic processing, ideas are analyzed and refined until matched with a word that has the correct meaning and nuance. Language disorders in the sensory limb therefore either affect processing of speech sounds to cause word deafness, or associations of sound with meaning to cause a sensory or Wernicke's aphasia. Patients with disorders of sound perception cannot deduce meaning from incoming verbal information whether it is written or spoken. Faulty input leads to faulty output. The characteristic output disorder of Wernicke's aphasia is the formation of word errors known as paraphasias. These errors represent faults in the pathway between idea analysis and word-sound analysis. Either the incorrect word is chosen if the wrong node in the idea analysis pathway is selected or an incorrect sound or syllable is inserted into the word if the word-sound analysis is faulty. Idea analysis can be faulty in several ways: If no meaning can be derived from the target word, a neologism is formed; if a word with a meaning not related to the target word occurs, a random paraphasia is created; or if a word very closely related in meaning to the target word is chosen, a semantic paraphasia develops. If in the word-to-sound analysis a nonexistent word is chosen, a neologism is formed, but if only a single sound or syllable is in error, a literal or phonemic paraphasia occurs. In addition to faulty output in the formation of individual words, the meaning that is derived from whole sentences is defective. Wernicke's aphasics produce grammatically correct, but semantically meaningless utterances (e.g., "I went to the store so tomorrow she'll see me up the stairs"). Inputs to the Wernicke's area are not only from external sources but also from internal sources in the form of feedback about the accuracy of an utterance so that conscious adjustments in output can occur in case an expression is faulty. Wernicke's aphasics lose feedback or conscious

knowledge about their language. As a result, they cannot monitor the speed of speech and often speak at a hyperfluent rate of greater than 100 words per minute (normal = 50 to 100 words per minute) and appear confused as to why other people are not responding in a predictable way to their queries or comments.

Disorders of Language: Motor Limb

Disorders of language output begin with lesions in the frontal lobe, anterior to the line formed by the Sylvian fissure and central sulcus in the motor portion of the left hemisphere: the frontal operculum, the posterior portion of the inferior frontal gyrus or Broca's area, the subjacent white matter, and central sulcus. Overall output is reduced, reflected by terse, telegraphic speech at lower than normal speech rates of 5 to 7 words per utterance or less than 50 words per minute. The output program for speech is created by syntax: the sequencing and ordering of words and ideas into sentences, the creation of relationships between words because of their order in the sentence, or the use of special grammatical words that imply sequence, order, or relationship.[13] For a Broca's aphasic, there is no disruption in the perception of externally or internally produced words and the analysis of their meaning, but the arrangement of the nouns and verbs and the use of words that provide ordering or sequencing, such as articles, prepositions, conjunctions, auxiliary verbs, and words implying physical location or relation are disarranged. Though it may be clear that a Broca's aphasic is speaking about Tom and Joe in an altercation, he or she cannot use word order to indicate subject and object so that we may deduce who hit whom by the sequence. The telegraphic quality of speech occurs because of the omission of grammatical words. Language output from the frontal lobe, like motor output from the frontal lobe, is voluntary; it is the propositional speech or purposeful action that is initiated at will that is affected by lesions in these areas. There are connections to language output areas that bypass voluntary areas of motor speech output and therefore allow sparing of certain kinds of utterances. Emotional speech, expletives, and exclamations arise from limbic areas of the brain, regions outside the Broca's area, and are therefore commonly expressed, whereas a factual explanation of how a person feels cannot be stated. Iterative, stereotyped, automatic speech such as lists of days, months, and numbers, greetings, or habitual remarks are processed by habit motor areas near the basal ganglia and can be used by a Broca's aphasic to access a statement of fact that requires a specific date or number, by allowing a recitation of the list until the desired fact or number is reached. Though intonation and stress changes cannot be used to indicate grammatical constructs such as the end of a sentence or commas, the inflections used to communicate emotions are still intact because the right hemisphere processes the prosody used to communicate internal mood states to others. Words connected to music in the form of singing are spared in Broca's as long as the right hemisphere area for music is intact. Melodic intonation therapy utilizes spared right hemisphere music-language pathways to help patients recover voluntary speech. Part of the motor function of the anterior portion of the frontal lobe is control of movement in the form of executive functions. These functions control attention to thinking or movement. An inability to shift attention is called perseveration. A prominent disorder of Broca's aphasia is the involuntary repetition of a single word or phrase despite an intent for a different word or phrase or the inability to change topics or thoughts, which are all forms of perseveration. The disorder is not specific to the aphasia but reflects the location of the aphasic lesion in the portion of the brain devoted to executive functions.

Just as in Wernicke's aphasia where input and output limbs are both affected by disruption of sensory processing, Broca's aphasics have difficulty in using syntax to decode incoming information. Broca's aphasics cannot follow commands where understanding depends on a preposition. In the following sentences, the patient may know that a spoon and a stone are to be handled, but they won't detect the differences in how they are to be handled.

> Pick up the stone and the spoon.

> Pick up the stone with the spoon.

Subject and object relationships cannot be discerned because only word order differs in these sentences:

> Sam likes Jan.

> Jan likes Sam.

In other varieties of aphasia, the characteristics of the language disorder are part of the overall disruption of other sensory or motor functions of that region. For transcortical motor aphasia, the reduced speech output is not primarily due to the extreme effortfulness in producing it as in Broca's aphasia, but the overall lack of initiative and motivation that occur with lesions to the supplementary motor area and medial frontal lobe that disrupt limbic circuits connecting emotional information to voluntary motor areas.[95] Apathy and lack of initiative can also be seen in their lack of initiative for starting any movement, project, or routine without an external structure to provide an impetus to act. Speech can even be evoked by provision of an external structure; transcortical motor aphasics can repeat or echo, even repetitively, the statements of others, but not initiate similar statements of their own. One of the executive functions that is impaired in the transcortical aphasias and other disorders, such as stroke, that involve lesions to the basal ganglia with extension to the cerebral cortex,[96] the thalamus with extension to the posterior limb of the internal capsule,[97] periventricular white matter or rostral midbrain is the inability to inhibit action that is started. This can be manifested as echolalia, the tendency to involuntarily repeat what others have said, or pallilalia, the spontaneous and multiple repetitions of one's own syllables, words, or phrases. In the latter, lesions tend to be bilateral and involve more of the medial thalamus,[98] subthalamic nuclei,[99] or combined frontal and parietal lobes.[100] Disinhibition, a frontal lobe disorder, may be reflected in more than repetitive speech. The uttering of profanities in Broca's aphasia, when lesions occur in the frontal operculum, represents a failure of inhibition of impulsive thoughts.

Sensory Specific Aphasias: Disconnection Disorders

Other aphasias, particularly the sensory specific aphasias such as color anomia, optic aphasia, word deafness, tactile aphasia, and word alexia are more easily conceptualized as combined disorders of language and its connections to other sensory portions of the cortex. All the sensory cortex behind the central sulcus is organized into concentric rings of hierarchical processing: primary processing areas (S1) where sensory information from the periphery is first registered into consciousness, secondary processing areas (S2) where attributes of a particular sense are analyzed separately, but simultaneously, and tertiary processing (S3) where all intramodal analyses in the other two regions are combined to form a complete sensory specific trace of a stimulus that then can be transferred to other regions of the brain. If connections from the intramodal visual cortex for color or shape to language areas becomes disrupted, color anomia or optic aphasia results. Loss of word image to word-meaning connections from associative visual cortex to language cortex causes word alexia. Tactile aphasia occurs with loss of somatosensory cortex connections to posterior temporal language cortex so that tactually presented shapes to either hand cannot be named while vision is occluded. Finger agnosia and loss of right-left body space discrimination are close relatives to tactile aphasia and can involve loss of the ability to name fingers as they are touched or the ability to label right and left halves of the body. Rather than strictly conceptualizing these as aphasias, they may be better understood as forms of associative agnosias (see horizontal axis).

Subcortical Aphasias

Subcortical aphasias result from lesions involving the caudate,[101] putamen, and thalamus[102,103] and other portions of the brain in the distribution of the anterior cerebral artery. Initially they present with mutism, hemiparesis, and/or hemisensory loss, and possibly ataxia. The latter symptoms result from interruption of descending fiber tracts of the motor and sensory cortices that become packed into tight bundles near and within deep gray matter areas. Speech characteristics mirror the limb motor deficits: ataxic and inarticulate due to disruption of ascending cerebellar efferents or spastic, high pitched, strained, and effortful, due to disruption of voluntary movement tracts. A characteristic quality of the dysarthria is hypophonia. This characteristic, along with a slow rate of speech, is similar to that seen in parkinsonism which causes bradykinesia, bradyphrenia, and a bradykinetic dysarthia. Paraphasias accompany the subcortical aphasias and are difficult to perceive because of the severe dysarthria.[96] Paraphasias lessen with repetition creating the clinical perception that repetition is relatively preserved in comparison to voluntary speech. Unlike the cortical aphasias with paraphasias, the subcortical aphasias have intact or well-preserved comprehension.

Language in Dementia

Dementias, especially Alzheimer's disease and Pick's frontotemporal degeneration, cause aphasic symptoms. These dementias affect the posterior parietal cortex, the area where sensory aphasias occur in acute lesions to the brain. Like the acute sensory aphasias, the components of the language disorder in dementias include fluent, but empty speech, paraphasias and jargon, and anomia.[105–107] Unlike the sensory aphasias, comprehension is better preserved than output, and the order of ap-

pearance of the symptoms is opposite to that of stroke: anomia, then paraphasias and jargon, and fluent but empty speech. As the degeneration of frontal lobes ensues, echolalia, pallilalia, and finally, mutism appear.

Right Brain: Visuospatial, Gestalt, and External Functions

While the left brain is specialized for language, analysis, and detail, the right brain is specialized for visuospatial processing and gestalt. The left brain listens to a story's adjectives and adverbs. Its recounting of a tale consists of the specifics: the vermilion of Little Red Riding Hood's cloak, the largeness of the wolf's fangs, the chronicle of steps from mother's kitchen to woods to Grandmother's house. The right brain, in contrast, gives the overview. Don't trust all that you see; things aren't always what they seem. This hemisphere puts detail in context and the story acquires a meaning. In addition to aphorisms, the right brain provides reaction.[108] We fear for the little girl's naiveté, share her stunned surprise at the wolf in grandmother's guise, and become tachycardic as she races out of the house. This display of emotion is demonstrated in gesture, facial expression, and prosodic overlay. It permits empathy and shared understanding. Subjectively, our words can express our feelings, but objectively our actions speak louder. The right hemisphere provides the physical changes in our body to communicate emotions outward to others. Internally, the left hemisphere still allows the words and experience of emotion, but without the right hemisphere, no one else can tell.

In the same way as with language, the right hemisphere pictorially makes one picture out of a thousand words. The right hemisphere contains contour maps of space that are internal and external to our body and organizes the individual steps of drawing, building, moving, and perceiving into a picture, a model, an activity, or a precept.[109] The right hemisphere conceives of the scaffolding of a house, while the left hangs the windows and hinges the doors.[110] Both right and left parietal lobes play a role in drawing and construction as both right and left perisylvian regions conspire in communication.[111] Like the organization of language, the organization of space also has both a sensory limb and a motor limb defined by localization anterior or posterior to the central sulcus.[112] On the sensory side, maps exist for the perception of stimuli on the body and in space. On the motor side, maps combine with hand and body movements for navigation and manipulation.

The disorders of sensory perception or imagination for stimuli in space are: astereopsis and stereoblindness, spatial disorientation, spatial inflexibility, and spatial misestimation.[113] The disorders of visual, auditory, or tactile stimulus localization on the body are: allesthesia or allochiria (finger mislocalization), autotopagnosia, and right-left disorientation. The motor disorders of spatial perception are weighted toward deficits in visual-motor integration since in sighted individuals, vision dominates the guidance of limb movement. Constructional disability causes inaccuracy in the making or drawing of a model and optic ataxia leads to faulty pointing or reaching for a target.

Stereopsis

Binocular vision allows for the perception of depth in space. Each eye views the same scene from a slightly different position and the disparity between what the two eyes see creates the impression of depth.[113] Lesions of the right parietal lobe, especially posterior to the central sulcus, interrupt the brain's ability to merge the divergent images from each eye into a single image that appears to have depth. When objects are viewed by both eyes, not only binocular disparity, but local (specific) features of the object's form, contour, and shading[114] contribute to the mental computation of depth. The disorder of the analysis of object features in depth perception is therefore termed local astereopsis. When viewing random patterns, there are no form, contour, or shading cues to aid in depth perception analysis and only binocular disparity information is available. The disorder of depth perception resulting from faulty binocular disparity alone is termed global astereopsis.[115] Patients may not be aware of their disturbed depth perception until it is tested. Testing is performed by viewing three-dimensional vectographs of objects: a housefly, a series of circles, and animals, or of random dots under a stereoscope.

Spatial Disorientation

Spatial disorientation causes impaired judgment of the real orientation of objects, lines, drawings, or tactile stimuli in space. This disorder can lead to loss of navigational ability, called topographical disorientation. People can lose their way even in familiar environments. In some patients, losing their way correlates with an inability to recognize prominent landmarks, such as buildings.[116] In others, knowledge of topographical landmarks is preserved, but the imagery of the spatial layout of the route is faulty.[117] There may be a disassociation between imagery of the visual features of landmarks and the spatial organization of landmarks in the environment.[118] Patients can navigate familiar routes yet not describe them, and as soon as they must concentrate on identifying and visually describing landmarks as they walk, they get lost.

Testing of spatial disorientation can be done with the Benton Judgement of Line Orientation Test.[119,120] This test asks patients to visually match and identify a target angle that corresponds exactly to one of three other angles. The Benton Judgement of Line Orientation Test identifies right posterior hemisphere lesioned patients,[121] which corresponds to the site of lesions for patients who cannot image the spatial orientation landmarks in the environment.

Topographical disorientation can be tested by constructing maps made up of evenly spaced dots that correspond to a route consisting of dots drawn or indicated on a floor.[13] Dots must be spaced several dot diameters apart to allow several steps to be taken in between each dot. Maps must indicate North at the top of the page and one wall of the room should be designated as being North. Patients are instructed to hold the map so that north is furthest away from their body. Routes on the map are indicated by a heavy black line that connects each dot and terminates at the end of the route with an arrow. Patients must traverse the path on the map without changing the orientation of the map relative to their body.

Spatial inflexibility results in the loss of the ability to mentally manipulate objects to imagine their movement in space, a change in their orientation or perspective, an alteration to the body of an object such as a fold, tear, separation, or twist, or to envision how many objects or pieces fit together as a whole.[122] The story of the blind men and the elephant illustrates the dilemma of a patient with this disorder; in turn, like each blind man in the story, an elephant could be portrayed as a leg, a trunk, an ear, standing to the rear, facing head on, profiled on the side, laying, marching, or batting flies, but never all at once and all together. Testing cannot be done at the bedside.

Spatial misestimation leads to an inaccurate estimation of the number of individual elements in an **array** of images, such as dots, blocks, or letters, when the computation is dependent on the spatial configuration of the array.[123] A bowler knows that a strike is dependent on hitting 10 pins based on the triangular orientation of the array. Unless allowed to count each pin individually, a person with spatial misestimation wouldn't aim for all 10 pins. Testing can be done by obliterating part of an array of objects and quickly asking for the patient to estimate the number of objects that make up the complete array. The array must conform to a predictable overall shape, such as a rectangle, circle, or triangle.

The relationships of body parts to one another and to the space around the body also results from right hemisphere lesions. Stimulus mislocalization (allesthesia and allochiria) leads to inaccuracy in locating the position of visual and auditory stimuli in the space around the body and inaccuracy in locating the position of tactile stimuli on the body.[124–126] Stimuli may be misperceived as being located at another position on the same side of the body or in a homologous area on the opposite side of the body. Bedside testing can be done by touching parts of the body while vision is occluded and asking the patient to identify the name of the body part stimulated and the localization right or left. Similarly, with eyes closed and assurance that hearing is adequate, sounds can be made from different locations around the patient and the patient must verbally identify or point to the localization of the sound.[127,128] Finger mislocalization occurs especially from parietal lobe lesions but from either hemisphere. The deficit in either or both hands leads to an inability to identify which finger has been touched by an examiner without the aid of visual feedback (i.e., eyes are closed). Body parts cannot be located to verbal command in autotopagnosia.[127] Though the person can name body parts pointed to by the examiner or indicate the actions or use of body parts, the person cannot localize arms, legs, and facial parts on his or her own body, an examiner's body, or on a scale model. Despite mislocalization to command, localization of the same parts of the body is possible during an overlearned act, such as drinking from a glass of water and being able to locate the lips. Similar to spatial disorientation, autotopagnosia leads to difficulty in verbally describing the relative positions of body parts. Right-left disorientation is the impairment in discriminating opposite sides of the body either in reference to one's own body or in relationship to another's. It results from left-sided or bilateral lesions of the parietal lobe, the thalamus, or from diffuse lesions, such as in dementias.[121] The Benton Right-Left Orientation Test[128] involves commands to patients to point to lateral parts of their bodies with either hand, ipsilateral hand, and the contralateral hand and to point to body parts of the examiner' body with either hand and then with a specified hand.

Disruption of the parietal lobes can also lead to constructional disability, the motor disorder of spatial misperception. In rendering a drawing or three-dimensional model, the right hemisphere relates individual parts to the whole in outline, perspective, and orientation.[86–88,110] The left hemisphere provides details organized into perfect alignment and proportion. Right parietal, basal ganglia, thalamic, frontal, and temporal-occipital lesions lead to drawings deficient in overall spatial alignment, but preserved relationship of parts. Left hemisphere lesions in similar areas cause simplification of drawings and models, incorrect placement of parts and their alignment, and omission of details, but preserved gestalt. The construction deficit remains regardless of which hand is used in its execution, but different errors may be made by each hand. Patients may detail the inaccuracy of their drawings verbally, but still be unable to remodel them. Testing can be done by asking patients to copy a complex drawing such as a house, draw a clock from memory,[22] or copy simple geometric figures, such as those from the Mesulam 3-Word, 3-Figure Test.[40] Drawings are analyzed for completeness and accuracy of overall outline and relationship of parts to wholes, lateralization of omitted parts (i.e., left or right neglect), omission of detail and simplification, impaired orientation or perspective, rotation, "closing-in" (drawing on or near the sample), or writing the name of the drawing instead of executing the drawing. On clock drawings, the planning and spacing of numbers, adherence of numbers to the borders of the circle, and placement of the hands to indicate the time 1:45, are evaluated.

Optic ataxia is the loss of the ability to visually guide the hand to a target in one or both sides of space. As it nears a target, the hand will begin to waver side to side in a searching movement with the palm open. Patients can accurately describe the location and orientation of objects, but still cannot reach for them.[128,129] The deficit may appear in one or both hands and be associated with an inability to move the eyes on demand (oculomotor apraxia) or an inability to perceive more than one stimulus at a time (simultanagnosia) called Balint's syndrome.[130] Parietal or occipital lobe lesions in this disorder interrupt occipital-frontal connections and disconnect the visual areas of the brain from the frontal eye fields and premotor areas of the frontal lobe responsible for manual exploration.

HORIZONTAL AXIS

The horizontal axis partitions the cortex into front and back halves at the central sulcus (Figure 12–7). Most functions localized anterior to the central sulcus are sensory in nature.

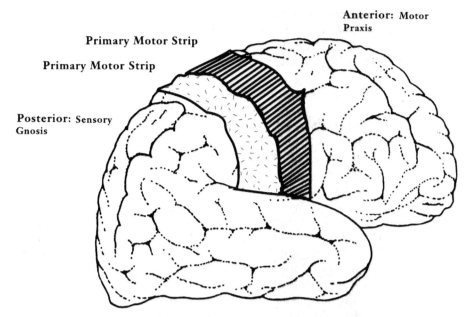

Figure 12–7. The horizontal axis.

At this cortical level, motor functions are termed praxis:[56] the ability to formulate, access, and sequence skilled movements of the face and hands. Abnormalities in these skills are termed apraxias. Besides anterior cortical structures themselves, lesions to the connections of these regions to subcortical nuclei, the basal ganglia and thalami, and sensory regions more posterior in the brain can result in defects of praxis.[131] Posterior to the central sulcus are the sensory cortices: temporal, auditory, parietal somatosensory, and occipital visual (Fig. 12–8). Knowledge of the outside world is through the senses; the Greek word for knowledge is *gnosis*. Agnosia, literally the lack of knowledge, is the disorder of sensory perception that results from injury to sensory cortices. Awareness is particularly linked to arousal and the anatomic regions for gnosis are intricately connected to the reticular activating system fibers of the vertical axis.[132,133] Disorders in level of consciousness resulting from disturbances in vertical axis reticular activating system function distort perception that can cause hallucinations, illusions, and delusions.

Apraxia

The frontal lobes, anterior to the central sulcus, plan, chart, execute, and regulate movement or action. Immediately anterior to the central sulcus, the central gyrus regulates simple voluntary movements of isolated parts of the limbs and face, especially the hand and distal muscles. The premotor regions codify combined and sequential movements and progressing more anteriorly the prefrontal regions provide intention systems or regulatory systems discussed earlier as executive functions. Premotor systems link individual movements into complex acts. The instruction or "how" of this system is termed praxis. Praxic programs provide three types of instructions[52]: (1) "how" to move in space based on inputs from the parietal spatial systems; (2) "how" to time the movement in terms of speed and the relationship of one movement to the other and; (3) "how" to order the components of an act. Disorders of this system are termed apraxias. Patients with apraxia, therefore, make errors in spatial orientation of limbs, hands, and fingers during movement, perform movements slowly or less fluidly, and may disorder and disorganize the proper sequences of movements in a complex act.

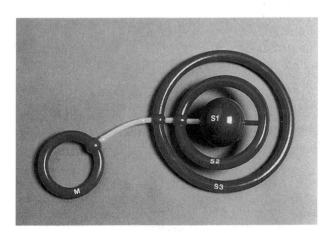

Figure 12–8. The organization of sensory cortex.

As is true with other functions (language, drawing, construction), right and left hemispheres may contribute different controls to the regulation of praxis.[134] As the complexity and cognitive demands of a movement or planning increases, the left hemisphere plays a greater regulating role. It may be the site for construction and storage of motor programs and contain the software for selection and retrieval of motor programs for sequential movement. The greater the number of steps that need to be strung together and the more rapid the sequential movement must be performed, the greater the left hemisphere seems to be involved. During fine movement, if sensory feedback is needed to monitory and modify accuracy (i.e., the shape of the movement), the left motor systems must be activated. Lesions of the left frontal lobe then cause qualitative deficits in the shape and sequence of movement and slow the overall pace of action. The right hemisphere contributes trajectory or spatial information—the where of action.[135] Sensory feedback provides on-line information about the accuracy of aim. Disorders of right frontal motor systems lead to spatially disoriented movements, such as flexing the palm in the direction of the body instead of away when waving good-bye.

Oral Apraxias

Buccofacial apraxia, buccolingual apraxia, and oral apraxia lead to incorrect movements or substitutions of a verbal response for pantomimed skilled movements of the lower face, lips, tongue, pharynx, or larynx. Instead of puckering the lips into a kiss, an apractic patient may blow air or just say "kiss." Imitation of the examiner's performance of the movement may be faulty, but with an actual object such as a straw or whistle or in the context of whistling for a dog, movements are performed accurately. Buccofacial apraxia is associated with anterior aphasias, especially Broca's or conduction aphasia and mutism. Lesions of anterior structures, the frontal operculum, anterior insula, lenticular nuclei of the basal ganglia, anterior limb of the internal capsule, and adjacent periventricular white matter lead to the apraxias of the face and larynx.

Ideomotor Apraxia

Ideomotor apraxia involves faulty sensorimotor integration for movement so that the plane of motion is faulty or incomplete and inaccurate programming of the movement so that the velocity, trajectory, and coordination of movement across different joints involved in the movement are distorted.[136] Thus, the act of brushing one's teeth is performed with a flattened hand oriented away from the face and lacking the characteristic up and down or side-to-side wiping of the brush on the teeth. Instead of orienting the hand in a grip for an imagined brush, the apractic patient may form a brush with their fingers, an error termed body part as object. Programs for movement may be difficult to access and some patients begin with elaborate descriptions of the context in which the act of brushing teeth occurs to aid in cueing the motor program: opening the cap on the toothpaste, squeezing it, turning on the water, and preceding the actual brushing movements with verbal descriptions: "I grip the toothbrush, bring it to my mouth, move it side to side and up and down." At times, no physical act follows or accompanies the verbal description, an error termed verbal substitution. At times, pantomime on demand is more impaired than imitation and object use.

Since more of the cortex is devoted for limb and speech structures, axial movements involving the head and trunk may be preserved despite the presence of apraxia for limb movements.[137] Axial movements are controlled more by subcortical motor systems, such as the basal ganglia, and may be spared in the cortical lesions causing limb apraxia.[138] After acute lesions, recovery from apraxia occurs first for object use, and then for imitation of movements, but usually a permanent deficit in pantomiming to command remains.[139]

In addition to faulty performance of complex movements, patients may be deficient in their ability to recognize the same movements performed by others. Outside the testing environment, apraxia may lead to difficulty in learning new motor skills. Lesions leading to ideomotor apraxia involve the origins of sensory input, the parietal lobe, especially the operculum and supramarginal and angular gyri, and its terminus in the premotor programming area, the supplementary motor cortex, and caudate and lenticular nuclei with occasional extension to the anterior limb of the internal capsule or thalamus.

Disorders of the sequencing of movement are termed ideational apraxia.[140] In the act of baking a cake, a person with ideational apraxia omits ingredients or steps, whips the eggs before separating the whites, and may incorrectly substitute mushrooms for chocolate chips. Despite the confusion for the sequential order of the steps, omission of one or more steps, or substitution of incorrect actions for one or more of the steps, an apractic can perform any individual step in isolation without error. Any lesion of the anterior insula, precentral gyrus, inferior and middle frontal gyri, supplementary motor area, the lateral temporal lobe, or inferior-posterior parietal lobe leads to bilateral impairments in sequential movement.

Gait consists of a complex series of limb, head, and trunk movements that are acquired over time just as in limb and oral-buccal-pharyngeal movements alone. The components of movement needed for walking can be incorrectly programmed to lead to gait apraxia. Frontal lobe disorders, such as Pick's dementia, normal pressure hydrocephalus, demyelinating disorders, gliomas, and stroke can cause hesitancy in initiating walking, inability to maintain an upright stance, slow short steps that appear meted out inch by inch and cleaved to the floor, and complete inability to walk.[12]

Apraxia is determined by requesting movements of each hand separately for a series of actions. Transitive limb movements involve the translation of movement onto an object: brushing teeth, eating soup, hammering a nail. Intransitive limb movements do not require real or abstracted objects; they are semiotic or gestural: waving good-bye, signaling to come, stopping traffic. The patient is asked to make each movement and errors are tallied as body part as object when the body part becomes the object instead of being shaped into the position for use of the object, verbal substitution when words are substituted for movement, verbal overflow when descriptions of context are needed to initiate the action, disorientation for movements that are disorganized in space, and omissions, substitutions, or confusion for the errors in sequencing a series of movements. In addition to pantomime to command, movement accuracy to imitation and real object use should be evaluated and rated for errors. Oral-buccal-lingual movements include real and imagined object use (blowing a whistle, sucking a straw) and semiotic gestures (kiss, wink, blink) like the transitive and intransitive limb movements. Errors are tallied as in limb movements. Gait apraxia is determined by observation of a person's ability to initiate walking, maintain an upright stance, accompany truncal movement with symmetric and coordinated arm and head swing, effect a narrow based stride and shift body movements across the foot from heel to lateral foot, then anteriorly across the ball of the foot (metatarsal heads) to the great toe alternately from right to left leg.

Agnosia

Agnosias result from the absence or improper processing of sensory information delivered to cortical sectors for vision, hearing, and touch from peripheral sensory receptors and tracts. Gnosis, knowledge of the outside world, depends on the serial processing of each component of a sensory trace in the cortex from registration of the stimulus (present or not present), to intramodal processing (analysis of within category characteristics), and finally intermodal processing (sharing of sensory information between senses and other areas of the brain). Each sensory-specific region can be conceptualized as being arranged in a grouping of three major concentric circles (Figure 12–8): S1, in the center where conscious registration of the stimulus occurs; in S2, stimulus is analyzed into component parts, such as for vision, shape, texture, color, orientation, figure-ground relationships; and then in S3 regions, information is collated from each of S2 substations to form a whole perception. Injuries to S2 and S3 regions give rise to material-specific amnesias, lack of knowledge of a particular sensory stimulus, termed agnosias. Though related to memory processing, if sensory information is disrupted at this level, the level of perception, it is considered as part of the defects of the horizontal axis rather than of the memory system of the vertical axis. The sensory cortex, located posterior to the central sulcus, is arranged anatomically to reflect the purposes of these areas. The sensory cortex that registers the presence of incoming sensory information is specified for each sense as A1 for hearing (Heschl's gyrus, area 41 or 42), V1 for vision (striate cortex, area 17), and S1 for somatosensory perception. Disorders of these primary regions give rise to loss of elemental sensations: absence of vision as cortical blindness or partial field loss (hemianopsia, quadrantanopsia), absence of cortical sensations of two-point tactile discrimination, touch localization, position sense, and stereognosis, or absence of sound localization. Intramodal processing areas, designated as V2 (area 18 and 19, 20, 21, and 37), S2 (area 5 and anterior area 7), and A2 (area 22) lead to deficits in the analysis of each component of a particular sensation. Perceptions are therefore distorted, not absent, and collectively disorders in these regions are known as apperceptive agnosias.

For vision, intramodal processing dissects images into its elements of motion, form, color, binocular disparity, texture, and pattern recognition. Lesions in V2 regions lead to achromatopsia, visual form imperception, and facial imperception. In somatosensory cortical association areas, touch cannot be analyzed in terms of spatial distribution, movement across the body and localization on the body, and form discrimination based on contour, texture, orientation, shape, weight, and temperature. Lesions in the superior and inferior parietal lobules lead to tactual form imperception: agraphesthesia or loss of three-dimensional form discrimination.

The auditory cortex parses sound into frequencies, intensity, rhythm, and timing and relates these to environmental, language, and musical sources. If distortion in sound analysis occurs, sounds will not be characteristic of the memory traces created of those sounds and therefore they will not be recognized. Auditory pattern imperception results, causing amusia and lack of ability to reproduce rhythms, environmental sound agnosia, and lack of phoneme discrimination and speech sounds perception. Finally, sensory traces are related to other regions of the brain to allow intermodal relationships—knowledge of an object or experience can be related to all the sensory stimuli it evokes, and the sensory information can be used singly or in combination to direct movement and action. Intermodal cortices allow for identification of an orange by its color and shape, visual characteristics, and its texture, a tactile characteristic. These areas also allow vision to direct movement for reaching and exploring by linking to premotor cortex, hearing to lead to word perception by connecting to language areas, and touch to connect to memory stores to allow recall of object identification.

The discussion of individual agnosias is beyond the scope of this chapter, but at the bedside several tests of vision and touch can help identify the presence of higher order processing deficits of agnosia. As associative agnosia can be demonstrated when:[13]

- There is a persistent inability to recognize previously familiar stimuli.
- The stimuli that aren't "recognized" can still be matched and discriminated from other stimuli.
- All alternative methods of demonstrating stimulus recognition have failed.

In patients with aphasia, naming of an object may be impossible but a description of use ("Egypt" for pyramid) or an associated fact (wheelchair—used in the hospital) is sufficient to demonstrate knowledge. Multiple-choice formats for aphasics can be employed to demonstrate recognition if verbal means fail. Head nodding or pointing to the correct target stimulus out of an array of objects or oral presentation of three stimuli can be done. If multiple-choice formats fail, object use pantomiming can be performed.

For visual object agnosia, a series of objects are presented: toothbrush, comb, pencil, scissors, hammer, and cup. Without touching and by preventing sounds from the object from cuing the patient, the examiner asks for the name of the object. If naming fails, multiple-choice options are given, and finally use of the object is asked. If the patient fails to recognize the object by any of the three methods (naming, multiple-choice option, pantomiming use), object agnosia can be inferred. The same procedure can be followed for forms: square, triangle, circle, cross, to determine visual form of recognition agnosia and for faces: presidents, photos of family members, or friends for prosopagnosia.

Tactile object agnosia can be demonstrated by the presentation of objects and alternately to right and left hands and asking for identification of the object after tactile manipulation only (vision is occluded). If the object cannot be named, multiple-choice options and object use are tested.

Amusia is evaluated by the presentation of a few bars of famous songs: *Happy Birthday, Row, Row Row Your Boat, Jingle Bells, Mary Had a Little Lamb, The National Anthem* and the name, description of the song (e.g., for the anthem—it's sung at baseball games), or multiple-choice options can be queried.

Apperceptive agnosia testing employs the same procedures as for associative agnosia, but the patient will have deficits in matching and discrimination of the objects. For visual apperceptive agnosia, pictures and real objects cannot be matched; objects with similar shapes or colors may not be discriminated, so that a pencil, toothbrush, and straw may all be identified as the same, or the patient won't be able to pick out the toothbrush from the other two similarly shaped objects. To test, different objects of similar shape (button, coin, tiddly wink; pencil, toothbrush, straw; cup, bowl, basin) are presented and the patient is asked to identify one item out of the group. Additionally, different examples of the same object (toothbrushes of different colors, brush shapes, and sizes), can be presented and the patient is asked to identify which are the same or different. The identical procedure is followed for visual forms, photos, colors, and line drawings for other types of visual apperceptive agnosia. The presentation of similarly shaped, but different objects can be used for tactile manipulation and determination of tactile apperceptive agnosia or environmental sounds. Songs can be presented serially, and patients can be asked if the songs are the same or different from a target refrain for musical apperceptive agnosia or auditory apperceptive agnosia.

SUMMARY

The mental status exam is an orderly, hierarchical evaluation of discrete cognitive functions that can be related to anatomical sites along three axes. Once each element of cognition is tested and sites of behavioral aberrations tallied, anatomic localizations of lesions can be inferred and used as a basis for extracting possible differential diagnoses. The vertical axis is always tested first since its function or dysfunction influences the accuracy of functioning in the lateral axes (language and visuospatial processing) and in the horizontal axis (praxis and gnosis). For example, delirium, the disruption of the vertical axis at its base (the level of overall arousal or activation of the whole brain), leads to a diffuse disorder of behavior—sleepiness alternating with agitation, inattentiveness and perseveration, loss of short-term memory and confabulation, paranoia or apathy, distortions in perception as visual, tactile, or auditory illusions and hallucinations, fragmented incomplete movements, anomia, and spatial disorientation. When present, medical or systemic disorders can be inferred as the cause of the disorder. Other lesions, may only affect certain nodes along the axes and cause partial or focal deficits in functioning. If fluent aphasia, ideomotor apraxia, simplification and loss of detail in drawing, and right-sided neglect are found, a left posterior parietal lesion is probable and the etiologies include stroke, hemorrhage, mass, or focal degenerative disease, such as a variant of Alzheimer's or "progressive" aphasia.

The axes approach to mental status exam also aids in understanding behaviors of the aphasias. Patients with Broca's aphasia exhibit other frontal motor and executive function deficits: apraxia, perseveration, and loss of initiative. Wernicke's aphasics lose negative sensory feedback and so are hyperfluent, disinhibited, and at times unaware of their disordered speech. Although each behavior is tested in isolation, brain function is coordinated and the axes are only an approximation in understanding the parallel, distributed, and collaborative processes that underlie human behavior.

STUDY QUESTIONS

1. Identify the components of the vertical axis and explain their relationships to the general function of alertness or alerting. What is the anatomical and biochemical basis of the system?

2. How do afferent (sensory) systems affect the neural pathways for different levels of consciousness? What are the efferent (motor) systems involved in interpreting the level of consciousness? How does testing these systems yield information about the level of brain functioning?

3. Explain the following terms related to memory:
   a. Long-term memory
   b. Middle-term memory
   c. Short-term memory
   d. Material specific memory
   e. Verbal memory
   f. Visuospatial memory
   g. Eidetic memory
   h. Cognitive memory
   i. Habit memory
   j. Spatial memory
   k. Recognition memory
   l. Anterograde memory
   m. Retrograde memory
   n. Global memory loss
   o. Sensory associative memory
   p. Habit memory
   q. Declarative memory

4. Explain the biochemical events supporting the development of short-term recall, medium-term recall, anesthesia resistant recall, and long-term recall. Explain the relationship of drill, rest, and repeated exposure to information in the formation of long term memory.

5. In testing memory, explain the significance of:
   Cueing
   Rehearsal
   Free recall
   Recognition

6. What is the significance of the observation of a flat facies?

7. What are executive functions and how do they affect interpretation of other mental status tests?

8. Why is delirium a global dysfunction of the brain? Name the behavioral and cognitive components of the syndrome.

9. Explain the following features of aphasia in terms of localization of the lesion along the three axes of function:
   a. Perseveration in Broca's aphasia
   b. Lack of speech in transcortical motor aphasia
   c. Moria and logorrhea in Wernicke's aphasia
   d. Melodic intonation therapy for Broca's aphasia
   e. Persistence of cursing, iterative, and emotional remarks in nonfluent aphasia

10. Explain the differences in right and left hemisphere functioning in drawing and storytelling.

REFERENCES

1. Smith DB, Craft BR: Sudden behavioral change: Guide to initial evaluation. In Green JB, ed., Symposium on the borderland between neurology and psychiatry. *Neurologic Clin* 1984; 2:3–22.

2. Moruzzi G, Magoun HW: Brainstem reticular formation and activation of the EEG. *Electroencephalogr Clin Neurophysiol* 1949; 1:455.

3. Plum F, Posner J: *Diagnosis of stupor and coma,* 3rd ed. F.A. Davis Co., Philadelphia, 1980.

4. Dekker JAM, Connor DJ, Thal LJ: The role of cholinergic projections from the nucleus basolis in memory. *Neurosci Behav Res,* 1991; 15:299–317.

5. Mesulam M-M: Cholinergic pathways and the ascending reticular activating system of the human brain. *Ann NY Acad Sci* 1995; 757:169–179.

6. Medina JL, Rubino FA, Ross E: Agitated delirium caused by infarctions of the hippocampal formation and fusiform and lingual gyri: A case report. *Neurology* 1974; 24:1181–1183.

7. Mesulam M-M, Waxman SG, Geschwind N, Sabin TD: Acute confusional states with right middle cerebral artery infarctions. *J Neurol Neurosurg Psychiatryt* 1976; 39:84–89.

8. Caplan LR, Kelly M, Kase CS, et al: Infarcts of the inferior division of the right middle cerebral artery: Mirror image of Wernicke's aphasia. *Neurology* 1986; 36: 1015–1020.

9. Mehler MF: The rostral basilar artery syndrome. *Neurology* 1989; 39:9–16.

10. Devinsky O, Bear D, Volpe BT: Confusional states following posterior cerebral artery infarction. *Arch Neurol* 1988; 45:160–163.

11. Talemichi TK, Desmond DW, Prohovnik I, et al: Confusion and memory loss from capsular genu infarction: A thalamocortical disconnection syndrome. *Neurology* 1992; 42:1996–1979.

12. Adams RD, Victor M: Principles of neurology, 4th ed. McGraw-Hill, New York, 1989.

13. Stringer AY: *A guide to adult neuropsychological diagnosis.* F.A. Davis Co., Philadelphia, 1996.

14. Halsband V, Passingham R: The role of premotor and parietal cortex in direction of action. *Brain Res* 1982; 240:368–372.

15. Mendez MF, Adams NL, Lewandowski KS: Neurobehavioral changes associated with caudate lesions. *Neurology* 1989; 39:349.

16. Belyi BI: Mental impairment in unilateral frontal tumors: Role of the laterality of the lesion. *Int J Neurosci* 1987; 32:799.

17. Nestor PG, et al: Divided attention and metabolic dysfunction in mild dementia of the Alzheimer's type. *Psychology* 1991; 29:379.

18. Kaplan E, et al: WAIS-RN1 Manual. WAIS-R as a neuropsychological instrument. The Psychological Corporation, New York, 1981.

19. Wale J, Geffen G: Focused and divided attention in each half of space with disconnected hemispheres. *Cortex* 1989; 25:33.

20. Woods DL, Knight RT: Electrophysiologic evidence of increased distractibility after dorsolateral prefrontal lesions. *Neurology* 1986; 36:212.

21. Stuss DT, et al: Subtle neuropsychological deficits in patients with good recovery after closed head injury. *Neurosurgery* 1985; 17:41.

22. Strub RL, Black FW: *The mental status examination in neurology,* 3rd ed. F.A. Davis Co., Philadelphia, 1993.

23. Connolly JB, Tully T: You must remember this: Finding the master switch for long term memory. *The Sciences* 1996; May–June:37–42.

24. Kapur N: *Memory disorders in clinical practice.* Butterworths, London, 1988.

25. Mishkin M, Appenzeller T: The anatomy of memory. *Scientific American* Special Report, 1987.

26. Murray A, Mishkin M: Amygdalectomy impairs crossmodal association in monkeys. *Science,* 1985; 228: 604–606.

27. Lilly R, Cummings JL, Benson DF, Frankel M: The human Klüver-Bucy syndrome. *Neurology,* 1983; 33: 1141–1145.

28. Aggleton JP, Mishkin M: The amygdala. Sensory gateway to the emotions. In Plutchik R, Kellerman H, eds., *Emotion; theory, research, and experience,* Vol 3. Academic Press, New York, 1985.

29. Smith ML, Milner B: The role of the right hippocampus in the recall of spatial location. *Neuropsychologia* 1981; 19:781–793.

30. Ungerleider LG, Mishkin M: Two cortical visual systems. In Igle DJ, Mansfield RJW; Goodale MS, eds., The analysis of visual behavior. Cambridge, MA, MIT Press, 1982, pp 549–286.

31. Rubenstein JH, Taybi H: Broad thumbs and toes and facial abnormalities: A possible mental retardation syndrome. *Am J Dis Child* 1968; 105:588.

32. Samuel W, Terry RD, DeTeresa R, et al: Clinical correlates of cortical and nucleus basalis pathology in Alzheimer dementia. *Arch Neurol* 1994; 51: 772–778.

33. DeKosky ST, Scheff SW: Synapse loss in frontal cortex biopsies in Alzheimer's disease: Correlation with cognitive severity. *Ann Neurol* 1990; 27:428–437.

34. Foster NL, Chase TH, Fedio P, et al: Alzheimer's disease: Focal cortical changes shown by positon emission tomography. *Neurology* 1983; 33:961–965.

35. Haxby J: Cognitive deficits and local metabolic changes in dementia of the Alzheimer type. In Papoport S, Petit H, Leys D, Christen Y, eds., *Imaging, cerebral topography and Alzheimer's disease.* Springer-Verlag, Berlin, 1990; pp:109–119.

36. Keilp J, Prohovnik I: Intellectual decline predicts the parietal perfusion deficit in Alzheimer's disease. *J Nucl Med* 1995; 6:1347–1354.

37. Delacoste Mc, White CL: The role of cortical connectivity in Alzheimer's disease pathogenesis—A review and model system. *Neurobiol Aging* 1993; 14:1–16.

38. Delaere P, Duyckerts C, Brion JP et al: Tau, paired helical filaments and amyloid in the neocortex: A morphometric study of 15 cases with graded intellectual status in aging and senile dementia of the Alzheimer's type. *Pathol* 1989; 77:645–653.

39. Corkins: Aging, age-related disorders and dementia. In Boller F, Grafmun J, eds., *Handbook of neuropsychology*. Elsevier, Amsterdam, 1991, vols 4,5.

40. Mesulam M-M, ed: *Principles of behavioral neurology*. F.A. Davis Co., Philadelphia, 1985.

41. Moosy J, Martinez J, Hanin I. et al: Thalamic and subcortical dementia. *Arch Neurol* 1987; 44:510.

42. Ryan C, Butters N, Montgomery K: Memory deficits in chronic alcoholics: Continuities between the "intact" alcoholic and the alcoholic Korsakoff patient. In Begleiter H, Kissin BV, eds., *Alcohol intoxication and withdrawal*. New York, Plenum Press, 1979.

43. Serdaru M, Hausser-Haun C, Laplane D, et al: The clinical spectrum of alcoholic pellagra encephalopathy. *Brain* 1988; 111:829.

44. Ross ED: The aprosodias. *Arch Neurol* 1981; 38:561–569.

45. Reisberg B, Borenstein J, Salob SP, Ferris SH, Franssen E, Georgotas A: Behavioral symptoms in Alzheimer's disease: Phenomenology and treatment. *J Clin Psychiatry* 1987; 48(Suppl):9–15.

46. Harinath M, Rosen J, Marin R: Neuropsychiatric sequelae of cerebrovascular disease. *The Neurologist* 1995; 1:219–231.

47. Robinson RG, Szetela B: Mood change following left hemisphere brain injury. *Ann Neurol* 1981; 9:447–453.

48. Hier DB, Mondlock J, Caplan LR: Behavioral abnormalities after right hemisphere stroke. *Neurology* 1983; 33:337

49. Syndulko K, Gilden ER, Hansch EC, Potvin AR, Tourtellotte WW, Potvin JH: Decreased verbal memory associated with antichoinergic treatment in Parkinson's disease patients. *Intern J Neuroscience* 1981; 14:61–66.

50. Ross ED, Rush AJ: Diagnosis and neuroanatomical correlates of depression in brain damaged patients. *Arch Gen Psych* 1981; 58:1344–1354.

51. Ross ED, Mesulam M-M: Dominant language features of the right hemisphere? Prosody and emotional gestures. *Arch Neurol* 1979; 36:144–148.

52. Passingham R: *The frontal lobes and voluntary action.* Oxford University Press, Oxford, 1993.

53. Stuss ET, et al: Subtle neuropsychological deficts in patients with good recovery after closed head injury. *Neurosurgery* 1985; 17:41.

54. Schiffer RB, Herndon RM, Rudick RA: Treatment of pathologic laughing and weeping with amitriptyline. *N Engl J Med* 1985; 312:1480–1482.

55. Benowitz LI, Bear DM, Rosenthal R, Mesulam M-M, Zaidel E, Sperry RW: Hemispheric specialization in nonverbal communication. *Cortex* 1983; 19:43–50.

56. Levin HS, Eisenberg HM, Benton AL, eds: *Frontal lobe function and dysfunction.* Oxford University Press, New York, 1991.

57. Sandson J, Albert MC: Perseveration in behavioral neurology. *Neurology* 1987; 37:1736–1741.

58. Kertesz A, Nicholson I, Canceiliere A, Kassa K, Black S: Motor impersistance. *Neurology* 1985; 35:662–666.

59. Verfaellie M, Heilman KM: Response preparation and response inhibition following lesions of medial frontal lobes. *Arch Neurol* 1987; 44:1265–1275.

60. Luria AR: *Higher cortical functions in man,* 2nd ed. Basic Books, New York, 1980.

61. Teasdale G, Jennett B: Assessment of impaired consciousness and coma. *Lancet* 1974; 2:81.

62. Mayer M: *There's a nightmare in my closet.* Dial Press, New York, 1968.

63. Johnson C: *Harold and the purple crayon.* Harper & Row, New York, 1955.

64. Reynolds FC III, Hoch CC, Stack J, Campbell D: The nature and management of sleep/wake disturbance in Alzheimer's dementia. *Psychopharm Bull* 1988; 24:43–48.

65. Cummings JL, Kaufer D: Neuropsychiatric aspects of Alzheimer's disease: The cholinergic hypothesis revised. *Neurology* 1996; 47:876–883.

66. Rubin EH, Drevets WC, Burke WJ: The nature of psychotic symptoms in senile dementia of the Alzheimer type. *J Geriatr Psychiatry Neurol* 1988; 1:16–20.

67. Lennox G: Lewy body dementia. In Rosser MN, ed., *Unusual dementias.* Balliere Tindall, London, 1992; 1:653–676.

68. Capgras J, Reboul-Lachaux J: Lillusion des "sosies" dans un delire systematise. *Bull Soc Clin Med Ment* 1923; 11:6–16.

69. Mendez MF, Martin RJ, Smyth KA, Whitehouse PJ: Disturbances of person identification in Alzheimer's disease: A retrospective study. *J Nerv Ment Dis* 1992; 180:94.

70. Kimura S: Review of 106 cases with the syndrome of Capgras. *Bibl Psychiatry* 1986; 164:121–130.

71. Courbon P, Fail G: Syndrome "d'illusion de Fregdi" et schizophrenie. *Ann Med Psychol* 1927; 85:289–290.

72. Jasper HH, Riggio S, Goldman-Rakic PS, eds: *Epilepsy and the functional anatomy of the frontal lobe. Advances in neurology,* Vol. 66. Raven Press, New York, 1995.

73. Cummings JL, Victoroff JL: Noncognitive neuropsychiatric syndromes of Alzheimer's disease. *Neuropsychiatry, Neuropsychol, Behav Neurol* 1990; 3:140–158.

74. Richter JA, Perry EK, Tomlinson BE: Acetylcholine and choline levels in post-mortem human brain tissue: Preliminary observations in Alzheimer's disease. *Life Sciences,* 1980; 26(20):1683–9.

75. Crystal D: *The Cambridge encyclopedia of language.* Cambridge University Prfess, Cambridge, 1987.

76. Peretz I: Processing of local and global musical information by unilateral brain-damaged patients. *Brain* 1994; 117:1185–1205.

77. Blumstein S, Cooper W: Hemispheric processing of intonation contours. *Cortex* 1974; 10:146–158.

78. Peretz I: Hemispheric asymmetry in amusia. *Rev Neurol* 1985; 141:169.

79. Mendez MF, Geehkan Jr GR: Cortical auditory disorders: Clinical and psychoacoustic features. *J Neurol Neurosurg Psychiatry* 1988; 51:1.

80. Pinek B, et al: Audio-spatial deficits in humans: Differential effects associated with left versus right hemisphere parietal damage. *Cortex* 1989; 25:175.

81. Mavlov L: Amusia due to rhythm agnosia in a musician with left hemisphere damage: A nonauditory supramodal defect. *Cortex* 1980; 16:331–338.

82. DeRenzi E, Perani D, Cartesimo GA, et al: Prosopagnosia can be associated with damage confined to the right hemisphere; An MRI and PET study and a review of the literature. *Neuropsychology* 1994; 32:8–902.

83. Tanaka JW, Farah MJ: Parts and wholes in face recognition. *QJ Exp Psychol* 19; 46A:225–245.

84. Patterson, K, Vargha-Khadem F, Polkey CF: Reading with one hemisphere. *Brain* 1989; 112:39–63.

85. Zaidel E, Peters AM: Phonological encoding and ideographic reading by the disconnected right hemisphere: Two case studies. *Brain Lang* 1981; 14:205–234.

86. Benton AL: Constructional apraxia and the minor hemisphere. *Confinia Neurologica* 1967; 29:1.

87. Kertesz A: Right hemisphere lesions in construction apraxia and visuospatial deficit. In Kertesz, A, ed., *Localization in neuropsychology.* Academic Press, New York, 1983:455–457.

88. Umiltd C, Bagnara S, Simon F: Laterality effects for simple and complex geometric figures and nonsense patterns. *Neuropsychologia* 1978; 16:43–49.

89. Delis DC, Wapner W, Gardner H, Moses JA Jr: The contribution of the right hemisphere to paragraphs. *Cortex* 1983; 19:43–50.

90. Dwyer JH III, Rinn WE: The role of the right hemisphere in contextual inference. *Neuropsychology* 1981; 19:479–482.

91. Springer, SP, Deutsch G: *Left brain, right brain.* WH Freeman & Co., San Francisco, 1981.

92. Guariglia C, Padovani A, Pantano A, Pizzamiglio, L: Unilateral neglect restricted to visual imagery. *Nature* 1993; 364:235–237.

93. Newcombe F, Russell WR: Dissociated visual perceptual and spatial deficits in focal lesions of the right hemisphere. *J Neurol Neurosurg Psychiatry* 1969; 32:73.

94. Boll TJ: Right and left cerebral hemisphere damage and tactile perception: Performance of the ipsilateral and contralateral sides of the body. *Neuropsychologia* 1974; 12:235.

95. Freedman M, Alexander MP, Naeser MA: Anatomic basis of transcortical motor aphasia. *Neurology* 1984; 34:409.

96. Wallesch CW: Two syndromes of aphasia occurring with ischemic lesions involving the left basal ganglia. *Brain Lang* 1985; 25:357.

97. Cappa SF, Vignolo LA: Transcortical features of aphasia following left thalamic hemorrhage. *Cortex* 1979; 15:121.

98. Pierrot-Deseillgny C, Gray F, Brunet P: Infarcts of both inferior parietal lobules with impairment of visually guided eye movements, peripheral visual in attention and optic ataxia. *Brain* 1986; 109:81–97.

99. Fenmore C, et al: Language and memory disturbances from mesencephalothalamic infarcts. A clinical and computed tomography study. *Eur Neurol* 1988; 28:51.

100. Diercky RA, et al: Evolution of technetium-99m-HMPAO SPECT brain mapping in a patient presenting with echolalia and palilalia. *J Nucl Med* 1991; 32:1619.

101. Mendez MF, Adams NL, Lewandowski KS: Neurobehavioral changes associated with caudate lesions. *Neurology* 1989; 39:349–354.

102. Fromm D, Holland AL, Swindell CS, Reinmuth OM: Various consequences of subcortical stroke. *Arch Neurol* 1985; 42:943–950.

103. Bladin PF, Berkovik SF: Strictocapsular infarction: Large infarcts in the lenticulostriate arterial territory. *Neurology* 1984; 1423–1430.

104. Wechsler AF, Verity M, Rosenchein S, Fied I, Scheibel AB: Pick's disease. *Arch Neurol* 1982; 39:287–290.

105. Rochford G: A study of naming errors in dysphasic and in demented patients. *Neuropsychology* 1971; 9:437–443.

106. Bayles KA, Tomoeda CK: Confrontation naming impairment in dementia. *Brain Lang* 1983; 19:98–114.

107. Bayles, KA, Tomoeda CK, Kaszniak AW, Stern LW, Eagans KK: Verbal perseveration of dementia patients. *Brain Lang* 1985; 25:102–116.

108. Dimond SF, Farrington L, Johnson P: Differing emotional response from right to left hemisphere. *Nature* 1976; 261:690–692.

109. Shuare M: Disturbance of visual-spatial thinking in patients suffering local brain lesions. *Neurosci Behav Physiol* 1982; 12:133.

110. Mack JF, Levine RN: The basis of visual constructional disability in patients with unilateral cerebral lesions. *Cortex* 1981; 17:515–532.

111. McFie J, Zangwill OLO: Visual-constructive disabilities associated with lesions of the left cerebral hemisphere. *Brain* 1960; 83:243–260.

112. Dee HL: Visuoconstructive and visuoperceptive deficits in patients with unilateral cerebral lesions. *Neuropsychologia* 1970; 8:305–314.

113. Carmon A, Bechtold HP: Dominance of right cerebral hemisphere for stereopsis. *Neuropsychology* 1969; 7:29–40.

114. Ramachandran VS: Perceiving shape from shading. *Sci Am* 1988; 259:76–83.

115. Kase CS, Troncoso JF, Court JE, et al: Global spatial disorientation. *J Neurol Sci* 1977; 34:267–278.

116. Landis T, Cummings JL, Benson DF, Palmer EP: Loss of topographic familiarity. *Arch Neur* 1986; 43(2):132–136.

117. Bornstein B, Kidron DP: Prosopagnosia. *J Neurol Neurosurg and Psych* 1959; 22:124–131.

118. Basso A, Bislach E, Luzatti C: Loss of mental imagery: A case study. *Neuropsychologia* 1980; 18:435–442.

119. Benton Judgement of Line Orientation Test. Oxford University Press, New York.

120. Benton AL, Varney HR, Hamserde K: Visuospatial judgment: A clinical test. *Arch Neurol* 1978; 35:364–367.

121. Benton AL, et al: *Contributions to neuropsychological assessment: A clinical manual.* Oxford University Press, New York, 1983.

122. Ratcliff G: Spatial thought, mental rotation and the right cerebral hemisphere. *Neuropsychologia* 1979; 17:49–54.

123. Warrington EK, James M: Tachistoscopic number estimation in patients with unilateral cerebral lesions. *J Neurol Neurosurg Psychiatry,* 1967; 30:468.

124. Posner MI, Walker JA, Friedrich FJ, Rafal R: Effects of parietal injury on covert orienting of visual attention. *J Neurosci* 1987; 4:1863–1874.

125. Baynes K, Holtzman HD, Volpe BT: Components of visual attention: Alterations in response pattern to visual stimuli following parietal lobe infarction. *Brain* 1986; 109:99–114.

126. Karnath HO: Disturbed co-ordinate transformation in the neural representation of space as the crucial mechanism leading to neglect. *Neurophyshol Rehabil* 1994; 4:147–150.

127. Klingon GH, Bontecou DC: Localization in auditory space. *Neurology* 1966; 16:879.

128. Perenin MT, Vighetto A: Optic ataxia: A specific disruption in visuomotor mechanisms. Different aspects of the deficit in reaching for objects. *Brain* 1988; 11:643.

129. Damasio AR, Benton AL: Impairment of hand movements under visual guidance. *Neurology* 1979; 29:170.

130. Husain M, Stein J: Rezso Balint and his most celebrated case. *Arch Neurol* 1988; 45:89–93.

131. Rosevold HE: The frontal lobe system: Cortical-subcortical interrelationships. *Acta Neurobiol Exp* 1972; 32:439–460.

132. Albert ML, et al: Cerebral dominance for consciousness. *Arch Neurol* 1976; 33:453.

133. Schwartz B: Hemisphere dominance and consciousness. *Acta Neurol Scaand* 1967; 43:513.

134. Haaland KY, Harrington DL: Hemispheric asymmetry of movement. *Curr Opin Neurobiol* 1996; 6: 796–800.

135. Fisk JD, Goodale MA: The effects of unilateral brain damage on visually guided reaching: Hemispheric differences in the nature of the deficit. *Exp Brain Res* 1988; 72:425–435.

136. Poizner H, Clark MA, Merians AD, Macauley B, Gonzalez Roth LJ, Heilman KM: Joint co-ordination deficits in limb apraxia. *Brain* 1995; 118:227–242.

137. Roland PE, Zilles K: Functions and structures of the motor cortices in humans. *Curr Opin Neurobiol* 1996; 6:773–781.

138. Graybiel AM: Building action repertoires: Memory and learning functions of the basal *Curr Opin Neurobiol* 1995; 5:733–741.

139. Weiller C, Chollet F, Friston KJ, Brooks DJ, Dolan RJ, Frackowiak RS: The functional anatomy of motor recovery after stroke in humans: A study with positron emission tomography. *Ann Neurol* 1991; 29:63–71.

140. Haaland KY, Harrington DL: Limb sequencing deficits after left but not right hemisphere damage. *Brain Cogn* 1994; 24:104–122.

Appendix A

Anatomy	Area of Inquiry	Mental Status Exam	Intervention
VERTICAL AXIS: alertness attention amnesia affect executive fxn			
RETICULAR ACTIVATING SYSTEM: generalized disturbance focal lesion of thalamus or brainstem	ALERTNESS: acute or subacute change in alertness, alteration in sleep/wake cycles	OBSERVE: alert and responsive lethargic obtunded comatose RESPONSE TO: name shaking epicritic pain (pin) protopathic pain (sternal rub, supraorbital pressure)	ALERT: continue mental status exam LETHARGIC: discontinue mental status exam; delirium is present MOST COMMON CAUSE OF DELIRIUM IS A MEDICAL CONDITION: UTI pneumonia hypoxia electrolyte disturbance medication effect TREAT AND REEVALUATE
THALAMUS	BRIEF ATTENTION	DIGIT SPAN: seven digits forward; backward	SIMPLE ONE-STEP COMMANDS
FRONTAL LOBE	SUSTAINED ATTENTION	serial 7 subtraction	TASKS DIVIDED INTO SHORT STEPS
MEDIAL TEMPORAL LOBE left temporal lobe	MEMORY VERBAL: orientation recall of new information tracking bills overdrawn accounts unpaid bills pots burning gas left turned on faucets left running repetition of queries and comments discussions limited to past events; mistaking son for brother, husband for father, etc.	INFORMAL: during interview, the accuracy and chronology of recent and past history FORMAL IMMEDIATE: recall of 3 words DELAYED: recall of 3 words after 5 minutes CUEING: semantic (category) phonemic (first sound) recognition (choose out of 3 foils)	SUPERVISION OF: activities, appointments, and medications SUPERVISION OF: financial and legal affairs APPLIANCES UNPLUGGED: meals on wheels home health aide COUNSEL: not purposeful COUNSEL: patient cannot reason and cannot be reoriented; concept of the yearbook

Anatomy	Area of Inquiry	Mental Status Exam	Intervention
right temporal lobe	NONVERBAL: losing way/uncertainty of direction when driving losing way in the house; losing way outside of the house wandering	FORMAL IMMEDIATE: recall of 3 figures DELAYED: recall of 3 figures after 5 minutes CUEING: semantic (category) phonemic (first sound) recognition (choose target out of 3 foils)	DRIVING RESTRICTED: driving evaluation; sell car, don't renew license; alternative transportation LIGHT THE WAY TO THE BATHROOM; LOCK DOORS TO THE STAIRS: baffle locks, supervision on walks MEDICAL ALERT; SAFE RETURN PROGRAM: from the Alzheimer's Association Aricept 5 mg to 10 mg
LIMBIC; LEFT FRONTAL; RIGHT POSTERIOR PARIETAL	AFFECT DEPRESSED	SELF-REPORT ask anhedonia flat facies psychomotor retardation MAY BE EARLIEST SIGN OF ALZHEIMER'S DISEASE, PARTICULARLY IF FIRST EPISODE AND >50 YEARS OLD: In depression alone, exam reveals a lack of effort, poor performance on motor tasks linear with the degree of psychomotor retardation, and answers "I don't know." In dementia with depression, patients struggle for answers and often give wrong answers. Depression is not pseudodementia if accompanied by apraxias, agnosias, aphasia, severe amnesia.	TREAT WITH 5HT RE-UPTAKE INHIBITORS (Prozac, Paxil, etc.) and reassess cognition in 6 months; if mood is improved, but cognition is same or worsened, then depression is part of the dementing syndrome

Anatomy	Area of Inquiry	Mental Status Exam	Intervention
		Vegetative signs; not as reliable as due to depression when co-occurring with dementia	Meals on Wheels
			Aide for cooking and shopping
		Weight loss in dementia can also be due to inability to shop, to cook, forgetting to eat, difficulty in using eating utensils.	Divide meals into six small portions.
			Ensure or Carnation Instant Supplements
			Multivitamins
		Wasting is characteristic of midstage A.D.	Check B_{12} and folate levels regularly.
		The preference for sweets in dementia is part of the agnosia for smell and taste or disinhibition of impulse for sweets.	Speech–language pathology consult
			Dynamic swallowing study
		Dysphagia	Avoid thin liquid or alter their consistency with thickening aids (Diafoods Thick-It).
		Choking on liquids versus solids	Avoid extremes of food temperatures.
		Regurgitation	Drink with a straw and give drinks in between bites of food.
		Frequent pneumonia	If dysphagia or inanition is severe, PEG tube.
		Presence of acute change in mental status, motor weakness, or dysarthia	
		Dysphagia can be due to corticobulbar dysfunction or appearance of frontal release signs and dysfunction in frontal lobe functions	

Anatomy	Area of Inquiry	Mental Status Exam	Intervention
		Alteration in sleep/wake cycles.	Set rigid sleep and wake times. Avoid napping. Bed should be used only for sleep and sex. Increase aerobic physical activity before 7 P.M. Avoid food before bed. Hot milk with or without chocolate before bed. Determine if other factors interrupt sleep, such as pain, urinary frequency, or nocturia. Hypnotic and barbiturate sedatives should be avoided since they worsen daytime functioning, are habit forming, and tolerance to therapeutic effect occurs. Ambien 5 mg to 10 mg may be tried to reinstate a regular sleep/wake cycle.
RIGHT FRONTAL	FLAT WITHOUT DEPRESSION APROSODIA: no vegetative signs or symptoms denies depression of face and voice no associated gestures	OBSERVE: expressionless face absence of gesture monotone voice "I went to the store to buy a loaf of bread." Change voice to make the sentence imply anger, happiness, or sadness (expression). Interpret the examiner's emotion from the sentence said angrily, happily, or sadly (comprehension). Imitate the examiner's expression of the sentence in the three emotions (imitation).	SPEECH THERAPY COUNSEL: family to interpret content of patient's expression and not judge emotional state by voice and expression. Encourage the patient to express how he or she feels in words.

Anatomy	Area of Inquiry	Mental Status Exam	Intervention
BASAL GANGLIA	PARKINSONISM: above plus hypophonia bradykinesia bradyphrenia rigidity, tremor, or postural instability	MOTOR EXAM: rigidity pill-rolling tremor cogwheeling stooped, shuffling, short-strided gait retropulsion, propulsion	SINEMET: not always helpful in the dysarthria, but will improve other motor symptoms SPEECH THERAPY: for Parkinsonian dysarthria DEPRESSION: can coexist in 33%; treatment for depression should be concurrent with dysarthria therapy.
BIFRONTAL SUBCORTICAL: progressive subranuclear palsy frontal glioma	ABULIA: flat aprosodic apathetic extreme lack of motivation and initiative	FRONTAL RELEASE SIGNS: grasp Meyerson's (glabellar tap) snout palmomental apractic gait	
BILATERAL CORTICOBULBAR TRACT INJURY: multi-infarct dementia multiple sclerosis cerebellar degeneration	POOR MODULATION PSEUDOBULBAR: lability sudden, exaggerated or inappropriate laughing or crying, not matched to degree of internal mood state; patient surprised and embarrassed by behavior.	If tearfulness occurs during an interview, especially >5 times, then pseudobulbar effect is likely. Crying is usually limited to a few seconds to a minute. Crying is more common than laughing.	Elavil 25–50 mg once daily
FRONTAL Pick's closed head injury alcohol abuse	EXCESS HIGH WITZELSUCHT: "jokeface" silly, inappropriately jocular and disinhibited affect and behavior	OBSERVE inappropriate gesture and comments	Counsel family that behavior is involuntary.
LIMBIC ALZHEIMER'S DISEASE	AFFECT DELUSIONS Simple persecutory: things and people after patients: "Someone is taking my money" "Someone is coming into my house at night" Othello syndrome: delusional jealousy, unfaithful spouse	OBSERVE	ANTIPSYCHOTICS: Risperdal 1 mg–1/2 to 1 bid Haldol 0.5 mg–bid Recheck need for drug or wean every 6 weeks Educate caretaker regarding need to monitor for: tremor rigidity stooped posture shuffling gait postural instability slowing of movement Wean soon or balance benefit versus side effects if Parkinsonian side effects occur

Anatomy	Area of Inquiry	Mental Status Exam	Intervention
LIMBIC ALZHEIMER'S DISEASE (continued)			Midstage A.D. M.M.S.E. score ~12.5 Transient, lasting months to a year
			Cannot reason with the patient regarding the unlikeliness or untrue nature of their beliefs
			Distraction by physical activity, especially an outing or drive, can allay the anxiety of needing to "go home"
			Supervision of activities
RIGHT FRONTAL-PARIETAL LESION	Capgras: The Impostor Syndrome Reduplicative paramnesia exact duplicate of spouse or house and its contents exists elsewhere; accompanied by the need to "go home" or "find the real husband/wife"	May have other right parietal dysfunction	Distraction by physical activity, especially an outing or drive, can allay the anxiety of needing to "go home" Supervision of activities
FRONTAL MANIA	Grandiosity: Claim to be Jesus Christ, the President, or a CEO. Delusion of immortality and invincibility		PSYCHIATRIC REFERRAL
SCHIZOPHRENIA STREET DRUG-INDUCED PSYCHOSES	Complex persecutory: bizarre, complex stories regarding persecution by the government, aliens, other officials, often with elaborate tales of wire tapping, spying, extraterrestrial visits Voices, audible urges to do harmful acts		PSYCHIATRIC REFERRAL
TOXIC-METABOLIC	HALLUCINATIONS Infestation: bugs crawling onto the body		Remove anticholinergic or sedative-hypnotic drugs
OCCIPITAL LOBE VASCULAR MIGRAINE	Visual: simple: positive or negative; light flashes, zigzag lines, scotomas		Mass or vascular etiology to be considered first: C.T. or M.R.I., carotid dopplers, echo, or T.E.E. (embolic cause is likely), monitor for Atrial fibrillation

Anatomy	Area of Inquiry	Mental Status Exam	Intervention
	complex: figures; most often due to Sinement overdose not to be confused with misidentification of a family member, i.e., referring to a spouse as a brother or father		Decrease dose of Sinemet Explain to family members that memory loss leads to a loss of referents for recent past and patient believes that the past is present
TEMPORAL LOBE SCHIZOPHRENIA	Auditory: Voices condemning patient or encouraging a violent harmful act		Psychiatry referral
A.D. OR M.I.D.	Patient responding to TV or an individual who is deceased or is not present		If not agitated or upset, counsel the family to remain calm and not to "correct" the false belief If agitated, treat as in delusions
MEDIAL TEMPORAL LOBE OR INSULA	Taste or smell: Usually disagreeable		Consider the presence of a temporal lobe mass or seizures: MRI and sleep-deprived EEG
FRONTAL LOBE	EXECUTIVE FUNCTION: Lack of initiative, "withdrawn," "lazy," "just sits there" Distractibility: Unfinished tasks Unfinished conversations Tangential speech Perseveration Response mode same despite change in task Same answer or answer type to different questions	Doesn't join in during the interview Responds to other environmental stimuli Discussion rambling	Counsel caretaker that the behavior is not on purpose and that the patient is not lazy Structure must be imposed for patient activities: daycare, home health aide Limit the number of activities in the patient's immediate environment; avoid simultaneous TV, radio, vacuum cleaner with discussions

Anatomy	Area of Inquiry	Mental Status Exam	Intervention
	Disinhibition and impulsiveness: Eating with hands, grabbing food off serving plate Inappropriate sexual advances, comments Answering question before question is finished ("automatic" yes or no)	Inappropriate comments during the interview Inappropriate behavior Automaticity in answers Frontal release signs	Limit the number of children and guests in the home One-on-one strategy at large gatherings Stop tasks and restart later
	Bradykinesia and Bradyphrenia Slow movement walking Slow responses	Slow response and movement times	
LATERAL AXIS Left Brain: Language and arithmetic Analysis Internal mood and cognitive states Right Brain: Visuospatial Gestalt External expression of mood and external world			
LEFT LATERAL TEMPORAL LOBE Early Alzheimer's disease Multi-infarct state Resolved aphasia Complex visuospatial deficits	LANGUAGE Anomia: difficulty with proper names; *is not aphasia* difficulty with names of objects; blocks on words with substitutions and circumlocutions; spontaneous recall of target word; effect of anomia on communicability; increasing frequency of word finding difficulties leads to a hesitant, halting, tangential speech: "*empty speech*"	OBSERVE in spontaneous speech PERFORMANCE ON THE BOSTON NAMING TEST: category or simplification; paraphasic error; visuospatial error	Encourage family and friends to fill in for gaps in word finding: don't make the person "try."

Anatomy	Area of Inquiry	Mental Status Exam	Intervention
LEFT POSTERIOR-TEMPORAL-PARIETAL Vascular (Wernicke's aphasia) Comprehension will be poor Alzheimer's disease Mid-stage or focal onset Comprehension will be preserved	PARAPHASIAS Characteristic of aphasias *Semantic:* one word substituted for another; may or may not be related to the target word e.g., door for table *Literal:* one phoneme, letter, or syllable of a single word substituted by another phoneme, letter, or syllable e.g., brofa for sofa		Do not correct patient Clarify with context or objects if meaning cannot be determined
FRONTAL Vascular Late stage Alzheimer's	ECHOLALIA: repetition of others' sentences or phrases PALLILALIA: reiteration of same sound or phrase e.g., Bdee, Bdee I think I can, I think I can		Counsel family regarding the involuntary nature of the behavior
RIGHT PARIETAL-TEMPORAL LOBE	VISUOSPATIAL Loss of ability to find way while walking, driving, traveling room to room Inability to locate places of or for common items Lack of attention to left side of space on plate, dressing, activities, or body Inability to position body into chair or bed Lack of initiative for speech, activity	CLOCK DRAWING HOUSE DRAWING SIMPLE FIGURES from the Mesulam 3 Word, 3 Figure test Position of writing on page Margins of lines in address Visual search for letters or figures Line bisection	See driving and memory loss Food presented to the right Caretaker guides left arm into sleeve or pant leg and then lets patient dress right side Place conversations and activities to be attended to on the patient's right side
RIGHT FRONTAL LOBE	Lack of expression of voice, gesture		Speech pathology referral (see affect)

Anatomy	Area of Inquiry	Mental Status Exam	Intervention
HORIZONTAL AXIS Anterior: praxis Posterior: gnosis FRONTAL PREMOTOR	APRAXIA: Inability to cook, do laundry, clean, complete projects, dress, walk	PANTOMIME: Oral-buccal: blink wink puff out cheeks blow out a candle whistle Verbal: pa, ga, la repeated pagala baseball player huckleberry Transitive: Brush teeth Hammer Eat soup Intransitive: Wave good-bye Signal to come Stop traffic Bilateral hands: Play piano Play the violin Eat corn on the cob Sequential: Mail a letter Bake a cake	Activities to be divided into a series of guided short steps Eventually, patient may need to be fed, dressed, bathed, carried, and all activities of daily living done by others
POSTERIOR PARIETAL LOBE	AGNOSIA: Tactile	FACE-HAND TEST: double simultaneous tap of the face and hand ipsilaterally and contralaterally; patient will extinct one side or the hands	See visuo-spatial

OCCIPITAL LOBE	Visual
	Not "seeing" things right in front of them
	Cannot locate a single item out of an array
	Failure to identify people visually
		On the Boston Naming Test, naming errors reflect visual perceptual deficits e.g., a wheelchair is called a bicycle
		Matching objects and drawings, photos, colors
		Visual object identification, form i.d., face i.d.:
		  naming
		  multiple choice i.d.
		  pantomime use
		Tactile object i.d.:
		  name
		  multiple choice
		  pantomime use
		Amusia:
		  sing songs
		  i.d. songs by melody	

13

Brain Imaging in Neurocommunicative Disorders

K. Paige George, Eric M. Vikingstad, and Yue Cao

CHAPTER OUTLINE

Brain Imaging Technologies

Brain/Language Relationships: The Influence of Neuroimaging

Future Trends and Conclusions

Brain Function and Language

Our understanding of human communication has relied largely on studies of patients with known brain lesions and their clinical manifestations. The lesion localization method has revealed the lesion sites associated with such disorders as aphasia, alexia, and agnosia. From these findings, models of the neural basis of language and associated disturbances have been developed. With advances in neuroimaging, however, our understanding of the neural basis for communication and its disorders has greatly increased. Over the past 25 years, computed tomography (CT) and magnetic resonance imaging (MRI) have enabled us to study *in vivo* the lesion locations associated with disturbances in speech and language. More recently, single photon emission tomography (SPECT), positron emission tomography (PET), and functional magnetic resonance imaging (fMRI) have allowed for the study of brain blood flow and metabolism in both normals and brain damaged individuals. These technologies have provided a valuable window into human brain structure and function. The relationship between the brain, human communication, and its disorders is being elucidated more rapidly than

ever before. These findings have significant implications for theoretical models and improved approaches to diagnosis, treatment, and prediction of prognosis.

This chapter provides a general overview of various neuroimaging technologies including CT, MRI, SPECT, PET and fMRI, describing technical aspects as well as clinical and research applications. The second section reviews how data from neuroimaging studies have shaped our understanding of the anatomy of language and the neuropathology of aphasia. The chapter concludes with a brief discussion about future directions for neuroimaging and its application to human communication disorders.

BRAIN IMAGING TECHNOLOGIES

Computed Tomography

Medical imaging was born in 1895 when Wilhelm Conrad Roentgen discovered X-rays while investigating the behavior of electron beams. The potential of X-rays in medicine was quickly realized, and plain film X-ray has been a mainstay of diagnostic medicine since that time. Plain film radiography, however, is of limited value in neuroimaging because in many cases it is not sensitive enough to reveal the subtle differences between normal and abnormal brain tissue. Despite its status as a subideal neuroimaging modality, until the early 1970s plain film X-ray and conventional angiography (a variant of plain film radiography in which an injected contrast agent is used to aid in the visualization of blood vessels) were the only noninvasive means of looking into the skull. In the late 1960s, Godfrey Hounsfield developed the first model of a computerized X-ray imaging device that allowed glimpses into the body that had never been possible before.[1] Several years later, in 1973, the first computed tomography scanners were installed at several hospitals in the United States.[2]

Principles

Computed tomography (CT) is an imaging technique in which X-rays are used to create cross-sectional pictures of the patient. Before we discuss the details of the CT scanner and CT image production, a few words about the interaction of X-rays in matter are appropriate. As an X-ray beam passes through tissue, it undergoes attenuation as some fraction of the X-rays interacts with electrons in the tissue. These interactions often produce scattered X-rays that can be detrimental to the CT image quality. The degree of attenuation of the beam is dependent upon the electron density of the matter, with different tissues exhibiting different attenuation properties. Bone, for example, has a high electron density and is quite opaque to X-rays (Figure 13–1). The CT scanner is able to measure how well certain tissues attenuate the X-ray beam by looking at the portion of the beam transmitted through the patient. The CT image, then, is simply a map of the degree of X-ray attenuation at each point in an axial slice of tissue.

CT scanners have undergone tremendous evolution since the first generation built in the early 1970s. Modern scanners normally consist of four components. These include: (1) an X-ray tube mounted on a track that circles the patient, (2) a ring of solid state X-ray detectors that also encircles the patient, (3) *collimators* (see Appendix A), which are located at the detector faces and help prevent the detection of scattered radiation, and (4) a computer for image reconstruction (Figure 13–2). The X-ray tube track and detector ring are coplanar and concentric, and their plane defines the section of the patient that will be imaged. The tube generates a fan-shaped X-ray beam with a maximum **energy** (see Appendix A) of about 120 keV that enters the patient at a thin slice of tissue. As the beam passes through the patient it under-

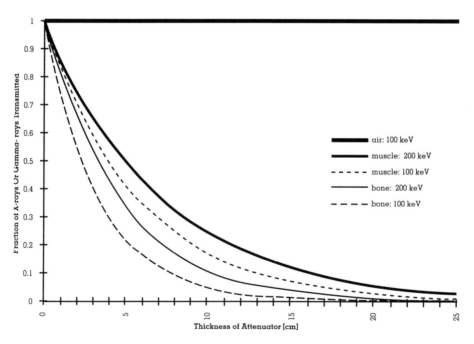

Figure 13–1. A demonstration of the effects of tissue type and photon energy on X-ray attenuation. Transmission of radiation decreases exponentially with attenuator thickness. The degree of attenuation increases as attenuator electron density increases and photon energy decreases.

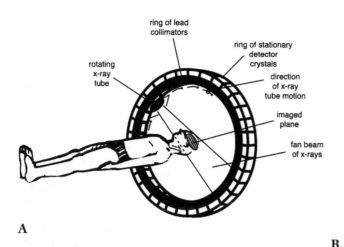

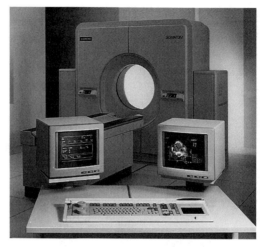

A

B

Figure 13–2. (A) A schematic drawing of a CT scanner. The ring of collimated detector crystals and the rotating X-ray tube are shown. **(B)** Photograph of a modern CT scanner. (Photograph courtesy of Siemens.)

goes nonuniform attenuation as some X-rays interact in the different tissues of the body. Those X-rays that are transmitted through the patient (i.e., do not interact in the patient) are recorded as a projection (Figure 13–3) by the collimated X-ray detectors opposite the X-ray source. Additional projections are taken at many angles as the X-ray tube moves on its track around the patient. The entire projection set is then fed into the computer system that reconstructs the CT image. A very rapid acquisition technique, called spiral CT, is available on modern scanners. In this technique the X-ray tube rotates

continuously as the patient is slowly moved through the plane of the detector ring, allowing the X-ray beam to describe a spiral path around the patient. Such an acquisition scheme will collect data from a volume of tissue, allowing images to be reconstructed in any plane and three-dimensional renderings to be generated.

As previously mentioned, the CT scanner records radiation transmitted through the patient. Since transmission and attenuation are directly related, the computer is able to use these projections to reconstruct a map of X-ray attenuation at each point in the slice of tissue. This map, in fact, is the CT image. Contrast in CT images arises because different tissues have different attenuation properties. Tissues with large differences in attenuation will also display a large degree of contrast (e.g., bone and gray matter), while those with very similar electron densities will be difficult to distinguish. It is often beneficial to artificially increase the electron density of a tissue to increase contrast and make a particular structure more visible. This is usually done by the injection of an iodinated contrast agent (NaI—sodium iodide) into the bloodstream. NaI will increase X-ray attenuation in the blood compartment, thereby making the vascular anatomy highly visible (Figure 13–4). It will also detect compromises of the blood brain barrier as evidenced by leakage of high contrast into the brain parenchyma (Figure 13–5).

CT scanner performance has improved significantly in the years since its inception. Modern spiral scanners are capable of acquiring an image in about one second, and spatial resolution is unrivaled by any other modality. In-plane resolutions

Figure 13–3. An example of a single X-ray projection taken through a phantom with regions of varying electron density. During the CT acquisition procedure, projections are recorded at many different angles and fed into the image reconstruction computer to generate the CT image.

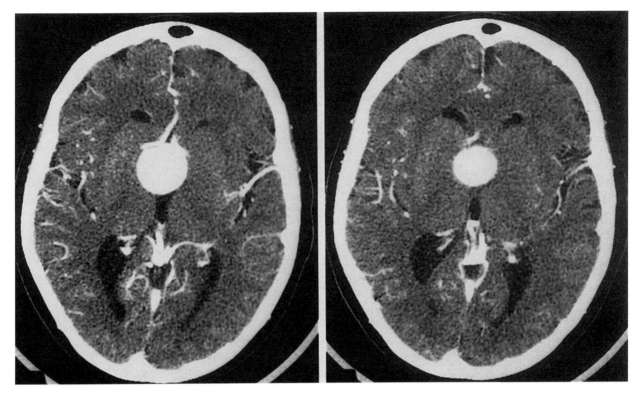

Figure 13–4. Axial CT angiography images from a patient with a midline aneurysm. Iodinated contrast material has been used to enhance the lesion and vascular structure. To aid in the diagnosis of vascular disease, vascular anatomy may be separated from the surrounding soft tissue by a technique called subtraction angiography (not shown) in which a pre-contrast scan is subtracted from the angiogram.

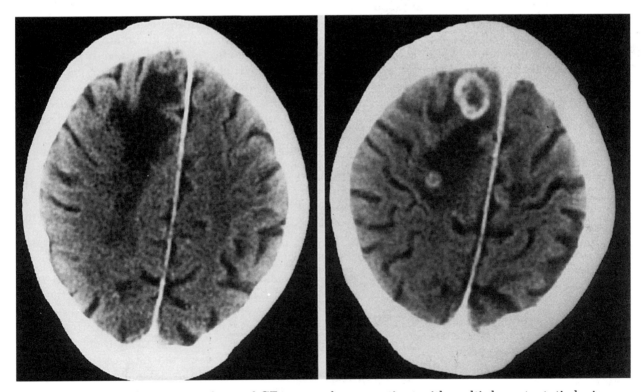

Figure 13–5. Axial contrast enhanced CT images from a patient with multiple metastatic lesions in the right frontal lobe. Notice the ring of enhancement around the larger anterior mass indicating a compromise of the blood brain barrier by the invasive tumor. The darker regions surrounding the lesion sites are indicative edema. (Images courtesy of David Hearshen.)

of 20 line pairs per cm (0.25 mm) are possible, and slices as thin as 0.5 mm can be taken. Such capabilities make CT a powerful tool for imaging anatomical features, and much of its use in the clinical and research environments is based upon its ability to detect changes in anatomy.

Clinical Applications

In the clinical arena, CT has seen widespread use, and is of diagnostic benefit in many diseases and in many different organ systems (Table 13–1). In the field of head and brain imaging, CT is an ideal modality for the detection of bone fractures and trauma to the skull. It plays an essential role in the evaluation of central nervous system (CNS) neoplasms including the detection of edema, hemorrhage, and calcification associated with the tumor (Figure 13–5). CT has also found a role in the diagnosis of CNS infections such as encephalitis and meningitis. Cerebrovascular disease is very commonly assessed by CT, and although magnetic resonance imaging is generally more sensitive to cerebral ischemia, a CT scan is usually the first step in evaluating a potential stroke victim (Figure 13–6). With the administration of iodinated contrast, CT angiography becomes an excellent technique for the detection of aneurysm, stenosis, and hemorrhage secondary to any number of conditions including neoplasm, trauma, arteriovenous malformation, hypertension, and coagulopathies (Figure 13–4).

Applications in Neuroscience Research

In the field of neuroscience research, CT has played a rather limited role when compared to other imaging modalities (Table 13–1). Even so, its present and potential contribution should not be ignored. CT's superior resolution and ability to accurately identify the position and extent of CNS lesions have made it a popular brain mapping tool over the past two decades. Lesion localization and lesion size measurements have been performed in patients suffering from a wide range of clinical disorders including aphasia,[3–6] memory impairment,[7] motor system dysfunction,[8] Parkinson's disease,[9] and many others. In addition to providing much information about the neural circuitry of these systems, lesion location and size measurements have also been examined as predictors of recovery following stroke.[3,5,10] In addition to its role in brain mapping, CT has proven useful in studying brain morphology in several psychiatric disorders including schizophrenia,[11–13] depression, and dementia.[14]

CT as a Functional Imaging Modality

One of the most interesting potential applications of CT lies in the measurement of cerebral perfusion. Measurements of regional cerebral blood flow (rCBF) and blood volume (rCBV) have been reported using injected iodinated contrast agents[15] and, more commonly, inhaled xenon contrast.[16] There is a generally accepted link between increased blood flow to a brain region and activation of that region. Thus, CT perfusion studies have the potential to reveal regions of functional activity, and xenon enhanced maps of rCBF have been obtained during motor tasks and sensory stimulation (Figure 13–7).[17] With CT being more widely available than any of the other perfusion imaging modalities, there is definite motivation to establish

Table 13–1. Applications of CT in Clinical Brain Imaging and Neuroscience Research

	Imaging Technique	Application
Clinical CNS applications	Anatomical imaging	Cerebrovascular disease Congenital malformation Infection Neoplasm Trauma
	Angiography	Aneurysm Arteriovenous malformation Vascular occlusive disease
Neuroscience applications	Anatomical imaging	Brain morphology studies Lesion localization studies
	Perfusion imaging	Activation studies Cerebrovascular disease

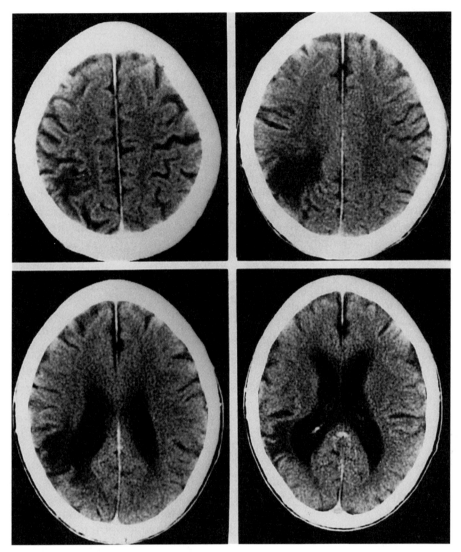

Figure 13–6. Axial CT images from a patient with an old right parietal lobe infarct. The image intensities of the lesion and the ventricle are comparable, indicating that the infarct has become cystic. Notice also a compensatory dilatation of the right lateral ventricle. (Images courtesy of David Hearshen.)

this technique. Particularly exciting are studies evaluating stroke risk in patients with carotid artery disease.[18,19] Other topics currently of interest in CT include the development of intraoperative stereotactic localization systems that utilize images generated by CT or magnetic resonance scanners to guide lesion excision during neurosurgery.[20,21] Such technology would help to limit craniotomy sizes in these surgeries.

Strengths and Limitations

Computed tomography is a powerful diagnostic imaging technique, though it does have limitations. Some of the strengths and weaknesses of this modality are listed in Table 13–2. CT scans provide excellent resolution, allowing the visualization of much anatomic detail. Contrast, on the other hand, between gray and white matter is not as striking as in magnetic resonance imaging. CT scans can be completed rapidly, thereby limiting motion artifacts and increasing patient comfort. The scan is entirely noninvasive, unless contrast is administered, making the procedure easy to perform, and relatively anxiety free. Of the imaging modalities discussed in this chapter, CT is the most widely available and the least expensive. The technique does, however, harbor some small risk for the patient. A CT scan exposes the patient to indirectly ionizing radiation in the form of X-rays.

Table 13–2. Summary of the Strengths and Weaknesses of CT, MRI, SPECT, and PET

Modality	Strengths	Weaknesses
CT	Excellent spatial resolution Excellent temporal resolution Excellent geometric accuracy Widely available	Radiation exposure Limited versatility
MRI	Low Risk Extremely versatile Excellent soft tissue contrast Excellent spatial resolution Moderate temporal resolution Quantitative measurements possible	Cannot image patients with metallic implants, artificial valves, etc. Possible mild geometric distortion
SPECT	Extremely versatile Potential for coincidence detection Widely available	Radiation exposure Poor spatial resolution Very poor temporal resolution Pseudo- or Nonquantitative measurements
PET	Extremely versatile Moderate spatial resolution Quantitative measurements possible	Radiation exposure Poor temporal resolution Low availability High cost

The X-rays deposit radiation dose in the patient's tissues and have the potential of causing damage to DNA through the production of free radicals. Radiation dose in a typical CT scan can range from 2 to 4 **rem** (see Appendix A). An additional drawback is that thrombotic and embolic strokes may not be visualized within the first few days of onset, and very small strokes are commonly missed. Other limitations of CT include motion sensitivity and difficulty in visualizing soft tissue near bone.

Magnetic Resonance Imaging

The phenomena of nuclear magnetic resonance (NMR) was discovered independently in 1946 by Felix Bloch and Edward Purcell.[22,23] The field of NMR spectroscopy grew rapidly over the next several decades and by the 1960s was firmly entrenched as one of the primary methods of determining the chemical structures of organic compounds. In 1971 Damadian discovered that the NMR signal could be used to distinguish cancerous tissue from normal tissue in rats[24] and further explorations into the medical application of NMR were quick to follow. In 1973 Paul Lauterbur, using the same image reconstruction theories that had been developed for CT, generated the first image from NMR signals[25] and the field of magnetic resonance imaging (MRI) was born. After another decade of development, the FDA approved the commercial production of MRI scanners in 1984.

Principles

Magnetic resonance imaging utilizes the magnetic properties of the hydrogen nucleus to generate a picture of a slice of tissue. The principles behind MRI are very complex and only a brief introduction to the subject is possible here. Certain atomic nuclei, including hydrogen whose nucleus consists of a single proton, possess an intrinsic **magnetic moment** (see Appendix A). Under normal conditions, the nuclear magnetic moments within a sample are randomly oriented. When they are placed within a strong external magnetic field, however, they tend to come into alignment with the field, resulting in a net magnetization. The external field will also cause each nuclei with a magnetic moment to **resonate** (see Appendix A) at a specific frequency. This resonant frequency is called the Larmor frequency, and is dependent upon the nuclear species and the strength of the external magnetic field. When the sample is subject to a **radio frequency** (see Appendix A) (RF) electromagnetic wave at the Larmor frequency, those nuclei which are resonating at that frequency will absorb the RF energy, and their net magnetization will be deflected away from the main magnetic field. Once deflected, the net magnetization will begin to precess about the external magnetic field in much the same way that the axis of a spinning top precesses about the Earth's gravitational field (Figure 13–8). As the net magnetization precesses, it will emit RF

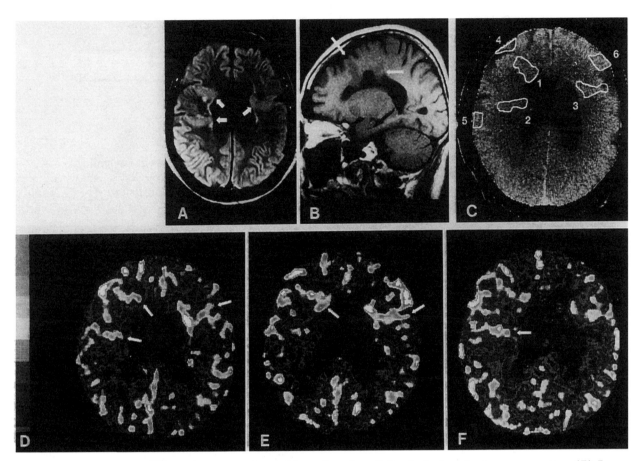

Figure 13–7. Xenon CT perfusion studies of functional activity in heterotopic gray matter. (**A**) Axial proton density, and (**B**) coronal T1 weighted MRI scans revealing the locations of the heterotopic gray matter; (**C**) CT scan showing regions of interest in the zones of heterotopic gray matter (**1–3**) and overlying cortex (**4–6**); (**D-F**) axial regional cerebral blood flow (rCBF) CT images during rest (**D**), voluntary movement of the left limbs (**E**), and sensory stimulation of left limbs (**F**). Motor activity induced rCBF increases in frontal heterotopic gray matter locations (arrows), while sensory stimulation induced a rCBF increase in the right parietal heterotopic gray matter site (arrow). (Reprinted with permission from: Shimodozono M, Kawahira K, Tanaka N: Functioning heterotopic grey matter? Increased blood flow with voluntary movement and sensory stimulation. *Neuroradiology* 1995; 37(6):440–442. Copyright 1995 Springer-Verlag New York, Inc.)

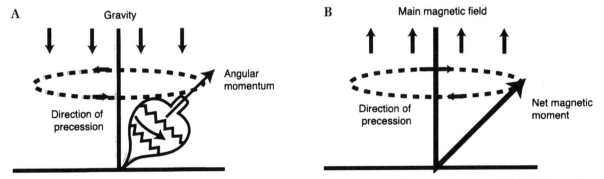

Figure 13–8. Illustration of a spinning top precessing in the earth's gravitational field (**A**), and a net nuclear magnetic moment precessing in the main magnetic field of the MRI scanner (**B**). While not entirely precise, this analogy provides a useful method of visualizing the motion of the net magnetic moment. Deflection of the net magnetic movement by a radiofrequency pulse will increase its angle with the direction of the main field.

energy and gradually return to its equilibrium position along the direction of the main magnetic field. The emitted energy is collected as the NMR signal. To reconstruct an MR image, NMR signals from the sample must be spatially documented. This is achieved by techniques called spatial encoding and Fourier transformation.

The basic components of the MRI scanner have not changed a great deal since the technique was first developed, although there have certainly been many refinements in scanner hardware and software. The scanner consists of five primary components (Figure 13–9): (1) a magnet capable of generating a large static magnetic field usually in the range of 0.1 to 3 **Tesla** (see Appendix A) which is used to align magnetic moments in the patient, (2) a RF transmitter coil used to manipulate the net magnetic moment, (3) a set of three orthogonal linear **gradient coils** (see Appendix A) used to spatially encode the magnetization in a sample, (4) a RF receiver coil used to detect the MR signal, and (5) a computer to control each part of the scanner and reconstruct images. The main field is generated by either a permanent magnet, an electromagnet, or a superconducting magnet. The RF transmitter and receiver are often contained in a single coil, although transmission and reception cannot occur simultaneously.

One of the greatest strengths of MRI is that it can produce tremendous variations in image contrast by utilizing the MR characteristics of different tissues (Table 13–3). This is achieved by special software, called a **pulse sequence** (see Appendix A), which manipulates power to the RF and gradient coils. The three tissue parameters most commonly used to generate contrast in an MRI are proton density (PD), T_1 (spin-lattice relaxation time), and T_2 (spin-spin relaxation time). The physical meanings of these terms are complex and beyond the scope of this chapter, however, tissues can be discriminated based upon differences in these parameters. For instance, in brain, white matter has a lower PD than grey matter, resulting in white matter having low intensity and grey matter having high intensity in a PD-**weighted** (see Appendix A) MR image (Figure 13–10). Similarly, white and gray matter can be discriminated by their T_1 and T_2 characteristics in T_1-weighted and T_2-weighted images (Figure 13–10). The same principle can be applied to contrast pathology from the surrounding normal tissue.

The capability of MRI extends beyond the production of these three types of contrast, however,

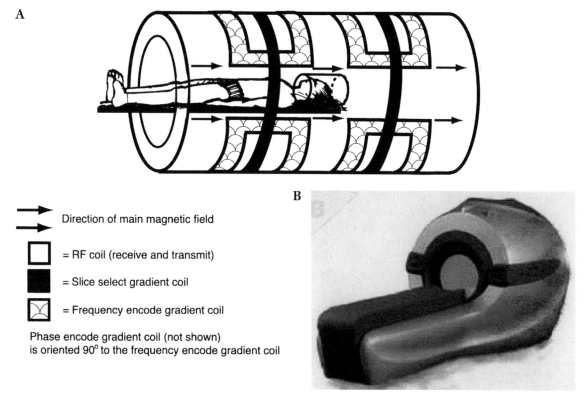

A

Direction of main magnetic field

☐ = RF coil (receive and transmit)

■ = Slice select gradient coil

▨ = Frequency encode gradient coil

Phase encode gradient coil (not shown)
is oriented 90° to the frequency encode gradient coil

B

Figure 13–9. (A) Schematic of an MRI scanner showing patient positioning and the locations of the gradient and RF coils. **(B)** Photograph of a modern MRI scanner. (Photograph courtesy of Elscint.)

Table 13–3. Applications of MR in Clinical Brain Imaging and Neuroscience Research

	Imaging Technique	Application
Clinical CNS applications	Anatomical imaging	Cerebrovascular disease Congenital malformation Infection Neoplasm Trauma White matter disease
	Angiogaphy	Aneurysm Arteriovenous malformation Vascular occlusive disease
Neuroscience applications	Anatomical imaging	Brain morphology studies Lesion localization studies
	Angiography	CNS pulsatility
	Diffusion imaging	Cerebrovascular disease Epilepsy Neoplasm
	Blood oxygenation imaging	Activation studies
	Perfusion imaging	Activation studies Cerebrovascular disease
	Spectroscopic imaging	Activation studies Alzheimer's disease Huntington's disease Migraine Neoplasm Parkinson's disease Schizophrenia

and the technique can measure several other physical and physiological properties of the tissue. MR image contrast can be made sensitive to water diffusion, tissue perfusion, chemical composition, blood flow, blood oxygenation, functional activity, and of course anatomy. It is also possible to artificially enhance the contrast in an image by introducing an exogenous contrast agent. Intravenous gadolinium is frequently administered in cases where blood flow to the cerebral tissues is to be studied. Gadolinium has the property of altering the T_1 and T_2 in blood as well as blood vessel-rich tissue, resulting in striking signal intensity differences between these regions and the surrounding tissue. These differences are especially useful for imaging brain vasculature and cerebral perfusion, and assist in revealing compromises of the blood brain barrier.

MRI offers a wide range of performance in terms of resolution and scan time. Depending upon the application, resolution can be chosen to be as high as 1 or even 0.5 mm, and slice thickness can be submillimeter. Of course there are tradeoffs when performing a high resolution scan—

namely increased scan times and decreased signal to noise ratio. Imaging time is affected by several choices, primarily the type of pulse sequence used, the acquisition method, and the resolution of the image. Conventional acquisition techniques may require anywhere from seconds to minutes to collect an entire image. Echo planar imaging (a very rapid acquisition technique), on the other hand, allows images to be acquired in tens of milliseconds.

Clinical Applications

MRI has played a diverse and successful role in the clinical arena. While used to image nearly every body system, MRI excels at neuroimaging. It has seen considerable use in the detection of brain neoplasms, both metastatic and primary, and in many cases is more sensitive than CT (Figure 13–11). Certain CNS infections including some forms of encephalitis, meningitis, and abscess can be visualized with MRI. Anatomical MR imaging has proven a powerful tool in the detection of cerebrovascular disease. It has the ability to reveal

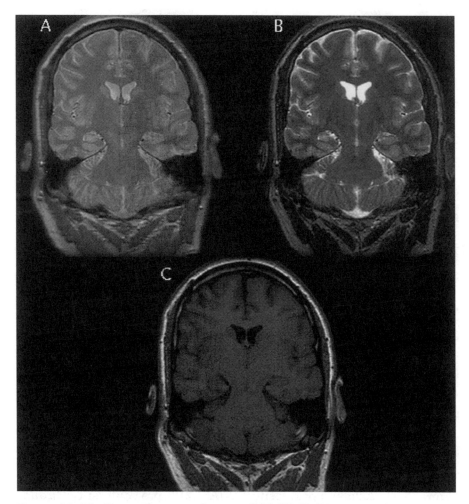

Figure 13–10. Coronal proton density (PD) (**A**), T_2 (**B**), and T_1 (**C**) weighted magnetic resonance images illustrating the various tissue contrasts achievable with MRI. In the PD and T_2 weighted images CSF, edema, and other fluids appear bright, while in the T_1 weighted image they are dark. (Images courtesy of Jeffrey Hasenau.)

cerebral infarction at an early stage, often within 6 hours of the stroke event, and is typically more sensitive than CT in the evaluation of a suspected stroke. Gadolinium may be administered to enhance detection of cerebrovascular disease, infection, and neoplasm. There has been considerable interest in using gadolinium perfusion imaging as an early indicator of stroke[26,27] (Figure 13–12). Perfusion maps can reveal areas of total or near total perfusion deficit very early in ischemia, and coupled with diffusion imaging (to be discussed later) these techniques provide a powerful means for the early detection of stroke or stroke risk. While MRI is a poor choice for imaging bone, the technique still has a role in diagnosing CNS trauma, especially shearing injury and intracranial hemorrhage, although CT may be preferable in cases of acute hemorrhage. Finally, MR imaging has made

dramatic contributions to the diagnosis of white matter diseases including the leukodystrophies, multiple sclerosis (Figure 13–13), and demyelination secondary to ischemia or infection (progressive multifocal leukoencephalopathy).

Applications in Neuroscience Research

The anatomical imaging capabilities of MRI have found applications in neuroscience research that closely parallel those of CT. MRI scanning has been used in brain mapping experiments by providing a tool for lesion localization and size measurement. As with CT, these lesion studies have been used to map several brain systems including vision,[28] memory,[29] and language.[30] Examination of brain morphology with anatomical MR images has been performed in the study of many

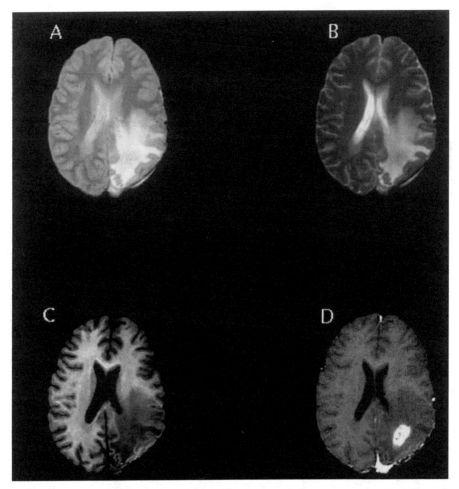

Figure 13–11. Axial proton density (PD) (**A**), T2 (**B**), pre-contrast T_1 (**C**), and post-contrast T_1 (**D**) weighted magnetic resonance images in a patient with a left parietal lobe tumor. The PD and T_2 images highlight the large region of edema associated with the tumor. In the contrast enhanced image, compromise of the blood brain barrier is clearly illustrated in the tumor core. (Images courtesy of Jeffrey Hasenau.)

diseases. For example, increased thickness of the corpus callosum and the absence of a leftward asymmetry in the planum temporale and perisylvian cortex have been associated with dyslexia[31,34] and many attempts have been made, with mixed results, to correlate alterations in brain morphology with schizophrenia.[32,33] Finally, much interest exists in developing intraoperative techniques that utilize anatomical MRI and CT scans to guide the neurosurgeon more accurately to the site of a lesion.

NMR methods for studying rates of molecular diffusion within a sample have been available for several decades.[35,36] Rather more recently, however, the first descriptions of diffusion weighted MR imaging were published.[37] In this technique images are obtained that are sensitive to the **diffusion coefficients** (see Appendix A) of water molecules within the slice of tissue. This sensitivity occurs because random diffusional motion results in a decrease in the MR signal. Thus, water molecules with low diffusion coefficients will contribute more to the MR signal than those with high diffusion coefficients, and in the image these regions of low diffusion will appear brighter. The diffusion of water is affected by cellular membranes that tend to restrict diffusion, as well as by the local macromolecular environment. Diffusion-weighted imaging has been used in the study of several major disease states. One of the more exciting applications of this technology is in the detection and assessment of focal cerebral ischemia.[38,39] Since diffusion imaging is highly sensitive to imbalances in intra/extracellular water homeostasis, diffusion

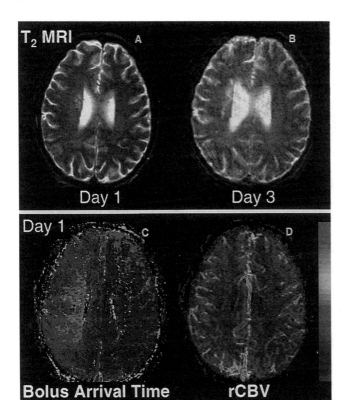

Figure 13–12. Axial T_2 weighted magnetic resonance images of a right hemisphere periventricular stroke at day one (**A**) and day three (**B**), and axial gadolinium injection perfusion weighted MR images of the same patient at day one showing arrival time of the gadolinium bolus (**C**) and regional cerebral blood volume (rCBV) (**D**). Note that at day one the perfusion images reveal a larger area of abnormal cerebral tissue than that detected by the T_2 weighted MRI. By day three, however, T_2 MRI demonstrates an enlarged lesion similar to that detected by perfusion imaging at day one. (Images courtesy of Peter Barker.)

weighted images have the ability to detect stroke at a very early point, sometimes within three hours of symptom onset (Figure 13–14). Early detection of stroke is becoming increasingly important, as certain new therapies have a very narrow administration time window. In addition to stroke, diffusion weighted imaging has been used as a tool to investigate other conditions including hydrocephalus,[40] brain neoplasms,[41] and epilepsy.[42]

Strengths and Limitations

For all its diagnostic and investigational power, MR imaging is a surprisingly low-risk procedure. Unlike most other medical imaging modalities,

MRI does not utilize ionizing radiation and is free of the dangers associated with X-rays and gamma rays. The large magnetic field of the scanner does pose a risk to those patients with pacemakers or metallic implants (including some heart valves, clips, and stents) and such individuals are not eligible for MR scanning. In addition, the noise output of the scanner is considerable, and requires the use of hearing protection during scanning. Advantages of MRI include excellent spatial and temporal resolution, especially with the utilization of rapid imaging techniques, and sensitivity to a diverse and widespread set of physical and physiological parameters. MRI is also superior to CT for the detection and localization of ischemic infarcts. It can demonstrate a lesion within a few hours of onset, while commonly a few days must pass before CT scanning detects infarction. CT, however, surpasses MRI in more reliably demonstrating an acute cerebral hemorrhage within the first 48 hours. Of course MRI has its drawbacks as well. MRI may be unbearable for the claustrophobic patient as the bore of a typical MRI scanner is rather narrow. In addition, MRI is susceptible to several artifacts, most notably patient motion, susceptibility effects, and metal artifact. Susceptibility artifacts arise most frequently near bony or air filled structures like the sinuses or the petrous part of the temporal bone where the MR signal is often minimized. Metal artifact arises when some sort of metallic object is overlooked during patient screening and is brought into the scanner. A large signal void will appear in the image at the site of the object. Table 13–2 lists some of the advantages and disadvantages of MR imaging.

Functional Magnetic Resonance Imaging

Principles

The advent of rapid imaging techniques, mainly echo planar imaging, has permitted the recent development of functional MRI (fMRI) techniques. This technique detects alterations in brain function or physiology associated with cognitive, motor, and sensory task performance. In 1991, the first pictures of functional activity in humans using gadolinium perfusion MRI were obtained during photic stimulation (Figure 13–15).[43] Such methods require repeated injections of gadolinium, however, and have fallen out of favor. Current fMRI studies are dominated by the blood oxygenation level dependent (BOLD) technique. The BOLD method takes advantage of the difference in magnetic properties of oxy- and deoxyhemoglobin to

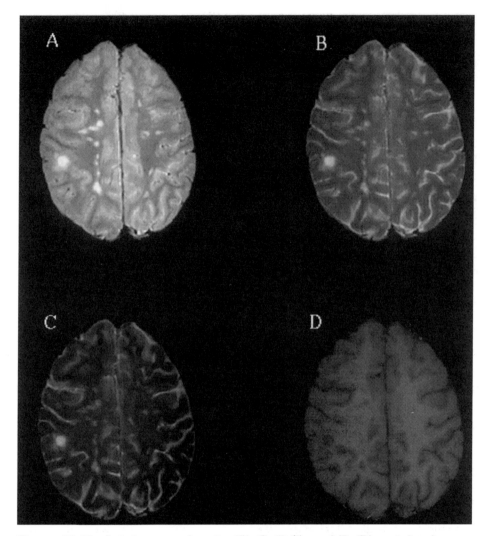

Figure 13–13. Axial proton density (**A**), T_2 (**B,C**), and T_1 (**D**) weighted magnetic resonance images of a patient with multiple sclerosis (MS). Magnetic resonance imaging has proven a powerful tool in detecting white matter disease, and in these images numerous right and left hemisphere MS plaques are clearly seen. (Images courtesy of Jeffrey Hasenau.)

generate images that are sensitive to the oxygenation level of blood. This effect was first observed by Ogawa in 1990, who discovered that deoxygenated blood can decrease MR signal intensity.[44] Since regional blood flow increases exceed increases in tissue oxygen extraction during neural activity, the oxygenation level of blood increases, and active brain areas (areas contributing to behavioral or cognitive processing) show increased signal on BOLD images.

Newer approaches to functional brain mapping with MRI have been developed, and one in particular—the arterial spin tagging approach—has shown considerable potential (Figure 13–16).[45,46] This method is similar to gadolinium injection techniques with the important difference that arterial blood water is "tagged" magnetically using an RF pulse rather than by Gd injection. This technique is capable of collecting functional signal from brain capillaries and parenchyma, thus measuring neuronal activity more accurately than the BOLD method. Arterial spin tagging also has the potential to perform quantitative measurements of regional cerebral blood flow, but suffers from a low signal-to-noise.

Clinical Applications

As a clinical tool, fMRI has seen limited use; however, there have been some preliminary attempts at using functional imaging to guide neurosurgery or radiation therapy in an effort to spare important functional tissue.[47]

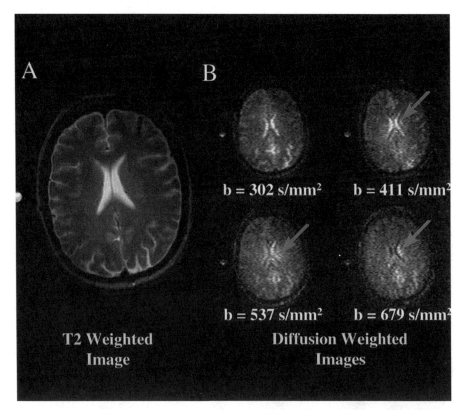

Figure 13–14. Axial T$_2$ (**A**), and diffusion (**B**) weighted magnetic resonance images of a stroke patient. Note that at 4.5 hours after the onset of stroke symptoms the left hemisphere periventricular stroke cannot be detected on the T$_2$ weighted scan, but is visible as a region of abnormal tissue diffusion in the diffusion weighted images (arrows). (Images courtesy of Vijaya Nagesh.)

Applications to Neuroscience Research

The first functional maps using the BOLD method were obtained during photic stimulation and motor task performance.[48,49] Since that time, BOLD fMRI has seen tremendous use in neuroscience research. It would be impossible to provide a comprehensive list of the many brain mapping studies performed with BOLD fMRI, but activation experiments have been performed to map the human visual[50,51] and motor systems,[52,53] as well as language lateralization,[54] word generation,[55] sentence comprehension,[56] and mental rotation of complex objects.[57] There has also been considerable interest in using BOLD fMRI to study brain activity in several disease states. Functional recovery of motor and language ability in stroke patients has been examined, and these studies seem to indicate that there are clear changes in functional organization following such injury (Figures 13–17 and 13–18).[58–60] Functional MRI has also been used to map regional changes in activity during epileptic seizures,[61] and to reveal altered activation patterns in schizophrenic patients during photic stimulation.[62]

Strengths and Limitations

The BOLD method has several advantages over other functional techniques, including a high signal-to-noise ratio allowing the study of individual subjects, the capability of imaging the entire brain, and good temporal and spatial resolution. Because fMRI does not impose the risk of radiation exposure or use radioactive tracers, it is ideal for studing patients repeatedly over time. This is particularly exciting as a means of examining progressive neurological diseases and neurological recovery following brain damage. Alterations in brain function associated with learning or pre- and post-speech–language treatment might also be demonstrated. The largest drawback of the BOLD fMRI scheme lies in questions about the true source of the BOLD effect. It has been shown that a fraction of the functional signal arises not from the brain capillaries and parenchyma (presumably at the site of activation), but rather from larger draining veins.[63] Certain techniques are available to minimize signal contributions from these veins in BOLD fMRI; however, this "brain-vein" dilemma somewhat

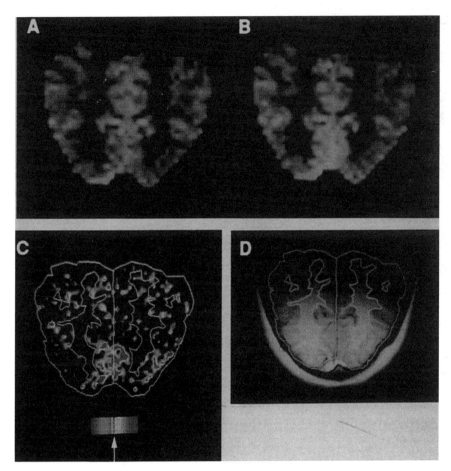

Figure 13–15. Oblique magnetic resonance images of functional activity in the occipital lobe during visual stimulation using the gadolinium injection method of perfusion imaging. (**A**) Regional cerebral blood volume (rCBV) image taken during rest. (**B**) rCBV image taken during 7.8 Hz photic stimulation. (**C**) Subtraction image of changes in rCBV induced by photic stimulation. Arrow points to the +2 standard deviation threshold. (**D**) Anatomic T_1 weighted magnetic resonance image taken through the same region as the images in **A–C**. A marked increase in rCBV (~24%) is localized in the anatomically defined primary visual cortex visual stimulation. (Reprinted with permission from Belliveau JW, Kennedy DN, McKinstry C, Buchbinder BR, Weisskoff RM, Cohen MS, Vevea JM, Brady TJ, Rosen BR: Functional mapping of the human visual cortex by magnetic resonance imaging. *Science.* 1991; 254(5032):716–719. Copyright 1991, American Association for the Advancement of Science.) See Color Plate 1.

limits the accuracy with which neural activity can be localized.

The Nuclear Medicine Techniques: Single Photon Emission Computed Tomography and Positron Emission Tomography

General Principles

Single Photon Emission Computed Tomography (SPECT) and Positron Emission Tomography (PET) belong to the nuclear medicine class of imaging modalities. These techniques are set apart from other radiological methods for the reason that image formation utilizes radioactive isotopes, called **radionuclides** (see Appendix A) (Table 13–4). Prior to scanning, a **radiopharmaceutical** (see Appendix A) is introduced into the patient's body by some means (frequently injection or inhalation), and allowed to distribute among the tissues. The SPECT or PET scanner is then used to reconstruct pictures of the distribution of the radiopharmaceutical as it decays within a slice (or volume) of tissue. The distribution of radioactivity in the patient is governed by interactions between the radiopharmaceutical

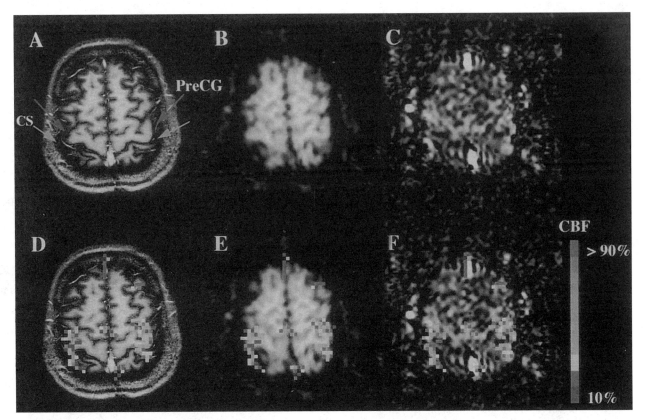

Figure 13–16. Axial magnetic resonance images of functional activity during bilateral finger movements using the arterial spin tagging method of perfusion imaging. (**A**) T_1 weighted anatomical image showing the locations of the precentral gyrus (PreCG) and the central sulcus (CS). (**B**) Slice selective inversion recovery image used in the generation of the perfusion weighted image. (**C**) Representative perfusion weighted image of regional cerebral blood flow obtained using arterial spin tagging. (**D–F**) Regions experiencing a relative increase in cerebral blood flow during finger tapping were color coded and overlaid on the images in (**A–C**). Notice that bilateral functional activity is observed in the area of the somatosensory cortex. (Reprinted with permission from Kim SG: Quantification of relative cerebral blood flow change by flow-sensitive alternating inversion recovery (FAIR) technique: application to functional mapping. *Mag Res Med* 1995; 34(3):293–301. Copyright 1995, Williams & Wilkins.) See Color Plate 2.

and the physiologic and biochemical processes in the body, including absorption, transport, metabolism, and excretion. The fundamental difference between PET and SPECT lies in the type of particle emitted as the radiopharmaceutical decays. In SPECT imaging, the radiopharmaceutical will always contain a gamma ray emitting radionuclide. PET radionuclides, on the other hand, always undergo positron (β^+) decay. Positrons (or anti-electrons) are particles identical to electrons except that they carry a positive charge.

Radiopharmaceuticals administered to patients in nuclear medicine studies can act as tracers, substances that follow a physiological or biochemical process. The use of tracers stems from a desire to gain information about how a process behaves normally and how changes in this normal pattern of be-

havior can be associated with certain conditions. Tracers may be naturally occurring substances, analogs of natural substances, or compounds that interact with specific biological processes. Radiopharmaceuticals have been developed that trace a tremendous number of diverse biochemical and physiological processes, several of which will be mentioned when we discuss the individual nuclear medicine modalities. An effective radiotracer will possess two important qualities. First, interaction between the tracer and the process must be known and predictable. Second, the radiotracer must be used in quantities small enough so as not to disrupt the process, yet large enough that there is sufficient activity to generate an image. In general, PET imaging is capable of yielding quantitative data about the process under study, while, for

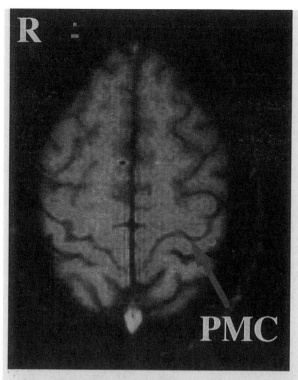

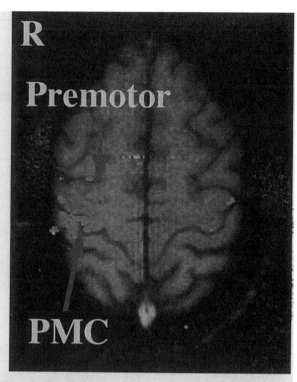

R Hand Movement

L Hand Movement

A

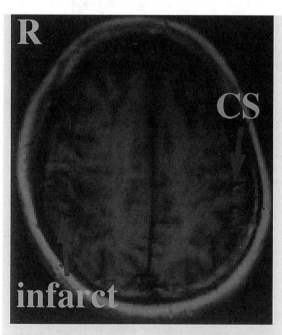

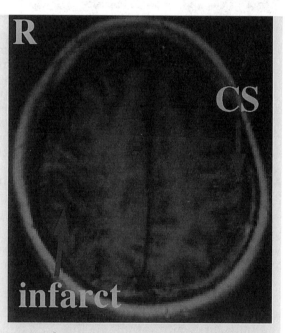

Normal (R) Hand Movements

Paretic (L) Hand Movements

B

Figure 13–17. Axial magnetic resonance images of functional activity during unilateral finger tapping using the blood oxygenation level dependent (BOLD) method. (**A**) Functional maps obtained from a normal volunteer overlaid on T_1 weighted anatomical images. Notice that finger tapping largely activates the primary motor cortex (PMC) and premotor areas of the contralateral hemisphere. (**B**) Functional maps obtained from a hemiparetic stroke patient overlaid on T_1 weighted anatomical images. During movement of the normal hand (ipsilateral to the stroke lesion), activity in the contralateral hemisphere is mainly observed; however, movement of the paretic hand results in primarily ipsilateral hemisphere activation. (Images courtesy of Yue Cao.)

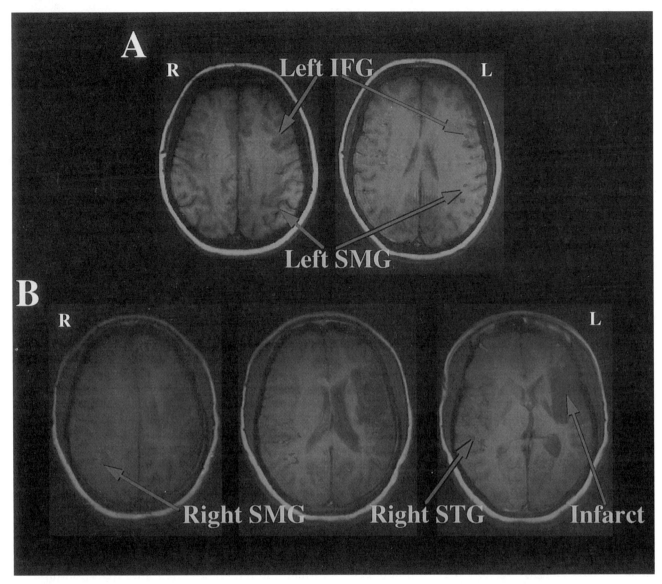

Figure 13–18. Axial magnetic resonance images of functional activity during a picture naming task using the blood oxygenation level dependent (BOLD) method. (**A**) Functional maps obtained from a normal volunteer overlaid on T_1 weighted anatomical images. Notice that in this subject picture naming is lateralized to the left hemisphere in the inferior frontal (IFG) and supramarginal gyri (SMG). (**B**) Functional maps obtained from a recovered aphasic stroke patient overlaid on T_1 weighted anatomical images. The patient's stroke lesion is visible in the left hemisphere. When this patient performs the picture naming task, extensive right hemisphere activity is observed in the right SMG and right superior temporal gyrus (STG).

reasons we will discuss later, SPECT is limited to qualitative or relative results.

Single Photon Emission Computed Tomography

The most commonly used SPECT detector was invented by Hal Anger in 1956 and is called an Anger or scintillation camera. This device had many applications outside tomographic imaging, and in fact it was not until the 1970s that the Anger camera was used in this capacity. Development of SPECT imaging during the 1970s paralleled that of CT, and in 1977 the first scintillation camera tomographic system was reported.[64] Since that time SPECT performance has improved steadily and the technique currently plays a significant and growing role in clinical and research settings.

Table 13–4. Common SPECT and PET Radiopharmaceuticals

	Radiopharmaceutical Class	Radiopharmaceutical	Radionuclides
SPECT	Blood brain barrier agents	DTPA, TlCl	^{99m}Tc, ^{201}Tl
	Cerebral perfusion agents	HMPAO, ECD, Xe	^{99m}Tc, ^{133}Xe
	Receptor binding agents	Acetylcholine, benzodiazepine, dopamine, and somatostatin receptor agents	^{111}In, ^{123}I
	Labeled antibodies	vs. Neoplasm, amyloid	^{99m}Tc, ^{123}I, ^{131}I
PET	Blood brain barrier agents	EDTA	^{68}Ga
	Cerebral perfusion agents	H_2O, CO, CO_2	^{15}O
	Receptor binding agents	Acetylcholine, benzodiazepine, dopamine, histamine, opium, and serotonin receptor agents	^{11}C, ^{18}F
	Metabolic tracers	Methionine, O_2, FDG	^{11}C, ^{15}O, ^{18}F
	Neurotransmitter tracers	L-Dopa	^{18}F
	Labeled antibodies	vs. Glioma	^{124}I

Principles

Several components of the SPECT imaging system are, in name, similar to those of the CT scanner. While those components with similar names may perform similar functions, they are by no means identical. The modern SPECT scanner consists of four major components (Figure 13–19): (1) between one and three gamma ray detectors, (2) a collimator that is attached to the detector face, (3) a pulse height analyzer to help discriminate **primary** (see Appendix A) and scattered radiation, and (4) a computer to control the scanner and reconstruct images. Unlike CT scanners, the radiation source for SPECT imaging is not a part of the scanner itself. The radioactive gamma emitters used in SPECT are produced in a radiopharmaceutical lab and then introduced into the patient prior to the scan. Some radionuclides finding frequent application in SPECT include ^{99m}Tc, ^{67}Ga, ^{201}Tl, ^{133}Xe, ^{123}I, and ^{131}I (Table 13–4). The specific radiopharmaceuticals incorporating these radionuclides are examined later.

As mentioned above, SPECT relies on the detection of gamma rays emitted by a radiopharmaceutical introduced into the patient's body. As these gamma rays leave the body and speed toward the Anger camera, they will first encounter a collimator mounted on the front face of the detector, which prevents the detection of scattered radiation. The collimator plays a large role in determining image resolution and limiting image noise. Modern scanners use between one and three detector cameras; multiple head systems offer several advantages over single head systems, including improvements in imaging time and the potential for coincidence detection (to be discussed later). The typical Anger camera consists of a single sodium iodide (NaI) scintillation crystal, which detects those gamma rays passing through the collimator and converts them into light photons. The Anger camera also contains an array of photomultiplier tubes (PMT) which converts the light emitted from the scintillation crystal into an electric signal with intensity proportional to the amount of light collected. The signal from the camera is fed into the next component of the SPECT system, the pulse height analyzer (PHA), which differentiates scattered or incompletely absorbed gamma rays from completely absorbed primary gamma rays. In modern scanners, the PHA may be set to accept counts in several energy windows to allow imaging with multiple radionuclides or with radionuclides that have several decay products. The filtered signal from the PHA is then sent to the computer and contributes to the reconstruction of the tomograph.

Data collection and image reconstruction in SPECT share some similarities with CT. In SPECT, the Anger cameras slowly rotate about the patient (reminiscent of X-ray tube motion in CT), collect-

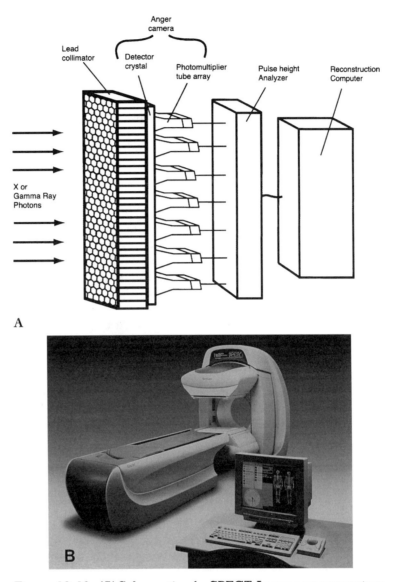

A

B

Figure 13-19. (A) Schematic of a SPECT Anger camera system showing the collimator, detector crystal, and photomultiplier tube array. **(B)** Photograph of a modern two-detector SPECT imaging system. In this photograph the heads are oriented opposite each other. (Photograph courtesy of Elscint.)

ing emission projections at many different angles. While a CT scanner typically acquires data from one slice at a time (unless it is operating in spiral mode), the Anger camera collects projections from a volume of tissue. The image reconstruction algorithms used in CT and SPECT are based in the same theory, and both utilize sets of projection data to assemble the tomographs. Slices may be reformatted in any direction (much like volume CT and MRI methods), and 3-D rendering of the volumetric data is also available.

In CT, the computer reconstructs a map of the X-ray attenuation values in the slice of tissue im-

aged. In SPECT, however, the reconstruction should represent the distribution of the administered radionuclide within the imaged slice. Since the gamma rays used in SPECT imaging are similar in energy to the X-rays used in CT, they are also subject to attenuation as they pass through the patient's body. This attenuation, however, is extremely undesirable in SPECT for it disturbs the pattern of radionuclide distribution observed by the Anger camera, making regions near the center of the patient seem "colder" than they truly are. The SPECT reconstruction computer goes through great lengths to correct for gamma ray attenuation, but currently these correction techniques are imperfect. The imperfect attenuation correction in SPECT imaging is a major limitation of the modality, and prevents accurate quantitative information (such as precise measures of radioactivity in specific tissues) from being obtained.

SPECT imaging is hampered somewhat by poor spatial and temporal resolution. Typical in plane resolution is on the order of 7.5 mm and is depth dependent, with system resolution being determined primarily by the collimator. Slice thicknesses in SPECT are variable depending upon how the volume data is reformatted, but the minimum attainable is about 1 cm. Imaging times in SPECT are usually in the neighborhood of 15 to 30 minutes, limiting somewhat the ability of SPECT to investigate rapidly changing processes.

Clinical Applications

Like MRI and CT, SPECT has found considerable clinical use in organ systems throughout the body. In this section we will briefly examine the applications of SPECT in the CNS (Table 13–5). In general, SPECT radiopharmaceuticals used for brain imaging can be divided into four classes: agents that assess blood brain barrier integrity, agents that assess cerebral perfusion, agents that bind to specific hormone or neurotransmitter receptors, and labeled antibodies directed at specific targets. SPECT has found a niche providing qualitative measures of cerebral perfusion, and these maps of regional cerebral blood flow (rCBF) are of diagnostic aid in several diseases. The radiopharmaceuticals most commonly used to image rCBF are ^{99m}Tc-HMPAO and ^{99m}Tc-ECD. Both are lipophilic compounds that cross the blood brain barrier and distribute in the brain tissue in a pattern proportional to tissue perfusion (Figure 13–20). These radiopharmaceuticals are administered intravenously, and must be given within 30 minutes of preparation. SPECT-acquired cerebral blood flow maps have established themselves as an effective technique in the detection of acute stroke, generally allowing identification of ischemic regions earlier than CT, though not quite as early as MRI. Other potential uses of SPECT in cerebrovascular disease include determination of stroke subtype, diagnosis of transient ischemic attacks, and identification of vasospasm following subarachnoid hemorrhage. In addition to cerebrovascular disease, SPECT-generated rCBF maps have been used to identify underlying disease processes in dementia cases (Figures 13–21 and 13–22), localize epileptic foci (Figure 13–23),[65,66] and detect abnormalities in cases of traumatic brain injury. SPECT studies of perfusion have been used on a more experimental basis in several diseases including Parkinson's disease,[70] obsessive compulsive disorder,[71] schizophrenia,[72] and depression.[73] The ^{99m}Tc perfusion mapping techniques have been used with mixed results in brain tumor imaging, and other SPECT techniques have proven more effective. One such method employs ^{201}T$_1$, which is readily taken up by a variety of tu-

Table 13–5. Applications of SPECT in Clinical Brain Imaging and Neuroscience

	Radiopharmaceutical Class	Application
Clinical CNS applications	Blood brain barrier agents	Assessment of brain death Detect compromise of BBB Neoplasm
	Cerebral perfusion agents	Cerebrovascular disease Dementing illnesses Epilepsy Trauma
	Receptor binding agents	Glioma, pituitary tumor
Neuroscience applications	Cerebral perfusion agents	Activation studies
	Receptor binding agents	Cerebrovascular disease Dementing illnesses Depression Epilepsy Migraine Schizophrenia
	Labeled antibodies	Alzheimer's disease Neoplasm

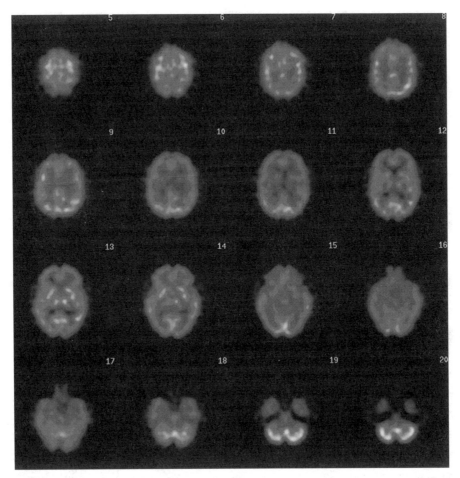

Figure 13-20. Axial SPECT images of cerebral perfusion in a healthy subject obtained using the radiopharmaceutical 99mTc-ECD. Notice that perfusion levels in the parietal cortex approach those of the occipital cortex and that the distribution of tracer appears rather smooth. (Images courtesy of David Wang.) See Color Plate 3.

mors, including some glioblastomas and intracerebral lymphomas in AIDS patients. Frequently, 201T$_1$ uptake is proportional to the malignant grade of the tumor. There are several radiopharmaceuticals designed to assess permeability of the blood brain barrier (BBB); the most widely used is 99mTc-DTPA. These agents help in highlighting lesions (tumor, hemangioma, etc.) that involve compromise of the BBB as well as in assessing brain death.

Applications to Neuroscience Research

SPECT imaging has proven a powerful tool in neuroscience research (Table 13-5). The ability to qualitatively measure rCBF provides SPECT with the means to map brain activity and, much like functional MRI, studies have been undertaken to examine activity patterns in a number of neurological processes in both normal brain and some disease states. These activation studies include in-

vestigations of thinking,[74,75] language,[74,76,77] and the motor[78] and somatosensory[79] systems. SPECT radiopharmaceuticals have been developed that bind specifically to certain receptors in the brain. One promising method of identifying some brain tumors is through the use of the radiopharmaceutical ^{111}In-octreotide, an analog of the hormone/neurotransmitter somatostatin. This radiopharmaceutical will localize in tissues expressing somatostatin receptors, and has shown an affinity for certain meningiomas, gliomas, and pituitary tumors.[80,81] Other receptor specific radiopharmaceuticals, most of which contain ^{123}I as their radionuclide, have been developed for use in SPECT imaging. Such pharmaceuticals include those with affinity for the muscarinic acetylcholine receptor with application to the study of Alzheimer's disease, dementia,[82] and epilepsy;[83] the benzodiazepine (GABA-A) receptor with application in the study of stroke[84] and epilepsy;[85] and certain dopamine

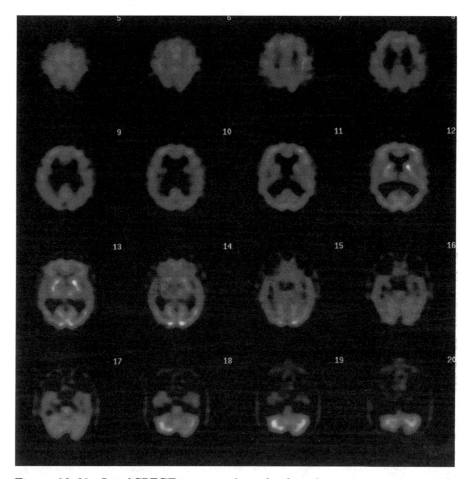

Figure 13–21. Axial SPECT images of cerebral perfusion in a patient with Alzheimer's dementia obtained using the radiopharmaceutical ⁹⁹ᵐTc-ECD. Perfusion in the parietal cortex is significantly reduced compared to that of the occipital cortex. This pattern of perfusion is typical in Alzheimer's type dementia, and is in clear contrast to that seen in healthy individuals (Figure 13–20). (Images courtesy of David Wang.) See Color Plate 4.

receptor subtypes that have been used to study depression,[86] schizophrenia,[87] migraine,[88] and Huntington's risk (Figure 13–24).[89] One additional area of radiopharmaceutical development with tremendous potential is the synthesis of radioactively labeled antibodies directed toward an antigen of interest. Labeling can be done with any of several radionuclides (⁹⁹ᵐTc, ¹³¹I, and ¹²³I are examples), and such antibodies have been raised against Alzheimer's amyloid protein[90] and several brain tumors (Figure 13–25).[91,92]

Strengths and Limitations

SPECT imaging has several strengths and weaknesses (Table 13–2). Since the technique employs radioactive pharmaceuticals, the subject will be exposed to ionizing radiation. Furthermore, the ra-

diation exposure is not limited to the imaged region, as the radiopharmaceutical will distribute throughout the body. The use of radiation also prevents the rapid repetition of experiments because radiation dose must be kept at an acceptable level and one must wait for the decay or elimination of radioactivity from previous scans before proceeding with the next. Current SPECT systems are unable to perform quantitative imaging due to imperfect attenuation correction. It is anticipated, however, that this limitation will be overcome in the near future. SPECT imaging does not possess the spatial or temporal resolution of MRI and CT; however, its ability to investigate a wide range of physiological and biochemical processes not available to conventional radiological techniques is a tremendous strength. While PET does offer many of the same imaging features

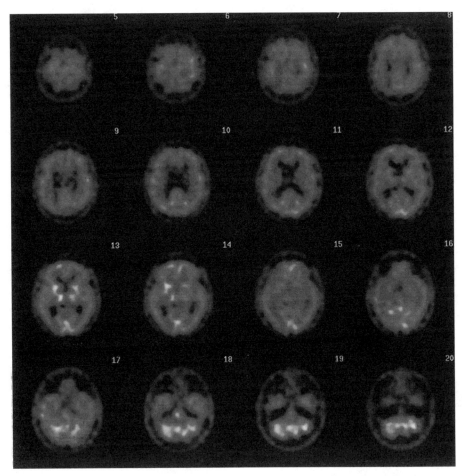

Figure 13–22. Axial SPECT images of cerebral perfusion in a patient with multi-infarct dementia (MID) obtained using the radiopharmaceutical ^{99m}Tc-ECD. Unlike the case of Alzheimer's type dementia (Figure 13–21), perfusion levels in the parietal cortex approach those of the occipital cortex. The pattern of perfusion, however, appears mottled when compared to the healthy scan (Figure 13–20), a trademark of MID. (Images courtesy of David Wang.) See Color Plate 5.

as SPECT, the SPECT scanning systems are considerably less expensive. Furthermore, modern SPECT scanners now have the ability to perform PET-like imaging with PET radiopharmaceuticals. This so called "high energy" or "coincidence detection" imaging tremendously broadens SPECT imaging potential.

Positron Emission Tomography

Positron emission tomography provided the first noninvasive look into the functional anatomy of the human brain. Many of the functional imaging experiments performed today, including fMRI and SPECT, have been guided by the rich PET literature that has already been available. The original PET scanners were built in the 1960s at several re-

search institutions and suffered from rather poor spatial resolution. The technology was improved over the next decade, and by the late 1970s the first PET scanners became commercially available. The spread of PET scanners into hospitals and research centers has been rather limited, however, by their high cost and limited clinical utility. Currently there are slightly more than 100 PET centers worldwide.

Principles

PET scanning belongs to the nuclear medicine class of imaging techniques. PET measures the activity distribution of injected or inhaled radioisotopes or radionuclides. Radionuclides commonly found in PET radiopharmaceuticals include

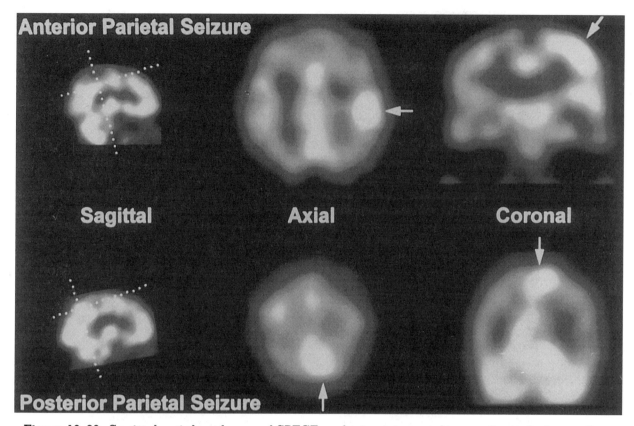

Figure 13–23. Sagittal, axial, and coronal SPECT perfusion images of two patients during epileptic seizures obtained using the radiopharmaceutical ^{99m}Tc-HMPAO. (**top**) Anterior parietal hyperperfusion in a patient whose seizure comprised tingling in the right hand followed by asymmetric bilateral dystonic posturing. (**bottom**) Posterior parietal hyperperfusion in a patient whose seizure comprised an experiential aura followed by psychoparetic complex partial seizure. (Reprinted with permission from Ho SS, Berkovic SF, Newton MR, Austin MC, McKay WJ, Bladin PF: Parietal lobe epilepsy: clinical features and seizure localization by ictal SPECT. *Neurology.* 1994; 44(12):2277–2284. Copyright 1994, Lippincott-Raven Publishers.)

^{15}O, ^{13}N, ^{11}C, ^{18}F, ^{68}Ga, ^{62}Cu, and ^{124}I (Table 13–4). Unlike SPECT in which the administered radiopharmaceutical emits gamma rays, PET radiopharmaceuticals are positron (positively charged electrons) emitters. These positron emitting isotopes are chemically incorporated into biologically active radiopharmaceuticals, enabling examination of a number of biochemical processes. The activity of these tracers in the patient is measured noninvasively by detectors arranged outside the body, and tomographic images are reconstructed. PET images should accurately reveal the distribution of the administered radiopharmaceutical in the region of the body being studied. In general, PET radiopharmaceuticals used in brain imaging fall into one of six categories: blood brain barrier agents, cerebral perfusion agents, tracers of metabolism, neurotransmitter tracers, agents that bind to specific CNS receptors, and labeled antibodies (Table 13–4).

PET scanners contain five basic components: (1) a ring of detector crystals, (2) a set of photo-

multiplier tubes (PMTs) attached to the detector ring, (3) a pulse height analyzer (PHA), (4) coincidence detection circuitry, and (5) a reconstruction computer (Figure 13–26). The PMTs, PHA, and computer perform functions identical to those described for SPECT systems. The detector ring of a PET scanner is composed of many small scintillation crystals, similar to the detector ring found in a CT scanner. The type of crystal used in PET imaging, however, is different from those found in either CT or SPECT. As with all nuclear medicine techniques, the radiation source used for imaging is not a part of the scanner, but is introduced into the subject in the form of a radiopharmaceutical.

When a PET radionuclide decays inside the subject's body an **annihilation** (see Appendix A) event will occur. The resultant 511 keV photons leave the site of decay in opposite directions, exit the subject's body (if neither are attenuated), and strike the crystal detector ring simultaneously at two different points. The scintillation light

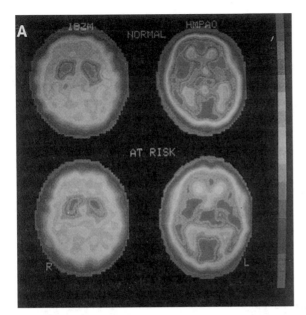

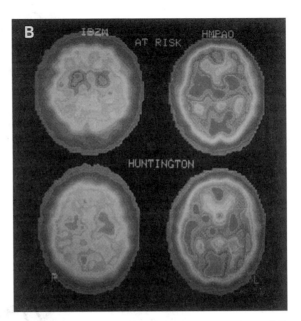

Figure 13–24. Axial SPECT dopamine receptor (DR) maps obtained using ^{123}I labeled IBZM, a DR ligand, and SPECT perfusion images obtained using ^{99m}Tc-HMPAO. (**A**) DR maps and perfusion images from a normal control (top) and an individual at risk for Huntington's disease (bottom). In this at-risk individual, striatal IBZM and HMPAO activities are similar to those of the control subject. (**B**) DR maps and perfusion images from an individual at risk for Huntington's disease (top) and a patient with Huntington's disease (bottom). In this at-risk individual, striatal IBZM uptake is reduced and HMPAO uptake is normal when compared to controls. Striatal IBZM and HMPAO uptake are both reduced in the patient with Huntington's disease. The results of this study indicate that ^{123}I-IBZM may provide a means of early diagnosis and preclinical detection of Huntington's disease. (Reprinted with permission from Ichise M, Toyama H, Fornazzari L, Ballinger JR, Kirsh JC: Iodine-123-IBZM dopamine D2 receptor and technetium-99m-HMPAO brain perfusion SPECT in the evaluation of patients with and subjects at risk for Huntington's disease. *J Nuc Med* 1993; 34(8): 1274–1281. Copyright 1993, Society of Nuclear Medicine, Inc. See Color Plate 6.

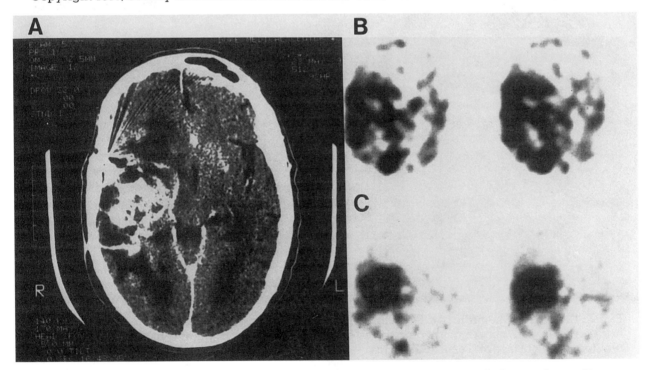

Figure 13–25. (**A**) Axial contrast enhanced CT of a patient with a large right hemisphere glioma. (**B,C**) Axial SPECT images of the same patient obtained using the radiopharmaceutical ^{123}I-81C6, an antibody raised against glioma tissue. SPECT images were obtained one hour (**B**) and 18 hours (**C**) following administration of the radiopharmaceutical. Reprinted with permission from Schold SC Jr, Zalutsky MR, Coleman RE, Glantz MJ, Friedman AH, Jaszczak RJ, Bigner SH, Bigner DD: Distribution and dosimetry of I-123-labeled monoclonal antibody 81C6 in patients with anaplastic glioma. *Invest Rad* 1993; 28(6):488–496. Copyright 1993, Lippincott-Raven Publishers.

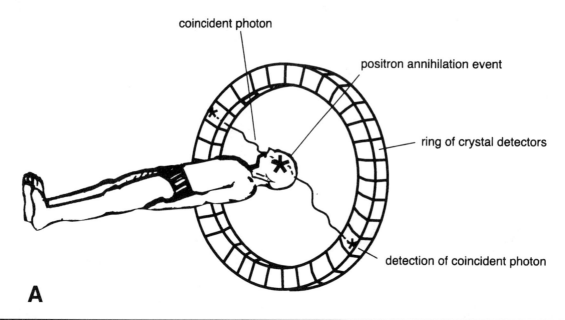

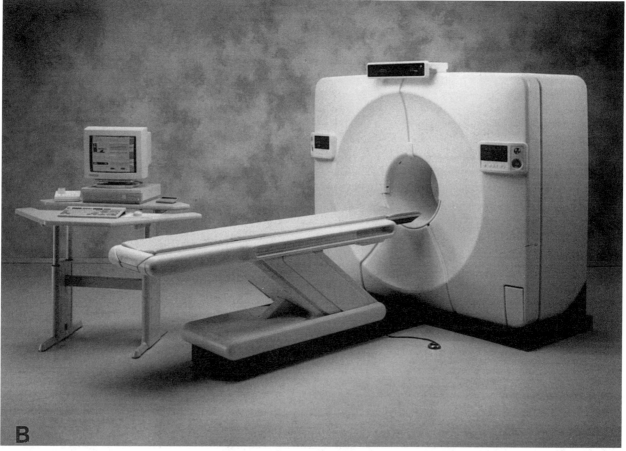

Figure 13–26. (**A**) Schematic of a PET scanner showing the ring of crystal detectors, and an annihilation even with subsequent coincidence detection. (**B**) Photograph of a modern PET scanner. (Photograph courtesy of General Electric.)

produced in each crystal is collected by the set of PMTs and converted into an electrical signal. This signal is measured by the pulse height analyzer to ensure that the detected photons are at the expected energy (511 keV). Lower energy photons, which likely result from scatter events, will be rejected by the PHA, and will not contribute to image formation. The PMT signal is also evaluated by the coincidence circuitry to ensure that only pairs of photons that were detected simultaneously (detected in coincidence) are allowed to contribute to the image. Coincidence detection can be performed in PET because we know that every positron decay and subsequent annihilation creates two coincident photons that will reach the detector ring at the same time. Single photons that arrive at the detector will either have originated outside the imaging region or will be the result of scatter. In this way, coincidence detection behaves in a manner similar to the collimator in CT and SPECT, and in fact is sometimes referred to as electronic collimation. Those PMT signals accepted by both the PHA and the coincidence circuits will then be fed into the reconstruction computer and the PET image is formed.

PET scanners in general perform better than SPECT systems in terms of resolution and scanning times. Modern PET scanners can attain in plane spatial resolution on the order of 3 to 5 mm, and slice thicknesses of approximately 1 cm. Scan time are still rather long, especially when compared to the faster functional MRI techniques, and a typical scan may require from 1 to 20 minutes to complete. This limits somewhat the ability of PET to examine rapidly changing processes.

Clinical Applications

The use of PET in clinical settings has been very slow to develop, and for most of its existence the technology has seen use primarily as a research tool (Table 13–6). Interest in the clinical application of PET is on the rise, however, and it is possible that the next several years will see PET blossom into a more widely appreciated clinical modality. Much of the current PET research reveals that this technique does have clinical relevance.[93]

Applications to Neuroscience Research

The history of functional imaging with PET is long, and an immense literature of activation studies has accumulated over the years. Recent PET functional

Table 13–6. Applications of PET in Clinical Brain Imaging and Neuroscience Research

	Radiopharmaceutical Class	Application
Clinical CNS applications	Metabolic tracers	Differentiation of recurrent tumor from radiation necrosis
Neuroscience applications	Cerebral perfusion agents	Alzheimer's disease Cerebrovascular disease Functional imaging
	Receptor binding agents	Alcoholism Alzheimer's disease Epilepsy Mood disorder Schizophrenia Parkinson's disease
	Metabolic tracers	Activation studies AIDS Alzheimer's disease Cerebrovascular disease Depression Epilepsy Neoplasm Parkinson's disease
	Neurotransmitter tracers	Parkinson's disease Schizophrenia
	Labeled antibodies	Glioma

imaging experiments have mapped the semantic processing of words and pictures,[94] REM sleep,[95] taste perception,[96] memory,[97] and learning (Figure 13–27).[98] PET studies of brain activity have also been performed in several disease states. Motor system reorganization following amputation[99] and the acquisition of hemidystonia[100] have been mapped, as have the neural systems of stuttering,[101] memory deficits in Alzheimer's disease,[102] Braille reading in the blind,[103] and auditory discrimination tasks in dyslexics.[104]

PET techniques have been used in baseline (non-activation) studies of cerebral perfusion and metabolism as well. In addition to the FDG tracer of glucose metabolism, radiopharmaceuticals have been developed that trace oxygen metabolism ($[^{15}O]O_2$), and amino acid metabolism ($[^{11}C]$methionine). The utility of such measurements in the assessment of several disease states has been investigated; a few of these results are mentioned here. Abnormal patterns of glucose metabolism have been reported in cases of depression,[105] Tourette's syndrome,[106] epilepsy,[107] anorexia nervosa,[108] congenital lactic acidosis,[109] Parkinson's disease,[110] and acquired immunodeficiency syndrome (AIDS).[111] There have been attempts at using amino acid and glucose metabolism to detect and grade certain tumors.[112] Such efforts have met with mixed success, although correlation of glucose metabolism with tumor aggressivity[113] and improved delineation of tumor extent with $[^{11}C]$methionine PET[114] have been reported. The differentiation of brain lymphoma from infection in AIDS patients has also been documented.[115] In cerebrovascular disease it was found that PET measures of perfusion and metabolism were of use in determining the degree of capillary recruitment in tissue recovering from stroke.[116] Combined cerebral blood flow and metabolism studies have also been used to elucidate the pathophysiology of hydrocephalus in infants[117] and reveal altered energy metabolism in Alzheimer's disease (Figure 13–28).[118]

Strengths and Limitations

PET scanning is a tremendously versatile technique. Radiopharmaceuticals have been developed that allow PET to trace physiological processes ranging from blood flow to energy and neurotransmitter metabolism. New pharmaceuticals are in constant development, and it is likely that PET and SPECT will both continue to find increasing application in clinics and research laboratories. This versatility is one of PET imaging's greatest assets. Other strengths of this technique include the ability to make quantitative physiologic measurements.

PET does have several drawbacks, however (Table 13–2). As with SPECT imaging, PET scanning will expose the subject to a radiation dose since a radioactive tracer is introduced into the body. The dose factor can limit how many times a procedure may be repeated. Repetition of experiments is also limited by the buildup of residual activity from previous scans. Some PET radiopharmaceuticals, however, have reasonably short half lives (especially ^{15}O), allowing repetition after a several minute delay. There are also some limitations in using PET during functional imaging studies. PET has a poor signal-to-noise ratio, and frequently PET data must be averaged over several subjects or several repetitions to attain the necessary signal-to-noise ratio. This makes individual studies difficult to perform; however, newer PET scanners are approaching the point where individual data may be considered reliable. PET activation studies also suffer from rather poor temporal resolution when compared to rapid fMRI techniques. PET scanning is easily the most expensive of the imaging modalities discussed in this chapter. With the introduction of less expensive coincidence detection SPECT systems capable of imaging positron emitting radiopharmaceuticals, one wonders if some day we might see the convergence of these two nuclear medicine technologies.

This concludes the discussion of CT, MRI, SPECT, and PET imaging technologies. The clinical and scientific applications of these modalities are summarized in Table 13–7. The remainder of this chapter will be devoted to the discussion of the role of neuroimaging in speech and language.

BRAIN/LANGUAGE RELATIONSHIPS: THE INFLUENCE OF NEUROIMAGING

Until 30 years ago, the understanding of the neurological basis of language depended largely on the neuropathological study of patients with aphasia. Remarkable advances were made through single case studies that correlated distinctive language disturbances with particular lesion locations. From these correlations, the classic models of aphasia first proposed by Broca, Wernicke, and Lichtheim in the nineteenth century were developed depicting the neural basis for the comprehension and production of language. These models were later extended in the twentieth century by Dejerine and Geschwind. According to the classical view, the peri-

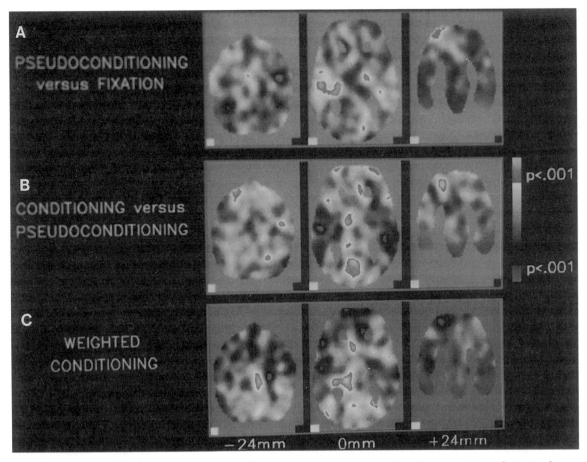

Figure 13–27. Axial PET ^{15}O-water perfusion images averaged across seven subjects showing regions of functional activation and deactivation during eyeblink conditioning. (**A**) Functional maps of pseudoconditioning (in which the presentation of a tone and delivery of air puff stimulation to the right eye were not correlated in time) relative to a visual fixation rest state. (**B**) Functional maps of conditioning (in which the presentation of a tone preceded airpuff stimulation by 400 ms) relative to pseudoconditioning. (**C**) Functional maps of conditioning experiments weighted by a behavioral learning measure relative to pseudoconditioning. Pseudoconditioning relative to rest elicited increases in regional cerebral blood flow (rCBF) in frontal and temporal cortex, basal ganglia, left hippocampus, and pons. Conditioning relative to pseudoconditioning elicited activation in bilateral frontal cortex, left thalamus, right hippocampus, left lingual gyrus, and pons; and decreases in rCBF in bilateral temporal cortex, right putamen, and right hippocampus. (Reprinted with permission from Blaxton TA, Zeffiro TA, Gabrieli JD, Bookheimer SY, Carrillo MC, Theodore WH, Disterhoft JF: Functional mapping of human learning: A positron emission tomography activation study of eyeblink conditioning. *J Neurosci* 1996; 16(12):4032–4040. Copyright 1996, Society for Neuroscience.) See Color Plate 7.

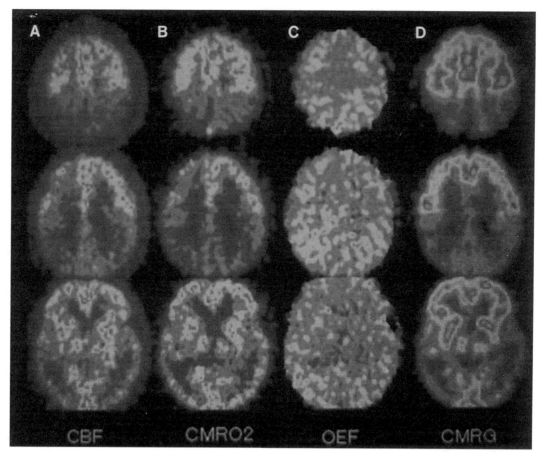

Figure 13–28. Axial PET images of (**A**) cerebral blood flow (CBF), (**B**) oxygen metabolism (CMRO2), (**C**) oxygen extraction fraction (OEF), and (**D**) glucose metabolism (CMRG) in a patient with Alzheimer's disease. Significant reductions of CBF and CMRG and moderate reduction of CMRO2 were noted in the parietotemporal region. A slight increase in OEF was observed in the same region. (Reprinted with permission from Fukuyama H, Ogawa M, Yamauchi H, Yamaguchi S, Kimur J, Yonekura Y, Konishi J: Altered cerebral metabolism in Alzheimer's disease: A PET study. *J Nucl Med* 1994; 35(1): 1–6. Copyright 1994, Society of Nuclear Medicine, Inc.) See Color Plate 8.

sylvian area in the left hemisphere contains the "zone of language." In this zone, cortical language centers exist that support specific language functions.

1. Wernicke's area, in the posterior superior temporal lobe, is involved in receptive language. Semantic associations are also aroused here and give meaning to receptive input.
2. Broca's area in the posterior inferior frontal region is specialized for motor aspects of speech, and receives input from Wernicke's area via the arcuate fasciculus.
3. The angular gyrus participates in cross-modal associations. Word reading requires the translation of visual input into an auditory code in the angular gyrus, and then meaning is subsequently accessed through Wernicke's area.[119]

Each of these centers is interconnected, and damage to any one or the connections between them can result in a specific aphasic syndrome. With the advent of radioisotope scanning in the 1960s and the introduction of CT in the early 1970s, our understanding of the neurology of language has greatly expanded. Using CT, and later MRI, lesion location could be identified *in vivo* and large-scale studies of brain-damaged patients with language disturbances began to be published. Recent advances in other neuroimaging techniques, such as PET, SPECT, and fMRI, have further enhanced our understanding of the neurophysiology of language and hold promise for understanding functional mechanisms of recovery following neurological insult. Neural evidence for brain/language relationships has come from three different sources: (1) lesion localization data; (2) blood flow and

Table 13–7. Summary of the Applications of CT, MRI, SPECT, and PET

Modality		Primary Applications
CT	**Clinical**	Cerebrovascular disease, congenital malformation, neoplasm, trauma, angiography
	Neuroscience	Lesion studies, brain morphology studies
MRI	**Clinical**	Cerebrovascular disease, congenital malformation, infection, neoplasm, white matter disease, angiography
	Neuroscience	Activation studies, cerebral perfusion studies, in vivo spectroscopy, diffusion imaging, lesion studies, brain morphology studies
SPECT	**Clinical**	Dementing illnesses, neoplasm, cerebrovascular disease, epilepsy
	Neuroscience	Activation studies, cerebral perfusion studies, receptor mapping studies
PET	**Clinical**	Differentiation of recurrent tumor from radiation necrosis
	Neuroscience	Activation studies, cerebral perfusion studies, baseline metabolic studies (glucose, oxygen, and amino acids), receptor mapping studies

baseline metabolism studies; (3) functional brain activation studies. This section reviews some of the major findings from neuroimaging studies and illustrates how our understanding of brain/language relationships and recovery from aphasia have evolved.

The Lesion Localization Method

Clinical-Anatomical Studies

CT studies began in 1973 and the first studies of CT and aphasia emerged in 1977.[120] Most early studies sought to correlate specific lesion locations with the classic aphasia syndromes, and several reviews from those efforts have been published.[121,122] Table 13–8 highlights the typical lesion locations of the classic aphasia syndrome. Another tenet supported by CT and MRI scan data has been the fluent and nonfluent dichotomy associated with pre-Rolandic and post-Rolandic lesions. A challenge to classic models, however, has been that the location of the lesion may predict the aphasia type, but the reverse does not always hold true. Furthermore, alternative lesion locations for classic aphasia syndromes have been found, which suggest the need to revise the classical language models.

Using CT, Basso et al.[123] examined 207 subjects with aphasia, and 36 presented with atypical find-

ings. Five patients with Wernicke's aphasia and 2 patients with transcortical sensory aphasia had lesions that spared the post-Rolandic area; 6 patients with lesions encompassing both Broca's and

Table 13–8. Lesion Location of Classic Aphasia Syndromes

Aphasia Classification	Lesion Location
Broca's	Left lateral frontal, prerolandic, suprasylvian regions (Broca's area) extending into the adjacent subcortical periventricular white matter
Wernicke's	Left posterior, superior temporal gyrus
Conduction	White matter pathways under supramarginal gyrus
Anomic	Angular gyrus; second temporal gyrus
Transcortical motor	Anterior and superior to Broca's area
Transcortical sensory	Posterior parieto-temporal, sparing Wernicke's area
Global	Large perisylvian, extending deep into subjacent white matter

Wernicke's areas had Wernicke's aphasia rather than global aphasia. There were also 7 cases of fluent aphasia and anterior CT lesions, and 6 cases of nonfluent aphasia and posterior CT lesions. Vignolo et al.[124] studied 37 patients with global aphasia and found nearly half of them had atypical lesion sites; 8 had purely anterior lesions, 3 purely posterior, and 4 deep lesions. These findings illustrate the problems that have been met by attempts to correlate aphasia syndromes with lesion sites and the limited success some researchers have had. These studies also challenge the method of correlating an entire aphasia syndrome with a specific lesion location. Use of the classical typology of aphasia has been criticized previously as being less than ideal for development of a theory of the structure of the processing components of normal language and their associated neural substrates.[125,126] It is readily agreed that macrofunctions such as language comprehension or expression are convenient ways of depicting mind and behavior, but are in fact composed of many subcomponents or mental processes. A more fruitful approach to understanding brain/language relationships may involve localization of specific symptoms or subcomponents of language, rather than whole syndromes.

The localization of symptoms or subcomponents is not new and was implemented by Mohr et al.[127] in the 1970s who shifted the focus of Broca's aphasia away from a study of the complete syndrome to its constituent elements. This type of study has been made possible with the increasing sensitivity of CT and MRI, allowing for more detailed anatomical-clinical correlations. Alexander et al.[128] examined lesions involving the frontal operculum (Broca's area). Three distinct functional systems were identified as a result of lesions involving or encroaching upon the frontal operculum. The following structures were correlated with these functions: (1) frontal operculum (initiation and formulation); (2) lower motor cortex (articulation and prosody); and (3) temporo-parietal to opercular connections (phonemic production). Each of these systems can be injured in isolation, but they operate in concert for language production. The pattern of injury to each of these structures determines the resulting language behavior. Other attempts to localize speech–language symptoms have met with some success. Dronkers[129] found that the insula was the common structure lesioned in 27 patients with apraxia of speech. Of 17 patients without apraxia of speech, all spared the insula, yet still had lesions involving most of the left hemisphere. Further analysis demonstrated that damage to the arcuate fasciculus results in severe production deficits. In patients with Broca's aphasia, a lesion to the arcuate fasciculus reduced verbal output to stereotypies. Sparing of the arcuate fasciculus resulted in less severe production deficits. These studies illustrate how the correlation of symptoms with lesion sites is a much more effective method for investigating the relationship between brain regions and speech and language disorders.

Subcortical Structures and Language

Clinical-anatomical studies have also demonstrated that atypical language syndromes may result from subcortical lesions.[130–132] In 1906, Marie proposed that lesions to subcortical structures could cause aphasia, but it was not until the advent of CT that more conclusive evidence was provided.[133] This finding has revised the notion that aphasia is purely a cortical manifestation and the primary neural substrate of language.

Damage to the thalamus, basal ganglia, and internal capsule has repeatedly been shown to cause aphasia.[134–137] Thalamic aphasia is characterized by preserved repetition, variable but relatively good auditory comprehension, reduced spontaneous speech, a predominance of semantic paraphasic errors, and anomia. Impaired attention and memory are also frequently reported. Naeser et al.[122] identified three additional subcortical aphasia syndromes: (1) capsular-putaminal (C/P) with anterior-superior extension; (2) capsular-putaminal with posterior extension; and (3) capsular-putaminal with both anterior-superior and posterior extension. Patients with C/P with anterior-superior extension had language that resembled Broca's aphasia with good comprehension and grammatical, but slow, dysarthric speech. C/P syndrome with posterior extension resembled a Wernicke's aphasia with poor comprehension and Wernicke-like fluent speech. C/P lesions with both anterior and posterior extension resulted in global aphasia. In all cases, patients had a lasting right hemiplegia. Since this study, Alexander et al[138] have developed a model that explains the various roles of subcortical structures in aphasia based on CT findings. The reader is also referred to Crosson[139,140] for further reviews of the subcortical structures involvement in language.

Using CT and MRI to Predict Outcome and Plan Treatment

Lesion localization data have been used to predict recovery and outcome in aphasia. Demeurisse et al.[141] found lesion volume in patients with cortical-subcortical lesions to correlate significantly with the ultimate severity of aphasia and associated verbal expression and auditory comprehensions deficits. Patients with deep lesions (no contact with cortex), however, had no significant correlation between size of lesion and clinical outcome. These findings demonstrate that the correlation between size of lesion and severity of aphasia holds true only for cortical-subcortical infarcts; the more intact brain tissue remaining, the less severe the language disorder. It also suggests that deep subcortical structures play an important role in language processing. Small lesions to deep structures can have significant consequences on language behavior. Despite these findings, most studies have shown that lesion *location*, more than lesion size is a better predictor of recovery.[5] Generally, this is true except in cases of very large or very small lesions, with very large lesions resulting in poorer outcomes.[142–144] For example, patients with global aphasia from a subcortical lesion have deficits as severe as those with much larger cortical infarcts, even when their infarct is half the size. This is because this smaller lesion associated with subcortical global aphasia undercuts the critical white matter pathways for speech and comprehension resulting in devastating consequences on communication.[145]

A number of studies have been conducted correlating lesion location with recovery of speech and language.[146–148] Naeser et al.[146] have found that combined lesions to the medial subcallosal fasciculus and the middle one-third of the periventricular white matter result in no recovery of spontaneous speech. Knopman et al.[147] discovered that persistent nonfluency is associated with damage to the left precentral gyrus. Additionally, oral naming, repetition, and sentence-length auditory comprehension remain impaired with damage to the left-posterior-superior temporal gyrus (Wernicke's area) and the inferior parietal lobe.[149] Finally, damage to greater than one-half of Wernicke's area has been associated with poor recovery of auditory comprehension.[143]

The response of patients with nonfluent aphasia to Melodic Intonation Therapy (MIT) has been correlated with CT scan localization data.[148,154] Patients who responded well to MIT had lesions involving Broca's area and/or the white matter deep to this area, plus large superior lesion extension into periventricular white matter deep to the lower motor cortex area for the face. The subjects with a good response did not have a large lesion in Wernicke's area, a lesion in the temporal isthmus, or the right hemisphere. Subjects with a poor response had bilateral lesions or lesions including Wernicke's area or the temporal isthmus.

These studies emphasize the importance of knowing the site of lesion for planning appropriate treatment interventions and providing accurate statements of prognosis. They also reinforce the idea that there are critical brain regions and highly focal areas that contribute to specific language functions. When these areas are lesioned, language pathways or networks are severely disrupted.

Lesion Localization Studies: Conclusions

CT and MRI have led to a number of valuable discoveries both in academic and clinical arenas. From the correlation of specific lesion locations with patterns of disturbed behavior, the classic localizationist model of aphasia has been generally upheld.[151,152] CT and MRI data have since been used to expand models of aphasia to include the basal ganglia and thalamus as critical to language functioning. The anatomic model of aphasia has its limitations, however. One shortcoming is that many patients with aphasia cannot be classified with this model. This limits the power of this model to delineate the neuropathology of language. As a result, studies have begun to correlate selected subcomponents as opposed to entire syndromes of language with particular lesion sites. This shift in focus has allowed for more precise understanding of brain/language relationships and accounted for the individual variations of disturbed language behavior observed. Lesion localization data can also be used to make predictions about potential for recovery of language and for planning appropriate treatment interventions. For example, patients who are not expected to regain functional spontaneous speech can be channeled into a nonverbal or augmentative treatment program, utilizing time and resources more effectively.

A significant limitation of lesion localization studies and CT and MRI data is that they only provide information about brain structure, not brain function. Functional neuroimaging technologies such as PET and SPECT have shown that anatomic information alone cannot supply a full understanding of normal or disordered language. The next section will review how neuroimaging studies of brain blood flow and metabolism have revised our thinking about brain/language relationships and aphasia.

BRAIN FUNCTION AND LANGUAGE

For many decades the primary means for understanding the organization of language in the brain was through the analysis of behavior patterns associated with focal brain lesions. One of the drawbacks of the lesion localization method is that the damaged brain may not process language like the nondamaged brain. A second problem with the lesion method is that it examines brain structure and not brain function (i.e., blood flow, glucose metabolism, oxygen metabolism). In many studies, brain function has been shown to correlate more closely with behavior than brain structure, making it an extremely important avenue of study.[153] These problems have been solved to some degree with the advent of the functional neuroimaging technologies: PET, SPECT, and fMRI. The neurophysiology of normal as well as brain damaged individuals can now be studied.

One of the primary techniques for studying brain function is to examine the brain at rest for patterns of blood flow and metabolism. These studies are referred to as baseline metabolism or "resting" state studies. Typically in these studies alterations in blood flow, oxygen metabolism, or glucose metabolism are measured. The second method is to engage subjects in a specific cognitive task and measure changes in blood flow and metabolism corresponding with the task. These are known as functional activation studies.

Baseline Brain Metabolism and Blood Flow

The technologies for studying brain metabolism and blood flow PET and SPECT have increased our understanding of the relationship between brain function and behavior. In brain damaged individuals, these technologies allow for investigation of brain function beyond the site of the structural lesion. New insights into the functional impact of brain damage have been gained largely from PET studies which have measured glucose metabolism. Because glucose is the main source of energy for the brain, alterations in its utilization or metabolism reflect change in the brain's functional capacity. Reduced glucose metabolism can be the result of structural damage to a region, a loss of information coming in from other regions, a loss of intrinsic functional capacity, a loss of information going out to other regions, or a change in the overall homeostasis of the region.[154] PET studies have repeatedly shown that metabolic depression extends beyond the site of the lesion, suggesting that structurally normal tissue may in fact be abnormal in function.[147] Focal brain damage can cause (1) diffuse functional changes with widespread alterations of brain physiology; (2) focal physiological changes in specific remote regions; or (3) a combination of these effects.[155] This results in changes in

areas distant from the structural damage and may alter the functional relationship between regions. Understanding these effects can increase our understanding of normal and disordered language.

Baseline Metabolism Studies in Normal Individuals

Normal values of brain metabolism have been calculated during the "resting" state. Different results have been obtained depending on the researchers' definition of a resting state. In resting studies with the subjects' eyes closed and the ears unoccluded, a strong degree of metabolic symmetry exists between homologous structures in the left and right hemispheres.[156,157] With increasing age, there is a small decline in global and cortical metabolism across all brain regions.[158] Changing the resting state to involve occlusion of the ears and covering the eyes has resulted in a significant right < left hemisphere asymmetry that was not observed when the ears and eyes were unoccluded.[156]

Metabolic Changes with Structural Brain Lesions

A number of studies have examined metabolic changes in brain regions as a result of a structural lesion. Two patterns have emerged:

- Remote brain effects from structural lesions that *exceed* the size of the lesion
- Structural lesions with *no* remote metabolic changes

Focal brain lesions are associated with diffuse, but generally predictable changes in brain metabolism and brain function.[159] Cortical lesions are typically associated with alterations in brain metabolism in the ipsilateral cortex adjacent to and distant from the lesion, ipsilateral basal ganglia and thalamus, and in the contralateral cerebellum.[160–162] Lacunar lesions in the subcortex result in metabolic abnormalities in cortical areas. These remote metabolic disturbances suggest that function in these regions may be abnormal. The effects of distant metabolic dysfunction may account for some of the aphasic language disturbances observed in patients with aphasia.

Another interesting finding is that clinically silent lesions exist that do not show distant metabolic effects, yet evidence of a lesion is seen on anatomic imaging studies. Even with a structural lesion, these individuals perform normally on neuropsychological testing. Metter[159] has suggested that for a structural lesion to be symptomatic, remote metabolic changes must occur. It has also been demonstrated that persistence of aphasic symptoms is associated with remote metabolic changes.[159]

Brain Metabolism and Blood Flow in Aphasia

PET and SPECT scanning have provided some valuable insights into patterns of brain metabolism in individuals with aphasia. Several important trends have been found:

- Metabolic depression extends beyond the zone of infarction, suggesting that structurally undamaged tissue may be abnormal.[163]
- Metabolic changes occur in the temporo-parietal regions in essentially all adults with aphasia regardless of the location of the structural lesion.[164]
- Lesions that densely damage or extend into the deep subcortical structures damage cortical-subcortical communication with disruption of cortical-basal ganglia-thalamic loops.[165]
- Correlations of aphasia type are stronger for regional metabolism than for lesion site location.[155]

Metter studied chronic Wernicke's, Broca's, and conduction aphasia patients using PET and CT and found abnormal metabolism in regions beyond the structural lesion.[163] The lesion localization data and glucose metabolic pattern were different for these three groups of patients. All patients showed a similar pattern of metabolic asymmetry in the temporoparietal region. Patients with conduction aphasia had slightly less hypometabolism at that site. The three syndromes differed, however, in the extent of metabolic abnormality in the prefrontal cortex, an area not typically associated with aphasic language disturbance. Patients with conduction aphasia exhibited no prefrontal abnormality with about half showing hypometabolism in Broca's area. Patients with Wernicke's aphasia had mild to moderate glucose hypometabolism in Broca's area and about half had prefrontal changes. Broca's aphasia patients demonstrated severe hypometabolism in the left frontal lobe, including prefrontal regions and Broca's area. The commonality among these three aphasic syndromes was temporoparietal hypometabolism reinforcing the role of this region in aphasia. These syndromes differed, however, in the extent of prefrontal involvement. It may be that hypometabolism in the prefrontal region influences an aphasia patient's overall language and behavioral functioning. For example, the feature of press of speech exhibited by Wernicke's aphasia patients may be a result of

prefrontal dysfunction; the patient shows a lack of awareness and self-monitoring over his or her own speech output. In Broca's aphasia patients, prefrontal involvement may be manifested as a slowness in responding and difficulty coordinating motor behavior and other complex sequences. This study highlights a number of different brain regions involved in normal language processing, including brain regions not typically associated with aphasia (i.e., prefrontal involvement in Broca's and Wernicke's aphasia patients) in the classic localizationist models of language. It also illustrates the interaction between brain structure and function in language processing and that the effects of brain damage extend well beyond the lesion site.

Another common finding in aphasia as mentioned earlier is the consistent metabolic abnormality in the temporo-parietal cortex. Using (F-18) fluorodeoxyglucose, Metter et al.[164] studied 44 aphasic patients with a variety of classic syndromes in a resting state to determine if consistent metabolic abnormalities existed. Ninety-seven percent showed decreased metabolism in the angular gyrus, 87% had abnormalities in the supramarginal gyrus, and 85% in the posterosuperotemporal (Wernicke's) area. With these temporoparietal regions combined, 100% of patients had left temporoparietal hypometabolism. These findings suggest that functional abnormality in the temporo-parietal region is essential for the acquisition of aphasia. What differentiates the syndromes is involvement of left frontal and subcortical regions either directly from structural damage or indirectly through remote metabolic effects. The nature and extent of aphasia depend on the interaction between the structurally damaged regions, their effects on temporoparietal function, and the rest of the brain.

Relationship Between Subcortical Structures and Aphasia

CT studies have demonstrated that lesions of subcortical structures including the basal ganglia and thalamus result in aphasia. In general, metabolic patterns associated with subcortical lesions correlate with the subcortical aphasia syndromes discussed earlier.[131,138,166] PET scanning data have been used to answer the question of whether subcortical damage has a direct role on the resulting language profile or whether the effect is indirect through metabolic depression in the cortex. Metter et al.[167] used pathway analysis to model the relationship of subcortical structural damage with cortical hypometabolism on behavior. Subcortical structural damage directly affected fluency, but not comprehension. Indirect effects were also found primarily through alterations in frontal lobe metabolism. The internal capsule contributed to these alterations. Damage here disconnected frontal regions from deeper subcortical structures, disrupting motor pathways that participate in the control and management of speech production. These findings provide support for the critical role of subcortical structures in language as more recent models propose.[140,168]

Blood Flow and Brain Metabolism in Recovery from Aphasia

Results from SPECT and PET scan studies have been used to make predictions about outcome and recovery in aphasia. In general, there is an inverse relationship between the size of rCBF defect and potential for stroke recovery.[169,170] Using SPECT, Mlcoch et al.[171] found that metabolism in the inferior frontal area significantly correlated with recovery of fluent speech in patients with nonfluent aphasia. Eight of 9 patients with good recovery of fluency had normal rCBF to the inferior frontal region while 4 of 5 patients with poor recovery showed hypoperfusion in this area. Tikofsky et al.[172] studied five patients with aphasia at one year poststroke. The three patients with improved language function had decreased, but not absent, rCBF in the left cortical language regions of the left hemisphere and a slight increase in rCBF in regions of the right hemisphere. In addition, aphasic individuals with poor outcome showed larger rCBF defects associated with the infarcted tissue. Metter et al.[155] found that changes in regional glucose metabolism of the left and right temporo-parietal regions significantly correlated with changes in the Western Aphasia Battery comprehension score.

The role of the right hemisphere in recovery of function has also been demonstrated. Patients with aphasia with a "good" prognosis have been shown to have increased rCBF in the area homologous to Broca's area in the right hemisphere.[173] Heiss et al.[174] examined 26 patients with aphasia, finding that resting glucose metabolism of the left cerebral hemisphere outside the infarct was the greatest predictor of improvement on Token Test performance. These studies demonstrate the importance of residual left hemisphere functioning for recovery of language comprehension and indicate that the right hemisphere also appears to assume some function. They also suggest that cell loss beyond the immediate infarct may be one cause for poor recovery.

In summary, brain-damaged patients with the greatest potential for recovery show patterns of increased blood flow and metabolism in *both* the left and right hemispheres, compared to normals and subjects with a poor prognosis. It has been suggested that the mechanism of recovery following brain damage is functional reorganization. Parts of the intact brain substitute for damaged parts, and homologous regions may take over to some extent as well, but usually not completely.[175] The patterns of blood flow and metabolism from these studies provide evidence for the possible functional reorganization of language.

Baseline Metabolism and Blood Flow Studies: Conclusions

There have been many valuable contributions to our understanding of brain/language relationships from studies examining baseline brain metabolism and blood flow. The extensive PET literature and work conducted by Metter and colleagues[159] have contributed immensely to these insights. First, the impact of remote effects of structural damage can be observed and are now known to greatly influence language behavior. These studies provide further evidence that both cortical-cortical connections and cortical-subcortical connections are critical for intact language functioning. Aphasia also appears to have a unifying pathophysiology as evidenced by decreased metabolism in temporo-parietal cortex in all individuals with aphasia. At the same time, different patterns of glucose metabolism, most notably in the prefrontal and subcortical regions, differentiate aphasic syndromes supporting theories of multiple types of aphasia. These findings illustrate that many brain regions operate in concert as a highly complex interactive system for normal language functioning. Disruption to one region interferes with normal functioning of connected regions both near and far. Finally, baseline studies have shown that recovery of language function correlates with specific patterns of rCBF and glucose metabolism. More is to be learned about brain function, however, by visualizing brain activity during task performance in both normals and brain damaged. The next section will discuss some of the findings from activation studies and how they have influenced our thinking about the neural correlates of language.

Functional Brain Activation Studies

Another technique used to correlate brain/language relationships is to control mental processing with specific activation tasks, and measure alterations in brain function, such as a change in blood flow, glucose metabolism, or oxygen metabolism. Brain activation has been studied most extensively with PET [176,177] and more recently with fMRI.[48,54,55] There are many benefits to brain activation studies compared to the lesion localization method. First, the lesion localization method correlates patterns of behavior with the site of lesion. As seen with baseline metabolism and blood flow studies, the extent of brain dysfunction is greater than the structural lesion. Furthermore, the lesion may disrupt not only the site of a particular language or cognitive function, but may also disturb that behavioral function's input or output connections resulting in a similar clinical picture.[178] Activation studies have the potential to capture several brain regions that participate in a particular language function. In addition, the brains of both normals and brain damaged can be studied during language and other task performance. These methods therefore allow for a more direct approach to brain/behavior correlation.

Methodology

The rationale behind activation studies is that performance of a task places information processing demands on the brain.[179] Each cognitive task can be analyzed into basic mental operations that are then localized to specific brain regions. For example, when reading a word, the component mental operations include: processing of the visual features of letters, orthographic processing, phonological processing, and processing of the word meaning (semantics). By measuring changes in brain metabolism or blood flow associated with task performance, certain brain regions or networks can be isolated that are thought to contribute to a particular cognitive operation.[180] Many basic operations are involved in a cognitive task resulting in a set of distributed functional areas

that must be coordinated for cognitive task performance. Language then is not localized to a particular Brodman area or lobe; a center that houses speech production or auditory comprehension does not exist. Instead, language functions such as auditory comprehension utilize a complex and distributed set of brain regions and networks that regulate their overall function.

Although activation studies have many benefits, they also entail many limitations and methodological challenges. When measuring language or mental processing, the first challenge is to isolate the process of interest. This is typically accomplished by developing an experiment with a hierarchical design where each level of task performance adds a higher level of information processing. It is not uncommon to have experiments with three to four different steps, each adding a small number of operations to those of its subordinate (control) state. In a study conducted by Petersen et al.,[176] this methodology was used to investigate processing of single words. To examine this, subjects were asked to give an appropriate action or use for a common noun. For example, when presented with the word, "cake," subjects might respond with "eat." This task was chosen because it could be broken down into a number of identifiable mental operations. Table 13–9 outlines the hierarchical design for this study. Each activation state is compared to the control state to isolate the process of interest. In the first comparison, the presentation of a word is compared to visual fixation on a crosshair, isolating sensory input and involuntary word-form processing. In the second step, repeating each presented word is compared to passive viewing of each word. This step isolates areas involved in output coding and motor control. In the final comparison, repeating each word is compared to generation of a use for each target noun.

Table 13–9. Hierarchical design of the Lexical Access Experiment

Control State	Activation State	Cognitive Operations
Fixation point only	Passive viewing of words	Passive sensory processing Automatic word-level coding
Passive viewing of words	Repeat words	Articulatory coding Motor programming and output
Repeat words	Generate verbs (uses and actions)	Semantic association Selection for action

Source: Adapted from Peterson SE, Fox PT, Posner MI, et al: Positron emission tomographic studies of the cortical anatomy of single-word processing. *Nature* 1988; 331:585–589; Posner MI, Raichle ME: Interpreting words. In *Images of Mind,* pp. 104–129. Scientific American Library, New York, 1994.

This comparison attempts to isolate semantic processing. With PET studies, typically the images obtained during the control state are subtracted from images of the same slice during the activation or experimental state to demonstrate brain regions associated with the process of interest. This method of data extraction is known as the subtraction method. Additional methods of data extraction include Fourier analysis and cross-correlation thresholding.[181]

The next challenge in brain activation studies is to interpret the patterns of brain activation visualized. An area of activation does not necessarily correspond to a particular cognitive or behavioral function. Metter[159] identified three different types of brain activation patterns. The first is a general increase in blood flow and metabolism related to task difficulty and the degree of attentional demand. As task complexity and attentional demand increase, brain activation may increase. The second type of activation pattern involves areas of little activation, even in areas traditionally thought to be associated with a given task. For example, during some language tasks the supramarginal gyrus and angular gyrus show little activation while lesion studies and cortical mapping have suggested an integral role in language processing. The third type of activation pattern is an increase or decrease in blood flow or brain metabolism that is task dependent (e.g., the activation of auditory cortex during auditory tasks). Another consideration in analyzing activation patterns is that increased activation may also be the result of one brain region inhibiting the function of another. These different patterns of activation can make image interpretation very difficult.

An additional problem with PET activation studies has been that data are generally intersubject averaged. Averaging data has been criticized because association and higher level cortical areas have greater anatomic variability, making intersubject averaging inappropriate.[182] A second criticism is that individual differences in cognitive processing might be blurred. Inherent problems in averaging data for brain-damaged patients also exist as their clinical profiles are usually not homogeneous. A benefit of fMRI is that data do not need to be averaged across subjects, allowing for the study of individuals.

Functional Activation Studies in Normal Individuals

The recent advances in functional brain imaging techniques have expanded present conceptions of brain/language relationships. This information has largely been gained from PET studies with normal subjects and more recently with fMRI. Studies of language have examined auditory speech perception,[183] single word reading,[184] verbal fluency,[185] language lateralization,[186] phonological processing,[187] the auditory and visual lexicons,[188] semantics,[189,91] and word finding.[190] From these studies it has been found that language involves a complex network of brain regions in the left and right hemispheres, including several subcortical structures, and the cerebellum contralateral to the dominant hemisphere. Compared to classic models, activation studies have shown that language involves many more brain regions in both the left and right hemispheres than were previously apparent from lesion localization studies.

One of the first studies of language activation that has since served as a model for future studies was completed by Petersen et al.[176,177,191] This study used a hierarchical design to examine single word processing in both the visual and auditory modalities at three distinct levels as described earlier (see Table 13–9). Separate brain regions were responsible for the processing of visual and auditory word forms. Passive listening to real words activated modality-specific primary and extraprimary sensory-processing areas including the belateral superior temporal gyri and a left-lateralized area in the temporoparietal cortex. Passive viewing of words presented visually activated several areas of extrastriate visual cortex in both hemispheres. During the repetition task, speech output produced activation of the primary sensorimotor mouth cortex, the supplementary motor area (SMA), and regions of the cerebellum. In addition, repetition of words presented in either the visual or auditory modality resulted in a set of activations around the Sylvian-opercular cortex and a left-lateralized region on the lateral surface of the frontal cortex encroaching upon Broca's area. The verb generation task activated two areas of cerebral cortex for both auditory and visual presentations. The left inferior frontal area (Brodman's area 47) was activated and thought to participate in processing of semantic associations. The second area was the anterior cingulate believed to be part of the selective attentional system. Thus, a number of brain regions were found to contribute to single word processing including the extrastriate visual cortex (visual presentation), temporal cortex (auditory presentation), lateral premotor areas, anterior cingulate, prefrontal areas, and the cerebellum.

Petersen et al.[177] further examined the processing of visual words and word-like stimuli with

PET. Four different sets of stimuli were presented: (1) single common nouns (real words), (2) pseudo-word strings/nonwords that followed the rules for English spelling (i.e., "FLOOP and TOGLO"), (3) orthographically irregular strings of letters (i.e., "JVJFC"), and (4) strings of letter-like forms or false fonts. PET imaging showed areas of activation in the left medial extrastriate visual cortex with visual presentation of both pseudowords that followed the rules of English spelling and real words. Of interest is that these areas were not activated by nonsense strings of letters or false fonts. Petersen et al. argued that the left medial extrastriate plays an integral role in single word recognition or storage of visual word forms. These word forms can be real English words or words that conform to English spelling rules. Another interesting finding was that the presentation of words, but not pseudowords, activated the left inferior frontal area. The left inferior frontal activation was attributed to general semantic processing. This region has been activated during other semantic tasks providing support for this region as being integral to semantic processing. This study demonstrated that subcomponent processes of language (basic sensory, orthographic, and semantic) can be isolated and localized to focal areas within the brain.

Not all of Petersen et al.'s findings have been replicated, however. Using PET, Howard et al.[185] studied changes in regional cerebral blood flow (rCBF) to examine the brain regions associated with spoken and visual word recognition. There were two experimental and two control conditions in this study: (1) reading aloud of single words, (2) repetition of spoken words, (3) presentation of false fonts—subject says same word on presentation of each stimulus (control task), and (4) presentation of real words rerecorded in reverse—subject responds with the same word on presentation of each stimulus (control task). Two distinct foci were found for the auditory and visual (Petersen's visual word form) lexicons. The auditory lexicon (repetition of words) involved Wernicke's area in the left superior temporal gyrus and the middle part of the left temporal gyrus. Processing of complex auditory stimuli (listening to words rerecorded in reverse) involved bilateral activation of both the primary and secondary auditory cortex. The visual lexicon (reading words aloud) activated an area in the left posterior middle temporal gyrus, approximately 16 mm away. Visual processing (viewing of false fonts) activated the striate and extrastriate cortex bilaterally. This finding is in contrast to Petersen's finding of activation in the left medial extrastriate for visual word forms. A trend for increased activation in the left medial extrastriate region was observed in this study, although it did not reach significance. Another interesting finding was that reading aloud and repetition resulted in a decrease in rCBF in the right hemisphere compared to the control conditions. This suggests that with linguistic tasks, the left hemisphere has an increase in rCBF accompanied by a decrease in the right hemisphere.

The difference in location of the visual word lexicons between these two studies demonstrates how slight variations in procedure can render different results. It was hypothesized that the discrepant outcomes might be the result of the rate and exposure duration of the target stimuli, the degree of noun concreteness of the target stimuli, or the presentation method of passive viewing verses words being read aloud to the subjects.[182] Recently, Price et al.[192] examined brain activity during reading to measure the effects of exposure duration and task. There were three different tasks: (1) reading aloud; (2) reading silently; and (3) lexical decision on visually presented words and pseudowords (saying "present" for a real word and "absent" for a pseudoword). The left middle and superior temporal regions were activated during reading aloud and reading silently. The lexical decision task involved the left inferior and middle frontal cortices and the supplementary motor area. Exposure duration also had a significant effect; greater brain activity was observed for shorter exposure durations (150 ms) than for longer exposure durations (1000 ms or 981 ms). Interestingly, shorter exposure durations activated a greater number of brain regions than longer durations. It was hypothesized that (1) additional cognitive processes may be involved with shorter durations, such as increased working memory or attentional demands and/or (2) with longer exposures, increased activation during word processing may be counterbalanced by subsequent decreases in activity. These findings demonstrate the need to better understand how small differences in experimental design can influence brain activity. Before a reliable account of the neuroanatomy underlying language processing can be developed these variations need to be better understood.

Other studies have been conducted demonstrating that many brain regions in both hemispheres contribute to language functioning. Friberg[74] measured rCBF during two different linguistic tasks: (1) a verbal description of pieces of furniture in a subject's living room, and (2) a conversation on a specified topic. In both tasks, increased rCBF was seen in the visual association areas: the posterior superior parietal cortex and the posterior inferior temporal cortex. This was related to visual memories being "stored" at that location. Activation was also observed in the superior prefrontal cortex, the mid-temporal areas, and the posterior inferior frontal areas (Broca's area and its right sided homologue). Speech output was associated with activation in the supplementary motor areas and the primary motor area of the mouth. Finally, there was activation of mid- and inferior prefrontal areas in the left hemisphere. This study illustrates the high degree of involvement of brain regions distributed throughout the brain in both the left and right hemispheres during two different language tasks.

Activation studies have also been used as a noninvasive measure of language lateralization. Using fMRI, Binder et al.[54] compared patterns of brain activation during two different auditory processing tasks. The first task ("tone monitoring") was a pure tone discrimination task where subjects heard clustered sequences of 3 to 7 tones of either low (500 hz) or high (750 hz) pitch. When any sequence contained two tones of high pitch, subjects signaled with their left finger. The second task was a semantic monitoring task. Subjects heard a list of the names of animals and signaled when an animal met a specified semantic criterion. The pure tone monitoring task activated the temporal lobe auditory areas and dorsolateral frontal regions bilaterally. When the pure tone task served as a control for the semantic monitoring task, brain activity was observed in distributed regions of the left hemisphere including the left lateral frontal lobe and left temporo-parieto-occiptial heteromodal areas. The exact location and extent of activity varied across subjects, although brain activation was left-lateralized for the semantic task. The activity in the left frontal lobe in semantic processing is consistent with Petersen et al.'s[176,177] findings as highlighted earlier. Activation was also seen in the left posterior heteromodal areas during semantic processing; this is more consistent with classic models of aphasia and lesion studies that demonstrate semantic deficits following dominant posterior temporal and temporo-parietal lesions. It has been hypothesized that both frontal and temporo-parietal regions participate in a distributed network controlling semantic processing. The more posterior regions "store" semantic information and the frontal regions enable access to this information.[186] A more recent study demonstrated a widely distributed semantic network consisting of many regions: the junction between parietal and temporal lobe, between fusiform and inferior temporal cortex, the left middle temporal gyrus, and the left

inferior frontal gyrus (Brodman's areas 11/47) providing support for participation of both anterior and posterior regions in semantic processing.[94]

Using PET, Demonet et al.[187] have examined semantic and phonological processing during an auditory comprehension task. There were three different tasks: (1) detection of a rising pitch within a series of tones (control task); (2) a phonological monitoring task where subjects were to detect the phoneme /b/ in nonwords following the phoneme /d/ in preceding syllables; and (3) a lexico-semantic task where subjects monitored for nouns of small animals with "positive" attributes in attribute-noun pairs (i.e., "kind mouse"). Phonological processing compared to the tone control tasks activated the left superior temporal gyrus (mainly Wernicke's area) and, to a lesser degree, areas 44 and 45 (Broca's area) in the left hemisphere, and the right superior temporal gyrus. Lesion studies of patients with aphasia support the role of the superior temporal gyrus for phonological processing. The activation seen in Broca's area was attributed to subjects' verbally rehearsing phoneme strings during the phoneme monitoring task. This is consistent with notions of a specialized verbal working memory system as proposed by Baddley.[193] Lexico-semantic processing resulted in more extensive activation of the left temporal lobe that included the left middle, inferior, and superior temporal gyri, the left inferior parietal region (supramarginal and angular gyri), and the left superior prefrontal region. Again, this study demonstrates how language processing is distributed across many brain regions that are all integral components of a neural system participating in language comprehension.

Another direction for functional activation studies is the use of PET and fMRI to examine the effects of learning and practice on patterns of blood flow and brain metabolism. Raichle[194] and Raichle et al.[195] observed changes in rCBF with practice during a verb–noun association task (i.e., say "kick" when shown "ball"). Over time, there was a progressive reduction in rCBF in the left prefrontal cingulate, cerebellar, and posterior temporal cortex; at the same time, an increase in rCBF was seen in the insular cortex bilaterally. This study has led to the hypothesis that two language networks might exist: one for learned, automatic language processing and one for more novel, unlearned language processing.[191]

In conclusion, these studies demonstrate that language organization is much more complex and involves many more brain regions in both the left and right hemispheres than previously thought from lesion localization studies. The left hemisphere specialization for language has also been upheld, as shown by increased left hemisphere activation for isolated linguistic tasks.

Functional Activation Studies in Patients with Aphasia

Functional brain activation studies have the potential to demonstrate brain plasticity and provide insights into mechanisms of language recovery following brain damage. Using PET, Knopman et al.[196] examined recovery of single word comprehension in patients with aphasia both in the early and late stages of recovery. Subjects participated in an auditory verbal comprehension task. Those with better overall recovery demonstrated diffuse right hemisphere activation early after the stroke. When imaged at a later session (approximately 100 days later), activation was seen in the left posterior brain regions, suggesting a restitution of the left posterior-temporal language region. This study suggests that the right hemisphere may play an important role in the early phases of recovery. Heiss et al.[174] measured glucose metabolism in 17 patients with aphasia while they spoke spontaneously for 30 minutes about a topic of personal interest. Subjects with glucose metabolism in the infarct zone, its contralateral mirror region, and Broca's area demonstrated the most improved language function. Activation in these regions demonstrated viable cells that later could contribute to recovery or reorganization of function. Using functional magnetic resonance imaging (fMRI), Vikingstad et al.[60] measured patterns of brain activation in recovered aphasic patients. A general trend for increased brain activation in the right hemisphere during completion of language tasks, compared to normal controls, has been found. In one patient with aphasia, 80% of total cortical activity was located in the right hemisphere for each language task. Increased percentages of total activation in specific regions compared to normals have also been noticed. For example, in one recovered aphasic patient the left supramarginal and angular gyri had a three-fold higher percentage of activation than normal females during a naming task and in tasks that engaged phonologic and orthographic processing. Figure 13–18 illustrates these different activation patterns. Using SPECT, Tikofsky examined brain activation during the Boston Naming Test in patients with aphasia and normals. Those subjects with good recovery demonstrated increased rCBF compared to normals, while aphasia patients with poor recovery had lower rCBF than

normals.[197,198] Demeurisse et al.[141] have demonstrated similar findings of a more favorable prognosis in patients with increased rCBF activation patterns in both hemispheres during a naming task. The finding of greater blood flow and metabolism during activation tasks compared to normals parallels the trend already found in baseline or resting state studies.

There is still much work to be done examining recovery of language in brain-damaged patients. A challenge in studying brain damaged patients has been the establishment of the brain activation patterns in normals for a variety of language tasks. Once there is uniform agreement about brain activation in normals, more studies of patients with brain damage are likely to emerge. A related concern in studying brain-damaged patients is how to best interpret the results. It is difficult to determine whether the changes in activation patterns are the result of another brain region "taking over" a specific cognitive function, related to increased attentional demands, or are because brain-damaged patients are using a different processing strategy to accomplish the same task (i.e., phonologically decoding each word versus reading each word "by sight.") Differences in processing strategies for the same task have been shown to result in different activation patterns.[199] The exact mechanism underlying different activation patterns needs to be further clarified. One can speculate, however, that some degree of functional reorganization of language is occurring.

Functional Activation Studies: Conclusions

The study of language through brain activation paradigms with PET and fMRI has provided some new insights and supported some long-held ideas. The neuroanatomy of language is relatively consistent with classic models; most brain activation with language tasks falls in the left hemisphere and perisylvian zone. As would be expected, the left inferior frontal and left posterior-temporal regions are activated most consistently in all the activation studies. The organization of language differs, however, from classic explanations. Three general principles about language organization have emerged:[200,201] (1) Language is organized in a number of regions throughout the brain; (2) subcomponents of language can be related to highly focal areas; and (3) language functioning involves networks of neurons widely distributed throughout the brain. These interactive networks operate in serial and parallel ways enabling language function.

The neuronal networks involve a number of regions in both the left and right hemispheres, and include cortical as well as subcortical structures. Some of these structures are near each other, providing the regional nature of language organization, while some are more distant, demonstrating the widely distributed character of language. These regional and distributed networks have multiple interconnections and operate in massively parallel ways.[200,202]

The classical "zone of language" has been demonstrated with activation studies. Within this zone many neural networks integrally related to language are superimposed. The classical notion of "centers" that store a particular language function have been replaced. These networks contain highly focal regions or "bottlenecks" for processing of particular language functions.[203] A lesion to one of the critical locations can result in a highly focal language disturbance.

Although activation studies in brain-damaged patients are few, there is preliminary evidence to demonstrate the plasticity of the human adult brain and the potential for functional reorganization of language function; regions in the right hemisphere and new regions in the left hemisphere are being utilized to accomplish a task. This can be explained as either the adoption of a different processing strategy that utilizes a pathway undamaged by brain injury and/or the recruitment of still viable neurons.

FUTURE TRENDS AND CONCLUSIONS

Neuroimaging has been invaluable to the study of human communication and its disorders. CT and MRI are clinically useful in showing underlying brain lesions associated with specific disorders, while PET, SPECT, and fMRI have revealed aberrant patterns of blood flow and brain metabolism associated with many disease processes. Neuroimaging has also led to new insights about the organization of language in the brain. Lesion localization, baseline blood flow and metabolism, and functional activation studies have provided different, although converging evidence of the neural correlates of language. Models of language have evolved to encompass many structures not traditionally thought to participate—including the subcortical structures and structures related to arousal and attention. The right hemisphere also appears to play a role. Language is now viewed as being part of a large distributed network of many brain regions and highly focal processing nodes

that operate in concert. This conception of language has enhanced our understanding of brain language relationships and the impact of brain damage on language functioning.

There is also much recent excitement about the use of PET, SPECT, and fMRI activation paradigms to shed light on many unanswered questions about language organization and recovery following brain injury. The primary direction for future neuroimaging studies will most likely place heavy emphasis on activation paradigms in both normals and communicatively impaired individuals. A particularly exciting application will be the examination of functional brain plasticity over time in different clinical populations and following different speech–language interventions. The neurophysiological mechanisms associated with learning and restitution of speech–language behavior have yet to be elucidated. The ability to conduct serial fMRI studies has great potential for answering these questions. While activation studies hold promise, there is still the challenge of developing activation paradigms to isolate the processes of interest and making accurate interpretations of the patterns of brain activation. The role of attention, arousal, task difficulty, exposure duration, and memory all appear to influence the results. Additional studies need to be developed to address these points before activation studies progress much further.

STUDY QUESTIONS

1. Name 3 clinical applications for each of the neuroimaging modalities.

2. Which neuroimaging studies would you recommend for a patient with a sudden onset of language deficits? a slowly progressive language impairment? Why?

3. What are the strengths and weakness of CT? MRI? PET? SPECT? fMRI?

4. How can structural imaging information facilitate with planning of speech–language treatment and prediction of prognosis?

5. What information do functional neuroimaging studies provide that anatomical imaging studies do not?

6. How have the classic models of language and the neuropathology of aphasia evolved? What brain structures and regions have been incorporated into more recent models?

7. How can functional neuroimaging data inform speech–language intervention?

8. What are the challenges involved in functional activation studies?

REFERENCES

1. Katz M: Principles and techniques of image reconstruction with CT. In Weisberg L, Nice C, Katz M, eds., *Cerebral computed tomography: A text atlas.* W.B. Saunders, Philadelphia, 1984.
2. Seeram E: *Computed tomography technology.* W.B. Saunders, Philadelphia, 1982.
3. Kertez A, Harlock W, Coates R: Computer tomographic localization, lesion size, and prognosis in aphasia and nonverbal impairment. *Brain Lang* 1979; 8:34–50.
4. Selnes OA, Niccum N, Knopman DS, et al. Computed tomographic scan correlates of auditory comprehension deficits in aphasia: A prospective study. *Ann of Neurology* 1983; 13:558–566.
5. Naeser MA, Palumbo CL: Neuroimaging and language recovery in stroke. *J Clin Neurophys* 1994; 11:150–174.
6. Willmes K, Poeck K: To what extent can aphasic syndromes be localized? *Brain* 1993; 116:1527–1540.
7. McMackin D, Cockburn J, Anslow P, et al: Correlation of fornix damage with memory impairment in six cases of colloid cyst removal. *Acta Neurochirurgica* 1995; 135:12–18.
8. Ebeling U, Huber P: Localization of central lesions by correlation of CT findings and neurological deficits. *Acta Neurochirurgica* 1992; 119:17–22.
9. Reider-Groswasser I, Bornstein NM, Korczyn AD: Parkinsonism in patients with lacunar infarcts in the basal ganglia. *Eur Neurology* 1995; 35:46–49.
10. Beloosesky Y, Streifler JY, Burstin A, et al: The importance of brain infarct size and location in predicting outcome after stroke. *Age and Aging* 1995; 24:515–518.
11. DeQuardo JR, Tandon R, Goldman R, et al: Ventricular enlargement, neuropsychological status, and premorbid function in schizophrenia. *Bio Psychiatry* 1994; 35:517–524.
12. Raz S: Gross brain morphology in schizophrenia: A regional analysis of traditional diagnostic subtypes. *J Consulting Clin Psych* 1994; 62:640–644.
13. Benson KL, Sullivan EV, Lim KO, et al: Slow wave sleep and computed tomographic measures of brain morphology in Schizophrenia. *Psychiatry Res* 1996; 60:125–134.
14. Wurthmann C, Bogerts B, Falkai P: Brain morphology assessed by computed tomography in patients with geriatric depression, patients with degenerative dementia, and normal control subjects. *Psychiatry Res* 1995; 61:103–111.
15. Hamberg LM, Hunter GJ, Halpern EF, et al: Quantitative-high resolution measurement of cerebrovascular physiology with slip-ring technology. *Am J Neurorad* 1996; 17:639–650.
16. Nambu K, Suzuki R, Hirakawa K: Cerebral blood flow: Measurement with xenon-enhanced dynamic helical CT. *Radiology* 1995; 195:53–57.
17. Shimodozono M, Kawahira K, Tanaka N: Functioning heterotopic grey matter? Increased blood flow with voluntary movement and sensory stimulation. *Neuroradiology* 1995; 37:440–442.
18. Yonas H, Smith HA, Durham SR, et al: Increased stroke risk predicted by compromised cerebral blood flow reactivity. *J Neurosurg* 1993; 79:483–489.
19. Webster MW, Makaroun MS, Steed DL, et al: Compromised cerebral blood flow reactivity is a predictor of stroke in patients with symptomatic carotid artery occlusive disease. *J Vasc Surg* 1995; 21:338–344.
20. Gerdes JS, Hitchon PW, Neerangun W, et al: Computed tomography versus magnetic resonance imaging in stereotactic localization. *Stereo Func Neurosurg* 1994; 63:124–129.
21. Otsubo H, Hwang PA, Hunjan A, et al: Use of frameless stereotaxy with localization of electroencephalographic electrodes on three-dimensional computed tomographic images in epilepsy surgery. *J Clin Neurophys* 1995; 12:363–371.
22. Bloch F, Hansen WW, Packard ME: Nuclear induction. *Physiol Rev* 1946; 69:127–128.
23. Purcell EM, Torrey HC, Pound CV: Resonance absorption by nuclear magnetic moments in a solid. *Physiol Rev* 1946; 64:37–38.
24. Damadian RV: Tumor detection by nuclear magnetic resonance. *Science* 1971; 171:1151–1153.
25. Lauterbur PC: Image formation by induced local interactions. Examples employing nuclear magnetic resonance. *Nature* 1973; 242:190–191.
26. Moseley ME, de Crespigny AJ, Roberts TP, et al: Early detection of regional cerebral ischemia using high-speed MRI. *Stroke* 1993; 24:I60–I65.
27. Reith W, Forsting M, Vogler H, et al: Early MR detection of experimentally induced cerebral ischemia using magnetic susceptibility contrast agents: Comparison between gadopentetate dimeglumine and iron oxide particles. *Am J Neurorad* 1995; 16:53–60.
28. Takayama Y, Sugishita M, Fukuyama H, et al: Localization in impaired spatial vision. *Clin Neur Neurosurg* 1995; 97:249–252.
29. Welch LW, Nimmerrichter A, Kessler R, et al: Severe global amnesia presenting as Wernicke-Korsakoff syndrome but resulting from atypical lesions. *Psych Med* 1996; 26:421–425.
30. DeVos KJ, Wyllie E, Geckler C, et al: Language dominance in patients with early childhood tumors near left hemisphere language areas. *Neuro* 1995; 45:349–356.
31. Rumsey JM, Casanova M, Mannheim GB, et al: Corpus callosum morphology, as measured with MRI, in dyslexic men. *Biolog Psych* 1996; 39:769–775.
32. Bullmore E, Brammer M, Harvey I, et al: Cerebral hemispheric asymmetry revisited: Effects of handedness, gender and schizophrenia measured by radius of gyration in magnetic resonance images. *Psych Med* 1995; 25:349–363.
33. Noga JT, Aylward E, Barta PE, et al: Cingulate gyrus in schizophrenic patients and normal volunteers. *Psych Res* 1995; 61:201–208.

34. Larsen JP, Hoien T, Lundberg I, Odegaard H: MRI evaluation of the size and symmetry of the planum temporale in adolescents with developmetnal dyslexia. *Brain Lang* 1990; 39:289–301.

35. Carr HY, Purcell EM: Effects of diffusion on free precession in nuclear magnetic resonance experiments. *Phys Rev* 1954; 94:630–638.

36. Sjeskal EE, Tanner JE: Spin diffusion measurements: Spin echoes in the presence of a time-dependent field gradient. *J Chem Phys* 1965; 42:288–292.

37. LeBihan D, Breton E, Lallemand D, et al: MR imaging of intravoxel incoherent motions: Application to diffusion and perfusion in neurologic disorders. *Radiology* 1986; 161:401–407.

38. Hoehn-Berlage M: Diffusion weighted NMR imaging: Application to experimental focal cerebral ischemia. *NMR in Biomedicine* 1995; 8:345–358.

39. Welch KMA, Windham J, Knight RA, et al: A model to predict the histopathology of human stroke using diffusion and T_2-weighted magnetic resonance imaging. *Stroke* 1995; 26:1983–1989.

40. Gideon P, Thomsen C, Gjerris F, et al: Increased self diffusion of brain water in hydrocephalus measured by MR imaging. *Acta Radiologica* 1994; 35:514–519.

41. Brunberg JA, Chenevert TL, McKeever PE, et al: In vivo MR determination of water diffusion coefficients and diffusion anisotropy: Correlation with structural alteration in gliomas of the cerebral hemispheres. *Am J Neurorad* 1995; 16:361–371.

42. Wang Y, Majors A, Najm I, et al: Postictal alteration of sodium content and apparent diffusion coefficient in epileptic rat brain induced by kainic acid. *Epilepsia* 1996; 37:1000–1006.

43. Belliveau JW, Kennedy DN, McKinstry C, et. al: Functional mapping of the human visual cortex by magnetic resonance imaging. *Science* 1991; 254:716–719.

44. Ogawa S, Lee TM, Kay AR, et al: Brain magnetic resonance imaging with contrast dependent on blood oxygenation. *Proceed Nat Acad Sci, USA* 1990; 87: 9868–9872.

45. Edelman RE, Siewert B, Darby DG, et al: Qualitative mapping of cerebral blood flow and functional localization with echo-planar MR imaging and signal targeting with alternating radio frequency. *Radiology* 1994; 192:513–520.

46. Kim SG, Tsekos NV: Perfusion imaging by a flow-sensitive alternating inversion recovery (FAIR) technique: application to functional brain imaging. *Magnetic Res Med* 1997; 37:425–435.

47. Jack CJ, Thompson RM, Butts RK, et al: Sensory motor cortex: Correlation of presurgical mapping with functional MR imaging and invasive cortical mapping. *Radiology* 1994; 190:85–92.

48. Kwong KK, Belliveau JW, Chesler DA, et al: Dynamic magnetic resonance imaging of human brain activity during primary sensory stimulation. *Proceed Nat Acad Sci, USA* 1992; 89:5675–5679.

49. Bandettini PA, Wong EC, Hinks PS, et al: Time course EPI of human brain function during task activation. *Mag Res Med* 1992; 25:390–397.

50. Sereno MI, Dale AM, Reppas JB, et al: Borders of multiple visual areas in humans revealed by functional magnetic resonance imaging. *Science* 1995; 268:889–893.

51. DeYoe EA, Carman GJ, Bandettini P, et al: Mapping striate and extrastriate visual areas in human cerebral cortex. *Proceed Nat Acad Sci, USA* 1996; 93: 2382–2386.

52. Nitschke MF, Kleinschmidt A, Wessel K, et al: Somatotopic motor representation in the human anterior cerebellum. A high resolution functional MRI study. *Brain* 1996; 119:1023–1029.

53. Rao SM, Binder JR, Hammeke TA, et al: Somatotopic mapping of the human motor cortex with functional magnetic resonance imaging. *Neurology* 1995; 45: 919–924.

54. Binder JR, Rao SM, Hammeke TA, et al: Lateralized human brain language systems demonstrated by task subtraction functional magnetic resonance imaging. *Arch Neur* 1995; 52:593–601.

55. Cuenod CA, Bookheimer SY, Herz-Pannier L, et al: Functional MRI during word generation, using conventional equipment: A potential tool for language localization in the clinical environment. *Neur* 1995; 45:1821–1827.

56. Just MA, Carpenter PA, Keller TA, et al: Brain activation modulated by sentence comprehension. *Science* 1996; 274:114–116.

57. Cohen MS, Kosslyn SM, Breiter HC, et al: Changes in cortical activity during mental rotation. A mapping study using functional MRI. *Brain* 1996; 119:89–100.

58. Cao Y, Vikingstad EM, Huttenlocher PR, et al: Functional magnetic resonance studies of the reorganization of the human hand sensorimotor area after unilateral brain injury in the perinatal period. *Proc Nat Acad Sci, USA* 1994; 91:9612–16.

59. Cao Y, D'Olhaberriague D, Levine SR: Brain reorganization during motor recovery from stroke in humans. *Stroke* 1996; 27:194.

60. Vikingstad EM, Cao Y, George KP, et al: Using BOLD functional magnetic resonance imaging to examine language systems in recovered aphasic stroke patients. 1997 meeting of the International Society of Magnetic Resonance in Medicine. Vancouver, B.C.

61. Jackson GD, Connely A, Cross JH, et al: Functional magnetic resonance imaging of focal seizures. *Neurology* 1994; 44:850–856.

62. Renshaw PF, Yurgelun-Todd D, Cohen BM: Greater hemodynamic response to photic stimulation in schizophrenic patients: An echo planar MRI study. *Am J Psych* 1994; 151:1493–1495.

63. Lai S, Hopkins AL, Haake EM, et al: Identification of vascular structures as a major source of signal contrast in high resolution 2D and 3D functional activation imaging of the motor cortex at 1.5T. *Mag Res Med* 1993; 30:387–392.

64. Keyes JW: The Humongotron: A scintillation-camera transaxial tomograph. *J Nuc Med* 977; 18:381–387.

65. Ho SS, Berkovic SF, Newton MR, et al: Parietal lobe epilepsy: Clinical features and seizure localization by ictal SPECT. *Neuro* 1994; 44:2277–2284.

66. Rodrigues M, Botelho MM, Fonseca AT, et al: Combined study of 99mTc-HMPAO SPECT and computerized electroencephalographic tomography (CET) in patients with medically refractory complex partial epilepsy. *Ann Nuc Med* 1996; 10:113–118.

67. Johnson KP, Mueller ST, Walshe TM, English RT, Holman L: Cerebral perfusion imaging in Alzheimer's disease. *Arch Neurol* 1987; 44:165–168.

68. Frachowiak RSJ, Pozzilli C, Legg NJ: Regional cerebral oxygen supply and utilization in dementia: A clinical and physiological study with oxygen- 15 and positron tomography. *Brain* 1981; 104:753–778.

69. Lee H, Kramer JH: Brain SPECT imaging in progressive aphasia. *Clin Nuc Med* 1992; 17(10):800–802.

70. Defebvre L, Lecouffe P, Destee A, et al: Tomographic measurements of regional cerebral blood flow in progressive supranuclear palsy and Parkinson's disease. *Acta Neurol Scand* 1995; 92:235–241.

71. Lucey JV, Costa DC, Blanes T, et al: Regional cerebral blood flow in obsessive-compulsive disordered patients at rest. Differential correlates with obsessive-compulsive and anxious-avoidant dimensions. *Brit J Psych* 1995; 167:629–634.

72. Rubn P, Hemmingsen R, Holm S, et al: Relationship between brain structure and function in disorders of the schizophrenic spectrum: Single photon emission computerized tomography, computerized tomography and psychopathology of first episodes. *Acta Psych Scand* 1994; 90:281–289.

73. Scott AI, Dougall N, Ross M, et al: Short-term effects of electroconvulsive treatment on the uptake of 99mTc-exametazine into brain in major depression shown with single photon emission tomography. *J Aff Dis* 1994; 30:27–34.

74. Friberg L. Brain mapping in thinking and language function. *Acta Neurol—Suppl* 1993; 56:34–39.

75. Baron-Cohen S, Rinh H, Moriarty J, et al: Recognition of mental state terms. Clinical findings in children with autism and a functional neuroimaging study of normal adults. *Brit J Psych* 1994; 165:640–649.

76. Tzourio N, Heim A, Zilbovicius M, et al: Abnormal regional CBF response in left hemisphere of dysphasic children during a language task. *Ped Neuro* 1994; 10:20–26.

77. Beversdorf D, Metzger S, Nelson D, et. al. Single-word auditory stimulation and regional cerebral blood flow as studied by SPECT. *Psych Res* 1995; 61:181–189.

78. Rascol O, Sabatini U, Chollet F, et al: Normal activation of the supplemantary motor area in patients with Parkinson's disease undergoing long-term treatment with levodopa. *J Neuro Neurosurg Psych* 1994; 57: 567–571.

79. Zifko UA, Slomka PJ, Young GB, et al: Brain mapping of median nerve somatosenory evoked potentials with combined 99mTc-ECD single-photon emission tomography and magnetic resonance imaging. *Euro J Nuc Med* 1996; 23:579–582.

80. Luyken C, Hildebrandt G, Scheidhauer K, et al: 111Indium (DTPA-octreotide) scintigraphy in patients with cerebral gliomas. *Acta Neuro* 1994; 127:60–64.

81. Ur E, Mather SJ, Bomanji J, et al: Pituitary imaging using a labelled somatostatin analog in acromegaly. *Clin Endocrin* 1992; 36:147–150.

82. Weinberger DR, Jones D, Reba RC, et al: A comparison of FDG PET and IQNB SPECT in normal subjects and in patients with dementia. *J Neuropsych Clin Neurosci* 1992; 4:239–248.

83. Muller-Gartner HW, Mayberg HS, Fisher RS, et al: Decreased hippocampal muscarinic cholinergic receptor binding measured by 123I-iododexetimide and single-photon emission computed tomography in epilepsy. *Ann Neuro* 1993; 34:325–328.

84. Hatazawa J, Satoh T, Shimosegawa E, et al: Evaluation of cerebral infarction with iodine 123-iomazenil SPECT. *J Nuc Med* 1995; 36:2154–2161.

85. Sjoholm H, Rosen I, Elmqvist D: Role of I-123-iomazenil SPECT imaging in drug resistant epilepsy with complex partial seizures. *Acta Neurol Scand* 1995; 92:41–48.

86. Ebert D, Feistel H, Kaschka W, et al: Single photon emission computerized tomography assessment of cerebral dopamine D2 receptor blockade in depression before and after sleep deprivation: Preliminary results. *Bio Psych* 1994; 35:880–885.

87. Pilowsky LS, Costa DC, Ell PJ, et al: D2 Dopamine receptor binding in the basal ganglia of antipsychotic-free schizophrenic patients. An 123I-IBZM single photon emission computerised tomography study. *Brit J Psych* 1994; 164:16–26.

88. Friberg L: In vivo neuroreceptor imaging by SPECT in migraine. *Cephalagia* 1995; 15:310–315.

89. Ichise M, Toyama H, Fornazzari L, et al: Iodine-123–IBZM dopamine D2 receptor and rechnetium-99m-HMPAO brain perfusion SPECT in the evaluation of patients with and subjects at risk for Huntington's disease. *J Nuc Med* 1993; 34:1274–1281.

90. Bickel U, Lee VM, Trojanowski JQ, et al: Development and in vitro characterization of a cationized monoclonal antibody against beta A4 protein: A potential proble for Alzheimer's disease. *Bioconj Chem* 1994; 5:119–125.

91. Arbit E, Cheung NK, Yeh SD, et al: Quantitative studies of monoclonal antibody targeting to disialoganglioside GD2 in human brain tumors. *Euro J Nuc Med* 1995; 22:419–426.

92. Schold SC Jr, Zalutsky MR, Coleman RE, et al: Distribution and dosimetry of I-123-labeled monoclonal antibody 81C6 in patients with anaplastic glioma. *Invest Radiol* 1993; 28:488–496.

93. Wagner, HN Jr: 1996 SNM annual meeting: Medical problem solving. *J Nuc Med* 1996; 37:11N–31N.

94. Vandenberghe R, Price C, Wise R, et al: Functional anatomy of a common semantic system for words and pictures. *Nature* 1996; 383:254–256.

95. Maquet P, Peters J, Aerts J, et al: Functional anatomy of human rapid-eye-movement sleep and dreaming. *Nature* 1996; 383:163–166.

96. Kinomura S, Kawashima R, Yamada K, et al: Functional anatomy of taste perception in the human brain studied with positron emission tomography. *Brain Res* 1994; 659:263–266.

97. Andreasen NC, O'Leary DS, Arndt S, et al: Short-term and long-term verbal memory: A positron emission tomography study. *Proceed Nat Acad Sci, USA* 1995; 92:5111–5115.

98. Blaxton TA, Zeffiro TA, Gabrieli JD, et al: Functional mapping of human learning: A positron emission tomography activation study of eyeblink conditioning. *J Neurosci* 1996; 16:4032–4040.

99. Kew JJ, Riddling MC, Rothwell JC, et al: Reorganization of cortical blood flow and transcranial magnetic stimulation maps in human subjects after upper limb amputation. *J Neurophys* 1994; 72:2517–2524.

100. Ceballos-Baumann AO, Passingham RE, Marsden CD, et al: Motor reorganization in acquired hemidystonia. *Ann Neurol* 1995; 37:746–757.

101. Fox PT, Ingham RJ, Ingham JC, et al: A PET study of the neural systems of stuttering. *Nature* 1996; 382: 158–161.

102. Valladares-Neto DC, Buchsbaum MS, Evans WJ, et al: EEG delta, positron emission tomography, and memory defect in Alzheimer's disease. *Neuropsychobiol* 1995; 31:173–181.

103. Sadato N, Pascual-Leone A, Grafman J, et al: Activation of the primary visual cortex by braille reading in blind subjects. *Nature* 1996; 380:526–528.

104. Hagman JO, Wood F, Buchsbaum MS, et al: Cerebral brain metabolism in adult dyslexic subjects assessed with positron emission tomography during performance of an auditory task. *Arch Neurol* 1992; 49: 734–739.

105. Mann JJ, Malone KM, Diehl DJ, et al: Demonstration in vivo of reduced serotonin responsivity in the brain of untreated depressed patients. *Am J Psych* 1996; 153:174–182.

106. Braun AR, Randolph C, Stoetter B, et al: The functional neuroanatomy of Tourette's syndrome: An FDG-PET study. II: Relationships between regional cerebral metabolism and associated behavioral and cognitive features of the illness. *Neuropsychopharm* 1995; 13:151–168.

107. Nagarajan L, Schaul N, Eidelberg D, et al: Contralateral temporal lobe hypometabolism on positron emission tomography in temporal lobe epilepsy. *Acta Neurol Scand* 1996; 93:81–84.

108. Delvenne V, Lotstra F, Goldman S, et al: Brain hypometabolism of glucose in anorexia nervosa: A PET scan study. *Biolog Psych* 1995; 37:161–169.

109. Duncan DB, Herholz K, Kugel H, et al: Positron emission tomography and Magnetic resonance spectroscopy of cerebral glycolysis in children with congenital lactic acidosis. *Ann Neurol* 1995; 37: 351–358.

110. Hirato M, Ishihara J, Horikoshi S, et al: Parkinsonian rigidity, dopa induced dyskinesia, and chorea: Dynamic studies on the basal ganglia-thalamocortical motor circuit using PET scan and depth microrecording. *Acta Neurochirurgica Suppl* 1995; 64:5–8.

111. Hinkin CH, van Gorp WG, Mandelkern MA, et al: Cerebral metabolic change in patients with AIDS: Report of a six month follow-up using positron emission tomography. *J Neuropsych Clin Neurosci* 1995; 7: 180–187.

112. Ogawa T, Inugami A, Hatazawa J, et al: Clinical positron emission tomography for brain tumors: Comparison of fludeoxyglucose F18 and L-methyl-^{11}C-methionine. *Am J Neurorad* 1996; 17:344–353.

113. Di Chiro G, Hatazawa J, Katz DA, et al: Glucose utilization by intracranial meningiomas as an index of tumor agressivity and probability of recurrence: A PET study. *Radiology* 1987; 164:521–526.

114. Ogawa T, Shishido F, Kanno I, et al: Cerebral glioma: Evaluation with methionine PET. *Radiology* 1993; 186:45–53.

115. Hoffman JM, Waskin HA, Schiffer T, et al: FDG-PET in differentiating lymphoma from nonmalignant central nervous system lesions in patients with AIDS. *J Nucl Med* 1993; 34:567–575.

116. Gjedde A, Kuwabara H: Absent recruitment of capillaries in brain tissue recovering from stroke. *Acta Neurochirurgica Supp* 1993; 57:35–40.

117. Shirane R, Sato S, Sato K, et al: Cerebral blood flow and oxygen metabolism in infants with hydrocephalus. *Child's Nervous System* 1992; 8:118–123.

118. Fukuyama H, Ogawa M, Yamauchi H, et al: Altered cerebral metabolism in Alzheimer's disease: A PET study. *J Nucl Med* 1994; 35:1–6.

119. Geschwind N: The organization of language in the brain. *Science* 1970; 170:940–944.

120. Mazzocchi F, Vignolo LA: Localization of lesions in aphasia: Clinical-CT scan correlation in stroke patients. *Cortex* 1979; 15:627–653.

121. Damasio AR, Geschwind N: The neural basis of language. *Ann Rev Neurosci* 1984; 7:127–47.

122. Naeser MA, Hayward RW: Lesion localization in aphasia with cranial computed tomography and the Boston diagnostic aphasia exam. *Neurol* 1978; 28: 545–551.

123. Basso A, Lecours A, Moraschini S, et al: Anatomoclinical correlations of the aphasias as defined through computerized tomography: Exceptions. *Brain Lang* 1985; 26:201–229.

124. Vignolo LA, Boccardi E, Caverni L: Unexpected CT-scan findings in global aphasia. *Cortex* 1986; 22: 55–69.

125. Caramazza A: The logic of neuropsychological research and the problem of patient classification in aphasia. *Brain Lang* 1984; 21:9–20.

126. Schwartz MF: What the classical aphasia categories can't do for us and why. *Brain Lang* 1984; 21:3–8.

127. Mohr J, Pessin M, Finkelstein S, et al: Broca aphasia: Pathologic and clinical. *Neurol* 1978; 28:311–324.

128. Alexander MP, Naeser MA, Palumbo C: Broca's area aphasias: Aphasia after lesions including the frontal operculum. *Neurol* 1990; 40:353–362.

129. Dronkers NF: Cerebral localization of production deficits in aphasia. National Center for Neurogenic Communication Disorders Telerounds #9, 1993.

130. Damasio AR, Damasio H, Rizzo M, et al: Aphasia with nonhemorrhagic lesions in the basal ganglia and internal capsule. *Arch Neurol* 1982; 39:15–20.

131. Naeser MA, Alexander MP, Helm-Estabrooks, et al: Aphasia with predominantly subcortical lesion sites— Description of three capsular/putaminal aphasia syndromes. *Arch Neurol* 1982; 39; 2–14.

132. Mega MS, Alexander MP: Subcortical aphasia: The core profile of capsulostriatal infarction. *Neuro* 1994; 44(10): 1824–1829.

133. Marie P: Revision de la question del l'aphasie. *Semaine Medicale* 1906; 21:241–247, 493–500, 565–571.

134. Gorelick PB, Hier DB, Benevento L, Levitt S, Tan W: Aphasia after left thalamic infarction. *Arch Neurol* 1984; 41:1296–1298.

135. Graff-Radford NR, Eslinger PJ, Damasio AR, et al: Nonhemorrhagic infarction of the thalamus: Behavioral, anatomic, and physiologic correlates. *Neurol* 1984; 34:14–23.

136. Mohr JP, Watters WC, Duncan GW: Thalamic hemorrhage and aphasia. *Brain Lang* 1975; 2:3–17.

137. Wallesch C-W, Kornhuber HH, Brunner RJ, Kunz T, Hollerbach B, Suger G: Lesions of the basal ganglia, thalamus and deep white matter: Differential effects on language functions. *Brain Lang* 1983; 20:286–304.

138. Alexander MP, Naeser MA, Palumbo CL: Correlations of subcortical CT lesion sites and aphasia profiles. *Brain* 1987; 110:961–991.

139. Crosson B: Subcortical functions in language: A working model. *Brain Lang* 1985; 25:257–292.

140. Crosson B: *Subcortical functions in language and memory.* Guilford Press, New York, 1992.

141. Demeurisse G, Capon A: Language recovery in aphasic stroke patients: Clinical, CT and CBF studies. *Aphasiology* 1987; 1(4):301–315.

142. Kertesz A, Harlock W, Coates R: Computer tomographic localization, lesion size and prognosis in aphasia and nonverbal impairment. *Brain Lang* 1979; 8:34–50.

143. Naeser MA, Helm-Estabrooks N, Haas G, et al: Relationship between lesion extent in "Wernicke's Area" on CT scan and predicting recovery of comprehension in Wernicke's aphasia. *Arch Neurol* 1987; 44: 73–82.

144. Yarnell P, Monroe P, Sobel L: Aphasia outcome in stroke: A clinical neuroradiological correlation. *Stroke* 1976; 7(5):516–522.

145. Naeser MA, Palumbo, CL: How to analyze CT/MRI scan lesion sites to predict potential for long-term recovery in aphasia. In HS Kirshner, ed., *Handbook of neurological speech and language disorders.* Marcel Dekker, New York, 1995, pp. 91–148.

146. Naeser MA, Palumbo CL, Helm-Estabrooks, et al: Severe non-fluency in aphasia: Role of the medial subcallosal fasciculus plus other white matter pathways in recovery of spontaneous speech. *Brain* 1989; 112:1–38.

147. Knopman DS, Selnes OA, Niccum N, et al: Longitudinal study of speech fluency in aphasia. CT correlates of recovery and persistent non-fluency. *Neurology* 1983; 33:1170–1178.

148. Naeser MA, Helm-Estabrooks: CT scan lesion localization and response to melodic intonation therapy with nonfluent aphasia cases. *Cortex* 1985; 21: 203–223.

149. Knopman DS, Selnes OA, Niccum N, et al: Recovery of naming in aphasia: Relationship to fluency, comprehension and CT findings. *Neurol* 1984; 34: 1461–1471.

150. Albert M, Sparks R, Helm, N: Melodic intonation therapy for aphasia. *Arch Neurol* 1973; 29:1130–131.

151. Benson DF: *Aphasia, alexia, agraphia.* New York: Churchill-Livingstone, 1979.

152. Benson DF, Geschwind N: The aphasias and related disturbances. In AB Baker, RJ Joynt, eds., *Clinical neurology.* Philadelphia, Harper & Row, 1991.

153. Metter EJ, Riege WH, Hanson WR, et al: Correlations of glucose metabolism and structural damage to language function in aphasia. *Brain Lang* 1984; 21:187–207.

154. Metter EJ, Jackson CA, Kempler D, et al: Temporo-parietal cortex and the recovery of language comprehension in aphasia. *Aphasiology* 1992; 6(4):349–358.

155. Metter EJ: Neuroanatomy and physiology of aphasia: Evidence from positron emission tomography. *Aphasiology* 1987; 1(1):3–33.

156. Mazziotta JC, Phelps ME, Carson RE, Kuhl DE: Tomographic mapping of human cerebral metabolism: Normal unstimulated state. *Neurol* 1981; 31:502–516.

157. Phelps ME, Huang SC, Hoffman EJ, Selin CS, Sokoloff L, Kuhl DE: Tomographic measurement of local cerebral metabolic rate in humans with (F-18) 2-flouro-2-deoxyglucose: Validation of method. *Ann Neurol* 1979; 6:371–388.

158. Kuhl DE, Metter, EJ, Riege WH, et al: Effects of human aging on patterns of local cerebral glucose utilization determined by the (18F) fluorodeoxyglucose method. *J Cereb Blood Flow Metab* 1982; 2:163–167.

159. Metter EJ: PET in aphasia and language. In HS Kirshner, ed., *Handbook of neurological speech and language disorders.* Marcel Dekker, New York, 1995, pp. 187–212.

160. Metter EJ, Wasterlain CG, Kuhl DE, et al: 18FDG positron emission computed tomography in a study of aphasia. *Ann Neurol* 1981; 10:173–183.

161. Martin WRW, Raichle ME: Cerebellar blood flow and metabolism in cerebral hemisphere infarction. *Ann Neurol* 1983; 14:168–176.

162. Metter EJ, Kempler D, Jackson C, et al: Cerebellar glucose metabolism in chronic aphasia. *Neurol* 1987; 37:1599–1606.

163. Metter, EJ, Jackson CA, Kempler D, et al: Glucose metabolic asymmetries in chronic Wernicke's, Broca's, and conduction aphasias. *Neurol* 1986; 36:317.

164. Metter EJ, Hanson WR, Jackson CA, et al: Temporo-parietal cortex in aphasia. Evidence from positron emission tomography. *Arch Neurol* 1990; 47: 1235–1239.

165. Metter EJ Riege WH, Hanson WR, et al: Comparisons of metabolic rates, language and memory in subcortical aphasias. *Brain Lang* 1983; 19:33–47.

166. Baron JC, D'Antona R, Pantano P, et al: Effects of thalamic stroke on energy metabolism of the cerebral cortex. *Brain* 1986; 190:1243–1259.

167. Metter EJ, Riege WH, Hanson WR, et al: Subcortical structures in aphasia: An analysis based on (F-18) fluorodeoxyglucose positron emission tomography, and computed tomography. *Arch Neurol* 1988; 45: 1229–1335.

168. Alexander MP, Naeser MA, Palumbo CL: Correlations of subcortical CT lesion sites and aphasia profiles. *Brain* 1987; 110:961–991.

169. Bushnell DL, Gupta S, Lmcoch AG, et al: Prediction of language and neurologic recovery after cerebral infarction with SPECT imaging using N-isopropylp-(1123) iodamphetamine. *Arch Neurol* 1989; 46: 665–669.

170. Giubilei F, Lenzi GL, Dipiero V: Predictive value of brain perfusion single photon emission computed tomography in acute ischemic stroke. *Stroke* 1990; 21:895–900.

171. Mlcoch AG, Bushnell DL, Gupta S, Milo TJ: Speech fluency in aphasia: regional cerebral blood flow correlates of recovery using single-photon emission computed tomography. *J NeuroImag* 1994; 4(1):6–10.

172. Tikofsky RS, Collier BD, Hellman RS, Sapena VK, Zielonka JS, Krohn L, Gresch A: Cerebral blood flow patterns determined by SPECT I-123 iodamphetamine (IMP) imaging and WAB AQs in chronic aphasia: A preliminary report. *Arch Neurol* 1985; 35:625–632.

173. Yamaguchi F, Meyer JS, Sakai F, Yamamoto M: Case reports of three dysphasic patients to illustrate r-CBF responses during behavioral activation. *Brain Lang* 1980; 9:145–148.

174. Heiss W-D, Kessler J, Karbe H, et al: Cerebral glucose metabolism as a predictor of recovery from aphasia in ischemic stroke. *Arch Neurol* 50 1993; 958–964.

175. Kertesz, A: What do we learn from recovery from aphasia. In Waxman SG, ed., *Advances in neurology. Vol. 47: Functional recovery in neurology disease.* Raven Press, New York, 1988, pp. 277–292.

176. Peterson SE, Fox PT, Posner MI, et al: Positron emission tomographic studies of the cortical anatomy of single-word processing. *Nature* 1988; 331:585–589.

177. Peterson SE, Fox PT, Snyder AZ, et al: Activation of extrastriate and frontal cortical areas by visual words and word-like stimuli. *Science* 1990; 249:1041–1044.

178. Wise R, Hadar U, Howard D, et al: Language activation studies with positron emission tomography. Exploring brain functional anatomy with positron tomography. In W Chichester, Ciba Foundation Symposium 163, 1991; 218–234.

179. Peterson SE, Fiez, JA: The processing of single words studied with positron emission tomography. *Ann Rev Neurosci* 1993:16:509–530.

180. Gur RC, Erwin RJ, Gur RE: Neurobehavioral probes for physiologic neuroimaging studies. *Arch Gen Psych* 1992;49:409–414.

181. Binder JR, Rao SM: Human brain mapping with functional magnetic resonance imaging. In Kertez A, *Localization and neuroimaging in neuropsychology.* Academic Press, New York, 1994, pp. 185–212.

182. Steinmetz H, Seitz RJ: Functional anatomy of language processing: Neuroimaging and the problem of individual variability. *Neuropsych* 1991; 29: 1149–1161.

183. Binder JR, Rao SM, Hammeke TA, et al: Functional magnetic resonance imaging of human auditory cortex. *Ann Neurol* 1994; 35:662–672.

184. Shaywitz BA, Shaywitz SE, Pugh KR, et al: Sex differences in the functional organization of the brain for language. *Nature* 1995; 373:607–609.

185. Yetkin FZ, Hammeke TA, Swanson SJ, et al: A comparison of functional MR activation patterns during silent and audible language tasks. *Am J Neurorad* 1995; 16:1087–1092.

186. Binder JR, Rao SM, Hammeke TA, et al: Lateralized human brain language systems demonstrated by task subtraction functional magnetic resonance imaging. *Arch Neurol* 1995; 52:593–601.

187. Demonet J-F, Chollet F, Ramsay S, et al: The anatomy of phonological and semantic processing in normal subjects. *Brain* 1992; 115:1753–1768.

188. Howard D, Patterson K, Wise R, et al: The cortical localization of the lexicons. *Brain* 1992; 115: 1769–1782.

189. Demb JB, Desmond JE, Wagner AD, et al: Semantic encoding and retrieval in the left inferior prefrontal cortex: A functional MRI study of task difficulty and process specificity. *J Neuro* 1995; 15(9); 5870–5878.

190. Frith CD, Friston KJ, Liddle PF, et al: A PET study of word finding. *Neuropsychol* 1991; 29(12): 1137–1148.

191. Posner MI, Raichle ME: *Interpreting words. Images of mind.* Scientific American Library, New York, 1994, pp. 104–129.

192. Price CJ, Wise RJS, Watson JDG, et al: Brain activity during reading: The effects of exposure duration and task. *Brain* 1994; 117:1255–1269.

193. Baddley AD: *Working memory.* Clarendon Press, Oxford, 1986.

194. Raichle ME: Memory mechanisms in the processing of words and word-like symbols. In Collins R, ed., *Exploring brain functional anatomy with positron tomography.* John Wiley & Sons, New York, 1991, pp. 198–217.

195. Raichle ME, Fiez J, Videen TO, Fox PT, Pardo JV, Peterson SE: Practice related changes in human brain functional anatomy. *Soc Neurosci Abs* 1991; 17:21.

196. Knopman D, Rubens A, Selnes O, et al: Mechanisms of recovery from aphasia: Evidence for serial xenon 133 blood flow studies. *Ann Neuro* 1984; 15: 530–535.

197. Tikofsky RS: SPECT brain studies: Potential role of cognitive challenge in language and learning disorders. *Adv Funct Neuroimaging* 1988; 1:12–14.

198. Tikofsky RS, Hellman RS, Collier BD, et al: Influence of a naming task on SPECT I-123 iodamphetamine (SPECT/IMP) brain imaging: Chronic aphasics vs normals. *J Nucl Med* 1987; 28:559–560 (abstr).

199. Pugh KR, Shaywitz BA, Shaywitz SE, et al: Predicting reading performance from neuroimaging profiles: The cerebral basis of phonological effects in printed word identification. *J Exp Psyc* (In press).

200. Bachman D, Albert ML: The cerebral organization of language. In A Peters, E Jones, eds., *Cerebral cortex.* Plenum, New York, 1990.
201. Mesulam M-M: Large scale neurocognitive networks and distributed processing for attention, language, and memory. *Ann Neurol* 1990; 28:597–613.
202. Helm-Estabrooks N, Albert ML: *Manual of aphasia therapy.* Pro-Ed, Austin, TX, 1991.
203. Damasio AR, Damasio H: Cortical systems for retrieval of concrete knowledge: The convergence zone framework. In C. Koch, ed., *Large-scale neuronal theories of the brain,* MIT Press, Cambridge, 1994, pp. 61–74.

Appendix A
Glossary of Highlighted Terms

1. A **collimator** is a device, commonly made of lead, that prevents undesirable X-rays or gamma rays from reaching a detector. Discrimination is based upon the direction of travel of the rays: only those rays moving in a specific direction are allowed to pass through the collimator—all others will be absorbed in the walls or septa of the collimator. Thus, scattered radiation whose direction has been altered will not be detected.

2. X-ray or gamma ray **energy** in commonly expressed in units of electron volts (eV). One keV is equal to 1000 eV, approximately 1.602×10^{-16} Joules.

3. The **rem** is a unit used to express the biological effect of energy deposited in a mass of tissue during an exposure to ionizing radiation. For X-rays, one hundred rem is equivalent to one Joule/kg. The average dose received by an individual from background radiation and other manmade radiation sources is 0.2 rem per year.

4. A nuclear **magnetic moment** can be visualized as a tiny bar magnet within the nucleus of an atom. When the north and south poles of all the tiny bar magnets line up together (as with a collection of hydrogen nuclei placed in a strong external magnetic field) their fields will add up to form a net magnetization.

5. **Resonance** refers to a phenomena where a system (in this case a collection of aligned nuclear magnetic moments) will absorb and transmit only that energy which falls within a very specific and narrow range.

6. The term **radio frequency** refers to a specific range of the electromagnetic spectrum. In addition to NMR signals, television and FM radio broadcasts also fall within this portion of the EM spectrum.

7. The unit of magnetic field strength is called the **Tesla**. One Tesla is equal to 10,000 Gauss, and is approximately 2000 times the size of the earth's magnetic field.

8. A **gradient coil** is nothing more than several loops of wire oriented in such a way that a linear magnetic field gradient is generated in a specific direction when a current is put through the wire. In an MR scanner, the three gradient coils are controlled independently and are in perpendicular directions. They are called the slice select, frequency encode, and phase encode gradients.

9. A **pulse sequence** controls the pattern of radiofrequency and gradient pulses that are used during the acquisition of the MR signal. This pattern, which includes the timing of pulses as well as their strengths and durations, will determine the type of contrast present in the resultant image. Two timing parameters are often used to describe a pulse sequence: TE (time to echo) refers to the length of time between the first RF pulse and the detection of the MR signal, while TR (time to repeat) refers to the time between successive repetitions of the pulse sequence.

10. **Weighting** in MRI refers to the type of contrast sensitivity exhibited in an image. Thus, a T_1 weighted image will be sensitive to differences in tissue T_1 values, while a diffusion weighted image will reveal rates of water diffusion.

11. The **diffusion coeficient** of a molecule provides a measure of how rapidly that molecule diffuses, or moves, within a solution or tissue. Molecules with higher diffusion coefficients move more rapidly than those with lower coefficients. Diffusion coefficients are usually reported in units of mm²/s.

12. The radioactive atomic isotopes used in nuclear medicine imaging are called **radionuclides**. A list of radionuclides commonly used in SPECT and PET is given in Table 13–3. All SPECT radionuclides emit gamma rays, while PET radionuclides are positron emitters.

13. **Radiopharmaceuticals** are radioactive molecules that are introduced into the body for the purpose of nuclear medicine imaging. The radiopharmaceutical always contains a radionuclide, and in some scanning procedures is simply an unmodified radionuclide. Often, though, the radiopharmaceutical is a larger molecule to which the radionuclide has been chemically bonded.

14. **Primary** radiation refers to those X-rays or gamma rays which did not undergo an interaction during their passage through the patient. Scattered photons have undergone interactions in the patient.

15. **Annihilation** refers to the complete conversion of mass to energy when a particle (an electron, for example) and its antimatter equivalent (a positron) collide. In the case of a positron and electron, the annihilation event produces two 511 keV photons that leave the point of annilihation in opposite directions.

14

Assessment and Diagnosis in Neurogenic Communication Disorders

ALEX F. JOHNSON, K. PAIGE GEORGE, AND JACKIE HINCKLEY

CHAPTER OUTLINE

Assessment and Diagnosis: General Principles

Activities of Assessment and Diagnosis

Using Diagnostic Information for Prediction and Planning

Diagnosis of speech–language disorders in patients with various neuropathologies provides for one of the more interesting experiences afforded the speech–language pathologist. Neurological diseases can result in disorders of speech, language, cognition, or swallowing. In addition, some of the more puzzling conditions present with combinations of these effects. It is important for the speech–language pathologist to have a basic understanding of neurological diseases including pathophysiology, natural course of the illness, predicted sequelae and outcomes, and speech and non-speech symptoms. A basic review of this information can be found in this text in Chapters 11 and 12. The chapter by Musson (Chapter 15) reviews the effects of neurological disease on the swallowing mechanism.

In addition to appreciating the significant havoc that impaired neurological function can impose on communication and swallowing, it is important for the speech–language pathologist to have skill and knowledge resulting in the compe-tent ability to conduct evaluation of communicative abilities and interpret the results of this evaluation. This chapter presents key features and principles of the diagnostic process, emphasizes key issues in the diagnostic interview and patient testing, and provides a framework for differentiation of the various disorders.

ASSESSMENT AND DIAGNOSIS IN MEDICAL SPEECH-LANGUAGE PATHOLOGY: GENERAL PRINCIPLES

In the practice of medicine, the physician conducts a careful interview with the patient, completes a physical examination, orders appropriate tests to address questions that became obvious in the first two activities, considers the various reasonable explanations for the presenting problem based on the data available, and ultimately states the diagnosis. The diagnosis being sought by the physician is the underlying cause of the presenting symptom(s). In medical speech–language pathology it is helpful to use this same model as a guide for the initial scope of interaction with patients. The SLP interviews the patient, family, and other care providers and reviews relevant data from the medical record. Following the gathering of some preliminary information, the clinician forms a clinical hypothesis regarding the possibilities that exist to explain the variant communication and/or swallowing patterns. The formal observation and data collection aspects of diagnosis are used to support or refute various possibilities. Finally, a statement of the diagnosis is made. This statement should always include the probable or possible causes of the speech–language disorder, the severity of the problem, the functional limitations exhibited by the patient, and a prognosis for potential outcome with appropriate follow-up.

Terminological and Conceptual Issues

As a topic within the field of speech–language pathology, the area of assessment and diagnosis has received considerable attention. Key texts in neurologic communication disorders have addressed diagnosis and differential diagnosis as a key professional function within the scope of practice for speech–language pathologists. Nation and Aram[1] carefully delineate the "Speech and Language Processing Model" as a framework for the consideration of key factors in the formulation of a diagnosis. They differentiated and defined the terms that are frequently used interchangeably with diagnosis including testing, examination, appraisal, evaluation, and assessment. These authors suggest that although these activities are subsumed under the concept of diagnosis, they are not synonymous. Identifying the elements of diagnosis as "determining the speech or language disorder, understanding causation, and proposing patient management," they cite limitations in the use of these other terms. For example, they note that "testing" merely involves the collection of data and thereby contributes to the establishment of the speech–language diagnosis, but does not necessarily contribute to the understanding of causation.

We find these distinctions helpful in clarifying the nature of the SLP's professional function in addressing the three major functions of diagnosis cited by Nation and Aram. For purposes of discussion, the following topics are proposed as descriptions of the basic functions that contribute to the establishment of a diagnosis: assessment, testing, and hypothesis testing.

Assessment

In the conduct of diagnostic activities, an orderly approach or system of activities is implied. Assessment, then, refers to the *process* of delivering the diagnostic service. The assessment process is determined by the setting in which the service is provided, the type of referral question that is being addressed, and the philosophy of the provider as the service is being delivered. A second aspect of assessment extends beyond the establishment of the diagnosis to include the decisions that are made across the continuum of service delivery over time. As patients are enrolled in treatment or as their conditions change, important questions must be continually addressed to continue to manage the patient's needs. Consider, for example, the 42-year-old woman with Amyotrophic Lateral Sclerosis (ALS), a degenerative disease of the nervous system. While the initial speech and swallowing diagnosis is established at the time of other diagnostic services, the role for the SLP is to continually monitor changes in patient function so that various appropriate interventions can be provided to the patient in a timely and meaningful way. Effective patient management over time requires that the clinician use a planned assessment approach to determine the stage of the patient's illness and initiate appropriate intervention.

The expert clinician will continuously address questions and adjust treatment, referrals, and patient/family education activities to accommodate the patient's needs and desires. Figure 14–1 presents a model showing some of the decisions that are indicated as the patient moves across the continuum of care in speech–language pathology. Review of this figure suggests that many important decisions are made by the clinician using some of the tools and techniques of assessment, well beyond the period of initial diagnosis. Failure to consider these types of issues as treatment or change in condition occurs will likely lead to a less than desirable patient outcome.

Testing

The function of testing (and clinical observation) is to generate sufficient data that can be used in assessment, diagnosis, and differential diagnosis. Clinicians in our field have a plethora of tools, instruments, protocols, and observation formats that can be helpful in eliciting information about their patients. The information provided by these various approaches and tools can be extremely useful

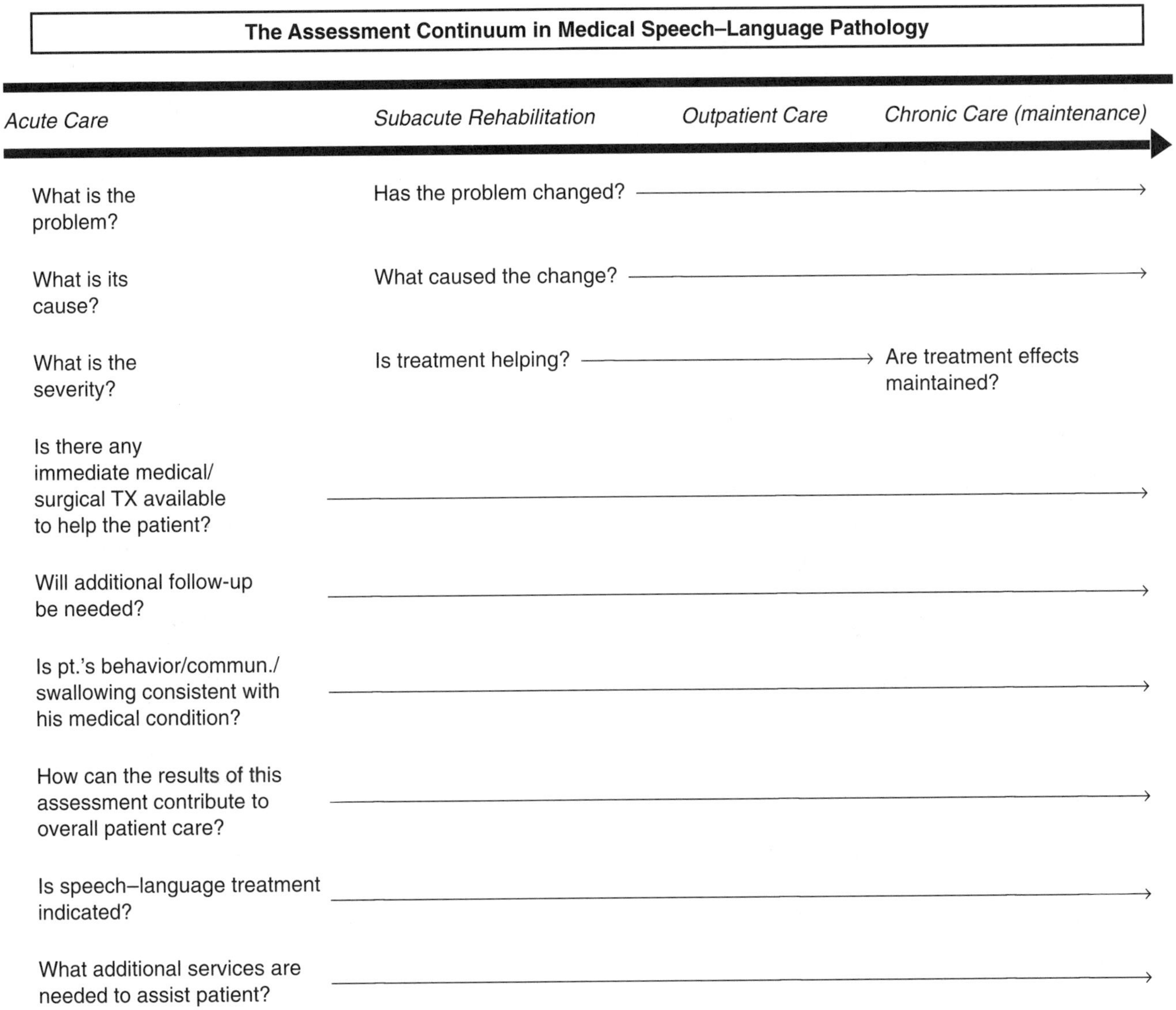

The Assessment Continuum in Medical Speech–Language Pathology

Acute Care	Subacute Rehabilitation	Outpatient Care	Chronic Care (maintenance)

What is the problem? — Has the problem changed? ————————————————→

What is its cause? — What caused the change? ————————————————→

What is the severity? — Is treatment helping? ————————→ Are treatment effects maintained?

Is there any immediate medical/surgical TX available to help the patient? ————————————————→

Will additional follow-up be needed? ————————————————→

Is pt.'s behavior/commun./swallowing consistent with his medical condition? ————————————————→

How can the results of this assessment contribute to overall patient care? ————————————————→

Is speech–language treatment indicated? ————————————————→

What additional services are needed to assist patient? ————————————————→

Figure 14–1. Assessment decisions across the continuum of care in speech–language pathology.

when obtained efficiently and reliably, and when the use of the tool is justified based on the referral question or the clinician's hypothesis about the disorder. Conversely, the use of extensive time, cost, or energy in obtaining test data is not justified unless it is necessary to lead to a diagnosis or provide a focus for treatment. Experienced clinicians usually find that they are able to generate sufficient information for formulating a diagnosis utilizing basic protocols based on the question of the referral source or the patient. Too little test or observation information is dangerous in that it presents the risk of generating insufficient information for support of a precise diagnosis. Too much testing is costly to the patient and the provider and may generate information that is redundant or superfluous.

A variety of approaches have been used to evaluate tests, clinical procedures, and protocols for observation and clinical analysis and these discussions can be found in a variety of texts on neurogenic communication disorders such as those by Helm Estabrooks,[2] Johns,[3] Duffy,[4] Bayles,[5] Tompkins,[6] and many others. General texts covering assessment and diagnosis[1,7,8] also present listings of test procedures and protocols. Many of the chapters throughout this text refer to specific procedures and protocols. Finally, a compendium of tests designed specifically for use by speech–language pathologists has been developed by the American Speech–Language-Hearing Association.[9]

A review of these resources demonstrates quickly that the problem for the diagnostician is rarely related to the availability of a tool or proto-col that can provide data. There are problems, however, that every clinician must consider. The clinician's dilemma is related to the choice of tools that are valid, reliable, efficient, and serve to best address the referral question or diagnostic characteristics.

The topics of clinical reliability and validity are discussed in every graduate diagnosis course and text, and thus basic knowledge of these areas is presumed for individuals reading this chapter. However, the challenges and dangers of violation of reliability and validity are rarely discussed in an explicit manner, especially as they relate to the practice in neurogenic communication disorders or medical speech–language pathology. Table 14–1 highlights these issues.

For us to evaluate the reliability and validity of a specific tool for a particular patient, we can take several approaches. Some guidelines that may be helpful to the clinician include:

1. *Review the test manual or published reviews and articles about the test.* Knowledge of statistical information about the test, as well as its stated purposes and limitations will allow the diagnostician to determine if the patient being tested fits the profile for which the instrument was designed. If the patient's problem or the referral question does not align with the stated purpose, or the demographic group (age, gender, disability type) on which the test was normed or other key variables, then the information obtained by using the instrument will have to be interpreted cautiously.

2. *Obtain skill in administering the test prior to using it for differential diagnosis.* Many

Table 14–1. Problems Associated with Poor Reliability and Validity of Testing and Observation Tools in Medical Speech–Language Pathology Practice

Limitations in interpretation of data

Generation of conflicting data among instruments or observers

Establishment of inaccurate or incomplete diagnosis

Establishment of inappropriate or ineffective treatments

Miscommunication of results to patient, family, referral source

Inaccurate prediction of course of the disorder

Inaccurate prognosis for recovery

tests used by speech–language pathologists are complex regarding their "rules" for administration, scoring of responses, and interpretation of results. Clinicians should never administer a test with an expectation of using results in differential diagnosis if they have not learned the overall requirements for administration and scoring or if they have not practiced the test items. Failure to become facile with the administration of a complex instrument will reduce the degree to which results can be comfortably and logically used.

3. *Select tests that align with the patient's behavioral styles and/or cognitive abilities.* Tests used in our discipline have been designed for a variety of age groups, intellectual levels, and patient types. Clinicians may choose to use a test because of previous experience, popularity of the instrument, or the amount of information that it is purported to generate. While these may be good reasons in general, if they violate the patient's sense of self-confidence, engender mistrust, or exceed the patient's attention or interest span, the results obtained may fail to reflect the patient's true ability. It is not uncommon for patients to perceive testing as an attempt to "trick" them or to make them look inferior or childish in some way. Clinicians need to use good judgment to be sure that the test instrument, as well as their own communication and clinical style, do not exacerbate any underlying feelings of uncertainty in the patient.

Note also that many of the procedures used to obtain valuable data with adult patients are not standardized. Observations made by the examiner in the interview with the patient, data obtained from observing the patient's interaction with others, information yielded from written or oral reports from other professionals, and results of "informal" testing with the patient all serve as essential data sources in the development of the diagnosis. Thus, clinicians need to develop extensive skill in reliably using these categories of information. While many of these "tools" are unpublished, the examiner can gain competence in completing these aspects of patient testing and observation by formalizing the process, developing specific forms or data sheets for recording information, and learning to carefully evaluate the results obtained prior to using the results in the formation of the diagnosis. Failure to follow this process of formalization may invalidate the use of the data obtained and can often lead to an inappropriate diagnosis. Again, many textbooks on diagnosis include interview formats, history forms, data sheets, observation protocols for various disorder types, and detailed approaches to informal assessment. In general, clinicians having less experience with a specific patient type can benefit from the attempt to formalize nonstandard approaches to testing.

Hypothesis Testing

Diagnostic activity is mental activity for the clinician. Miller and Groher state: "Development of the skill of early hypothesis testing is at the crux of the differential diagnostic process. This skill is usually achieved only after the clinician has had exposure to a wide variety of communication disorders and referrals from various medical disciplines" (p. 175).[10]

Hypothesis testing refers to the formulation of a thoughtful, logical, and probable classification of the observed behavior and then using the combined set of data available to determine if the hypothesis is accurate. The hypothesis should be based in the presenting information about the patient, the patient's condition and available history, as well as the SLP's extensive knowledge of the discipline. The hypothesis is then tested using the data collected from the patient. This approach is implicit to the diagnostic process and when done well facilitates efficient and appropriate patient care. It should be noted that this approach to diagnosis is highly individualized; without a reasonable hypothesis to be tested in diagnostic activity, the clinician is likely to expend time in unnecessary testing.

In summary, diagnosis is typically the first professional interaction that occurs between a patient and the speech–language pathologist. In some ways, it is the most important clinical activity because it provides the focus for therapy, supplies the baseline information from which measurement of change over time with treatment will be measured, and generates information that will be used by other professionals as well as the SLP. Assessment includes the set of measurement observations and actions that occur in the development of the diagnosis, as well as the ongoing measurement activities that occur over time to evaluate the effects of treatment. For the skilled diagnostician, the decision process that leads to a diagnosis is fluid and becomes almost automatic. For the novice clinician, however, this process should be taught as a deliberate and formal process. Diag-

nostic utility and reliability are increased when new practitioners have the opportunity to gauge their diagnostic decisions and interpretation against those of more expert professionals.

THE ACTIVITIES OF ASSESSMENT AND DIAGNOSIS

The process and techniques of diagnosis are accomplished through a series of actions that must be individualized for each patient. A routine "cookbook" approach to the steps of diagnosis is not feasible for all patients with neurologic communication disorders. The complexities of the human communication system call for a problem-oriented approach. This method has been described in neurologic diagnosis.[11] In the formulation of the hypothesis about the patient's presenting difficulty, the clinician must choose activities for measurement and observation that will test the hypothesis. This results in an individualized approach for each patient. The steps in arriving at a diagnosis in neurology (Table 14–2) are, in many ways, parallel to those used in speech–language pathology (see Table 14–3). The process outlined in Table 14–3 will be used to organize the discussion of the steps in the diagnostic process for neurogenic communication disorders.

Careful Planning for the Assessment

Planning for the session includes a variety of activities that focus on important features of the evaluation to be completed. These areas of focus include (1) the patient, (2) the environment where the session will occur, and (3) clinical skills and resources. Patient-focused aspects of assessment planning involve an attempt to understand and appreciate at a very detailed level the reason for the referral and the scope of features that may be presented by the patient. Important information sources for this aspect include the referral question or statement, any preliminary information available from the medical records or from other sources outside the immediate clinical setting, and—perhaps most important—the clinician's fund of knowledge about neurogenic communication disorders. A planning checklist for patient-related assessment planning is found in Table 14–4.

History and Interview

Table 14–5 provides an outline for a comprehensive case history checklist for neurogenic communication disorders. The examiner needs to be sure

Table 14–2. Steps in Arriving at a Neurologic Diagnosis.

Process	Concepts	Skill	Knowledge
History	Anatomic and pathologic concept of the disorder [A]	Interrogative skill	Basic neuroscience and neuropathology
Physical signs	Anatomic and functional localization [B]; confirm or refute [A]	Clinical examination	Interpretation of physical signs to localize and assess dysfunction
Differential diagnosis	Confirm or refute [A] or [B]	Discriminative	Knowledge of sensitivity and predictability of tests
Final diagnosis			

Source: Reprinted with permission from Olson WH, Brumback RA, Iyer V, Gascon, G: *Handbook of symptom oriented neurology,* (2nd ed), p. 475. St. Louis, MO, Mosby, 1994.

that the appropriate information is collected from the patient or the family. This basic information regarding the "facts" of the patient's health, social, psychological, and communication history guides the subsequent aspect of the interview.

The interview can be elucidating in appreciating the patient's problem, especially as the examiner attempts to understand the patient's attitudes and perspectives. Through this interview, the clinician learns of the presenting communication difficulties and observes the patient's communication "on-line." In most cases the interview process allows the clinician to "know" whether or not a communication disorder is present. It is also this information that leads to a clinical hypothesis about potential cause–effect relationships.

There are general guidelines that should be followed throughout the interview process so that the

interview will run smoothly and efficiently. The interviewer should have a sense of the direction for the interview to proceed, determine the information that is needed, and know different ways of eliciting case history for documentation purposes.

There are three general goals for the interview process: (1) establish rapport, (2) obtain information, and (3) make preliminary judgments about communication and/or swallowing functions.

Establish Rapport

Development of a trusting relationship with the patient is key to a successful evaluation. By giving the patient undivided attention, actively listening to his or her complaints and concerns, and showing genuine concern, a favorable clinician–patient relationship is typically established. The inter-

Table 14–3. Steps in Arriving at a Diagnosis in Speech–Language Pathology

Process	Concepts	Skill	Knowledge
History	Anatomic and pathologic concept of the disorder [A]	Interrogative skill	Basic understanding of language, cognition, communication, and their underlying physical and psychozlogical systems
Physical and behavioral signs	Anatomic and functional correlates; behavioral characteristics [B]; confirm or refute [A]	Clinical examination	Interpretation of physical and behavioral signs assess dysfunction and clarify the problem
Differential diagnosis	Confirm or refute [A] or [B]	Discriminative	Knowledge of sensitivity and predictability of tests; appreciation of significance of various findings among types of disorders
Final diagnosis			

Source: Adapted with permission from Olson WH, Brumback RA, Iyer V, Gascon G: *Handbook of symptom oriented neurology,* (2nd ed.), p. 475. St. Louis, MO, Mosby, 1994.

Table 14–4. Assessment Checklist: Patient-focused Planning

Referral information	Who is the referral source?
	What is the referring diagnosis?
	Why is the patient being referred?
	What is the stated referral question?
	Is the patient's (or family's) referral statement or question the same as the referring physician's?
Information from other sources	What other testing has been completed?
	What information is available from physician or hospital records?
	Is there other information available from previous speech–language hearing testing?
	Are there other important (essential) data sources missing?
	What steps need to be taken to obtain missing information that could be crucial to diagnosis?
Clinician's knowledge of patient's problems	Does clinician have experience with other patients with this disorder type?
	Does the clinician have knowledge of the characteristics, causes, and variations associated with this disorder?
	Does the clinician understand the disease process and its implications for the patient?
	Does the clinician have necessary background about the patient's communication needs and desires and the social-vocational context of the patient?

view should always be conducted at an unhurried pace so that the patient is cooperative and relaxed.

Obtain Information

The interview enables the clinician to complete the case history. The clinician collects additional information about the patient's speech–language concerns, medical and psychosocial history, and daily functioning not found in the medical record. The skill of the interviewer often determines the quality of information elicited. Strauss[12] has described the types of questions that are most useful in the assessment interview. Table 14–6 presents the various question types and provides examples that might be used in neurogenic communicative disorder assessments.

Make Preliminary Judgments about Speech, Language, and Cognition

The interview provides a conversation sample from which preliminary judgments about aspects of communication can be made. The patient who independently offers an accurate and complete account of speech–language deficits and medical history is very different from one whose spouse must provide all this information. Generally the clinician can narrow the differential diagnosis drawn to a few possibilities at the completion of the interview. The clinician can then decide which method of assessment and testing will clarify the diagnosis, determine the patient's potential benefit from treatment, and assist in making a judgment of prognosis.

Observation of the Patient

In addition to the more direct sources of information (case history; formal testing), the clinician needs to take time to spend observing the patient. The medical setting affords many opportunities for this—on the ward or in the waiting room, interacting with family and staff, during meals or social interactions, or while family members or other persons are providing information. These nondirected observations of the patient can serve as another valuable data set. As the clinician observes the patient in these various situations, the following questions should be addressed:

1. How well does the patient perform tasks involved in communication, swallowing and eating, nonverbal interaction, or activities of daily living?
2. Does the patient spontaneously initiate interaction?
3. Is the patient attentive and responsive?
4. How do others react to the patient?
5. Is the patient aware of the communication needs of others?
6. How do patient responses vary in quality and quantity among various situations?

The answers to these questions provide an important reliability check for inferences drawn from

Table 14–5. The Comprehensive Patient History in Neurogenic Communicative Disorders

Demographic Information:

    Name, Address, Phone No.

    Age, gender, marital status, occupation

    Religion

Source of Referral/Specialty:

Statement of Referral/Referral Question:

Sources of Information (medical chart, family, patient, other):

Chief Complaint: State in the patient's own words if possible

    History of communication problem: Precipitants, onset, course, duration; symptoms and signs; effects on environment; family, job, friends/relationships effects

    Previous therapy

General Medical History:

    Concurrent medical problems

    Current medications

    Past medical history

    Allergies

    Medical review of systems

    Psychological or psychiatric issues including substance abuse

Neurological History:

    Details of current illness and its course

    CT, MRI, other neuroimaging findings

    Family history of neurologic or communication disorders

    Neurologic symptoms: Motor, sensory, cognitive, language, speech, other

    Episodic disorders: Seizures, alterations of consciousness, headaches, intermittent communication disturbances

    Identification of referring neurologist

Marital History (or other significant relationships):

    If married: description of relationship with spouse; history of marriage

    If divorced or remarried: length of previous marriage

    If children: ages and relationship with parent

Social History:

    Young to middle age adults: Education, work, responsibilities, military service, social relations, recreational and avocational pursuits, goals

    Older adults: Career status and changes, losses, aging issues, family issues.

more structured observations and formal testing. Also, when the clinician suspects a psychogenic component to the communication disturbance, valuable information about the consistency of the patient's behavior can be made from these observations.

Testing and Differential Diagnosis

Each of the neurogenic disorders of communication has specific characteristics and signs, associated conditions and behaviors, and a course of recovery, stabilization, or deterioration. In the di-

agnostic process, the clinician is attempting to elicit observable, reliable data and supporting information to classify and distinguish the patient's disorder. It is useful to approach the process from the perspective of a series of questions that, when answered, lead to a limited number of diagnostic possibilities and usually to a definite diagnosis.

Disorders of Language

The most common language disorder in neurologic illness is, of course, aphasia. The features that con-

Table 14–6. Types of Questions Used in the Interview Process

Open-Ended Questions:

These encourage an open-ended reply and are useful when it is desirable to elicit a lengthier response.

> *Example:* Tell me what happened when you were in the hospital.

Closed-Ended Questions:

These tend to encourage a shorter response. They should be used for efficiency or for eliciting a response from a patient who is confused or expressively impaired.

> *Example:* Did you come to the hospital on Thursday or Friday?

Echo questions:

The clinician repeats part of what the patient said to encourage him or her to continue elaborating on a certain idea or point.

> *Example:* The patient states—"I'm afraid I'm going to lose all my friends because it takes so long to get the words out." Clinician—"Because it takes so long to get all your words out. . . ."

Probe questions:

These are requests for specific details or examples.

Example: Give me an example of what you have trouble remembering.

---

firm the presence of aphasia include difficulty with language formulation and comprehension. Virtually all patients with aphasia have some degree of naming deficit, and varying abilities in comprehension, repetition, conversation, reading, and writing. From a diagnostic perspective it is important to emphasize that in aphasia the patient's language abilities are the area of primary difficulty and surpass degree of deficit in other higher cortical functions. When aphasia is suspected by history or observation, the speech–language pathologist should complete a comprehensive aphasia examination battery such as the *Boston Diagnostic Aphasia Examination,*[13] *Western Aphasia Battery,*[14] or the *Multilingual Aphasia Examination*[15] to determine the language subsystems that are implicated, the degree of overall impairment, and the relative pattern of impairment that leads to the classification of aphasia type. When the patient's impairment is so severe that it becomes difficult to obtain useful information from these tests, the *Boston Assessment of Severe Aphasia*[16] should be considered. On the other hand, careful testing early on with some stroke patients may reveal a subtle aphasia. With these patients it may be useful to use language tasks and tests that are more difficult than the typical aphasia test. This is essential when the patient was premorbidly a high-level communicator. Appropriate tasks are those that emphasize the integrative and communicative aspects of language. Formal testing with subtests of the *Woodcock-*

Johnson Psychoeducational Battery[17] and informal testing with measures of discourse or higher level reading and writing tasks may help determine the extent and/or impact of the presenting mild aphasia symptoms.

Once it is determined that the patient has aphasia, the question of type becomes important. Type of aphasia can be ascertained through analysis of the presenting language profile and history. Cortical and subcortical aphasias should be differentiated using their characteristic profiles of language behavior.[2] In addition, primary progressive aphasia can be elucidated based on the patient's history of gradual worsening of language symptoms over time.

In addition to demonstrating the type of aphasia and its clinical severity, it is important to determine the level of functional impairment. This can be accomplished through use of a scale or measure that is directed at looking at communication use in the environment where the patient typically communicates. The recent publication of *the ASHA Functional Assessment of Communication Skills (FACS)*[18] complements some of the tools that have been use for a longer period of time such as the *Communication Activities of Daily Living*[19] or the *Communication Effectiveness Index (CETI).*[20]

From the perspective of differentiation, it is important to distinguish aphasia (a "pure" language disorder) from the various cognitive-language disturbances (dementia, right-hemisphere syndrome, post-traumatic cognitive impairment). Aphasia can be differentiated from dementia by its typical pattern of presentation, which is sudden onset after a stroke, and by its relative sparing of nonlinguistic cognitive functions. The key distinguishing characteristic of aphasia from right hemisphere syndrome is the typical sparing of essential linguistic functions in right hemisphere syndrome. Finally, when diffuse injury to the brain occurs as is common in traumatic brain injury, the patient usually exhibits confusion, disorientation, and multiple cognitive deficits in addition to language symptoms.

Disorders of Speech

Various disorders of speech production are known to be associated with various neurologic conditions. Duffy[4] defines motor speech disorders as "disorders of speech resulting from neurologic impairment affecting the motor programming or neuromuscular execution of speech. They encompass apraxia of speech and the dysarthrias" (p. 4). These two disorders are considered together because they both affect the acoustic output of speech that in town affects the quality and intelligibility of the sound generated by the speaker. While other communication disorders, especially those of language, may co-occur with motor speech disorders, the underlying mechanisms and pathophysiology are distinct.

The specific etiologies that cause motor speech disorders can be associated with focal or diffuse damage to the nervous system, and many disease processes can result in dysarthria and apraxia. In addition, lesions in various levels of the nervous system produce perceptually identifiable patterns of speech disturbance. For a complete review of the clinical pathophysiology of motor speech disorders, the reader is referred to Duffy's *Motor Speech Disorders: Substrates, Differential Diagnosis, and Management*.[4]

When the clinician detects the presence of a speech disturbance or the patient's complaint is one of difficulty producing speech or maintaining intelligibility, the diagnostician should focus on examination for motor speech disorders. The first task is to determine whether or not the patient has a speech disturbance and second to determine if the problem is neurogenic or non-neurogenic. The major non-neurogenic causes of speech disturbance are associated with developmental speech disturbances (i.e., articulatory or phonological disorders) that have persisted into adulthood or psychogenic

disorders. Persistent developmental problems are identified by taking careful historical information from the patient or from others who have known the person since childhood. Psychogenic disorders are suspected when the patient's history does not give evidence of associated neurogenic disease; when there are environmental or psychological precipitants; when the presenting symptoms are not consistent with the neurologic diagnosis; or when the patient's speech fluctuates significantly from session to session without clear explanation. The reader interested in psychiatric abnormalities and especially psychogenic disturbances of speech is referred to Section V of this text.

Once it has been established that the patient's speech difficulty is likely to be a neurogenic speech disturbance, it becomes the challenge of the diagnostician to determine if the problem is one of dysarthria or apraxia of speech. This is accomplished by completing a careful history, taking a conversational speech sample, completing an examination of the speech production mechanism, and using a variety of speech tasks including diadochokinetic rates, alternating motion rates, vowel prolongation, and assorted voice and/or articulation measures. In addition, to completing these tasks, the examiner needs to assess the general communication abilities (functional communication skills) of the patient. To complete the assessment, the clinician must interpret the speech data obtained using perceptual analysis. A commonly used procedure for making perceptual rating has been outlined by Duffy.[4]

Dysarthria

Dysarthria is defined by Hedge as:

> . . . a group of motor speech disorders resulting from disturbed muscular control of the speech mechanism due to damage of the peripheral or central nervous system; oral communication problems due to weakness, incoordination, or paralysis of speech musculature; physiologic characteristics include abnormal or disturbed strength, speed, range, steadiness, tone, and accuracy of muscle movements; communication characteristics include disturbed pitch, loudness, voice quality, resonance, respiratory support for speech, prosody, and articulation (p. 180).[21]

From a diagnostic perspective, the clinician confirms the presence of dysarthria by demonstrating that the presenting speech disturbance is associated with weakness, paralysis, or incoordination, or neuropathologies that affect the motor system (e.g., Parkinson's disease, amyotrophic lateral sclerosis), exhibits fairly consistent error types and patterns, and may exhibit respiratory, phonatory, resonance, and articulatory problems.

Apraxia

Apraxia of speech is a neurogenic speech disorder that typically manifests itself primarily with errors in articulatory production, has associated prosodic characteristics, and is usually associated with lesions in Broca's area and the supplementary motor area of the left cerebral hemisphere.[4,9] The presence of apraxia of speech is confirmed by demonstration of speech characteristics in articulation and prosody, observation and documentation of inconsistency of productions, and also demonstration of struggling and groping during speech attempts. It is well documented that apraxia of speech can occur with aphasia, especially Broca's type.

Once the classification in type of motor speech disorder (dysarthria vs. apraxia of speech) is made, further assessment is indicated to differentiate among the various types of dysarthria or the characteristics of apraxia of speech. The dysarthrias are classified based on their perceptual characteristics, with varying patterns of characteristics being associated with one of the types of dysarthrias that have been described by Darley, Aronson, and Brown.[22] Classification of dysarthria is important from a neurodiagnostic perspective, and speech–language pathologists should document whether the presenting dysarthria is consistent with the neurological diagnosis, if it is known. Classification of dysarthria by the SLP can be important information for the neurologist who is struggling with a difficult diagnosis, or when the speech problem is the primary or first symptom noted in the course of an illness.

In assessment of apraxia, it is important to characterize the presenting symptoms, determine the severity and functional impairment of the patient in his or her daily life communication activities, and determine which strategies will be helpful in treatment. Because for many patients there is an accompanying oral or limb apraxia, it is important to test for these dysfunctions.

Only one standardized test, *Apraxia Battery for Adults*[23] has been widely used as a formal measure of apraxic characteristics in adult speech. Helm-Estabrooks[24] has developed a standardized assessment tool for measurement of performance oral (non-speech) and limb movements. In addition, most standard aphasia batteries include measures of speech, oral, and limb apraxia. It is

important to use one of the standardized measures to obtain scores that can be comparable over time for assessment of patient change.

Cognitive-Communication Disorders

A group of disorders that have significant effects on language and communication have received increased attention in the literature. These disorders generally fall into three categories that reflect their major etiologies: right hemisphere dysfunction, dementia, and traumatic brain injury. Typically, when these patients present to the speech–language pathologist they come with multiple complaints that reflect their problems in memory, attention, judgment, orientation, perceptual abilities, decision making, or executive functions in addition to their problems in language. Because the communication problems of these patients are frequently not well understood by referral sources, the patients are often referred to as being aphasic. Thus, this becomes the first important distinction to be made. These three groups of patients differ from each other by history, initial presentation, and natural course of their problem.

Right hemisphere dysfunction occurs primarily as a result of stroke, although other etiologies that produce focal right hemisphere damage can be etiologic. Because stroke is a common etiology for both right and left hemisphere disorders, patients with aphasia and right hemisphere syndrome are sometimes confused. Typically, the neurological exam and behavioral testing of cognitive areas and language provides evidence of those features that distinguish the patient from those with other language disorders. Major distinguishing features include absence of significant problems in naming, fluency, comprehension, and reading. In addition, these patients may exhibit significant problems in visuospatial perception. Left-sided neglect becomes obvious to the clinician when patients fail to produce details on the left side of an object they are building or drawing or omit letters from the left side of a word, and occasionally when they dress or groom only one-half of their body. Again, the major difference noted between patients with aphasia and those with right hemisphere syndrome will be the prominence of nonverbal deficits in the non-aphasic patient and the relative sparing of the communication functions classically affected in those with aphasia.[6,9]

Standardized tests commonly used in SLP assessment include the *Rehabilitation Institute of Chicago Right Hemisphere Battery*[25] or the

Mini-Inventory of Right Brain Injury.[26] For symptoms that need additional assessment or description, consider administering measures of neglect (*Behavioral Inattention Test*[27]) or testing of the patient's ability to interpret higher level language (humor, sarcasm, metaphor). If the patient shows signs of specific linguistic disturbance, administer tests to determine the nature and extent of the linguistic deficits that are present. Another area that has received additional attention is the area of discourse and conversational abilities in right hemisphere patients.[28] This area of observation and assessment is important for addressing the patient's functional communication and has significant implications for treatment planning.

The language of dementia is observed in patients with a variety of neurological diseases that produce generalized cognitive impairment. Common types of dementia include those that are associated with cortical dysfunction (Alzheimer's disease, Pick's disease), those seen in subcortical dysfunction (Parkinson's disease, Huntington's chorea, progressive supranuclear palsy), and the mixed dementias (multi-infarct dementia, Creutzfeldt-Jakob disease, Korsakoff's syndrome).[29]

The most common dementia seen by the speech–language pathologist are observed in patients with Alzheimer's disease (AD), Parkinson's disease (PD), and multi-infarct stroke patients (MID). The language symptoms of each of these types has now been fairly well documented. In AD the initial presentation includes mild naming and memory problems that progress over several years to severe language disturbance crossing all modalities of communication. In the subgroup of patients with PD who are also demented, language problems are usually less notable than in those with AD. In addition, patients with AD are not likely to exhibit speech production difficulties. In MID, the onset of problems is abrupt, with sudden (stepwise) changes that occur over time as new infarcts occur. Again, the various dementias are distinguishable from aphasia based on pattern of communication at onset (aphasia vs. AD; aphasia vs PD); pattern of change over time (improvement vs. decline); and of course primacy of language disturbance vs. generalized cognitive dysfunction with a language component.

Patients with traumatic brain injury (TBI) are easily distinguishable from those with other conditions because the etiology is obvious and abrupt. Depending on the site and extent of brain injury, patients may exhibit disorders of both speech and language in addition to their typical cognitive deficits. TBI patients have been monitored for recovery from the time of their accident/injury for purposes of developing predictive tools and models. This has led to the development of tools that are useful in describing the patient's level of responsiveness[30] and also his or her level of cognitive-linguistic functioning.[31]

While differentiation of language problems secondary to TBI from other language disorders is rarely difficult, the challenge in assessment and diagnosis lies in the area of differentiation and clarification of the symptoms. The rapid change that occurs in these patients, along with their more common behavioral difficulties, can make lengthy complex testing sessions difficult and at times unreliable. Most approaches to testing that are documented in the literature have included batteries of tests designed to tap into cognitive, social, linguistic, and general behavioral domains. In addition, two tests have been developed by speech–language pathologists specifically for sampling behavior in the TBI population.[32,33] Kennedy and Deruyter[34] have provided detailed guidelines for patient assessment throughout the recovery stages outlined by Hagen.[31] These guidelines should be helpful to the clinician attempting to assess TBI patients across the continuum of care.

USING DIAGNOSTIC INFORMATION FOR PREDICTION AND PLANNING

Determination of a language of speech diagnosis contributes to the medical management of the patient, and at times may aid the physician in establishing medical diagnosis or a locus for the lesion. In addition, the diagnosis, as we noted previously, provides a roadmap to the determination of important decisions about speech–language follow-up and therapy. However, some information beyond the diagnosis is needed for predicting outcome and making decisions regarding appropriate treatment.

Outcome

An Outcome Perspective

Outcome has been simply defined as "when all is said and done, what happened to the patient?"[35] Outcome can be conceptualized on four levels. The first is physiological outcome, which includes the medical stability of the patient. The next three levels have been described by the World Health Organization (WHO) in International Classification of Impairments and have been used by the American

Speech–Language-Hearing Association for the development of functional outcome measures. Behavioral outcome refers to the measurement of speech, language, or cognitive impairments through the use of traditional assessment tools. Functional outcomes measure the ability of the patient to handle communication issues within the context of daily activities, and to complete daily activities that depend on communication. Finally, the WHO's handicap level refers to the social consequences of the language impairment and is measured through tools that address such issues as quality of life and wellness. These four levels are intended to address the full spectrum of measurable aspects of a patient's functioning after a serious medical event. They reflect the types of issues that are important to the patient while moving across the continuum of care.

Prognosis

Numerous factors are known to contribute to an attainable outcome. Factors from the individual patient and from the immediate and extended environment interact with each other to contribute to the patient's outcome. Although no equation exists that accounts for these variables and adequately predicts an outcome, we do have evidence about the importance of various factors. The master clinician must depend on experience to combine information about these factors to predict behavioral, functional, or quality-of-life outcomes.

Factors to be Used in Prediction

The starting point for establishment of the prognosis is the endpoint of the initial diagnostic speech–language-cognitive evaluation. In addition to providing a diagnosis, the evaluation yields a behavioral profile about preserved abilities, type and severity of impairments, spontaneously produced compensatory strategies, and error types. The combination of these factors leads to the prognosis.

Unfortunately, we do not have clear guidelines from the research literature regarding the significance of all the predictor variables that we use in the evaluation of neurogenic communication disorders. Consequently, the clinician must readjust relative importance of particular factors depending on the patient's premorbid status, family life, and personal history. These factors and their importance must be considered for each patient on an individual basis.

The Disease Process

The underlying disease that has caused the speech or language disorder and its process is a critical factor to consider. Various categories of disease may have generally different effects on prognosis and management in neurogenic communication disorders. *Progressive* diseases (e.g., Alzheimer's disease, Pick's disease, ALS) typically have a progressive downhill course. It should be noted that in most neurodegenerative diseases the course is typically slow. While this lengthy downward spiral is difficult for patients and their families, the time course does allow the SLP to develop specific assessment and treatment protocols consistent with the stage of the disease. *Traumatic* injuries are typically worse at onset or immediately after and then have a course of ongoing improvement. *Systemic* diseases, such as cancer or metabolic disorders, may affect the nervous system as well as other body systems. *Sporadic* diseases (e.g., multiple sclerosis, epilepsy) have fluctuating courses and are difficult to deal with in the prognostic puzzle because of their limited predictability.

Age, Gender, and Occupation

Most recent studies investigating the role of age, gender, and occupational level in outcome or recovery have not supported these variable as good prognosticators. There have been early reports that older patients are less likely to be independent and in general to have poorer outcomes. However, when there are controls for general medical status and other chronic diseases, age no longer emerges as a good predictor. Older individuals are more likely to have one or more chronic diseases, and it may be the presence of these diseases, and general medical status, that is predictive of outcome, rather than age alone. There is no evidence that gender or occupational status predicts recovery or outcome.

Cognitive Status

The etiology of a communication disorder may affect other aspects of the cognitive system equally, as in the dementias, or the sequelae may be essentially limited to the communication system. In both cases, overall cognitive status is an important predictor of outcome and should be considered in our choice of treatment approach. When cognition is affected, along with language as a result of diffuse pathology, assessment will reveal the behavioral impairments that reflect the loss of executive function, memory, or learning. In the case of focal lesions, which result in more specific language loss, cognitive assessment may unveil relatively preserved strengths in reasoning, new memory, self-monitoring, and learning. These assessment results can direct choice of treatment. Since we are dependent on the learning system of the individual for intervention success and for ultimate ability to problem solve communication breakdowns, severity of cognitive dysfunction is negatively correlated to positive outcomes.

Executive Function

Executive function includes the ability to self-monitor, self-analyze, reason, perform meta-cognitive and metalinguistic tasks, and engage in prospective memory (knowing that you need to remember something). The *Western Aphasia Battery*[15] includes a measure of nonverbal reasoning. Other neuropsychological tests, such as the *Wisconsin Card Sorting Test*,[36] are also commonly used to measure the patient's ability to learn rules. When patients can demonstrate that they have intact executive function, the diagnostician can use this information as a positive predictor of the patient's long-term ability to adapt to their communication disability and lead a full and productive life.

Patients with executive dysfunction may have difficulty adapting to the common therapeutic strategy of recalling and applying a particular strategy or technique. Consequently, the number and type of therapeutic options become reduced.

Memory

Many patients with neurogenic communication disorders experience impairment of "working memory," which is the temporary storage location for incoming information. This information is rehearsed in working memory and then encoded into long-term memory. If incoming information cannot be held in working memory long enough to be encoded, due to a disorder, then the presentation of new information will not be stored for retrieval and use on future occasions. The severity of the memory disorder will determine the extent to which encoding may occur. In milder impairments, additional repetitions or mnemonic strategies such as visual imagery may enhance encoding. In severe cases, these strategies are typically not beneficial.

Psychosocial Factors

The psychological status of the patient and the social support provided make up the context in which the communication impairments will be interpreted. Ability to function in daily living tasks, and ultimately to lead a fulfilling lifestyle, will largely be determined by the patient's psychological adjustment to the communication impairments, as well as the adjustment of important members of the support system.

Psychological Status

Reactive depression can be a consequence of adjusting to residual deficits. A majority of patients with aphasia experience depression and are most likely to do so during the period 9 to 18 months post onset. When a patient is undergoing a depressive period, it is wise for the clinician to recommend and assist in prioritizing appropriate psychological services.

In general, depression should be viewed as a negative prognostic factor. Patients for whom depression has been managed with appropriate medical or psychological interventions may be ready to focus on functional and long-term goals in language or speech intervention.

Planning Management

Besides establishing the communication diagnosis and prognosis, we must consider the question of potential treatment benefit and the focus of such treatment. Based on projected outcomes and the cognitive, psychosocial, and demographic factors described above, the clinician can use a hierarchical series of questions to determine the usefulness of further management. These questions are listed in Table 14–7. This table emphasizes the series and order of questions that can be used to guide clinicians in selection of appropriate treatment goals for patients.

SUMMARY

This chapter has described a framework for diagnostic decision making in patients with neurologically based communication disorders, provided highlights of differential diagnosis and prognosis, and prevented some considerations for preliminary patient management. Successful application of each of these areas is crucial to patient management. Errors in this vital aspect of patient decision making will undermine the good intentions of the speech–language pathologist and the hopes of the family and the patient. Failure to provide critical diagnostic information limits understanding for

Table 14–7. Hierarchy of Patient Management Questions for Use after the Diagnosis is Established

1. Is the patient medically stable?
   YES: Proceed to Question 2
   NO: Will ongoing assessment contribute to the medical management of the patient?
      (a) If no, recheck after an appropriate interval
      (b) If yes, continue with periodic re-assessments

2. Is the patient entering a period of rapid recovery?
   YES: Initiate treatment to facilitate improvement
   NO: Proceed to Question 3

3. Is the patient at the peak of communication abilities with expected future decrease in function?
   YES: Initiate appropriate education or intervention program
   NO: Proceed to Question 4

4. Is the patient experiencing psychiatric or psychological complications?
   YES: Refer for appropriate services
   NO: Proceed to Question 5

5. Could a course of intervention significantly alter the patient's vocational or independent living status?
   YES: Initiate appropriate treatment
   NO: No direct treatment indicated; consider support or maintenance program

the patient, his or her family, and for other professionals who may be providing service. Inaccurate prognostication (over- or underestimation) will lead to an inappropriate allocation of services for a given patient. Finally, poor decision making about patient management can lead to misdirections in therapy that are both costly and ineffective. By applying the principles outlined in this chapter, such errors can be reduced.

CASE ONE—APHASIA VS. PSYCHOGENIC DISTURBANCE

The patient was referred for evaluation of his language disturbance that had resulted in chronic difficulties communicating with the family and inability to coordinate activities of daily living. The patient was 10 years post-onset of a single left-hemispheric stroke, with no residual hemiparesis. He resided at home with his wife, a mental health professional. At the time of the evaluation his medical records were not available. Standardized aphasia testing using the *Boston Diagnostic Aphasia Examination,* conversational analysis, and informal observations was completed. During the course of the evaluation, the patient described the existence of two "selves," one

who he called "Michael," who did not experience communication difficulty; the other was "Mike," who could only speak telegraphically.

Language diagnosis was completed to determine whether language symptoms were consistent with aphasia or were more consistent with language disturbance observed in some psychotic patients. Results of language testing showed naming errors (i.e., semantic paraphasias) under all conditions, with no literal paraphasias. Auditory comprehension was mildly impaired. Performance on silent reading comprehension tasks alternated between explicit matching of single words to apparent ability to comprehend text including morphosyntactical relations. The patient wrote with his dominant right hand legibly. "Michael" was able to write complete grammatical sentences with minimal errors, and "Mike" was only able to string single content words together in spontaneous writing. Verbally, "Michael" was very fluent, verbose, and made occasional uncorrected naming errors. "Mike" produced telegraphic single content words, no functors at all, with relatively few paraphasic errors in this condition of any type. Repetition skills were relatively good under every condition.

Although the patient's language system was certainly abnormal, it was judged that the patient did not present a language profile consistent with the typical aphasia syndromes; rather the profiles were more consistent with language of psychogenic disturbance. The patient and his family were provided with suggestions for behavioral management at home, suggestions about family communication, and referral to a psychiatric clinic for additional follow-up.

CASE TWO—APPROPRIATE ASSESSMENT LEADS TO FUNCTIONAL TREATMENT

The patient, a 63-year-old male, was referred for evaluation of chronic aphasia. He was 10 years post-onset of single large left hemispheric occlusive stroke that had resulted in a large fronto-parietotemporal lesion. He had residual paresis of his right upper extremity but was able to ambulate well without aid. He had been at home since his initial discharge from speech therapy, and spent his time watching television. He engaged in no other activities of any sort, and was not an active participant in the family system.

Evaluation revealed severe Broca's aphasia with oral–verbal apraxia. The patient comprehended oral directions, and could match single written words to pictures. His speech output was limited to "no," "yes," and "OK." He had some preserved drawing ability of word shape and length and could indicate this by slotting.

A course of treatment was provided that focused on the types of tasks that this patient was likely to be able and to want to do in his home environment. A system of multimodality communication, combining drawing, gesture, written first letters, and a word–picture notebook was trained. This patient had the cognitive capabilities to learn these strategies and deploy them appropriately. Functional outcome for this patient was significantly changed because he was able to take and pass his driver's examination and drive independently for the first time in ten years, and hold down a volunteer position in the mail services department of his previous company, which gave him the opportunity to regularly see friends and acquaintances of many years. His contribution and role in the family also expanded.

STUDY QUESTIONS

1. What are key components in patient diagnosis?

2. Explain the use of the term "hypothesis testing" as it relates to diagnosis and assessment.

3. Compare diagnosis in speech–language pathology to diagnosis in neurology.

4. Provide differentiating characteristics among the following disorders:
   a. Aphasia and dementia
   b. TBI and aphasia
   c. Right and left hemisphere infarcts
   d. Neurogenic and psychogenic speech disorders
   e. Dysarthria and apraxia
   f. Apraxia and aphasia

5. Outline a brief protocol for assessment and diagnosis in motor speech disorders.

6. Outline a brief protocol for assessment and diagnosis in cognitive-linguistic disorders.

7. Explain your philosophy of diagnosis for patients with neurogenic communication disorders.

8. How should nonlanguage variables be used in prognosis?

9. How does the process of diagnosis relate to patient outcome?

REFERENCES

1. Nation JE, Aram DM: *Diagnosis of speech and language disorders* (2nd ed.) St. Louis, MO, Mosby, 1984.

2. Helm-Estabrooks NH, Albert ML: *Manual of aphasia therapy.* Austin, TX, Pro-Ed, 1991.

3. Johns, D: *Clinical management of neurogenic communication disorders* (2nd ed.) Boston, Little, Brown, 1985.

4. Duffy JR: *Motor speech disorders: Substrates, differential diagnosis, and management.* St. Louis, MO, Mosby Year Book, Inc., 1995.

5. Bayles KA, Kaszniak AW: *Communication and cognition in normal aging and dementia.* Austin, TX, Pro-Ed, 1987.

6. Tompkins C: *Right hemisphere communication disorders: Theory and management.* San Diego, CA, Singular Publishing, 1995.

7. Meitus IJ, Weinberg B: *Diagnosis in speech–language pathology.* Baltimore, MD, University Park Press, 1983.

8. Negde MN: *Pocket guide to assessment in speech–language pathology.* San Diego, CA, Singular Publishing Group, Inc., 1996.

9. ASHA: *Director of speech–language pathology assessment instruments.* Rockville, MD, American Speech–Language-Hearing Association, 1995.

10. Miller RM, Groher ME: *Medical speech pathology.* Rockville, MD, Aspen Publisher, 1990.

11. Olson WH, Brumback RA, Iver V, Gascon, G: *Handbook of symptom oriented neurology* (2nd ed.) St. Louis, MO, Mosby, 1994.

12. Strauss GD: Diagnosis and psychiatry: Examination of the psychiatric patient. In HI Kaplan and BJ Sadock, eds. *Comprehensive textbook of psychiatry VI.* (1995). Baltimore: Williams & Wilkins.

13. Goodglass H, Kaplan, E: *Assessment of aphasia and related disorders.* Philadelphia, Lea and Febiger, 1972.

14. Kertesz A: *The Western aphasia battery.* New York, Grune & Stratton, 1982.

15. Benton AI, deS.Hamsher K, Sivan AR: *Multilingual aphasia examination.* Iowa City, IA, AIA Associates Inc., 1994.

16. Helm Estabrooks N: *Boston assessment of severe aphasia.* Chicago, Riverside Publishing, 1989.

17. Woodcock RW, Johnson MB: *Woodcock Johnson psychoeducational battery—revised.* Allen, TX, DLM Teaching Resources, 1989.

18. Frattali, CM, Thompson CK, Holland AL, Wohl, CB, Ferkefic, MM, *Functional Assessment of Communication Skills for Adults.* Rockville, MD: ASHA, 1995.

19. Holland A: *Communication Activities of Daily Living.* Baltimore, MD: University Park Press, 1980.

20. Lomas J, Pickard L, Bester S, Elbard H, Finlayson A, Zoghiab C: The communication effectiveness index: Development and psychometric evaluation of a functional communication measure for adult aphasia. *Speech Hear Dis* 54, 113–124, 1989.

21. Hedge MN: *Pocket guide to assessment in speech–language pathology.* San Diego, CA, Singular Publishing Group, Inc., 1996.

22. Darley F, Aronson A, Brown J: *Motor speech disorders.* Philadelphia, W.B. Saunders, 1975.

23. Dabul B: *Apraxia battery for adults.* Austin, TX, Pro-Ed, 1979.

24. Helm-Estabrooks N: *Test of oral and limb apraxia,* Chicago, Riverside Publishing Co., 1992.

25. Halper AS, Cherney LR, Burns MS: *Clinical management of right hemisphere dysfunction.* Gaithersburg, MD, Aspen Publication, 1996.

26. Pimental PA, Kingsbury NA: *Mini-inventory of right brain injury.* Austin, TX, Pro-Ed, 1989.

27. Wilson BA, Cockburn J, Halligan P: *Behavioral inattention test.* Bury St. Edmunds, Suffolk, England, Thames Valley Test Company, 1987.

28. Brookshire RH: *An introduction to neurogenic communication disorders* (4th ed.) St. Louis, MO, Mosby Year Book, 1992.

29. Ripich DN: Language and communication in dementia. In D. Ripich, ed., *Handbook of geriatric communication disorders.* Austin, TX, Pro-Ed, 1991.

30. Teasdale G, Jenette B: Assessment of coma and impaired consciousness. *Lancet,* 1974; 2, 81.

31. Hagen C: Language disorders in head trauma. In A. Holland, (ed.), *Language disorders in adults.* San Diego, College-Hill Press, 1984.

32. Helm-Estabrooks N: *The brief test of head injury (BTHI).* Chicago, Riverside Press, 1992.

33. Adamovich B, Henderson J: *Scales of cognitive ability for traumatic brain injury* (SCATBI), Austin, TX, Pro-Ed, 1992.

34. Kennedy MR, Deruyter F: Cognitive and language bases for communication disorders. In D. Beukelman and K. Yorkston, eds., *Communication disorders following traumatic brain injury: Management of cognitive, language, and motor impairments.* Austin, TX, Pro-Ed, 1991.

35. Reinertson, JL: Outcomes management and continuous quality improvement: The compass and the rudder. *Qual Res Bull,* 1993; January 5–7.

36. Grant DA, Berg EA: *Wisconsin card sorting test.* Odessa, FL, Psychological Assessment Resources, Inc., 1993.

15

An Introduction to Neurogenic Swallowing Disorders

NAN D. MUSSON

CHAPTER OUTLINE

Data Collection

Acquired Neurogenic Disorders: Common Symptoms and Physical Signs Associated with Feeding and Swallowing Disorders

Establishing the Goals of Dysphagia Intervention

People rarely concentrate on the actual act of eating. Most people focus on the pleasure of eating and experiences related to the eating environment. In reality, eating (self-feeding and swallowing) is an extremely complex and integrated neuromuscular process that synchronizes volitional and automatic movements to provide adequate nutrition and hydration for keeping the human body functioning and healthy. Although normal swallowing can be described as a continuous sequence of events, the process of swallowing may be separated into two to four distinct phases. When there is a breakdown in one or more of these phases, the impaired swallowing may be labeled dysphagia. When the dysphagia is suspected to have a neurogenic etiology, the terms neurogenic dysphagia or neurogenic swallowing disorder have been used.[1] Dysphagia can be categorized into one of two types: oropharyngeal (pre-esophageal) or esophageal,[2] depending on the site of the dysfunction.[3] Although some neurological diseases may impair the smooth muscles in the esophagus, the majority of neurogenic conditions cause oropharyngeal dysphagia or interfere with the transfer of the bolus prior to entry to the esophagus.[1,3,4]

Virtually any disease or trauma to the neurological system has the potential to cause a breakdown or disorder in the feeding and swallowing process; this in turn will impact on the safety and efficiency of oral intake and the individual's health status. The accurate identification of communication and swallowing disorders often provides confirmation of a specific disease or neurological diagnosis, may offer evidence to question a neurological diagnosis, or signal the need for further assessment. Neurogenic dysphagia may be identified as one of a variety of neurological symptoms or as an initial symptom of a neurological syndrome or process.[1] In other words, the patient with a known neurologic disease may have symptoms of dysphagia (e.g., Parkinson's disease) or neurogenic dysphagia may be an initial symptom of an unrecognized or undiagnosed neurologic disease (e.g., amyotrophic lateral sclerosis).

Speech–language pathologists are often charged with the task of ruling out a possible feeding or swallowing disorder, establishing a diagnosis of dysphagia, identifying an etiology, confirming a previous diagnosis with observed behaviors, and establishing an intervention plan. This chapter introduces the reader to a holistic approach to patient intervention, particularly for those individuals with suspected or known neurogenic swallowing disorders.

Intervention for patients with suspected neurogenic swallowing disorders requires a systematic collection of biographical, medical, and behavioral data to make a diagnosis, formulate a prognosis, and, when appropriate, implement a treatment or management program. Gathering an accurate history, completing a neurological and communication screening, and cautiously observing feeding and swallowing behaviors are the first three steps of the decision-making process for successful dysphagia intervention. These steps are designed to assist the clinician in clearly defining the swallowing problem and establishing a realistic prognosis. Once the diagnosis and prognosis are established, the professional(s) and patient/surrogate can delineate the choices for intervention and weigh the risks and benefits of those choices. At that time, the actual plan of intervention may be established, implemented, and periodically assessed and revised as needed.

DATA COLLECTION

Through the history and clinical examination, the speech–language pathologist may determine the signs and physical symptoms of the dysphagia or underlying neurological disorder, identify the time of onset and course of the swallowing problem, localize the disease process, confirm a potential site of lesion, or unveil a previously undiagnosed medical, psychological, or social problem. Finally, the speech–langauge pathologist should assess the degree of disability, judge the potential for restoration of function, and influence the intervention process for individuals with feeding and swallowing disorders. These broad steps are the basis of the clinical process and offer a wide choice in the order by which information is collected and interpreted. Although cause, site of lesion, symptoms, and course are common ways of describing a neurogenic disease or feeding-swallowing disorder, there are also limitations to using each individually rather than collectively or as an integrated approach.[5,6] (Tables 15–1, 15–2).

Causes of Neurogenic Dysphagia

Classifying feeding and swallowing disorders on the basis of a cause is a common approach used by health care professionals. Any cause that might affect the swallowing center of the brainstem or the cranial nerves that modulate the process (CNS V, VII, IX, X, and XII) or disturb the striated muscles of the oropharynx can cause oropharyngeal dysphagia and any disease or disorder that interferes with the cognitive status of the patient may interfere with the eating process.[1,3] Many causes will lead to similar symptoms or disorders of swallowing, and some causes may affect more than one area of the neurological system.[1,5,6] For example, a stroke, neoplasm, or head trauma may all result in pharyngeal stage dysphagia depending on the site of lesion. The speech–language pathologist must be aware that a known cause may lead to an assumption and should be cautious to confirm the symptoms with observations rather than assign a treatment plan based on a cause of the neurogenic disorder.[5] In addition, there may be more than one cause for an oropharyngeal dysphagia with a variety of symptoms or physical signs. Each of the etiologies may carry a different prognosis. Common causes associated with communication and swallowing disorders are listed below.

- *Genetic disorders:* Genetic disorders originate from a defect or defects in the inherited genetic material within cells. In some cases, a genetic disorder may occur as a result of a mutation of a gene. Genetic disorders may appear at birth or in adult years. Examples: Huntington's chorea, Joseph's disease, Wilson's disease.
- *Developmental disorders:* Developmental disorders originate from abnormal fetal development (not from defective genes). Known causes include viral infections or use of alcohol, nicotine, or drugs by the mother. Examples: Cerebral palsy, hydrocephalus, anencephaly, microcephaly.
- *Impaired blood and oxygen supply:* Anything that interferes with the brain's blood supply or prevents oxygen from entering the blood can cause brain damage. Examples: stroke, asphyxiation, drowning, strangulation, electrocution.
- *Neurotransmitter disturbance:* Brain and nervous system disorders can arise from altered production of a neurotransmitter (chemical secreted by nerve cells to communicate with each other), altered sensitivity of a specific

receptor site, or selective loss of nerve cells that contain a neurotransmitter. Examples: Parkinson's disease, schizophrenia, depression.

- *Tumors:* Tumors can occur in any part of the brain, spinal cord, or their coverings. Tumors can directly destroy tissue or compress other structures as they grow within a confined space or may spread (metastasize) from sites elsewhere in the body. Tumors may be cancerous (malignant) or noncancerous (benign). Examples: brain tumor, base of skull tumor, acoustic neuroma, metastasis to the brain.

- *Physical injury:* The brain and spinal cord are vulnerable to injury. Injury may occur from a motor-vehicle accident, sports injury, bullet wound, surgical trauma, fall, or any other physical trauma. Examples: skull fracture, spinal cord injury, severed nerves, crushed nerves.

- *Nerve compression:* Compression or entrapment of a nerve or nerve root by surrounding structures can cause pain, numbness or weakness in the area supplied by the nerve. Examples: disc prolapse, carpal tunnel syndrome.

Table 15–1. Comprehensive Clinical Examination of Swallow Function

I. History
  A. Medical history including significant past treatment and medication history
  B. Current medical diagnosis
    1. Coexisting medical problems
    2. Current medical treatment
    3. Medications
    4. Respiratory status
      (pulmonary disease, history of aspiration pneumonia, respiratory rate, presence of a tracheostomy tube or ventilator)
  C. Current nutritional, dietary, and hydration status
    1. Recent progressive weight loss
    2. Method and amount of nutritional intake
    3. Laboratory values
      (serum sodium, serum albumin, total protein, prealbumin, total lymphocyte, BUN)
    4. Special dietary concerns and preferences
  D. General physical condition

II. Description of the problem as perceived by the patients or significant other
  A. Progressive sudden onset of dysphagia
  B. Date of onset of other medical problems
  C. Duration of the problem
  D. Frequency of the problem (intermittent vs. constant)
  E. Exacerbating factors (food types, postures, etc.)
  F. Sensation of obstruction
  G. Sensation of pain
  H. Heartburn or reflux (time observed)
  I. Coughing or choking
  J. Mouth odor
  K. Xerostomia
  L. Drooling
  M. Change in food tastes
  N. Appetite change
  O. Nasal regurgitation
  P. Awareness of speech or voice change(s)

III. Clinical observation and mental status assessment
  A. Speech, language, and voice status
  B. Cognitive status (attention, memory, judgment, etc.)

IV. Oral mucosa and dentition

Table 15–1. (*continued*)

    V. Sensory motor examination of oral facial structures
        A. Oral Sensation
            1. Lips, tongue, and buccal mucosa
            2. Observations of pathological reflexes
        B. Symmetry and strength of facial muscles
        C. Range of motion, symmetry, and strength of muscles of mastication
        D. Range of motion, strength, speed, and tone of the tongue and lingual muscles
        E. Pharynx (at rest and on gag)
        F. Palate (at rest, during phonation, and on gag)
        G. Larynx
            1. Extrinsic muscles of the larynx
               (laryngeal elevation noted on palapation during swallows)
            2. Intrinsic larynx
               (vocal fold mucosa, vocal fold and arytenoid positions, and potential ability to
               protect the airway (vocal cord closure, throat clearing, and cough)
    VI. Speech and voice analysis
        A. Voice quality
        B. Resonance
        C. Articulation
        D. Respiratory support
    VII. Test swallow observations
        A. Time required to manage the oral phase
        B. Time required to initiate the pharyngeal stage
        C. Observable oral residue
        D. Cough, throat clearing, or changes in voice quality
        E. General environment observations
        F. Self-feeding/feeding observations
        G. Dietary/meal tray observations
   VIII. Selection of instrumental studies/examinations
        A. Videofluoroscopic
        B. Endoscopic (rigid and flexible fiberoptic)
        C. Ultrasound
        D. Other studies

Source: From Clinical Examination of Oropharyngeal Swallowing Function, Department of Veteran Affairs, 1B 141–86, Sept. 1991.

- *Infection:* Almost any microorganism (virus, bacteria, fungus, yeast) can affect the brain and spinal cord. Infections may enter the nervous system directly from a penetrating wound, spread from a local infection, or travel from another site by the bloodstream. Examples: meningitis, poliomyelitis, syphilis, acquired immuno-deficiency syndrome.

- *Disorders of body systems:* The brain and nerves depend on nutrients or closely controlled levels of acidity and constituents of the blood. Disorders of other body organs can lead to breakdown of a balance state for the body. Examples: diabetes mellitus, thyroid dysfunction, kidney failure, liver failure.

- *Poisoning:* Acute or chronic poisons can damage the brain and nervous system. Ex-

amples: drug or alcohol abuse, lead or mercury poisoning, arsenic, botulism.

- *Degenerative disorders:* Several disorders are characterized by gradual, progressive degeneration of part of the nervous system. The etiology of many degenerative disorders is unknown. Examples: amyotrophic lateral sclerosis (ALS), Alzheimer's disease.

- *Iatrogenic disorders:* Unfortunately, iatrogenic illnesses may contribute to a decline in self-feeding and swallowing and even mimic or mask a neurogenic disorder. For example, hospitalized patients may become deconditioned and as a result lose the functional abilities present prior to hospitalization. Polypharmacy or adverse drug reactions may influence behaviors observed during a clinical

Table 15–2. Anatomy and Physiology of Feeding and Swallowing Function

FEEDING
    Definition: voluntary placement of food in the mouth
    Structures: upper extremities, sensory input, oral cavity
    Function: part of the eating process, placing food in the mouth
    Cognitive: cognitive status impacts on self-feeding skills
    Manifestations: weight loss, nutritional compromise, feeding assistance required, time
       required for feeding
    Assessment: clinical observation
ORAL PREPARATORY (included in the horizontal subsystem)
    Definition: voluntary mastication and preparation of food into a bolus
    Structures:
      Bone/cartiledge: hard palate (maxilla and palatine bone), mandible, 32 teeth
      Muscles: Muscles of lips (orbicularisaris, risorius)
        Cheek muscles (buccinator)
        Mandibular muscles
          Open mouth
          Lateral pterygoid
          Geniohyoid
          Anterior belly of digastric
          Upward force for biting and chewing
          Masseter
          Medial pterygoid
          Temporalis
        Tongue muscles (tip, blade, dorsum, root)
          Intrinsic lingual muscles
          Superior longitudinal
            Shortens tongue and curls tip and sides up
          Inferior Longitudinal
            Shortens tongue and curls tip and sides down
            Vertical—flattens tongue
            Transverse—narrows and extends tongue
          Extrinsic lingual muscles
          Genioglossus—pulls tongue into a trough
          Styloglossus—draws tongue posteriorly and superiorly
          Hyoglossus (paired)—pulls down side of dorsum
          Palataloglossus (paired)—pulls side of tongue dorsum upward and lowers soft palate
        Soft palate muscles
          Velopharyngeal closure—tensor palatine, levator palatani, palatoglossal
          Pull velum downward—palatopharyngeus, palatopharyngeus, muscularis uvlus
      Nerves: Oral sensation—V, VII (taste anterior ⅔),
      IX (taste posterior ⅓, touch, pain and temperature),
      X (general taste and sensation from the base of tongue)
      Motor—V, VII, XII, XI
      Glands: parotid, submaxilary, and sublingual saliva glands
      Cavities: oral cavity, nasal cavity
      Spaces: anterior sulcus, lateral sulcus
    Function: acceptance and containment of food in the oral cavity, mastication of food, and initial
      chemical breakdown of the material in the oral cavity.
    Cognitive: cognitive status impacts on voluntary mastication and compensatory strategies.
    Manifestation: anterior spillage, pocketing of bolus, impaired mastication, nasal reflux, posterior spillage
    Assessment: clinical observation, clinical examination, videofluoroscopy, ultrasound

Table 15–2. (*continued*)

ORAL PHASE (included in the horizontal subsystem)
  Definition: voluntary movement of the bolus from the tip of the tongue to the anterior tonsillar pillars
  Structures:
    Bone/cartiledge: (same as above)
    Muscles: (same as above)
    Nerves: (same as above)
    Cavities: oral cavity, nasal cavity
    Spaces: anterior sulcus, lateral sulcus
  Function: propels the cohesive bolus from the front of the oral cavity to the top of the pharynx, the tongue elevates and
    rolls posteriorially making sequential contact with the hard and soft palate.
    Generates a positive oropharyngeal pressure.
  Cognitive: cognitive status impacts upon voluntary movement of the bolus and compensatory strategies for disordered
    swallow
  Manifestations: delayed transition of bolus, posterior spillage, aspiration, nasal reflux
  Assessment: clinical observation, clinical examination, videofluoroscopic studies, ultrasound
PHARYNGEAL PHASE (included in the vertical subsystem)
  Definition: reflexive passage of the bolus from the oral cavity into the upper esophagus
  Structures:
    Bone/cartilage: mandible, bony framework of the hard palate, hyoid, laryngeal cartilages (epiglottis, thyroid,
      arytenoid, cricoid), tracheal rings
    Muscles: suprahyoid muscles
      extrinsic laryngeal elevators
        digastric, geniohyoid, hyoglossus, mylohyoid
      extrinsic movement downward
        digastric, stylohyoid
        aryepiglottic, thyroepiglottic muscles
      extrinsic laryngeal muscles
        sternothyroid, thyrohyoid, sternohyoid, omohyoid
      intrinsic laryngeal muscles
        thyroidarytenoids—vocal fold adduction
        cricothyroids—increase vocal fold length and tension
        lateral cricoarytenoids—movement of arytenoid
        posterior cricoarytenoids—abduct the vocal folds
        transverse arytenoid—arytenoid approximation
        oblique arytenoid—adduct vocal folds
      peristaltic action
        superior, middle, and inferior constrictor muscles
        palatopharyngeus, stylopharyngus, salpingopharyngus
    Nerves: V, VII, X, XI, XII
    Cavities: nasal cavity, oral cavity, pharynx
    Spaces: valleculae, laryngeal vestibule, pyriform sinuses
  Function: The tongue makes sequential contact with the posterior wall of the pharynx. Concurrently the pharyngeal
    constrictors contract and intrinsic laryngeal muscles approximate the arytenoid and epiglottis, close the false cords,
    and adduct the true cords assisting in prevention of aspiration. The hyolaryngeal complex is lifted upward and for-
    ward and assists in deviating the bolus laterally around the airway and opening the upper esophageal sphincter.
    Generates a negative hypopharyngeal suction pump.
  Cognitive: normal swallow—reflexive
    disordered swallow—cognitive abilities may assist in compensatory strategies
  Manifestations: nasal regurgitation, aspiration, voice quality
  Assessment: clinical examination, videofluoroscopic studies, endoscopic and fiberoptic examinations, manometry,
    electromyographic studies

Table 15–2. (*continued*)

UPPER ESOPHAGEAL PHASE (included in vertical subsystem)
  Definition: reflexive passage of the bolus through the upper esophageal sphincter down the esophagus
  Structures:
    Muscles: cricopharyngeus
    Nerves: X
    Cavities: None
  Functional: The transition of the bolus between the pharynx and esophagus. This transition involves three forces: the
    momentum of the bolus from lingual and pharyngeal compression, peristaltic action, and gravity.
  Cognitive: normal swallow—reflexive
    disordered swallow—cognitive abilities may assist with compensatory strategies
  Manifestations: food sticking, aspiration, heartburn
  Assessment: clinical history, radiographic studies, endoscopic studies, manometry

examination. Another iatrogenic problem is that of unnecessary diagnostic and therapeutic procedures, which have associated costs and morbidity. Diagnostic tests, including those used to identify dysphagia, should only be performed when the results will change the way the patient is to be treated.

Lesion Sites in Neurogenic Dysphagia

The cause, course, and severity of the dysphagia may vary based on the site and extent of the neurological lesion. Classification of communication disorders (e.g., aphasia, apraxia, dysarthria) based on the neuroanatomic area or system involved has been a common scientific and clinical approach to assessment and intervention for speech–language pathologists. Researchers and clinicians also search for common symptoms of swallowing disorders based on the site of lesion. Lesions that interrupt or disrupt the movement patterns of striated muscles of the oral pharyngeal mechanism may cause oropharyngeal dysphagia.[3] For example, lesions in the brain stem or cranial nerves V, VII, IX, X or XII can interfere with the swallowing process.[3] However, localization as a means of classifying neurogenic communication and swallowing disorders breaks down when the injury is diffuse (e.g., traumatic brain injury) or when there are mixed disorders (e.g., an individual with Parkinson's disease who suffers a stroke).[5,7] In addition, the localization of a particular lesion does not necessarily mean that a particular swallowing disorder will be present.[5] For example, a lesion to the vagus nerve (CN X) may cause reduced vocal cord mobility and as a result interfere with adequate airway protection before or after a swallow; yet an individual with a lesion of CN X (unilateral or bilateral) may not present with symptoms of dysphagia due the ability of the system to adapt with adequate hy-

olaryngeal elevation and epiglottic inversion to protect the airway during oral intake. Examples of peripheral nerve disorders, brainstem, and cortical lesions and the potential impact on disruption in swallowing are described below.

Acquired Peripheral Disorders

Cranial nerves V, VII, IX, X, XI, and XII are involved in the swallowing process, and a pathology of one or more nerves may result in dysphagia.[7] Damage to the facial nerve (CN VII) may significantly interfere with maintenance of the bolus in the oral cavity while paralysis of one vocal cord (CN X) may impact on the ability of the individual to protect the airway before or after the swallow. Impairment to CN VII, CN IX, and CN X may result in the inability to maintain oral intake or to expel material from the laryngeal vestibule.[8] Damage to the last four cranial nerves (IX, X, XI, and XII) may result in combinations of symptoms including disorders of resonance and voice quality, dysphagia, and aspiration.[7] Causes of acquired peripheral nerve disorders may vary. For example, cerebellopontine angle tumors may cause compression of cranial nerves V and VII while acoustic neuromas may impact upon CNS VII and VIII.[7]

Brainstem

A swallowing disorder associated with brainstem involvement is the failure of hyoid-laryngeal elevation or cricopharyngeus muscle relaxation during swallowing with pharyngeal retention or residue after the swallow and, in some cases, nasal regurgitation.[7,9] Brainstem involvement may be associated with a variety of causes including: bulbar palsy following vascular interruption, poliomyelitis, trauma, tumors, amyotrophic lateral sclerosis, or syringobulbia.[1,7] The brainstem is densely packed with important tracts and nuclei including the corticobulbar tracts, the nuclei solitarii, the nuclei ambigui in the medulla and the adjacent medullary centers.[1,10] Unilateral vascular cerebral lesions often spare the brainstem,[7] while brainstem strokes may be extremely discrete and oropharyngeal dysphagia may be the only symptom.[1,11]

Cortical Lesions

The clinical effects of cortical lesions may be grouped into categories of physical or neurological signs and syndromes of the brain.[12] For example, a patient with a right frontal lobe lesion may present with symptoms of left hemiplegia, elevation of mood, loss of initiative, difficulty in adaptation, and, in some cases, instinctive grasp reflex, while a patient with a left occipital lobe lesion may present with a right homonymous hemianopsia, alexia, color-naming deficits, and visual object agnosia.[12] The higher cortical symptoms or signs may interfere with the ability of the individual to purchase or select foods, cook, self-feed or significantly impact the ability to compensate for a swallowing disorder. Unilateral cortical lesions that result in apraxia or agnosia may interfere with the voluntary movements or series of movements associated with self-feeding. Left hemisphere strokes appear to impact function of the oral phase of the swallow while right hemisphere strokes tend to compromise pharyngeal phase function.[1,13,14] Unilateral hemispheric lesions may spare swallowing because there is bilateral representation in the brainstem. Consequently, bilateral lesions often have more severe effects.[1,7,8] Bilateral corticobulbar lesions may result in dysphagia, dysarthria, drooling, impaired gag reflex, reduced emotional threshold, and frontal release signs.[8] Lacunar infarcts, as in multi-infarct dementia, may potentially influence cognitive communication behaviors and influence the individual's ability to learn new information to compensate for a swallowing problem or learn self-feed strategies.[8]

Symptoms and Clinical Signs

The speech–language pathologist may not always have an accurate history that identifies the cause or site of lesion and may be the first person to identify the possibility of a dysphagia with a neurological etiology. On the other hand, the symptoms or physical signs observed or reported by the clinician after an initial assessment are often used to confirm the cause or site of lesions. Common symptoms of dysphagia include: coughing or frequent throat clearing during meals, "wet" hoarse voice quality after oral intake, change in respiratory patterns during eating, drooling, refusal to accept foods or fluids, or slow chewing or swallowing patterns requiring significant amounts of time to consume meals.[15] The common symptoms associated with dysphagia may assist the clinician in the identification of a specific stage of swallowing disorder or cause of the disorder.[16] For example, drooling or oral spillage of food and liquids may direct the clinician to further examine the facial nerve (CN VII) and its impact on the oral preparatory or oral phase of the swallow or the ability of the patient to obtain and maintain labial closure.[7] These symptoms and physical signs may be recognized as highly characteristic of a particular syndrome or disease process, such as Bell's palsy, and narrow the range of possible etiologic factors.

However, different disease processes may cause identical symptoms, which is understandable in view of the fact that the same parts of the nervous system may be affected by several diseases.[1,5] For example, a breathy voice may focus the assessment on the larynx and identify the reason for a cough after all trials of oral intake. While changes in vocal quality may indicate a peripheral nerve lesion, altered voice quality can occur in carcinoma, infection such as herpes zoster, trauma to the vocal folds or larynx, and vocal fold edema associated with gastroesophageal reflux disease or chronic coughing.[7] Additional symptoms such as odynophagia (pain on swallowing) may reflect a need for referrals or additional medical assessment.[8]

A general neurological examination may assist the speech–language pathologist or health care professional with clinical data collection for individuals with suspected neurogenic swallowing disorders. The neurological examination begins with an observation of the patient while the history is obtained and includes informal or formal assessment of cortical functions (mental status and language skills), cranial nerves, motor function, reflex function, sensory function, gait and stance, and nutritional or trophic changes.[17,18]

Observations of Higher Cortical Functions

Although there is a tendency to assess and treat oropharyngeal dysphagia in isolation, it is imperative to also assess the cognitive and communication behaviors that will impact on self-feeding and intervention. Mental status changes are frequently identified in patients with neurological disease(s), and a general understanding of them is helpful for differential diagnosis and selection of appropriate treatment or management strategies for dysphagia.[17,18,19] An accurate assessment of the human communication process is important whether the problem presents as an impairment of swallowing or as other communication disorders of voice, motor speech, fluency, language, or cognition.[18] Observation or assessment of higher cortical functions will identify whether or not a communication or cognitive disorder exists, identify effective communication modalities for teaching compensatory strategies, and determine the potential of the individual to learn new information.[18,19] The assessment of higher cortical functions will assist the speech–language pathologist in differentiating those patients who will benefit from behavioral treatment strategies from those who will require direct feeding management.[18,19]

Many examples of cognitive and communication functions may be obtained during the patient interview or medical chart review and, when necessary, confirmed during formal assessments.[17,18] General behaviors (appearance, cooperation, posture), mood (anxiety, apathy, irritability, depression), orientation and insight into current medical problems, and cognitive skills (attention, speed of response, concentration, short-term memory) should all be assessed.[17] An assessment of cognitive processes usually includes observations of attention and vigilance, auditory memory, visual perception, visual memory, and ideation.[19] Impairments of attention and vigilance are often seen in patients with diffuse brain dysfunction.[16] Traumatic brain injury, multiple infarcts, cerebral atrophy, postsurgical states, and systemic infections are included in this group.[18] Aphasia, dysarthria, apraxia, and agnosia are communication disorders that present with symptoms associated with specific neurological disorders. Aphasia is used to refer to language disturbances caused by brain lesions but not those caused by cognitive deficits, disturbances of sensory organs, or paralysis of the muscles essential for speech.[5,12] Lesions of certain areas of the dominant cerebral hemisphere are prone to be associated with aphasia. Aphasia affects all elements of the function of language, auditory input, verbal output, reading, writing, and gesturing.[5,17] Dysarthria is due to paresis of the muscles used in speaking while apraxia is the inability to carry out, on request, a complex or skilled movement not related to a paralysis, ataxia, sensory change, or confusion.[17] Auditory and visual memory assessments define the limits of the

patient's memory and assist in the development of a treatment plan and the need for appropriate physical prompts or cues.[17] Nonlanguage observations of visual-motor perception are also important in the assessment of feeding and swallowing disorders and will help to identify performance breakdowns in nonverbal cognitive functions.[19] Agnosia refers to the failure to recognize familiar objects perceived by the senses.[17] Agnosias are usually considered to be caused by disturbances in the association function of the cerebral cortex.[17] After the major input and output modalities of attention, language, construction, and memory are assessed, the clinician should determine the patient's ability to manipulate these modalities for abstract thinking and problem-solving abilities.[19]

The presence of coexisting communication and swallowing disorders is common.[20,21] For example, functions of the larynx affect not only the pharyngeal stage of the swallow, but also the associated functions of phonation and respiration. Neurogenic oropharyngeal dysphagia is rarely an isolated finding and may be one symptom with a variety of coexisting communication disorders.[20,21] Coexisting communication disorders will also influence the type, frequency, amount, or timing of intervention recommended.[1,19] For example, an individual with a moderate to severe cognitive-communication decline will not be able to remember safe swallow strategies independently and will require direct assistance for cues or prompts during mealtimes. Decreased alertness and cognitive function impact on the individual's ability to self-feed. Patients with poor judgment, sensory deficits, or poor motor coordination from brain damage may not possess the vigilance and physical ability to handle their food intake safely.[15]

Motor Movements and Tone

The brain is the central regulating mechanism concerned with initiating and integrating muscle movements.[17] Motor disturbances include weakness and paralysis, which may result from lesions of the voluntary pathways or the muscles themselves. Lower motor neuron lesions interrupt the final pathway through which neural impulses reach the muscle, and as a result, signs or symptoms include flaccid paralysis of the involved muscles or muscle atrophy.[8,17,19] Diseases that affect the lower motoneurons of the brainstem or their peripheral connections to the muscles involved in swallowing may render the muscles either weak or paretic.[8] The upper motor neuron lesions interfere with the impulses from the motor area of the cerebrum and signs or symptoms include spastic paralysis or paresis of the involved muscle with little or no muscle atrophy.[17,19] The musculature for swallowing may be weak and uncoordinated.[8] The pharyngeal phase of the swallow may be retained even though it may be difficult to stimulate or initiate voluntary movements.[8] Normal muscle tone may be increased (hyperactive) or decreased (hypotonia).[17] In spasticity, there is an increased resistance to sudden passive movements, and after the initial resistance there may be muscle relaxation. In rigidity, there is increased resistance to passive motion and steady contraction of the muscles. Hypotonic muscles feel soft and flabby and offer less than normal resistance to passive movements. Signs of disturbed tone and increased movement may be observed in patients with tremors, spasms, and movement disorders (choreiform, athetoid, dystonia, tics, myoclonus, hemiballism). Lesions of the cerebellum or its pathways may interfere with a coordinated integrated action between muscle groups. Symptoms or signs of cerebellar disorders include: ataxia, adiadochokinesia, dysarthria, dysmetria, and nystagmus.[17]

From a functional standpoint, neurogenic causes of swallowing disorders (i.e., upper motoneuron, lower motoneuron) may produce different patterns in the speed and duration of swallow and as a result difficulty with a variety of food and liquid consistencies.[8,22] In general, patients with lower motoneuron damage or dysphagia paralytica should avoid foods that fall apart or stick as they pass through the pharynx.[8] Since many patients with lower motor neuron involvement retain cognitive functions and some voluntary control (upper motoneuron) control of the muscles of swallowing, behavioral intervention may be offered to assist in airway protection.[8] Surgical options such as enteral tube feedings or tracheostomy tubes may need to be considered for those patients with severe dysphagia and poor airway protection or for those with progressive diseases requiring preventative intervention.

Patients with pseudobulbar dysphagia (upper motorneuron) dysphagia often complain of difficulty swallowing liquids.[8] This is compatible for a swallowing mechanism with disruptions in timing and delayed initiation of the pharyngeal stage of the swallow.[8] Semisolid foods and thickened liquids appear to assist in the prevention of aspiration in patients with pseudobulbar dysphagia.[23] Patients with pseudobulbar palsy are at risk for impairments in cognitive-communication and, as a result, need a structured environment with partial or total feeding assistance.[8]

Variations of lower motoneuron and upper motoneuron characteristics are seen in neurological diseases such as myasthenia gravis, amyotrophic lateral sclerosis (ALS), Parkinson's disease, and Huntington's chorea. Patients with myasthenia gravis experience muscle fatigue after repeated exercise and, as a result, patients may masticate and swallow well at the beginning of a meal and then deteriorate at its end.[8,24] ALS is a progressive disease of the upper and lower motor neurons of unknown cause. Patients with bulbar involvement show combined symptoms of flaccid and spastic muscle movements.[8] The muscles of mastication develop fatigue, the facial muscles become weak and drooling is common, lingual muscles are weakened with muscle fasciculations and eventually become paralyzed, and vocal cord abduction and adduction are impaired.[8] Patients with ALS confined to muscles supplied by the spinal cord exhibit dysphagia related to loss of respiratory muscle support.[8] Patients with Huntington's chorea exhibit feeding and swallowing disorders related to choreatic movements.[8] Patients first lose the ability to self-feed and symptoms of dysphagia emerge as involuntary movements become more frequent and uncontrollable.[8] Patients with Parkinson's disease exhibit a variation of pseudobulbar symptoms, and when rigidity is the prominent feature of the muscle movements, dysphagia appears as a symptom.[8]

Sensation

Sensation may be divided into three groups: superficial, deep, and combined.[17] Superficial sensation is concerned with touch, pain, and temperature and is commonly assessed by the speech–language pathologist. Patients with reduced sensation in the oral cavity, pharynx, or larynx are often not aware of residue in the valleculae, laryngeal vestibule, or pyriform sinuses after an initial swallow and make no effort to clear the residue. Deep sensation is concerned with muscle and joint position, muscle pain, and vibration sense. Both superficial and deep sensory mechanisms are involved in the ability to recognize familiar objects and localize stimuli. Pain is subjective and may be described as local or diffuse, constant or intermittent, sharp, dull, burning, or shooting. Parasthesia consists of abnormal sensations such as numbness or tingling. Individuals with pain on swallowing or odynophagia require additional medical assessment or treatment. Types of sensation identified during a clinical examination may assist in the identification of characteristics common to localization or cause.

The speech–language pathologist must remember that eating (feeding and swallowing) is a holistic sensory process involving a combination of sensory cranial nerve fibers. Prior to food entering the mouth, the optic nerves (CN II) transmit visual images received by the retina, the oculomotor nerves (CN III) change the pupil size and adjust the lens shape for near vision, and the olfactory nerve fibers (CN I) are activated by odors and stimulate receptors in the nose. When the food enters the mouth the facial (CN VII) and glossopharyngeal (CN IX) nerves transmit information from the face and mouth about taste, while the trigeminal nerves transmit information about sensations in the head and face during chewing, and the vagus nerves (CN X) convey information from the larynx and trachea. The pharyngeal phase of the swallow is initiated by sensory impulses transmitted as a result of stimulation to the receptors on the posterior faucial pillars, tonsils, soft palate, base of tongue, and posterior pharyngeal wall.[25] These sensory impulse reach the medulla primarily through CNS VII, IX, and X.[25]

Reflexes

Reflexes are innate stimulus-response mechanisms that are important in the diagnosis and localization of neurologic lesions. Reflexes may be classified according to the level of their central representation (i.e., spinal, bulbar, midbrain, cerebellar) or into one of the following four groups: superficial (skin and mucous membrane) reflexes, deep reflexes, visceral (organic) reflexes, and pathologic (abnormal) reflexes.[17] Superficial reflexes commonly assessed by a speech–language pathologist are the pharyngeal (or gag) reflex and the uvular (or palatal) reflex. Retching or gagging when the pharynx is irritated is absent in lesions of the ninth or tenth cranial nerves or their nuclei. The ninth and tenth cranial nerves also play an important role in the raising of the uvula in phonation or sensation of the mucous membranes. The gag reflex is diminished or absent in patients with lower motor neuron lesions and hyperactive in patients with upper motor lesions.[8] The maxillary (jaw jerk) reflex is an example of a deep reflex that is manifested by a sudden closure of the jaw on striking the middle of the chin when the mouth is slightly open. The blink reflex, which occurs when there is an unexpected approach of an object toward the eyes causes closure of the eyelid, is an example of a visceral reflex.[17] Pathological reflexes are found when there is separation of the lower motor neuron from the higher cerebral centers. Pathologic reflexes of the head include: Babinski's platysma sign, glabella reflex, snout reflex, and head retraction reflex.[17] Pathologic reflexes are present in patients with pseudobulbar palsy and generally absent in patients with bulbar palsy.[15]

Nutritional or Trophic Changes

Nutritional or trophic changes are symptoms associated with neurologic disorders. The signs or symptoms may appear in the skin, nails, subcutaneous tissue, muscles, bone, and joints. For example: mucosal inflammation in the oral cavity may be apparent in infections such as herpes zoster, candidiasis, reflux esophagitis, or as a result of radiation or chemotherapy. Neurogenic control, disuse of muscles, blood supply, nutritional elements (vitamins), lymph drainage, and endocrine activities are all factors that influence trophic changes.[17] Denervated tissue loses the vitality of normal tissues and muscles and inactivity or disuse atrophy following prolonged immobilization can impact on muscle fiber electrical response and cause bone atrophy. Adequate blood supply is essential to the nutrition and oxygenation of tissue and changes may be evident in the appearance of the skin and nails.[17] Food intake must be sufficient to prevent cachexia and general weight loss.[17] Avitaminoses cause specific trophic changes seen in beriberi and scurvy. They also cause glandular disturbances that impact on growth functions.[17]

The Course of the Neurologic Disorder

The time of the onset of the neurological disorder and the anticipated course of the disease will influence the potential for rehabilitation. Information about the disease course will guide decisions about the individual's potential for improvement with and without treatment and appropriate timing for implementation of an intervention. The course of the disease process may be classified as: acute (e.g., progressive improvement anticipated during spontaneous recovery following a head injury), chronic (e.g., stable condition with a plateau 8 months after a stroke), degenerative (e.g., progressive decline as with amyotrophic lateral sclerosis), or exacerbating (e.g., brief decline followed by remission as in multiple sclerosis).

Setting dysphagia treatment or management goals and objectives that are consistent with the prognosis of the neurological disorder is particularly important. For example, very different goals may be established for a patient with a stable neurological condition (i.e., left hemisphere stroke) than for an individual who is likely to experience progressive deterioration (i.e., Parkinson's disease). Potential for improved motor movement is often related to the pathophysiology of the disorder. Patients with amyotrophic lateral sclerosis may expect a progressive decline in speech and swallowing. Oral motor strengthening exercises for patients with myasthenia gravis are contraindicated because muscles fatigue and cannot recover.[8] Prognosis for recovery from a traumatic brain injury is an extremely complex issue.[16] Patients who have a specific focal brain lesion such as in a right hemisphere stroke are generally regarded as more apt to develop compensations during a rehabilitation program than those who have generalized diffuse impairments.[16] A complete cure or resolution of a swallowing disorder may be an unrealistic goal while maintenance of nutrition and hydration by assistance is often an appropriate one. In severely impaired or terminally ill populations, prevention of complications and comfort, rather than improvements in function, may be the focus of care.[19]

ACQUIRED NEUROGENIC DISORDERS: COMMON SYMPTOMS AND PHYSICAL SIGNS ASSOCIATED WITH FEEDING AND SWALLOWING DISORDERS

There is a tendency to attach a neurological diagnosis to symptoms of dysphagia. Yet, the current state of knowledge indicates that clinical and instrumental observations of symptoms and physical signs of dysphagia tend to overlap substantially among patients with neurological disorders.[1] At present, feeding and swallowing disorders and the patient's ability to adapt or compensate must be evaluated in the context of all features of an underlying neurologic cause or lesion and course.[1,17,19] The following outline will attempt to list frequently encountered neurological diseases and their course along with the common syndromes or signs associated with feeding and swallowing disorders. This outline is only a guide for the reader based on limited knowledge regarding neurogenic swallowing disorders and cognitive communication behaviors that will interfere with oral intake. The reader should never lose sight of the fact that each disease process may affect patients in different ways, and intervention must be individualized to meet patient needs.[8]

I. STROKE SYNDROMES/VASCULAR DISORDERS: Stroke syndromes are numerous and confusing based on upper or lower motor neuron involvement.[8] Brainstem strokes are more likely to result in oropharyngeal dysphagia than hemispheric strokes, even though hemisphere-specific strokes are much more common.[1,10,26] Hemorrhagic strokes may be more devastating than ischemic strokes and more likely to cause dysphagia although an embolic stroke involving the middle cerebral artery has been known to cause dysphagia.[1]

A. Left Hemisphere Stroke

CAUSE: hemorrhagic or ischemic stroke

LESION: left hemisphere

COURSE: presents abruptly and resolves gradually and spontaneous improvement may be observed within days to months after the stroke unless there are coexisting medical or neurological problems that complicate the recovery process[1]

COMMUNICATION: potential for impaired language (aphasia) or reduced speech intelligibility (dysarthria or apraxia)[8]

COGNITIVE: cognitive communication usually remains intact with the potential to learn new information.[8] In some cases, the patient may become overwhelmed and confused while attempting to eat with a left hand due to a right sided hemiparesis may be aphasic[27,28]

SELF-FEEDING: right hemiparesis may impair the ability to self-feed

SWALLOWING: pharyngeal phase of the swallow is often intact but breakdown may occur with the oral phase or voluntary involvement[1,8]

RESPIRATION: respiratory complications may be observed due to oropharyngeal swallowing disorders[1]

NUTRITION: nutritional decline may be observed secondary to functional skills, self-feeding ability, or neurogenic swallowing disorders

INTERVENTION: there is often potential to benefit from behavioral treatment[8,19]

B. Right Hemisphere Stroke

CAUSE: hemorrhagic or ischemic strokes

LESION: right hemisphere

COURSE: presents abruptly and resolves gradually; spontaneous improvement may be observed within days to months following the stroke unless there are coexisting medical or neurological problems that complicate the recovery process[1]

COMMUNICATION: potential for reduced speech intelligibility (dysarthria)[8]

COGNITIVE: potential for impaired right hemisphere cognitive processes including difficulty focusing attention and impulsivity, perceptual and temporal deficits, reduced visual memory skills, difficulty with problem solving, and poor judgment[27]

SELF-FEEDING: potential for praxis,[28] left hemiparesis, visual field cut, or neglect and impaired cognitive behaviors may interfere with motor sequences involved with self-feeding

SWALLOWING: pharyngeal phase may be impaired[1,10]

RESPIRATION: respiratory complication may be observed secondary to pharyngeal phase function and aspiration[1,10]

NUTRITION: nutritional decline may be observed secondary to functional skills, self-feeding ability, or neurogenic swallowing disorders

INTERVENTION: potential to benefit from structured behavioral treatment and management strategies

C. Bilateral Upper Motor Neuron Involvement (pseudobulbar palsy)

CAUSE: bilateral hemorrhagic or ischemic strokes

LESION: bilateral upper motoneuron involvement (right and left hemispheres)[8]

COURSE: an abrupt onset, and after the stroke or the acute phase some improvement may occur although total recovery is not expected.[8] In some cases there may be a stepwise deterioration and decline in functional skills[30]

COMMUNICATION: harsh or unintelligible speech (spastic dysarthria) and aphasia may be observed in some cases[8,15]

COGNITIVE: cognitive communication may be impaired interfering with the potential to learn new information; there may be confusion, disorientation, spatial/perceptual impairments reduced ability to make sound judgments, and lowered emotional threshold or lability may be present.[1,8,15] Some patients may be diagnosed with vascular dementia[30]

SELF-FEEDING: impaired cognitive-communication, perceptual skills, motivation, and upper extremity limitations may result in inability to sequence the motor act for self-feeding[8,30]

SWALLOWING: reduced speed and coordination of the oral and pharyngeal phases of the swallow with varying degrees of laryngeal vestibule penetration and aspiration and residue after the initial swallow are often exacerbated by cognitive impairments[8]

RESPIRATION: respiratory complications may be observed secondary to the swallow function and aspiration[1,10]

NUTRITION: nutritional decline may be observed secondary to functional status, need for partial or total feeding assistance, and supervision for safe oral intake[8]

INTERVENTION: may not benefit from individual treatment, but there is the potential need for ongoing management strategies (feeding assistance) to maintain nutrition and hydration status and to prevent a decline in general health status[8]

D. Brainstem Stroke

CAUSE: large or small vessel disease in the brainstem[1]

LESION: involvement of lower motor neurons, brainstem tracts, and nuclei involved in the control of swallowing: notably the nuclei tract solitarii, the nuclei ambigui in the medulla, and medullary swallowing centers[1]

COURSE: presents abruptly with spontaneous improvement over days to months unless coexisting neurological or medical complications are present[1]

COMMUNICATION: speech may be impaired (flaccid dysarthria, weak voice), language remains intact[8,15]

COGNITIVE: cognitive-communication skills often remain intact[8]

SELF-FEEDING: self-feeding skills often remain intact[8]

SWALLOWING: reduced hyoid laryngeal elevation may interfere with cricopharyngeal relaxation and result in pharyngeal residue[7,9]

RESPIRATION: the central respiratory mechanism may be affected and when swallow and cough are affected a tracheostomy may be placed to adequately control secretions or depending on severity or the lesion, some cases require mechanical ventilation[8,29]

NUTRITION: some cases may require alternate enteral tube feeding[8]

INTERVENTION: patients may benefit from behavioral treatment strategies and in severe cases surgical intervention may be an option[8]

II. DEGENERATIVE/PROGRESSIVE NEUROLOGICAL DISEASES

A. Probable Alzheimer's Disease

KEY CHARACTERISTICS: cortical dementia with steadily progressive worsening of memory and cognitive functions[30]

CAUSE: cerebral cortical neuronal degeneration[30]

LESION: cortical mantel atrophy most pronounced in the temporoparietal and anterior frontal regions while areas of the cortex subserving primary motor, somatosensory, and visual functions are relatively spared and subcortical structures do not become involved until late in clinical course.[30] (*Note:* there must be an absence of systemic or other brain diseases capable of producing a dementia syndrome to use the label of probable Alzheimer's disease)

COURSE: intellectual deterioration usually described in three stages Stage I (Early) with average duration of 1 to 3 years, Stage II (Mid) with an average range of duration from 2 to 10 years, and Stage III (Late) with an average duration of 8 to 12 years[30]

COMMUNICATION: anomia is observed in the early stages, with breakdown in content in the mid stage and at the end stage no functional communication is apparent. Motor speech may be normal in the early stages and with significant rigidity in the end stages[30]

COGNITIVE: impaired ability to learn new information or short-term memory disturbance is nearly always the feature that heralds the onset of the disease exacerbated by poor judgment, spatial and temporal disorientation, indifference, occasional irritability, and suspiciousness;[30] in the mid stage of the disease recent and remote recall are severely impaired, and finally in the terminal stage there is impairment of all intellectual capacities[30]

SELF-FEEDING: independent feeding is a significant problem in the mid stages of the disease with a eventual loss of ability to self-feed in the late stages of the disorder[1]

SWALLOWING: delays in the oral preparatory or oral transition phase of the swallow in the mid stages with pharyngeal stage involvement late in the course of the disease[30]

RESPIRATION: respiratory complications may be observed secondary to delays in the oral and pharyngeal phases of the swallow and potential risk to aspirate[1,10]

NUTRITION: risk for decline in the early stage due to loss in ability to complete independent activities of daily living (i.e., shopping, prepare meals) and particularly in the mid and late stages due to changes in self-feeding exacerbated by delays in the oral preparatory and oral stage of the swallow and cognitive functions to participate in the eating process[30,31]

INTERVENTION: there is no curative therapy for dementia of the Alzheimer's type;[30] burden is on the caregivers and encompasses management strategies to maintain nutrition and hydration and may include alternate enteral tube feeding for partial or total nutrition and hydration;[1,31] tranquilizers should be used with precaution as they often increase confusion and further impair cognitive and motor functions

B. Parkinson's Disease

KEY CHARACTERISTICS: complex motor system disturbance including bradykinesia, rigidity (cogwheel rigidity), tremor (pill rolling), masked facies, decreased and slowed (rigid) limb movements, micrographia and disturbances of gait (shuffling), posture (stooped with reduced stability), and equilibrium[1,30,32,33]

CAUSE: idiopathic or unknown etiology[1,30,32]

LESION: involving multiple brainstem and subcortical areas, especially the dopamine-producing neurons of the substantia nigra and midbrain[1,30]

COURSE: slow progressive degenerative disorder with mean duration of 8 years (range 1 to 30 years); certain medications may decrease the severity of the symptoms and assist with preventive decline in health status[8,30,32]

COMMUNICATION: hypokinetic dysarthria with reduced loudness and monopitch significantly interfering with speech production for the listener; speech may decline and eventually become inaudible; auditory comprehension remains intact until the late stages of the disease; progressive micrographia is an initial complaint[30,32]

COGNITIVE: over 55 % of Parkinson's patients may display symptoms of dementia and the occurrence of dementia in the older patient with more severe rigidity and hypokinesia suggests that dementia becomes more prevalent and severe as the disease advances[30,32]

SELF-FEEDING: decreased or slowed limb movements interfere with amount of time required and ability to self-feed[30]

SWALLOWING: approximately 50 to 95% present with dysphagia with varying combinations of oral preparatory delay, prominent oral transition phase abnormality, pharyngeal impairment, and esophageal disorders;[1,8,32,33] dysphagia is not an early or predominant symptom of Parkinson's disease;[1] patients are frequently not aware of their swallowing problems[32,33]

RESPIRATION: pneumonia related to recurrent aspiration is a leading cause of death in the late stages of the disease[1,30,32]

NUTRITION: Delays in self-feeding and swallowing may interfere with the amount or oral intake and place the patient at risk for nutritional decline

INTERVENTION: dopaminergic medications should be given to coincide with mealtimes;[8,32] although dopaminergic agonists may alleviate some limb movement disorders (resting tremor, slowed movements) they do not prevent the progression of Parkinson's disease;[1] feeding management and varying the amount and frequency of meals may be of benefit; in some cases if the ability to learn compensatory strategies is intact, treatment may be provided; eventually in the late stages of the disease alternate enteral nutrition is an option[32]

C. Progressive Supranuclear Palsy

KEY CHARACTERISTICS: extrapyramidal syndrome characterized by supranuclear gaze paresis (loss of volitional downward gaze), pseudobulbar palsy, axial/truncal rigidity, ataxic gait and dementia[30,32]

CAUSE: neuropathologic alterations in the subthalamic nucleus, red nucleus, substantia nigra, pedanculopontine nucleus, superior colliculus, periaqueductal gray matter, globus pallidus, dentate nucleus of the cerebellum, and oculomotor, trochlear, and abductens nuclei[30,32]

LESION: known as one of the "Parkinson's plus" syndromes with multisystem atrophies or changes noted in the brainstem, basal ganglia, cerebellar nuclei, midbrain, and pontine tegmentum[1,32]

COURSE: onset initially may have symptoms similar to Parkinson's disease yet progression is more rapid with death in 5 to 10 years[32]

COMMUNICATION: dysarthria (hyperkinetic or spastic-ataxic features) with eventual mutism[32]

COGNITIVE: intellectual deterioration may be mild until the mid to late phases of the illness[30]

SELF-FEEDING: decline in self-feeding observed as decline in upper extremity motor skills and cognitive status is identified

SWALLOWING: oral and pharyngeal dysfunctions are observed in the mid to late stages of the disease and are often more prominent and profound than in Parkinson's disease[1]

RESPIRATION: decline in respiration may be expected with decline in swallowing and potential risk for aspiration

NUTRITION: as with other progressive diseases a decline in self-feeding skills will directly impact on the amount of calories consumed and should diet modifications be required nutrition and hydration are at risk

INTERVENTION: preventative approaches with management strategies and at the end stages alternate enteral nutrition may be an option

D. Huntington's Disease

KEY CHARACTERISTICS: chorea, dystonia (involuntary movements), incoordination, changes in personality[1,32]

CAUSE: inherited autosomal dominant disease[1,32]

LESION: atrophy of striated bodies and cortical atrophy[32]

COURSE: slowly progressive disease with death occurring in 15 to 20 years from onset[32]

COMMUNICATION: involuntary movements interfere with speech production (hyperkinetic dysarthria) and simple assistive or augmentative communication may be of use as the disease progresses[32]

COGNITIVE: cognitive changes are observed early in the disease with reduced orientation, judgment, and concentration; patients may be easily distracted; reduced insight to the disorder may be evident, subcortical dementia may be described, and uncontrollable outbursts of temper may be observed[1,8,32]

SELF-FEEDING: problems in self-feeding and manipulation of utensils are observed early in the disease due to choreic movements, although patients may be able to continue self-feeding with finger foods;[8] as the frequency of choreic movements intensifies moderate to total feeding assistance is required and unpredictable movements may interfere significantly with the feeding process including significant delays in oral intake and anterior loss of foods[8,32]

SWALLOWING: choreiform disorder that may affect the coordination of swallowing; swallowing during the early stages is usually functional, and as the disease progresses dysphagia is noted secondary to unpredictable speed and timing of the swallowing; sudden movements during the oral transition or pharyngeal phases of the swallow compromise protection of the airway[8,32]

RESPIRATION: oropharyngeal dysphagia with uncontrolled airway protection may lead to terminal pulmonary complications[1,32,35]

NUTRITION: difficulty with oral intake exacerbated by excessive energy needs may result in reduced nutritional intake to meet the caloric needs of the patient[8]

INTERVENTION: dopamine antagonists (neuroleptics) may be used to control chorea in some cases;[1] patients may benefit from head and trunk positioning or restraints during oral intake to assist in maintaining postures; feeding assistance and management strategies may be required and feeders should allow the patient to take the food from the spoon rather than place the spoon in the patent's mouth; in some cases the patient may continue self-feeding with finger foods;[8] alternate enteral tube feeding is an option

E. Dystonia and Dyskinesia

KEY CHARACTERISTICS: uncontrollable focal muscle contraction[1]

CAUSE: spontaneous onset or precipitated by prolong use of dopamine antagonists (neuroleptics)[1]

LESION: subcortex or brainstem[1]

COURSE: variable depending on use of medications or elimination of medication side effects

COMMUNICATION: speech may be impaired and in some cases characteristics of hyperkinetic dysarthria may be present

COGNITIVE: usually intact; some cases may have a psychiatric history that was the reason for neuroleptic medications

SELF-FEEDING: usually intact unless there an overlapping cognitive component or the dystonic movements are in the upper extremity muscles

SWALLOWING: dystonias of the head and neck may interfere with compromised postures during swallowing or contractions and incoordination of muscles during swallowing[1]

RESPIRATION: usually not impaired; in some cases the coordination of respiration, phonation, and swallowing compromise the airway requiring a tracheostomy tube

NUTRITION: usually not a significant risk for decline

INTERVENTION: botulinum toxin may impair neuromuscular transmission in overactive muscles and improve function;[1] medication reviews to eliminate neuroleptic medications may be warranted; feeding management strategies may be utilized

F. Amyotrophic Lateral Sclerosis (ALS)

ALS is a progressive neurological disease of upper and lower motoneurons of unknown cause. Degeneration of motor units as a result of involvement of upper and lower motoneurons causes spastic and flaccid symptoms of cranial, spinal, and peripheral musculature.[1,8,32] The symptoms may be divided into one of two ALS syndromes based on whether the spinal nerves involving the extremities are initially impaired or the bulbar nerves involving the speech and swallowing are initially identified.[32]

1. ALS with bulbar features

KEY CHARACTERISTICS: ALS with clinical syndrome of bulbar features[1,32]

CAUSE: unknown etiology[1,32]

LESION: central and peripheral nervous system pathology with predominately involved lower motor neurons in the pons and medulla[1,32]

COURSE: rapidly progressive

COMMUNICATION: mixed dysarthria often requiring augmentative communication or assistance from a familiar listener to anticipate needs;[1,8,32] linguistic functioning is usually intact[29]

COGNITIVE: cognitive functioning is usually intact in the early stages but may develop cognitive decline as the disease progresses[8,32]

SELF-FEEDING: progressive decline in self-feeding is observed with the need for total feeding assistance at the end stages of the disease[8]

SWALLOWING: oropharyngeal dysphagia may be an early symptom, with fatigue during mastication, drooling, reduced lingual movement, reduced sensation in the pharynx, and reduced respiratory support and poor cough to protect the airway creating significant risks for aspiration during oral intake;[8,32] oral feeding will eventually become inefficient and unsafe as the disease progresses.[8,32]

RESPIRATION: progressive respiratory insufficiency (hypoventilation) and weakness of abdominal muscles or diaphragmatic paralysis result in progressive respiratory and speech deterioration and reduced ability for a productive cough;[8,29] oral, pharyngeal, and laryngeal dysfunction also interrupts the upper airway protection;[29] a tracheostoma or mechanical ventilation may be offered during the course of the disease;[8,29] repeated aspiration-related pulmonary infections and respiratory failure due to reduced diaphragmatic movements are the leading cause of mortality[29]

NUTRITION: nutritional decline may be expected without early intervention.[8]

INTERVENTION: intervention should be ongoing and focus upon early prevention of nutritional decline with careful monitoring of weight, nutritional status, and hydration; education may be offered at all stages of the disease with modification of food and fluids consistencies as needed; compensatory strategies may only be a temporary solution as the disease progresses; enteral tube feeding may be an option for partial or total nutrition and hydration[8,32]

2. ALS with upper motor neuron features

KEY CHARACTERISTICS: ALS with clinical syndrome of upper motor neuron symptoms (spinal nerves)[1,32]

CAUSE: unknown etiology[1,32]

LESION: upper motor neurons of the corticobulbar tracts are primarily involved[1]

COURSE: slow progressive decline[1]

COMMUNICATION: mixed dysarthria (spastic/flaccid)[32]

COGNITIVE: the person usually has good cognitive functioning during the early stages but may develop cognitive decline as the disease progresses;[32] lowered emotional threshold may be observed[1]

SELF-FEEDING: self-feeding may be impaired in the early to mid stages in the disease process

SWALLOWING: dysphagia is usually late in onset of the disease with coexisting loss of respiratory support[8]

RESPIRATION: there is reduced respiratory support late in the disease[8]

NUTRITION: a decline may be observed as independent skills in daily living decline

INTERVENTION: education and early management strategies to prevent decline in nutrition, hydration and health status[32]

III. IMMUNE-MEDIATED DISEASES

A. Multiple Sclerosis

KEY CHARACTERISTICS: loss of spinal and cortical input that often is manifested initally by loss of bladder control, gait abnormality, lower extremity weakness, and visual changes (optic neuritis)

CAUSE: immune-mediated attack that occurs for unclear reasons[1]

LESION: demyelinating disease of the white matter of the central nervous system that causes formation of plaques in the brain and spinal cord with multifocal central nervous system deficits[1,29,32]

COURSE: symptomatic relapses and remissions over days to weeks; general progressive decline over years[1]

COMMUNICATION: may affect speech (mixed dysarthria/spastic-ataxic)[29,32]

COGNITIVE: may affect cognitive functions[29,32]

SELF-FEEDING: often requires partial to moderate feeding assistance in the mid to late stages

SWALLOWING: dysphagia may be present when brainstem involved[1]

RESPIRATION: respiratory problems occur late in the disease process from plaque development in the cervical spine and as respiratory musculature is affected, respiratory failure may result[29]

NUTRITION: patients are at risk for nutritional decline based on ability to complete independent tasks of daily living and to self-feed

INTERVENTION: corticosteroids or beta-interferon are potential treatments;[1] education and preventative management should be offered throughout the disease process; feeding assistance and strategies are often needed; enteral tube feeding is an option at the end stages of the disease or if the eating process is not a pleasure[32]

B. Guillian-Barré Syndrome

KEY CHARACTERISTICS: rapid physical-motor deterioration[29]

CAUSE: immune-mediated demyelination[1]

LESION: peripheral and cranial nerves[1]

COURSE: acute onset and rapid deterioration of muscle function followed by spontaneous recovery[1,29]

COMMUNICATION: linguistic abilities are spared; speech is impaired in severe cases with respiratory impairment[29]

COGNITIVE: cognitive abilities are usually spared

SELF-FEEDING: initially self-feeding may be impaired

SWALLOWING: pharyngeal phase function may be impaired[1]

RESPIRATION: the disease may lead to impaired respiratory muscle function with acute respiratory failure in at least 25% of all cases;[1,29,35] the majority of cases who receive support may be weaned within weeks; however, some patients with axonal involvement do not recover respiratory function and require long-term ventilatory support[29]

NUTRITION: during the acute stage or in severe cases enteral tube feeding may be necessary[1]

INTERVENTION: treatment enhanced by use of plasmaphoresis or intravenous immunoglobulin and supportive medical care may be warranted[1]

IV. MISCELLANEOUS DISEASES

A. Myasthenia Gravis

KEY CHARACTERISTICS: muscle fatigue after exercise or exertion[8]

CAUSE: production of autoantibodies that bind and degrade acetylcholine receptors[1]

LESION: involves the striated musculature[1,8]

COURSE: fluctuation of weakness over hours and muscle fatigue brought about by sustained exertion[1]

COMMUNICATION: mild to severe decline in speech production (dysarthria) that may be fluctuating

COGNITION: no significant problem with cognitive-communication behaviors

SELF-FEEDING: patients maintain self-feeding skills

SWALLOWING: fatigue noted during the oral transition phase of the swallow[8]

RESPIRATION: no significant respiratory decline expected

NUTRITION: decline may be observed if fatigue interrupts adequate oral intake

INTERVENTION: anticholinesterase-producing medication may be coordinated with eating/meal times;[8] conservation of energy is recommended by monitor physical activity prior to oral intake[1,8]

POLIOMYELITIS AND SYSTEMIC INFECTIONS: Dysphagia may be a primary symptom of tetanus, herpes zoster may cause facial and in some cases laryngeal paralysis, botulism may cause a temporary paralysis of oral, pharyngeal, laryngeal, or respiratory musculature, and diptheria may impact on brainstem functioning.[1,8] Infections and peri-infections in herpes, diphtheria, and botulism that may cause dysphagia or dysphonia require acute/emergency medical attention.[8] Reversibility is possible with medical intervention.

V. GLOBAL NEUROLOGICAL DISORDERS

A. Traumatic Brain Injury

CAUSE: variable

LESION: minimal to diffuse cortical and brainstem involvement

COURSE: after the acute onset spontaneous recovery may be expected with variability based on the amount and severity of brain damage and coexisting medical complications

COMMUNICATION: coexisting communication disorders may be expected and vary widely based on amount and type of brain damage (dysarthria, apraxia, language, voice and cognitive disorders)

COGNITIVE: coexisting cognitive impairments may be present and may significantly interfere with intervention plans[1]

SELF-FEEDING: self-feeding skills are often impaired; the patient may require alternate enteral tube feeding during the recovery process

SWALLOWING: any traumatic injury to the brain, brainstem, or cranial nerves may produce oropharyngeal dysphagia with similar characteristics of post-stroke dysphagia[1]

RESPIRATION: trauma to the brainstem or spinal cord may cause restrictive lung disorders due to the impairment of respiratory muscles;[29] severing the cervical spinal cord above the fourth cervical vertebra renders respiratory musculature nonfunctional if the diaphragm becomes totally or partially paralyzed; cervical nerve damage below the fourth cervical vertebra spares the diaphragm, but other muscles of inspiration and expiration are impaired and as a result interfere with the ability to produce an effective cough[29]

NUTRITION: patients are at ongoing risk for nutritional decline based on cognitive, self-feeding, and swallowing abilities; alternate enteral nutrition may be a part of the nutrition program during acute or transitional phases

INTERVENTION: treatment and management strategies are varied and based on the individuals cognitive-communication skills and swallowing disorder; the rehabilitation process may be slow[1]

B. Tumors and Neoplasms

CAUSE: primary brain tumors including gliomas (intrinsic), meningiomas and neuromas (extrinsic), or chrodoma and nasopharyngeal carcinoma[1]

LESION: progressive invasion of brainstem tracts or compression of the brainstem or cranial nerves[1]

COURSE: course and prognosis dependent on lesion, location, response to medical treatment (surgery, radiation, and chemotherapy) and potential side affects of medical treatment[1]

COMMUNICATION: potential risks for dysarthria or voice disorders

COGNITIVE: potential risk for cognitive impairments

SELF-FEEDING: may remain intact based on lesion, location, and medical intervention

SWALLOWING: potential for odynophagia and oropharyngeal swallowing disorders based on lesion and medical treatments

RESPIRATION: may be impaired based on site of lesion, medical intervention, and ability to maintain a safe open airway; tracheostomy tubes or mechanical ventilation may be required for short intervals during medical management or for those with terminal disease processes

NUTRITION: parenteral or enteral tube feeding options may be needed based on the lesion and medical intervention process

INTERVENTION: may involve surgery, radiation therapy, or chemotherapy and as a result multifactorial education, treatments, and management programs may be of benefit based on lesion and prognosis for recovery[1]

ESTABLISHING THE GOALS OF DYSPHAGIA INTERVENTION

The overall goal of dysphagia intervention is to provide safe, efficient nutrition while preserving optimum quality of life for the individual. To accomplish this task the professional will need to address three major goals of dysphagia intervention:

Goal 1: To maintain or improve nutrition and hydration

Goal 2: To prevent or reduce the risk of aspiration

Goal 3: To maintain or restore highest level of functioning and maximize quality of life

With these three goals in mind the dysphagia specialist(s) can provide input for establishing the direction of the intervention (treatment or management) plan, set realistic patient-focused goals, outline the goals of prevention or rehabilitation, and assist the patient, family, surrogate, or guardian with

a benefit and burden analysis. Education for the patient, caregiver, and professional/nonprofessional staff is a constant and ongoing process. Because dysphagia intervention is multifactorial, a comprehensive approach may require a number of health care professionals to fully diagnose and treat the patient.[1,8,19,37,38]

Maintaining or Improving Nutrition and Hydration

There is no disease process or disorder that benefits from starvation. Starvation impacts on body protein and fat for energy and sets up the individual for a potential cycle of malnutrition and dehydration. Adequate nutrition is essential for good health at any age. The health care provider should be alert and assist in the early identification and prevention of a decline in nutrition and hydration and provide aggressive treatment for the malnourished patient. In many cases, the success of dysphagia intervention will be measured by weight gain, the efficiency of the feeding process, and the amount of calories consumed during a meal. The health care professional must also recognize those individuals who are too severely malnourished to benefit from intervention.

Parenteral and Enteral Feeding

Alternate nutrition devices (e.g., intravenous [IV], nasogastric [NG] tube, esophagostomy, percutaneous endoscopic gastrostomy [PEG], gastrostomy, jejunostomy) provide hydration and nutrition if patients with disordered swallowing are unable to eat orally without risk of medical complications.[39–41] Tables 15–3 and 15–4 provide the reader with a list of parenteral and enteral tube feeding definitions and types of enteral tubes. Provision of some or all nutrients by means other than the gastrointestinal tract is usually evaluated and monitored by the physician, dietitian, pharmacist, and nurse or nutritional support team. Central parenteral nutrition is delivered through a large diameter vein while peripheral nutrition is delivered through a peripheral vein, usually of the hand or forearm.[39–41] The speech–language pathologist may monitor such patients for potential for oral intake and initiate intervention for patients with rehabilitation potential. In addition, the speech–language pathologist may recommend parenteral nutrition for individuals unable to maintain adequate enteral (oral or tube feeding) nutrition.

Enteral nutrition is offered when the gut is functioning normally. Nutrition provided through

Table 15–3. Enteral and Parenteral Nutrition Options

ENTERAL NUTRITION
Nutrition provided via the gastrointestinal tract

  ENTERAL ORAL NUTRITION
  Enteral nutrition taken by mouth

  ENTERAL TUBE FEEDING
  Enteral nutrition provided through a tube or catheter that delivers nutrients distal to the oral cavity

  COMBINED ENTERAL NUTRITION
  Nutrition provided by mouth and tube feedings simultaneously.
    Example: Oral nutrition for food and tube feedings for liquids

PARENTERAL NUTRITION
Provision of some or all nutrients by means other than the gastrointestinal tract (usually intravenous)

  PERIPHERAL
  Parenteral nutrition delivered through a peripheral vein, usually the hand or forearm.

  CENTRAL
  Parenteral nutrition delivered through a large diameter vein, usually the superior vena cava via the subclavian or jugular vein.

COMBINED NUTRITIONAL APPROACHES

  ENTERAL NUTRITION
  Nutrition and hydration provided by mouth and tube feedings.
  Example: Food taken by oral intake and liquids supplied by tube feedings

  ENTERAL AND PARENTERAL NUTRITION
  Nutrition and hydration provided by enteral and parenteral routes.
  Example: Food taken by mouth and fluids provided via a peripheral vein.

  TRANSITIONAL FEEDING
  Progression from one mode of feeding to another while attempting to maintain or achieve estimated nutrient requirements.
    Example #1: Dysphagia individual one month post right cerebrovascular accident progressing from tube feedings to oral intake.
    Example #2: Dysphagic individual with a history of amyotrophic lateral sclerosis decreases amount of oral intake as enteral tube feeding is increased.

Table 15–4. Enteral Tube Feeding Options

Invasive, Nonsurgical Procedures

Name	Location	Time Considerations
Orogastric	mouth/esophagus	each feeding (individual)
Nasogastric	nose/stomach	less than 30 days
Nasojujunal	nose/jejunum	less than 30 days

Surgical, Radiographic or Endoscopic Procedures

Name	Location	Time Consideration
Pharyngostomy	pharyngeal stoma/stomach	greater than 30 days
Esophagostomy	esophageal stoma/stomach	greater than 30 days
Gastrostomy (PEG, PEJ)	stomach stoma/stomach	greater than 30 days
Jejunostomy (PEJ)	jejunum stoma/stomach	greater than 30 days

Additional issues include:

speed of delivery to the gut
type and amount of formula
amount of hydration needed
comfort to individual

a tube or catheter distal to the oral cavity is referred to as enteral tube feeding.[39,40] Enteral tube feeding options are based on the area of entry to the system (mouth, nose, esophagus, gut) and where the tube delivers the formula and fluids is usually based on the risk of gastric reflux and lower esophageal function (stomach, jejunum). Additional variables include: life expectancy, surgical candidacy, and projected length of tube feeding required. The dietitian recommends appropriate formula and hydration needs of the patient and determines appropriate delivery (bolus, continuous drip or gravity drip), frequency, time, and amount of feedings. Enteral tube feeding variables include route of feeding, time of feeding, rate of feeding, type of formula, care setting, and prevention of complications. The speech–language pathologist assists with the dysphagia evaluation, determines the prognosis for oral intake, and, when appropriate, provides behavioral treatment.

Transitional or Combined Feeding

Transitional feeding is the progression from one mode of feeding to another, while attempting to maintain or achieve estimated nutrient requirements. Transitional feeding may be provided during dysphagia rehabilitation from enteral tube feeding to oral intake or during progressive decline in swallowing from oral intake to enteral tube feeding. The dietitian is responsible for monitoring the dietary intake of the patient during each stage of transitional feeding while the speech–language pathologist provides behavioral treatment or teaches management strategies to caregivers.

Trial, Withdrawal, or Refuse Feeding

The patient, surrogate health care provider, or guardian has the option to refuse alternate feedings, withdrawal alternate feedings, or agree to a trial period of parenteral or enteral tube feedings. Each option should be carefully reviewed with the individual and the decision may be reversed at any time. Trial parenteral or enteral tube feeding refers to a preset time of offering intervention to observe for changes in overall nutritional and health status of the individual while withdrawal refers to removal of alternate tube feedings. Both professional and nonprofessional caregivers should be counseled regarding the prognosis for improvement or decline and assist in monitoring the status of the individual with dysphagia. When the individual elects not to accept the recommendation for parenteral or enteral tube feeding, the multidiscipli-

nary or interdisciplinary team may choose to combine recommendations for the safest oral nutrition consistency and diet.

Preventing or Reducing the Risk of Aspiration

Aspiration is a generic term that indicates the entry of material into the airway below the level of the true vocal folds.[42] Entry of material into the laryngeal vestibule but not below the true vocal folds is not considered aspiration. To reduce the risk of aspiration, it is important to identify the structural or functional etiology defined during the assessment.[16]

Aspiration may occur for variety of reasons including: reduced tongue control of the bolus during chewing or during the oral transport of the bolus; delayed or absent initiation of the pharyngeal phase of the swallow; reduced pharyngeal peristalsis; unilateral or bilateral pharyngeal dysfunction; incomplete laryngeal vestibule or glottic closure; reduced speed or maintenance of laryngeal elevation; and cricopharyngeal dysfunction.[16,27] Aspiration may occur from reflux from the gut or esophagus after the swallow has occurred.

It is also important to assess the individual's ability to protect the airway from aspiration and observe response to aspirated material.[16] These may include reflex responses, voluntary adaptation, or automatic compensation.[16,42,43] A gag and a cough are reflexes that protect the entrance of the airway from foreign material or aspiration.[42] Foreign material may penetrate the laryngeal vestibule or trachea, but the patient's cough may be productive and material is expectorated. Silent aspiration is a term used to describe aspiration without a response or an absent cough reflex. Choking implies obstruction of the airway.

Strategies to protect the airway from aspiration may be subdivided into three major categories: medical/surgical intervention, behavioral or indirect intervention, and direct intervention. Medical, surgical, or dental options are approaches provided by the physician, psychiatrist, surgeon, or dentist. Medical/surgical or dental intervention usually prepares the patient for safe nutrition. Referral for medical intervention may be the initial step of swallowing treatment, or it may be the last stage after behavioral/indirect oral management strategies fail. Behavioral or indirect treatment options prepare the dysphagic patient for oral intake without food or with small controlled amounts of food and fluid.[42] Behavioral intervention may be provided by the speech–language pathologist, occupational therapist, physical therapist, or psychologist. Speech–language pathologists have knowledge of the anatomy and physiology of the vocal tract for speech and swallowing and are trained to provide behavioral treatment, which may complement or substitute surgical or medical treatment. Direct interventions are strategies selected for use during oral intake of food and fluids. Such options may be recommended by the clinician and implemented by the patient or caregiver. Table 15–5 provides a partial list of medical, surgical, and dental intervention and behavioral or indirect treatment options by structure or swallow function and Table 15–6 provides a list of common management or direct feeding strategies. Goals of intervention vary based on physical potential for change or the ability of the individual to learn new behaviors and to change.[19]

Table 15–5. Examples of Behavioral and Medical Treatment Options

	Behavioral	Medical Intervention

Feeding	Cognitive rehabilitation
	Visual (field, focus)
	Establish communication
	   hearing, auditory
	Upper extremity movement
	Positioning
	   trunk
	   neck
	   head
	Utensils/adaptive equipment
		Acute or secondary to a recent
		   trauma, illness
		Control of pain
		Psychiatric
		   depression
		   anorexia

Oral Preparatory
Oral Stage
	Oral motor
	   tone
	   strength
	   speed
	   range
	   isometrics/coordination
	   reflexes
	Sensory stimulation
		Dental/oral treatment
		   Xerostomia
		   Thrush/candida
		   Oral hygiene
		   Dentures
		Maxillary prosthesis
		   Plastic surgery
		   Surgical reconstruction
		   Palatal obturator
		Palatal prosthesis
		Tongue prosthesis

Laryngeal/Pharyngeal Stage	Sensory stimulation
	Glottic closure (adductor)
	Voice/pitch exercises
	Laryngeal elevation
	Patterning
	Coordinated respiration and swallowing patterns
	Positioning
	   Head/Neck
	      neck rotation
	      neck flexion
	   Trunk
	      up/down
		Pulmonary/respiratory
		Tracheostomy
		Vocal fold augmentation
		   gelfoam
		   teflon
		   silastic
		   bioglass
		Laryngeal suspension
		Supraglottic or glottic closure
		Tracheoesophageal diversion
		Laryngeal separation
		Laryngectomy

Cricopharyngeal/Esophageal Stage	Laryngeal elevation	Enteral tube feeding
		Parenteral nutrition
		Medication
		   Botox
		   reflux
		Dilation
		Myotomy
		Laryngeal suspension

Note: Behavioral intervention strategies include target behaviors, appropriate communication, ability to learn, and feedback for the individual.

Table 15–6. Examples of Direct Intervention or Management Options

Always initiated with education and counseling

Modify the environment
    Type of setting and amount of assistance available

Delivery of Meals and Snacks (frequency and time of day)

Positioning/Posture
    Feeding strategies (trunk, neck, head, extremities)
    Swallowing strategies (trunk, neck, head)

Equipment
    Sensory (hearing aid, glasses)
    Utensils or fingers
    Adaptive (spoons, plateguards)
    Prosthetic devices (dental prosthesis)

Bolus and Modifications (viscosity of food and liquid)
    Liquids: thin, thick, ultra thick
    Foods: puree, soft, regular, crunchy
    Strategies to modify consistencies (commercial, mixes, blenderized)
    High calorie boluses and supplements
    Cultural differences

Feeder
    Professional staff
    Spouse or family caregiver
    Volunteer

Feeding Assistance
    No assistance
    Partial assistance
    Moderate assistance
    Total assistance

Feeding Strategies
    Speed of feeding (time pressures and rate of feeding/swallowing)
    Alternate bolus consistencies (solid/liquid)
    Alternate bolus taste(s) and texture(s)
    Alternate temperature(s) (warm/cold)
    Multiple swallows per bolus
    Placement of the bolus in the mouth
    Cues/prompts
        verbal cues (auditory input)
        physical cues (touch)
        physical prompts
        Additional compensatory strategies (taught by clinician or
          therapist)

Oral status (pre- and post-oral intake)

Medication (pre- and post-oral intake)

Safety (how much and when/observations and equipment)

Defining Types of Intervention

Treatment

Treatment, remediation, or therapy implies that intervention is offered to patients who demonstrate on examination that they are capable of modifying impaired functions either by eliminating the disability, by improving the quality or efficiency of associated behaviors, or by developing compensations to minimize the effects of the impairments. *Patients must have demonstrated their potential for change on the basis of either their physical findings or learning potentials.*[19]

Management

Management refers to an intervention that is chronic, intractable, or has an undetermined prognosis. Patient and family education, recommendations for nursing care, and evaluative management (diagnostic therapy) are some of the contributions to support management.[19]

Combined Treatment and Management

Treatment and management may overlap or be intermittently introduced for some cases.[19] For example, an individual status post head trauma may not initially benefit from treatment strategies due to acute medical or cognitive conditions and management strategies may be employed. Once the individual's cognitive status improves the treatment program may be initiated.

No Intervention

The diagnosis of dysphagia or the desire for treatment does not automatically indicate that the individual is a candidate for intervention. If the dysphagic individual is not medically stable or has a negative attitude regarding treatment, postponement of treatment may be indicated. The person's financial considerations or living arrangements may necessitate management in lieu of treatment. If the potential for improvement is judged poor, the patient should be scheduled for a follow-up evaluation to assess any changes in medical, cognitive, or psychosocial status that mitigated treatment at the present time.

Maintaining or Restoring the Highest Possible Level of Functioning

Physical conditions, psychological factors, and socioeconomic issues can contribute, as well as interact with each other, to affect overall functional abilities to consume adequate oral intake. Small changes in the environment, social support, or function may make major differences in the quality of life. Regaining the ability to oppose the thumb to the other fingers after a stroke may enable the individual to become independent in feeding, or positioning the head may allow the individual to maintain oral intake.[44]

Patient-Focused Approach

The goals of intervention should be agreed on by patient and clinician. The patient and professional or family caregiver should participate in all aspects of the treatment and discharge planning and receive instruction regarding their role(s) in this implementation. Self-determination is defined as the right of the competent individual to freely make choices concerning medical care. Health care professionals have a duty to respect persons and their right to independent self-determination regarding the course of their lives and issues concerning the integrity of their bodies and minds.[44]

Common dilemmas such as determining patient or surrogate decision-making capacity or deciding whether to forgo life-sustaining nutritional treatment are a part of patient care.[44] Learning to identify and handle these issues while communicating with patient, family, and other involved health care providers are essential skills for the speech–language pathologist. Decisions about intensity of treatment such as enteral tube feeding should be made prospectively, especially in patients with progressive neurological diseases. Advanced directives or living wills are important tools in practice. If the desire for treatment from the patient or the patient's guardian is present, treatment may be initiated. If the patient or guardian is uninterested in receiving treatment at the present, a follow-up evaluation should be offered to reassess the motivation for treatment at a later time.

Dysphagic individuals commonly have multiple medical problems that are medical, functional, socioeconomic, cognitive, or emotional. Their complicated care often requires multidisciplinary or interdisciplinary interactions with a variety of health care professionals.[44] Teams may be preestablished within a medical setting or established on an as needed basis as determined by the medical center or patient needs. Speech–language pathologists, rehabilitation therapists (physical and occupational therapists), dietitians, dentists, respiratory therapists, psychologists, social workers, and pharmacists often join nurses and a variety of physician specialists (otolaryngologists, gastroenterologists, radiologists, neurologists, oncologists, geriatricians, or psychiatrists) in the care of the dysphagic individual. The role of the speech–language pathologist may vary considerably based on the setting and availability of other health care professionals.

Intervention for dysphagic individuals may occur in a variety of settings such as medical/surgical hospitals (acute care, intermediate care, chronic care, teaching hospital, specialized center), extended care facilities (long-term care or nursing homes), outpatient clinics, and home care. Regardless of the setting the goals should include: (1) providing a safe supportive environment, (2) preserving autonomy of the individual, (3) preventing medical and iatrogenic problems, and (4) maintaining or restoring the highest possible level of functioning to maximize quality of life.

Implementing and Monitoring the Plan

Short- and long-term functional treatment goals and specific objectives are determined from assessment and represent the framework for treatment. Quantitative and qualitative data should be maintained and reviewed periodically to determine appropriateness.

The success of treatment should be measured at the conclusion of each treatment paradigm to determine if there has been satisfactory improvement. If improvement has been satisfactory, the patient may be discharged from treatment and seen for follow-up examination. When improvement is unsatisfactory the clinician attempts to determine the reason for failure to improve and either initiates new therapy or refers the patient to other health care professionals for additional testing or treatment. Criteria for measurement of success and termination of treatment are determined during the initial assessment. Success criteria are based on knowledge of anatomy and potential change through treatment.[19]

When no measurable change is observed or the patient is dissatisfied with results, progress is considered unsatisfactory. If improvement is unsatisfactory, suspect that inappropriate treatment or instructions have been provided, the patient is unmotivated or unable to follow the treatment regimen, the patient and clinician goals are mismatched, or concomitant medical problems need to be resolved.

The patient should be periodically reassessed with standardized, valid, and reliable measures that will reflect changes that need to be made in the focus of the treatment or the decision to terminate treatment. The duration of the time between the assessments depends on a number of patient variables, including, but not limited to, the time after onset, motivation, complicating medical, social, or psychological illnesses, and frequency or quality of treatment. If the swallow and nutrition status are maintained/improved, the patient may be terminated from the program. If the swallow has regressed, a review treatment program is instituted and follow-up is performed on a more frequent basis until the target is maintained to both the clinician's and patient's satisfaction.

CASE ONE—AMYOTROPHIC LATERAL SCLEROSIS

A 42-year-old male with history of amyotrophic lateral sclerosis (ALS) was admitted to a nursing home.

The diagnosis of ALS was made three years prior to admission to the long-term care facility and the patient required assistance with all activities of daily living. He presented with mixed dysarthria and oropharyngeal dysphagia and required total feeding assistance due to limited upper extremity mobility. The patient had been issued an electric wheelchair operated by a joy stick switch. He had received individual speech treatment for one month before admission and a palatal lift had been made by a prosthodontist. The initial speech/communication assessment supported a diagnosis of mixed dysarthria with significantly reduced speech intelligibility requiring a skilled or familiar listener to interpret. A videofluoroscopic examination of swallow function was scheduled to assess the safety of a variety of food and liquid consistencies combined with strategies for protecting the airway. A language and cognitive communication assessment revealed auditory comprehension and visual input/reading to be within normal limits. The patient demonstrated good attention, concentration, and memory skills. He was able to participate in humor and demonstrated good pragmatic skills. During the interview, the patient indicated a preference for drinking liquids from a straw, noted that the palatal lift did not significantly change speech output or ease of swallowing and interfered with the "feeling in his mouth," and had an advanced directive requesting no enteral tube feedings or mechanical ventilation. A formal assessment revealed that the palatal lift was too short to significantly impact on velopharyngeal closure for speech or swallowing. The palate elevated during swallowing and there was no nasal reflux. He had significantly delayed oral preparatory and oral transition phases of the swallow for soft mechanical and pureed consistencies. Food coated the palatal lift and the patient was not able to clear the residue. As reported during the interview, he was able to drink thick and thin liquids from a straw with the head tilted slightly down. While drinking from a straw he had good maintenance of hyolaryngeal elevation during consecutive swallows. There was no aspiration during consecutive swallows. The patient was counseled and provided with educational materials regarding tube feeding options due to anticipated decline in ability to maintain oral intake. Intervention for communication incorporated assessment and selection of an augmentative communication device. Management for oral intake included modification of meals to include high-calorie thick and thin liquids offered by straw and total feeding assistance by staff and volunteers. Adaptive cups and straws were provided. The patient has been a resident in the nursing home for 7 years. During that time he has not had pneumonia and continues to receive oral intake with total feeding assistance. He has maintained an appropriate body weight with expected loss of muscle mass.

This clinical example offers several lessons and reinforces the importance of including the patient in the decision-making process. This example of a progressive neurological disease reinforces the need to assess and manage both communication and swallowing. Identification of functional verbal and nonverbal communication modalities was important in allowing the patient the freedom to participate in planning his medical care. The palatal lift was initially provided as a medical/dental intervention to modify resonance or speech output and possibly assist in swallowing; however, the prosthesis was too short to change the patient's speech (Figure 15–1), and palatal elevation was not a problem during the swallow. As a result, the prosthesis was not functional for the patient and only created discomfort. This emphasizes the need for careful selection of an intervention strategy. A second lesson from this case focuses on the ability of the patient to maintain laryngeal elevation while drinking thin liquids from a straw. Figure 15–2 is a still photograph from a fluoroscopic study of the patient drinking thin liquids from a straw and demonstrates good palatal and hyola-

ryngeal elevation during consecutive swallows. Without careful clinical and instrumental examination, a typical diet for a patient with neurogenic dysphagia would be pureed foods. Liquids would be thickened or eliminated altogether. In this case the patient was able to maintain nutrition via liquids. It is also important to note the the health care team honored the patient's wish not to have enteral tube feeding placed. Figure 15–3 is a photograph of the patient with a volunteer providing total feeding assistance.

Although he did not have individual speech treatment or tube feedings, a management program, with feeding assistance, was established in the nursing home to offer a preventative approach to reduce the risk of health or nutritional decline.

CASE TWO—PROBABLE ALZHEIMER'S DISEASE

A 67-year-old male was diagnosed with probable Alzheimer's disease five years prior to admission to a sub-acute unit. The patient was a non-functional communicator and relied on others for all input and communication needs. The patient needed total assistance with activities of daily living. The patient's spouse was an active caregiver and came to the facility four times a week to assist with daily care. The wife provided total feeding assistance for the

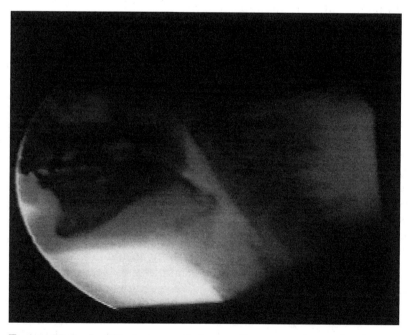

Figure 15–1. A still photograph from a fluoroscopic study of a patient with ALS. Note that the short palatal lift does not assist the patient with palatal elevation during speech production.

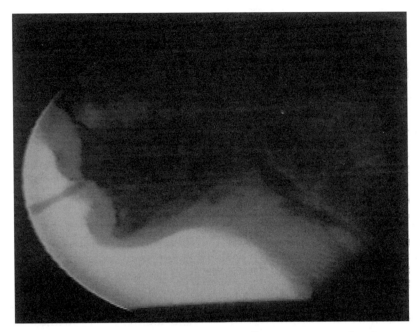

Figure 15–2. A still photograph from a fluoroscopic study of a patient with ALS. The patient is drinking thin liquids from a straw and functional palatal elevation and hyolaryngeal elevation occur during consecutive swallows.

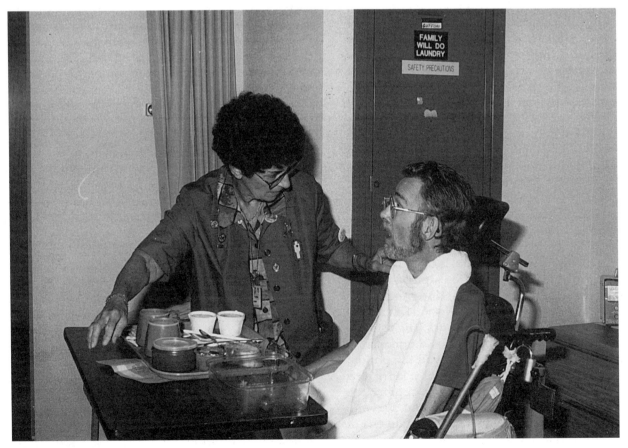

Figure 15–3. A volunteer provides feeding assistance as part of a management program for a patient with ALS.

noon and evening meals and snacks. The professional caregivers had indicated that the patient refused to accept foods offered from a spoon, particularly during evening meals. Clinical assessment supported a diagnosis of severe cognitive-communication decline. The patient was able to feed himself finger foods (e.g., crackers, cheese, chicken nuggets, dry cereal) with minimal cues or prompts from the examiner. He accepted cold and sweet boluses (e.g., ice cream and Italian ice) from a spoon during a clinical examination. Radiographic/videofluoroscopic assessment of the oral pharyngeal mechanism during swallowing revealed reduced rotary chew (munch pattern), multiple chews per bolus even when mastication was not required, and delayed initiation of the pharyngeal stage of the swallow. The bolus rested in the valleculae prior to the initiation of the swallow reflex. Once the swallow was initiated there was no aspiration and no residue after the swallow. A slow progressive weight loss had been documented by the staff and confirmed by the wife. The patient was considered at moderate nutritional risk. The patient had outlined an advanced directive prior to the decline in cognitive status and opted not to have enteral tube feedings. Intervention included modification of the meals and snacks to include a variety of finger foods, cold and sweet foods to be offered during feeding by a caregiver, increased calories during the morning and noon meal with fewer total calories needed for the evening meal, and training in feeding for the spouse and staff. The patient obtained his ideal body weight within a six-month interval and continued total oral intake for the remainder of his life, which was also an important social interaction for the spouse.

CASE THREE—MULTI-INFARCT DEMENTIA

A 69-year-old male with a diagnosis of multi-infarct dementia and a history of recurrent episodes of aspiration pneumonia over the past three years was referred for a dysphagia work-up. He had been a resident of a nursing home for two years. The communication assessment supported a diagnosis of moderate stage cognitive decline, and the patient was not able to retain new information or learn new tasks. The patient had many socially appropriate verbal and nonverbal behaviors (smiling, waving, laughing when others laughed, appropriate use of "please" and "thank you") that were endearing to the staff at the nursing home. He required assistance with all activities of daily living including partial feeding assistance. He was cooperative during feeding and accepted all food and fluids offered. The clinical observation of the swallow indicated delayed initiation of hyolaryngeal elevation. Videofluoroscopic examination of swallow function revealed good oral transition with delayed onset of the pharyngeal stage of the swallow. There was silent aspiration of thin liquids prior to initiation of the swallow with no cough reflex, and the cough to command was inconsistent and not productive to clear the airway. The patient did not maintain head positioning without physical prompts. The patient was at 90% of his ideal body weight, and laboratory values for nutrition were low, placing the patient at moderate nutritional risk. Management of the patient focused on liquid consistency modification, and extensive education for all staff involved. Due to current nutritional status and expected decline in both cognitive and swallowing function, tube feeding options were offered as a preventative approach to the overall care of the patient. The legal guardian elected to have a percutaneous endoscopic gastrostomy (PEG) placed. The patient was given a combined approach to enteral nutrition with oral intake for pureed and soft mechanical foods supplemented by tube feeding for fluids and nutrition as needed. Transition to increased tube feedings occurred as a decline in oral intake was observed. The patient's overall nutritional and hydration status improved and there was no skin breakdown or infections over a three-year interval. He expired from a cardiac arrest.

The two clinical examples demonstrate the importance of cautious clinical and instrumental examination of feeding and swallowing function even though both individuals presented with a diagnosis of dementia. Although individual treatment was not offered to either of these patients due to the lack of ability to learn new information, a program was established and incorporated the family and staff as important care providers in the management of the patients. These cases also emphasize the differences between a cortical dementia (probable Alzheimer's disease) and a multi-infarct dementia in regards to swallowing and feeding behaviors. The patient with probable Alzheimer's disease had obvious delays in the oral preparatory and oral transition phase of the swallow while the patient with multi-infarct dementia had primarily pharyngeal phase impairments with sensory loss and silent aspiration. Figure 15–4 is a still photograph from videofluoroscopy of the patient with

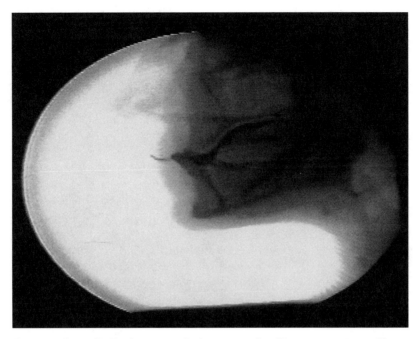

Figure 15–4. Still photograph from a videofluoroscopic swallowing study of a patient with probable Alzheimer's disease showing the pureed bolus just after deposit in the oral cavity.

probable Alzheimer's disease accepting a bolus and Figure 15–5 shows the same patient swallowing 26 seconds after the bolus was presented. Figure 15–6 provides an example of the patient with multi-infarct dementia swallowing pureed consistencies and Figure 15–7 demonstrates silent aspiration after drinking thin liquids from a cup. Each patient had different reactions to feeding assistance. The patient with Alzheimer's disease had intervals of refusing feedings but would self-feed

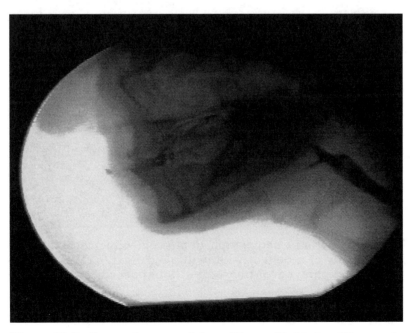

Figure 15–5. Same photograph from Figure 15–4 taken 26 seconds later during the pharyngeal phase of the swallow.

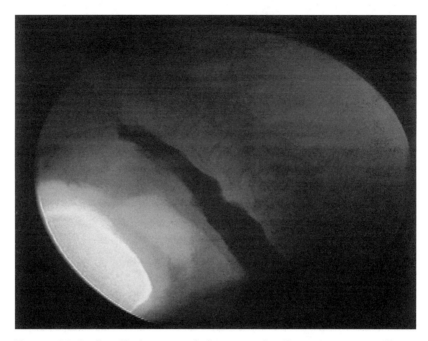

Figure 15–6. A still photograph from a videofluoroscopic swallowing study of a patient with multiple cortical strokes demonstrating the pharyngeal phase of a pureed consistency swallow.

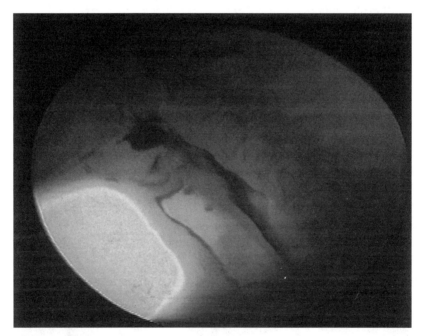

Figure 15–7. A still photograph from a videofluoroscopic swallowing study of a patient with multiple cortical strokes demonstrating the pharyngeal phase of a liquid consistency swallow with silent aspiration.

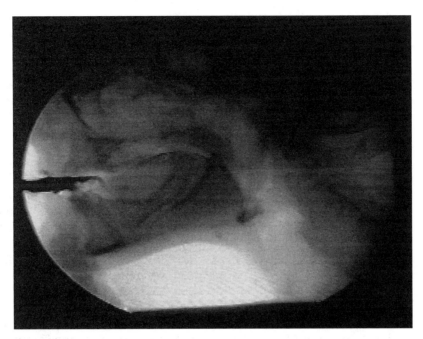

Figure 15–8. A still frame from a videofluoroscopic study showing a patient with probable Alzheimer's disease self-feeding finger foods during the study.

when finger foods were provided; this was utilized as a management strategy for enhanced caloric intake. Figure 15–8 shows the patient self-feeding finger foods during the videofluoroscopic study. While the patient with multi-infarct dementia had positive social skills and accepted all food that was offered, these behaviors were a considered a risk or burden requiring all staff to be familiar with his history of silent aspiration with liquids. These cases also demonstrate issues regarding decisions for tube feeding made in advance and those made by a health care surrogate or guardian. The patient with multi-infarct dementia was able to use combined enteral oral and tube feeding and transitioned to increased tube feeding as his condition progressed. Both patients demonstrate the successful outcome of a management program when issues such as weight and incidence of infections are monitored.

CASE FOUR—RIGHT HEMISPHERE STROKE

A 58-year-old male was admitted to a rehabilitation unit with a diagnosis of a right hemisphere stroke. The onset was 5 days prior to admission to the medical center. The patient exhibited mild left facial weakness with no significant lingual weakness or impaired articulatory precision. There was a breathy voice quality. Impulsive behaviors were noted dur-

ing self-feeding tasks. The patient complained of odynophagia (pain on swallowing) during the clinical examination. A videofluoroscopic examination of swallow function was completed 2 days after admission to the unit. The study revealed osteophytes along the vertebra of the cervical spine at the level of the cricopharyngeal sphincter and irregular tissue along the posterior larynx and upper esophagus. An endoscopic examination by an otolaryngologist revealed a lesion in the esophagus, and a biopsy confirmed a malignant tumor. Treatment was changed to a medical/surgical focus, and the patient was followed by oncology. The patient agreed to placement of a percutaneous endoscopic gastrostomy (PEG) during medical/surgical intervention.

The speech–language pathologist must remember that disorders of the nervous system can have a wide variety of symptoms, and swallowing disorders may be only one indication of a potential or co-existing nervous system disorder. The assessment and intervention of potential dysphagia require thorough attention to identifying and optimally treating reversible and treatable conditions. Symptoms of dysphagia should not automatically be attributed to a neurogenic etiology, and it is imperative to seek potentially reversible causes of the symptoms rather than simply attribute them to a neurogenic causes. Case Four reinforces the need to follow this rule. In Figure 15–9 liquid barium outlines the areas of irregular tissue during a videofluoroscopic study of swallow function. In this case the breathy voice quality might be due to the tumor rather than the stroke. The complaint of odynophagia was a significant symptom that was considered a key component in differential diagnosis during the clinical examination.

CASE FIVE—NEUROLOGICAL SWALLOWING DISORDER FOLLOWING SURGICAL TRAUMA

A 76-year-old male was referred for a dysphagia evaluation 3 weeks status post a right radical neck dissection and biopsy to rule out a malignancy. The surgeon suspected cranial nerve damage. The patient had a nasogastric tube in place immediately after surgery that was removed one week prior to the assessment. All language and cognitive communication assessments were within normal limits. His verbal speech output was imprecise with excessive vocal loudness used as a compensation technique. The assessment of swallowing revealed poor ability to transfer the bolus from the anterior to posterior oral cavity with significant residue along the blade of the tongue. There was reduced base-of-tongue to posterior pharyngeal wall contact and laryngeal vestibule penetration existed in all trials. The patient had an automatic cough that was productive for clearing the airway. The communication and swallowing assessments confirmed the suspicion of peripheral nerve damage (CNS IX, XI, and XII). The patient was enrolled in individual treatment, and behavioral treatment was initiated to address compensatory lingual movements and safe swallow strategies. The patient agreed to placement of a percutaneous endoscopic gastrostomy (PEG) for primary nutrition and hydration to be transitioned as oral intake improved. After six sessions of treatment, the patient indicated that it was no longer a pleasure to eat, eating out socially was not an activity prior to the surgery, and he would continue the PEG feedings. The patient was reassessed every 6 months over a 7 year period until he moved to another city. Although he had the PEG, he had experienced two episodes of suspected aspiration pneumonia. His weight and nutritional status remained within normal limits. The patient returned to pre-morbid social activities (playing cards) and hobbies (carpentry, wood working).

When there is damage to more than one cranial nerve involved in swallowing, a neurogenic dysphagia may be expected. In this case it was secondary to surgical trauma or iatrogenic in nature. The poor ability to manipulate the bolus in the oral cavity is shown in Figure 15–10. Perhaps the most

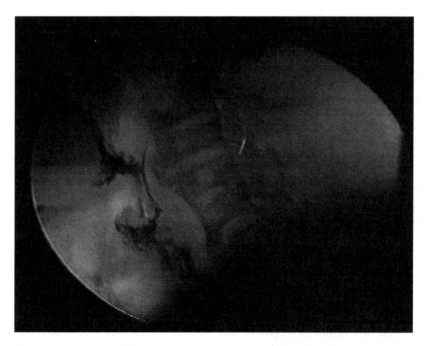

Figure 15–9. A still frame of a videofluoroscopic swallowing study demonstrating the irregular outline of the barium along the posterior larynx and upper esophagus. A biopsy confirmed a malignant tumor.

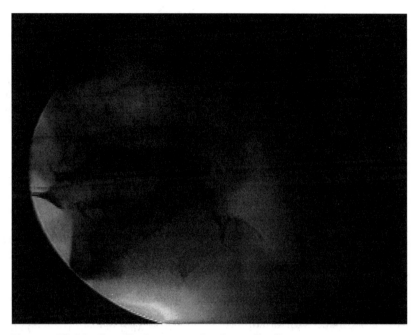

Figure 15–10. A still photograph of a videofluoroscopic examination of the swallow for a patient with CNS IX, XI, and XII surgical trauma. The residual effects of nerve damage are demonstrated during the oral transition phase of the swallow.

striking issue of this clinical example was the lack of pleasure in eating when compensatory strategies were employed and the patient's subsequent decision to continue total enteral tube feeding while engaging in social activities. This case also highlights the fact that tube feeding does not prevent aspiration.

SUMMARY

Dysphagia is not a problem that routinely occurs in isolation, and a multifactorial approach to assessment and intervention is critical. The speech–language pathologist should be familiar with the common causes of neurogenic disorders, the potential impact of a variety of lesions on communication and swallowing, symptoms associated with neurogenic disorders, and the course of a disease or syndrome. The incidence of co-existing communication and swallowing disorders is high, and cognitive-communication behaviors should always be a focus of the speech–language pathologist's assessment. The speech–language pathologist can be the leader in planning a holistic approach to safe oral intake. When a patient has a progressive neurological disease, the clinician may need to plan a program designed to prevent a decline in nutrition, hydration, and health status rather than

attempting a curative approach that ultimately will be nonproductive. In addition, the speech–language pathologist will be a part of the health care team for monitoring the outcome of the treatment or management program. Although health care professionals have access to medical and surgical technology, consideration of the individual patient's wishes for intervention is paramount and should be the focus of the patient care planning.

STUDY QUESTIONS

1. Which of the following statements is true?
   a. Patients with right hemisphere strokes have cricopharyngeal dysfunction.
   b. Dysphagia may be an early symptom of bulbar type ALS.
   c. Dysphagia may be a symptom of a trauma to the brainstem.
   d. Dysphagia may be a symptom of a tumor.

2. Which of the following statements is false?
   a. Dysarthria and dysphagia may be co-existing problems.
   b. A breathy voice and dysphagia may co-exist.
   c. Cognitive-communication disorders and dysphagia may co-exist.
   d. Patients with voice disorders also have swallowing disorders.

3. Which statement is true?
   a. Patients with myasthenia gravis should practice oral-motor exercises prior to meals to assist with swallowing.
   b. Oral-motor exercises are contraindicated in patients with myasthenia gravis.

4. Which statement is true?
   a. ALS patients benefit from starvation.
   b. ALS patients may be offered alternate enteral tube feeding as an option to prevent decline in nutrition and hydration.

5. Which statement is false?
   a. Patients with a history of bilateral strokes are at risk for symptoms of cognitive decline that may interfere with self-feeding and the ability to learn new information with treatment for swallowing disorders.
   b. Patients with a history of a unilateral cerebrovascular accident have impairment with cricopharyngeal sphincter opening.

6. Which statement is false?
   a. Patient with complaints of odynophagia should be placed on peripheral tube feedings.
   b. Patients with complaints of odynophagia may required additional medical assessment or intervention.

7. Which of the following statements is true?
   a. A spouse may participate in feeding management.
   b. A nurse may provide feeding management three times a day.
   c. A speech–language pathologist should provide individual treatment for all patients with neurogenic dysphagia.

8. Which of the following statements is false?
   a. A patient with Alzheimer's disease will have a progressive decline in cognitive and memory.
   b. The cause of ALS is unknown and a progressive decline is expected.
   c. Patients with Parkinson's disease have periods of exacerbation and remission, and as a result some weeks they will be able to eat all types of food consistencies.

REFERENCES

1. Buchholz DW, Robbins JA: Neurologic disease affecting oropharyngeal swallowing. In Perlman AL, Schulze-Delrieu K, eds., Deglutition and its disorders, pp. 319–342. Singular Publishing Group, San Diego, 1997.
2. Hurwitz AL et al: Oropharyngeal dysphagia. *Am J Dig Dis* 1975; 20:313.
3. Castell DO: Eating and swallowing disorders. In Hazzard WR, Bierman EL, Blass JP, Ehinger WH, Halter JB (Editors): *Principles of geriatric medicine and gerontology.* McGraw-Hill, New York, NY, 1994.
4. Bosma JF: Sensorimotor examination of the mouth and pharynx. *Front Oral Physiol* 1976; 2:78.
5. Wertz RT: Neuropathologies of speech and language: An introduction to patient managment. In Johns DF, ed., *Clinical management of neurogenic communicative disorders,* pp 1–101. Little, Brown, Boston, 1978.
6. Adams RD, Victor M, Ropper AH: *Principles of neurology,* 6th ed. McGraw Hill, New York, 1997.
7. Morrell RM: Neurogenic disorders of swallowing. In Groher ME, ed., *Dysphagia disgnosis and managment,* 2nd ed. Butterworth-Heinemann, Boston, 1992.
8. Miller RM, Groher ME: General treatment of neurologic swallowing disorders. In Groher ME, ed., *Dysphagia diagnosis and management,* 2nd ed. Butterworth-Heinemann, Boston, 1992.
9. Schultz A, Niemtzow P, Jacobs S, Naso F: Dysphagia associated with cricopharyngeal dysfunction. *Arch Phys Med Rehabil* 1979; 60:381–386.
10. Horner J, Buoyer FG, Alberts MJ, Helms MJ: Dysphagia following brain stem stroke: Clinical correlates and outcome. *Arch Neurology* 1991; 48:1170–1173.
11. Bucholz DW: Clinically-probable brainstem stroke presenting primarily as dysphagia and nonvisuallized by MRI. *Dysphagia* 1993; 8:235–238.
12. Adams RD, Victor M, Ropper AH: Neurologic disorders caused by lesions in particular parts of the cerebrum. In *Principles of neurology.* McGraw-Hill, New York, 1997.
13. Logemann JA, Shanahan T, Rademaker AW, Kahrilas PJ, Lazar R, Halper A: Oropharyngeal swallowing after stroke in the left basal ganglion/internal capsule. *Dysphagia* 1993; 8:230–234.
14. Robbins JR, Levine RL, Maser AM, Rosenbeck JR, Kempster GK: Swallowing after unilateral stroke of the cerebral cortex. *Arch Phy Med Rehabil* 1993; 74: 1295–1300.
15. Schulze-Delrieu KS, Miller RM: Clinical assessment of dysphagia: In Perlman AL and Schulze-Delrieu KS: *Deglutition and its disorders.* Singular Publishing Group, San Diego, CA, 1997.
16. Logemann JA: *Manual for the videofluorographic study of swallowing,* 2d ed. Pro-Ed, Austin, TX, 1993.
17. Chusid JG: Principles of neurodiagnosis (Section III). In Chusid JG, *Correlative neuroanatomy and functional neurology.* Lange Medical Publications, Los Altos, CA, 1970.
18. Miller RM, Groher ME: The mental status examination. In Miller RM, Groher ME, *Medical speech pathology.* An Aspen Publication, Rockville, MD, 1990.
19. Miller RM, Groher ME: Principles of treatment and management. In Miller RM and Groher ME, *Medical speech pathology.* An Aspen Publication, Rockville, MD, 1990.
20. Martin BJW, Corlew MM: The incidence of communication disorders in dysphagic patients. *J Speech Hearing Dis,* 1990; 55:28–32.

21. Musson ND: Dysphagia: evaluation and management of geriatric nursing home residents. Unpublished paper presented at American Speech, Language, and Hearing Association Convention, Los Angeles, CA, 1993.

22. Logemann JA, Boshes B, Blonsky RE, Fischer: Speech and swallowing evaluation in the differential diagnosis of neurological disease. *Neurol-Neurocirugia-Psiquiatria,* 1977: 18:71–78.

23. Groher ME: Bolus managment and aspiration pneumonia in patients with pseudobulbar dysphagia. *Dysphagia,* 1987; 1:215–216.

24. Merritt HH. *A textbook of neurology.* Lea & Febiger, Philadelphia, 1967.

25. Bass NH, Morrell RM: The neurology of swallowing. In Groher ME, *Dysphagia diagnosis and management,* 2nd ed. Butterworth-Heinemann, Boston, 1992.

26. Teasell RW, Bach D, McRa M: Prevelance and recovery of aspiration poststroke: A retrospective analysis. *Dysphagia,* 1994; 9:35–39.

27. Miller RM: Clinical examination for dysphagia: In Groher ME, *Dysphagia diagnosis and managment,* 2nd ed. Butterworth-Heinemann, Boston, 1992.

28. Larsen GL: Chewing and swallowing: In Martin N, Holt N, Hicks DJ, eds., *Comprehensive rehabilitation nursing.* McGraw Hill, New York, 1981.

29. Dikeman KJ, Kazandjian MS: *Communication and swallowing management of tracheostomized and ventilator-dependent adults.* Singular Publishing Group, Inc, San Diego, CA, 1995.

30. Cummings, JL, Benson, DF: *Demenita: A clinicial approach,* 2nd ed. Butterworth-Heinemann, Boston, 1992.

31. Horner J, Alberts M, Dawson D, Cook G: Swallowing in Alzheimer's disease. *Alzheimers Dis Rel Dis* 1994; 8:1–13.

32. Yorkston KM, Miller RM, Strand EA: *Management of speech and swalowing in degenerative diseases.* Communication Skill Builders, Tuscon, AZ, 1995.

33. Hoehn MM, Yahr M: Parkinsonism: Onset, progression and mortality. *Neurology,* 1967; 17:427–442.

34. Robbins JA, Logeman J, Kirshner A: Swallowing and speech in Parkinson's disease. *Ann Neurol* 1986; 19: 283–287.

35. Kagel MC, Leopold NA: Dysphagia in Huntington's disease: A 16 year retrospective. *Dysphagia* 1992; 7: 106–114.

36. Scanlan CL, Gupta TL: Synopsis of cardiopulmonary diseases. In Scanlan CL, Spearman CB, Sheldon RL, ed., *Egan's fundamentals of respiratory care.* Mosby, St. Louis, MO, 1990.

37. Musson ND, Kincaid J, Ryan P, Glussman B, Varone L, Gamarra N, Wilson R, Reefe W, Silverman M: Nature, nurture, nutrition: Interdisciplinary programs to address the prevention of malnutrition and dehydration. *Dyphagia* 1990; 5:96–101.

38. Musson ND: Dysphagia team management: Continuous quality improvement in a long-term care setting. *Amer Speech Lang Hear Assoc Qual Improv Dig* 1994; Winter:1–10.

39. *American Society of Parenteral and Enteral Nutrition Guidelines and Standards.* American Society for Parenteral and Enteral Nutrition National Office, Silver Springs, MD, 1993.

40. ASPEN Board of Directors: Guidelines for the use of enteral nutrition in the adult patient. *J Parenteral Enteral Nutr* 1987; 11:435–439.

41. ASPEN Board of Directors: Guidelines for use of total parenteral nutrition in the hospitalized adult patient. *J Parenteral Enteral Nutr* 1986; 10:441–445.

42. American Speech–Language-Hearing Association: Knowledge and skills needed by speech–language pathologists provinding services to dysphagic patient/clients. *ASHA* 1990; 32 (Suppl 2):7–12.

43. Jones B, Donner MW: Normal and abnormal swallowing: *Imaging in diagnosis and therapy.* Springer-Verlag, New York, 1991.

44. Kane RL, Ouslander JG, Abrass IB: *Essentials of clinical geriatrics,* 3d ed. McGraw-Hill, New York, 1994.

16

Post-Acute Clinical Management: The Rehabilitation of the Patient with Neurologic Communication Disorders

CARL COELHO

CHAPTER OUTLINE

Definitions

Overview of Communicative Interventions

Treatment Planning

This chapter reviews the rehabilitation of patients with neurologic communication disorders. The discussion begins by defining rehabilitation, continuum of care, and the multidisciplinary rehabilitation team. Next, specific issues related to the management (assessment, treatment planning, discharge, and organization of treatment) of individuals with neurologic communication impairments are presented. Finally, case studies of three patients with neurologic communication disorders are given to illustrate clinical management principles with this population.

DEFINITIONS

Rehabilitation

Rehabilitation has been defined as the development of the individual to the fullest physical, psycholog-

ical, social, vocational, avocational, and educational potential consistent with his or her physiological or anatomical impairment and environmental limitations.[1] Rehabilitation may also be considered from the perspective of the World Health Organization's (WHO) classification of the consequences of disease or a disorder, in which three levels are specified: (1) *Impairment,* defined as "any loss or abnormality of psychological, physiological or anatomical structure or function"[2] (p. 27); (2) *Disability,* defined as "any restriction or lack (resulting from impairment) of ability to perform an activity in the manner or within the range considered normal for a human being"[2] (p. 28); and (3) *Handicap,* defined as "a disadvantage, for a given individual, resulting from an impairment or a disability, that limits or prevents the fulfillment of a role that is normal (depending on age, gender, and social and cultural factors) for that individual"[2](p. 29). Historically, rehabilitation has focused on impairment and disability issues following neurologic disease or injury. However, the ultimate determination of successful rehabilitation is the reintegration of the individual into the community in a meaningful social role.[3–5]

Continuum of Care

The rehabilitation process involves a continuum of care. This continuum consists of five distinct stages in which a variety of services are provided on the basis of the individual's needs. The typical rehabilitation continuum stages are: acute care, subacute care, inpatient rehabilitation, outpatient rehabilitation, and community reintegration (Table 16–1). It should be kept in mind that throughout this chapter when the terms individual or patient are used they will be referring to individuals or patients with neurologic communication disorders.

Acute Care

Acute care takes place while the individual is in the acute hospital. It is that point in the treatment continuum where the primary goals are, by necessary, more medically oriented. However, the benefits of early and aggressive interventions (including speech–language pathology services) during acute hospitalization have been documented and recommended.[6–9] For example, MacKay and colleagues compare outcome data for a group of traumatic brain injury (TBI) patients who were involved in an early intervention program that included assessment and therapy being provided in the intensive care unit with a second group that did not undergo this treatment. Findings indicated that the early intervention group had significantly shorter rehabilitation stays. Furthermore, the early intervention group was discharged with higher levels of cognitive functioning and had a significantly higher percentage of discharges home versus discharges to extended care facilities. Therefore, for the purposes of the present discussion, acute care is considered the beginning point of the rehabilitation continuum.

Once life-threatening issues have been addressed and medical stability has been achieved, the patient no longer requires the level of care provided

Table 16–1. Characteristics of the Rehabilitation Continuum of Care and the Responsibilities of the Speech–Language Pathologist in the Management of Neurologic Communication Disorders

Level of Care	Primary Objective	Function of Speech–Language Pathologist
Acute care (acute hospital)	Achieve medical stability following neurologic event (e.g., CVA, TBI, exacerbation of disease) as quickly as possible	Differential diagnosis of communication disorder, initiate diagnostic treatment
Subacute care (extended care facility)	Provision of medical care and rehab. services on a less intensive basis for patients who are medically complicated or slower to recover	Assessment and treatment of communication disorder, therapy may be provided on a less rigorous schedule (3×/week vs. 5, or half-hour sessions vs. hour).
Inpatient rehabilitation (rehab. hosp. or unit)	Provision of intensive multidisciplinary rehab. and to discharge patient to least restrictive environment given limited length of stay (usually <4 weeks)	Assessment and treatment of communication disorder, therapy provided as intensively as patient is able to tolerate, regular interdisciplinary team meetings, targeting behaviors that will increase patient's functional status to the greatest extent in the designated time frame.
Home Care (patient's home)	Provision of short-term rehab. care in patient's home usually until patient can ambulate or has sufficient mobility to be transported to outpatient care	Assessment and treatment of communication disorder in real-world context of home, identification of significant communication handicaps that can be addressed over an extended period in outpatient therapy if necessary
Outpatient Rehabilitation (rehab. center)	Provision of extended rehab. (often interdisciplinary), duration often determined by insurance coverage vs. need	Assessment and treatment of handicap posed by communication disorder, focus is on community reintegration

in the acute medical setting and is discharged to one of three settings: a subacute care facility, an inpatient rehabilitation facility, or home.

Subacute Care

When discharged to a subacute care facility, the patient may be medically stable, but too weak or unable to fully participate in and benefit from an aggressive inpatient rehabilitation program [e.g., one or more hours of physical therapy (PT), occupational therapy (OT), and speech–language therapy per day]. Subacute facilities provide skilled nursing care as well as the full complement of therapy services, which are offered on a less intensive basis (e.g., half an hour of PT, OT, and speech–language three times per week). The typical length of stay in subacute facilities is generally longer than in inpatient rehabilitation hospitals. Patients in subacute facilities may eventually be discharged to inpatient rehabilitation facilities or home. Subacute facilities are typically organized to deliver services via a multidisciplinary team of professionals (Table 16–2). The concept of multidisciplinary rehabilitation is discussed later in this chapter.

Inpatient Rehabilitation

Inpatient rehabilitation hospitals or units are intended to provide intensive multidisciplinary rehabilitation. Although several years ago the average length of stay in such facilities was much longer, currently stays may range from, for example, one to five weeks for stroke patients and three to ten weeks for patients with TBIs. To be a candidate for intensive inpatient rehabilitation, an individual must actively be involved in a minimum of three hours of therapy per day and have ongoing goals in at least two services (PT, OT, and/or speech–language pathology). An integral part of this phase of the rehabilitation process is the weekly interdisciplinary team meeting to establish and discuss the individual's rehabilitation goals, prognosis, and discharge plan. In all instances the rehabilitation program designed for a given individual depends on his or her appropriate short- and long-term goals, and the targeted outcome. A patient may be discharged from the inpatient rehabilitation facility to a subacute care facility if the individual has not progressed rapidly and is not ready to return home but is still considered a candidate for ongoing inpatient services. Under ideal circumstances the individual is discharged home.

Home and Outpatient

The patient who is discharged home continues rehabilitation on an outpatient basis or through a homecare agency. Outpatient rehabilitation services will generally be comparable to what the individual was provided with on an inpatient basis but at different intensities. For example, an individual may

Table 16–2. Interdisciplinary Team

Primary Professionals	Function	Mode
Physical therapists	Work with patients to restore mobility, either through independent walking, use of wheelchair, or cane.	Involves improving strength and range of motion of muscles of the trunk, and upper and lower extremities.
Occupational therapists	Work on improving patients' sensory-motor, perceptual, and neuromuscular functions needed for independent performance of activities of daily living (ADLs) such as personal grooming, dressing, and feeding.	Involves improving strength and coordination of upper extremities, use of compensatory strategies and adaptive equipment.
Neuropychologists	Administer and interpret tests of cognitive and mental functions.	Information regarding a patient's attentional and memory functions as well as learning potential is determined and shared with other team members as they formulate treatment plans.
Social workers	Address patient and family issues related to their psychosocial adjustment to their injury or disease.	Through individual or group meetings. Also facilitate discharge planning and assist with referrals to community resources.

continue to receive services from PT, OT, and speech–language pathology but only two or three times per week. Conversely, an individual may be enrolled in an outpatient day treatment program involving five hours of interdisciplinary services five days per week. Once again the rehabilitation services are ideally determined by the individual's needs, but may also be dictated by the resources available in a given facility or region. Chapter 8 has a detailed discussion of rehabilitation services delivered through home care systems.

For outpatient rehabilitation, the individual is transported from home to the outpatient facility for rehabilitation services and then returns home each day. When the individual receives services through a home care agency, rehabilitation services are provide in the home by professionals. These services are usually of short duration and end as soon as the individual is ambulatory or mobile enough to be safely transported to an outpatient rehabilitation facility. One particular advantage to providing rehabilitation in the individual's home is that the service providers can see firsthand the everyday real-world obstacles that the patient must overcome or compensate to decrease his or her handicap.

Community Reintegration

The end point of the rehabilitation continuum of care involves community reintegration. Although in this discussion it is presented last, we must emphasize that successful community reintegration must begin early in the rehabilitation process. All therapy goals should be influenced by the specific long-term expectations for a given individual. Regardless of whether the ultimate goal is for an individual to return home and to his or her previous job, or to live in supervised housing and work in a sheltered workshop, those skills necessary for the successful return to that environment must be identified and addressed in every treatment session.[4,10–13] Obviously community reintegration will be different for each individual with a neurologic communication disorder. For example, an individual with a TBI may require a highly structured environment including job coaches and supervision at home to provide prompts and cues that will help that individual compensate for cognitive impairments and communicative difficulties. On the other hand, an individual with a significant dysarthria secondary to a degenerative disease may require support involving augmentative and alternative communication devices and education of those individuals who communicate with the individual so they know how to facilitate successful interactions.

Interdisciplinary Rehabilitation

A rehabilitation team is a group of professionals who work together to improve the functional abilities and quality of life of an individual. The team and its purpose are defined by the problems and needs of the patient. Members of an interdisciplinary team collaborate on identification of treatment goals and establishment of an optional treatment plan for a patient. The team goals will always supersede the goals of an individual discipline.[14] Team composition will vary from program to program (and patient to patient) but generally will always include the patient and family, several professionals, and supporting disciplines. Primary professionals are almost always involved in one way or another with direct patient care. Included in this category are such disciplines as PT, OT, SLP, psychology, social work, nursing, and medicine. There are also a number of professionals on the rehabilitation team who serve in a supporting capacity—that is, they may be called on to address specific needs of certain patients. A brief description of each discipline is included in Table 16–2 to help clarify the roles of the various team members.

OVERVIEW OF COMMUNICATIVE INTERVENTIONS

In this section management principles for neurologic communication disorders are presented. Specifically, we will discuss issues pertinent to assessment, treatment, and discharge of patients along the rehabilitation continuum. Although acute care was noted as the first step of the rehabilitation continuum, no information related to the management of neurologic communication disorders in the acute care setting is presented in this chapter—the reader is referred to Chapters 5 and 6 for information related to that topic.

Assessment

Linebaugh[15] has noted that information obtained from a test of aphasia may be employed for a variety of general purposes: (1) differential diagnosis; (2) localization of lesion; (3) determination of patient's level of functional communication; (4) establishment of a prognosis; (5) focusing of treatment, and (6) assessment of recovery and efficacy of treatment. Although Linebaugh's discussion pertains specifically to aphasia, it can be meaningfully applied to the assessment of all neurologic communication disorders. Each of these six general purposes is discussed below.

Differential Diagnosis

The first task in the assessment process with a neurologic communication disorder is to make a series of differentiations. One must first determine whether the individual's communication skills are impaired or within normal limits. If communication is impaired, the next determination is whether it is language specific (i.e., aphasia) or a reflection of some other primary disturbance (e.g., TBI or dementia). Finally, it must be determined whether the impairment is limited to only language processes (i.e., morphology, phonology, syntax) or it involves motor planning and programming or execution for speech (i.e., apraxia of speech or dysarthria). These differentiations are critical not only for their contribution to the medical diagnosis, but for their implications for determining whether the patient is a candidate for therapy and, if so, the nature of that therapy.

A number of factors contribute to the differential diagnosis process. These include:

1. The fluency with which a patient produces speech, which can be determined by using an assessment protocol that provides for the elicitation of verbal responses encompassing a wide range of length.
2. Degree of impairment of specific communicative abilities, for which the assessment protocol should include tasks in all language modalities covering a wide range of difficulty to provide adequate data for differentiating among various aphasic and nonaphasic communication impairments.
3. The patient's response patterns on nonlanguage tasks, which are included to assess specific processes that subserve language (i.e., attention and memory, whose integrity are necessary prerequisites to successful performances on speech and language tasks).
4. The type of responses produced by the patient, which requires a detailed analysis of the patient's responses, from which we seek to infer the mediating process by which the responses were produced.
5. The relevance of the patient's responses to test stimuli, because errors of relevance involve bizarre responses that appear unrelated to the stimulus.
6. Awareness of errors and the ability to self-correct.

Duffy[16] describes several general guidelines with regard to differential diagnosis of motor speech disorders that should be kept in mind during the assessment of any patient with a neurologic condition:

1. A speech examination should always lead to an attempt at diagnosis: the better the problem is understood the better it can be treated.
2. When a diagnosis cannot be made on the basis of the findings from the assessment, the reasons should be clearly stated.
3. A diagnosis should not be stated when one cannot be determined
4. A diagnosis should be related to the suspected or known neurologic diagnosis.
5. Different speech (and language/cognitive-communicative) disorders may co-occur.
6. A diagnostic label is a convenient shorthand for communicating information to other professionals.

Localization

Particular pattern of speech and language impairment may be related to involvement of specific regions of the central nervous system. The development of increasingly sophisticated neuroradiologic procedures (e.g., computed tomography scans, magnetic resonance imaging, positive emission tomography, etc.) have alleviated the need for making an inferential leap between behaviors and specific brain regions. However, careful description of an individual's speech and language impairment and delineation of error patterns will significantly contribute to the overall process of either reaching or confirming a neurologic diagnosis. The reader is referred to Chapter 13 of this text for a thorough discussion of the application of brain imaging to neurologic communication disorders.

Determining Level of Functional Communication

Attempts at determining a patient's performance in natural communicative situations may involve predicting such performance from scores of standardized tasks employed in formal testing. For example, in the Aphasia Severity Rating Scale from the Boston Diagnostic Aphasia Examination,[17] the portion of communicative burden is carried by the listener. A second more direct strategy is to assess performance in tasks approaching natural communication situations such as Communication Abilities in Daily Life[18] or through the use of rating scales such as the Functional Communication Profile[19] or the Communicative Effectiveness Index,[20] in which functional communication is rated by the clinician or other care providers. A third approach for determining functional performance involves any of a variety of functional status measures that are currently being used by most rehabilitation centers to determine outcomes of extended rehabilitation for neurologic patients. Such measures include the Functional Independence Measure,[21] the Patient Evaluation and Conference System,[22] the Rancho Rehabilitation Outcome Evaluation,[23] and the Rehabilitation Institute of Chicago-Functional Assessment Scales,[24] in which communication skills are one dimension of a patient's "functional status" that are rated. A major limitation of all these data management systems used for measuring rehabilitation outcomes is that, at the present time, they are not sophisticated or sensitive enough to detect small increments of functional change, particularly in the area of communication skills. In response to speech–language pathologists' concern with these functional outcomes scales, the Functional Assessment of Communication Skills for Adults (ASHA FACS) was developed and recently validated on both head-injured and aphasic inpatients.[25] Preliminary finding have indicated that this measure is sensitive for detecting improvement in functional outcome during inpatient speech intervention.

Prognosis

Perhaps one of the most challenging clinical endeavors is predicting the eventual extent of an individual's recovery. Patient variables such as age, time of post-onset, and extent of lesion are considered predictive in certain neurologic conditions, while length of coma, initial degree of impairment in auditory comprehension, overall severity of communicative impairment, or severity of left neglect are thought to be predictive in others.

Focusing Treatment

The most important use of the information derived from speech and language testing is that it be reliably employed for focusing treatment. Whether it be a list of psycholinguistic or information processing factors for an aphasic patient, or an analysis of components of normal speech production for a dysarthric patient, this assessment protocol should determine the level of breakdown (i.e., that point at which the patient begins to experience difficulty) and identify those components that, if addressed in therapy, will have the greatest impact on improving communication function.

Assessing Recovery and Efficacy of Treatment

For performance to be compared across time (i.e., pre- to post-treatment) some form of standard score must be used that utilizes a sensitive scoring system that reflects subtle changes in the patient's performance over time and also has a high degree of stability. Such scores include the aphasia quotient (AQ) of the Western Aphasia Battery,[26] overall score from the Porch Index of Communicative Ability,[27] overall score from the Arizona Battery for Communication in Dementia,[28] overall score on the Scales of Cognitive Ability in Traumatic Brain Injury,[29] or intelligibility scores from the assessment of Intelligibility of Dysarthric Speech.[30]

Whenever possible, traditional assessment procedures should be supplemented by functional assessment techniques. Such procedures include observation, questionnaires, checklists, and rating scales. Functional assessment determines current level of functioning and assists in the determination of optimal approaches to intervention. Giles[31] notes that functional assessment is central to the selection of goals and target behaviors required for the rehabilitation team's integrated treatment plan. Functional assessments should be conducted under conditions as close as possible to those the individual will experience following rehabilitation. The rigorous control of extraneous variables that is necessary for standardized assessments is sacrificed in favor of ecologic validity. There are many variables that may influence performance in real world situations, including setting (where the individual is at a particular point in time), cues (events that facilitate the production of a behavior), or environmental conditions (who else is present, level of activity, time of day, etc.). Patient observation enables clinicians to identify skills that appear to be intact or functional in the sterile clinical setting, but are actually nonfunctional in a home or work environment.[32]

Ongoing Assessments

In the acute rehabilitation setting the patient has usually stabilized medically and is strong and alert enough to participate in intensive rehabilitation. However, if there is a question on admission of whether a patient is ready for that particular setting, the patient may be admitted for a trial evaluation period. In either instance, this may be the first opportunity for the patient's communication skills to be comprehensively evaluated. Depending on the presenting diagnosis, the focus of the assessment may be on speech only (e.g., dysarthria); speech and language (e.g., left hemisphere stroke in which aphasia, dysarthria, and/or apraxia of speech are suspected); or speech, language, and cognitive abilities (e.g., TBI). If recent test results are available from the acute care medical setting, they may be used as baseline measures. However, if the test results are incomplete or unavailable, or if the patient appears to have changed since the tests were administered, a complete evaluation will be necessary.

Although scheduling practices and procedures may vary in different facilities, a comprehensive evaluation is usually completed by all the primary professionals and their findings incorporated into discipline-specific evaluation reports within 48 hours of admission. This enables an interdisciplinary team meeting to be scheduled during which team goals and length of stay are established, all within the first week of admission. In general, the nature of the goals will determine the length of stay. For example, if only one discipline recommends an extended period of treatment, the patient's stay will be brief. On the other hand, if two or more services (e.g., PT, OT, and speech–language pathology) have active short-term goals, it may be recommended that the patient stay, depending on the diagnosis, for two to eight weeks of intensive treatment.

Once the patient has been discharged from the acute rehabilitation setting, subsequent assessments will be utilized primarily for the purpose of documenting recovery and measuring effectiveness of ongoing treatment. In the case of the patient who has returned home or to some other long-term care living arrangement (e.g., a supervised apartment or transitional living unit), clinical staff have a greater opportunity for conducting functional assessments in the person's permanent "real-world" living environment.

TREATMENT PLANNING

Assessment has been described as the process of gathering data about the impairment (the underlying neurologic disorder), the disability (the decreased functional communicative ability resulting from the impairment), and the handicap (the decreased ability of the individual to communicate in the context of expected social roles). Decisions about the clinical course of action are made on the basis of that information. Treatment planning, therefore, may be viewed as the outcome of the assessment process.[33]

Treatment planning is a highly complex process. It begins with an evaluation of the individual's communication strengths and weaknesses using standardized and informal measures. Because each patient brings a diverse combination of factors to the clinical setting, these must also be considered during the planning process, apart from a communicative diagnosis and etiology. Such factors include age, motivation, vocational/educational history, and family support. Consideration of assessment findings without placing that information within the context of their circumstances yields an intervention approach that is generic, impersonal, and ineffective. Furthermore, such an approach to treatment planning will most likely be focused at the impairment and disability levels as opposed to the handicap. For example, two individuals with similar mild dysarthrias present with comparable communicative disabilities. However, suppose that one individual is a greenskeeper and the other a school teacher. From that perspective, the relatively mild disability might be a minor handicap for the greenskeeper and a potentially devastating one for the teacher. Treatment plans for these two individuals should be very different, even though they both have mild dysarthria.

Treatment Candidacy

A very important issue related to the treatment planning process is determining who is a candidate for treatment. Merely recognizing that a patient has a communication disorder does not help the clinician decide how important it is to treat an individual. To a large extent the idiosyncratic circumstances of each patient, as opposed to simply their communicative diagnosis, will determine their candidacy. Urgency of treatment does not depend solely on the impairment or disability but rather on the resulting handicap.[33]

Apart from degree of handicap, initial severity has been suggested as being an important factor in determining candidacy for treatment. Brookshire[34] has noted that not all aphasic patients are capable of recovering functional communication. The presence of such symptoms as verbal stereotypes, inability to match identical objects or pictures to objects, unreliable yes/no responses, or jargon and empty speech without self-correction are all signs of irreversible aphasia, and typically such patients are not candidates for extended treatment. However, Holland and colleagues[35] have noted that there is conflicting literature regarding the effectiveness of treatment for global aphasia, suggesting that the extent to which severity of aphasia influences the effectiveness of treatment is unclear.

Age has also been cited as a factor for determining candidacy for treatment. Although it has been suggested that, in the absence of health-related complications, elderly individuals with aphasia benefit just as much from treatment as younger patients,[36,37] Holland and Bartlett[38] note that elderly individuals who are not medically compromised to some degree following their strokes are rare and that such patients typically do not make as full a recovery as younger patients.

Finally, the issue of heterogeneity of the brain-injured population also needs to be considered. Individual differences most relevant to recovery include location of lesion, extent of neurologic damage, time post-onset, age at injury, rate of improvement immediately following injury, and a variety of factors related to pre-morbid level of functioning such as socioeconomic status and drug or alcohol abuse.

General Characteristics of Brain-Injured Patients

Brookshire[34] has observed that most brain-injured individuals demonstrate behaviors that aggravate their communicative impairments. Included here are such behaviors as: (a) decreased response flexibility (patient has difficulty changing response sets when the requirements of the task change); (b) impulsivity (patient responds quickly without taking time to fully appreciate the intended meaning of stimuli; such behavior is particularly evident in TBI and right hemisphere damaged patients and less so in patients with aphasia); (c) excessive caution (patient is reluctant to respond, lacking confidence in his perceptions of stimuli presented); (d) perseveration (patient repetitively produces responses when they are no longer appropriate); (e) decreased self-monitoring (patient has an impaired ability to monitor her own performance and lacks awareness of errors); and (f) delayed responses (delays may range from a few to several seconds between perception of the stimuli and the patient's response) (see Table 16–3).

Regardless of the nature of the communicative deficit, the effect of any of these co-existing behaviors will need to be considered and addressed in the treatment program. As an example, Horner and LaPointe[39] characterized brain-injured patients' tendency toward either impulsivity or cautiousness as variations in cognitive style. Furthermore, patients' cognitive styles should always be factored into the treatment plan. A patient who displays a more cautious style will progress through tasks slowly and have response delays but usually produce few errors. Conversely, a patient with a more impulsive style responds rapidly, at times prior to the completion of stimulus presentation, making frequent errors. A clinician's approach to each patient would need to be different, encouraging the cautious patient to respond more rapidly but not to the point of error generation, and attempting to slow down the impulsive patient in an effort to decrease error rate by increasing self-monitoring.

Table 16–3. Characteristics of Brain-Injured Patients

Behavior	Comments
Decreased response flexibility	Patient has difficulty changing response sets when the requirements of the task change.
Impulsivity	Patient responds quickly without taking time to fully appreciate the intended meaning of stimuli. Such behavior is particularly evident in TBI and right hemisphere damaged patients and less so in patients with aphasia.
Excessive caution	Patients reluctant to respond, lacking confidence in his or her perceptions of stimuli presented
Perservation	Patient repetitively produces responses when they are no longer appropriate
Decreased self-monitoring	Patient has an impaired ability to monitor his or her performance and lacks awareness of errors
Delayed responses	Delays may range from a few to several seconds between perception of the stimuli and the patient's response

Primary Treatment Goals

Although each patient with a neurologic communication disorder will have a host of very specific treatment objectives, certain primary goals that are common to all such patients will also be part of the plan. Such goals include maximizing the effectiveness, efficiency, and naturalness of the patients communication.[33,40] Duffy[16] notes that attaining these goals involves the following efforts: (a) restoration of lost function or reduction of impairment, although full restoration is typically an unrealistic goal, ["some degree of recovery occurs for many patients and may be enhanced with treatment, especially when etiology is an acute vascular or traumatic event or other etiology in which full or partial physiologic recovery can be expected" (p. 372)]; (b) compensation through the use of residual function (e.g., modifications to rate or prosody of speech or use of an appointment book to facilitate memory); and (c) reduction of the need for lost function through such things as vocational adjustments (modifications to the work environment or responsibilities) or lifestyle adjustments (interacting with individuals or small groups).

Treatment Context

Throughout the treatment planning process the issue of context must be carefully considered. Context, which is closely tied to the conception of ecologic validity previously discussed, refers both to the content of what a particular individual needs and to the setting or physical environment that the individual requires to function optimally. Decontextualized treatment activities that take place in artificial environments and involve tasks the individual will never be called on to perform may not constitute effective intervention.[41–43] Treatment programs vary depending on the stage of recovery as well as treatment setting. To facilitate carryover of treatment objectives to nonclinical environments, contextualization of treatment activities should take place as soon as feasible. For example, the patient could practice using an augmentative and alternative communication device on the telephone or on public transportation, or return to work with a job coach or some other type of support.

Treatment Setting

The treatment planning process and the issue of treatment candidacy may also be influenced by the setting where the individual with a neurologic communication disorder is receiving treatment. In the acute medical setting, treatment may be minimal, with the speech–language pathologist's primary goal being to complete an assessment and make a differential diagnosis prior to discharge. Those findings contribute to the decision about where the patient goes for the next level of care. In the acute rehabilitation setting, treatment is apt to be of short duration (i.e., 2 to 4 weeks), diagnostic in nature, and focused on reestablishing or identifying functional modes of communication. The patient's length of stay in this type of setting may also be abbreviated by a lack of progress. In the subacute setting, treatment is directed toward the same goals as in the acute rehabilitation setting but in a less aggressive fashion and over a longer period of time (i.e., typically longer length of stay).

The outpatient setting is often the only point along the treatment continuum where the clinician can pause and consider long-term objectives. The treatment planning at the outpatient stage involves consideration of several factors, each discussed individually below.

Recovery—Compensation

All outpatient treatment planning falls somewhere along a recovery-compensation continuum.[44] At one end of the continuum is recovery, whether it be linguistic or cognitive for aphasic or TBI patients, or normal speech production for individuals with dysarthria or apraxia of speech. At the other end of the continuum is communicative compensation—treatment that focuses on developing strategies for communicating the message regardless of the way that message is presented. Thus, a patient may use writing or gesture in social situations, rather than speech. Additional compensations may involve training the listener to ask appropriate questions, using an augmentative communication device, or simply modifying rate of speech or respiration/phonation dynamics. The skilled clinician is able to focus treatment at an optimal point along this continuum and modify the recovery-compensation focus whenever the patient does better or worse than anticipated. Changes in this focus may also be influenced by such factors as prior treatment, reimbursement issues, and type and severity of communicative disability.

Prior Treatment

Outpatients with neurologic communication disorders often present with one or a combination of the following treatment histories: (a) no previous treatment; (b) acute care hospitalization with or without speech–language intervention; (c) acute rehabilitation; (d) skilled nursing facility treatment; or (e) treatment through a home health agency. Generally, patients with more severe communicative impairments have received some type of speech and language treatment prior to being referred for outpatient services. Patients with milder motoric deficits (e.g., fluent aphasia) often are referred for outpatient treatment directly from the acute medical center. Such patients and their families have often had minimal education or counseling about their communicative impairment. Therefore this becomes the immediate priority in the treatment planning process.

Reimbursement

Reimbursement is another factor that impacts treatment planning. With the dramatic changes that are currently occurring in health care, fewer sessions are being authorized by insurance companies and health maintenance organizations. For example, it is not unusual to receive a treatment authorization for fewer than ten sessions to rehabilitate an individual with aphasia. Unfortunately in these cases, reimbursement may drive the selection process of treatment goals.[44] Obviously, when a minimal number of treatment sessions are authorized, the speech–language pathologist is unable to focus on recovery with regard to the recovery-compensation continuum. Rather, compensation for the communicative impairments, family education, and home programs become the treatment options.

Severity

Another factor that will certainly influence treatment planning is severity of the communicative impairments. Although factors such as age and motivation cannot offset the consequences of a very severe disability (e.g., global aphasia) they will certainly determine the perspective from which the treatment candidacy decision was made. For example, a trial period of therapy is typically warranted for all individuals with aphasia, regardless of severity. Those individuals who respond well to the trial period are then scheduled for ongoing treatment. Individuals who are not felt to have benefited from the trial period of treatment are recommended for a different type of intervention, perhaps less intensive or administered by a family member and monitored by the speech–language pathologist. Although this is a reasonable alternative for a retired individual who may be 74 years old, if the severely aphasic individual is a 21-year-old college student, the decision regarding treatment candidacy is far less straightforward.

Individuals with mild communicative impairments may present the greatest challenge to speech–language pathologists. Such individuals have the ability to select and prioritize their treatment goals. They also have the best potential for returning to their pre-morbid vocational, educational, personal, and recreational pursuits. These individuals may benefit the most from an emphasis on the recovery end of the recovery-compensation continuum.

Nature of Neurologic Diagnosis

The nature of the underlying neurologic impairment will also impact the treatment planning process. Treatment goals for an individual with a dysarthria secondary to a progressive neurologic disease such as Parkinson's will certainly be different from those established for an individual with dysarthria resulting from a stroke. Generally speaking, goals for the first are likely to focus on temporary compensations, listener training, and environmental modifications, whereas those for the stroke patient may focus more on recovery. Severity of the communicative impairment would also influence the treatment planning process for both individuals.

Discharge Planning

One of the most important aspects of the treatment planning process is the decision of when treatment should end. Ideally, discharge planning should begin as soon as the individual is scheduled for treatment. Thus, the speech–language pathologist should always have in mind criteria for what the individual needs to attain in terms of functional status or specific skills for treatment to be no longer necessary. A number of factors will influence the discharge decision, including the nature of the treatment objectives, the individual's potential for improved communicative functioning, and various factors external to the individual such as transportation, family support, and insurance coverage.

As discussed previously, the nature of the treatment objectives is determined by the extent of handicap resulting from the communicative impairment. For example, an individual with potential for returning to work will have a potentially longer and more involved course of treatment than an individual residing in a skilled nursing facility. Potential for improvement is determined in large measure by severity of the communicative impairment. In most instances the extent of brain damage will determine an individual's capacity to reacquire previous skills or learn compensatory strategies for accomplishing former skills in a different manner. External factors may also dictate discharge decisions. For example, despite excellent potential for improvement, if an individual does not have access to a facility where services are provided, or a family or significant other willing to reinforce or in some instances carry out treatment activities at home, ongoing treatment will not effective. Limited financial resources will also frequently determine when treatment must end.

Organization of Treatment

Management Approaches

Duffy[16] discusses several management approaches including medical, prosthetic, behavioral, and counseling and support groups. Although not all these approaches will be appropriate for all individuals with neurologic communication disorders, management of most patients will fall into one or more of these categories. (It should be noted that, although Duffy's discussion of these management categories is in the context of dysarthria, I have taken the liberty of applying this classification system to all interventions for neurologic communication disorders.)

Medical Approaches

Medical interventions may be categorized as either surgical or pharmacological. Medical management should always precede or be provided in conjunction with other interventions. Examples of surgical interventions directed toward the improvement of speech include medialization laryngoplasty, teflon injection, recurrent laryngeal nerve resection, and pharyngeal flap. Pharmacological interventions are typically directed the reduction of symptoms. Such treatments involving treating the underlying disease process as opposed to improving speech (e.g., use of levadopa for an individual with Parkinson's disease), but if the symptoms of the disease are decreased, speech may also improve.

Prosthetic Approaches

Prostheses may be broadly defined as any device that can be used to facilitate speech or communication. Such devices range from a palatal lift prosthesis used to assist palatal elevation in an effort to decrease nasality in a dysarthric patient, to some type of an augmentative and alternative communication device for an individual with minimal functional speech, to an electronic organizer for individual with memory problems. Use of prosthetic devices may be temporary until additional recovery takes place or becomes permanent.

Behavioral Approaches

Behavioral management includes all interventions not categorized as medical or prosthetic.[16] Behavioral interventions may be classified as either speaker-oriented or communication-oriented approaches. Speaker-oriented approaches include those in which improvement of some aspect of the speaker's speech or language skills is the target (e.g., improving speech intelligibility, word retrieval, auditory comprehension of sentences, etc.), with the overall goal of improving communication. Communication-oriented approaches are those in which treatment is focused on improving

communication even in the absence of improvement in speech and language skills. This approach to treatment is consistent with Yorkston's[45] adaptation of the concept of comprehensibility, defined as "the extent to which a listener understands utterances produced by a speaker in a communication context"[46](p. 32), which involves modifications to the communication environment (e.g., decreasing background noise and other distractions, facing the speaker, etc.), as well as listener training (e.g., establishing context for what is being said, asking yes/no questions, encouraging the use of communication supplements such as an alphabet board, picture books, or drawing).

Counseling and Support Groups

Counseling is an integral aspect of the clinician's responsibilities in the management of any patient with a neurologic communication disorder. Educating the patient and family regarding the nature of the communicative dysfunction, its etiology, and the prognostic implications—or in the case of a progressive condition the expected course of progression and the implications to communication skills—is a critical component of a comprehensive rehabilitation program. Another important responsibility of the clinician is to assist the patient and family in accessing community support groups. The function of such groups (e.g., National Aphasia Association, Multiple Sclerosis Society, National Head Injury Foundation, etc.) may be educational in nature while also providing a vehicle by which patients and their families can meet other individuals who are experiencing the same situation and help to develop a network for emotional support.

Determining What to Treat

How clinicians decide what to treat is more art than science, resulting from a combination of the clinician's conceptions or what the patient's communicative impairment represents, attitudes about what is important, opinions about the nature of therapy, and previous success and failures with patients who resemble the current patient"[34](p. 129).

Several approaches have been described by Brookshire[34] as to how clinicians decide what to treat in patients with neurologic communication disorders. For example, the clinician can assess the relative level of impairment, in which a patient's test performance is analyzed to identify particular "peaks" (areas in which impairments are less pronounced) and "valleys" (areas of relative impairments). The peaks and valleys are then focused on in treatment, with clinicians typically targeting the performance peaks. Assessing the patient by means of a fundamental abilities approach, in which clinicians attempt to identify impaired process or abilities underlying linguistic or communicative skills, allows the clinician to focus on the underlying process as opposed to the communicative symptoms. (A related notion to this approach is to identify the specific aspect of speech, language, or communication that will have the greatest impact on the overall system. For example, if an individual with a moderate dysarthria presents with problems in articulation resonance, and a severe problem with mild phonation, treating phonation will have a greater impact on overall speech intelligibility than will working on articulation or resonance, if phonation can be improved.) The third approach is the functional abilities approach, in which the clinician identifies skills that will be important for the patient in his or her everyday life in the home or work environment and then focuses treatment on improving those skills. In most instances the resulting treatment protocol is a combination of all three approaches.

General Guidelines for Treatment

The structure of treatment sessions for any patient with a neurologic communication disorder will be determined by the nature of the goals selected, the point along the rehabilitation continuum at which a particular patient may be, and the patient's physical status and endurance.

Type of Treatment

Type of treatment selected (i.e., individual versus group) is very much dependent on the treatment objectives. If the recommended treatment requires extensive drill activities (e.g., work on articulation or language stimulation), individual therapy (i.e., one-on-one with a clinician) would be optimal. However, if the focus is more communicatively based (e.g., increasing topic initiations in conversation), group therapy would be a better alternative because it requires more natural interactions and multiple participants. In many instances clinicians opt to enroll patients in a combination of individual and group therapies.

Session Length and Frequency

The actual length of treatment sessions will depend on the patient's physical endurance. Individual sessions may range from 10 to 15 minutes at bedside in the acute care setting to one hour of individual sessions followed by one hour group sessions on an outpatient basis. Frequency of treatment sessions will again be determined by the point along the rehabilitation continuum at which the patient currently is. During inpatient rehabilitation treatment may be quiet intensive (e.g., two one-hour individual sessions per day supplemented by computer-assisted therapy or therapy groups). On an outpatient basis therapy may consist of three one-hour sessions per week. Unfortunately, intensity of therapy, particularly outpatient therapy, may be dictated by insurance coverage and have nothing to do with treatment objectives or need.

Organization of a Treatment Session

Brookshire[34] has described a typical treatment session as consisting of five segments. The first segment has been termed the "hello segment" during which the clinician may informally estimate a patient's overall communicative status and establish rapport with the patient. The next segment is referred to as the "accommodation segment" in which the patient is warmed up for the main treatment activities through the presentation of activities that the patient has achieved a high level of success (90 to 95%) on during previous sessions. The third phase is the "work segment" during which more difficult and challenging tasks are presented; rate of success should be between 60 to 80%. The next segment is termed the "cool-down segment," which is intended to help the patient relax after the more difficult work segment. Again, tasks are presented in which the patient can respond with a higher level of accuracy (as in the warm-up segment). The final segment is the "good-bye segment" in which the clinician and patient are engaged in conversation, perhaps reviewing the day's activities and plans for the next session.

Facilitating Generalization

"Treatment of communication disorders should not be considered successful if the therapeutic changes achieved in the clinic do not transfer to the patient's daily life"[34](p 140). A number of procedures for facilitating generalization have been described and are currently being incorporated into many treatment studies for patients with neurologic communication disorders. Stokes and Baer[47] have noted that even though the literature shows many instances of generalization, it is still frequently observed that when a change in behavior has been accomplished through experimental contingencies, that change is manifest where and when these contingencies operate and is often seen only in transitory forms in other places and at other times. These authors describe several procedures for facilitating generalization, including (a) making use of natural maintaining contingencies (i.e., targeting behaviors that when they occur will elicit positive consequences in the patient's everyday life) (b) training sufficient exemplars, which may involve training the targeted behavior in many different settings so that the behavior will generalize to more than one setting, or training a class of responses, consisting of several representatives, as opposed to a single response; (c) loose training, which involves varying the stimuli used to elicit the targeted response, accepting a variety of predefined responses, and varying the nature and schedule of response contingencies (feedback); (d) using indiscriminable contingencies, which involves choosing contingencies similar to those expected in the patient's natural environment; and (e) programming common stimuli, which involves altering the context in which the targeted behavior is trained so that it resembles the context in which the behavior is generalized.

Treatment Efficacy

With the ongoing changes in our health care system, clinicians are being called on to demonstrate the effectiveness of their interventions with patients demonstrating neurologic communication disorders. Treatment efficacy is a general term that addresses a variety of questions relating to treatment effectiveness (i.e., does treatment work?), treatment efficiency (i.e., does one treatment work better than another?), and treatment effects (i.e., how does treatment change behavior?).[48] Efficacious treatment yields communicative improvements beyond those expected to result from spontaneous recovery.[35] The issue of treatment efficacy in neurologic communication disorders was recently addressed in a series of papers that reviewed and summarized the available scientific and clinical evidence.[35,49,50] Conclusions from these reviews were that there is currently a body of evidence, derived from group-treatment studies, single-subject studies, and case reports, supporting the effectiveness of speech and language intervention for aphasia, dysarthria, and specific cognitive deficits (e.g., attention, memory, executive functions) and of social skills training.

The usefulness of single-subject designs for documenting the effectiveness of interventions for individuals with neurologic communication disorders is well established.[51–54] Multiple-baseline designs are particularly well suited for intervention research because they are able to deal with one of the primary confounding variables in determining the effects of intervention: spontaneous recovery. Only by demonstrating greater improvement in a trained skill area than in a non-trained skill area can intervention effects be inferred. The multiple-baseline-across-behaviors design allows for this sequential intervention and evaluation.[55] Furthermore, use of multiple-baseline designs permit clinicians, in the context of a fee-for-service setting with high productivity expectations, to access the efficacy of their treatment and appropriately modify their interventions, online, without the need for additional clinical time or cost.[56]

Reimbursement Issues

Because financial and reimbursement issues have become increasingly important in terms of treatment and discharge planning, clinicians have had to become well versed in terms of how insurance companies review claims for speech–language pathology services. For example, according to Busch[57] when an intermediary (an insurance company under contract to Medicare in a particular state) receives a Medicare claim, it is reviewed at three levels. At the first level clerical employees make decisions regarding the number of visits or days of treatment coverable without review for different communicative disorder diagnosis on the basis of predetermined criteria. At the second level, experienced professionals, typically physical therapists or nurses who are trained to interpret and implement Medicare policy, review claims that are beyond the allowable criteria for number of visits. Coverage decisions are based on Medicare policy. If these reviewers are unsure about a coverage decision, the claim may be passed on to a third level, which in approximately 25 states is a speech–language pathologist, but also may be a nurse or physician. Coverage decisions at the second and third levels are based on Medicare policies[58] that include the following principles:

1. Services must be necessary to diagnose and treat communication disabilities and swallowing disorders and must be based on a specific written plan.
2. The following conditions must be met for the services to be considered reasonable and necessary:[58]

- The services must meet accepted standards of practice for specific and effective treatment for the diagnosis.
- The services must be of such complexity that requires the expertise of a qualified speech–language pathologist.
- There must be expectation of significant improvement in a reasonable time period, or the services must be necessary to establish a safe and effective maintenance program.
- The amount, frequency, and duration of services must be reasonable under accepted standards of practice.

In most instances inpatient speech–language pathology services for all patients are covered by insurance companies with minimal review. However, appropriateness of outpatient services for an individual with a neurologic communication disorder will depend on adequate documentation (i.e., for those insurance companies that cover outpatient speech–language pathology services). Careful documentation of medical history and assessment findings is critical.[57] Important information from the medical history includes pertinent medical and communicative disorders diagnosis, date of onset or of recent change, and description of the individual's level of communicative functioning prior to onset or change, and a summary of previous evaluations or treatment services from other speech–language pathology providers. Assessments are considered appropriate when they are reasonable and necessary to determine candidacy for treatment. Treatment candidacy is determined by medical history, baseline data derived from the assessment, and whether overall findings indicate rehabilitation potential. In the case of recent onset of the communicative disorder, at least a trial period of therapy is appropriate. If the communicative disorder is chronic, there must be adequate justification for initiating or reinitiating treatment services, such as a recent change in medical, communicative, or cognitive function. Coverage decisions are based on the timely submission of thorough documentation.[57]

For those individuals considered to be treatment candidates a plan of treatment must be developed. The plan should include the following: type and nature of treatment to be provided; functional goals and estimated rehabilitation potential; treatment objectives (short and long term); and frequency and estimated duration of treatment.[59] Medicare guidelines stress that the goals must be of a functional nature: "Functional goals must be

written by the speech–language pathologist to reflect the level of communicative independence the patient is expected to achieve outside of the therapeutic environment. The long term functional goals must reflect the final level the patient is expected to achieve, be realistic, and have a positive effect on the quality of the patient's everyday functions"—that is, on the individual's ability to "communicate basic physical needs and emotional states" and "carry out communicative interactions in the community"[60](pp. 4–487).

Rehabilitative services are covered only for improvement and making significant functional gains in communication. Progress that has been documented within the structured treatment tasks should be compared with and related to any changes in real-life communication activities. When there has been no generalization from the treatment setting to the individual's everyday environment coverage for treatment will be stopped. Establishment of a maintenance program, including providing education for the individual, family, and support staff, should be completed by the time treatment is completed.

SUMMARY

This chapter reviewed issues related to rehabilitation of individuals with neurologic communication disorders and stressed the importance of considering rehabilitation from the perspective of the World Health Organization's classification of handicap versus simply disability. The differences in patient management along the rehabilitation continuum of care were also discussed, as were the varied roles of the interdisciplinary team members. An overview of communicative interventions, including assessment, differential diagnosis, treatment and discharge planning, was presented, followed by a discussion of how these processes may vary depending on the setting or where along the rehabilitation continuum of care the individual happens to be. Reimbursement issues were also reviewed, specifically how insurance companies review claims for speech–language pathology services for neurologic communication disorders.

CASE ONE

A 45-year-old male, WC, was employed as a chemist in research and development with a pharmaceutical firm when he suffered a single thromboembolic stroke in the left hemisphere. CT scan revealed a lesion in the temporoparietal region. WC was initially hospitalized for one week in a large acute care hospital and then was transferred to an acute rehabilitation hospital. At approximately 10 days post-onset, he presented with a mild right-sided hemiparesis that affected his right arm and hand to a greater degree than his leg, and a moderate to severe fluent aphasia. Because he was ambulatory, his inpatient rehabilitation stay was limited to two weeks. At the family conference, which was held four days after his admission, the main concern voiced by his wife was how soon WC would be able to return to work. In as much as his physical limitations were minor, the primary disability was aphasia. It was decided that, in view of his relatively young age, his high level of motivation, strong family support, excellent insurance coverage for outpatient speech and language therapy, and an employer who wanted WC back at work whenever he was ready, he should be scheduled for an intensive outpatient speech and language rehabilitation program.

The speech and language intervention involved daily sessions (five days per week) consisting of one hour individual sessions, one hour group sessions, and two hours of independent work that included reading and writing drills and work on a computer. This routine continued for six months and was then reduced to three days per week, two days per week and eventually one day per week. As intervention was decreased at the hospital, independent activities at home were increased with the assistance of WC's wife, a brother, and friends. After approximately three months of therapy, the primary clinician contacted WC's employer (with WC's permission and that of his family) and arranged for a meeting to discuss the nature of WC's job responsibilities and whether a colleague could be recruited to be a coach for WC's eventual return to work. The employer was initially hesitant regarding having WC back at work in a lesser capacity than prior to his stroke. After ongoing discussions and some education, the employer identified a colleague from WC's section who was willing to help in any way he could to facilitate WC's return.

With the help of WC's colleague, treatment activities from that point on were tailored to working on job-related activities, including use of technical manuals for reading activities, as well as simulation of job assignments. Eventually, however, because these simulations were limiting, WC's employer was again approached about having WC return to work in a part-time, unpaid capacity as an assistant to his colleague. WC's employer agreed to this arrangement and WC worked initially two half-days a week and gradually increased to three full days per week. The advantage to this arrangement was that although the clinician was not permitted to come to the company to observe WC, his colleague and WC were able to report to the clinician all difficulties WC was having and these could then be addressed in therapy activities.

After approximately six months, WC had resumed many of his former responsibilities at work but continued to have certain aspects double-checked by his "coach." Once WC's employer was comfortable that WC could handle many aspects of his job despite his aphasia, WC continued to work part-time and undergo speech and language treatment for the next several months. At approximately three years post-onset WC was working full-time in a paid capacity. He continued to demonstrate a mild to moderate aphasia. At that time his primary complaint was the length of time it took him to write monthly projects summaries; otherwise he was content with his performance, as was his employer.

CASE TWO

A 25-year-old male, MD, was employed as a cabinet maker when the motorcycle he was driving was struck by a car. He was not wearing a helmet and suffered a severe closed head injury. On admission to an acute care hospital, MD was unconscious and CT scans revealed multiple bilateral cerebral contusions to the frontal, temporal, and occipital lobes. In addition he sustained numerous orthopedic and facial injuries and a collapsed lung. He remained comatose for approximately five weeks, and once he emerged from coma, he remained in a confused and agitated state (Rancho Los Amigos Level IV [61]) for nearly three months. MD eventually progressed to RLA Level V (confused-nonagitated) and remained at that level for nearly six months; he never progressed beyond RLA Level VI (confused-appropriate).

At approximately two months post-onset MD was transferred to a rehabilitation hospital where he remained for the next six months. On admission, cognitive-communicative assessment was difficult because of his agitation; however, with time it became apparent that he did not have dysphagia, dysarthria, or aphasia, but demonstrated cognitive-communicative deficits characterized by very severe deficits in all aspects of attention, memory, reasoning, problem solving, and executive functions. MD also demonstrated significant problems with balance, gait, and visual perception. Interdisciplinary treatment was initially focused on management of his agitation, while diagnostic therapy probed for cognitive abilities that could be used to develop compensatory strategies for circumventing MD's significant cognitive-communicative impairments. Over the course of a few weeks it was discovered that MD had enjoyed rock music and this was incorporated into treatment as a positive reinforcement. Once MD had passed through the agitated stage of his recovery, it was apparent that his communicative abilities were moderately limited. Conversational speech was characterized by frequent confabulations, poor topic management, and frequent disruptive topic shifts. Functional auditory comprehension was limited.

At approximately six months post-onset MD was discharged to the home of his mother, from whom he had been estranged since he dropped out of high school at the age of 16. MD's mother was obviously concerned about his well-being and took on his care and supervision. MD continued to come to the hospital for an outpatient interdisciplinary TBI day treatment program that met five days per week. Over the next six months MD demonstrated very little progress in the cognitive-communicative domains but grew steadily stronger and began a series of job trials within the hospital. His performance in these trails was poor but with moderate supervision he was able to complete tasks. Eventually, his former employer, a furniture maker, asked if MD could return to work with him. Although staff were not optimistic, a job trial was arranged for MD at his former job site. It soon became apparent that MD had no safety awareness in handling tools and was unable to complete even the most basic tasks, such as sweeping the workshop, because of distractibility. Although his employer wanted to keep him, MD's inappropriate social skills and disinhibition around customers finally lead to the employer's deciding that the arrangement was a failure.

At approximately two years post-onset MD's mother passed away. MD, who had continued with a modified day treatment program focusing on vocational and social skills training, was placed in a supervised apartment and began work in a sheltered workshop. At three years post-onset his status was essentially unchanged but he was being evaluated for more independent jobs in the workshop.

CASE THREE

A 69-year-old male with Parkinson's disease at the age of 59 was employed as a salesman and also ran a diner with his brother. Early in the course of the disease his primary limitations were physical, and

he had difficulty maintaining the long days he had managed for many years—opening the diner at 5:00 A.M., cooking until 7:30 A.M., then heading out for a full day of appointments as a paper goods salesman, and returning to the diner at 4:30 P.M. to work the supper shift. When he first sought assistance for his speech, he presented with mildly reduced breath support, weak phonation with decreased loudness and pitch variation, and mild articulatory distortions, all consistent with a mild hypokinetic dysarthria. Intervention at that point was focused on increasing respiratory/phonatory effort and education regarding his disease and the course of the dysarthria. This stage of intervention was for approximately two months and consisted of two sessions per week. RH made good use of these sessions, practiced activities at home, and was satisfied with the outcome. He was encouraged to return in approximately three months for a follow-up session.

RH was not seen again for nearly 18 months. At that time his speech was noted to have deteriorated significantly and regular intervention was again initiated. As before, the primary feature of RH's dysarthria was the respiratory-phonatory component with quite limited loudness and pitch variation. Articulatory accuracy was inconsistent and rigidity apparent in the jaw, along with a pronounced lingual weakness. A trial period of therapy indicated that increasing respiratory-phonatory forced helped overall intelligibility, but to a lesser degree than during the pervious therapy, and it appeared that RH needed more prompting to sustain this effort consistently. RH's physical condition had also suffered with the progression of his disease and he was no longer working. His wife reported that she was having more difficulty managing his physical needs at home and that she was getting regular assistance from RH's brother and neighbors. Additional family education was provided regarding prompting RH for increasing phonatory force and the potential usefulness of a vocal amplifier particularly for talking on the phone. It was recommended that RH return to the hospital for a follow-up in eight to ten weeks.

Approximately 12 months after the second course of treatment, RH was admitted to a veteran's home for permanent placement because his wife could no longer manage his physical needs at home. In that setting RH received regular PT for exercise and periodic speech therapy for his dysarthria. Over the next five years his speech continued to deteriorate and his attempts at speech were supplemented with various augmentative communication devices such as a letter/work board.

Most of the speech intervention was focused on training his caregivers to prompt his efforts at increasing phonatory effort, positioning RH in his bed or chair for maximum breath support, and questioning strategies when they could not understand what he was attempting to say. The most recent complication was the apparent onset of dementia, which was limiting his memory and retention session to session.

STUDY QUESTIONS

1. Distinguish between the World Health Organization's three levels for classifying the consequences of disease or disorder (impairment, disability, handicap).

2. What are the basic distinctions between the five levels described along the continuum of care for rehabilitation?

3. What distinguishes the services provided by an interdisciplinary rehabilitation team from those offered by a group of autonomous clinicians?

4. As discussed by Linebaugh, what could information obtained from a test of aphasia be used for?

5. Why is treatment planning viewed as the outcome of the assessment process?

6. Discuss ecologic validity with regard to assessment of neurologic communication disorders.

7. Why is it important to consider treatment context during the treatment planning process?

8. What are some factors that influence treatment planning for outpatients?

9. Describe the general categories of treatment management approaches discussed by Duffy.

10. What techniques may be used for measuring treatment effectiveness?

REFERENCES

1. Whyte J, Rosenthal M: Rehabilitation of the patient with head injury. In DeLisa JA, ed., *Rehabilitation: Principles and practice,* pp 246–259. J.P. Lippincott, Philadelphia, 1988.
2. World Health Organization International Classification of Impairment, Disabilities, and Handicaps. Geneva. 1980.
3. Finlayson MAJ, Garner SH: Challenges in rehabilitation of individuals with acquired brain inury. In Finlayson MAJ & Garner SH, eds., *Brain injury reha-*

bilitation: *Clinical considerations,* pp 3–10. Williams & Wilkins, Baltimore, 1994.
4. Kreutzer JS, Wehman P: *Community reintegration following traumatic brain injury.* Paul H. Brookes, Toronto, 1990.
5. Ylvisaker M, Gobble EM, eds: *Community re-entry for head injured adults.* Litte, Brown, Boston, 1988.
6. Belanger SA: Genral considerations for managing the aphasic patient in the acute medical setting. *Am Speech–Lang-Hear Assoc Div 2 Newsletter,* 1994; 4:2–5.
7. Caplan LR: *Stroke: A clinical approach.* Butterworth-Heinemann, Boston, 1993.
8. Cope DN, Hall KH: Head injury rehabilitation: Benefit of early intervention. *Arch Phys Med Rehab* 1982; 63:433–437.
9. MacKay LE, Bernstein, BA, Chapman PE, et al: Early intervention of severe head injury: Longterm benefits of a formalized program. *Arch Phys Med Rehab* 1992; 73, 635–641.
10. DePompei R, Blosser JL: Functional cognitive-communicative impairments in children and adolescents: Assessment and intervention. In Kreutzer JS & Wehman PH, eds., *Cognitive rehabilitation for persons with traumatic brain injury: A functional approach,* pp 215–236. Paul H. Brookes, Baltimore, 1991.
11. Kneipp S: Cognitive remediation within the context of a community re-entry program. In Kreutzer JS & Wehman PH, eds., *Cognitive rehabilitation for persons with traumatic brain injury: A functional approach,* pp. 239–250. Paul H. Brookes, Baltimore, 1991.
12. Story TB: Cognitive rehabilitation in home and community settings. In Kreutzer JS & Wehman PH, eds., *Cognitive rehabilitation for persons with traumatic brain injury: A functional approach,* pp 251–268. Paul H. Brookes, Baltimore, 1991.
13. Wehman PH: Cognitive rehabilitation in the workplace. In Kreutzer JS & Wehman PH, eds., *Cognitive rehabilitation for persons with traumatic brain injury: A functional approach,* pp 269–288. Paul H. Brookes, Baltimore, 1991.
14. Kimbarow ML: Interdisciplinary team intervention. In Chapey R, ed., *Language intervention strategies in adult aphasia,* pp 584–588. Williams and Wilkins, Baltimore, 1994.
15. Linebaugh CW: Assessing the assessments: The adequacy of standardized tests of aphasia. *Clin Aphasiol* 1979; 9:8–22.
16. Duffy JR: *Motor speech disorders: Substrates, differential diagnosis, and management.* Mosby, St. Louis, 1995.
17. Goodglass H, Kaplan E: The Boston diagnostic aphasia examination. Lea & Febiger, Philadelphia, 1972.
18. Holland AL: Communicative abilities in daily living. University Park Press, Baltimore, 1980.
19. Sarno MT: The functional communication profile: Manual of directions. (Rehabilitation Monograph 42). New York University Medical Center, Institute of Rehabilitation Medicine, New York, 1969.
20. Lomas J, Pickard L, Bester S, et al: The communicative effectiveness index: Development and psychometric evaluation of a functional communication

measure for adult aphasia. *J Speech Hear Disord* 1989; 54:113–124.

21. State University of New York at Buffalo: *Functional Independence Measure (FIM) (Uniform Data System for Medical Rehabilitation).* Buffalo, 1990.

22. Harvey R, Jellinek H: *Patient evaluation conference system (PECS).* Marianjoy Rehabilitation Center, Wheaton, IL, 1979.

23. Rancho Los Amigos Medical Center: *Rancho Rehabilitation Outcome Evaluation (RROE).* Downey, CA, 1993.

24. Heinemann A: *Rehabilitation Institute of Chicago Functional Assessment Scales (RIC-FAS).* Rehabilitation Institute of Chicago, Chicago, 1993.

25. Frattali C, Thompson CK, Holland A, et al: *Functional assessment of communication skills for adults (ASHA FACS).* American Speech–Language-Hearing Association, Rockville, MD, 1995.

26. Kertesz A: *Western aphasia battery.* Grune and Stratton, New York, 1982.

27. Porch BE: *Porch index of communicative ability.* Consulting Psychologists Press, Palo Alto, CA, 1981.

28. Bayles KA, Tomoeda C: *Arizona battery for communication disorders of dementia.* Canyonlands Publishing, Tucson, 1991.

29. Adamovich BLB, Henderson JA: *Scales of cognitive ability for traumatic brain injury.* Riverside Publishing, New York, 1992.

30. Yorkston KM, Beukelman DR: *Assessment of intelligibility of dysarthric speech.* C.C. Publications, Tigard, OR, 1981.

31. Giles GM: Functional assessment and intervention. In Finlayson MAJ & Garner SH, eds., *Brain injury rehabilitation: Clinical considerations,* pp. 124–156. Williams & Wilkins, Baltimore, 1994.

32. Starch S, Falltrick E: The importance of home evaluation for brain injured clients: A team approach. *Cog Rehab* 1990; 8:28–32.

33. Yorkston KM, Beukelman DR, Bell KR: *Clinical management of dysarthric speakers.* Little Brown, Boston, 1988.

34. Brookshire RH: *An introduction to neurogenic communication disorders.* Mosby-Year Book, St. Louis, 1992.

35. Holland AL, Fromm DS, DeRuyter F, et al: Treatment efficacy: Aphasia. *J Speech Hear Res* 1996; 39: S27–S36.

36. Sarno MT: Language rehabilitation outcome in the elderly aphasic patient. In Obler L & Albert M, eds., *Language and Communication in the Elderly,* pp 191–204. D.C. Health, Lexington, MA, 1980.

37. Wertz RT, Dronkers N: Effects of age on aphasia. Proceedings of the Research Symposium on Communication Sciences and Disorders and Aging (ASHA Reports 19, pp. 88–98). American Speech–Language-Hearing Association, Rockville, MD, 1990.

38. Holland AL, Bartlett C: Age and spontaneous recovery from asphasia. In Ulatowska H, ed. *The aging brain,* pp. 57–73. College Hill Press, San Diego, CA, 1985.

39. Horner J, LaPointe LL: Evaluation of learning potential of a severe aphasic adult through analysis of five performance variables. In Brookshire RH, ed., *Clinical aphasiology Conference Proceedings,* pp. 101–114. BRK, Minneapolis, 1979.

40. Rosenbek JC, LaPointe LL: The dysarthrias: description, diagnosis, and treatment. In Johns DF, ed., *Clinical management of neurogenic communication disorders.* Little Brown, Boston, 1985.

41. Klonoff P, O'Brien L, Prigatano G: Cognitive retraining after traumatic brain injury and its role in facilitating awareness. *J Head Trauma Rehab* 1989; 4: 37–45.

42. Lawson M, Rice D: Effects of training in use of executive strategies on a verbal memory problem resulting from closed head injury. *J Clin Exper Neuropsych* 1989; 11:842–854.

43. Singley M, Anderson JR: *The transfer of cognitive skill.* Harvard University Press, Cambridge, MA, 1989.

44. Elman RJ: Aphasia treatment planning in an outpatient medical rehabilitation center: Where do we go from here? *Amer Speech–Language-Hearing Assoc Div 2 Newsletter* 1994; 4:9–13.

45. Yorkston KM, Strand EA, Kennedy MRT: Comprehensibility of dysarthric speech: Implications for assessment and treatment planning. *Amer J Speech–Lang Path* 1996; 5:55–66.

46. Barefoot SM, Bochner JH, Johnson BA, et al: Rating deaf speakers' comprehensibility: An exploratory investigation. *Amer J Speech–Lang Path* 1993; 2: 31–35.

47. Stokes TF, Baer DM: An implied technology of generalization. *J Appl Behav Anal* 1977; 10:349–367.

48. Olswang LB: Treatment efficacy: The breadth of research. In Olswang LB, Thompson CK, Warren SF, et al., eds., *Treatment efficacy research in communication disorders.* American efficacy research in communication disorders American Speech–Language-Hearing Association, Rockville, MD, 1990.

49. Coelho CA, DeRuyter F, Stein M: Treatment efficacy: Cognitive-communicative disorders resulting from traumatic brain injury in adults. *J Speech Hear Res* 1996; 39:S5–S17.

50. Yorkston KM: Treatment efficacy: Dysarthria. *J Speech Hear Res* 1996; 39:S46–S57.

51. Kearns K: Response elaboration training for patient-initiated utterances. In Brookshire R, ed., *Clinical aphasiology Conference Proceedings,* pp. 196–204. BRK, Minneapolis, 1985.

52. Sohlberg MM, Mateer CA: Effectiveness of an attention training program. *J Clin Exper Neuropsych* 1987; 9: 117–130.

53. Whitney JL, Goldstein H: Using self-monitoring to reduce dysfluencies in speakers with mild aphasia. *J Speech Hear Dis* 1989; 54:576–586.

54. Thompson CK, Shapiro LP, Roberts MM: Treatment of sentence production deficits in aphasia: A linguistic-specific approach to Wh-interrogative training and generalization. *Aphasiology* 1993; 7:11–133.

55. Franzen MD, Harris CV: Neuropsychological rehabilitation: Application of a modified multiple baseline design. *Brain Inj* 1993; 7:525–534.

56. Sohlberg MM, Sprunk H, Metzelaar K: Efficacy of an external cueing system in an individual with severe frontal lobe damage. *Cog Rehab* 1988; 6:36–41.

57. Busch C: How is a treatment plan for an aphasic patient reviewed in terms of Medicare policy and guidelines? *Am Speech–Language-Hearing Assoc Div 2 Newsletter* 1994; 4:14–17.

58. Department of Health and Human Services, Health Care Finance Administration: *Medicare Part A: Intermediary Manual* (Transmittal No. 942). Washington, DC, 1981.

59. Department of Health and Human Services, Health Care Finance Administration: *Medicare Hospital Manual* (Transmittal No. 565). Washington, DC, 1989.

60. Department of Health and Human Services, Health Care Finance Administration: *Medicare Intermediary Manual* (Transmittal No. 1424). Washington, DC,1989.

61. Hagan C, Malkmus D, Burditt G: Levels of cognitive functioning. In *Rehabilitation of the head injured adult: Comprehensive physical management.* Professional Staff Association, Rancho Los Amigos Hospital, Downey, CA, 1979.

17

Neurogenic Communicative Disorders of Childhood

KEITH J. GOULDEN AND MEGAN HODGE

CHAPTER OUTLINE

Overview of Developmental Issues

Conditions Not Specific to Childhood

Conditions Unique to Childhood

The view is widely accepted that the course of speech and language development is a correlate of cerebral maturation and specialization.[1] Brain weight increases dramatically from about 3 months gestational age to 5 years postnatally, with continuing less rapid increases extending into adolescence and early adulthood.[2] There are two major differences between adult and pediatric neurogenic communicative disorders, both based on the fact that the brain and the behaviors that it controls develop during childhood. A brain injury of similar nature to that seen in adults (e.g., trauma, stroke, acquisition of HIV) will result in different communicative symptoms depending on the child's pre-morbid developmental stage. Thus, speech–language assessment and management for children must include developmental considerations as well as issues specific to the acquired brain injury. Other neurogenic conditions affecting communication present *only* in childhood as the brain develops. These can be infrequent and severe (e.g., autism, cerebral palsy, mental retardation, acquired epileptic aphasia, neurodegenerative disorders) or more frequent and less severe (e.g., specific language impairment,

language-based learning disabilities). Congenital or acquired impairment of special sense organs for hearing (and vision) may also affect communication, but a discussion of childhood sensorineural hearing impairment is beyond the scope of this chapter.

Table 17–1 provides examples of neurogenic conditions that may either present with a communication disorder or by definition are characterized by a communication disorder. These conditions are classified by whether they have their onset (1) any time during childhood or adulthood or (2) only during childhood. Those conditions in the second category may be present from birth (congenital) or acquired either during or following the primary period of speech–language development (up to 4 years). Child neurology textbooks[3–5] or specialized texts[1,6–8] provide descriptions of pathology, clinical manifestations, neurologic diagnoses, and medical treatments specific to each condition. The introductory chapter of several of these texts may offer an overview of the neurologic examination (history and physical) and neurodiagnostic procedures used with infants and children. It is of interest to note that prematurity/low birthweight is

Table 17–1. Examples of Neurogenic Conditions Associated with Communication Disorders Classified by Time of Onset

Congenital (Specific to childhood and present from birth)	Late Degenerative (Appearing after the primary period of communication development)	Acquired (Consider pre-morbid communication skills)
Impaired development of skill (in one or more areas)	*Ongoing loss of skill (may be in all or only some areas of development)*	*Acute loss of skill (with recovery to full or impaired developmental velocity)*
Specific language impairment	Juvenile Huntington's disease	Stroke
Autism/pervasive developmental disorder	Duchenne's muscular dystrophy	Traumatic brain injury
Cerebral palsy	Friedreich's ataxia	Acquired epileptic aphasia
Spina bifida/myelodysplasia	Mitochondrial disorders	Meningitis/encephalitis
Congenital infections	Leukodystrophies	Hypoxic/ischemic-encephelopathy
Intrauterine teratogen (e.g., FAS)		Brain tumors
Developmental apraxia of speech		Toxins: e.g., lead
Childhood suprabulbar paresis		
Various syndromes:		
Retts		
Williams		
Fragile X		

not included as a major causal condition for communication disorders, despite widespread concern about morbidity associated with it. This is because recent studies[9] show that prematurity is not a direct risk factor for abnormal language development; it acts rather via other biologic factors such as perinatal brain injury.

Like adults, children with neurogenic communication disorders are typically served by a team of health care professionals. In the medical setting, speech–language pathologists work closely with pediatricians as this medical specialty often represents the entry point into health care for children. Given their knowledge of disorders common to children, pediatricians also make referrals to other specialists such as developmental pediatricians, child neurologists, or physiatrists.

This chapter begins with an overview of developmental issues to consider when providing speech and language services to children with neurogenic communication disorders. Tracheostomy, stroke, and traumatic brain injury will then be briefly reviewed as examples of conditions that affect both adults and children and result in communicative disorders. Following this, conditions specific to childhood that may be encountered by speech–language pathologists working in acute care or rehabilitation hospitals and that have implications for long-term communicative functioning will be reviewed. These include: acquired epileptic aphasia (Landau-Kleffner syndrome); developmental language disorders (e.g., autism, specific language impairment); cerebral palsy (which can be associated with language and/or speech disorders); and developmental motor speech disorders (e.g., childhood suprabulbar palsy, Moebius syndrome, developmental apraxia of speech). Each condition will be reviewed with a focus on the manner in which the neurologic impairment influences communicative functioning. Suggested resources for speech and language assessment and treatment are provided for each neurologic condition where relevant.

OVERVIEW OF DEVELOPMENTAL ISSUES

Childhood is a time of great change, particularly in processes related to overall communication (e.g., sensory, perceptual, motor, cognitive, socioemotional) and more specifically to speech and language (linguistic) function. As a newborn the infant is presumed to have a brain capable of developing full adult function but demonstrates essentially no verbal communication output.[10] Receptively, newborns have a universal ability to discriminate verbal input, which is as yet unconstrained by the phonemic contrasts of their language environment.[11] During infancy the range of vocalizations that will be included in the child's later spoken language repertoire emerges, followed by words in the ambient language. The preschool period is marked by the acquisition of the rules of verbal and nonverbal communication (though these are not always followed). Elementary school children learn to communicate with each other under the guidance of adults, while adolescents achieve independent social communication in groups and then one on one. This entire process can be very variable, with familial, cultural, and individual patterns. Individual temperament, for example, can influence whether a child *approaches* a given social situation or *withdraws* from it, and will affect that child's language learning as a result.

Brain injury acquired during this complex developmental process will lead to both a loss of skill and limitations in further gains. Similar brain injuries will therefore look very different in children of differing ages. Even the division between "acquired" and "congenital" is arbitrary, as a prenatal "injury" may lead to dysgenesis or damage (or both) depending on timing.[12] Dysgenesis (faulty construction at a cellular level) of a critical brain area may not manifest until many years after birth, giving the impression of "acquisition" (particularly if onset of symptoms is tied to an "event" such as a seizure).

The assessment of developmental differences involves an understanding of the range of normal development, and cultural, familial, and individual influences. It also involves an understanding of the concepts of *delay*, *deviance*, and *dissociation*[13]; while children vary in their timing of skill acquisition, disorders are recognized by deviation from normal developmental patterns or by discrepant development in one skill area in comparison with others (dissociation). Although there is controversy over the meaning and importance of language *delay* (a temporal lag in otherwise typical development),[14] language *disorders* require both explanation and intervention.

An assessment of communication begins with a history or exploration of presenting complaints, usually by health nurses or primary physicians.[15] Screening for communication disorders can be performed informally in this way, or proceed more formally by using standardized instruments such as the Early Language Milestone Scale.[16] Hearing should always be assessed formally in children with communication delays or disorders. Further diagnostic assessment of communication abilities should take place for any child in whom a significant speech and/or language delay or disorder is present. Table 17–2 provides specific suggestions for speech–language assessment tools by developmental age and disorder. A list of assessment and treatment resources specifically for children with motor speech disorders appears in Appendix A. It is obviously important that evaluators use instruments that are appropriate and with which they are familiar and comfortable. They must recognize both the advantages and limitations of their chosen instruments, keeping in mind the necessity for meaningful outcome measures and evidence-based practice.

This chapter will review two situations relative to neurogenic conditions associated with communication disorders in childhood: those similar in nature to disorders seen in adults whose manifestations are different because of developmental considerations (e.g., stroke, traumatic brain injury); and those presenting uniquely in childhood (cerebral palsy, acquired epileptic aphasia, autism, specific language impairments, and several conditions characterized by developmental motor speech disorders) that are also seen in adults who have "grown up" with them. Both groups of conditions are relevant to practitioners seeing adults or children, since they involve life-long disabilities.

CONDITIONS NOT SPECIFIC TO CHILDHOOD

Tracheostomy

Acute neurogenic conditions in either children or adults may give rise to the need for a tracheostomy—an artificial opening between the cervical trachea and neck that permits passage of air in and out of the lungs for life-sustaining purposes and, when needed, mechanical ventilation. Bleile[17] provides an excellent overview of characteristics of children with long-term tracheostomy (in place greater than 28 days) and issues regarding their care. Children with tracheostomies have a serious communication disorder and require support for both oral and nonvocal communication so that their developmental needs can be met.[18]

Stroke in Childhood

Stroke is a relatively rare event in childhood, with an incidence of 2.7 per 100,000.[19] No definite etiology is found for one-third of children with

Table 17–2. Suggested Resources for Language Assessment in Children

Age Range (yrs)	Test Instrument
0–3	Rossetti Infant-Toddler Language Scale. LinguiSystems, East Moline, IL, 1990
0.8–2.6	MacArthur Communication Development Inventories. (Fenson L, Dale PS, Reznick JS et al) Psychol Corp, San Antonio, TX, 1993
0.4–4	Sequenced Inventory of Communicative Development—Revised (Hedrick D, Prather E, Tobin A). Western Psychol Serv, Los Angeles, CA, 1984
0–6.11	Preschool Language Scale—3 (Zimmerman I, Steiner V, Pond R). Psychol Corp, San Antonio, TX, 1992
0.8–2.0 (age equiv)	Communication and Symbolic Behavior Scales (Wetherby A, Prizant B). Riverside Publishing, Chicago, IL, 1993 (suspected autism)
3–6.11	Clinical Evaluation of Language Fundamentals—Preschool (Wiig EH, Secord W, Semel E). Psychol Corp, San Antonio, TX, 1992
1–6	Reynell Developmental Language Scales (Reynell JK, Gruber CP). Western Psychol Serv, Los Angeles, CA, 1990
3–Adult	Test for Auditory Comprehension of Language—Revised (Carrow-Woolfolk E). Pro-Ed, Austin, TX, 1985
5–16+	Clinical Evaluation of Language Fundamentals—Revised ((Semel E, Wiig EH, Secord W). Psychol Corp, San Antonio, TX, 1987
3–12	Token Test for Children (DiSimoni F). Pro-Ed, Austin, TX, 1978
5–18.11	Test of Language Competence—Expanded Edition (Wiig E, Secord W). Psychol Corp, San Antonio, TX, 1989
12–80	Test of Adolescent/Adult Word Finding (German DJ). Pro-Ed, Austin, TX, 1990

ischemic stroke,[20] while the remaining two-thirds with ischemic and most children with hemorrhagic stroke have an identifiable underlying cause. Some of these causes involve diseases recognized to be risk factors for stroke (such as sickle cell disease or childhood cancer), while others are only discovered by investigation following the event. Unless there is an underlying cause that contributes to the disability or leads to recurrent strokes, long-term prognosis is usually quite reasonable for overall functioning. On the other hand, the condition of "acute infantile hemiplegia"[21] involves an idiopathic middle cerebral artery stroke in early childhood, and leaves sequelae indistinguishable from congenital hemiplegic cerebral palsy.

In the initial period following a unilateral cerebrovascular event,[22] the child is usually mute, with a combined expressive and receptive aphasia. Recovery is usually rapid, with progress through a period of paraphasia and dysarthria. Even relatively minor sequelae can interfere in long-term learning, particularly given the acute onset of difficulties and previous lack of concern in this area.

These children require both acute assessment and long-term follow-up by a speech–language pathologist. The psychosocial aspects of children and families who have gone through a traumatic and (often) unexpected event can also lead to long-term negative consequences that need to be recognized and dealt with. The speech–language pathologist has a key role in educating family members, other health care providers, peers, and teachers about appropriate expectations for the child's language comprehension and production and in modeling appropriate communicative interaction techniques for significant others in the child's home, school, and other social environments, as well as in health care settings.

CASE ONE

Kim, a right-handed 3 year old, was playing with a friend when she suddenly fell to the ground. She was alert but not speaking, and she would not get up. On examination in the emergency room she had a flaccid right hemiparesis with hemianopsia (loss of right visual field), was mute and without apparent comprehension of verbal language, and had no gag reflex. Over the next few days, she had negative investigations for cardiac, hematologic, metabolic, and connective tissue diseases. On angiography, she was found to have a complete occlusion of the left middle cerebral artery.

During this time, she began to respond to verbal input, and developed some single word output, although many words were unintelligible or jargon. Throughout, she was very frightened and withdrawn, requiring the continuous presence of a parent to get through procedures or even daily care. Despite an aggressive "range of motion" program, she developed increasing spasticity of the right arm and leg, with involvement of the face. After 3 days she recovered sufficient oral—pharyngeal motor control to be fed carefully by mouth. A communication system was implemented using her parent for verbal input with head movements for yes/no and a pointing system (she was pre-literate), but this required considerable speech—language pathology input to help hospital staff to understand and use.

Two years later she has a mild right hemiparesis that has not changed her hand preference. She continues to have mild word-finding difficulties, and has had trouble establishing reading-readiness skills for kindergarten despite involvement in early education programming and speech—language pathology input to the family. Her speech is intelligible to familiar listeners in context, but is distorted and produced at a slower than normal rate. She remains overly dependent on her parent, with notable difficulty in novel situations (in contrast to her premorbid style).

Traumatic Brain Injury

Traumatic brain injury (TBI) is the major cause of death and disability in children.[23] Although it has previously been assumed that children are more resilient to TBI because of their age, more recent findings do not support this assumption. The young child may be at greater risk because the immature skull is thinner and has limited protective covering, brain myelinization is incomplete, and increased intracranial pressure causing secondary brain injury is more likely than in adults. The younger the child, the greater the long-term cognitive impairment (due to immature neuroanatomy and lack of previous learning). TBI in children may affect areas of the brain that are still developing, so deficits may not be evident for years afterward. Even relatively minor TBI in school-aged children may lead to difficulty with new learning.

A disproportionate number of children/adolescents with TBI have pre-injury disorders such as learning disabilities or behavior disturbance.[24] Like adults, processes that are important for communication such as motor function, cognition, attention, long- and short-term memory, organizational skills, reasoning, and problem solving, may be affected by TBI in childhood, but children are more likely to be involved in new learning. Deficits associated with TBI may interfere in family function or in the child's function within a group-learning environment (i.e., school). The transition from acute care to rehabilitation to the community requires careful planning, and communication is an important aspect of the child's ability to adapt to new environments. Because deficits may not emerge for many years after injury, the family requires ongoing support or access to future support services. There are several recent reviews of TBI in childhood, including Blosser & DePompei[24] and Lees.[25] References on TBI rehabilitation include in Ylvisaker[26] and Freund et al.[27]

CASE TWO

Tim, a 12 year old, was riding his bicycle across a city street when he was hit by a car. He was unconscious at the scene, and remained in a coma for 4 days. He had several fractures and lacerations, as well as brain swelling on CT scan but no focal hemorrhage. On transfer to the rehabilitation hospital 2 weeks after the event, he was awake with variable alertness and responsiveness. At worst, he would become quite agitated and aggressive, with screaming and flailing. His casts seemed to confuse and upset him. At best, he seemed interested in the speaker but unable to comprehend, with a lot of semipurposeful motor behavior and unintelligible jargon. He fatigued easily and therapy sessions had to be short.

Over the next three months he made a good recovery, with ability to function independently in the familiar setting. He remained confused by new situations or events, with a tendency to become perseverative or even aggressive when under pressure. His memory continued to be poor, but he was able to use external cues or prompts (if offered gently). His attention was quite short, but had been improved somewhat with a small dose of stimulant medication. Language assessment showed him to have significant difficulties with word finding and auditory-verbal processing. His family continued to hope for "full recovery," and had great difficulty adapting to Tim's behavior, particularly as he had been a quiet and polite boy before his TBI. Although his school was eager to have him back, staff had difficulty understanding his changed needs, and even more difficulty obtaining resources to meet them.

CONDITIONS UNIQUE TO CHILDHOOD

Acquired Epileptic Aphasia

The syndrome of acquired epileptic aphasia (AEA), also called the Landau-Kleffner syndrome, involves a loss of language skills in association with epilepsy.[28] Although temporary loss of language skills following a seizure is also possible, the diagnosis is reserved for those situations in which there is a progressive loss of receptive language over days to months.[29] The most usual language disorder that develops is a verbal-auditory agnosia (VAA) or "word deafness," in which phonologic decoding is the major deficit. There may also be regression in social skills, leading to a clinical picture indistinguishable from autism.[30] This is a rare disorder, but is of interest because it may be specifically treatable.

Untreated, the prognosis is more guarded than for other acquired aphasias: While the seizures (if present) and electroencephalogram (EEG) almost always return to normal, there are long-term language deficits in almost all affected children.[31] There is some evidence that treatment with anticonvulsants, steroids, or even seizure surgery[32] may improve language outcome,[33] so the pattern of progressive loss of language (with or without regression in other skills) is worth investigating with an EEG during sleep and neurologic assessment.

Lees[34] provides a list of speech and language tests in the areas of auditory-verbal comprehension, confrontation naming, association naming, short-term auditory verbal processing and memory, and expressive language for use in children with acquired aphasias. She also outlines a protocol for the study of children with acquired aphasias that would be applicable for children with AEA as well as stroke, TBI, or other causes.

CASE THREE

Jim is a 4-year-old boy who gradually stopped speaking over a period of several months. Some family stresses were occurring at the same time, but there was definitely no specific triggering event. Jim stopped responding to voice (even for his name), but continued to respond to the theme music of his favorite television shows, the doorbell when his father came over, babies crying, and so on. He had no

recognized seizure, and he remains socially interactive and interested. His audiogram is normal, but EEG show bitemporal epileptiform discharges, which become almost continuous during sleep.

Trials of various anticonvulsants and steroids were unsuccessful in making major improvement, but over the next few years he slowly improved in his communication skills. He uses a combination of sign and single word output and has developed a remarkable facility to read and write (copying but not dictation). He remains largely "word-deaf."

Developmental Language Disorders

Developmental language disorders (DLD) are disorders of language that arise during the developmental period, whether or not associated with neurologic deficits. DLD are sometimes called developmental dysphasias,[35] and this term may also include phonologic disorders (because it may be impossible to separate these in the first 18 months of life). Various definitions are used by different authors, ranging from the "narrow" definition of specific language impairment (see that section) to a much broader one that overlaps with developmental motor speech disorders. Using a definition that excludes isolated motor speech disorders, DLDs are still among the most common disabilities seen, with a prevalence in young children of 8[36] to 12%.[37] Follow-up studies suggest that there is a long-term risk for ongoing language disorder,[38] learning disability,[39,40] and/or psychiatric disorder (of the order of 50%[41,42]). Many adults, therefore, will manifest DLDs and their sequelae.

Autism

Pervasive developmental disorder or autism is a "high severity/low incidence" developmental language disorder involving both verbal and nonverbal social communication. It is more easily recognizable in the presence of stereotyped repetitive, ritualistic behavior and/or anxiety in novel situations. There is frequently an association with obsessive-compulsive disorder, sensory sensitivities, and/or mental retardation. The prevalence is around 1 per 1000[43], with an additional number having "high-functioning autism" or Asperger syndrome.[44]

A number of neurologic conditions may cause the functional impairment in communication recognized as autism, ranging from genetic conditions such as tuberous sclerosis to congenital infections such as rubella to metabolic disorders such as phenylketonuria.[45] It is now accepted that autism has a neurologic basis, and most children with autism will have identifiable brain damage or dysfunction.[46] Epilepsy is frequent in children with autism, although it is not clear whether the risk is increased because of the autism or other associated conditions.[47] A small number of children with autism have a history of regression in communication during the second year of life; of these, some will meet clinical or EEG criteria for acquired epileptic aphasia (and a trial of anticonvulsant treatment may be justified).

The Communication and Symbolic Behavior Scales (Wetherby and Prizant, see Table 17–2) is an example of an instrument developed specifically to assess young children with suspected autism. Although the "age range" is quite narrow (8 mo to 2 yrs), this is a developmental level, and the instrument is useful for many preschool children with autism. The use of videotape with this instrument greatly enhances its reliability and usefulness as a teaching tool for parents.

Apart from treatment of an underlying disorder such as phenylketonuria, or of associated conditions such as obsessive-compulsive disorder, there is no specific treatment for autism. The management of this life-long disability involves a combination of communication enhancement and behavior modification. Numerous communication enhancement strategies have been advocated, depending somewhat on the level of communicative function of the individual. Approximately 50% of children with autism will fail to develop useful spoken language, and will remain dependent on alternate strategies such as sign, picture-symbol, or caregiver inference from subtle behavioral cues.

Of the children with autism who will develop useful spoken language, all continue to have some differences in their language use. High-functioning individuals with fewer language difficulties may fit a description of "Asperger syndrome,"[44] which is probably continuous with the autistic spectrum of disorders. Apart from social interaction difficulties, these individuals have an all-absorbing narrow interest and some motor clumsiness. Their communication difficulties involve both nonverbal (social) impairments and "language usage" problems: pragmatics, prosody, semantics. Both assessment and communication enhancement should be provided in a social setting, using strategies such as "scripting" or role-playing. Such children can be taught "social reading,"[48] which may greatly enhance both their communication and socialization.

Because communication and social functioning are almost essential elements of adult life, children with even mild disabilities in these areas will have significant long-term problems. They may need support within education settings, particularly in higher education, which is less formally structured. These individuals may also need assistance with structure to function in the workplace or for independent living. Adults with language-usage disorders are at risk for misunderstanding and psychiatric sequelae, and helping their colleagues to understand their disability may minimize these problems.

CASE FOUR

Sim is an 8-year-old boy referred for assessment of "attention problems." He had a speech–language assessment at age 3 because of delayed expressive language development and had been noted to be "somewhat odd and perseverative" during that assessment. He had speech–language therapy via an early education program for two years at preschool, but had developed sufficient expressive output by school entry to be discharged from speech–language pathology services. He is recognized by his parents and teacher to have persistent difficulties in language use, with problems in turn-taking and perseveration on certain topics (e.g., he loved to talk about dinosaurs). He has no friends, and gets along poorly at recess time. He has a number of abnormal sensory sensitivities—for example, he is upset by certain musical styles but attracted to others. He is also quite upset by novelty and has a very narrow range of preferred activities, foods, and so on. His attention was "over-focused" on certain activities, but very poor for verbal interactions unless he was allowed to talk about dinosaurs. Even a discussion on this topic was not interactive: He appeared to misunderstand specific "wh–questions," with some word-finding difficulties (despite knowing the scientific names of all the dinosaurs). Sim was judged by the team that assessed him to have atypical autism with normal cognitive function. Further communication enhancement was recommended following speech–language assessment in the classroom setting.

Specific Language Impairments

Specific language impairments (SLI) have been defined as "delayed acquisition of language skills, occurring in conjunction with normal functioning in intellectual, social-emotional, and auditory domains and without evidence of frank neurologic deficits or severe articulation/phonological deficits."[49] There is considerable diversity in the extent of linguistic impairment, range of linguistic subsystems (semantics, syntax, pragmatics, phonology) involved, and in modality (receptive and/or expressive) involved. SLI is a diagnosis of exclusion: It implies the absence of another identifiable cause for the child's communication difficulties. (This is somewhat arbitrary, however, since VAA of early onset is called "developmental" and is therefore classified as a SLI, while later onset would be recognized as an acquired aphasia; see AEA above.)

Because "normal" development of communication may have a wide range, the identification of a disorder requires either the presence of deviance in language use or a clear dissociation between verbal and nonverbal skills. A variety of classifications for SLI exist, with general recognition that there is an isolated expressive language disorder (sometimes associated with phonological or fluency problems) and a mixed receptive and expressive language disorder[50] (often associated with phonological, fluency, and other coordination difficulties). Theoretically, an isolated receptive language/comprehension disorder is also possible (as seen in adult aphasia[51] or other models[52]), but because these are developmental disabilities, children with "isolated" receptive problems will also have at least a delay in expressive skills (and usually a disorder as well).

The differentiation of speech disorders from language disorders may be difficult, but is important because of the difference in outcome[53] (phonologic competence alone does not predict outcome, but language competence does). There is controversy about the cost effectiveness of intervention, particularly for "language delay" or phonologic disorders.[54] Interventions that address behavioral issues or are aimed at the child with severe impairment are more easily justified. The long-term negative outcomes for SLI in learning and behavior, however, would suggest that intervention has significant potential for benefit (even if this cannot immediately be measured).

Cerebral Palsy

Cerebral palsy (CP) is defined as a group of nonprogressive disorders of movement or posture due to a defect or lesion of the developing brain.[55] The prevalence ranges from 2 to 3 per 1000 live births,[56] but there is a wide range of severity of CP, and of the type of limitation in function seen. Communication disorders in children with CP include developmental language disorders (such as autism or a more "specific" disorder), developmental motor

speech disorders, or a combination of both. Although there has been great interest in the complications of prematurity and/or perinatal asphyxia as causes of CP, these problems represent only a very small proportion of the total.[27]

Children with spastic tetraplegia have involvement of all limbs, with increased tone, decreased strength, and limited range of motion. This is the most extensive type of CP, although there is still a wide range in severity of impairment between children with the same condition. Frequently, there is involvement of the oromotor apparatus—for example, a "suprabulbar paresis" resulting in feeding difficulties, drooling, or dysarthria. Such children may also have either cognitive impairment or language disorder because of their extensive brain injury/dysgenesis, so it may be difficult to sort out the relative contribution of multiple disabilities. As children with CP are also at risk for visual and hearing impairment, there may be additional contributing disabilities.

Spastic hemiplegia involves the arm and leg on one side of the body, following pre- peri-, or early post-natal injury to the opposite cerebral hemisphere. Children with spastic hemiplegia involving their dominant hemisphere may have subtle language disorders, but these are not nearly as significant as those seen in children with acquired hemiplegia of later onset (after age 18 mo to 2 yrs). The brain is sufficiently "plastic" at this early age that language usually develops in the opposite hemisphere. These children do not have major oromotor problems either.

Children with the (now much less prevalent) problems of movement control involved in dyskinetic cerebral palsies (athetoid, choreiform, or dystonic) often have difficulties in oromotor control.[57] The type of speech difficulty depends somewhat on the global movement disorder.

Assessment of communication in children with CP involves distinguishing disabilities due to motor function from disabilities directly caused by the underlying brain injury (i.e., cognitive-linguistic). It also involves recognition of other contributing disabilities such as hearing or visual impairments. Frequently, they all are present to some degree. The management of these disabilities is life-long, and has as its focus the optimization of functioning. This is accomplished either by improving the function of specific systems or by avoiding the impact of disability in that system by alternate strategies.

The management of CP is a multidisciplinary process, with interdependence of those disciplines: for example, an augmented communication system designed to minimize the motor disability is dependent on the ambulation system, as the person must "free-up" motor systems from ambulation to use them for communication. Fatigue is an important factor in the functioning of individuals with motor impairment, particularly as they become older. Abnormal drooling is a symptom that is socially quite undesirable, and can be very difficult to manage.[58] New technology offers major opportunities for improving the functional outcome for children with even quite severe motor impairment, particularly in the area of communication.[59,60]

CASE FIVE

Lim is a 6-year-old girl with severe spastic tetraplegic CP who is totally dependent for ambulation on an adapted stroller (her family has not wanted her in a wheelchair). She has reasonable receptive abilities but is severely dysarthric. She is fed by gastrostomy tube and drools continuously. At school and at home, she uses a picture board to identify a range of meaningful ideas, including food preferences, yes/no, preferred companions or activities, and so on. The use of electronic communication devices has been limited because of family income (they do not qualify for assistance but cannot afford a home computer), her drooling (this is particularly an issue at school), and her positioning: She needs to sit forward to access a keyboard. The physical rehabilitation team has been working with the family to help them understand the advantages to Lim of having a wheelchair (better physical position to minimize deformity and access communication devices, potential for independent [motor] operation), but also the costs (financial, emotional: acceptance of long-term nature of Lim's severe disability and realization that ambulatory and communicative independence will allow "normal" childhood separation from parents).

Developmental Motor Speech Disorders

Developmental motor speech disorders are secondary to diagnosed or suspected nervous system [central (CNS) or peripheral (PNS)] or neuromuscular damage, either congenital or acquired during the primary period of speech development (preschool years). They may be manifested as:

1. Weakness, slowness, and reduced movement, accuracy and coordination of speech mechanism components, when primary cortical motor areas and subcortical motor systems are involved (childhood dysarthrias).
2. A speech motor learning disability, when speech motor cortical association centers are involved (i.e., developmental apraxia of speech [DAS]).
3. A combination of DAS and dysarthric characteristics (mixed developmental motor speech disorder).

In the United States, the incidence of dysarthria among children is estimated to be 1 to 2 per 1000,[61] with a 3 to 5% prevalence of speech delay associated with DAS among children referred for assessment of phonologic disorders.[62]

Childhood motor speech disorders are associated with a variety of neurological conditions such as CP, genetic syndromes, neuromuscular disorders, acquired brain injuries, or brain dysgenesis. The resultant speech disability is characterized by reduction in the rate and quality of speech development, the frequency of speech use, and the intelligibility, acceptability, and efficiency of speech production. The severity of the speech disability can range from mild (imprecise speech produced at slightly slower than normal rate) to profound (no functional speech). Some children with motor speech disorders have no other apparent neurologic impairment with intact ability to understand spoken language, while others have one or more additional impairments of motor, sensory, cognitive, or receptive language abilities. The degree of speech disability, the child's expected communication roles, and the attitudes of significant others all interact to determine the degree of handicap that the child suffers as a result of a motor speech disorder.[63]

Developmental motor speech disorders may occur as an isolated communication disorder or in conjunction with language delays or disorders. Early differential diagnosis is complicated by limited speech output. If no multiword utterances are present, then voice, resonance, prosody, and fluency are difficult to assess. As more speech is produced, additional impairments may be identified. Neurologic damage affecting speech motor control typically delays speech development; it is also expressed in specific disturbances of motor planning, programming, and/or execution. In many cases it is difficult to differentiate sensorimotor immaturity from neuromotor impairment, and motor planning or programming impairments from motor execution impairments. All are involved in speech motor learning. The diagnosis of developmental apraxia of speech cannot be made until the child is at least 3.5 to 4 years old.[64] It may be advisable to describe the profile of the child's speech mechanism impairment and speech behaviors and label the condition as a "developmental motor speech disorder" or "suspected developmental motor speech disorder"[65] until sufficient information can be obtained to make a more specific diagnosis. This category is particularly recommended where signs of slowness, weakness, movement inaccuracies, reduced postural control, tone abnormalities, or reduced coordination in the oral-articulatory, laryngeal, velopharyngeal, and/or respiratory musculature are observed, and these signs cannot be explained by immature motor development alone.

Childhood Dysarthrias

Cerebral palsy (discussed previously) is the most frequent neurologic condition in childhood that is associated with dysarthria, where deficits in speech motor control are reflected in more global motor control deficits. In contrast, "childhood suprabulbar paresis"[1] also called Worster-Drought syndrome[66] is characterized by congenital, isolated paresis of the oral musculature without major signs in the trunk or extremities. The corticobulbar fibers to one or more of the facial, velopharyngeal, laryngeal, and/or lingual musculature are affected, resulting in articulation errors, hypernasality, dysphonia, and other signs of oral motor problems such as dysphagia and drooling.

Möbius' syndrome is an example of a condition affecting communication development where there are specific disturbances in cranial nerve function due to agenesis or hypogenesis of selected cranial nerve nuclei and/or their efferent fibers. In this case the abducens (VI) and facial (VII) nerves are involved by definition, and there may be variable involvement of other cranial nerves. Bilateral facial paresis adversely affects labial articulation and facial expression for affective communication. The reduced lip function may also affect growth of dental structures and tongue posture/function. The syndrome presents with an expressionless face and dysarthria, but there may be additional disabilities secondary to acquired hypoxic brain injury or associated brain dysgenesis.

CASE SIX

Mim is a 6-year-old female diagnosed shortly after birth with a facial diplegia and bilateral abducens palsy (i.e., Möbius' syndrome). She had feeding difficulties in early infancy, but has learned to compensate for her incomplete lip closure. She still uses a tongue thrust swallowing pattern.[67] She has an associated mild sensorineural hearing loss bilaterally, which is treated with amplification. She has significant orthodontic problems, with an open bite and anterior tongue position. She has ongoing difficulties with speech intelligibility, although language function is judged to be normal. She recently underwent facial reanimation surgery,[68] in which a muscle is implanted into the face with neural attachment to another motor cranial nerve, and now requires intensive speech therapy to take advantage of her mildly improved (and quite unphysiologic) facial movements for social communication purposes. Her parents have also required significant support to carry them through the decision-making process around the surgery, and to help the family deal with the long-term implications of this visibly disfiguring disability.

Developmental Apraxia of Speech

Developmental apraxia of speech (DAS) is characterized by a limited speech sound repertoire and difficulty in volitional positioning of the articulators to initiate and sequence speech sounds in the absence of neuromuscular or sensory deficits.[64,69,70,71] Language comprehension skills are significantly better than speech production skills. The diagnosis of DAS is made by exclusion of "childhood dysarthrias" (i.e., "in the absence of obvious disturbance of the speech mechanism"[72]), although a group with mixed symptoms of both disorders exists. Hayden[64] described a protocol to differentially diagnose childhood motor speech disorders into four categories, those owing to 1) global motor involvement, 2) specific oromotor involvement (childhood suprabulbar paresis would be an example), 3) oral and speech sequencing disability (DAS), and 4) phonological disorder. According to Hayden's model, to be assigned to the DAS category, speech movement sequencing disruptions must occur in the absence of sensory, cognitive and language disruptions. If speech movement sequencing problems occur in conjunction with global or specific oromotor involvement, the child would be diagnosed with dysarthria rather than DAS. Children with characteristics of DAS may also exhibit an oral or buccofacial apraxia/dyspraxia characterized by reduced ability to volitionally position the articulators for nonspeech movements. Children with motor speech disorders resulting from acquired brain injury, for example, often show characteristics of both apraxia of speech and dysarthria.

Assessment and Treatment

The assessment of children with motor speech disorders includes information about the structure and function of the child's speech mechanism (for both speech and non-speech tasks); their articulatory ability, phonetic repertoire, and phonological system; their speech intelligibility, rate, and prosody, and non-speech communication behaviors in both structured and spontaneous speech tasks;[74,75] their metaphonological skills; and an estimate of the handicapping effect of their speech disorder on their day-to-day social interactions.[65,76]

Treatment approaches for childhood motor speech disorders include:

1. Augmentative communication modes (e.g., gestures and sign, picture, or alphabet boards).[77]
2. Behavioral training to develop consistent skills in producing a basic repertoire of speech movements and combining these in sequences to communicate meaning in contexts that facilitate semantic, grammatical, syntactical, and pragmatic aspects of expressive language and includes auditory-perceptual training if indicated.[66,78,79,80] If needed, work on increasing strength and/or postural and movement control of articulators is incorporated in this training (e.g., tongue placement and mobility exercises) in a way that complements speech training activities.[72,81,82]
3. Compensatory strategies to increase speech intelligibility (e.g., rate control,[83] "silent" rehearsal of phonetically complex words, self-cueing techniques). "Intelligibility drill" activities may be useful here, such as barrier games and so on where a response is contingent on understanding the message.
4. Maximizing speech acceptability through behavioral training to minimize prosodic, laryngeal and resonance abnormalities. (Computer training systems such as IBM's SpeechViewer III can be very useful when working on prosody.)
5. Counseling and educating the child, caregivers, and frequent communication partners about how to communicate effectively, increase the frequency of communicative interactions, and decrease the frequency of communication breakdowns.
6. Developing phonological awareness and metaphonological skills in analyzing spoken and written language.
7. Increasing the child's self-esteem and self-confidence in communicating.

As with other neurogenic communicative disorders of childhood, team management for children with develomental motor speech disorders is essential.[84] Examples of published assessment and treatment tools useful for children with motor speech disorders are provided in Appendix A.

SUMMARY

Children with neurogenic communication disorders may have similar problems to adults, but they manifest themselves differently because of the developmental tasks of childhood,[85] or may have conditions unique to childhood. Because children grow up to become adults, these disorders are of importance whether or not one's practice involves children directly. Childhood communication disorders may continue to present similar problems in adulthood (e.g., the older person with autism or acquired aphasia may continue to have a significant need for communication enhancement), or they may present more complex problems because of secondary overlay. For example, 28% of a group of preadolescents referred for psychiatric assessment had a previously undiagnosed language disorder,[86] and no doubt a similar or greater proportion of adult psychiatric patients would be found to have language disorders. Children with learning disabilities become adults with learning disabilities, who may be less obvious because of their ability to avoid structured learning situations (most of the time). Many of the adult clients seen for speech therapy following a stroke or head injury have a history of childhood communication disorder (epidemiology predicts 8 to 12%). The potential impact of pre-injury communication deficits on these adults' response to therapy post-injury should not be overlooked.

STUDY QUESTIONS

1. In developmental motor speech disorders, what are the critical factors for consideration by the diagnostician?

2. What is a "typical" course of recovery in a child who has sustained a stroke?

3. What are the reasons that a young child is at greater risk than older children for serious sequellae to traumatic brain injury?

4. Describe the characteristics of the Landau-Kleffner syndrome.

5. How is a diagnosis of specific language impairment made?

6. What is the pathophysiology and symtomatology of Möbius' syndrome?

7. Explain the various treatment options for children with motor speech disorders.

REFERENCES

1. Love RJ, Webb W: *Neurology for the speech language pathologist,* 2nd ed. Butterworth-Heinemann, Boston, 1992.
2. Capone GT: Human brain development. In Capute AJ, Accardo PJ: *Developmental disabilities in infancy and childhood,* 2nd ed., pp 25–75. Paul H Brookes, Baltimore, 1996.
3. Menkes JH: *Textbook of child neurology,* 5th ed. Williams & Wilkins, Baltimore, 1995.
4. Aicardi J: Diseases of the nervous system in childhood. *Clin Dev Med No.* 115/118. Cambridge University Press, New York, 1992.
5. Fenichel GM: *Clinical pediatric neurology: A signs and symptoms approach,* 2nd ed., W.B. Saunders, Philadelphia, 1993.
6. Molnar GE: *Pediatric rehabilitation,* 2nd ed. Williams & Wilkins, Baltimore, 1992.
7. Njiokiktjien C: *Pediatric behavioural neurology, Vol 1: Clinical principles.* Suyi Publ, Amsterdam, 1988.
8. Darby JK, ed: *Speech and language evaluation in neurology: Childhood disorders.* Allyn and Bacon, Boston, 1985.
9. Menyuk P, Liebergott JW, Schultz M: *Early language development in full-term and premature infants.* Lawrence Erlbaum, Hillsdale, NJ, 1995.
10. Kent R, Hodge M: The biogenesis of speech: Continuity and process in early speech and language development. In Miller J, ed: *Research on child language disorders: A decade of progress,* pp 25–53. Pro-Ed, Austin, TX, 1991.
11. Best C: The emergence of native-language phonological influences in infants: A perceptual assimilation model. In Goodman JC, Nusbaum HC, eds., *The development of speech perception,* pp 167–224. MIT Press, Cambridge, MA, 1994.
12. Sarnat HB: Cerebral dysplasias as expressions of altered maturational processes. *Can J Neurol Sci* 1991; 18:196–204.
13. Capute AJ, Accardo PJ: A neurodevelopmental perspective on the continuum of developmental disabilities. In Capute AJ, Accardo PJ: *Developmental disabilities in infancy and childhood,* 2nd ed. Vol I, pp 1–22. Paul H Brookes, Baltimore, 1996.
14. Whitehurst GJ, Fischel JE: Practitioner review: Early developmental language delay: What, if anything,
15. should the clinician do about it? *J Child Psychol Psychiatr* 1994; 35:613–648.
15. Klein SK: Evaluation for suspected language disorders in preschool children. *Pediatr Clin N Amer* 1991; 38: 1455–1467.
16. Coplan J: *Early language milestone scale,* 2nd ed. Pro-Ed, Austin, TX, 1993.
17. Bleile K, ed: *The care of children with long term tracheostomies.* Singular Publishing Group, San Diego, CA, 1993.
18. McGowan J, Bleile K, Fus L, Barnas E: Communication disorders. In Bliele K, ed: *The care of children with long term tracheostomies,* pp 113–140. Singular Publishing Group, San Diego, CA, 1993.
19. Broderick J, Talbot A, Prenger E, et al: Stroke in children within a major metropolitan area: The surprising importance of intracerebral hemorrhage. *J Child Neurol* 1993; 8:250–255.
20. Roach ES: Cerebrovascular disorders and trauma in children. *Curr Opin Pediatr* 1993; 5:660–668.
21. Aicardi J, Amsili J, Chevrie JJ: Acute hemiplegia in infancy and childhood. *Dev Med Child Neurol* 1969; 11:162–173.
22. Lees JA: Unilateral cerebral lesions of vascular origin. In Lees JA: *Children with acquired aphasias,* pp 25–43. Singular Publishing Group, San Diego, CA, 1993.
23. Schoenbrodt L, Smith R: *Communication disorders and interventions in low incidence pediatric populations.* Singular Publishing Group, San Diego, CA, 1995.
24. Blosser JL, DePompei R: *Pediatric traumatic brain injury: Proactive intervention.* Singular Publishing Group, San Diego, CA, 1994.
25. Lees JA: Head injury. In Lees JA: *Children with acquired aphasias,* pp 44–63. Singular Publishing Group, San Diego, CA, 1993.
26. Ylvisaker M, ed: *Head injury rehabilitation: Children and adults.* College-Hill Press, Boston, MA, 1985.
27. Freund J, Hayter C, MacDonald S, et al: *Cognitive-communication disorders following traumatic brain injury: A practical guide.* Communication Skill Builders, Tucson, AZ, 1995.
28. Gordon N: Acquired aphasia on childhood: The Landau-Kleffner syndrome. *Dev Med Child Neurol* 1990; 32:267–274.
29. Lees JA: Landau-Kleffner syndrome: In Lees JA: *Children with acquired aphasias,* pp 79–98. Singular Publishing, San Diego, CA, 1993.
30. Roulet-Perez E, Davidoff V, Despland PA, Deonna T: Mental and behavioural deterioration of children with epilepsy and CSWS: Acquired epileptic frontal syndrome. *Dev Med Child Neurol* 1993; 35:661–674.
31. Soprano A, Garcia EF, Caraballo R, Fejerman N: Acquired epileptic aphasia: Neuropsychologic follow-up of 12 patients. *Pediatr Neurol* 1994; 11:230–235.
32. Morrell F, Whisler WW, Bleck TP: Multiple subpial transection: A new approach to the surgical treatment of focal epilepsy. *J Neurosurg* 1989; 70:231–239.
33. Zardini G, Molteni B, Nardocci N, et al: Linguistic development in a patient with Landau-Kleffner syndrome: A nine-year follow-up. *Neuropediatr* 1995; 26:19–25.

34. Lees JA: *Children with acquired aphasias.* Singular Publishing, San Diego, CA, 1993.

35. Njiokiktjien C: Developmental dysphasia. In Njiokiktjien C: *Pediatric behavioural neurology, Vol 1: Clinical principles,* pp 286–310. Suyi Publ, Amsterdam, 1988.

36. Silva PA: The prevalence, stability and significance of developmental language delay in preschool children. *Dev Med Child Neurol* 1980; 22:768–777.

37. Beitchman JH, Nair R, Clegg M, Patel PG: Prevalence of speech and language disorders in 5-year-old kindergarten children in the Ottawa-Carleton region. *J Speech Hearing Disord* 1986; 51:98–110.

38. Tomblin JB, Freese PR, Records NL: Diagnosing specific language impairment in adults for the purpose of pedigree analysis. *J Speech Hearing Res* 1992; 35:832–843.

39. Pennington BF: Dyslexia and other developmental language disorders. In Pennington BF: *Diagnosing learning disabilities: A neuropsychologic framework,* pp 45–81. Guilford Press, New York, 1991.

40. Catts HW: The relationship between speech–language impairments and reading disabilities. *J Speech Hearing Res* 1993; 36:948–958.

41. Beitchman JH, Nair R, Clegg M, et al: Prevalence of psychiatric disorders in children with speech and language disorders. *J Am Acad Child Psychiatr* 1986; 25:528–535.

42. Baker L, Cantwell DP: A prospective follow-up of children with speech/language disorders. *J Am Acad Child Adol Psychiatr* 1987; 26:546–553.

43. Wing L: The definition and prevalence of autism: A review. *Eur Child Adol Psychiatr* 1993; 2:1–14.

44. Gillberg IC, Gillberg C: Asperger syndrome—Some epidemiological considerations: A research note. *J Child Psychol Psychiatr* 1989; 30:631–638.

45. Gillberg C, Coleman M: *The biology of the autistic syndromes,* 2nd ed. Clin Devp Med No. 126. Cambridge University Press, New York, 1992.

46. Steffenburg S: Neuropsychiatric assessment of children with autism: A population-based study. *Dev Med Child Neurol* 1991; 33:495–511.

47. Tuchman RF, Rapin I, Shinnar S: Autistic and dysphasic children. II: Epilepsy. *Pediatrics* 1991; 88:1219–1225.

48. Gray CA: Teaching children with autism to "read" social situations. In Quill KA: *Teaching children with autism: Strategies to enhance communication and socialization.* Delmar Publishers, New York, 1995.

49. Watkins R: Specific language impairments in children: An introduction. In Watkins R, Rice M, eds., *Specific language impairments in children,* pp 1–15. Paul H Brookes, Baltimore, 1994.

50. Task Force on DSM-IV: *Diagnostic and statistical manual of mental disorders,* 4th ed., pp 55–61. American Psychiatric Association, Washington, DC, 1994.

51. Rapin I, Allen DA: Syndromes in developmental dysphasia and adult aphasia. In Plum F, ed., *Language, communication and the brain,* pp 57–75. Raven Press, New York, 1988.

52. Korkman M, Hakkinen-Rihu P: A new classification of developmental language disorders (DLD). *Brain & Lang* 1994; 47:96–116.

53. Bishop DV, Edmundson A: Language impaired 4 year olds: Distinguishing transient from persistent impairment. *J Speech Hearing Disord* 1987; 52:156–173.

54. Whitehurst GJ, Fischel JE: Practitioner review: Early developmental language delay: What, if anything, should the clinician do about it? *J Child Psychol Psychiatr* 1994; 35:613–648.

55. Bax M: Terminology and classification of cerebral palsy. *Dev Med Child Neurol* 1964; 6:295–307.

56. Stanley FJ, Blair E: Cerebral palsy. In Pless IB, *The epidemiology of childhood disorders,* pp 473–497. Oxford University Press, New York, 1994.

57. Molnar GE: Cerebral palsy. In Molnar GE, *Pediatric rehabilitation,* 2nd ed., pp 481–533. Williams & Wilkins, Baltimore, 1992.

58. Blasco PA, Allaire JH, participants of the Consortium on Drooling: Drooling in the developmentally disabled: Management practices and recommendations. *Dev Med Child Neurol* 1992; 34:849–862.

59. Beukelman D, Mirenda P: *Augmentative and alternative communication: Management of severe communication disorders in children and adults.* Paul H Brookes, Baltimore, 1992.

60. Goosens C: Aided communication intervention before assessment: A case study of a child with cerebral palsy. *Augmentative Alternative Communication* 1989; 5:14–26.

61. Ad Hoc Committee on Communication Processes and Nonspeaking Persons: Nonspeech communication: A position paper. *ASHA* 1980; 22:267–272.

62. Shriberg, LD: Five subtypes of developmental phonological disorders. *Clin Commun Disord* 1994; 4:38–53.

63. Hodge M, Hancock H: Assessment of developmental apraxia of speech: A procedure. *Clin Commun Disord* 1994; 4:102–118.

64. Hayden D: Differential diagnosis of motor speech dysfunction in children. *Clin Commun Disord* 1994; 4:119–141.

65. Crary M: Clinical evaluation of developmental motor speech disorders. *Semin Speech Lang* 1995; 16(2):110–125.

66. Crary M: *Developmental motor speech disorders.* Singular Publishing Group, San Diego, 1993.

67. Hanson M, Barrett R: *Fundamentals of orofacial myology.* Charles C Thomas, Springfield, IL, 1988.

68. Zuker RM, Manktelow RT: A smile for the Moebius' syndrome patient. *Ann Plast Surg* 1989; 22:188–194.

69. Hall P, Jordan L, Robin D: *Developmental apraxia of speech: theory and clinical practice.* Pro-Ed, Austin, TX, 1993.

70. Marquardt T, Sussman H: Developmental apraxia of speech: theory and practice. in Vogel D, Cannito M (eds): *Treating disordered motor control: for clinicians by clinicians,* pp. 341–390. Pro-Ed, Austin, TX, 1991.

71. Hodge M: Assessment of developmental apraxia of speech: A rationale. *Clin Commun Disord* 1994; 4:91–101.

72. Love RJ: *Childhood motor speech disability.* Maxwell Macmillan Canada Toronto, 1992.

73. Hodge M: Assessing early speech motor function. *Clin Commun Disord* 1991; 1:69–85.

74. Kent R, Miolo G, Bloedel S: The intelligibility of children's speech: a review of evaluation procedures. *Am J Speech–Lang Pathol* 1994; 3 (2):81–95.

75. Shriberg LD: Four new speech and prosody-voice measures for genetics research and other studies in developmental phonological disorders. *J Speech Hear Res* 1993; 36:105–140.

76. Hodge M, Hancock H: Assessment of developmental apraxia of speech: a procedure. *Clin Commun Disord* 1994; 4:102–118.

77. Dowden PA: Augmentative and alternative communication decision making for children with severely unintelligible speech. *AAC Augmentative and Alternative Communication* 1997; 13:48–58.

78. Bernhardt B: Phonological intervention techniques for syllable and word structure development. *Clin Commun Disord* 1994; 4(1):54–65.

79. Klick S: Adapted cueing technique: Facilitating sequential phoneme production. *Clin Commun Disord* 1994; 4 (3):183–189.

80. Mitchell P: A dynamic interactive developmental view of early speech and language production: Application to clinical practice in motor speech disorders. *Semin Speech Lang* 1995; 16(2):100–109.

81. Hayden D, Square P: Motor speech treatment hierarchy: a systems approach. *Clin Commun Disord* 1994; 4 (3):162–174.

82. Strand E: Treatment of motor speech disorders in children. *Semin Speech Lang* 1995; 16(2):126–139.

83. Rosenthal J: Rate control therapy for developmental apraxia of speech. *Clin Commun Disord* 1994; 4 (3): 190–200.

84. Mitchell P, Mahoney G: Team management for young children with motor speech disorders. *Semin Speech Lang* 1995; 16(2):159–172.

85. Murdoch BE, ed: *Acquired neurological speech/ language disorders in childhood.* London, Taylor and Francis, 1990.

86. Cohen NJ, Davine M, Meloche-Kelly M: Prevalence of unsuspected language disorders in a child psychiatric population. *J Am Acad Child Adol Psychiatr* 1989; 28: 107–111.

Appendix A
Assessment and Treatment Tools for Children with Motor Speech Disorders

ASSESSMENT TOOLS

Dysarthria Examination Battery (Older children)
Author: S.S. Drummond (Manual and Forms)
Publisher: Communication Skill Builders, 3830 E Bellvue/P.O. Box 42050, Tucson AZ 85733

Dworkin-Culatta Oral Mechanism Exam—Treatment (D-COME-T)
Authors: J. Dworkin & R. Culatta (1995)
Publisher: Edgewood Press Inc, P.O. Box 811, Nicholasville KY 40356
(Bite Blocks available too)

Early Motor Control Scales (8–30 months; older if delay present)
Authors: D.A. Hayden, A.M. Wetherby & B.M. Prizant
Publisher: Applied Symbolix, 16 West Erie, Suite 300, Chicago IL 60610

Pre-speech Assessment Scale (0–2 Years)
Author: S. Evans-Morris (1982)
Publisher: J.A. Preston Corp, 60 Page Rd, Clifton NJ 07012

Prosody-Voice Screening Profile
Author: L. Shriberg, J. Kwiatkowski & C. Rasmussen (1991)
Publisher: Communication Skill Builders, 3830 E Bellvue/P.O. Box 42050, Tucson AZ 85733

Screening Test for Developmental Apraxia of Speech
Author: R. Blakeley (1980)
Publisher: C.C. Publications Inc, P.O. Box 23699, Tigard OR 97223

TREATMENT MATERIALS

Apraxia of Speech Stimulus Library
Treatment Program and Stimulus Materials (Text with Pictorial Supplement)
Author: J. Thresher
Publisher: Communication Skill Builders, 3830 E Bellvue/P.O. Box 42050, Tucson AZ 85733

Easy Does It For Apraxia-Preschool (Ages 2–6 Yrs.)
Manual and Materials Book
Publisher: LinguiSystems Inc, 3100 4th Ave, East Moline IL 61224–9700

Easy Does It For Apraxia and Motor Planning (Ages 4–12 Yrs.)
Manual and Materials Book
Publisher: LinguiSystems Inc, 3100 4th Ave, East Moline IL 61224–9700

Moving Across Syllables: Training Articulatory Sound Sequences (3–10 Yrs.)
Test Booklet and Training Program with Reproducible Pictures for 1, 2 and 3 Syllable Words
Publisher: Communication Skill Builders, 3830 E Bellvue/P.O. Box 42050, Tucson AZ 85733

Workbook for the Verbally Apraxic Adult (Suitable for School Age Children)
Reproducibles for Therapy and Home Practice
Publisher: Communication Skill Builders, 3830 E Bellvue/P.O. Box 42050, Tucson AZ 85733

Voice Therapy for Children
Author: M. Andrews (1986)
Publisher: Longman Inc, 95 Church St, White Plains NY 10601

Voice Therapy for Adolescents
Author: M. Andrews (1988)
Publisher: College-Hill, Little, Brown & Co, Boston, MA

40,000 Selected Words: Organized by Letter, Sound and Syllable
Authors: V. Blockolsky, J. Frazer & D. Frazer
Publisher: Communication Skill Builders, 3830 E Bellvue/P.O. Box 42050, Tucson AZ 85733
(Also available in software program for the Apple)

Book of Words: 17,000 Words Selected by Vowels and Diphthongs
Author: V. Blockolsky
Publisher: Communication Skill Builders, 3830 E Bellvue/P.O. Box 42050, Tucson AZ 85733

Working with Dysarthric Clients (Suitable for Older Children)
Author: S. Robertson & F. Thomson (1986)
Publisher: Communication Skill Builders, 3830 E Bellvue/P.O. Box 42050, Tucson AZ 85733

Prosody Management of Communication Disorders
Authors: P.M. Hargrove and N.S. McGarr
Singular Publishing Group Inc, San Diego CA

MINIMAL PAIR MATERIALS

Contrasts: The Use of Minimal Pairs in
  Articulation Training
Authors: M. Elbert, B. Rockman & D. Saltzman
Publisher: Pro-Ed, 8700 Shoal Creek Blvd,
  Austin TX 78757–6897

RULES: Remediating Unintelligible Linguistic
  Expressions of Speech
A Phonological Approach for Remediating the
  Speech of Unintelligible Children
Authors: J.C. Webb & B. Duckett (1988)
Publisher: The Speech Bin Inc, 231 Clarksville
  Rd, P.O. Box 218, Princeton Junction NJ
  08550–0218

Picture Pairs and More Picture Pairs: Board and
  Card Games Based on Minimal Pairing
Language Age 4–10 Years
Publisher: Communication Skill Builders, 3830
  E Bellvue/P.O. Box 42050, Tucson AZ 85733

Frequent Errors Pairs (d/g; f/th; t/s; w/r; s blends)
More Frequent Error Pairs (t/k; p/f; s/sh; th/s; l
  blends)
Publisher: Communication Skill Builders, 3830
  E Bellvue/P.O. Box 42050, Tucson AZ 85733

18

Language and Its Management in the Surgical Epilepsy Patient

Anne Marie Valachovic, Brien Smith, Kost Elisevich, Gary Jacobson, and John Fisk

The surgical treatment of epilepsy began over 100 years ago when in 1886 Sir Victor Horseley resected a region of the motor cortex injured 15 years earlier by a depressed skull fracture in a 22-year-old patient with focal motor seizures. Interest in the surgical approach to epilepsy grew in the ensuing years, particularly in mainland Europe. Cortical stimulation for motor mapping was routinely used following exposure of focally injured brain in epileptic patients, many of whom were wounded during World War I. In the late 1920s Wilder Penfield, an American, secured the support of the Rockefeller Foundation and McGill University in Montreal to establish a neurosurgical practice with an emphasis in the surgical treatment of epilepsy and ultimately to found the famed Montreal Neurological Institute (MNI) that would become the center of such treatment in North America for many years.

In 1934 the MNI opened its 50-bed hospital for neurological disorders and research center to which many trainees and associates from around the world were attracted. Many subsequently returned to the United States and elsewhere to establish similar programs. In 1937 electroencephalography (EEG) was introduced at the MNI, and in 1939 an EEG laboratory was annexed to aid in patient selection for operative consideration and provide electrocorticographic localization of the epileptic focus during surgery (Figure 18–1).

The cortical localization of language and other functions became a central theme in the intraoperative study of patients by Penfield and his

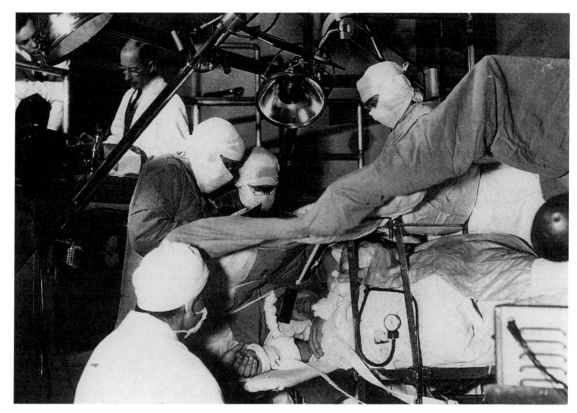

Figure 18–1. Surgical amphitheater at the Montreal Neurological Institute. Penfield is operating and Jasper is analyzing electrographic data during a recording session. (From Feindel W: Toward a surgical cure for epilepsy. In Engel J Jr, ed. *Surgical treatment of the epilepsies.* New York, Raven Press, 1993, p 7. Reprinted with permission.)

successor, Theodore Rasmussen. Sites of language processing were outlined with the aid of electrical stimulation in numerous patients (Figure 18–2). Over time, temporal lobe resection became the most frequent surgical treatment of epilepsy. As a consequence, language mapping and the study of language representation in the temporal lobe have continued to the present day.

The surgical treatment of medically intractable epilepsy has steadily increased through the years and is currently performed at numerous neurosurgical centers throughout North America. Because of the increasing number of surgically treated epilepsy patients and the need for language assessment and management, the services of the speech–language pathologist in this area are of great importance and have become an integral part of the epilepsy surgery process.

This chapter is organized into sections: The first section provides a general overview of epilepsy and the epilepsy patient, the second focuses on the battery of presurgical tests and the surgery itself, and the third section reports on surgical outcomes and the importance of follow-up treatment.

THE EPILEPSIES

Incidence and Prevalence

Epilepsy is a disorder of the central nervous system (CNS) whose main symptom is recurrent seizures unprovoked by any known proximate cause. The prevalence of epilepsy has been assessed in numerous populations and has ranged from 5 to 8 per 1000.[1] Based on a 1980 prevalence in Rochester, MN, of 6.66 per 1000, the number of people estimated to have epilepsy in the United States in 1990 was 1.7 million.[2] The cumulative incidence over a lifespan calculated from the Rochester data suggests that about 3% of the population will have epilepsy at some time during their lives. Although the highest incidence of epilepsy is believed to occur during early childhood, more recent studies have shown a higher peak in the elderly as the average lifespan in our population has increased.[3] These figures make epilepsy the third most common neurological disorder, following stroke and Alzheimer's disease.[4]

A INTERFERENCE WITH SPEECH

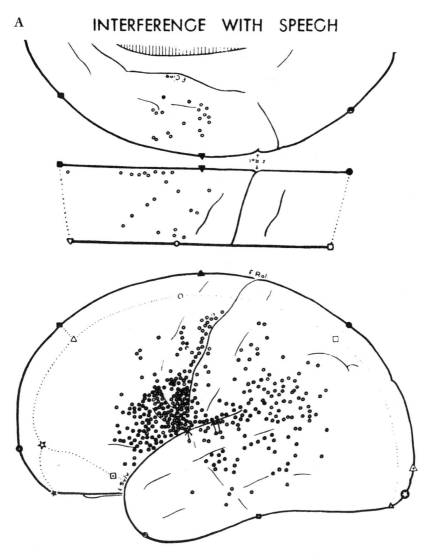

Figure 18–2. (**A**) A composite brain map of Penfield's showing stimulation points associated with speech interference. Although widespread over the cerebral convexity and medial cerebral surface, a dense cluster of points appears in the inferior frontal and precentral gyri. The parietotemporal area represents a second language-associated region. (From Roberts L: The evidence from cortical map. In Penfield W, Roberts L, eds: *Speech and brain mechanisms.* Princeton, Princeton University Press, 1959, p 122. Reprinted with permission.)

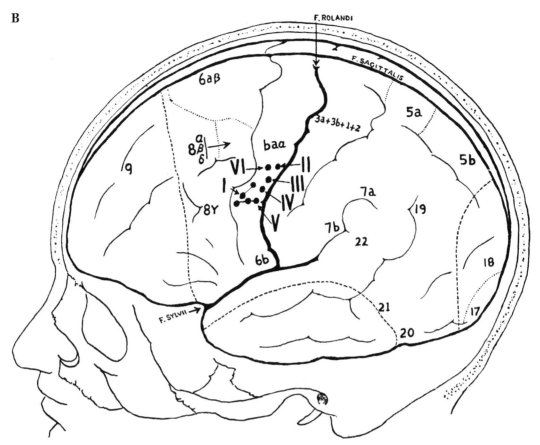

Figure 18–2. (B) Schematic illustration by Penfield showing localization of points where vocalization was produced in 6 cases (I–VI). (From Penfield W: The cerebral cortex in man. The cerebral cortex and consciousness. *Arch Neurol Psychiatr* 1938; 40:417–442. Copyrighted 1938, American Medical Association. Reprinted with permission.)

Seizure Definitions

Historically, the term "seizure" has been used in a broad and rather vague context to refer to any sudden, catastrophic event. This chapter will focus only on epileptic seizures and not other non-epileptic conditions (i.e., syncope, pseudoseizures) frequently discussed in the differential diagnosis. An epileptic seizure is the clinical manifestation of excessive and/or hypersynchronous, usually self-limited, abnormal activity of neurons in the cerebral cortex.[5] This clinical event may consist of an alteration in behavior including a change in motor activity, autonomic function, consciousness, or sensation.[6] The clinical manifestations of seizures are variable and are determined not only by the initial region(s) of brain involved but also by the speed, pathway, and extent of propagation (spread) of the abnormal electrical discharge.

Classification and Terminology

The various forms of epilepsy and epileptic syndromes cover a wide spectrum of clinical manifestations. To help organize the appropriate diagnosis and treatment of these various conditions, a clas-sification scheme with standardized terminology was created. In 1981 the Commission on Classification and Terminology of the International League Against Epilepsy proposed a revised clinical and electroencephalographic classification of epileptic seizures[7] (Table 18–1) and subsequently in 1989 proposed the reclassification of epilepsy and epileptic syndromes[8] (Table 18–2). Previous terms including petit mal, grand mal, and psychomotor seizures have been replaced by terms such as absence, generalized tonic-clonic, and complex partial seizures. These classification schemes emphasize the difference between the two major types of epilepsy: partial versus generalized. Such a classification provides guidance in selecting appropriate medical therapy and helps determine possible etiology, potential candidacy for surgical intervention, and long-term prognosis.

Etiology

Only about one-third of all cases of epilepsy can be considered secondary to definitive etiologies. The most common presumed etiologies of epilepsy in-

Table 18–1. Epileptic Seizures: Classification and Characteristics

I. Partial seizures (focal seizures)
  A. Simple partial seizures
    1. With motor signs
    2. With somatosensory or special sensory signs
    3. With autonomic symptoms
    4. With psychic symptoms
  B. Complex partial seizures
    1. Simple partial onset followed by impairment of consciousness
    2. With impairment of consciousness at the onset
  C. Partial seizures evolving to secondarily generalized seizures
    1. Simple partial seizures evolving to generalized seizures
    2. Complex partial seizures evolving to generalized seizures
    3. Simple partial seizures evolving to complex partial seizures evolving to generalized seizures

II. Generalized seizures (convulsive or nonconvulsive)
  A. 1. Typical absence seizures (petit mal)
     2. Atypical
  B. Myoclonic seizures
  C. Clonic seizures
  D. Tonic seizures
  E. Tonic-clonic seizures (grand mal)
  F. Atonic seizures

III. Unclassified epileptic seizures
  Includes all those seizures that cannot be classified because of incomplete data or because they defy classification into the above categories.

IV. Status epilepticus

Source: *Epilepsia* 1981; 22:489–501; used with permission.

clude cerebrovascular disease (13.2%), developmental disorders (5.5%), head trauma (4.1%), brain tumor (3.6%), infection (2.6%), degenerative CNS disease (1.8%), and other causes (0.5%). The cause of the remaining 70% of cases of epilepsy is unknown.[1] These percentages will vary depending on the age of the population being analyzed and the type of epilepsy (partial versus generalized). Although most epilepsies appear to result from multiple factors, the majority of partial epilepsies result from acquired insults whereas generalized epilepsies result from a hereditary/genetic predisposition. The two most common regions involved in patients with medically intractable partial epilepsy include the temporal (56 to 74%) and frontal (11 to 18%) lobes.[9,10]

Criteria for Surgical Candidacy

Approximately 20 to 30% of patients with chronic epilepsy are inadequately controlled with antiepileptic therapy.[11] These are the patients who are referred as possible candidates for surgical treatment. Patients considered appropriate candidates for epilepsy surgery are those with medically intractable partial epilepsy or those who have a sur-

gically remediable lesion.[12] Although there is some variation in defining intractability, it generally refers to those patients who continue to have seizures despite treatment with the first-line antiepileptic medications (phenytoin, carbamazepine, and valproic acid) in monotherapy or polytherapy over at least two years. The presence of a surgically remediable lesion may modify the approach considerably and may support early surgical intervention even if a patient is well controlled with low dose monotherapy.

THE PATIENT WITH EPILEPSY

Language Functioning

Epilepsy is associated with language abnormalities, but most patients have normal language function or only mild deficits.[13] Language abnormalities are generally more common when seizures originate in the dominant hemisphere. At times language dysfunction is the sole manifestation of a seizure (sometimes called "paroxysmal aphasia").[14,15,16,17]

Language function may be disrupted during the seizure (the ictal state), in the minutes to hours following the seizure (the post-ictal state), and in

Table 18–2. International Classification of Epilepsies and Epileptic Syndromes

1. Localization-related (focal, local, partial) epilepsies and syndromes
   A. Idiopathic with age-related onset
      a. Benign childhood epilepsy with centrotemporal spikes
      b. Childhood epilepsy with occipital paroxysms
   B. Symptomatic
      Based on anatomical localization, clinical features, seizure types, and etiology

2. Generalized epilepsies and syndromes
   A. Idiopathic, with age-related onset, listed in order of age
      a. Benign neonatal familial convulsions
      b. Benign neonatal convulsions
      c. Benign myoclonic epilepsy in infancy
      d. Childhood absence epilepsy (pyknolepsy)
      e. Juvenile absence epilepsy
      f. Juvenile myoclonic epilepsy
      g. Epilepsy with grand mal seizures on awakening
      h. Other generalized idiopathic epilepsies
   B. Idiopathic and/or symptomatic (in order of age of appearance)
      a. West's syndrome (infantile spasms)
      b. Lennox-Gastaut syndrome
      c. Epilepsy with myoclonic-astatic seizures
      d. Epilepsy with myoclonic absences
   C. Symptomatic
      a. Nonspecific etiology
         Early myoclonic encephalopathy
      b. Specific syndromes
         Diseases in which seizures are a presenting or predominant feature

3. Epilepsies and syndromes undetermined as to whether they are focal or generalized
   A. With both focal and generalized seizures
      a. Neonatal seizures
      b. Severe myoclonic epilepsy in infancy
      c. Epilepsy with continuous spike waves during slow wave sleep
      d. Acquired epileptic aphasia (Landau-Kleffner syndrome)
   B. Without unequivocal focal or generalized seizures
      All cases where clinical and EEG findings do not definitively permit classification as clearly focal or generalized

4. Special syndromes
   A. Situation-related seizures
      a. Febrile convulsions
      b. Seizures related to other identifiable situations such as stress, hormonal changes, alcohol, drugs, or sleep deprivation
   B. Isolated, apparently unprovoked epileptic events
   C. Epilepsies characterized by specific modes of seizure precipitation
   D. Chronic progressive epilepsia partialis continua of childhood

Source: Epilepsia 1989; 30:389–399; reprinted with permission.

the time between seizures (the interictal period). Ictal and post-ictal language assessment is beneficial to the epileptologist in that it may provide information regarding the hemispheric lateralization of seizure onset.[14,17–20] The speech–language pathologist is concerned with the evaluation and treatment of interictal language dysfunction or the linguistic deficits patients exhibit while in their usual state of health.

The language differences seen in patients with epilepsy may be multifactorial in etiology: frequent seizures involving excessive bursts of abnormal cerebral electrical activity, subclinical epileptiform discharges,[21] structural lesions, effects of antiepileptic medications, and psychosocial factors such as limited communicative opportunities and independence.

Because the temporal lobes are the most common site of epileptogenicity, patients with temporal lobe epilepsy have been the most extensively studied. In Hermann and Wyler's[22] investigation of the performance of patients with temporal lobe epilepsy, those with seizures of dominant temporal lobe origin performed worse on six of the seven subtests of the Multilingual Aphasia Examination than those patients with seizures of nondominant origin. These findings were felt to represent a mild generalized impairment of language function in patients with dominant temporal lobe seizures.

Several types of interictal language impairment have been documented in patients with chronic epilepsy. Deficits have been found in the areas of naming, verbal fluency, comprehension, reading/writing, and expressive language.

Naming

In the literature, the most commonly reported symptom of language disturbance in the adult with epilepsy is impaired naming.[23–30] Not surprisingly, word-finding difficulty is probably the single most common language-related complaint reported by adults with dominant hemisphere epilepsy. In a group of 435 patients with epilepsy who completed a memory questionnaire, the most common daily "memory" problem was the feeling that a word was on the "tip of the tongue."[31] A selective anomia may be the only language disturbance in some patients.[28] Studies have shown significant superiority of patients with right nondominant epilepsy over left dominant epilepsy on the Boston Naming Test.[29] Mayeux et al.[27] found a striking impairment in confrontation naming in a group of patients with left temporal lobe epilepsy compared to patients with right temporal or generalized epilepsy. Significant correlations existed between naming ability on the Boston Naming Test and scores on the Wechsler Memory Scale. The authors proposed that the anomia seen in patients with left temporal epilepsy may contribute to the poor verbal memory and recall performance so often observed in these patients. Hermann et al.[32] investigated this hypothesis and confirmed that the degree of language impairment was a powerful predictor of memory and learning performance on the California Verbal Learning Test in their sample of patients with dominant temporal lobe epilepsy.

Verbal Fluency

The verbal output of patients with epilepsy is fluent, although deficits have been found in tasks of timed associative word fluency. Left dominant patients with left hemisphere seizure foci have performed significantly lower than age-matched controls on measures of phonemic word fluency.[26] In an investigation of the word fluency performance in patients with both left and right temporal lobe epilepsy, patients were required to generate words based on phonemic criteria (words beginning with a particular letter) and semantic-based criteria (words belonging to a given semantic category).[33] All subjects performed more poorly than normal controls and the left temporal group performed significantly worse than the right temporal group.

Comprehension

Auditory comprehension appears to be relatively unaffected in patients with epilepsy. The hypothesis that patients with left hemisphere seizure foci would have an impaired performance on verbal comprehension tasks was not confirmed in a recent study.[34] A group of patients with left temporal seizure foci did not perform in a significantly different fashion than normal controls on the Complex Ideational Material subtest of the Boston Diagnostic Aphasia Examination.[28]

Reading/Writing

Reading impairment may be more common in patients with epilepsy than the general population. In an investigation by Schachter et al.,[35] patients with epilepsy were four times more likely to have a history of dyslexia than age-matched controls (9% versus 2.3%). Of the patients with epilepsy, dyslexia was disproportionately high in left-handed females and in males with seizure onset by age 12. Several possible explanations have been suggested for an association between dyslexia and epilepsy: (1) cortical lesions may be epileptogenic and may involve the neural systems of reading, (2) subclinical epileptiform discharges may interfere with reading, (3) dyslexia and epilepsy may be genetically linked (although such an association has not been reported to date), and (4) anticonvulsant toxicity may impair reading.[36]

Agraphia has been documented to occur during seizures,[17] although most of the literature regarding the interictal writing abilities of patients with dominant temporal epilepsy is related to the occurrence of hypergraphia, or excessive and almost compulsive writing.[37–41]

In our experience, the written language of adults with epilepsy is widely variable and ranges from above average, sophisticated writing skills to marked disturbances in grammar, syntax, and spelling.

Expressive Language

Recently we found that discourse abilities of patients with dominant temporal seizure foci are reduced as compared to controls matched by age, education, and gender (Valachovic, unpublished data). Using Nicholas and Brookshire's[42] method of Correct Information Unit (CIU) analysis, patients with intractable left temporal epilepsy had significantly lower %CIU and CIUs per minute on all three of the discourse tasks studied: narrative picture description, procedural picture sequence description, and story retelling. The total number of CIUs produced did not differ significantly. Therefore, the core information in each task was present and accurate but was conveyed in a more time-consuming and wordy manner. This pattern of scores was felt to represent reduced communicative efficiency in this group of patients.

A long duration of left or bitemporal epilepsy has been associated with the verbal trait of "viscosity," the behavioral tendency to talk repetitively and circumstantially.[43] Patients with a long-standing history of complex partial seizures with left temporal foci have been found to be more verbose with increased circumstantiality based on responses to the "cookie theft" picture of the Boston Diagnostic Aphasia Examination.[44] Rao et al.[43] speculated that viscosity was a result of a critical deficit in the temporal lobe epilepsy patient's ability to perceive verbal and nonverbal social cues in conversation.

Verbal Memory

Much evidence exists documenting an association between seizure disorders and memory impairment. Investigations at the Montreal Neurological Institute in the 1950s demonstrated that bilateral damage to medial temporal structures could result in severe memory loss.[45,46] In general, investigations have shown that disturbance in verbal memory is more prominent in patients suffering left temporal epileptogenicity,[47,48] whereas lesions in the right temporal lobe are more likely to impair free recall of nonverbal material such as faces, music, and figural stimuli.[49] However, most of these investigations studied patients suffering from intractable epilepsy and inferences regarding the nature of memory disturbances were often based on postsurgical results.[50] Further, many early investigators failed to control for other factors known to have an impact on memory function such as seizure frequency and severity, onset and duration of the disorder, and medication effects. In fact, some investigators have failed to demonstrate consistent laterality effects.[51,52]

Memory, however, is not a unitary concept. Mnestic disturbance can reflect a variety of underlying impairments in cognition including defective attentional deployment, deficiencies in encoding, a defect in new learning (i.e., anterograde amnesia), problems with retrieval of specific information, and state dependent effects (e.g., medication effects). In short, a number of sources of variance contribute to the strength of memory traces.[53] Nevertheless, damage to the left temporal lobe structures is likely to result primarily in deficits in verbal memory. These deficits are characterized mostly by anterograde amnesia—disturbance in the ability to encode new verbal information such as word lists, connected discourse, and verbal associations.[54–56]

Psychosocial Factors

Disturbances in behavioral and personality functioning have long been associated with epilepsy. Indeed, considerable research effort has been directed toward identifying the nature of the relationship between epilepsy and mood disorder.[57–59] Unfortunately, no definitive clinical picture has emerged regarding the emotional-psychological phenomenology associated with different aspects of seizure states or different forms of epilepsy.

A variety of factors, in addition to seizures, contribute to the emotional-psychological status of epileptic individuals including neurobiological factors, treatment and medication effects, and psychosocial variables. Hermann and Whitman[60] have proposed that, aside from possible direct biological and pharmacological effects, psychosocial factors (financial stress, unemployment, discrimination, social isolation, etc.) that afflict many epileptic patients may lead directly to pathological behavior. These investigators examined the relationship between psychosocial factors and psychiatric distress in 102 cases of confirmed epilepsy and concluded that: (1) psychosocial factors are important in understanding the psychiatric status in epileptic patients, (2) financial status and general adjustment to epilepsy are particularly powerful factors, and (3) biological and medical variables are surprisingly poor predictors of psychiatric status. Clearly, epilepsy is associated with a wide variety of problems in living, particularly in the more severe and chronic cases. For example, Thompson and Oxley,[61] using the Social Problems Questionnaire to investigate socioeconomic problems in 92 patients with intractable epilepsy, found that 71% reported problems with employment, 73% with social activities, 37% with finances, and 29% with housing. Chaplin et al.[62] found that chronicity was also an important variable in a study of 62 individuals with either recently diagnosed or chronic epilepsy. The only significant difficulty reported by recently diagnosed subjects was fear of seizures. In contrast, chronic subjects reported worry regarding their social life and leisure activities. They displayed a more negative outlook on life, were concerned regarding their future, and were more likely to feel socially isolated.

For epilepsy patients being considered for surgical treatment, preoperative psychological adjustment is an important predictor regarding overall postoperative psychosocial outcome.[63] Basically, the more well adjusted the patient presurgically, the better the psychosocial adjustment postsurgically. Sperling et al.[64] found a reduction in postsurgical unemployment and underemployment in a study of 86 epilepsy surgery patients at 3.5 to 8 years follow-up. Further analyses revealed that favorable employment outcome was positively related to the degree of seizure relief obtained postsurgically. Conversely, patients who continued to suffer from significant seizures postoperatively also experienced increased unemployment.

Interictal Behavior Syndrome of Temporal Lobe Epilepsy

Some patients with temporal lobe epilepsy exhibit a distinct cluster of behavioral features that may constitute an interictal behavior syndrome. The behavioral features have been reported to include increased concern with philosophical, moral, or religious issues; alterations in sexual behavior (usually hyposexuality); hypergraphia; impulsivity/irritability; deepened emotionality; sense of personal destiny; circumstantiality and viscosity; anger/aggression; guilt; and humorlessness.[65,66,67] Personality changes usually appear several years after the onset of seizures.[37] This is a behavioral syndrome, not a behavioral disorder, and many patients who exhibit characteristics of the syndrome remain fully functional and productive.[66]

The presence of this syndrome in patients with temporal lobe epilepsy has been attributed to limbic system dysfunction, specifically, sensory-limbic hyperconnection.[66,67] The syndrome is not highly common.[65]

Handedness and Language Localization

Initial reports regarding language representation compared handedness and language dominance in epileptic patients with or without an early cerebral injury who were suspected of having atypical language lateralization.[68] These studies have shown

that handedness and language dominance may not be as strongly linked as previously suspected.

There is strong evidence that patients with epilepsy have an increased incidence of atypical language representation. Approximately 95% of right-handers and 70% of left-handers in the general population are left-hemisphere dominant for language.[69] In a series of 130 patients with medically intractable focal epilepsy, only 70% were completely left-hemisphere language dominant, 23% had bilateral or incomplete left hemisphere dominance, and 7% were completely right hemisphere dominant.[69] Similar results were reported by Strauss et al.[70] and by Loring et al.[71]

In normally developing right-handed individuals, hemispheric lateralization of language function may be complete by age 5.[72] This is consistent with reports that early onset of focal left brain injury (prior to age 6 years) is associated with an atypical pattern of left hemisphere language representation.[68,73] Damage to either Broca's area or the posterior parietotemporal language area in infancy may cause a functional reorganization of the brain in which dominance for language is assumed by the right hemisphere or bilaterally.[68] In some cases, a dissociation of receptive and expressive language functions may occur so that only one of these functions is assumed by the right hemisphere.[74] In cases of left posterior temporal injury, there may be an upward displacement of the posterior language area to include a larger area of parietal cortex.[68] Left-handed or ambidextrous patients with epilepsy have a high incidence of bilateral speech representation.[68] When language is not solely mediated by the left hemisphere, for reasons such as handedness or early brain injury, bilateral language representation is more common than pure right hemisphere representation.[71] The occurrence of right hemisphere dominance for speech without an early left hemisphere lesion is rare.[68,75]

Transfer of Language Function

The transfer of language function from the left to the right hemisphere is thought to occur secondary to either an early left hemisphere cerebral injury or a left temporal seizure focus. The presence of dominant temporal lobe seizure foci during language development is associated with a more widespread or diverse distribution of temporal language areas, with more anteriorly distributed temporal language representation.[24] Language functions may be displaced from the temporal lobe into the parietal lobe when a long-standing temporal seizure focus is present since early childhood.[76] Thus, early left frontal or parietal brain injury appears to displace language functions partially or completely to the right hemisphere,[68] and early left temporal epilepsy may displace language within the left hemisphere[24] or to the right hemisphere.[69,77] The transfer of language to the right hemisphere may occur at a considerable price to language functioning.[26,69]

Some early left hemisphere lesions or seizure foci result in a shift of language dominance and not in handedness.[68,73,77] Language dominance and hand preference are more likely to shift together in an early lesion onset (probably before age 3), while shift in language dominance alone is more likely to occur in a later onset lesion, usually before age 6.[73]

Factors that may influence the transfer of language function include handedness (nondextral > dextral),[68,78] gender (women > men),[79] age of injury (greatest when less than 5 to 6 years old),[68,75,78] location of injury (frontal and parietal speech areas > posterior temporal lesions),[68,80] and severity of injury (greater when lesion causes hemiparesis).[80]

Many of these investigations have been referenced as representative of language lateralization in the general public, but many have limitations due to selection bias.[80] Clearly, information regarding language localization in patients with focal epilepsy may not be reliably generalized to the normal population. Abou-Khalil[81] has suggested that groups of consecutive patients with late onset epilepsy and no history of early brain injury may be most representative of the normal population.

EPILEPSY SURGERY PROGRAM

The members of an epilepsy surgery program specifically evaluate in a comprehensive manner those patients with medically intractable focal epilepsy to determine whether the surgical approach is a valid therapeutic option. The intent is to improve a patient's quality of life with elimination or reduction of seizures with a minimal chance of morbidity or mortality. This requires a multidisciplinary team approach with trained professionals in many subspecialties (Table 18–3) who have appropriate experience and the ability to interact productively with patients and other members of the team on a regular basis.

Presurgical Evaluation

The presurgical evaluation consists of an initial outpatient evaluation (usually by an epileptologist) to determine whether the patient is an appropriate candidate for surgical intervention. This is followed by outpatient studies including a baseline EEG and magnetic resonance imaging (MRI) of the brain. These two studies provide significant data not only in distinguishing focal versus generalized epilepsy but also in determining the epileptogenic zone or seizure focus (the area of the brain that requires surgical resection to achieve a seizure-free status). Although epilepsy is an electrical disorder of the brain, the detection of an anatomical structural lesion frequently is concordant with, or the actual cause of, the electrical disturbance. Other studies that are used by most centers in the presurgical evaluation include functional neuroimaging and neuropsychological testing. Positron emission tomography (PET) and single photon emission computed tomography (SPECT) are the two forms of neuroimaging that have assisted in delineating the epileptogenic zone by defining abnormal regions of brain characterized by hypometabolism (PET) or altered cerebral perfusion (SPECT). The "gold standard" in delineating the epileptogenic zone continues to be the actual recording of the electrical onset of typical seizures (ictal onset zone) with scalp electrodes or directly from the surface or depth of the brain. This is usually done in an Epilepsy Monitoring Unit (EMU) where a patient is under continuous video/EEG surveillance. When this has been completed, a determination can be made whether the patient is a surgical candidate and whether cortical mapping is needed to define neighboring regions of eloquent cortex (cortex responsible for a specific function, such as motor and language cortex). Other studies including an intracarotid amobarbital procedure (Wada test), baseline language assessment, and visual field examination are done to determine the functional status of memory, language, and vision prior to a final decision on a surgical resection.

PRESURGICAL STUDIES

Electroencephalography (EEG)

Since epilepsy is an electrical disorder, the EEG is the most useful test in the evaluation, classification, and surgical monitoring of an epileptic patient. The EEG is a neurodiagnostic study that measures the difference in the electrical potential between various points on the head. It is generated by inhibitory and excitatory postsynaptic potentials of cortical nerve cells. These potentials summate in the cortex and extend through the coverings of the brain to the scalp. Synchronous involvement of at least 6 cm^2 of cortex is required to record scalp

Table 18–3. Epilepsy Surgery Evaluation

Outpatient Evaluation
Initial comprehensive evaluation
  Explanation and orientation to program (clinical nurse specialist)
  History and physical (epileptologist/epilepsy surgeon)
Baseline EEG (epileptologist)
MRI brain—epilepsy surgery protocol (neuroradiologist)
Functional neuroimaging—SPECT/PET (nuclear medicine radiologist/physicist)
Neuropsychological battery (neuropsychologist)
Psychiatric evaluation (psychiatrist)
Language assessment (speech–language pathologist)
Other—ME spectroscopy (MRS), magnetoencephalography (MEG)

Inpatient Evaluation (Phase I)
Prolonged video/EEG monitoring with scalp and sphenoidal electrodes (epilepsy monitoring unit, multidisciplinary team)
Ictal SPECT (nuclear medicine)

Presurgical Outpatient Testing
Intracarotid amobarbital procedure (Wada) (neuroradiologist, neuropsychologist, epileptologist)
Visual field study (ophthalmologist)
Functional mapping studies (MRI, PET, MEG)

Inpatient Evaluation (Phase II) - (if indicated)
Prolonged video/EEG with intracranial electrodes (epilepsy monitoring unit, multidisciplinary team)
Extraoperative cortical stimulation/functional mapping (epilepsy monitoring unit, multidisciplinary team)

Surgical Resection
Intraoperative mapping
  Electrocorticography (ECOG)
  Evoked potentials (EP)
  Intraoperative cortical stimulation/functional mapping (if indicated)

EEG changes.[82] There are two types of EEG recordings: extracranial, in which electrodes record the electrical activity of the brain from outside the cranium, and intracranial, in which electrodes are surgically placed inside the cranium to record electrical activity directly from the surface of the brain.

Extracranial EEG

With standard scalp EEG recording, a number of electrodes are applied to the scalp surface in a symmetrical distribution (International 10-20 System)[83] to provide comprehensive coverage. Under certain instances, twice as many electrodes may be applied to the scalp surface (10-10 System) in an attempt to localize the epileptogenic focus.[84] Other surface electrodes including inferolateral temporal scalp (T1, T2, F9, F10) and supraorbital (SO1, SO2) electrodes are regularly used to maximize localizing data recorded from the frontotemporal head regions.

The first step in evaluation of the patient with epilepsy is to obtain a baseline EEG lasting approximately 30 minutes. However, this initial study will only yield epileptiform abnormalities in 50 to 60% of patients due to the limited length of recording and because only 20 to 70% of cortical spikes are recorded at the scalp surface.[85] Therefore, most surgical candidates may require prolonged video/EEG monitoring with sphenoidal electrodes that are placed directly with a needle into the infratemporal fossa to record epileptiform discharges emanating from medial and basal temporal surfaces, a common site of epileptogenicity giving rise to intractable seizures. (See Figure 18–3B.)

Interictal Activity

Epileptiform abnormalities recorded in the period between seizures may consist of discharges classified as spike, polyspike, or sharp waves as determined by morphology and duration (see Figure 18–3A). These discharges suggest abnormal cortical excitability or irritability but are not diagnostic of the condition. Both focal and generalized epileptiform discharges have been recorded in patients with no history of seizures. This reinforces the fact that the EEG is an extension of the neurologic evaluation and that the diagnosis of epilepsy is a clinical one.

Ictal Activity

The recording of a seizure by video/EEG monitoring is considered most beneficial when attempting to verify that an epileptic seizure has occurred and in localizing the epileptogenic region that must be resected for a successful outcome (see Figure 18–3B). In the majority of patients, the scalp EEG in combination with other noninvasive studies (MRI, PET, SPECT and neuropsychological battery) provides the necessary concordant data for localizing the region of seizure onset (epileptogenic region) and offering a surgical option. These patients may then proceed directly to the surgical resection, without the need for intracranial recording. However, certain regions of the brain are not well sampled (i.e., medial surfaces, extratemporal areas) by scalp electrodes, so that some partial seizures arising from deeper limbic structures or small regions of the neocortex with minimal propagation may show no EEG changes. Therefore, for those patients whose clinical history strongly supports intractable partial epilepsy but whose scalp EEG data are insufficient, intracranial electrode placement for further sampling will be necessary prior to surgery.

Intracranial EEG

The surgical placement of intracranial electrodes to record typical seizures directly from the surface of the brain is necessary when (1) the scalp ictal EEG is poorly localizing, (2) noninvasive data are discordant, (3) clinical data suggest nonlesional extratemporal lobe epilepsy, (4) the possibility of independent temporal or extratemporal foci exists, or (5) there is possible involvement of eloquent cortex requiring functional cortical mapping.

Subdural electrodes and depth electrodes are commonly used intracranial electrodes in most surgical centers (Figure 18–4). Subdural electrodes are stainless steel conductors of electrical activity that are surgically placed under the dura to directly record electrical activity from the underlying cerebral cortex. Electrodes are placed over the region of the brain that is suspected to be the epileptic region. The type of electrode(s) used varies and selection is frequently based on the physician's experience. More centers are electing to use a combination of these electrodes depending on the clinical presentation and probable epileptogenic region. Although all intracranial electrodes have limitations in sampling and carry a small risk of complications/morbidity when implanted, the type of electrode used may depend on the region requiring coverage (temporal, extratemporal, neocortical, and medial cortical surfaces) and whether extraoperative functional mapping is indicated.

Wada Procedure

The intracarotid amobarbital test (Wada procedure) is performed as part of the presurgical evaluation in most epilepsy surgery centers. This study was initially developed by Wada in 1949[86] to determine hemispheric dominance for language prior to surgical resection. Its clinical use was later expanded by Rasmussen and Milner[68] to determine the risk of severe memory loss after a temporal resection.

The goals of the Wada test for the epilepsy surgery evaluation are to establish cerebral representation of language function(s), to predict patients who are at risk for developing a postsurgical amnestic syndrome, and to identify lateralized dysfunction to help confirm seizure onset laterality.[87] The determination of language dominance is important since approximately 70% of patients who are considered surgical candidates have seizures that arise from the left or right temporal lobe. Although there are numerous issues related to the assessment of memory and other behavioral functions, this discussion will be limited to the analysis of language function.

The study is performed by an epileptologist and/or neuropsychologist in cooperation with a neuroradiologist. A cerebral angiogram is initially undertaken to analyze the cerebral vasculature. After completion of the angiogram, sodium amobarbital is injected into the internal carotid artery to pharmacologically inactivate regions supplied by the cerebral arteries. The pertinent areas affected by this injection include the hippocampus (memory), Wernicke's area, Broca's area, and the basal temporal area (language). In addition to producing transient aphasia in areas with language representation, this injection usually will result in a myriad of transient neurobehavioral disturbances including contralateral hemiplegia, hemianesthesia, homonymous hemianopia, and neglect[86] among other functions.[88] Depending on the dose administered (50 to 200 mg), these changes will last a few minutes, allowing time for multiple cognitive tasks to be administered.

Before conclusions from the Wada procedure can be drawn, the criteria used to determine

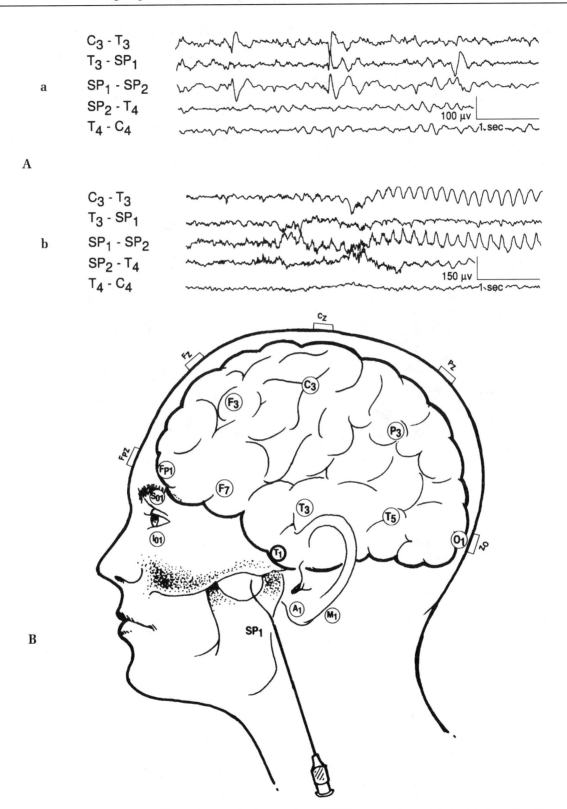

Figure 18–3. (A) (a) Electroencephalographic (EEG) examples of interictal epileptiform discharges; (b) ictal EEG recording of a partial seizure. Both examples are recorded maximally over the left temporal head region (electrodes SP_1 and T_3). **(B)** Schematic representation of standard scalp (International 10–20 System) and sphenoidal electrode coverage over the left hemisphere.

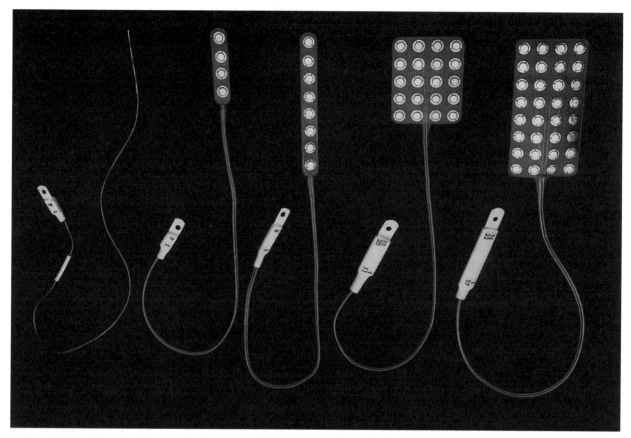

Figure 18–4. Depth electrodes (far left) and subdural electrodes. Subdural electrodes are arranged in single rows (strips) or in multiple rows (grids), which are chosen based on the size and location of the cerebral area to be covered.

whether linguistic function has been impaired with the injection must be defined. Generally, right-handed patients will stop speaking (i.e., counting and naming) after left hemisphere injection and will be able to continue speaking after right hemisphere injection. Snyder et al.[89] surveyed 55 epilepsy surgery centers on the methodology used with Wada testing and found that the criteria used to determine speech lateralization for the dominant hemisphere included naming (93%), counting ability (80%), unspecified aphasic signs (78%), unfamiliar word/phrase repetition (65%), and familiar word/phrase repetition (61%). The presence of paraphasic errors may be the most direct evidence of cerebral language representation.[90] When determining whether there is language representation in the nondominant hemisphere, the criteria used have been more variable, resulting in reports of bilateral language representation ranging from 0 to 60%. Exclusive right cerebral language dominance is rare and bilateral language representation is more commonly demonstrated with the appropriate testing.[70]

Some centers that limit the resection to anterior temporal structures may choose not to perform the Wada test.

Baseline Language Assessment

In those patients with a dominant hemisphere seizure focus, a comprehensive language assessment should be performed by the speech–language pathologist before surgery to measure baseline language functioning and again within the first postoperative week to delineate any acute changes. Testing may be repeated at 6 to 12 months after surgery to determine long-term language outcome. Table 18–4 provides a recommended baseline language assessment protocol.

The following considerations should serve as guiding principles for testing:

1. Evaluate all language modalities (verbal expression, auditory comprehension, reading comprehension, and written expression) to detect any baseline language deficits. This data becomes critical during postoperative

Table 18–4. Baseline Language Assessment Protocol

Boston Diagnostic Aphasia Examination (BDAE)[91]

Boston Naming Test[92]

Discourse samples
  Nicholas and Brookshire discourse analysis[42]
  Aesop's fables[93]

Written language samples
  Procedural (patient writes down his/her typical daily routine or writes the
    steps in performing a familiar action)
  Narrative (patient writes a response to a question such as, "What is your job
    description?" or "How do you hope surgery will affect your future?")

Fluency/word generation task
  Controlled Oral Word Association Test[94]
  Normative data for animal naming in BDAE[91]
  FAS test[95]

Supplementary:

Token Test[96]

Test of Adolescent/Adult Word Finding[97]

Western Aphasia Battery[98]

Multilingual Aphasia Examination[94]

Woodcock Reading Mastery Tests[99]

Woodcock-Johnson Tests of Cognitive Ability/Achievement[100]

testing when attempting to differentiate between new and preexisting deficits.

2. Administer highly sensitive language tasks because most patients have subtle deficits that may surface only on complex testing. In our experience, naming and writing are sensitive language measures in these patients and appear to be susceptible to subtle changes resulting from surgery.

3. Perform a profile analysis of the patient's linguistic strengths and weaknesses that may highlight any patterns or areas of relative deficit. This is particularly important for those patients with normal baseline test performance.

CORTICAL STIMULATION

Many patients with intractable focal epilepsy are found to have the focus of their seizures located in the dominant hemisphere. Although the success of the surgical intervention is determined by the degree of postoperative seizure control, preoperative language abilities should not be compromised to achieve this goal. In the attempt to strike the ideal balance between the maximal resection and minimal risk of postoperative language deficits,

language areas may need to be localized via extra-operative cortical stimulation.

The aim of electrical stimulation of cortical regions is to localize motor, sensory, and language areas so that these areas may be identified and spared at the time of surgical resection of the seizure focus. The purpose of the Wada procedure is to lateralize language function, whereas the purpose of cortical stimulation is to localize language function. Cortical stimulation for language localization, or language "mapping," identifies those areas that must be excluded from surgical resection to preserve preoperative language abilities. The determination whether the epileptogenic region encompasses language cortex is critical as presurgical assumptions of language representation may lead to inadvertent resection of language cortex and render a highly functioning patient aphasic as a result of surgery.

Electrical stimulation of the cortex is considered the most definitive method available to map areas of the brain that have language representation. In some cases, accepted neuroanatomical boundaries may be used to guide the extent of a dominant hemisphere resection rather than functional mapping, although this approach is usually reserved for straightforward cases in which the epileptogenic zone has been localized to the anterior or medial temporal regions. For those cases with the epileptogenic zone localized to the dominant midtemporal neocortex, or, in which a structural lesion may have rearranged the classical cerebral language representation, cortical mapping is indicated to define language localization.

Intraoperative vs. Extraoperative Cortical Stimulation

Direct cortical stimulation and language mapping can be done either intraoperatively prior to surgical resection or extraoperatively (in the EMU) after intracranial electrodes have been implanted by the neurosurgeon. Historically, most of the data collected to create the functional maps of the human brain (e.g., motor and sensory homunculus) were obtained intraoperatively.[101,102,103] More recently, many epilepsy surgery centers complete cortical mapping extraoperatively using intracranial electrodes as this method provides days to weeks to obtain and analyze data. This continues to be a topic

of debate because of multiple factors including methodology, cost, and potential morbidity.

Extraoperative Cortical Stimulation

Clinical Setting

The elements required for extraoperative cortical mapping include an electrical stimulus generator, EEG, a cooperative patient, and the appropriate personnel (see Figure 18–5). The aim of cortical stimulation is to identify the function of selected cortical regions (i.e., motor, sensory, language). Limitations of this technique may include induction of seizures, development of afterdischarges, poor patient cooperation, or production of pain when the dura or branches of the trigeminal nerve are stimulated.[104]

Ideally, cortical mapping should be performed after the initial discomfort attributed to intracranial implantation has subsided and the patient is cooperative and energetic. In patients who require

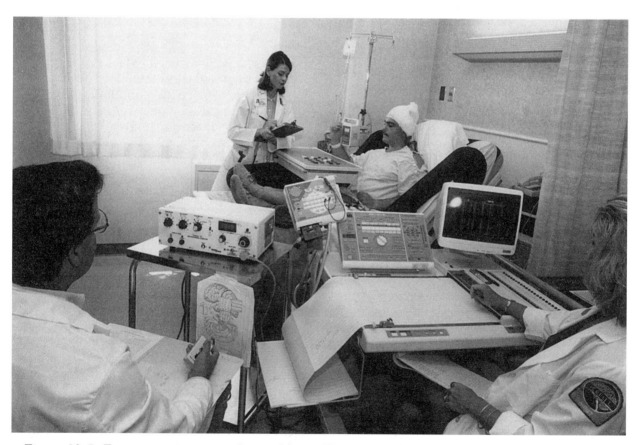

Figure 18–5. Extraoperative cortical stimulation: The epileptologist (far left) regulates the intensity and timing of the electrical stimulus as the EEG technician monitors the EEG for afterdischarges. The speech–language pathologist (standing) administers an auditory comprehension task.

intracranial recording of their typical seizures to determine the epileptogenic zone, antiepileptic medications are reduced or withheld causing the patient to be more susceptible to seizures when electrically stimulated. Mapping done later during the recording period, after the resumption of antiepileptic therapy, will often be more productive.

Stimulus Parameters

The same intracranial (usually subdural) electrodes for recording cerebral electrical activity are used during cortical stimulation to transmit the electrical stimulus into the cerebral cortex. The electrical stimulus used conventionally is a biphasic rectangular pulse with an intensity (I) between 0.5 and 15 mA and a pulse duration (D) of 0.3 msec. The pulses are usually delivered at a rate of 50/sec in trains lasting 2 to 5 sec.[105] In children, stepwise increments of stimulus intensity and duration above the accepted limits for adults may be needed to elicit responses in a brain with nonmyelinated nerve fibers.[106]

Electrocorticography/Afterdischarges

EEG recording during cortical stimulation is required for the monitoring of afterdischarges and subclinical seizure activity. Afterdischarges represent persistent epileptiform discharges elicited by electrical stimulation that occur at one or more electrodes. Stimulation with intensities above the afterdischarge threshold tends to produce clinical seizures. When an afterdischarge is elicited, it may not be accompanied by clinical changes or it may produce transient dysfunction. The clinical changes that may occur should not be used to construct the final map of cortical representation since the degree and extent of its propagation are unknown.

Procedure for Extraoperative Cortical Stimulation

Application of an electrical current to a circumscribed area of the brain can either activate or block a response. The effect of electrical stimulation differs depending on the cortical region being stimulated.[107]

Primary Efferent/Afferent Areas

The main stimulation effect to primary motor and sensory areas is "positive" in that the stimulation activates a response. Stimulation to the primary motor area results in contralateral muscle twitches or flexion, while stimulation to the primary sensory area elicits contralateral paresthesias. Simple visual or auditory phenomena are elicited on stimulation of the respective sensory areas. Motor phenomena are readily seen by the observer, and sensory responses are reported by the patient to the examiner. The patient is highly aware of stimulation that results in a positive effect, and the effect lasts only as long as the duration of the stimulus.

Association Areas

Stimulation of cortical association areas, such as that representing language, will block a response, producing exclusively "negative" signs. The stimulation may have no outward effect while the patient is at rest; the negative effect only becomes apparent when the patient attempts to perform a specific function that requires the action of the stimulated cortex. Therefore, the patient must be engaging in a language task in order for language interference to occur. Table 18–5 provides a list of language tasks administered during cortical stimulation. The inability to perform the function lasts only as long as the stimulus duration, and the patient is able to resume the function once the stimulus has ended. "Stimulation acts on complex systems such as language generally like a temporary lesion, as though noise were introduced into the system."[113] Stimulation intensities below 5 to 10 mA usually do not elicit negative effects in language cortex.[114] The degree of disruption of language is a function of the stimulus intensity.[107] For example, at a lower stimulus intensity (8 mA) the patient may experience difficulty reading or following complex commands, and at a higher intensity (14 mA) the patient may be completely unable to read aloud or follow even simple commands. Language-related errors that have been observed during electrical stimulation of cerebral cortex are outlined in Table 18–6.

At the completion of cortical mapping, significant findings are plotted onto a schematic brain map displaying the patient's subdural electrode array (Figure 18–6) to guide the neurosurgeon in planning the surgical resection of the epileptic focus.

Intraoperative Cortical Stimulation

Cortical stimulation in the intraoperative setting requires a modification of the extraoperative protocol to accommodate for the brief amount of time, position of the patient, and the testing environment.

Table 18–5. Language Tasks Administered During Cortical Stimulation

Reading aloud as the screening measure at all electrode sites (continuous reading aloud of any material at patient's reading level)

Confrontation naming (naming can also be used as the screening measure at all sites)

Automatic speech: counting aloud, days of week, months of year, alphabet

Responsive naming (i.e., "What tells time?")

Reading comprehension (following written commands or answering written questions)

Auditory comprehension: modified Token Test, following verbal commands

Repetition of words/sentences

Writing: to dictation, copying, spontaneous writing

Drawing/copying of figures, shapes, designs

Calculations (solve mental math problems presented visually or auditorially)

Spontaneous speech (describe pictures, objects, events)

Phrase completion (i.e., "The coldest season of the year is ____")

Comprehension and production of oral spelling

*Specific test items to be administered during cortical stimulation are individualized for each patient after baseline language testing is completed. The patient should be able to perform all test items accurately in the absence of stimulation. This ensures that errors are the result of stimulation and not due to inappropriate selection of tasks too difficult for the patient.

*All tasks must conform to the 5 second stimulus duration, so each item must require only a few seconds for a response.

Source: Cleveland Clinic protocol.[107–112]

Table 18–6. Language-Related Errors Elicited by Cortical Stimulation

Distortion of speech, similar in character to upper motor neuron dysarthria

Speech arrest (patient is essentially mute during the stimulation)

Confusion of numbers while counting

Impaired repetition of words/sentences

Anomia (inability to name with retained ability to speak)

Incorrect naming

Paraphasias

Circumlocutions

Neologisms

Perseveration

Slow, effortful reading

Fluent reading with mistakes or paraphasias

Impaired auditory comprehension

Impaired reading comprehension

Written language errors

Source: Compiled from Penfield, Roberts 1959;[150] Ojemann, Sutherling et al 1993;[116] Lüders et al 1986.[111]

The tasks administered in the operating room are the same as those during extraoperative stimulation; however, naming is used as the screening measure instead of continuous reading aloud as it is administered more easily in this setting. Task modifications are also necessary because of the shorter duration of electrical stimulus trains (1 to 3 sec) and a shorter time available overall for intraoperative testing.

Electrical stimulation of association cortex for mapping of language function is performed over multiple sites in the exposed cortex. The speech–language pathologist administers the language tests and informs the neurosurgeon of the accuracy of each response provided by the patient. Object naming is tested at each cortical site. Three trials of stimulation are applied at each site, and those sites with repeated naming errors are considered essential for language.[115] When electrical stimulation elicits consistent naming errors at a specific site, additional language tasks are administered at that site. Language mapping of perisylvian cortex requires about 20 to 30 minutes (maximum of 60 minutes) of testing. Refer to the section on surgical technique for a comprehensive description of the surgical process.

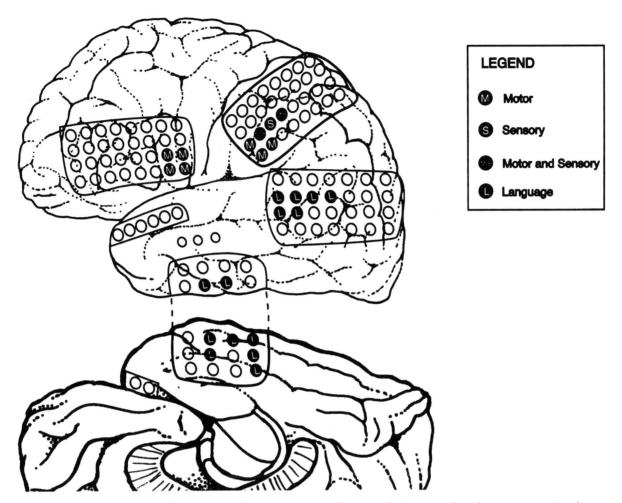

Figure 18–6. A schematic brain map that represents the cumulative results of extraoperative functional cortical mapping in a 32-year-old right-handed female with medically intractable complex partial epilepsy. Note that multiple electrodes in the basal temporal region elicited language interference on stimulation.

Several investigators have reported findings that emphasize the validity of cortical stimulation in localizing essential language areas.[107,116,117] A left anterior temporal lobectomy within 2 cm of a cortical site with consistent naming errors has been associated with an increase in errors on the Wepman Aphasia Battery on retesting one month after surgery. No changes on the test battery occurred in those patients whose resection avoided sites with naming errors by over 2 cm. There was no association between increased errors on the test battery and preoperative language abilities, extent of surgical resection (outside the 2 cm limit), or postoperative seizure control.[116] Haglund et al.[117] reported that a group of patients with normal preoperative language function and permanent postoperative language deficits all had their resection margins less than 1 cm from an identified language area. In those patients with language areas greater than 1 cm from the margins of the resection, preoperative language function returned within the first postoperative week. The Cleveland Clinic group[107] has reported that their standard practice is to avoid functional cortical areas by at least 1 cm. In those cases in which this was not possible, neurological deficits were present. These reports present a clear validation of the sensitivity and specificity of functional language mapping.

Techniques measuring blood flow or metabolism (such as PET)[118–120] often show a greater area of cortex involved in language than cortical stimulation. These methods may indicate those regions that participate in language function, whereas functional mapping with cortical stimulation may show those areas that are essential for it.[121]

Language Areas Identified with Cortical Stimulation

Frontal Language Area

During cortical stimulation, complete speech arrest will localize Broca's area anterior to the face region of the motor cortex.[122] It is differentiated from stimulation to the face motor cortex by the absence of evoked movement.[123] Stimulation mapping of Broca's area produces both motoric arrest of speech and naming errors with retained ability to speak.[113] The small motor speech area is considered Broca's area, which in turn constitutes only a small portion of the frontal naming area.[113] The remaining adjacent area eliciting changes in naming is considered the frontal language area.[113] Thus, the frontal language area has Broca's area (the motor speech area) within it, and Broca's area is just one component (the motor component) of the frontal language area.

Electrical stimulation of Broca's area can elicit a severe receptive and expressive aphasia.[110] Despite classical views of relatively intact comprehension in Broca's aphasia, stimulation of Broca's area may elicit a written and spoken language comprehension deficit[110] similar to the comprehension deficit elicited by stimulation of Wernicke's area.[124] Broca's area also contains a writing center.[109]

Based on results of cortical stimulation, it has been concluded that the posterior inferior frontal region integrates speech and other complex motor acts, and lesions to this region may result in functional apraxias.[109] To summarize, "the pre- and post-Rolandic cortex in the vicinity of the Rolandic head area seems to be the point at which the language system interfaces with the motor speech system."[113] This area has been called the "final motor output pathway for language."[125]

The frontal language area, however, is not limited to the inferior frontal gyrus, but may extend into the middle frontal gyrus and the lower part of the superior frontal gyrus.[110] Stimulation of the supplementary motor area can elicit speech arrest caused by a negative motor effect rather than a pure language deficit.[108,114]

Posterior Language Area

Stimulation of the left posterior temporal lobe (Wernicke's area) results in comprehension deficits, and, at some sites, deficits occur only as information becomes more complex.[124] Stimulation to Wernicke's area may cause speech arrest during oral reading—the opposite of what is expected as lesions in this area typically result in fluent speech. Lesser et al. speculated that due to the transient nature of the electrical stimulation, the brain does not utilize alternative language areas and pathways that enable fluency to supervene in the event of a chronic lesion to Wernicke's area.[124]

Naming errors have been elicited on stimulation within 3 cm of the temporal pole,[122] a region that is included in a standard temporal lobectomy (Figure 18–7). Stimulation of the parietal operculum and adjacent parietal portions of the supramarginal gyrus has elicited naming errors.[23] The insula has also been found to be part of the perisylvian language zone.[113]

Basal Temporal Language Area

A third language area, the basal temporal language area (BTLA), was discovered by Lüders et al. in 1986 during cortical stimulation of an epileptic patient with basal temporal subdural electrodes.[111] The BTLA is located in the dominant basal temporal fusiform (occipitotemporal) gyrus, 3 to 3.5 cm posterior to the temporal pole[111,126] (Figure 18–8). It may extend into the inferior temporal or parahippocampal gyri.[127,128] A BTLA was found in 8 of 22 epilepsy patients with subdural electrodes under the dominant temporal lobe; Broca's area was identified in 15 of 22 patients and Wernicke's area in 14 of 22.[126] Electrical stimulation of the BTLA elicits both receptive and expressive deficits including anomia, agraphia, alexia, and impaired repetition. Deficits elicited during stimulation have been similar to that of Wernicke's area, suggesting a functional link between the two areas. In fact, some connectivity is apparent between the two areas.[126] The BTLA is not an extension of Wernicke's area, as the two areas have been found to be separated by at least 4 cm of cortex. It has been suggested that resection of the BTLA may not be associated with a lasting neurological deficit or language disturbance.[126] However, Malow et al.[129] reported persistent responsive naming deficits 2 years following resection of the BTLA in one patient who showed normal performance on this measure prior to surgery.

To summarize, naming sites have been found far beyond the traditional boundaries of Broca's and Wernicke's areas.[121] In fact, Ojemann[130] reported that the variability in localization of essential language areas for naming exceeds the variability of cortical morphology. The significance of this is twofold: (1) a resection in the dominant hemisphere without stimulation mapping may include language areas outside the classical language areas; and (2) in some patients with no language function

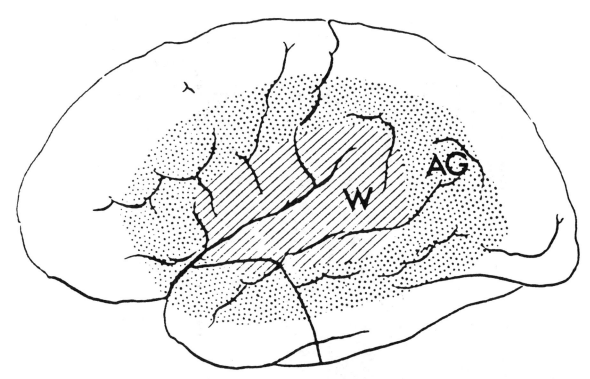

Figure 18–7. Diagram of left cerebral hemisphere indicating zone where pathology results in aphasia. Diagonal lines represent areas where pathology invariably results in aphasia; stippling represents areas where pathology frequently results in aphasia. Solid line indicates resection margin of a standard left temporal lobectomy for epilepsy. W: Wernicke's area, AG: Angular gyrus. (Reprinted with permission from Rausch R: Effects of temporal lobe surgery on behavior. In Smith D, Treiman D, Trimble M, eds., *Advances in neurology*, Vol 55, pp 279–292. Raven Press, New York, 1991. Original source: Benson DF. Aphasia. In Heilman KM, Valenstien E, eds., *Clinical neuropsychology*. New York, Oxford University Press, 1985, pp. 17–47.).

in the classical areas, this particular cortical area can be resected without risk to language for a more beneficial result.

SURGICAL TECHNIQUE

Temporal lobectomy is the most frequently performed surgery for the treatment of focal epilepsy, particularly complex partial focal epilepsy. It is performed under general anesthesia in most institutions. There are four main types of temporal lobectomy for epilepsy; the particular type selected for a given patient is based on the localization of the epileptogenic region to be resected. The first type, the classical resection (standard resection), establishes a posterior margin of 5 cm from the pole of the temporal lobe on the left side and a variable posterior margin of 7 to 9 cm on the right side. The resected volume commonly includes the amygdala and anterior hippocampus. The second type, a tailored resection, allows for a more limited removal of the neocortex by establishing the loca-

tion of epileptogenicity through intraoperative electrocorticography. In the third type, a strictly lateral cortical removal is carried out preserving the medial structures entirely. Finally, a selective amygdalohippocampectomy accomplishes the removal of the medially situated structures while preserving the lateral temporal cerebral convexity.

Preoperative Anesthesia

Most surgeries for the resection of an epileptic focus are performed under general anesthesia. The strongest indication for surgery performed with the patient awake ("awake anesthesia") is in the case of an intended resection in the language area where language mapping is a prerequisite. In children, much of this mapping can be performed extraoperatively using electrodes implanted intracranially under general anesthesia. This avoids the need to subsequently expose the brain under local anesthesia and reduces the overall level of anxiety in a younger individual less well equipped to tolerate a lengthy procedure.

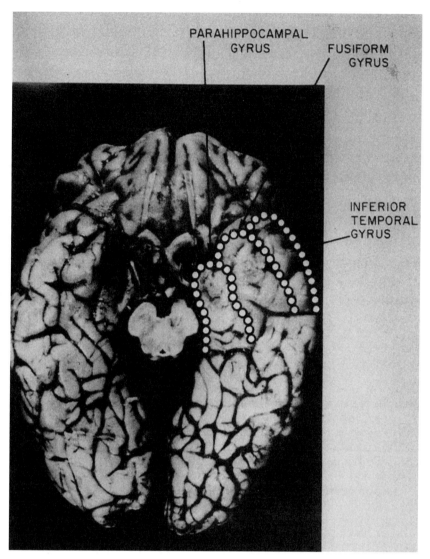

Figure 18–8. Photograph of base of brain illustrating the region of the basal temporal language area: the fusiform (occipito-temporal) gyrus. (Reprinted with permission from Lüders H, Lesser R, Hahn J, et al: Basal temporal language area demonstrated by electrical stimulation. *Neurology* 1986; 36:505–510.).

Cortical language mapping requires the attention and cooperation of the patient to obtain as comprehensive an evaluation as possible prior to defining the borders for resection. To this end, a variety of measures are undertaken to establish a comfortable environment for the patient. Prior to entry into the operating room, the scalp on the side of the intended surgery is regionally anesthetized. This is followed by infiltration of the scalp along the line of the incision with 0.33% bupivacaine (60 ml). The protocol allows for sufficient analgesia to carry out the entire operative procedure including skin closure without the need for further local anesthetic infiltration.

Following preparation of the operative site, a surgical instrument table is positioned over the patient and the drapes are configured in such a manner as to allow relatively wide visual access to the surroundings for the patient. Space in this area is created for the speech–language pathologist and a slide projector unit to carry out language testing.

In the final stages of preparation, both peripheral venous and arterial catheters are implanted and a urinary catheter is placed. Cardiac leads are positioned for electrocardiographic monitoring. Systemic arterial pressures, heart rate and rhythm, fluid intake and output, and blood gases along with serum electrolytes are assessed periodically. Sedation is provided intravenously with propofol and can be reversed quickly by discontinuing the drip.

Operative Procedure

Surgical exposure to the level of the dura is accomplished in 60 to 90 minutes. At this point, additional xylocaine (1%) is instilled into the dural envelope adjacent to the middle meningeal artery as it passes in the area of the pterion to anesthetize the dura, which itself is pain sensitive. Cerebral tissue is insensitive to pain. Electrocorticography (electrical recording of the exposed brain surface) is then performed to define the probable epileptogenic territory. This is accomplished with a combination of tower-based individually fitted spring-loaded electrodes with 3 degrees of freedom and electrode contacts mounted within a thin plastic housing that can be advanced along the skull base to record from the basal cerebral surface (see Figure 18–9). The recording is carried out with a standard EEG machine using referential and bipolar montages to appreciate points of origin of electrographically abnormal features such as spikes, polyspikes, slow waves, and spike-wave discharges. A resection margin is created encompassing the region of abnormality.

At this point, the patient is awakened and language testing is initiated. Electrical stimulation of the cortical surface is performed in the manner outlined below using a current source (i.e., Ojemann Cortical Stimulator, OCS-1, Radionics Co.,

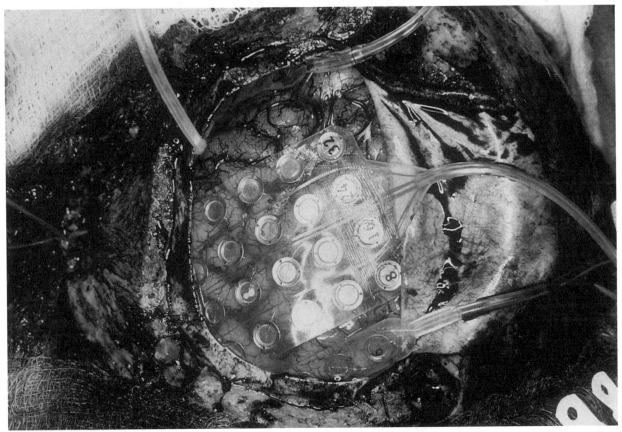

A

Figure 18–9. Operative exposure of the left frontal lobe in a 21-year-old male with an intractable seizure disorder. Extraoperative recording with implanted subdural electrodes of the cerebral convexity was required with stimulation mapping of the language area. (**A**) The frontal convexity has been re-exposed following a 2-week period in the epilepsy monitoring unit. Subdural strips and a grid are evident and specific electrode locations are marked by paper labels on the cerebral surface to identify sites of epileptogenic activity. (**B**) Superior view of operative exposure showing the electrode tower fastened to the cranium to provide additional electrographic information and allow a finer delineation of the surgical resection. (**C, D**) Labels are added to the cerebral surface to mark sites of electrographic abnormality, combining information from prior extraoperative recording with that of operative electrocorticography. (**E**) A corticectomy has been carried out (darkened area) in the posterior portion of the middle frontal gyrus immediately above the motor speech area.

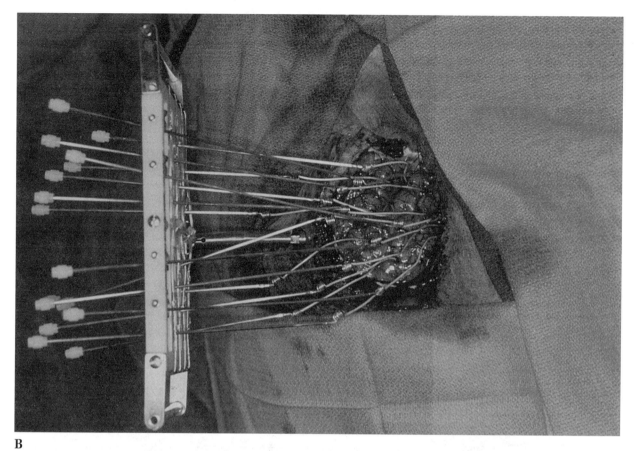

B

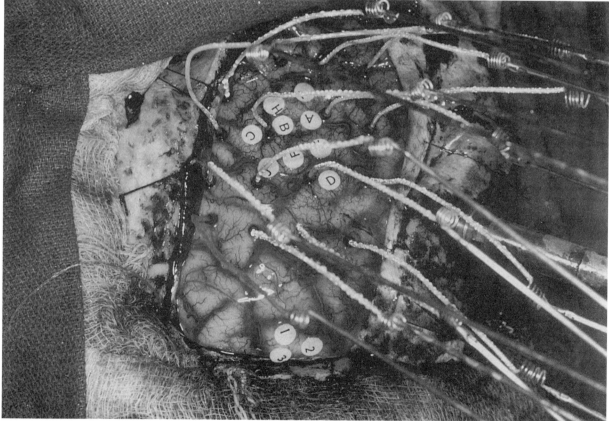

C

Figure 18–9. (continued)

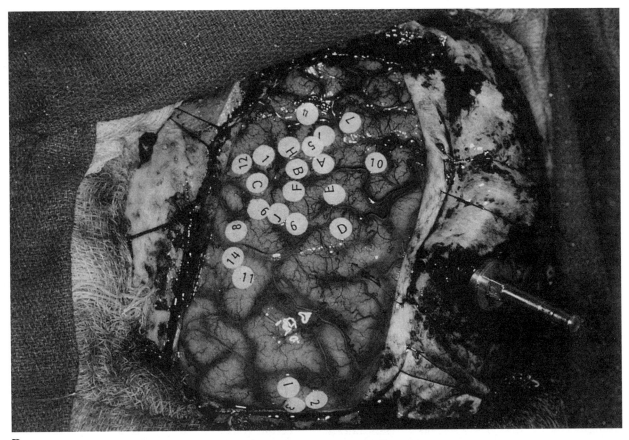

D

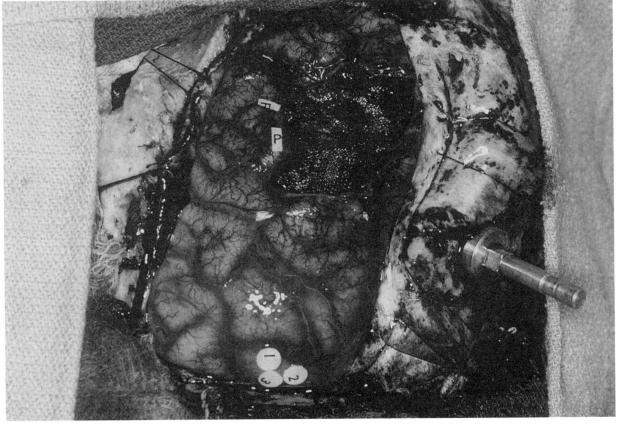

E

Figure 18–9. (continued)

Burlington, MA). The stimulating current should be raised incrementally in each functional area to prevent the induction of a seizure. Stimulation parameters vary commonly within the following ranges: frequency, 10 to 50 Hz; pulse duration, 0.4 to 1.0 ms; and train duration, 1 to 3 sec. Any positive responses demonstrated by the movement of a limb, a sensory phenomenon, or negative response such as the interruption of a language function are followed in random fashion by stimulation in the same area to reproduce the impression and by sham stimulation to judge its authenticity.

Stimulation of the posterior (temporal) speech area requires higher currents than are needed for rolandic (sensorimotor) responses and will also result in the arrest or alteration of spontaneous speech, serial counting, or naming. An absolute anomia may manifest with a confrontation naming task or interruption in the cadence of serial counting may be apparent. A negative response may not absolutely indicate the absence of function,[131] although elevation of the electrical current to levels 5 to 10 times that required to elicit threshold responses in the sensorimotor areas without speech disturbance is accepted with reasonable assurance to declare the given area is unlikely to influence spontaneous speech. This may be further confirmed by proceeding with removal of the area, should it be necessary for seizure control, while the patient is engaged in spontaneous dialogue. Negative responses to the stimulation of the speech area appear to be more common in both female and ambidextrous patients and in those found to have bilateral speech representation.[132] Removal of cerebral tissue extrinsic to functional cortical areas is carried out with adherence to certain surgical principles. A subpial removal of tissue is performed taking into account the sulcal landmarks in the vicinity. In such a way, the anatomical plan of resection closely approximates the demarcated area of epileptogenicity and yet preserves the circulation of immediately adjacent tissues.

In those cases where language areas may overlap with epileptogenic sites, there is an absolute indication to proceed with cerebral exposure under local anesthesia to allow language mapping. Following electrocorticography, cortical stimulation and resection of allowable tissues, areas of epileptogenicity may remain within the designated language cortex. Repeat electrocorticography following the initial resection may confirm this notion. Under such circumstances where repetitive persistent spiking activity remains despite resection of adjacent cerebral tissue, some groups have undertaken multiple subpial transections of the cerebral cortex in an attempt to se-

quester regions of epileptogenicity by limiting the lateral spread of discharge. Morrell et al.[133] first reported the safety and efficacy of this technique that undertakes a series of shallow cuts through the gray matter orthogonal to the axis of a given gyrus. This approach ostensibly spares vertically oriented fibers, thus preserving the functional integrity of the tissue. Experience with multiple subpial transection of the posterior language area indicates that a period of global aphasia may persist for a number of days postoperatively with improvement to baseline or beyond noted in a variety of language-related tasks over the remaining months of the first year. Continued difficulties have been noted in such tasks as reading, writing, naming, and repetition.[134]

On completion of the multiple subpial transections during which time the patient is asked to engage in conversation, the final stage of surgery is undertaken. Hemostasis is ensured prior to closure of the dura. The craniotomy segment is returned and sutured to the cranium followed by reapproximation of the muscle, fascia, and the scalp in two layers.

OUTCOMES

The success or failure of a surgical resection in any patient with a medically intractable seizure disorder must be determined not merely in regard to the elimination or reduction of seizures but with attention to any improvements that the surgery has rendered in the patient's quality of life. Surgical complications resulting in a temporary or permanent neurological deficit and the psychosocial needs of dependency on family or society will detract from the obvious benefit of being seizure-free and ultimately rid of antiepileptic medication. Quantitative measures to assess postoperative quality of life are currently being considered and will be part of the standard regimen of assessment in the near future.

Table 18–7 gives a frequently used scale for judging the success of surgery concerning the alteration of a seizure disorder. Seizure occurrence may subside over a number of months or years following surgery or it may stop entirely for years and then return. A postoperative follow-up may therefore be lengthy, requiring a dedicated physician–patient commitment. Outcomes after 10 years in those patients found initially to be seizure-free for 1 to 2 years postoperatively indicate that about 60% remain so. In a review of 1579 operations between 1929 and 1980 at the Montreal Neurological Institute, 30% of patients were found to be seizure-free for 2 years or more and 43% of these had subsequent late seizures. In 41% of cases, the recurrence

Table 18–7. Classification of Postoperative Outcome

Class I: Free of disabling seizures[a]
   A. Completely seizure free since surgery
   B. Nondisabling simple partial seizures only since surgery
   C. Some disabling seizures after surgery, but free of disabling seizures for at least 2 years
   D. Generalized convulsion with antiepileptic drug withdrawal only

Class II: Rare disabling seizures ("almost seizure free")
   A. Initially free of disabling seizures but has rare seizures now
   B. Rare disabling seizures since surgery
   C. More than rare disabling seizures after surgery, but rare seizures for at least 2 years
   D. Nocturnal seizures only

Class III: Worthwhile improvement[b]
   A. Worthwhile seizure reduction
   B. Prolonged seizure-free intervals amounting to greater than half the follow-up period, but not less than 2 years

Class IV: No worthwhile improvement[b]
   A. Significant seizure reduction
   B. No appreciable change
   C. Seizures worse

---

[a] Excludes early postoperative seizures (first few weeks).
[b] Determination of "worthwhile improvement" will require quantitative analyses of additional data such as percent seizure reduction, cognitive function, and quality of life.
Source: From Engel J, Van Ness PC, Rasmussen TB, Ojemann LM: Outcome with respect to epileptic seizures. In J Engel Jr, ed., *Surgical treatment of the epilepsies,* 2nd ed. Raven Press, New York, 1993, pp 609–621.

was in the form of 1 to 3 isolated seizures followed by a seizure-free status for a prolonged time.

When the analysis is confined to temporal lobe resections, the seizure-free outcome approaches 70% with improvement noted in a further 24% of patients. Strictly neocortical resections involving temporal and/or extratemporal territories and avoidance of medial temporal structures have been shown to yield less favorable results with a seizure-free status rendered in 45% of patients and improvement noted in a further 35%. When resection involved removal of an associated epileptogenic lesion (i.e., tumor, angioma, etc.), seizure-free outcomes were seen in 67% of cases and improvement noted in a further 22%.

Parameters used in predicting the success of surgery are undergoing refinement. Most lesion-associated seizure disorders likewise have a high probability of elimination with surgery. Postoperative outcome batteries will ultimately require an amalgamation of parameters that take into consideration not only an alteration of the seizure disorder but the reintegration of the patient into society with all of its benefits and burdens.

Outcome: Language

The long-term outcome of language after the surgical treatment of intractable epilepsy has not been as extensively investigated as that of verbal memory, although substantial evidence exists to confirm that surgery of the dominant hemisphere poses a risk to language functioning. Anomia is the most commonly reported postoperative deficit in patients after left temporal lobectomy for intractable epilepsy.[135–144] Rausch has asserted that "a mild depression in confrontational naming is a sequela of left temporal lobectomy."[142] Indeed, in our experience anomic aphasia is the most common type of aphasia after dominant temporal lobectomy, followed by conduction aphasia, and much less frequently by Wernicke's aphasia, each of which rapidly evolve into anomic aphasia.

Frequently, no changes in language are apparent after surgery. However, "the absence of a frank aphasia does not mean that language function is normal"[138] (p. 565). As is well known, many patients with anomic aphasia are not readily detected through interview alone. Therefore, highly complex language tests must be administered to detect subtle changes postoperatively. In some patients, language deficits after surgery represent an exacerbation of preexisting deficits,[145] emphasizing the importance of baseline language assessment.

Acute Language Changes

Immediately after left temporal lobectomy with cortical mapping, changes have been observed in confrontation naming, descriptive naming, repetition, reading, and writing.[140,144] This indicates that acute postoperative language deficits may result from left temporal lobectomy despite functional language mapping, possibly due to edema and diaschisis (loss of function of areas distant to a cerebral lesion but neuronally connected to it) in the preserved left hemisphere structures.[140] Postoperative language deficits are usually at a maximum 48 hours after surgery, when brain swelling due to surgery is greatest.[122] In a series of 29 patients after left temporal lobectomy with extraoperative cortical mapping, 5 (17%) developed a mild postoperative aphasia that did not resolve completely by the time of discharge from the hospital and was attributed to unplanned surgical injury to nearby speech areas.[146]

Patients tested one week after left anterior temporal lobectomy have shown significantly reduced formal (phonemic) and semantic (category) word fluency production,[33] and neuropsychological testing 2 weeks after left temporal lobectomy has revealed a specific decline in naming abilities.[147]

Age at onset of epilepsy may play a significant role in postoperative language outcome.[28,135,136] Several weeks after standard left temporal lobectomy, patients without early risk factors for seizures have shown an overall language decline (in phonemic and semantic fluency, repetition, comprehension, naming, and reading) with changes most pronounced on the Boston Naming Test.[28] None of the patients with early risk factors experienced a decline in naming. Patients with no known early risk factors for seizures are more likely to show acute postoperative anomia than those with early risk factors, and the anomia may still be present at the one-year follow-up assessment.[135] This may be due to atypical cerebral representation for naming in patients with early risk factors, before complete lateralization of language.[135] These studies indicate that functional language mapping may be most critical in those patients with later onset of epilepsy.

Long-Term Language Changes

In an early investigation, 4 of 10 patients after left temporal lobectomy exhibited anomic aphasia at testing 6 months postoperatively.[137] This led the investigators to conclude that in some patients the uncomplicated resection of the anterior temporal lobe may be associated with anomic aphasia. Testing has revealed a significant decline in scores on the Boston Naming Test 6 to 12 months following dominant temporal lobectomy.[24] Evidence of postoperative long-term language impairment in ver-

bal reasoning and problem-solving was found in a group of 64 patients with a mean follow-up of 7.7 months after standard left anterior temporal lobectomy.[148]

A group of patients tested 1 to 21 years after left anterior temporal lobectomy were significantly impaired in object naming and classifying objects as living or man-made (a verbally mediated process). Classifying objects as larger or smaller than a chair (a nonverbal process) was normal, although size classification was a more difficult task for the control subjects.[143]

Language Outcome of Resection with Versus without Cortical Language Mapping

The majority of centers provide surgical treatment of epilepsy under general anesthesia without intraoperative language mapping. Hermann and Wyler[149] reported a prospective investigation of language outcome after left temporal lobectomy under local anesthesia with intraoperative language mapping (n = 13) and under general anesthesia without language mapping (n = 13). At 6 months postoperatively, patients who had general anesthesia were more likely to be seizure free, although they demonstrated a mild persistent anomia. In another investigation, postoperative aphasia occurred after temporal lobectomy without functional mapping in 29 of 56 patients (52%), but proved to be transient in 24 patients and persistent in 5 (9%).[139] Penfield and Roberts[150] reported a lower incidence of aphasia with intraoperative cortical stimulation mapping immediately postoperatively in 22 of 273 operations (8%) involving the left hemisphere (frontal and/or temporal resections). Hermann and Wyler[149] reported results of dominant temporal lobectomy in 15 patients, 13 of whom underwent tailored resection with intraoperative cortical mapping. Six months after surgery, no significant changes from baseline were observed on the Multilingual Aphasia Examination. These results suggest that cortical stimulation mapping of language function may result in fewer cases of postoperative anomia and aphasia than standard temporal lobectomy without language mapping.

Language Outcome of Amygdalohippocampectomy

In some cases, the seizure focus is reasonably well localized to the mesial temporal lobe structures. This requires aggressive resection of mesial temporal structures, or amygdalohippocampectomy, with complete or near complete preservation of the lateral temporal neocortex. In such cases, language has been found to be relatively preserved and functional language mapping may not be warranted. Investigations of patients 6 to 12 months after left medial/anterior temporal lobectomy without language mapping have shown no significant decline in language as compared to baseline.[138,151]

Variables Related to Language Outcome

Several investigators have found no correlation between extent of cortical resection and postoperative aphasia.[22,141,146] Even small temporal resections that encroach on more anterior temporal naming areas have been followed by a persistent language disturbance.[125] Language deficits after dominant temporal lobectomy may therefore result from atypical or variable language localization in individual patients, rather than from the extent of the surgical resection.[146] Higher performance on preoperative language testing has been associated with a larger decline in postoperative performance,[152] suggesting that patients with high-level language functioning may be more at risk for language deficits after dominant temporal lobectomy than those with lower preoperative language performance. Patients at a younger age at the time of surgery have shown the greatest degree of postoperative cognitive improvement.[145]

Counseling on Language Outcome

Lutsep et al.[141] reported on a series of 25 patients who underwent standard left temporal lobectomy. Based on results of formal testing, 9 (36%) were aphasic in the immediate postoperative period; 4 (16%) remained aphasic 4 months later. Quantitative analyses after 4 months revealed no significant group differences from preoperative baselines, although 4 patients were persistently mildly or moderately aphasic. The authors recommended that the following points be made when counseling surgical candidates on the language risks associated with dominant temporal lobectomy: (1) approximately one-third of patients may experience a decline in performance on language examinations in the immediate postoperative period; (2) as a group, those patients with acute language deficits will recover by 4 months postoperatively; and (3) 16% of individuals may continue to have mild to moderate language difficulty 4 months after left temporal

lobectomy.[141] This emphasizes that there are individual negative language outcomes within the context of an overall group positive language outcome after left temporal lobectomy for epilepsy.[136]

Outcome: Verbal Memory

Although dramatic improvement in seizure control is the expected outcome of temporal lobectomy, unfortunately this can be accompanied by alterations in memory, language, visual/spatial abilities, and other cognitive/intellectual functions. Research over the past four decades clearly shows that deterioration in memory functioning constitutes the principle neuropsychological morbidity associated with unilateral temporal lobectomy.[145,148,153] Although postsurgically there may be a transient lowering of psychometric intelligence, recovery over the course of the next several months to presurgical levels is almost always observed.

In general, a left temporal resection results in decrements in verbal learning and memory whereas the right temporal lobectomy patient typically experiences a reduction in performance on measures designed to evaluate the encoding and/or retrieval of nonverbal stimuli. Performance decrements in left temporal lobe subjects have been shown with respect to the recall of connected prose,[154] learning and recall of word lists,[148,155,156] verbal paired associate learning,[157] and semantic memory.[143]

Improvement in specific domains of neurocognitive function has been reported in some cases.[158] In these instances, improvement in cognitive functioning is suggested to be secondary to the release of the intact hemisphere from the irritative seizure focus. However, a precise explanation for such improvements is speculative at best since a variety of other factors may also lead to improved function—for example, test-retest effects, improved emotional status, and reduced medication effects.

In this context, the pattern of postoperative memory change is related to the specific functional significance of the tissue removed.[142] Indeed, in the case of left temporal lobectomy, recent investigations have demonstrated that certain factors are predictive of outcome with respect to postoperative decrements in verbal memory function. In a retrospective study of 47 patients who underwent left temporal lobectomy, Wolf et al.[159] demonstrated that there was no difference in cognitive outcome between groups defined by extent of medial and/or lateral resection. However, associated data analyses revealed a negative correlation between cognitive change and age of seizure onset. Trenerry et al.[160] found a significant positive correlation between postoperative memory change and difference in MRI hippocampal volume (right minus left). Hermann et al.[161] demonstrated a relationship between degree of medial temporal sclerosis and cognitive outcome because patients without left hippocampal sclerosis reported significantly worse postsurgical memory function as compared to those subjects with significant sclerosis. In a retrospective study, Kneebone et al.[162] discovered that left temporal lobe resection subjects who performed well on the contralateral Wada test experienced significantly greater verbal memory deficits postoperatively than those subjects who had failed the test.

It appears that the earlier the age of seizure onset, the greater the degree of medial temporal sclerosis, and the smaller the hippocampal volume, the better is the outcome with respect to postsurgical memory decrement. This inverse relationship implies that removal of pathological tissue has relatively little impact on subsequent memory function. In contrast, removal of functional tissue, as in patients without evidence of hippocampal asymmetry and/or sclerosis, leads to greater morbidity regarding cognitive outcome. Thus, early onset of dominant temporal lobe seizure foci (i.e., greater pathology) appears to lead to more widespread distribution of language and memory areas.

Outcome: Auditory Function

Despite the number of years that cortical resections of the temporal lobe have been performed as a treatment for intractable seizures, there have been few systematic observations of the effects of these surgical interventions on audition. Investigations of auditory function in patients with temporal lobe epilepsy have been approached in three ways: (1) the temporal lobe has been stimulated electrically perioperatively and patients asked to report any auditory sensations; (2) sensitized speech and nonspeech dichotic tests of central auditory function have been administered pre- and postoperatively to patients undergoing temporal lobe resection to determine whether resection of the anterior temporal tip was associated with decrements in central auditory function; and (3) auditory evoked potentials have been recorded pre- and postoperatively from the scalp surface in an attempt to determine whether resection of the anterior temporal lobe was associated with changes in these evoked responses (i.e., loss of an evoked response might be expected to result in the loss of some characteristic of auditory processing).

The results of these investigations generally have shown that resections of the anterior temporal lobe are not associated with changes in hearing sensitivity unless the primary auditory cortex is breeched.[163,164] However, resections of the anterior temporal lobe are associated with decrements in auditory perceptual tasks for stimuli presented to the ear opposite the resected anterior temporal lobe. These deficits include impaired recognition of the order of presentation of paired pure tones differing in pitch and interstimulus interval,[165] impaired gap detection thresholds[166] (e.g., subjects requiring longer intervals between paired stimuli for detection of two stimuli to occur), deficits in spatial localization in the auditory hemispace opposite the resected anterior temporal lobe,[167] reduction in the capacity to selectively attend to one of multiple spatially separated simultaneous sound sources,[167] and a reduction in performance on dichotic speech tasks for the ear contralateral to the temporal lobectomy. Electrical stimulation of the medial temporal lobe[168] has resulted in deficits of phonemic discrimination, phonemic identification, and auditory comprehension.

Speech Stimuli

The understanding that speech processing predominates in the left hemisphere and processing of melodic patterns occurs predominately in the right hemisphere for right-handed individuals resulted from a series of pioneering dichotic hearing investigations of normal individuals by Kimura.[169,170] Oxbury and Oxbury[171] evaluated the performance of patients before and following temporal lobectomy either sparing or including Heschl's gyrus. Subjects participated in the dichotic digits task developed by Kimura.[169] The investigators reported that when the primary auditory cortex was spared, patients undergoing left temporal lobectomy reported digits presented to the left ear (right cortex) first more frequently than those presented to the right ear. A right temporal lobectomy sparing the primary auditory cortex did not alter performance on the dichotic digits task. Subsequent investigations of performance on dichotic materials of patients who underwent anterior temporal lobectomy have yielded stable[172–174] or degraded[173,175,176] contralateral ear performance (with reference to the resected hemisphere). In similar work, Berlin et al.[175–177] reported their observations of speech sound perception in epilepsy patients who had undergone either anterior temporal lobectomy or hemispherectomy. They found that performance on dichotic consonant vowel materials was poorer for the ear contralateral to the lobectomy or hemispherectomy.

Interestingly, ipsilateral ear performance on dichotic listening tasks has been reported to improve in some patients following anterior temporal lobectomy.[174,176] Additionally, auditory function on dichotic listening tasks has been reported to improve following right anterior temporal lobectomy and to worsen following left anterior temporal lobectomy.

In a landmark investigation, Boatman et al.[168] evaluated auditory perception during electrical stimulation of three patients with epilepsy who had multichannel subdural electrode arrays. Stimulation was conducted between adjacent electrode contacts of an implanted electrode grid placed over the temporal cortex. The auditory tasks included phonemic discrimination, phonemic identification, and auditory comprehension. The investigators found that stimulation of sites along the superior temporal gyrus resulted in auditory perceptual deficits. Additionally, the auditory deficits could involve auditory comprehension sparing auditory discrimination and identification, and auditory comprehension and identification sparing auditory discrimination, and could result in global auditory perceptual deficits across all forms of speech perception. The authors suggested that the findings argued against a top-down mode of speech perception.

OUTPATIENT TREATMENT OF LANGUAGE DEFICITS

Language deficits that persist beyond the acute postoperative period are usually mild. Anomic aphasia is perhaps the most common type of language disturbance treated in the outpatient setting after left temporal lobectomy for epilepsy. Postoperative deficits may represent an exacerbation of preoperative deficits, in which case the goal of treatment is the return to the *baseline* level of functioning. Outpatient speech–language treatment is most often short term, although some patients may need more long-term treatment focusing on anomia and exacerbated baseline reading and writing impairments. Most patients are optimistic and highly motivated to improve, as they consider mild changes in language after surgery a worthwhile exchange for control of their seizures. Table 18–8 provides guidelines for postoperative follow-up and treatment referral.

The purpose of surgery for epilepsy is to improve the patient's lifestyle by freeing the patient

Table 18–8. Postoperative Language Assessment

Objectives of acute postoperative inpatient testing:

1. Repeat preoperative baseline test battery (within 3 to 4 days after surgery).
2. Report results of testing and impressions in terms of change from baseline.
3. Determine whether treatment after discharge is warranted.
   a. Some patients will show no change from baseline when tested in the acute postoperative period and do not need outpatient treatment.
   b. Some patients will show mild change in one or two language parameters (most commonly naming and writing) that may only be apparent on formal testing. Short-term outpatient treatment is recommended. (This is perhaps the category in which most patients fall after surgery.)
   c. Some patients may experience more significant changes in language that may be apparent in conversation as well as formal testing. An outpatient treatment referral is indicated.

Most patients return to work or school approximately 2 months after surgery. Even those who exhibit transient naming deficits can benefit from outpatient treatment within the first few months after surgery, especially if anomia has not resolved by the time they return to work/school. Patients whose deficits are not transient may need longer term treatment.

from disabling seizures. Following surgery, patients may take on greater educational and vocational demands, so increased communication skills become important. Baseline communication skills may have been sufficient to meet previous needs, but for those patients who may be working or going to school for the first time, treatment is needed to help them meet the demands of novel communicative environments.

Patients who require treatment of language deficits after surgery generally fall into three main subtypes of therapy:

1. Traditional therapy: for patients who may have had more significant baseline language deficits, focusing on traditional language treatment.
2. Education-oriented therapy: strategy-based therapy for students, focusing on successful studying skills and school-related language use.
3. Vocational-specific therapy: strategy-based therapy for people who need to work on vocationally related language skills prior to returning to work after surgery.

Treatment involves many metalinguistic processes and begins with the awareness and recognition of the need for treatment and compensatory techniques. Whether a decline in language abilities on formal testing is functionally meaningful for a given patient may "depend on the patient's capacity for cognitive compensation, the nature and extent of environmental demands on these abilities, and psychosocial resources and support systems."[152] For many patients, postoperative deficits will ultimately resolve, but treatment is beneficial in the interim, especially if deficits have not resolved before their return to work or school.

Anomia

The anomia most commonly exhibited by patients after dominant temporal lobectomy is the *word-selection anomia* described by Benson.[178] In this type of anomia, the problem in word retrieval occurs at the point of accessing the phonological output lexicon.[179] The patient is able to access the semantic representation (the meaning of the object to be named), but is unable to retrieve the corresponding phonological representation (the sound of the word that represents the object). This results in the inability to name an object to confrontation with preserved ability to demonstrate semantic knowledge by gesturing or providing a description of the object. Patients will always recognize the target word once it is provided and can point to the target from an array of choices when the name is given. In addition, these patients invariably demonstrate an anomia for proper nouns.[180] Miceli et al.[181] provide a detailed account of a patient with impaired access to the phonological and orthographic output lexicons 10 years after left temporal lobectomy for intractable seizures.

Treatment of anomia focuses on the use of compensatory strategies for two purposes: (1) to aid retrieval of the desired word from the lexicon, and (2) to prevent anomia from resulting in pauses, hesitations, or complete halting of communication that often occurs when a speaker cannot find a specific word. The goal of treatment is to have the patient proficiently and *independently* utilize a number of compensatory strategies to improve word retrieval and prevent communication breakdown when anomia occurs. Treatment is focused on improving access to phonological representation from semantic knowledge through the use of retrieval strategies.

During the initial evaluation, a naming test such as the Boston Naming Test[92] should be administered as a formal measure of confrontation naming. Next, the patient is videotaped while engaging in conversation and while performing a variety of discourse tasks to assess on-line word-finding ability. As a baseline measurement for each task, the examiner counts the number of anomic episodes that are *apparent* in verbal expression and analyzes how the patient attempts to manage or compensate for the anomia. Typically, a patient may stop when speaking and make a comment such as, "I can't think of the word," followed by a long pause while trying to retrieve a specific word. This disrupts the flow of communication and therefore adversely affects the speaker's ability to convey the message, especially when this occurs several times in one conversation. Measurement of the outward occurrence of anomia provides an index of its functional impact on communication.

The next several sessions are devoted to educating the patient on compensatory strategies for anomia (Table 18–9). A strategy takes the place of the intended word in a sentence and provides information so that the listener understands the message without the patient necessarily saying the specific word. The strategy functions as a substitute for the intended word as well as a self-cue that may help the patient retrieve the desired word. In structured treatment tasks, the patient has a set of stimulus items (a stack of pictures or a stack of index cards with a single word written on each card) that are unable to be seen by the clinician. Unlike many other treatment programs in which

Table 18–9. Compensatory Strategies for Anomia

Gesture or pantomime to convey the meaning of the word

Substitute the target word with another word or phrase that has the same meaning

Describe the function or use of the item

Describe the appearance or physical attributes of the item

Provide a definition of the word

Describe the location of where the item is usually found

Associate the word with a referent familiar to the listener

Substitute the target word with the name of its superordinate category (rose—flower)

Formulate a phrase to be completed with the target word as a self-cuing strategy (i.e., "Please pass the salt and _____")

Think of the first letter of the word as a phonemic self-cueing strategy

Attempt to write the word as a graphic cueing strategy

Draw the object

the patient is required to provide the name of an object, the patient is explicitly instructed *not* to give the name of the object, even if able to think of the object name. The patient must use a strategy well enough to enable the clinician to name each of the target stimulus items. Each of the strategies is systematically learned and practiced through the complete hierarchy of stimulus items (Table 18–10).

Approximately five sessions are needed to educate the patient on all strategies. A patient may find greater success with certain strategies than others, in which case the preferred strategies should be practiced and utilized the most in treatment. Several more sessions are then needed to practice the strategies in discourse tasks and ultimately conversation. Home practice will help internalize the use of strategies.

Once all strategies have been learned using each type of stimulus item in the hierarchy, videotaping of conversation and discourse tasks is repeated and the occurrence of overt anomic episodes is counted for assessment of post-treatment word-finding disruptions in verbal expression. At this point the patient may use any strategy in the event of anomia. The goal is for patients to have an arsenal of strategies at their disposal whenever an episode of anomia occurs in spontaneous speech, so that they are able to readily compensate for the anomia and produce fluent, seamless verbal expression. The outcome measure is the change in the number of *overt* anomic episodes in on-line verbal expression.

This program for the compensation of anomia may be coupled with more traditional treatment approaches that focus on naming as the goal of treatment, such as the "lexical focus" approach described by Linebaugh[182] and the "semantic treatment" approach outlined by Howard and colleagues.[183]

Table 18–10. Hierarchy of Stimulus Items

Objects

Pictures of objects

Written words (concrete/imageable) presented on index cards (i.e., money, scissors, hanger)

Written words (abstract/nonimageable) (i.e., cheap, lie, opportunity, communication)

Words related to job, school, personal interests (i.e., overtime, midterm, meeting)

Proper names of people or places (famous or familiar people/places)

Discourse

In addition to treatment of anomia, many patients may require treatment of discourse abilities. Verbal expression is usually fluent and functional for communication but may need improvement in clarity, relevance, vocabulary, and organization of main concepts. Patients are encouraged to explicitly introduce new topics in conversation so that the listener establishes a clear understanding of context to facilitate comprehension of information. A patient who relies heavily on compensatory strategies may demonstrate discourse with a greater amount of total words, but qualitatively improved expression with less pauses, disruptions, and hesitations. Overall content of verbal output will be increased and the message will be conveyed more fluently. Patients may benefit from "scripting" of discourse topics for specific events or conversations. This has been used successfully by patients with mildly disorganized discourse structure. Patients do not read the script to the listener, but use it as a framework for verbal expression. Scripts should address core vocabulary and provide a format for the main ideas related to a given topic.

Reading Comprehension

Some patients may have a history of reading disturbance or developmental dyslexia. Indeed, we have found several patients who exhibited characteristics of surface dyslexia on preoperative testing. For such patients, more traditional or formal treatment approaches of reading comprehension, such as the approaches presented by Nickels[184] and Webb and Love,[185] may be indicated. Few patients experience newly acquired postoperative changes in reading function, which are usually mild and respond well to treatment focusing on compensatory strategies (Table 18–11).

It is helpful to obtain an inventory of the reading demands the patient had preoperatively for their occupation, schooling, and leisure, as well as an outline of the plans the patient has for the future. After surgery, some patients may acquire greater responsibilities that require stronger reading and writing skills, such as entering college or living independently for the first time. Most patients may begin treatment at the paragraph level. The length and semantic or syntactic complexity of paragraphs are gradually increased before working on multi-paragraph text. To assess comprehension, the patient is asked to retell what was read or answer spoken/written questions about

Table 18–11. Reading Comprehension Strategies

Read information twice

Take notes as you read lengthy text

Paraphrase written material in your own words

Periodically summarize (in writing or mentally) what you have read

Check your comprehension intermittently as you read

Identify and focus on the main concepts of written material

Underline important words/concepts

Discriminate essential facts or concepts from less critical, supporting information

Read aloud to hear the information in addition to seeing the words

Break paragraphs into component sentences

Break complex sentences into component parts

Use context to try to predict what might come next in the text, and then read to see if your comprehension of material was adequate in predicting subsequent information

Use the dictionary to determine the meaning of unfamiliar words to increase comprehension

Make charts or graphs to nonverbally represent what you have read

what was read (in verbal or written response). Questions should address both explicit and inferential information.

Written Expression

As with reading comprehension, patients may have written language disturbances preoperatively, such as surface/lexical dysgraphia. These patients may benefit from the types of treatment approaches reviewed by Hillis.[186] After surgery, changes in writing are fairly common, occurring second only to naming deficits. Fortunately, newly acquired postoperative writing impairments are usually mild and respond well to treatment focusing on the "postwriting," or editing, stage of writing.[187] In this approach, the patient generates written paragraphs and then concentrates on editing and proofreading skills. Patients are encouraged to develop an outline to guide and organize written expression. In the postwriting stage, skills are learned for editing and revising for meaning, content, cohesion, and organization. Proofing and correcting of errors in spelling, syntax, grammar, and punctuation are also learned and practiced.[187]

CONCLUSION

The surgical treatment of epilepsy has become increasingly successful and widely practiced since it was first attempted over a century ago. Patients with epilepsy may be candidates for surgical intervention if their seizures are poorly controlled by medications and an extensive battery of electrophysiological, neurobehavioral, and neuroimaging studies indicate a focal region of epileptogenicity. Often these patients experience difficulties in aspects of memory, language, and psychosocial functioning. Cortical stimulation for mapping of language and cognitive processes may be performed prior to surgery to safeguard against changes in preoperative abilities. The surgery for epilepsy involves resection of the epileptic focus, most commonly located in one of the temporal lobes. The outcome of surgery is judged in terms of the degree of reduction in or elimination of seizures, with a more recent emphasis on improvement of overall quality of life. Patients may experience postoperative declines in memory and language functioning, which may prove to be permanent in some cases. Speech–language therapy is recommended for those patients with postoperative language deficits.

STUDY QUESTIONS

1. What are the two major types of epilepsy and what is the most common cause of each type?

2. What are the main language disorders seen preoperatively in patients with dominant hemisphere epilepsy?

3. Which psychosocial factors are associated with a positive postsurgical psychosocial outcome?

4. How might an early cerebral insult influence language lateralization or localization?

5. Name the two main purposes of the intracarotid amobarbital test (Wada procedure).

6. How has cortical stimulation mapping increased our knowledge of human language processes?

7. In a classical temporal lobectomy, what are the resection margins and which temporal lobe structures are commonly included in the resection?

8. What are the reported long-term effects of left temporal lobectomy on language abilities?

9. What are the differential effects of left versus right temporal lobectomy on memory function?

10. What are some of the compensatory strategies for anomia that have been successfully utilized by patients with left temporal lobectomy?

REFERENCES

1. Annegers JF: The epidemiology of epilepsy. In Wyllie E, ed., *The treatment of epilepsy: Principles and practice.* Philadelphia, Lea & Febiger, 1993, pp 157–164.

2. Hauser WA, Annegers JF, Kurland LT: The prevalence of epilepsy in Rochester, Minnesota, 1940–1980. *Epilepsia* 1991; 32:429–455.

3. Hauser WA, Hesdorffer DC: *Epilepsy: Frequency, causes, and consequences.* New York; Demos Publications/Epilepsy Foundation of America, 1990.

4. Leppik IE: *Contemporary diagnosis and management of the patient with epilepsy.* Newtown, Penn. Associates in Medical Marketing Co., Inc. 2nd Edition.

5. Engel J, Jr: *Seizures and epilepsy.* Philadelphia, F. A. Davis, 1989.

6. Gumnit RJ, Leppik IE: The epilepsies. In Rosenberg R, ed., *Comprehensive neurology.* New York, Raven Press, 1991, pp. 311–336.

7. Commission on Classification and Terminology of the International League Against Epilepsy: Proposal for revised clinical and electroencephalographic classification of epileptic seizures. *Epilepsia* 1981; 22: 489–501.

8. Commission on Classification and Terminology of the International League Against Epilepsy: Proposal for the classification of epilepsy and epileptic syndromes. *Epilepsia* 1989; 30:389–399.

9. Rasmussen T: Focal epilepsies of non-temporal and non-frontal origin. In Wieser HG, Elger CE, eds., *Presurgical evaluation of epileptics: Basics, techniques and implications.* Berlin, Springer Verlag, 1987, pp 344–351.

10. Olivier A: Risk and benefit in the surgery of epilepsy: Complications and positive results on seizure tendency and intellectual function. *Acta Neurol Scand* 1988; 78(117):114–121.

11. Sperling MR: Who should consider epilepsy surgery? Medical failure in the treatment of epilepsy. In Wyler AR, Hermann BP, eds., *The surgical management of epilepsy.* Stoneham, MA, Butterworth-Heinemann, 1994, pp 26–31.

12. Engel J Jr, Shewmon DA: Overview: Who should be considered a surgical candidate? In Engel Jr, ed., *Surgical treatment of the epilepsies.* New York; Raven Press, 1993, pp 23–34.

13. Devinsky O, Vazquez B: Behavioral changes associated with epilepsy. *Neurol Clin* 1993; 11:127–149.

14. Hamilton NG, Matthews T: *Aphasia: The sole manifestation of focal status epilepticus. Neurology* 1979; 29:745–748.

15. Racy A, Osborn M, Vern B, Molinari G: Epileptic aphasia: First onset of prolonged monosymptomatic status epilepticus in adults. *Arch Neurol* 1980; 37:419–422.

16. Wells, C, Labar D, Solomon G: Aphasia as the sole manifestation of simple partial status epilepticus. *Epilepsia* 1992; 33:84–87.

17. Lebrun Y: Ictal verbal behavior: A review. *Seizure* 1994; 3:45–54.

18. Gabr M, Lueders H, Dinner D, et al: Speech manifestations in lateralization of temporal lobe seizures. *Ann Neurol* 1989; 25:82–87.

19. Koerner M, Laxer K: Ictal speech, postictal language dysfunction, and seizure lateralization. *Neurology* 1988; 38:634–636.

20. Privitera M, Morris G, Gilliam F: Postictal language assessment and lateralization of complex partial seizures. *Ann Neurol* 1991; 30:391–396.

21. Aarts J, Binnie C, Smit AM, Wilkins AJ: Selective cognitive impairment during focal and generalized epileptiform EEG activity. *Brain* 1984; 107:293–308.

22. Hermann B, Wyler A: Effects of anterior temporal lobectomy on language function: a controlled study. *Ann Neurol* 1988; 23:585–588.

23. Ojemann G: Individual variability in cortical localization of language. *J Neurosurg* 1979; 50:164–169.

24. Devinsky O, Perrine K, Llinas R, et al: Anterior temporal language areas in patients with early onset of temporal lobe epilepsy. *Ann Neurol* 1993; 34: 727–732.

25. Mateer C, Dodrill C: Neuropsychological and linguistic correlates of atypical language lateralization: Evidence from sodium amtyal studies. *Human Neurobiology* 1983; 2:135–142.

26. Strauss E, Satz P, Wada J: An examination of the crowding hypothesis in epileptic patients who have undergone the carotid amytal test. *Neuropsychologia* 1990; 28:1221–1227.

27. Mayeux R, Brandt J, Rosen J, Benson F: Interictal memory and language impairment in temporal lobe epilepsy. *Neurology* 1980; 30:120–125.

28. Saykin A, Stafiniak P, Robinson L, et al: Language before and after temporal lobectomy: Specificity of acute changes and relation to early risk factors. *Epilepsia* 1995; 36:1071–1077.

29. Davies KG, Maxwell R, Jennum P, et al: Language function following subdural grid-directed temporal lobectomy. *Acta Neurol Scand* 1994; 90:201–206.

30. Lesser RP, Lueders H, Dinner D, et al: The location of speech and writing functions in the frontal language area: Results of extraoperative cortical stimulation. *Brain* 1984; 107:275–291.

31. Thompson P: Memory function in patients with epilepsy. In Smith D, Treiman D, Trimble M, eds., *Advances in neurology,* Vol 55, pp 369–384. Raven Press, New York, 1991.

32. Hermann BP, Wyler A, Steenman H, Richey E: The interrelationship between language function and verbal learning/memory performance in patients with complex partial seizures. Cortex 1988; 24:245–253.

33. Martin R, Loring D, Meador K et al: The effects of lateralized temporal lobe dysfunction on formal and semantic word fluency. *Neuropsychologia* 1990; 28(8):823–829.

34. Schneider SK, Nowack W, Fitzgerald J, et al: WAIS performance in epileptics with unilateral interictal EEG abnormalities. *J Epilepsy* 1993; 6:10–14.

35. Schachter SC, Galabuda A, Ransil B: A history of dyslexia in patients with epilepsy: Clinical associations. *J Epilepsy* 1993; 6:267–271.

36. Schachter SC, Galaburda A, Ransil B: Associations of dyslexia with epilepsy, handedness, and gender. *Ann NY Acad Sci* 1993; 682:402–403.

37. Waxman SG, Geschwind N: Hypergraphia in temporal lobe epilepsy. *Neurology* 1974; 24:629–636.

38. Sachdev HS, Waxman SG: Frequency of hypergraphia in temporal lobe epilepsy: An index of interictal behaviour syndrome. *J Neurol Neurosurg Psych* 1981; 44:358–360.

39. Hermann BP, Whitman S, Arnston P: Hypergraphia in epilepsy: Is there a specificity to temporal lobe epilepsy? *J Neurol Neurosurg Psych* 1983; 46:848–853.

40. Hermann BP, Whitman S, Wyler A, Richey E, Dell J: The neurological, psychosocial and demographic correlates of hypergraphia in patients with epilepsy. *J Neurol Neurosurg Psych* 1988; 51:203–208.

41. Roberts JKA, Robertson M, Trimble M: The lateralising significance of hypergraphia in temporal lobe epilepsy. *J Neurol Neurosurg Psych* 1982; 45:131–138.

42. Nicholas L, Brookshire R: A system for quantifying the informativeness and efficiency of the connected speech of adults with aphasia. *J Speech and Hearing Res* 1993; 36:338–350.

43. Rao SM, Devinsky O, Grafman J, et al: Viscosity and social cohesion in temporal lobe epilepsy. *J Neurol Neurosurg Psych* 1992; 55:149–152.

44. Heoppner JB, Garron D, Wilson R, et al: Epilepsy and verbosity. *Epilepsia* 1987; 28:35–40.

45. Scoville WB, Milner, B: Loss of recent memory after bilateral hippocampal lesions. *J Neurol Neurosurg Psych* 1987; 20:11–21.

46. Penfield W, Milner B: Memory deficits produced by bilateral lesions in the hippocampal zone. *Arch Neurol Neurosurg* 1958; 79:475–497.

47. Milner B: Laterality effects in audition. In V. B. Mountcastle, ed., *Interhemispheric relations and cerebral dominance*. Baltimore, John Hopkins Press, 1962.

48. Hermann BP, Wyler AR, Richey ET, Rea JM: Memory function and verbal learning ability in patients with complex partial seizures of temporal lobe origin. *Epilepsia* 1987; 28:547–554.

49. Milner B: Visual recognition and recall after right temporal lobe excision in man. *Neuropsychologica* 1968; 6:191–209.

50. Bennett TL: Cognitive effects of epilepsy in anticonvulsant medications. In TL Bennett, ed., *The neuropsychology of epilepsy*. New York, Plenum Press, 1992.

51. Berent S, Giordani B, Sackellares JC, O'Leary D, Boll TJ: Cerebrally localized epileptogenic foci and performance on a verbal and visual graphic learning task. *Perceptual and Motor Skills* 1983; 56:991–1001.

52. Glowinski H: Cognitive defects in temporal lobe epilepsy: An investigation of memory functioning. *J Nerv Ment Dis* 1973; 157:129–137.

53. Bauer RM, Tobias D, Valenstein E: Mnestic disorders. In KM Heilman, and E Valenstein, eds., *Clinical neuropsychology*, 3rd ed. New York, Oxford University Press, 1993.

54. Hermann BP, Wyler AR, Somes G, Dohan FC, Berry AD 3rd, Clements L: Declarative memory following anterior lobectomy in humans. *Behav Neurosci* 1994; 108(1):3–10.

55. Raines GD, Milner B: Verbal recall and recognition as a function of depth of encoding in patients with unilateral temporal lobectomy. *Neuropsychologica* 1994; 32(10):1243–1256.

56. Saling MM, Berkovic SF, O'Shea MF, Kalins RM, Darby DG, Bladin PF: Lateralization of verbal memory in unilateral hippocampal sclerosis: Evidence of task specific effects. *J Clin Exper Neuropsych* 1993; 15(4):608–618.

57. Mendez MF, Cumming JL, Benson DF: Depression in epilepsy: Significance and phenomonology. *Arch Neurol* 1986; 43:766–770.

58. Betts TA: Depression, anxiety, and epilepsy. In EH Reynolds and MR Tremble, eds., *Epilepsy in psychiatry*. New York; Churchill-Livingston, 1981, pp 60–71.

59. Robertson, MA, Tremble MR, Townsend HRA: The phenomonology of depression in epilepsy. *Epilepsia* 1987; 28:364–372.

60. Hermann, BD, Whitman S: Neurobiological, psychosocial, and pharmacological factors in underlying inter-ictal psychopathology in epilepsy. In DB Smith, DM Treiman, and MR Tremble, eds., *Neurobehavioral prob epilepsy* 1991; 55:439–452.

61. Thompson, PJ, Oxley J: Socioeconomic accompaniments of severe epilepsy. *Epilepsia* 1988; 29(SI): F9–S18.

62. Chaplin JE, Shorvon FD, Floyd M, Lasso R: Psychosocial factors in chronicity of epilepsy. *J Neurology Neurosurg Psych* 1995; 58:112–113.

63. Hermann BP, Wyler AR, Somes G: Preoperative psychological adjustment and surgical outcome are determinants of psychosocial status after anterior temporal lobectomy. *J Neurology Neurosurg Psych* 1992; 55(6):491–496.

64. Sperling MR, Saghen AJ, Roberts FD, French JA, O'Connor MJ: Occupational outcome after temporal lobectomy for refractory epilepsy. *Neurology* 1995; 45(5):970–977.

65. Benson DF: The Geschwind syndrome. In Smith D, Treiman D, Trimble M, eds., *Advances in neurology*, Vol 55. Raven Press, New York, 1991.

66. Waxman SG, Geschwind N: The interictal behavior syndrome of temporal lobe epilepsy. *Arch Gen Psych* 1975; 32:1580–1586.

67. Hermann BP, Riel P: Interictal personality and behavioral traits in temporal lobe and generalized epilepsy. *Cortex* 1981; 17:125–128.

68. Rasmussen T, Milner B: The role of early left-brain injury in determining lateralization of cerebral speech functions. *Ann NY Acad Sci* 1977; 299:355–369.

69. Helmstaedter C, Kurthen M, Linke D, Elger C: Right hemisphere restitution of language and memory functions in right hemisphere language-dominant patients

with left temporal lobe epilepsy. *Brain* 1994; 117: 729–737.

70. Strauss E, Wada J, Goldwater B: Sex differences in interhemispheric reorganization of speech. *Neuropsychologia* 1992; 353–359.

71. Loring D, Meador K, Lee G, et al: Cerebral language lateralization: evidence from intracarotid amobarbital testing. *Neuropsychologia* 1990; 28:831–838.

72. Krashen S: Lateralization, language learning, and the critical period: Some new evidence. *Lang Learning* 1973; 23:63–74.

73. Satz P, Strauss E, Wada J, Orsini D: Some correlates of intra-and interhemispheric speech organization after left focal brain injury. *Neuropsychologia* 1988; 26: 345–350.

74. Kurthen M, Helmstaedter C, Linke D, et al: Interhemispheric dissociation of expressive and receptive language functions in patients with complex-partial seizures: An amobarbital study. *Brain Lang* 1992; 43: 694–712.

75. Strauss E, Wada J: Lateral preferences and cerebral speech dominance. *Cortex* 1983; 19:165–177.

76. Ojemann G, Whitaker H: Language localization and variability. *Brain Lang* 1978; 6:239–260.

77. Rausch R, Walsh G: Right-hemisphere language dominance in right-handed epileptic patients. *Arch Neurol* 1984; 41:1077–1080.

78. Branch C, Milner B, Rasmussen T: Intracarotid sodium amytal for the lateralization of cerebral speech dominance: Observations in 123 patients. *J Neurosurg* 1964; 21:399–405.

79. Silfvenius H, Christianson SA, Nilsson LG, Salsa J: Preoperative investigation of cerebral hemisphere speech and memory with bilateral intracarotid amytal test. *Acta Neurol Scand* 1988; 117:79–83.

80. Woods RP, Dodrill CB, Ojemann GA: Brain injury, handedness and speech lateralization in a series of amobarbital studies. *Ann Neur* 1988; 23:510–518.

81. Abou-Khalil B: Insights into language mechanisms derived from the evaluation of epilepsy. In Kirshner H, ed., *Handbook of neurological speech and language disorders*, pp 213–275. Marcel-Dekker, New York, 1995.

82. Cooper R, Winter AL, Crow HJ, Walter WG: Comparison of subcortical, cortical and scalp activity using chronically indwelling electrodes in man. *Electroenceph Clin Neurophys* 1965; 18:217–228.

83. Jasper HH: The 10–20 electrode system of the International Federation. *Electroenceph Clin Neurophys* 1958; 10:370–375.

84. Morris HH, Lüders H, Lesser RP, Dinner DS, Klem GH: The value of closely spaced scalp electrodes in the localization of epileptiform foci: A study of 26 patients with complex partial seizures. *Electroencephal Clin Neurophys* 1986; 63:107–111.

85. Abraham D, Ajmone-Marsan C: Patterns of cortical discharges and their relation to routine scalp electroencephalography. *Electroencephal Clin Neurophys* 1958; 10:447–461.

86. Wada J, Rasmussen T: Intracarotid injection of sodium amytal for the lateralization of cerebral speech dominance: experimental and clinical observations. *J Neurosurg* 1960; 17:266–282.

87. Loring DW: Wada testing. Paper presented at the European Conference of the International Neuropsychological Society, Angers, France, June 22, 1994.

88. Terzian H: Behavioural and EEG effects of intracarotid sodium Amytal injection. *Acta Neurochirurgica* 1964; 12:230–239.

89. Snyder PJ, Novelly RA, Harris LJ: Mixed speech dominance in the intracarotid sodium amytal procedure: Validity and criteria issues. *J Clin Exp Neuropsy* 1990; 12:629–643.

90. Loring DW, Meador KJ, Lee GP, King DW: Amobarbital effects and lateralized brain function: The Wada test. New York, Springer-Verlag, 1992.

91. Goodglass H, Kaplan E: *The assessment of aphasia and related disorders,* 2nd ed. Lea and Febiger, Philadelphia, 1983.

92. Kaplan E, Goodglass H, Weintraub S, Segal O: Boston Naming Test. Lea and Febiger, Philadelphia, 1983.

93. Ulatowska H, Sadowska M, Kordys J, Kadzielawa D: Selected aspects of narratives in Polish-speaking aphasics as illustrated by Aesop's fables. In Brownell H, Joanette Y, eds., *Narrative discourse in neurologically impaired and normal aging adults,* pp 171–190. Singular Publishing, San Diego, 1993.

94. Benton AL, Hamsher K: *Multilingual aphasia examination.* Oxford University Press, New York, 1983.

95. Spreen O, Benton A: Neurosensory center comprehensive examination for aphasia. Neuropsychology Laboratory, Department of Psychology, University of Victoria, Victoria, BC, 1977.

96. DeRenzi E, Vignolo L: The token test: A sensitive test to detect receptive disturbances in aphasics. *Brain* 1962; 85:665–678

97. German D: Test of adolescent/adult word-finding. DLM Teaching Resources, Allen, TX, 1990.

98. Kertesz A: *Western aphasia battery.* Grune and Stratton, New York, 1982.

99. Woodcock R: Woodcock reading mastery tests—Revised. American Guidance Service, Minnesota, 1987.

100. Woodcock RW, Johnson MB: Woodcock-Johnson psycho-educational battery—Revised. DLM Teaching Resources, Allen, Tx, 1989, 1990.

101. Penfield W, Boldrey E: Somatic motor and sensory representation in the cerebral cortex of man as studied by electrical stimulation. *Brain* 1937; 60: 389–443.

102. Penfield W, Gage L: Cerebral localization of epileptic manifestations. *Arch Neur Psych* 1933; 30:709.

103. Penfield W: Epilepsy and surgical therapy. *Arch Neur Psych* 1936; 36:449–484.

104. Lesser RP, Lüders H, Klem G, Dinner DS, Morris HH, Hahn J: Ipsilateral trigeminal sensory responses to cortical stimulation by subdural electrodes. *Neurology* 1985; 35:1760–1763.

105. Lesser RP, Lüders H, Klem G, Dinner DS, Morris HH, Hahn JF, Wyllie E: Extraoperative cortical functional localization in patients with epilepsy. *J Clin Neurophysiol* 1987; 4:27–53.

106. Jayakar P, Alvarez LA, Duchowny MS, Resnick TJ: A safe and effective paradigm to functionally map the cortex in childhood. *J Clin Neurophysiol* 1992; 9:288–293.

107. Lüders H, Lesser R, Dinner D, et al: Commentary: Chronic intracranial recording and stimulation with subdural electrodes. In Engel J, ed., *Surgical treatment of the epilepsies,* pp 297–321. Raven Press, New York, 1987.

108. Lüders H, Lesser R, Dinner D, et al: Localization of cortical function: New information from extraoperative monitoring of patients with epilepsy. *Epilepsia* 1988; 29 (Suppl 2):S56–S65.

109. Lesser R, Lüders H, Dinner D, et al: The location of speech and writing functions in the frontal language area. *Brain* 1984; 107:275–291.

110. Schaffler L, Lüders H, Dinner D, et al: Comprehension deficits elicited by electrical stimulation of Broca's area. *Brain* 1993; 116:695–715.

111. Lüders H, Lesser R, Hahn J, Dinner D, et al: Basal temporal language area demonstrated by electrical stimulation. *Neurology* 1986; 36:505–510.

112. Morris H, Lüders H, Lesser R, et al: Transient neuropsychological abnormalities (including Gerstmann's syndrome) during cortical stimulation. *Neurology* 1984; 34:877–883.

113. Ojemann G, Whitaker H: Language localization and variability. *Brain and Lang* 1978; 6:239–260.

114. Lüders H, Awad I, Wyllie E, Schaffler L: Functional mapping of language abilities with subdural electrode grids. In Wyler A, Hermann B, eds., *The surgical management of epilepsy,* pp 70–77. Butterworth-Heinemann, Boston, 1994.

115. Ojemann G: Intraoperative electrocorticography and functional mapping. In Wyler A, Hermann B, eds., *The surgical management of epilepsy,* pp 189–196. Butterworth-Heinemann, Boston, 1994.

116. Ojemann G, Sutherling W, Lesser R, et al: Cortical stimulation. In Engel J, ed., *Surgical treatment of the epilepsies,* pp 399–414. Raven Press, New York, 1993.

117. Haglund M, Berger M, Shamseldin M, et al: Cortical localization of temporal lobe language sites in patients with gliomas. *Neurosurgery* 1994; 34:567–576.

118. Petersen E, Fox P, Posner M, et al: Positron emission tomographic studies of the cortical anatomy of single-word processing. *Nature* 1988; 331:585–589.

119. Leblanc R, Meyer E, Bub D, et al: Language localization with activation positron emission tomography scanning. *Neurosurgery* 1992; 31:369–373.

120. Friberg L: Brain mapping in thinking and language function. *Acta Neurochirurgica* 1993; [Suppl.] 56: 34–39.

121. Ojemann G, Ojemann J, Lettich E, Berger M: Cortical language localization in left, dominant hemisphere: An electrical stimulation mapping investigation in 117 patients. *J Neurosurg* 1989; 71:316–326.

122. Berger M, Ojemann G: Intraoperative brain mapping techniques in neuro-oncology. *Stereotactic Functional Neurosurg* 1992; 58:153–161.

123. Ojemann G: Models of the brain organization for higher integrative functions derived with electrical stimulation techniques. *Human Neurobiol* 1982; 1: 243–249.

124. Lesser R, Lüders H, Morris H, et al: Electrical stimulation of Wernicke's area interferes with comprehension. *Neurology* 1986; 36:658–663.

125. Ojemann G: Brain organization for language from the perspective of electrical stimulation mapping. *Behav Brain Sci* 1983; 6:189–230.

126. Lüders H, Lesser R, Hahn J, et al: Basal temporal language area. *Brain* 1991; 114:743–754.

127. Burnstine T, Lesser R, Hart J, et al: Characterization of the basal temporal language area in patients with left temporal lobe epilepsy. *Neurology* 1990; 40:966–970.

128. Schaffler L, Lüders H, Morris H, Wyllie E: Anatomic distribution of cortical language sites in the basal temporal language area in patients with left temporal lobe epilepsy. *Epilepsia* 1994; 35:525–528.

129. Malow B, Blaxton T, Sato S, et al: Cortical stimulation elicits regional distinctions in auditory and visual naming. *Epilepsia* 1996; 37:245–252.

130. Ojemann G: Organization of language cortex derived from investigations during neurosurgery. *Sem neurosci* 1990; 2:297–305.

131. Rasmussen T: Cortical resection in the treatment of focal epilepsy. *Adv Neurol* 1975; 8:139.

132. Girvin JP: Neurosurgical considerations and general methods for craniotomy under local anesthesia. *Internat Anesthesiology Clin* 1986; 24:89–114.

133. Morrell F, Whisler WW, Bleck TP: Multiple Subpial transection: A new approach to the surgical treatment of focal epilepsy. *J Neurosurg* 1989; 70:231–239.

134. Devinsky O, Perrine K, Vazquez B, Luciano DJ, Dogali M: Multiple subpial transections in the language cortex. *Brain* 1994; 117 (pt 2):255–265.

135. Stafaniak P, Saykin A, Sperling M, et al: Acute naming deficits following dominant temporal lobectomy: Prediction by age at first risk for seizures. *Neurology* 1990; 40:1509–1512.

136. Hermann B, Wyler A, Somes G, Clement L: Dysnomia after left anterior temporal lobectomy without functional mapping: frequency and correlates. *Neurosurgery* 1994; 35:52–57.

137. Heilman K, Wilder B, Malzone W: Anomic aphasia following anterior temporal lobectomy. *Trans Am Neurol Assoc* 1972; 97:291–293.

138. Hermann B, Wyler A, Somes G: Language function following anterior temporal lobectomy. *J Neurosurg* 1991; 74:560–566.

139. Falconer M, Serafetinides E: A follow-up study of surgery in temporal lobe epilepsy. *J Neurol Neurosurg Psychiat* 1963; 26:154–165.

140. Loring D, Meador K: Effects of temporal lobectomy on generative fluency and other language functions. *Arch Clin Neuropsych* 1994; 9:229–238.

141. Lutsep H, Duffy J, Cascino G: Frequency, risk factors, and characterization of aphasia following left temporal lobectomy. *J Med Speech Lang Path* 1995; 3: 191–198.

142. Rausch R: Effects of temporal lobe surgery on behavior. In Smith D, Treiman D, Trimble M, eds., *Advances in Neurology,* Vol 55, pp. 279–292. Raven Press, New York, 1991.

143. Wilkins A, Moscovitch M: Selective impairment of semantic memory after temporal lobectomy. Neuropsychologia 1978; 16:73–79.

144. Loring DW, Meador K, Martin R, Lee G: Language deficits following unilateral temporal lobectomy. *J Clin Exp Neuropsych* 1989; 11:41 (abstract).

145. Hermann B, Wyler A: Neuropsychological outcome of anterior temporal lobectomy. J Epilepsy 1988; 1: 35–45.

146. Katz A, Awad I, Kong A, et al: Extent of resection in temporal lobectomy for epilepsy. II. Memory changes and neurologic complications. *Epilepsia* 1989; 30: 763–771.

147. Saykin A, Sperling M, Kester D, et al: Acute neuropsychological changes following temporal resection: Laterality effects for memory, language, and music. *Epilepsia* 1988; 29:669 (abstrac).

148. Ivnik R, Sharbrough F, Laws E: Anterior temporal lobectomy for the control of partial complex seizures: Information for counseling patients. *Mayo Clin Proc* 1988; 63:783–793.

149. Hermann B, Wyler A: Comparative results of dominant temporal lobectomy under general or local anesthesia: Language outcome. *J Epilepsy* 1988; 1: 127–134.

150. Penfield W, Roberts L: *Speech and brain mechanisms.* Princeton University Press, Princeton, 1959.

151. Davies K, Maxwell R, Beniak T, et al: Language function after temporal lobectomy without stimulation mapping of cortical function. *Epilepsia* 1995; 36: 130–136.

152. Chelune G, Naugle R, Lüders H, Awad I: Prediction of cognitive change as a function of preoperative ability status among temporal lobectomy patients seen at 6-month follow-up. *Neurology* 1991; 41:399–404.

153. Dodrill CD, Hermann BP, Rausch R, Chelune G, Oxbury JM: Use of neuropsychological tests for assessing prognosis following surgery for epilepsy. In J Engel, ed., *Surgical treatment of the epilepsies,* 2nd ed., pp 263–271. New York: Raven Press, 1993.

154. Milner G: Psychological defects produced by temporal lobe excision. *Assoc Nerv Mental Dis* 1958; 36: 244–257.

155. Dennis M, Farrell K, Hoffman HJ, Hendrick EB, Becher LE, Murphy EG: Recognition memory of item, associative, and serial order information after temporal lobectomy for seizure disorder. *Neuropsychologica* 1988; 26:53–65.

156. Raines GD: Incidental verbal memory as a function of depth of encoding in patients with temporal-lobe lesions. *J Clin Exp Neuropsych* 1987; 9:18.

157. Myer V, Yates AJ: Intellectual changes following temporal lobectomy for psychomotor epilepsy. *J Neurol Neurosurg Psych* 1955; 18:44–52.

158. Tuunainen A, Nousiainen U, Hurskainen H, Leinonen E, Pilke A, Mervaala E, Vapalahti M, Partanen J, Riekkinen P: Preoperative EEG predicts memory and selective cognitive functions after temporal lobe surgery. *J Neurol Neurosurg Psych* 1995; 58(6): 674–680.

159. Wolf RL, Ivnik RJ, Hirschorn KA, Sharbrough FW, Cascino GD, Marsh WR: Neurocognitive efficiency following left temporal lobectomy: Standard vs. limited resection. *J Neurosurg* 1993; 79(1):76–83.

160. Trenerry MR, Jack CR, Jr, Ivnik RJ, Sharbrough FW, Castino CD, Hirschorn KA, Marsh WR, Kelly PJ, Myer FV: MRI hippocampal volumes and memory functioning before and after temporal lobectomy. *Neurology* 1993, 43(9):1800–1805.

161. Hermann BP, Seidenberg M, Dohan FC, Jr, Wyler AR, Haltiner A, Bobholz J, Perrine A: Reports by patients and their families of memory change after left anterior temporal lobectomy: Relationship to degree of hippocampal sclerosis. *Neurosurgery* 1995; 36(1), 39–44.

162. Kneebone AC, Chelune GJ, Dinner DS, Naugle RI, Awad IA: Intercarotid amobarbitol procedure as a predictor of material-specific memory change after anterior temporal lobectomy. *Epilepsia* 1995; 36(9): 857–865.

163. Kileny PR, Paccioretti D, Wilson AF: Effects of cortical lesions on middle-latency auditory evoked responses (MLR). *Electroenceph Clin Neurophysiol* 1987; 66:108–120.

164. Jacobson GP, Privitera M, Neils JR, Grayson AS, Yeh H-S: The effects of anterior temporal lobectomy (ATL) on the middle-latency auditory evoked potential (MLAEP). *Electroenceph Clin Neurophysiol* 1990; 75: 230–241.

165. Sherwin I, Efron R: Temporal ordering deficits following anterior temporal lobectomy. *Brain Lang* 1980; 11:195–203.

166. Efron R, Yund EW, Nichols D, Crandall PH: An ear asymmetry for gap detection following anterior temporal lobectomy. *Neuropsychologia* 1985; 23: 43–50.

167. Efron R, Crandall PH, Koss B, Divenyi PL, Yund EW: Central auditory processing. III. The "cocktail party" effect and anterior temporal lobectomy. *Brain Lang* 1983; 19:254–263.

168. Boatman D, Lesser RP, Gordon B: Auditory speech processing in the left temporal lobe: An electrical interference study. *Brain Lang* 1995; 51:269–290.

169. Kimura D: Some effects of temporal lobe damage on auditory perception. *Can J Psychol* 1961; 15:156–165.

170. Kimura D: Left-right differences in the perception of melodies. *J Exp Psych* 1964; 14:355–358.

171. Oxbury JM, Oxbury SM: Effects of temporal lobectomy on the report of dichotically presented digits. *Cortex* 1969; 5:3–14.

172. Sussman HM, Macneilage PF: Dichotic pursuit auditory tracking after anterior temporal lobectomy. *Arch Otolaryngol* 1975; 101:389–391.

173. Olsen WO: Dichotic test results for normal subjects and for temporal lobectomy patients. *Ear Hear* 1983; 4:324–330.

174. Collard ME, Lesser RP, Luders H, Dinner DS, Morris HH, Hahn JF, Rothner AD: Four dichotic speech tests before and after temporal lobectomy. *Ear Hear* 1986; 7:363–369.

175. Berlin CI, Lowe-Bell SS, Jannetta PJ, Kline DG: Central auditory deficits after temporal lobectomy. *Arch Otolaryngol* 1972a; 96:4–10.

176. Berlin CI, Lowe-Bell SS, Cullen JK, Thomson CL, Stafford MR: Is speech "special"? Perhaps the temporal lobectomy patient can tell us. *J Acoust Soc Am* 1972b; 52:702–705.

177. Berlin CI, Porter RJ, Lowe-Bell SS, Berlin HL, Thomson CL, Hughes LF: Dichotic signs of the recognition of speech elements in normals, temporal lobectomies, and hemispherectomies. *IEEE Trans Audio Electroacoust* 1973; AU-21:189–195.

178. Benson DF: Anomia in aphasia. *Aphasiology* 1988; 2:229–236.

179. Caramazza A: The structure of the lexical system: Evidence from acquired language disorders. In Brookshire RH, ed., *Clinical aphasiology*, Vol 16, pp 291–301. 1986. Pro-Ed Austin, Tx.

180. Lucchelli F, DeRenzi E: Proper name anomia. *Cortex* 1992; 28:221–230.

181. Miceli G, Guistolisi L, Caramazza A: The interaction of lexical and nonlexical processing mechanisms: Evidence from anomia. *Cortex* 1991; 27:57–80.

182. Linebaugh C: Treatment of anomic aphasia. In Perkins C, ed., *Current therapies for communication disorders: Language handicaps in adults.* Thieme-Stratton, New York, 1983.

183. Howard D, Patterson D, Franklin S, et al: Treatment of word retrieval deficits in aphasia. *Brain* 1985; 108:817–829.

184. Nickels L: Reading too little into reading? Strategies in the rehabilitation of acquired dyslexia. *Euro J Dis Comm* 1995; 30:37–50.

185. Webb W, Love R: Treatment of acquired reading disorders. In Chapey R, ed., *Language intervention strategies in adult aphasia*, 3rd ed. pp 446–457. Williams and Wilkins, Baltimore, 1994.

186. Hillis AE: Facilitating written production. *Clin Comm Disord* 1992; 2:19–33.

187. Amster W, Amster J: Treatment of writing disorders in aphasia. In Chapey R, ed., *Language intervention strategies in adult aphasia*, 3rd ed, pp 458–466. Williams and Wilkins, Baltimore, 1994.

Appendix A
Language and Its Management in the Surgical Epilepsy Patient
Case Study—GD

HISTORY

Case History: GD is a 45-year-old male with a Master's degree in accounting. He is employed full-time as a partner in an accounting firm. GD is left-handed for writing but right-handed for many sports activities. Both of his parents and all four of his siblings are right-handed.

Past medical history: Significant for complex partial epilepsy. The patient experienced his first seizure in association with a high fever as an infant. He then experienced a seizure-free period for many years before the seizures resumed at age 35. At that time, they usually occurred as the patient was falling off to sleep. There was a pattern to his seizures in that they occurred in clusters; several weeks without a seizure were followed by several days with up to 10 seizures per day. The longest period of time without a seizure was 2 months, and they appeared to be increasing in frequency over time.

Preoperative medications: Dilantin 600 mg per day.

PRE-ADMISSION DIAGNOSTIC TESTS

MRI: Atrophic region in the left hippocampus with increased signal intensity on T_2-weighted images.

Baseline language assessment: Within normal limits based on the Boston Naming Test and the Boston Diagnostic Aphasia Examination.

Neuropsychological assessment: Wechsler Adult Intelligence Scale-Revised estimated IQ scores were in the superior to high average range. Figural memory was superior to verbal memory, and both were lower than expected given his high level of intelligence. He exhibited mediocre or low average ability to learn new verbal information over repeated trials on the Rey Auditory Verbal Learning Test.

PHASE I ADMISSION

Phase I Evaluation: Scalp EEG detected predominantly left hemispheric epileptogenicity, possibly concentrated in the temporal lobe, but not particularly well localized; not as well localized as the MRI indicated. Phase II for further evaluation and localization of seizure onset with intracranial electrode recording was warranted.

Ictal SPECT: Hyperperfusion in the left hemisphere with a focus of activity in the left temporal region.

Interictal SPECT: No areas of abnormal radiotracer activity throughout the brain.

PREOPERATIVE TESTING

WADA: Left hemisphere language dominance.
     Bilateral memory dysfunction.

PHASE II ADMISSION

Phase II Evaluation: Subdural electrodes were surgically placed over the cortex in the frontotemporal and parietooccipital distribution. The origin of the electrographic activity was found to be in the left medial temporal region, specifically in the middle and posterior aspects of the parahippocampal gyrus.

Cortical stimulation for functional language and sensorimotor mapping revealed language areas in the middle to posterior region of the superior temporal gyrus, as indicated by the inability to read upon stimulation. Auditory phenomenon (such as the feeling of voices moving from right to left) were reported upon stimulation to areas just posterior to the language area.

OPERATIVE INFORMATION

Surgical resection: Left anterior temporal lobectomy (3.5 to 4.0 cm from the temporal pole) that included the left amygdala and hippocampus.

Pathology Report: Focal loss of neurons and gliosis in the tissue sample from the hippocampus.

POSTOPERATIVE INFORMATION

Postoperative language assessment: Two days after surgery, the patient exhibited a decrease in score on the BNT from +56 to +27. Errors were predominantly semantic paraphasias. On the BDAE, the patient experienced a mild decline in scores on the following subtests: Complex Ideational Material, Repeating Phrases, Written Formulation, and Visual Confrontation Naming. Overall, his language profile was consistent with an anomic aphasia.

At one week after surgery, the patient exhibited mild agraphia and moderate anomia. Outpatient treatment was recommended.

The patient attended a short course of therapy focusing on word-retrieval and complex written expression. He returned to work within two months after surgery.

At the time of discharge from therapy (3 months after surgery), a minimal anomia persisted. The patient was able to compensate for any word-finding difficulties in conversation, and this has not prevented him from engaging in any of his preoperative activities, including work activities.

Neuropsychological assessment: Scores were not significantly different from baseline to 12 months after surgery on the Wechsler Adult Intelligence Scale-Revised and the Rey Auditory Verbal Learning Test.

Postoperative medications: Lamictal 300 mg per day.

Seizure status: GD has been free of seizures since his surgery over one year ago.

Color Plates

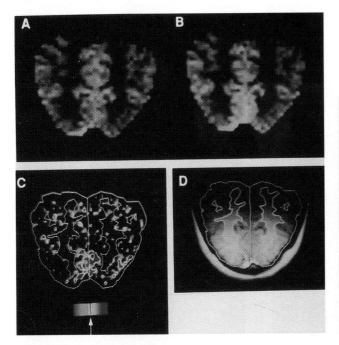

Color Plate 1. See page 300.

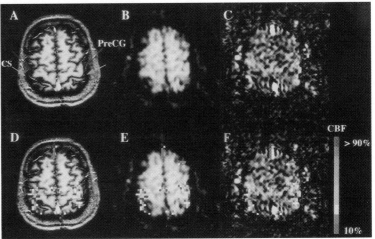

Color Plate 2. See page 301.

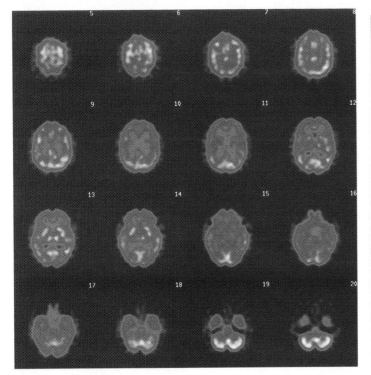

Color Plate 3. See page 307.

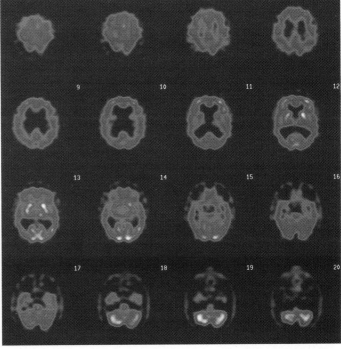

Color Plate 4. See page 308.

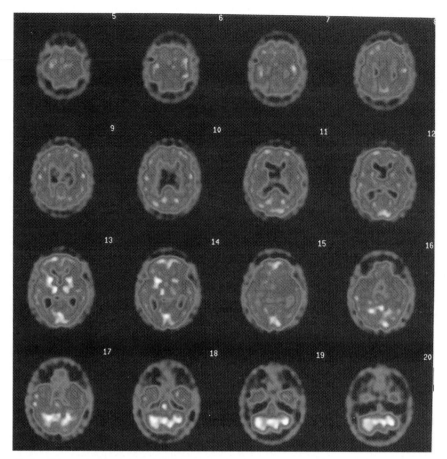

Color Plate 5. See page 309.

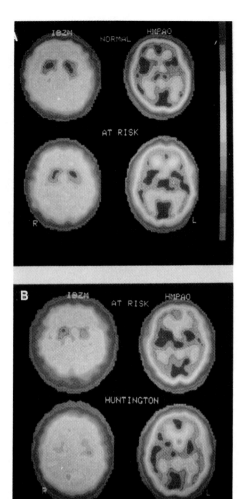

Color Plate 6. See page 311.

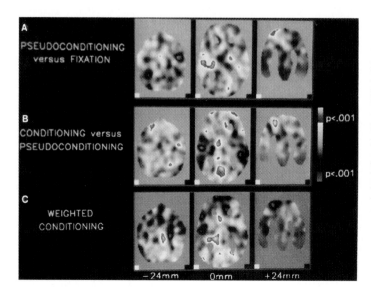

Color Plate 7. See page 315.

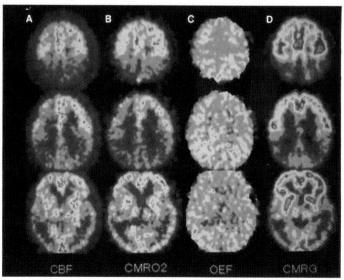

Color Plate 8. See page 316.

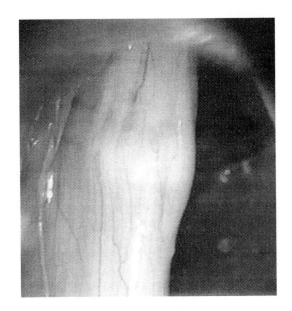

Color Plate 9. See page 513.

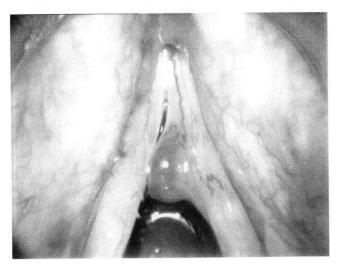

Color Plate 10. See page 514.

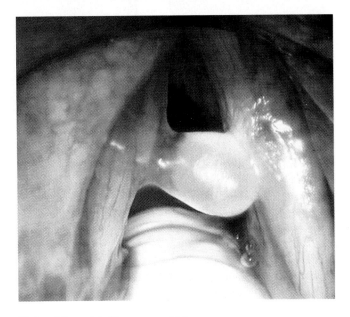

Color Plate 11. See page 514.

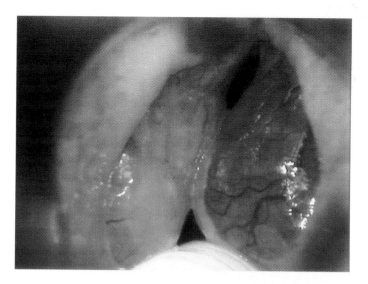

Color Plate 12. See page 514.

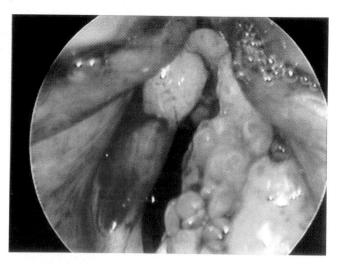

Color Plate 13. See page 515.

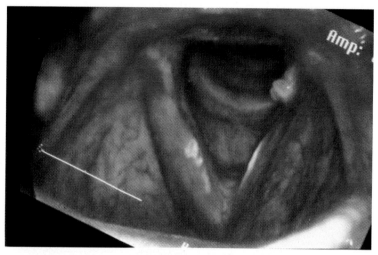

Color Plate 14. See page 516.

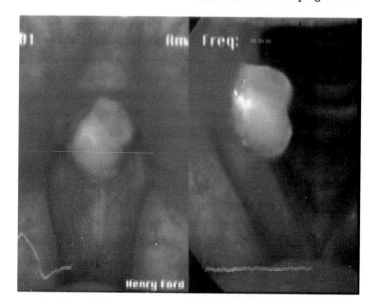

Color Plate 15. See page 516.

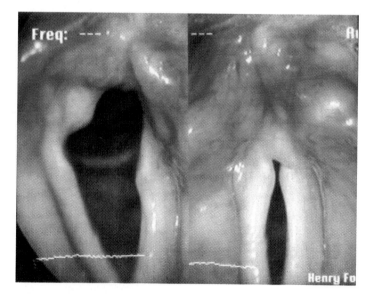

Color Plate 16. See page 517.

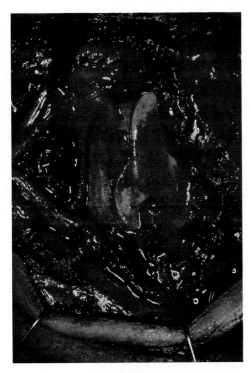

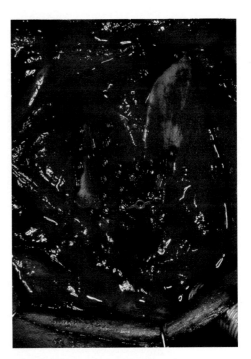

Color Plate 17. See page 521.

Color Plate 18. See page 521.

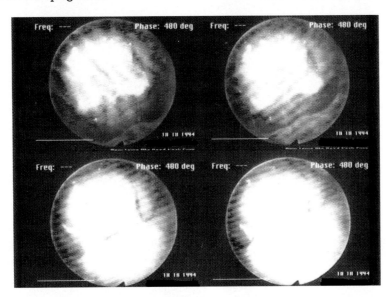

Color Plate 19. See page 565.

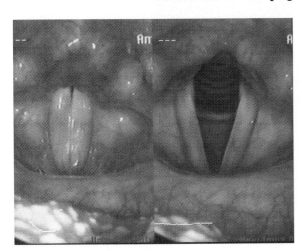

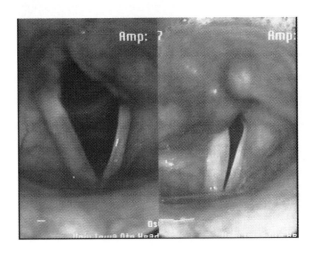

Color Plate 20. See page 569.

Color Plate 21. See page 570.

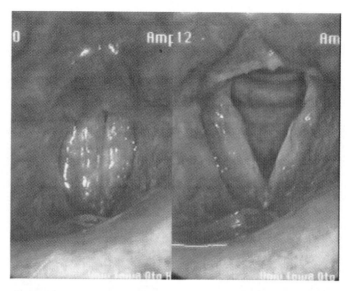

Color Plate 22. See page 571.

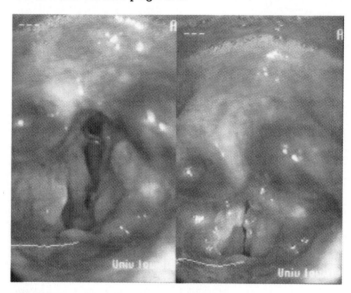

Color Plate 23. See page 571.

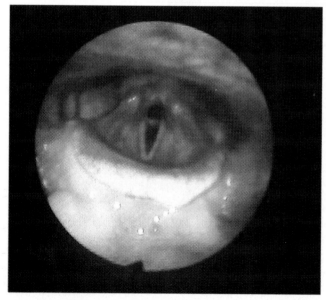

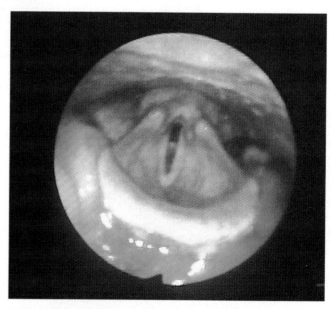

Color Plate 24. See page 578.

Color Plate 25. See page 579.

19

Dementia: A Review for the Speech–Language Pathologist

DANIELLE N. RIPICH AND ELAINE ZIOL

CHAPTER OUTLINE

Cognitive Changes and Normal Aging

Dementia Types and Associated Disorders

Language and Dementia

Assessment and Diagnosis

Intervention for Persons with Dementia

Dementia is not a disease but a symptom complex for a variety of diseases that affect an estimated four million adults in the United States and touches one in three families.[1] The prevalence of dementia increases later in life from 1 percent at age 60, doubling every five years so that 30 to 50 percent are affected by age 85,[2,3] but it is not inevitable. The estimate for residents in extended care with cognitive impairments (most often dementia) ranges from 50 to 67%.[4] Looking toward the millennium, Evans[5] has projected that the number of persons with dementia in the United States over age 65 will range from a low projection of 7.5 million to a high range of 14.4 million in the year 2050. A sevenfold increase in the oldest age group (over 85 years) compared to 1980 will account for most of the projected increase, placing heavy demands on services for this aging population with a growing need for communication services. It is essential that speech–language pathologists (SLPs) and others who work with persons with dementia are prepared to meet the communication needs of both cognitively impaired persons and their care providers.

The primary goal of this chapter is to provide organizing schemas that can be used clinically to meet the needs of this rapidly growing population. Initially, we will consider neurobehavioral/cognitive changes in normal aging. Next, a framework describing the dementias and related disorders is presented to provide a basis for differential diagnosis with an emphasis on the most common dementias. Then patterns of language and communication in dementia are presented and organized by levels of language processing: pragmatics, semantics, syntax, and phonology. We describe an approach to assessment and diagnosis based on this model. Finally, we give information for direct and indirect intervention for persons with dementia.

COGNITIVE CHANGES AND NORMAL AGING

Neurobehavioral/Cognitive Changes

There is marked variability among individuals with regard to cognitive changes in aging.[6–8] Birren and Birren[9] describe normal aging as orderly or regular changes that occur over the life span. A general cognitive decline is noted in most cohorts beginning in the sixth decade, with verbal abilities maintaining until the eighth decade.[10] However, the areas of memory, abstraction, language, visuospatial ability, and attention all eventually show a decline with normal aging.[11,12]

Studies suggest that although several types of memory are affected in normal aging, the elderly are compromised little in everyday life.[13] Primary (or short-term) memory shows little change in capacity. An example of a test of primary memory is the immediate recall of a list of words or numbers. However, when working memory is required for temporary storage or manipulation of information, age-related differences are apparent.[14] Normal aging has effects on secondary (or long-term) memory, probably due to shallow encoding, reduced organization, or deficits in visual elaboration.[15] Information in long-term memory has been divided into episodic or semantic.[16] Episodic memory is composed of information related to a temporal context or experiences in time such as a first train ride or what a person has eaten for breakfast that morning. Semantic memories, on the other hand, are organized by concepts, world knowledge, and word meaning, such as the features of a canary or the rules of syntax. Episodic memory shows age decrements, whereas semantic memory remains stable and even increases with age.[17] Tertiary (or remote) memory of personal information and events is not impaired in normal aging.

The term "benign senescent forgetfulness"[18] has been replaced by descriptions such as "age-associated memory impairment" (AAMI), defined as "mild memory loss occurring in the elderly unassociated with other cognitive deficits or with any identifiable illness that may be causing memory difficulty."[19] These individuals, who are usually over 50 years of age, display memory loss that does not interfere with daily lives, but can be noted by themselves and others. They show preserved intellectual function with performance on standardized memory tests that is one standard deviation below that of a younger group.[11]

Abstraction, the ability to understand and relate concepts as tested by proverb interpretation and tests of word similarities, decreases by the seventh decade,[12] though this can occur later in persons with higher educational status.[20] Although there does appear to be changes in language use during the seventh and eighth decades, complete agreement does not exist regarding the effects of aging on language.[11] Bayles and Kaszniak[21] suggested that "age effects on linguistic knowledge, if they exist, appear to be subtle and somewhat illusory" (p. 150). Generally, the aging process does not interfere with the individual's functional ability to communicate. Older persons show poorer performance in tests of visuospatial ability, although removing time constraints improves scores.[11] Finally, McDowd and Birren[22] reported some decrease of inhibitory attentional processes with aging, along with some decrease in ability to divide attention.

DEMENTIA TYPES AND ASSOCIATED DISORDERS

Definition of Dementia

The term *dementia* is used here to refer to (a) impairment in memory, (b) at least one of the following cognitive disturbances—aphasia, apraxia, agnosia, or disturbance in executive functioning, and (c) resultant impairment in occupational or social functioning that represents a decline from previous higher functioning.[23] There are both reversible and irreversible dementias. All possible causes of reversible dementias must be ruled out in the diagnostic process before moving to an identification of irreversible dementia. Reversible or treatable dementias include those that result from drug toxicity, metabolic imbalances, infections, tumors, normal-pressure hydrocephalus, alcohol abuse, neurosyphilis, and epilepsy. Geriatric depression (pseudodementia) is classified as a reversible dementia in some diagnostic models.[24] However, probably less than 10% of dementias are reversible, with more than two-thirds having drug toxicity, depression, or metabolic disorder as the cause.[25] Irreversible dementias include Alzheimer's disease (AD), multi-infarct dementia (MID) or vascular dementia (VaD), Pick's disease or frontal lobe dementia, and those dementias associated with Parkinson's disease, Huntington's disease, Wilson's disease, supranuclear palsy, Creutzfeldt-Jakob disease, Korsakoff's disease, and human immunodeficiency virus (HIV).

Alzheimer's Disease

Of the irreversible dementias, AD is by far the most common, accounting alone or in combination with other illnesses for 70% of all dementias.[19] AD is the fourth or fifth most common cause of death.[26] In addition to the basic dementia criteria previously described, the *Diagnostic and Statistical Manual of Disorders-IV (DSM-IV)*,[23] published by the American Psychiatric Association, has identified the following additional criteria for dementia of the Alzheimer's type:

- Insidious onset with a generally progressive deteriorating course
- Exclusion of all other specific causes of dementia by history, physical examination, and laboratory studies
- Deficits not occurring exclusively during the course of delerium
- Symptoms not accounted for by other major disorders such as a major depressive disorder or schizophrenia

AD presents with classical clinical symptoms of memory loss, decline in ability to perform routine tasks, impaired judgment, disorientation, personality changes, difficulty learning, and loss of language abilities.[27,26] AD may be accompanied by depression, delusions, and/or more rarely delirium, or may be diagnosed as uncomplicated if its onset shows none of these features.

Characteristic neuropathological changes include: helical neurofibrillary tangles,[28] senile plaques,[29] granulovacuolar degeneration,[30] and amyloid angiopathology.[31,32] Research has also indicated losses of neurons,[33] neurotransmitters,[34] and neuropeptides[35] as significant indicators of AD.[36] Recent research has identified genetic, clinical, and pathological heterogeneity in the presentation of AD with cases of sporadic and familial forms, of early and late age of onset, of early and prominent language impairment, myoclonus, or rigidity.[37] A confirmed diagnosis of AD can presently only be made on autopsy.

Vascular Dementia (also termed Multi-Infarct Dementia)

The *DSM-IV* criteria[23] for vascular dementia (VaD) include the basic dementia criteria with the addition of evidence of cerebrovascular disease (CVD). These are:

- Focal neurological signs and symptoms such as exaggeration of deep tendon reflexes, extensor plantar response, pseudobulbar palsy, gait abnormalities, or weakness of an extremity
- Laboratory evidence such as computed tomography (CT) or magnetic resonance imaging (MRI) showing multiple vascular lesions of the cortical and subcortical structures.

VaD includes dementing syndromes other than multiple infarcts resulting from CVD occurring over time and therefore has been expanded from the previous term, "multi-infarct dementia (MID)." Examples of vascular disorders other than stroke that can cause dementia include autoimmune vasculitides such as systemic lupus erythematosus or infectious vasculitides such as Lyme disease.[38] In this chapter, the terms VaD/MID will be used for this symptom complex. VaD/MID is the second most common subtype of dementia but occurs much less frequently than AD. This dementia accounts for approximately 20% of all persons with dementia and occurs concurrently with AD in another 15%.[39]

When the etiology of VaD/MID is multiple infarcts, symptoms present with abrupt onset and stepwise course of "patchy" losses of function depending on the areas damaged by the infarcts. To differentially diagnose VaD/MID, Roman et al.[40] detailed the relevant imaging of CVD through CT or MRI to include multiple large vessel infarcts, a single strategically placed infarct, or lacunae in the white matter or periventricular white matter. In addition to the focal neurological signs listed above in the criterion for VaD/MID, cognitive functions such as memory, abstract thinking, judgment, impulse control, and personality are nearly always affected.[24] This disorder is more common in males[41] and is without a documented familial pattern. It appears to have arterial hypertension, extracranial vascular disease, and valvular disease of the heart as predisposing factors.[42]

Hachinski et al.[43] developed an ischemic scoring system of 13 items designed to create two distinct nonoverlapping groups for differentiating between VaD/MID and AD. A study by Wagner et al.[44] evaluated the validity of the ischemic score as a differential diagnostic tool. Results indicated that the ischemic score was of major importance in differentiating VaD/MID from AD and depression. Molsa et al.[45] also found good discrimination (70% accuracy) between patients with VaD/MID and those with AD using the Hachinski scoring method.

Perhaps because of the heterogeneity of the language problems and the "patchy" nature of the loss of cognitive functioning in VaD/MID patients, there have been no large-scale studies of language loss in VaD/MID.[21] A comparison study of speech and language alterations between AD and VaD/MID patients[46] revealed that the verbal output of these two groups differed in several ways. The VaD/MID patients demonstrated greater motor speech disruption, whereas the AD patients showed more difficulty in language (i.e., empty speech and marked anomia). These results are noteworthy in that they revealed differences in these two syndromes despite the heterogeneity of the symptom complexes of AD and especially VaD/MID. VaD/MID is a subtype of dementia that warrants additional research and documentation of patterns of loss, as well as comparisons to other forms of dementia. (See Tables 19–1 and 19–2 for characteristics of VaD/MID and a comparison of VaD/MID with AD.)

Frontal Lobe Dementia (and Pick's Disease)

Patients demonstrating the symptom complex dementia of the frontal lobe type show impairment in executive functioning and disinhibited behavior with normal or minimally impaired performance on cognitive tasks.[47] These patients may not always exhibit distinctive pathological changes associated with Pick's disease. Personality rather than cognitive changes characterize those with frontal lobe dementia along with obsessive traits, apathy or jocularity, lack of empathy, disinhibition, and poor attention (Table 19–3). Neary and colleagues[48] suggest that dementia of the frontal lobe type may possibly represent a form of Pick's disease.

Pick's disease, a relatively rare progressive neurological disorder, causes deterioration of the frontal and/or temporal lobes due to loss of neurons, gliosis, and neuronal inclusions called Pick bodies.[49] The pattern of neuronal degeneration (i.e., primarily frontal lobe atrophy), including the inferior motor area and anterior temporal lobes and

Table 19–1. Characteristics of Vascular/Multi-Infarct Dementia (VaD/MID)

Assessment	Hachinski Scale Features[43]
	Abrupt onset[a]
	Stepwise deterioration
	Fluctuating course[a]
	Nocturnal confusion
	Relative preservation of personality
	Depression
	Somatic complaints
	Emotional incontinence
	History of hypertension
	History of strokes[a]
	Evidence of atherosclerosis
	Focal neurological symptoms[a]
	Focal neurological signs[a]
Clinical features	Weakness
	Slowness
	Dysphagia
	Small-step gait
	Emotional lability
Cognition	Reduced spontaneity
	Decreased speed of processing
	More preserved recent memory compared to AD
Language	Less characteristic speech/language profiles
	Dysarthria (pseudobulbar more common)
	Simplification of structural aspects of sentences
	Sentence fragments
	May show partial recovery of function

[a]Feature more heavily weighted.

Table 19–2. Distinctions Between Vascular/Multi-Infarct Dementia (VaD/MID) and Alzheimer's Disease (AD)

	VaD/MID	AD
Onset	May be abrupt	Insidious
Course	Stepwise and paroxysmal	Gradual and progressive
Gender	Men more frequent	Women slightly more frequent
Focal neurological signs	Frequent	Generally absent
Pathology at autopsy	Cerebral softening with multiple areas of infarction; cardiovascular arteriosclerosis	Neurofibrillary tangles, senile plaques; granulovacuolar degeneration; increased dendritic spine loss
Associated medical pathology	Strokes and other cerebral vascular accidents; myocardial infarction; angina pectoris and other cardiac pathology; hypertension; TIAs; peripheral vascular disease, diabetes mellitus; obesity	Vulnerable to numerous medical problems at late stages secondary to excessive cognitive disability
Genetic	Some genetic vascular risk factors	Some autosomal dominant forms (Chromosone 21, 1, 14) A genetically susceptible locus (Chromosone 19)
Bioelectric (EEG)	May show focal or lateralized slow activity over area of infarct	EEG activity inversely proportional to severity of memory impairment
Diagnostic Imaging CT scans	Focal and asymmetric pathology—best for acute lesions	Symmetrical atrophy and ventricular enlargement related to severity of the dementia
MRI	Sensitive to white matter lacunar strokes	May detect subtle atrophy
Regional cerebral blood flow	Less decrease in blood flow compared to metabolic decrease in area of infarct	Decreased blood flow compared with age-matched controls
PET scans	Promising studies underway	Promising studies underway
Treatment	Aspirin and agents with decreased platelet aggregation and clotting; antihypertensives; possibly anticoagulants	Cholinesterase inhibitors (e.g., tactrine)

Table 19–3. Characteristics of Frontal Lobe Dementia (and Pick's Disease)

Behavioral characteristics	Reduced spontaneity, inactivity
	Reduced insight, reduced executive function
	Disinhibition
Cognition	Relative sparing of cognitive areas (i.e., math, memory, visual spatial)
Language	Early language abnormalities
	Reduced spontaneous output
	Logorrhea, palilalia, echolalia (Pick's)
	Possible mutism even at middle stages (Pick's)
	May show sparing of specific language modality

sparing of the posterior cingulate gyrus and parietal lobes, differs from the diffuse pattern found in AD. However, the amygdaloid nucleus and hippocampus are involved in both disorders.[50] These patients display altered behavior including lack of spontaneity, inappropriate laughter, impaired insight and judgment, and early language deficit.[51] Compared to patients with AD, patients with Pick's disease can be distinguished by language features including early presentation of language symptoms,[52] logorrhea, reduced spontaneous speech output, echolalia, and mutism beginning even at middle stage of the disease.[53] Pick's disease is reported to begin at an earlier age than AD (40 to 60 years)[54] and is more common in women. In later stages, Klüver-Bucy syndrome (hyperoral behavior), hypersexuality, and visual agnosia have been reported.[55,56] Pick's disease is reported to occur from 1 to 10 percent as often as AD.[52,57,58]

Slowly Progressive Aphasia (also termed Primary Progressive Aphasia)

Mesulam[59] identified a group of six patients presenting with a slowly progressive aphasic disorder (SPA) without the additional intellectual and behavioral disturbances of dementia (Table 19–4). The pattern of symptoms in these patients suggested the presence of a selective degeneration of the perisylvian region of the left hemisphere, distinct from AD or Pick's diseases. Mesulam's patients were all right-handed. Heath et al.[60] confirmed the clinical entity of SPA in a left-handed patient.

As researchers began to study progressive aphasia a variety of theoretical and methodological questions were raised. Wechsler et al.[52] reported that a patient, previously described as manifesting a focal aphasic syndrome as the primary symptom of presenile dementia,[61] was found at autopsy to have pathologically confirmed Pick's disease and an apparently unique basilar dendritic pattern consisting of unusually long unbranched basilar dendrites. These findings suggested that progressive aphasia may be an unusual presentation of Pick's disease.

Concern regarding the comprehensiveness of Mesulam's assessment was voiced by Foster and Chase.[62] These authors stated that a more quantifiable neuropsychological assessment would provide convincing evidence that the progressive aphasia patients were not cognitively impaired. Related to this line of thinking was a position taken by Kirshner et al.[63] They pointed out that, in at least a subset of SPA patients, the language disturbance may be only an initial (if quite isolated) manifestation of a more generalized syndrome of cognitive deterioration. Although this view of progressive aphasia as a precursor to dementia has been upheld by other researchers,[64–66] Kirshner and colleagues[67] disputed the original report in a subsequent article that revealed postmortem autopsy results from the cases reported in the 1984 paper. Two patients from the 1984 study were reclassified as having SPA with no evidence of associated dementia. Mesulam[68] redefined SPA as primary progressive aphasia (PPA). This syndrome is characterized by aphasia with a relative or total sparing of activities of daily living, judgment, insight, and overall comportment. This aphasia does not neatly fit into existing classification schemes; however, anomia is the most common feature.

The focus of research in progressive aphasia to date has been in determining the presence of neuro-

Table 19–4. Characteristics of Slowly Progressive Aphasia (Primary Progressive Aphasia)

Behavioral characteristics	Able to continue with daily functional activities
Cognition	Progressive language impairment without generalized dementia at least at early stages
Language	Diverse language profiles; fluent aphasia more commonly reported
	Nonfluent with apraxias also reported
	Pragmatics more intact compared to AD
	Neuro-imaging shows L-hemisphere focal atrophy
	Possible motor speech involvement
	Research suggests positive effects for behavioral + pharmacological TX (maintenance difficult to disambiguate from disease progression)

pathologies that may precipitate SPA/PPA[69,70] and in determining that neuropsychological testing assures that subtle cognitive deficits found in dementia and other syndromes are noted.[71,65] Relatively little attention has been given to the careful and comprehensive examination of the dissolution of language in this syndrome. Reports of language deficits are often anecdotal.[61,64] A comprehensive protocol that includes a measure of functional communication as well as linguistic evaluation has not been used with SPA/PPA patients. The confusion surrounding the basis and manifestation of progressive aphasia has contributed to the unsystematic measurement of language decline in this syndrome.

Dementia Syndrome of Depression (Pseudodementia)

Depression, a common symptom, cause, and consequence of poor health in the elderly,[72] often co-occurs with dementia, and is sometimes termed pseudodementia[73] or dementia syndrome of depression[74] because the symptoms exhibited are quite similar. As a result, differential diagnosis of these two disorders is sometimes difficult. A 30% chance of misdiagnosis of the elderly person who presents with cognitive impairments, difficulty sleeping, appetite changes, and depressed affect has been reported by Jarvik[75] and Cummings and Benson.[51] A comprehensive history is useful in discriminating between these disorders. Accurate diagnosis is essential because appropriate drug therapy and intervention generally are successful in improving affect and cognitive symptoms associated with true depression. Differential diagnosis may be particularly difficult when depression co-occurs with a dementing disorder, particularly AD or Parkinson's disease. The person may be referred for depression and then found to have a primary diagnosis of dementia.[76]

Based on a review of available literature, Wells[77] developed a method of comparing and contrasting dementia and pseudodementia based on the (a) history; (b) clinical behavior and complaints; and (c) memory, cognitive, and intellectual performance. The following contrasts illustrate discernable differences in these disorders. In pseudodementia there is a definitive onset with rapid occurrence of most symptoms. This is in contrast to true dementia with its gradual onset and slow progression of symptoms. Patients with pseudodementia make little effort to perform clinical tasks, whereas dementia patients in the early stages often make every effort to prove themselves adequate. The pseudodementia patient's performance is highly variable on tasks of similar difficulty, whereas the dementia patient's poor performance is consistent across similar tasks.

LANGUAGE AND DEMENTIA

Aphasia

The relation between aphasia and dementia has been debated in the literature. Cummings et al.[78] reported that all 30 AD subjects they tested demonstrated aphasia and that aphasia should be included as a diagnostic criteria for AD. However, Bayles et al.[79] listed five criteria to differentiate aphasia and dementia. First, the rate of onset is sudden in aphasia and slow in AD. Second, decline is continuous in AD but not in aphasia. Next, AD results in diffuse brain atrophy whereas aphasia results from focal lesions. Further, they contend that dementia affects a range of cognitive abilities and aphasia does not. Finally, aphasic patients' performance on verbal and nonverbal tasks is dissociated, but dementia patients show simultaneous decline in these performances.

More recently Bayles and Kaszniak[21] have acknowledged that it is difficult to develop strict criteria for this differentiation. Au et al.[80] hold that studying all language function impairments in ways that lead to the development of a comprehensive model of brain-language relationships is more useful than using a differential approach. These authors, in contrast to Bayles and Kasz-niak,[21] Wertz,[81] Horner,[82] and others, propose that the language breakdown in dementia be viewed as a variation of the classical aphasia syndrome. This view appears to come from the same broad theoretical basis as Whitehouse's[83] argument against separating cortical and subcortical dementia. In both cases the argument is that there is more to be gained from examining commonalities than from developing a differentiating perspective (Table 19–5). Faber-Langendoen et al.[84] studied aphasia in demented patients and concluded that aphasia is a common feature of AD and identifies a subgroup with a more rapid progression of dementia. Furthermore, they contend that aphasia represents a specific dysfunction beyond the global cognitive impairment of AD. Both the differentiating and commonality perspectives are valid and depend on whether aphasia is defined as a result of "focal" brain damage or generalized brain damage. Shut[85] reports several cases in which a single vascular infarct, a homorganic stroke, produced part or all the

Table 19–5. Comparison of Characteristics of Aphasia and AD

	Aphasia	AD
Onset	Sudden	Gradual
Etiology	CVA Tumor Trauma	Diffuse damage 　neurofibrillary tangles 　senile plaque 　granulovacuolar degeneration
Course	Reversible Spontaneous recovery	Progressive, irreversible
Language	Impaired across all levels Speech not impaired	Semantics and pragmatics impaired 　early; syntax and phonology impaired 　later; speech impaired very late
Memory	Not impaired	Impaired early Worse for recent events
Performance characteristics	Poorer on language-based 　than nonlanguage tasks	Tries to perform; alert; consistent 　level of performance
Physical characteristics	May show right hemipare- 　sis; or hemiplegia	Normal; some pacing

symptoms of the dementia complex. The etiologic relationship between cerebrovascular disease and dementia warrants further study.

Bayles et al.[86] reported on a group of neuropsychological tests that differentiated AD patients (early and middle stages) from fluent and nonfluent aphasics (classified on the basis of word fluency measures). Memory tasks such as delayed spatial recognition, delayed verbal recognition, and delayed story retelling showed significant differences between AD patients and both groups of aphasics, with aphasics performing better. Mild AD patients performed better than nonfluent aphasics on the word fluency measure. Possibly the most difficult language differentiations among these language impairments are between early stage AD and the empty language of fluent and anomic aphasia.[87] Evaluation of memory performance can assist in this differentiation.

Communication Deficits in Dementia

The relationship between thought and language has long been debated by researchers and various theoretical positions have been developed. This debate has fostered numerous recent investigations into language breakdown in dementia. In addition, theoretical views of language have shown a dramatic shift from a formalist linguistic to a functionalist pragmatic perspective.[21,88,89] The shift to a functional perspective requires that we

view pragmatics, rather than syntax, as central to and regulative of the language system.[90] When we view pragmatics as central to the language system we must also view communicative competence as more basic than linguistic competence and structure our models accordingly. This perspective is particularly relevant to investigation of AD in that decline in pragmatics appears to be critical to the loss of functional communication in these patients.

Minimal normative data for evaluating the performance of individuals with AD on functional communication tasks is available.[91–93] Whereas declines in phonology, syntax, and semantics have been well documented,[86,94–96] the degree of decline in communication abilities seems to exceed the decline in these specific language areas.[91,97,98] Therefore, a complete description of the communication competence rather than linguistic knowledge is necessary for assessment in dementia. This broadened perspective requires analysis of communication units beyond the sentence level.

Existing data describe the linguistic abilities of persons with dementia on selected tasks for one of three purposes: (a) identification of dementia when it may be in question as a diagnosis,[99] (b) differentiation of dementia and other neurogenic communication disorders,[100–105] and (c) descriptions of the unique features of the language of dementia.[96,106–109]

Language Processing Levels

The following is a summary of the information gleaned from previous research on the four levels of language processing.

Pragmatics

Although this area appears to contribute most to the communicative deficit in AD and measures of pragmatics appear to be the most sensitive to interetiologic discrimination,[100] the documentation of the pragmatic deficits is limited.[110] In the early stage of dementia these deficits take the form of poor topic maintenance, briefer but more frequent turns, more directives, and breakdowns in cohesion and coherence;[97,111–114] in the middle stage as vague speech; and the final stage as difficulty in maintaining eye contact and conversational turns.

In addition, the discourse of AD speakers is described as confusing, lacking coherence,[106] and less cohesive than the speech of normal elderly speakers.[97] Bayles[115] anecdotally reports that requests are often missing in early to middle stages of the disease. However, confirmation and clarification requests have been reported to occur more frequently in the speech of early AD patients when compared to normal elderly by Ripich et al.[114] Other discourse differences identified in AD include high use of indefinite reference[97,108,112,116] and disordered and diminished content.[71,94]

The *Discourse Ability Profile (DAP)*[89] was used to examine and organize the discourse of early to middle stage AD patients on a variety of discourse tasks. Results showed significantly poorer overall discourse performance by AD patients.[117] The procedural discourse task, requiring instruction giving, was the poorest, and narrative abilities were somewhat poorer than those of age and education matched cohorts. However, conversational skills showed no differences. These results suggest that the pragmatic deficits noted in AD patients may depend on the nature of the discourse genre and task.[118] Further systematic examination of discourse as an aspect of communicative functioning may lead to a better understanding of the relative contribution of linguistic and discourse impairments to the dissolution of communication in AD.

Nicholas et al.[87] examined the relationship between the linguistic impairment of anomia assessed by the *Boston Naming Test*[119] and the discourse impairment measured by the Cookie Theft Picture on the *Boston Diagnostic Aphasia Examination*[120] in performances of persons with AD. They concluded that the naming deficits did not underlie the emptiness of the discourse content. However, some of the referential errors may have resulted from anomic difficulties. Methodologically, we are beginning to develop creative ways of systematically tapping natural language in ecologically valid contexts. These methodologies will allow us to determine the reliability and validity of what to date must be viewed as tentative findings in pragmatic communication.

Semantics

Semantics is thought to be a highly disordered linguistic level in AD. Deficits are characterized by limited vocabulary[121,122] and naming difficulty,[123–126] both likely caused by breakdown in cognitive processing perhaps at the prespeech level.[96,106,127–131] Anomia has been the subject of the most research in language and dementia.[71,79,106,132,133] Even so, the nature of the anomic disorder in AD and the impact of perceptual and linguistic factors on it remains controversial.[134] The majority of researchers appear to support the view that the primary breakdown in anomia is cognitively based as opposed to perceptual. However, a dispute remains regarding the nature of the cognitive deficit as either a processing limitation or degrading, or a failure of the underlying lexical representation.[96,135]

Syntax

Many investigators report relatively intact syntax in dementia.[96,99,106,108,109] However, Constantinidis[136] reported missing phrases and sentences, as well as breakdown in phrase markers and grammatical agreement. Irigaray[129] described poor noun choice and incorrect verb tense in AD patients. This discrepancy has not yet been resolved. However, it appears that comprehension of syntax is relatively more impaired than production.[137,138] One theory for the presence of this disparity is that the automatic natures of syntactic structures do not require a great deal of attention by the speaker and so are maintained; thus, syntax maybe a relatively automatic cognitive function that is preserved in the midst of a more general cognitive decline.[139] Further support for this view comes from Whitaker's[109] case study of a demented woman (not AD) who spontaneously corrected errors of syntax and phonology when repeating sentences even though her language was restricted to echolalia, and she was unresponsive to commands.

Phonology

Although phoneme errors have been reported in several investigations,[122,136] these appear to be indicative of a "higher" semantic or syntactic problem, and not a problem with the individual "speech sounds" or morphophonemics (individual language units signaling a change in meaning). However, there have been no firm findings to support this possibility. Table 19–6 shows breakdown in stages of AD summarized for language processing levels.

ASSESSMENT AND DIAGNOSIS

Comprehensive assessment and correct diagnosis of AD and other forms of dementia are critical for prognosis, treatment, and case management. The initial diagnostic work-up and assessment precedes intervention; however, assessment must be viewed as a dynamic and ongoing process.[140] Because the rate of change is variable and the symptom complex heterogeneous, systematic reassessment is required. In addition, because dementia is a symptom complex that includes physical, social, cognition,

Table 19–6. Communication Changes in Alzheimer's Disease

Early Stages (Aware)	
Pragmatics	Able to maintain conversations. Some difficulty with giving instructions and storytelling. Some breakdown in pronominal referencing. Frequent requests for clarification and confirmation. May have difficulty understanding humor, analogies, sarcasm, abstract expressions. May fail to initiate or may initiate inappropriately. May drift from topic. Reduced ability to generate series of meaningful sentences. Vague. Questions refer to concepts within and beyond immediate environment. Uses compliments. Expresses appreciation.
Semantics	Word fluency and word finding compromised. Circumlocution, gesture, or associated word used as strategy for word-finding deficit. Difficulty with comprehension of abstract and/or complex concepts.
Syntax	No errors generally
Phonology	No errors
Middle Stages (Less Aware)	
Pragmatics	Poor topic maintenance, poor use of pronominal reference and other cohesion devices. Knows when to talk. Responds to questions. Loss of sensitivity to conversational partners. Frequently repeats ideas, forgets topic. Talks about past events or trivia. Fewer ideas. Reliance on stereotypical, automatic utterances ("I'm fine, dear. How are you? Aren't you sweet!"). Rarely corrects mistakes.
Semantics	Poor word fluency and confrontation naming; diminished vocabulary. Circumlocutions, unrelated word substitutions, and empty speech frequently used.
Syntax	Occasional grammatical errors. Some difficulty with comprehension of complex structures.
Phonology	No errors
Late Stages (Unaware)	
Pragmatics	Lack of coherence, prosody intact. Difficulty maintaining eye contact and conversational turn-taking. Mutism in final stage. Output may be meaningless or bizarre. Few to no related ideas. Fewer words and utterances. Perseveration.
Semantics	Paraphasia, echolalia, palilalia. Comprehension poor. Jargon. Poor vocabulary.
Syntax	Grammar generally preserved with some use of elliptical clauses. Sentence fragments common. Poor comprehension of grammatical structures.
Phonology	Errors more frequent, but no non-native language sound combinations.

and communication features, multiple perspectives are required for adequate diagnosis and assessment. These perspectives can only be provided by an interdisciplinary team of professionals from medicine, nursing, social work, psychology, speech–language pathology, and audiology. A complete/exhaustive evaluation for dementia should include (a) careful and thorough case history, (b) neurological and medical diagnostic studies and examination, (c) behavioral assessment, and (d) language and communication assessment. The following sections detail important considerations in each of these areas of assessment.

Case History Interview

No peripheral marker for AD is presently known. Diagnosis depends on a variety of different kinds of information that allows for the exclusion of other possible causes for the presenting symptoms. Therefore, it is crucial that the history be fully developed because of the role the information plays in the diagnosis. Historical data is important to the SLP in the assessment process in that it provides information describing the communication contexts and communicative demands encountered by the patient on a daily basis. History taking with demented patients is difficult because of the memory, attention, and language problems associated with this disorder. A family member, caregiver, or close friend must serve as the informant or co-informant along with the patient.

A complete history should include information in the areas of health, psychological and cognitive, and social and communication status as well as any special problems that may be occurring. An *Alzheimer Dementia Risk Questionnaire* developed by Breitner and Folstein[141] is a useful guide for conducting a full history of education, work, family, course of AD, and present symptoms. The interview segment dealing with communication status involves questions regarding hearing, communication environment, speech and language abilities, and functional communication. The basic questions asked in speech and language adult case histories are appropriate for these patients (see Chapey[142]).

Neurological and Medical Evaluation

In combination with a careful history, a physical and neurological examination should be completed by the patient's primary physician, geriatrician, or a neurologist. The examination should include a series of diagnostic laboratory studies with certain ancillary studies when appropriate.[143,144] These results serve to rule out a variety of systemic diseases and disorders, as well as cerebrovascular diseases and conditions that may produce symptoms similar to those associated with AD.

Behavioral Assessment

Behavioral assessment can be best completed using three approaches: (1) performance on neuropsychological tests; (2) observation of behavior in naturalistic contexts; and (3) reports from family members, friends, and caregivers regarding the patient's behavior. These three approaches offer a multimodal perspective of behavior. They allow for a comprehensive assessment as well as provide data for cross-checking performance by looking for confirming evidence across multiple behavior assessment methods.

Behavioral assessments conducted by neuropsychologists normally generate considerable direct information concerning orientation, memory, attention and concentration, abstract thinking, and more cursory information regarding communication, language, and speech. A complete neuropsychological assessment should also evaluate executive function, problem solving, visual acuity field and perception, praxis, hearing acuity, and discrimination. In contrast, SLPs comprehensively assess communication, language, and speech functions and more generally examine the domains of overall cognitive status. The overlap and separation of assessment domains should be acknowledged and discussed by the professionals and a working alliance developed to optimize patient care.[145]

Language and Communication Assessment

The assessment battery presented here is designed to address the communication abilities of dementia patients based on conceptual models of language processing that include "top down" (knowledge driven) and "bottom up" (data driven) organization.[146,147] These models are relevant to the study of dementia because they consider the language features more vulnerable to cognitive dissolution (i.e., knowledge based pragmatics and semantics), as well as those that are better maintained (i.e., data driven syntax and phonology).

A comprehensive evaluation of communication in dementia should include a standardized test of linguistic competence that assesses oral and written language production and comprehension, as well as additional tests for specific language problems in pragmatics, semantics, syntax, and phonology, and finally a language memory task. Table 19–7 lists recommended assessment tools for measuring these communication abilities. This language and communication assessment battery is designed to be administered in approximately two hours. It may be completed across several sessions if necessary. It is critical that a supportive test atmosphere be developed for dementia patients.

Comprehensive Language Tests

Standardized tests of aphasia (e.g., *Boston Diagnostic Aphasia Examination* [*BDAE*],[120] *Western Aphasia Battery*,[148] *Porch Index of Communicative Ability*,[149] etc.) provide an evaluation of breakdowns in linguistic functioning across domains in receptive and expressive contexts. A discussion of patterns of performance of persons with AD on these tests is found in Bayles and Kaszniak.[21]

The *Arizona Battery for Communication Disorders of Dementia* (*ABCD*)[150] is a battery of linguistic and nonlinguistic based subtests that examines communication problems in dementia. The *ABCD* expands the language measures of most standardized aphasia tests in that it evaluates memory, linguistic reasoning, and visuospatial construction abilities. The relationship of these

tasks to those of primarily linguistic offers valuable information regarding language and cognitive status. Furthermore, the subtests that assess verbal episodic memory are appropriate for screening. These are the recall and recognition components of the Word Learning subtest and the Story Retelling subtest.

Pragmatics

Discourse analysis is offering new techniques for assessment and monitoring of pragmatic function throughout the course of progressive dementia, as well as for planning and describing outcome.[151] The *Discourse Abilities Profile* (*DAP*)[89] serves as a format for organizing and recording observations of patients during various discourse interactions. The *DAP* is divided into four sections. Three sections correspond to three genres of discourse—narrative, procedures, and spontaneous conversation. In each of these sections specific discourse features of the genre are tallied. In addition, the examiner indicates an overall rating of the patient's performance within the genre (excellent, good, adequate, fair, poor). The fourth section of the *DAP* corresponds to three general discourse features (paralinguistic behavior, nonlinguistic behavior, and coherence) that are required for successful dis-

Table 19–7. Language and Communication Assessment Measures for Use with Dementia Patients

Level	Behavior	Measure
I. Comprehension	Receptive and expressive Oral and written language	*Arizona Battery for Communication Disorders of Dementia*[150] *Boston Diagnostic Aphasia Examination*[120] *Western Aphasia Battery*[148]
II. Pragmatics and Discourse	1. Schemata 2. Turn-taking 3. Topic management 4. Conversational repair 5. Speech act use 6. Paralinguistic 7. Nonlinguistic 8. Cohesion and coherence	*Discourse Abilities Profile*[89]
III. Semantics	Lexical comprehension Confrontation naming Word fluency	*Peabody Picture Vocabulary Test—Revised*[152] *Boston Naming Test*[119] *FAS Word Fluency Measure*[154]
IV. Syntax	Sentence comprehension Sentence formulation	*Shortened Token Test*[158] *Auditory Comprehension Test of Sentences*[157] *Reporter's Test*[160]
V. Phonology	Word production	*Boston Diagnostic Aphasia Examination* (Subtest III)[120]
VI. Memory and Language	Delayed story retelling Word-list learning	*Wechsler Memory Scale-Revised* (Logical Memory Subtest)[162] *Rey Auditory Verbal Learning Test*[161]

course regardless of genre. Performances within these domains are also rated as either excellent, good, adequate, fair, or poor. Samples can then be analyzed, baselines established, and intervention individualized with more functional discourse behavior as the outcome.[151] Additional information regarding descriptive abilities can be obtained using a picture description task with complex stimuli such as a Norman Rockwell illustration.

Semantics

Assessment of semantic abilities using the *Peabody Picture Vocabulary Test* (*PPVT*),[152] the *Boston Naming Test* (*BNT*),[119] and a word fluency measure is recommended. The *PPVT* is a recognition task sensitive to the kinds of recognition difficulties persons with AD experience. Bayles and associates[86] found the *PPVT* to be one of the most discriminating measures between normal elderly and persons with mild AD. Expressive naming difficulties are an early presenting and persistent problem in persons with AD.[21] Confrontation naming as examined by the *BNT* necessitates the recognition of the stimulus, recall of its linguistic elements, and production of the target item. Research shows confrontation naming errors result from disruptions in the semantic network.[153] In addition, tests of verbal fluency are valuable as a diagnostic and assessment tool to measure speed of access to lexical and semantic information. Category fluency (e.g., naming animals in a category or items in a supermarket) has been shown to be superior to letter fluency (*FAS Word Fluency Measure*)[154] as a discriminator between those with and without AD due to its dependence on semantic structure, which deteriorates early in AD.[155,156]

Syntax and Phonology

Although syntax and phonology are relatively well preserved in the early stages of dementia, additional information regarding expression and comprehension performance on these levels may be useful for some patients.[136] Comprehension at the syntactic level for persons with AD shows a greater deficit initially on the *BDAE* subtests and the *Auditory Comprehension Test of Sentences* (*ACTS*),[157] both initially and over time, as compared to single word comprehension scores on the *PPVT*.[21] The *ACTS* systematically varies word frequency, sentence length, and syntactic complexity. The short version of the *Token Test*,[158,159] also a measure of sentence comprehension, allows for assessment of mild syntactic errors and can be administered

quickly. The *Token Test* is sensitive to the mild auditory comprehension problems demonstrated in early dementia. The *Reporter's Test*,[160] an expressive language task, is a measure of language formulation abilities. This test uses the test stimuli from the *Token Test* and can elicit mild syntactic errors. Phonology can be assessed in the context of the words and sentences from subtest III on the *BDAE*.

Memory and Language

A delayed recall task is an excellent way to assess the extent to which memory problems are impinging on language functioning. Across a period of approximately one hour patients can be asked to retell a 70- to 100-word story as a way of assessing functional memory. Bayles et al.[86] found that after a lapse of one hour persons with AD remembered only 2% of a novel story compared to 96% of story features recalled by normal elderly during a delayed story retelling task. Word learning lists (i.e., *Rey-Auditory Verbal Learning Test*[161]) and paired-associate word learning are also sensitive to dementia. The *Wechsler Memory Scale-Revised*[162] has subtests for both delayed story recall and paired word learning.

Specialized/Screening Geriatric Tests

A recent addition to test batteries performed on the older population is the *Ross Information Processing Assessment—Geriatric* (*RIPA-G*),[163] which was developed specifically to test cognitive-linguistic function in geriatric residents of skilled nursing facilities, hospitals, and clinics. This test provides data on memory; orientation to space, time, and environment; higher level and concrete reasoning; auditory processing; and comprehension, as well as supplemental subtests for naming and functional oral reading. Results are valuable for the team in developing rehabilitation goals.

A useful screening tool for the elderly is the *Middlesex Elderly Assessment of Mental State* (*MEAMS*),[164] which was designed to detect gross impairment of specific cognitive skills. The test items are easy, and cut-off scores suggest which patients should be referred for more extensive cognitive-linguistic evaluation.

Our challenge in clinical work in dementia is in the realm of assessment and intervention. Because all dementias are treatable, at least psychosocially, making an accurate diagnosis to initiate appropriate treatments and provide information to the patient and family about prognosis, possible genetic risks, and health care planning to the patient and the family is essential.[38] Many dementias occur secondarily to other disorders, so that the dementia may initially be masked. The heterogeneity of the symptom presentation in dementia subtypes further complicates the assessment and intervention process.

INTERVENTION FOR PERSONS WITH DEMENTIA

Ethical Issues in Treating Persons with Dementia

Quality of life and quality health care are rights of every individual including those who suffer from dementing disease. The components of quality of life include physical, mental, and spiritual health; cognitive ability; family and social relations; work and hobby activities; economic success; and subjective well-being.[165] Social interaction and continuing interpersonal relations have been closely linked to quality of life[166–168] and are affected by behavioral approaches to treatment of dementia. An innovative and flexible treatment program designed for persons with dementia will address these quality of life issues.

Arguably, it is the ethical responsibility of professionals involved in the care of persons with dementia to communicate as effectively as possible. For example, using complex, compound sentences when discussing plans for case management may be unethical if the patient becomes confused but could follow a discussion if simple subject-verb-object constructions were used. This is a position that places the bulk of the communication burden on the professional—the more competent communicator.

A considerable need exists for SLPs and other health care professionals to shift from a more traditional medical model based on assessing pathology and restoring function to a more holistic model based on maintaining function and preventing excessive response to disability.[169] The American Speech–Language and Hearing Association (ASHA) has two position statements on the general role of SLPs and audiologists in the extended care setting. The papers stress the need for increasing involvement in the assessment and management of persons with AD and related disorders, providing programs to maintain functional communication for as long as possible, and improving the quality of life/quality of care.[170,171]

Reimbursement Issues in Dementia Treatment

Obtaining reimbursement for services to persons with dementia is a challenge due to the progressive nature of the disease and the changing guidelines for coverage. Glickstein and Neustadt[172,173] have addressed reimbursement concerns by developing a model that describes reimbursable consultative and direct services with the goals of functional maintenance and reducing loss of abilities over time. For Medicare reimbursement, the SLP needs to be familiar with coverage requirements, specify length and frequency of treatment, clearly document a functional outcome, indicate the skilled intervention required, base assessments on standardized measures if possible, and use appropriate terminology. These issues will continue to be problematic and dynamic with changes in the health care system. However, SLPs can affect the communication functioning of the person with dementia with appropriate goal setting and documentation.

Direct Intervention for Persons with Dementia

With a direct approach, the communication specialist works with persons with dementia in groups or in individual sessions with the goals of maintaining residual functional communication and preventing excessive response to disability from occurring.[169] In this section, we will discuss a number of direct approaches that have been used in treating persons with dementia.

Reality Orientation (RO)

RO, first developed in 1958 by Dr. James Folsom for use at a veterans administration hospital, consists of two types: (1) the basic approach, with each encounter an opportunity to reinforce awareness and (2) formal RO classes in small groups.[174] Although sometimes criticized through the years, it has been frequently taught, and some techniques are still used. In the 24-hour one-on-one basic approach, there is attention to aspects of communication including awareness of barriers in the environment, correction for sensory deficits, attention to nonverbal communication, and structuring communicative exchanges by the caregiver. For the group approach, signs and information boards are recommended with activities that are structured for success. RO is used to begin and end the session.

RO has been criticized for having little theoretical basis,[175] no value,[176] showing no generalization to other areas of behavior,[177] and being too rigid, boring, and unstimulating.[178] However, single case studies have found that individual goals are attainable with training.[179–181] Numerous studies have shown an increase in verbal orientation[182–184] although this may not be reflected in functional behavioral changes. Greene and colleagues[185] reported improved affect in patients in RO groups and decreased mood in caregivers when RO groups were discontinued. (See Holden and Woods[186] for an extensive evaluation of the program.)

RO can be multifaceted and adapted to many settings and individuals while respecting the individuality and dignity of the person with dementia. Respectfully calling the person's attention to upcoming holidays and events can promote activity and interest.[187] As in any treatment method, the attitudes, values, and principles of the caregivers will determine how effective the approach is in a client-centered environment.

Reminiscence and Life Review

Reminiscence can provide a valued and enjoyable experience for persons with dementia in day care settings and extended care facilities. Instead of being seen as regression, stories from the past are thought to be beneficial for elderly especially during stress and transition. Reminiscence is the vocal or silent review of events in one's life. This approach may be particularly appealing for persons with dementia as an opportunity to communicate with others because it focuses on long-term memory.[188] This contrasts somewhat from the life-review process that encompasses reviewing, organizing, and evaluating the overall picture of one's life. Life review requires more structure and guidance. Triggers such as music, food, poems, faces, colors, objects, and smells can be useful for recall. Reminiscence can be encouraged informally by requesting advice, looking at family photographs, paging through old magazines such as *Life*, discussing hobbies, military experiences, and past jobs. Artifacts such as tools and household objects borrowed from a local museum have been used in a group to provide sensory stimulation and recall competencies and achievements from the past.[188]

Reminiscence in a group has many benefits: developing relationships, entertaining peers, enhancing status of participants, assisting with identify formation, facilitating resolution, reorganization, and reintegration of one's life, and establishing a sense of personal continuity.[189] Attendance at reminiscence sessions was reported by Baines and colleagues[182] to be higher when compared to RO sessions. In this crossover design the group who participated in RO sessions first, followed by reminiscence sessions, showed significant increase on a number of behavioral and cognitive scales. In another study, Kiernet[190] reported improvement on behavioral scales following twice weekly reminiscence sessions after 10 weeks. Furthermore, reminiscence has been associated with improved self-esteem in nursing home residents.[191]

Memory/Communication Compensations

Holden and Woods[186] reviewed evidence that aspects of learning may be maintained in dementia if supported and reinforced in the environment. Training in memory and communication strategies and compensations is appropriate particularly in early stages of dementia. A memory notebook with autobiographical information, calendar, and sections for things to do, maps, and daily logs[192] can draw on more intact procedural memory abilities to compensate for short-term memory failure. Bourgeois[193] demonstrated the use of developing memory wallets with pictures and sentences about familiar persons, places, and events. Persons with dementia improved conversational content with some subjects demonstrating improvements for up to 30 months following intervention.

The use of external strategies such as written "post-it notes," alarms, daily pill organizers, or audio- and videotapes can help maintain independent function for as long as possible. At early stages during which persons with dementia are more aware of communication breakdown, the SLP can reassure and train the client to ask for repetition or review of the topic and compensate with circumlocution, gesture, and associated words for semantic deficits. More recently, treatment using discourse tasks has addressed impairments in topic maintenance, organization, turn-taking, and cohesion. Furthermore, discourse measures can show functional outcomes and measurable changes from baseline.[151]

Engaging persons with dementia with collections of pictures of familiar categories (i.e., flowers, boating, fishing, golfing, home decorating, local landmarks, etc.) can decrease agitated behavior and increase interaction (Denis, personal communication, August 16, 1996). These "Look Books," strategically placed within the environment, can be used informally to distract or serve as a focus for reminiscence in a group setting. The SLP can help staff develop these materials and train in their use.

The following case study illustrates collaborative assessment and direct intervention with a patient presenting with a dementing syndrome.

CASE ONE

When referred for speech–language evaluation, Mrs. V. was a 70-year-old, right-handed woman who had been experiencing deteriorating language skills over the past 18 months. The referring physician indicated that her parents had a history of memory problems (diagnoses of probable Alzheimer's disease for her father and possible Alzheimer's and possible Parkinson's disease for her mother). Magnetic resonance imaging (MRI) of the brain showed mild parenchymal volume loss with focal parenchymal volume loss in the left frontal region in the location of Broca's area.

Mrs. V. was a college graduate who majored in English, piano, and physiology; she was married to a physician, had three children, and several grandchildren. The patient was a calm, dignified, well-dressed woman and stated that she maintained her regular daily activities of shopping, cooking, housekeeping, driving, banking, target shooting, fox hunting, and traveling extensively. She stated, however, "I'm slowing down now. I like my home."

Mrs. V. said that she read the newspapers and periodicals such as *Audubon* and *Smithsonian*. She said she had recently finished a popular novel, but was unable to recall its name or provide any information about the content. She reported a history of dyslexia. She also disclosed that lately she had difficulty remembering when reading and that her mind wandered. She did little writing with the exception of shopping lists. She denied other problems with episodic or long-term memory.

Neuropsychological evaluation suggested that Mrs. V. was of above average intelligence, scoring in the normal to above average range on most measures administrated. There was generally no evidence of cognitive impairment in areas of memory, executive functions, perceptual organizational skills and abstract reasoning. Mild difficulty for attention and concentration was noted.

Initial Speech–Language Evaluation

The patient was tested via the *Boston Diagnostic Aphasia Examination (BDAE), Boston Naming Test (BNT), Token Test, Reporters Test, Discourse Abilities Profile (DAP)*, and informal measures. She had no difficulty identifying single words, body parts, or concepts of R-L. She followed intermediate level commands and was 100% accurate answering yes/no questions, but 63% accurate answering yes/no questions after listening to paragraphs.

Mrs. V. scored 57 of 60 on the *BNT*. Repetition was generally accurate with occasional literal paraphasic errors for multisyllabic words or phrases. Responsive naming and oral reading were good. She generated 22 items in the animal category to test word fluency. Breakdown was most evident, however, in discourse as assessed in the *DAP* and a picture description task. The patient was nonfluent with numerous hesitations and mazes (restarts, fillers, repairs). Language was telegraphic with omission of functor words and with syntactic errors. Occasional cohesion errors resulted from pronoun substitutions ("And he had a puppy dog and he gave them to me.") Utterances ranged from single words to nine words in length, averaging five words per utterance. Oral motor structure and function were within normal limits. A mild verbal apraxia was indicated. Speech was somewhat monotone. Prosody was significantly impaired due to nonfluent language. Rate of speech was slightly slow. Functionally, Mrs. V. could converse about most everyday situations and ideas through words, phrases and sentences of simple syntax. Initiation was reduced and she was unable to expand or continue topics.

Reading showed breakdown for longer, more complex inferential material. Writing was legible with 90% spelling accuracy for dictated words. She could provide only one basic sentence when asked to write a paragraph about a familiar topic. Capitalization was accurate; punctuation was omitted.

Overall, Mrs. V. presented with at least mild deficits across all language modalities with oral expression showing most impairment. Although not tested formally, the patient's interview and behavior in the testing setting showed no evidence of cognitive involvement at this time.

Diagnosis and Treatment Plan

Medical, neuropsychological, and language assessment resulted in the diagnosis of a progressive aphasia. The treatment plan included providing the patient and her family with information about the disorder, individual psychotherapy aimed at strengthening adaptive coping skills, a program of speech–language therapy, and drug intervention.

Speech–Language Therapy

The initial course of treatment was for the patient to be seen on a weekly basis as her travel schedule allowed. The long-term goal at that time was to maintain communication skills with family and peers for as long as possible using compensatory strategies as needed. Speech therapy included standard aphasia treatment in all language modalities, training in compensatory strategies, and completion of hierarchical tasks on a syntax stimulation program. Following four months of consistent weekly treatment, Mrs. V. showed slight improvement in discourse abilities. (She provided 27 information content units on the Cookie Theft picture compared to 17 on initial evaluation, and she reduced utterances with mazes from 56% to 44%. Mean length of utterance, however, declined from five to four words.)

We also counseled Mrs. V.'s husband to spend 30 minutes each evening engaging her in conversation about her day and current events. We suggested other family members be encouraged to arrange a schedule of brief visits for the purpose of maintaining conversation and provided them with topic suggestions. Because Mrs. V. was described as withdrawing from conversations and social events, we provided her with a notebook with questions to cue herself to initiate and continue conversations with friends. These recommendations were part of a plan to keep her socially engaged. We further suggested subscribing to more visually oriented magazines such as *Travel and Leisure* since Dr. and Mrs. V. had continued to travel extensively.

Drug Intervention

Throughout the time this patient was followed (over two years) a number of therapeutic drugs were tried. A brief trial of Cognex was discontinued secondary to side effects. A trial of Deprenyl showed little improvement. A trial with acetylcarnitine, a drug shown to have some beneficial effect in younger Alzheimer's patients and approved in Italy but not yet in the United States, was also attempted with little effect. Most recently Mrs. V.'s physician prescribed Aricept, a drug similar to Cognex but with fewer side effects, which was approved by the Federal Drug Administration in 1996. Effects of this drug on progressive aphasia are not yet known.

Progress and Treatment

Because of her travel schedule, Mrs. V.'s treatment sessions were inconsistent, averaging 12 visits per year. Although she made progress shortly after she had begun therapy, language continued to deteriorate over time. Interestingly, this was reflected less in test scores than in actual discourse measures. The subtests or test measures that showed most change over evaluations every six months were a reduction in word fluency from naming 22 animal to 12 to 14 animals in subsequent test sessions and her ability to repeat sentences (decreasing in accurate repetition from 8 to 3 sentences). During the time this patient was followed, motor speech perfor-

mance became more impaired and discourse became significantly agrammatic. Prosody became progressively more impaired. Over the two years the patient's severity level increased from mild to moderately severe.

Throughout, in addition to tasks to facilitate language and decrease apraxia, training and structured drills were provided to encourage compensatory strategies such as gesture, drawing, writing, use of the environment, and a communication notebook. Alternate communication modalities and family education became more important as language deteriorated. Although Mrs. V. agreed that these options were helpful, she rarely spontaneously used them. She was most successful with writing single words or drawing, but required cueing for utilization. She declined attending group sessions to practice strategies. The patient's husband participated in several sessions for training as a communication partner.

Summary

The primary role for the speech–language pathologist in this case study was to provide the patient with information, help maintain speech skills for as long as possible, identify communication strengths, introduce and encourage alternative modalities for communication, and to offer support. In addition, the speech–language pathologist served on the team, reporting any changes in language performance noted with drug interventions and progress in therapy to the rest of the team. Continuing followup was recommended. The patient may be more amenable to communication options as her language continues to deteriorate. Further neuropsychological reevaluation was scheduled to monitor changes.

Group Treatment

Teaching strategies and discussing problems in group sessions for persons with similar memory problems can help maintain a positive and supportive atmosphere and foster communicative interaction. Group treatment even at more advanced stages of dementia provides opportunities to interact socially in a structured and supportive environment. Facilitators need to be familiar with communication level of participants to engage group members in the activity, cue appropriately, and promote interaction. Group treatment, consisting of simple, informative reminiscence sessions that review previous life experiences (discussions of traditional foods and celebrations, hobbies, school experiences, songs, and pets), has been shown to be successful for persons in the moderate stages of AD.[194] Group sessions can also include basic cognitive or sensory activities structured for success such as identifying textures and scents, and word, object, and melody recognition tasks. Ziol et al.[195] developed a group program with a variety of communication activities that incorporate aspects of RO, reminiscence, and training in compensations for those at mild and moderate stages with suggested variations in the activities for those at later stages.

The SLP treating persons with AD in group sessions will need to measure baseline communicative abilities and determine outcome measures (e.g., initiation, verbal and nonverbal responses, total words, total utterances, content, generalization, affect, interaction with other residents, interaction with staff, etc.). Goals should be realistic, functional, tailored to the cognitive level of the group participant, and focused on optimal functioning and maintenance of communicative skills.

Indirect Intervention: Training Caregivers of Persons with Dementia

Caregivers of persons with dementia can be family members and friends or professionals such as nurses or home health care staff. Communication breakdown is consistently listed among the top stressors in caregiver surveys of stress, strain, and burden.[196–198] Santo Pietro et al.[199] examined conversations between SLPs and persons with AD and found that certain communication strategies were effective in facilitating conversation whereas others were detrimental. Researchers report that family caregivers are sensitive to their relatives' communication problems and can identify the progression of the symptoms.[200,201] It would appear that caregiver training in facilitating strategies could provide useful tools to the caregiver communication partner. "Front line" care of persons with AD could be improved significantly by enhancing the communication skills of caregivers. The ability of caregivers to draw on strategies and techniques for dealing with communication problems in these persons would reduce their own stress and frustration and improve their competence in delivering quality care. In addition, caregivers would be better able to promote the use of residual functional communication abilities, provide appropriate social communication opportunities, and possibly to keep family members at home longer. Nurses and nursing assistants could also benefit from improved communication with their patients with AD. Several caregiver training programs will be discussed in the remainder of the chapter.

Validation Therapy

Naomi Feil developed validation therapy over 30 years ago as a response to the negative reaction to RO with the goals of stimulating verbal and nonverbal communication, restoring dignity and well-being, and resolving meaning in life for the person with dementia, particularly for those in later stages.[202] Rather than confront or correct persons with dementia the caregiver empathically "validates" or confirms their emotional states. Validation therapy assumes that the speech of the disoriented person has an underlying meaning and that the person with dementia returns to the past to resolve underlying conflicts.[203] In this approach, Feil[204] describes four stages (malorientation, time confusion, repetitive motion, and vegetation) and discusses appropriate interactions at each stage.

Empirical support for the program is limited to nonpublished, nonspecific reports of improved affect or positive effects[205–208] or inconsistent results when measuring communicative interaction while receiving validation therapy in a group setting.[203] However, validation therapy is reported to be used in over 500 institutions in the United States.[209] The techniques, which are expressions of empathy and emphasize nonverbal interactions, may best serve individuals at late stages in extended care facilities.

Training Caregivers: The FOCUSED Program

To improve communication with persons with dementia, Ripich and Wykle developed the *Alzheimer's Disease Communication Guide: The FOCUSED Program for Caregivers*.[210–212] This seven-step program uses the acronym FOCUSED to identify the major elements for communication maintenance and help the caregivers recall the strategies. This program was based on an interactive discourse model of conversational exchanges.[89] The key points of the program are:

F Face-to-face communication
O Orient to topic of conversation
C Continue topic of conversation
U Unstick communication blocks
S Structure with yes/no and choice questions
E Exchange conversation
D Direct, short, simple sentences

This program consists of didactic materials to better prepare family and professional caregivers to communicate with persons with AD. These materials include:

- Trainer's Manual—a word-for-word text of the program information with group discussion questions, role-play activites, and home practice assignments.
- Caregiver's Guides—outlines of topics and key information in easy-to-read format.
- Transparencies—reproducibles to present on an overhead.
- Pre- and Post-Assessments—tests of knowledge of AD and attitudes about communication satisfaction.
- FOCUSED Cards—cards containing the acronym FOCUSED with key ideas to serve as reminders of the communication principles.
- Videotape Vignettes—segments developed for the research protocol illustrating various communication problems caregivers encounter with persons with AD and demonstrations of appropriate use of techniques.
- Program Evaluations—forms completed at the end of training by participants to provide feedback to the trainer.

The training program is divided into five (or six) two-hour modules for family or professional caregivers with a section on cultural differences as an option for professional caregivers:

Module 1. Alzheimer's disease and the associated communication and language decline. This module discusses characteristics, pathology, and incidence of AD. The components and processes of language are presented. Participants learn how physicians make a diagnosis of probable AD and how language in aphasia and AD differ.

Module 2. The differences between memory decline in normal aging and AD and the effects of depression on the person with AD. In this module the caregiver is taught to understand changes in memory in the normal elderly, recognize symptoms of depression, and differentiate these symptoms from those of dementia. Discussion of the effects of depression on the person with AD's already decreasing ability to communicate with others is included.

Module 3. Interpersonal skills and the value of effective communication skills in the care of persons with AD. The critical importance of social communication to keep the person with AD engaged in communication to prevent excessive functional decline and maintain abilities is discussed. Participants learn verbal and nonverbal approaches to good communication. A discussion of empathy provides a foundation for promoting sensitive interpersonal exchanges that demonstrates respect for the person with dementia and supports the self-esteem of both the caregiver and the person with AD.

Module 4. The FOCUSED strategies to promote effective communication with persons with AD. This is a critical module that outlines the seven-point program. The program incorporates numerous strategies into a framework that is easy to recall and apply. A series of role-play exercises and videotaped vignettes (for the research protocol) are used to demonstrate the seven points of this communication enhancement program. Table 19–8 outlines the communication techniques.

Module 5. The stages of AD and concurrent communication characteristics including how to assess and recognize the person with AD at each stage and maximize his or her communication. Though fully aware of the heterogeneity of the progress of AD and the fact that dividing the progression into stages is an arbitrary device, the literature repeatedly reports three main levels of language deterioration designated as mild, moderate, and severe (see Table 19–6). In Module 5 these stages are described, the seven points of the FOCUSED program are reviewed, and the implementation of the strategies and communication goal at each stage are discussed.

Optional Module for Professional Caregivers: Cultural considerations in communicating with persons with AD. Cultural considerations are extremely important issues in helping the professional caregiver care for the person with AD. The conflicts that arise in a caregiving situation may be further complicated by the differences in cultural and socioeconomic backgrounds of extended care residents and nursing assistant staff. The resultant disparity in values and interpersonal dynamics accentuates the communication difficulties that are characteristic of persons with AD. Therefore, didactic and experiential content that enhances the caregivers' understanding of cultural considerations affecting that interpersonal communication process is presented.

In a pilot project using FOCUSED training for 17 nursing assistants results of pre- and post-test knowledge measures showed increased knowledge across all areas with significant ($p < .001$) gains in Modules 4 and 5, which present the FOCUSED program. This is somewhat predictable given the specific nature of the FOCUSED training information. Nevertheless, results suggested marked gains in information regarding communication strategies. Results of the attitude survey generally indicated improvement in attitudes of nursing assistants toward persons with AD. Their newly acquired skills reportedly made it more likely they

Table 19–8. FOCUSED Communication Strategies

F = Face
Face the person with AD directly
Call his or her name
Touch the person
Gain and maintain eye contact

O = Orient
Orient the person with AD to the topic by repeating key words several times
Repeat and rephrase sentences
Use nouns and specific names

C = Continue
Continue the same topic of conversation for as long as possible
Restate the topic throughout the conversation
Indicate to the person with AD that you are introducing a new topic

U = Unstick
Help the person with AD become "unstuck" when he or she uses a word incorrectly
    by suggesting the intended word
Repeat the sentence the person said using the correct word
Ask, "Do you mean . . . ?"

S = Structured
Structure your questions so that the person with AD will be able to recognize and
    repeat a response
Provide two simple choices at a time
Use yes/no questions

E = Exchange
Keep up the normal exchange of ideas we use in everyday conversation
Keep conversations going with comments such as, "Oh, how nice," or "That's great"
Do not ask "test" questions
Give the person with AD clues as to how to answer your questions

D = Direct
Keep sentences short, simple, and direct
Put the subject of the sentences first
Use and repeat nouns (names of persons or things) rather than pronouns (he, she, it,
    their, etc.)
Use hand signals, pictures, and facial expressions

would try to communicate with a person with AD instead of ignoring or patronizing him or her. The new enthusiasm of the nursing assistants regarding the importance of good communication was noted by a number of their supervisors.

A FOCUSED training project for African-American and white family caregivers of persons with AD (supported by National Institute on Aging grant #AG-08012-06) is being conducted to study the effects of communication skills training on communication patterns and stress and burden of these family caregivers. Preliminary results show similar positive effects for family caregivers in increasing knowledge about communication and AD, furthering positive affect, and reducing the hassles of caregiving. Family caregivers have com-

mented that "strategies were helpful in everything" and "role playing was very helpful in carrying out the strategies."

Other Caregiver Training Programs

Clark and Witte[213] developed "Making Family Visits Count," a communication training program for family members to improve quality and satisfaction in visits to relatives in nursing homes. In small practice groups, family members view prepared videotapes, taking note of facilitative communicative techniques and learning how to individualize strategies. In a communication stress management program for caregivers, Clark[214] teaches family members to understand the nature and progression of language changes in AD and increase and apply problem-solving skills to reduce caregiver stress and burden. As in the FOCUSED program, caregivers learn appropriate expectations and the importance of maintaining the person with dementia in communicative situations.

Communication training for caregivers can increase knowledge, improve communication satisfaction, and decrease hassles related to communication breakdown. Education in specific communication strategies can alter attitudes toward persons with AD. Providing adequate training to caregivers is essential to quality of life issues. Additional benefits may be caregivers' greater satisfaction and sense of accomplishment in their critical day-to-day activities. Caregivers can benefit from training in communication strategies and this training may improve the quality of life for persons with AD.

Continual Reassessment in Intervention

A final consideration in discussing treatment and intervention is the importance of continual reassessment as a part of the intervention process in this highly variable and heterogeneous symptom complex. Evaluation at six month intervals provides information regarding change and/or maintenance of competencies. Results of minimal or no change can be a very encouraging factor for many persons with dementia and their families. Identification of further decline in an area can focus and structure case management. Furthermore, the intervention process must ideally be multidisciplinary to address the scope of problems arising from this disorder. A collaborative perspective on the person with dementia, caregiver and family counseling, education, and communication treatment provide the optimal opportunity for comprehensive support of all aspects of intervention.

SUMMARY AND CONCLUSION

In summary, AD is the most frequently occurring type of dementia, followed by VaD/MID. AD is classified as a cortical dementia along with frontal lobe dementia and Pick's disease. We have included a discussion of slowly progressive aphasia, which continues to invite controversy in the literature as a distinct disease entity. (We did not include a dis-cussion of subcortical dementias [Parkinson's disease, Huntington's disease, Wilson's disease, and supranuclear palsy] or mixed dementias [Korsakoff's disease and Creutzfeldt-Jakob disease], which occur as a part of a more extensive symptom complex. For a more complete discussion of these dementias, consult Ripich,[215] "Language and Communication in Dementia," in the *Handbook of Geriatric Communication Disorders*.) We have included a discussion of the relationship of aphasia and the language of dementia. The basis of disagreement in terminology appears to be whether aphasia is defined as resulting from focal brain damage, or more broadly as resulting from any brain damage. It is important to note that aphasia and other related disorders may co-occur with dementia. Careful comparisons across neuropsychological and language measures are necessary for accurate diagnosis and assessment.

Finally, communication intervention must be viewed in the broadest possible terms and include education and counseling for all those in the communicative environment. In this way creative programs can be designed to assist patients in "staying in the communication game" as long as possible. For example, if we view the person with AD as being a weak player in the tennis match, by hitting the ball directly to him we help him "stay in the game." Using these premises to guide our intervention we can explore the complex challenge of case management with persons with dementia.

Developing the communication skills of professionals such as nurses, social workers, and physicians as well as direct caregivers can enhance the quality of life for the person with dementia. As a result of the degenerative nature of AD, these persons are initially cared for by family and eventually need institutionalization for long-term-care. It is important that all those who care for this increasing patient population have adequate training to communicate effectively with them. Primary caregivers of persons with AD report a gradual erosion of sociability, and maintain that communication is the single most distressing problem they face.[216,217] The goal of quality caregiving, therefore, should clearly be to prolong and promote communication between these patients and primary caregivers for as long as we can and on as high a level as possible.[214]

A review of the dementias, how language is affected in dementia, aspects of assessment and diagnosis, and intervention approaches for dementia have been addressed. This chapter challenges professionals working with persons with dementia to continue, through research and expanded clinical services, to meet the complex needs of these persons.

Acknowledgment

The preparation of this manuscript was supported by a grant from the National Institutes of Health/ Institute on Aging, #AG-08012. We wish to thank Peter J. Whitehouse, M.D., Ph.D., Director of the Alzheimer Center of University Hospitals of Cleveland, for his advice and assistance.

STUDY QUESTIONS

1. What changes in the following areas are noted in the normal aging process: memory, abstraction, language, visuospatial abilities, and attention?

2. What is "age-associated memory impairment"? Is it inevitable in aging?

3. Differentiate in type and etiology between the dementias that are reversible versus those that are irreversible.

4. How does slowly progressive aphasia differ from progressive dementias?

5. Why is it difficult to distinguish between pseudo-dementia and a true dementia?

6. How does aphasia differ from Alzheimer's disease (AD) with consideration to onset, etiology, course of the disease, language characteristics, memory, and physical characteristics?

7. Describe the stages of language changes through the course of AD.

8. What four areas should be included in a complete diagnostic evaluation for dementia?

9. Describe a speech–language assessment battery for a dementia patient based on a model of language processing that is "top down" (knowledge driven) and "bottom up" (data driven). Which processes would you expect to be more vulnerable to dissolution vs. those that are better maintained in AD?

10. Discuss appropriate compensations and treatment methods for persons with dementia (direct intervention).

11. You have been asked to give an inservice to nursing assistants in an extended care facility. Develop an outline for the 2-hour presentation.

12. Why is it important for the medical SLP to have a good understanding of cognitive impairment in the elderly?

13. What are ethical considerations for the SLP in treating persons with dementia?

REFERENCES

1. Advisory Panel on Alzheimer's Disease: Third Report of the Advisory Panel on Alzheimer's Disease, 1991 (DHHS Publication No. ADM 92–1917). U. S. Government Printing Office, Washington, DC, 1992.

2. Evans DA, Funkenstein HH, Albert MS, et al: Prevalence of Alzheimer's disease in a community population of older persons: Higher than previously reported. *JAMA* 1989; 262:2551–2556.

3. White LR, Cartwright WS, Cornoni-Huntley J, et al: Geriatric epidemiology. *Ann Rev Gerontol Geriatr* 1986; 6:215–311.

4. Lombardo NE: Policy implications of nature of cognitive impairment for service design. In Keenan MP, ed., *Issues in the measurement of cognitive impairment for determining eligibility for long-term care benefits,* pp 52–71. Public Policy Institute, Washington, DC, 1990.

5. Evans DA: Estimated prevalence of Alzheimer's disease in the United States. *Milbank Q* 1990; 68:267–289.

6. Albert ML: *Clinical neurology of aging.* Oxford University Press, New York, 1984.

7. Katzman R, Terry R: *The neurology of aging.* FA Davis, Philadelphia, 1983.

8. Koss E, Haxby JV, deCarli C, et al: Patterns of performance preservation and loss in healthy aging. *Dev Neuropsychol* 1991; 7(1):99–113.

9. Birren JE, Birren BA. The concepts, models, and history of the psychology of aging. In Birren JE, Schaie KW, eds., *Handbook of the psychology of aging,* 3rd ed., pp 3–20. Academic Press, San Diego, 1990.

10. Schaie KW: The hazards of cognitive aging. *Gerontologist* 1989; 29:484–93.

11. Oxman TE, Baynes K: Boundries between normal aging and dementia. In Emery VO, Oxman TE, eds., *Dementia: Presentations, differential diagnosis, and nosology,* pp 3–18. Johns Hopkins University Press, Baltimore, 1994.

12. Albert MS, Heaton RK: Intelligence testing. In Albert MS, Moss MB, eds., *Geriatric Neuropsychology,* pp 13–22. Guilford Press, New York, 1988.

13. Maxim J, Bryan K: Language and language change in the normal eldery population. In Maxim J, Bryan K, eds., *Language of the elderly: A clinical perspective,* pp 28–53. Singular Publishing Group, San Diego, 1994.

14. Craik FIM, Rabinowitz JC: The effects of presentation rate and encoding tasks on age-related memory deficits. *J Gerontol* 1985; 40:309–315.

15. Kazniak AW, Poon LW, Riege W: Assessing memory deficits: An information-processing approach. In Poon

LW, ed., *Handbook for clinical memory assessment*, pp 168–188. American Psychological Association, Washington, DC, 1986.

16. Tulving BG: Episodic and semantic memory. In Tulving E, Donaldson W, eds., *Organization of memory*. Academic Press, New York, 1972.

17. Smith AD, Fullerton AM: Age differences in episodic and semantic memory: Implications for language and cognition. In Beasley DS, Davis GA, eds., *Aging: Communication processes and disorders*, pp 139–155. Grune and Stratton, New York, 1981.

18. Kral VA: Senescent forgetfulness: Benign and malignant. *Can Med Assoc J* 1962; 86:257–260.

19. Mayeux R, Foster NL, Rossor M, et al: The clinical evaluation of patients with dementia. In Whitehouse PJ, ed., *Dementia*, pp 92–129. F. A. Davis, Philadelphia, 1993.

20. Schaie KW: The Seattle longitudinal study: A 21-year exploration of psychometric intelligence in adulthood. In Schaie KW, ed., *Longitudinal studies of adult psychological development*, pp 64–135. Guilford Press, New York, 1983.

21. Bayles KA, Kaszniak AW: *Communication and cognition in normal aging and dementia*. College Hill Press, Boston, 1987.

22. McDowd JM, Birren JE: Aging and attentional processes. In Birren JE, Schaie KW, eds., *Handbook of psychology of aging*, 3rd ed., pp 222–233. Academic Press, San Diego, 1990.

23. American Psychiatric Association: *Diagnostic and statistical manual of mental disorders*, 4th ed.—rev., pp 133–155. American Psychiatric Association, Washington, DC, 1994.

24. Tonkovich JD: Communication disorders in the elderly. In Shadden BB, ed., *Communication behavior and aging: A sourcebook for clinicians*, pp 197–215. Williams & Wilkins, Baltimore, 1988.

25. Clairfield AM: Diagnostic procedures for dementias II: Reversible dementias from gross structural lesions. In Emery VO, Oxman TE, eds., *Dementia: Presentations, differential diagnosis, and nosology*, pp 64–76. Johns Hopkins Univerisity Press, Baltimore, 1994.

26. Katzman R: Alzheimer's disease. *N Eng J Med* 1986; 314:964–1973.

27. McKhann G, Drachman D, Folstein M, et al: Clinical diagnosis of Alzheimer's disease: Report of the NINCDS-ADRDA work group under the auspices of the Department of Health and Human Services Task Force on Alzheimer's Disease. *Neurology* 1984; 34,939–944.

28. Wisniewski HM, Narang HK, Terry RD: Neurofibrillary tangles of paired helical filaments. *J Neurol Sci* 1976; 17:173–181.

29. Wisniewski HM, Merz GS: Neuropathology of the aging brain and dementia of the Alzheimer's type. In Gaitz CM, Samorajski T, eds., *Aging 2000: Our health care destiny*, Vol. 1, *Biomedical Issues*, p 231. Springer-Verlag, New York, 1985.

30. Woodward J: Clinico-pathological significance of granulovascular degeneration in Alzheimer's disease. *J Neuropathol Exp Neurol* 1962; 21:85–91.

31. Wegiel J, Wisniewski HM, Lach B, et al: Amyloid angiopathy ultrastructural studies. *J Neuropathol Exp Neurol* 1991; 50:314.

32. Wisniewski HM, Wegiel J, Wang KC, et al: Ultrastructural studies of the cells forming amyloid in the vessel wall in Alzheimer's disease. *Acta Neuropathol (Berl)* 1992; 84:117–127.

33. Terry RD, Peck A, De Teresa R, et al: Some morphometric aspects of the brain in senile dementia of the Alzheimer's type. *Ann Neurol* 1981; 10:184–192

34. Bartus RT, Dean RL, Beer B, et al: The cholinergic hypothesis of geriatric memory dysfunction. *Science* 1983; 217:408–417.

35. Bissette G, Reynold GP, Kilts CD, et al: Corticotropin-releasing factor-like immunoreactivity in senile dementia of the Alzheimer's type: Reduced cortical and striatal concentrations. *JAMA* 1985; 245: 3067–3069.

36. Hollander E, Mohs RC, Davis KL: Antemortem markers of Alzheimer's disease. *Neurobiol Aging* 1986; 7:367–387.

37. Wisniewski HM, Wegiel J, Morys J, et al: Alzheimer dementia neuropathology. In Emery VO, Oxman TE, eds., *Dementia: Presentations, differential diagnosis, and nosology*, pp 79–94. Johns Hopkins University Press, Baltimore, 1994.

38. Geldmacher DS, Whitehouse PJ: Evaluation of the patient with suspected dementia. *JAMA* (in press).

39. Tomlinson BE: Morphological changes and dementia in old age. In Smith WL, ed., *Aging and dementia*, pp 25–56. Spectrum Publications, New York, 1977.

40. Roman GC, Tatemichi TK, Erkinjuntti T, et al: Vascular dementia: Diagnostic criteria for research studies: Report of the NINDS-AIREN International Workshop. *Neurology* 1993; 43:250–260.

41. Butler RN, Lewis MI: *Aging and mental health*. A Plume Book, New York, 1983.

42. Cohen D, Eisdorfer C: Risk factors in late life dementias. In Wertheimer J, Marois M, eds., *Senile dementia: Outlook for the future*, pp 221–237. Alan R. Liss: New York, 1984.

43. Hachinski VC, Iliff LD, Zilhka E, et al: Cerebral blood flow in dementia. *Arch Neurol* 1975; 32:632–637.

44. Wagner O, Oesterreich K, Hoyer S: Validity of the ischemic score in degenerative and vascular dementia and depression in old age. *Arch Gerontol Geriatr* 1985; 4:333–345.

45. Molsa PK, Paljarvi L, Rinne JO, et al: Validity of clinical diagnosis in dementia: A prospective clinicopathological study. *J Neruol Neurosurg Psych* 1985; 48: 1085–1090.

46. Powell AL, Cummings JL, Hill MA, et al: Speech and language alterations in multi-infarct dementia. *Neurology* 1988; 38:717–719.

47. Heston LL, White JH, Mastri AR: Pick's disease—Clinical genetics and natural history. *Arch Gen Psych* 1987; 44:409–411.

48. Neary D, Snoden JS, Northen B, et al: Dementia of frontal lobe type. *J Neurol Neurosurg Psych* 1988; 51; 353–361.

49. Kirshner HS: Progressive aphasia and other focal presentations of Alzheimer disease, Pick disease, and other degenerative disorders. In Emery VO, Oxman TE, eds., *Dementia: Presentations, differential diagnosis, and nosology,* pp 108–122. Johns Hopkins University Press, Baltimore, 1994.

50. Brun A, Englude E: Regional pattern of degeneration in Alzheimer's disease: Neuronal loss and histopathological grading. *Histopath* 1981; 5:549–564.

51. Cummings JL, Benson DF: *Dementia: A clinical approach.* Butterworth, Boston, 1992.

52. Wechsler AF, Verity A, Rosenschein S, et al: Pick's disease: A clinical, computed tomographic and histological study with golgi impregnation observations. *Arch Neurol* 1982; 39:287–290.

53. Maxim J, Byran K: Language pathology in non-Alzheimer's dementia. In Maxim J, Bryan K, eds., *Language of the elderly: A clinical perspective,* pp 150–172. Whurr Publishers, London, 1994.

54. Lishman WA: *Organic psychiatry: The psychological consequences of cerebral disorder,* 2nd ed. Blackwell Scientific, Oxford, 1987.

55. Cummings JL, Duchen LW: The Kluver-Bucy syndrome in Pick's disease. *Neurology* 1981; 31:1415–1422.

56. Gustafson L, Nilsson L: Differential diagnosis of presenile dementia on clinical grounds. *Acta Psychiatr Scand* 1982; 65:194–209.

57. Jervis GA: Alzheimer's disease. In Minkler J, ed., *Pathology of the nervous system,* Vol. 2, pp 1385–1395. McGraw-Hill, New York, 1971.

58. Mendez MF, Zander BA: Dementia presenting with aphasia: Clinical characteristics. *J Neurol Neurosurg Psych* 1991; 54:542–545.

59. Mesulam MM: Slowly progressive aphasia without generalized dementia. *Ann Neurol* 1982; 22:533–534.

60. Heath PD, Kennedy P, Kapur N: Slowly progressive aphasia without generalized dementia. *Ann Neurol* 1983; 13(6):507–515.

61. Weschler AF: Presenile dementia presenting as aphasia. *J Neurol Neurosurg Psych* 1977; 40:303–305.

62. Foster NL, Chase TN: Diffuse involvement in progressive aphasia. *Ann Neurol* 1983; 13(2):224–225.

63. Kirshner HS, Webb WG, Kelly MP, et al: Language disturbance: An initial symptom of cortical degenerations and dementia. *Arch Neurol* 1984; 41:491–496.

64. Assal G, Favre C, Regli F: Aphasia as a first sign of dementia. In Werthheimer J, Marois M, eds., *Senile dementia: Outlook for the future.* Alan R. Liss, New York, 1984.

65. Poeck K, Luzzatti C: Slowly progressive aphasia in three patients: The problem of accompanying neuropsychological deficit. *Brain* 1988; 111:151–168.

66. Sapin LR, Anderson FH, Pulaski PD: Progressive aphasia without dementia: Further documentation. *Ann Neurol* 1989; 25:411–413.

67. Kirshner HS, Tanridag O, Thurman L, et al: Progressive aphasia without dementia: Two cases with focal spongiform degeneration. *Ann Neurol* 1987; 22:527–532.

68. Mesulam MM: Primary progressive aphasia—Differentiation from Alzheimer's disease. *Ann Neurol* 1987; 22(4):533–534.

69. Morris JC, Cole M, Banker BQ, et al: Hereditary dysphasic dementia and the Pick-Alzheimer spectrum. *Ann Neurol* 1983; 16:455–466.

70. Mandell AM, Alexander MP, Carpenter S: Creutzfeldt-Jacob Disease Presenting as Isolated Aphasia. *Neurology* 1989; 39:55–58.

71. Kirshner HS, Webb WG, Kelly MP, et al: Language disturbance: An initial symptom of cortical degenerations and dementia. *Arch Neurol* 1984; 41:491–496.

72. Cooper B: Psychiatric disorders among elderly patients admitted to general hospital wards. *J R Soc Med* 1987; 80:13–26.

73. Wells CE: Pseudodementia. *Am J Psych* 1979; 36:895–899.

74. Folstein MF, McHugh PR: Dementia syndrome of depression. In Katzman R, Terry RD, Bick K, eds., *Alzheimer's disease: Senile dementia and related disorders.* Raven Press, New York, 1978.

75. Jarvik LF: Pseudodementia. *Consultant* 1982; 22:141–146.

76. Feinberg T, Goodman B: Affective illness, dementia, and pseudodementia. *J Clin Psych* 1984; 45:95–103.

77. Wells CE: The diffrential diagnosis of psychiatric disorders in the elderly. In Cole J, Barrett J, eds., *Evaluation of appraisal techniques in speech and language pathology.* Raven Press, New York, 1980.

78. Cummings JL, Benson DF, Hill MA, et al: Aphasia and dementia of the Alzheimer type. *Neurology* 1985; 35:394–397.

79. Bayles KA, Tomoeda CK, Caffrey JT: Language in dementia producing diseases. *Commun Dis* 1983; 7:131–146.

80. Au R, Albert ML, Obler LK: The relationship of aphasia to dementia. *Aphasiology* 1988; 2(2):161–173.

81. Wertz RT: Neuropathologies of speech and language: An introduction to patient management. In Johns DF, ed., *Evaluation of appraisal techniques in speech and language pathology.* Addison-Wesley, Reading, MA, 1978.

82. Horner J: Language disorder associated with Alzheimer's dementia, left hemisphere stroke, and progressive illness of uncertain etiology. In Brookshire RH, ed., *Clinical Aphasiology Conference Proceedings,* pp 149–158. BRK Publishers, Minneapolis, 1985.

83. Whitehouse PJ: The concept of subcortical and cortical dementia: Another look. *Ann Neurol* 1986; 19:1–6.

84. Faber-Langendoen K, Morris JC, Knesevich JW, et al: Aphasia in senile dementia of the Alzheimer type. *Ann Neurol* 1988; 23(4):365–370.

85. Shut LJ: Dementia following stroke. *Clin Geriat Med* 1988; 4(4):767–784.

86. Bayles KA, Boone DR, Tomoeda CA, et al: Differentiating Alzheimer's patients from the normal elderly and stroke patients with aphasia. *J Speech Hear Disord* 1989; 54(1):74–87.

87. Nicholas M, Obler LK, Albert ML, et al: Empty speech in Alzheimer's disease and fluent aphasia. *J Speech Hear Res* 1985; 28:405–410.

88. Bates E, MacWhinney B: A functionalist approach to the acquisition of grammar. In Ochs E, Schiefflin B, eds., *Developmental pragmatics.* Academic Press, New York, 1982.

89. Terrell B, Ripich D: Discourse competence as a variable in intervention. *Sem Speech Lang Dis* 1989; 24:77–92.

90. Prutting C, Kirchner D: Applied pragmatics. In Gallagher T, Prutting C, eds., *Pragmatic assessment and intervention issues in language.* PRO-ED, Austin, TX, 1983.

91. Fromm D, Holland A: Functional communication in Alzheimer's disease. Paper presented at the American Speech–Language-Hearing Association Conference, New Orleans, LA, 1987.

92. Fromm D, Holland A: Functional communication in Alzheimer's disease. *J Speech Hear Disord* 1989; 54: 535–540.

93. Holland A: *Language disorders in adults.* PRO-ED, Austin, TX, 1984.

94. Bayles KA: Language function in senile dementia. *Brain Lang* 1982; 16:265–280.

95. Murdoch BE, Chenery HJ, Wilks V, et al: Language disorders in dementia of the Alzheimer's type. *Brain Lang* 1987; 31:122–137.

96. Schwartz M, Marin O, Saffran E: Dissociations of language function in dementia: A case study. *Brain Lang* 1979; 7:277–306.

97. Ripich D, Terrell B: Patterns of discourse cohesion and coherence in Alzheimer's disease. *J Speech Hear Disord* 1988; 53:8–15.

98. Ulatowska HK, Haynes SM, Donnell AJ, et al: Discourse abilities in dementia. Paper presented at the American Speech–Language-Hearing Association Conference, Detroit, MI, 1986.

99. Bayles KA, Boone DR: The potential of language tasks for identifying senile dementia. *J Speech Hear Disord* 1982; 47:210–217.

100. Bayles KA: Management of neurogenic communication disorders associated with dementia. In Chapey R, ed., *Language intervention strategies in adult aphasia,* 2nd ed., pp 462–473. Williams & Wilkins, Baltimore, MD, 1986.

101. Deal J, Wertz R, Spring C: Differentiating aphasia and the language of generalized intellectual impairment. In *Clinical aphasiology conference proceedings,* pp 166–173. BRK Publishers, Minneapolis, 1981.

102. Halpern H, Darley F, Brown J: Differential language and neurological characteristics in cerebral involvement. *J Speech Hear Disord* 1973; 38:162–173.

103. Holland A, McBurnery DH, Mossy J, et al: The dissolution of language in Ack's disease with neurofibrillary tangles: A case study. *Brain Lang* 1985; 24:36–58.

104. Horner J, Heyman A: Language changes associated with Alzheimer's dementia: A discussion section. In Brookshire RH, ed., *Clinical aphasiology conference proceedings,* pp 330–336. BRK Publishers, Minneapolis, 1981.

105. Watson J, Records L: The effectiveness of the Porch index of communicative abilities as a diagnostic tool in assessing specific behaviors of senile dementia. *Clinical Aphasiology Conference Proceedings.* BRK Publishers, Minneapolis, 1978.

106. Appell J, Kertesz A, Fisman M: A study of language functioning in Alzheimer's patients. *Brain Lang* 1982; 17:73–91.

107. Barker MG, Lawson JS: Nominal aphasia in dementia. *Br J Psych* 1968; 114:1351–1356.

108. Obler LK: Review of *Le langage des dements* by L. Irigary, 1973. The Hague: Mouton. *Brain Lang* 1983; 12:375–386.

109. Whitaker HA: A case of the isolation of language function. In Whitaker H, Whitaker H, eds., *Studies in neurolinguistics,* Vol. 2. Academic Press, New York, 1976.

110. Kempler D: Language changes in dementia of the Alzheimer's type. In Lubinski R, ed., *Dementia and communication,* pp 98–114. Singular Publishing Group, San Diego 1995.

111. Hutchinson JM, Jensen MA: A pragmatic evaluation of discourse communication in normal and senile elderly in a nursing home. In Obler L, Albert M, eds., *Language and communication in the elderly,* pp 59–64. D.C. Heath, Lexington, MA, 1980.

112. Irigaray L: *Le langage des dements.* Mouton, The Hague, 1973.

113. Ripich D, Terrell B, Spinelli F: Discourse cohesion in senile dementia of the Alzheimer's type. In Brookshire RH, ed., *Clinical Aphasiology Conference Proceedings,* pp 316–321. BRK Publishers, Minneapolis, 1983.

114. Ripich DN, Vertes DR, Whitehouse P, et al: Conversational discourse patterns in senile dementia of the Alzheimer's type. Paper presented at the American Speech–Language-Hearing Association, Boston, 1988.

115. Bayles KA: Language and dementia. In Holland A, ed., *Language disorders in adults.* Pro-Ed, Austin, TX, 1984.

116. Kempler D: Lexical and pantomine abilities of Alzheimer's disease. *Aphasiology* 1988; 2:147–159.

117. Ripich DN, Carpenter B, Ziol E: Cohesion in conversational discourse in men and women with Alzheimer's disease: A longitudinal study. (Manuscript in preparation.)

118. Kimbarow ML, Ripich DN: Task influences on discourse production in adults. Paper presented at the annual conference of the American Speech–Language-Hearing Association, St. Louis, 1989.

119. Kaplan E, Goodglass H, Weintraub S: *Boston Naming Test.* Lea & Febiger, Philadelphia, 1983.

120. Goodglass H, Kaplan E: *Boston Diagnostic Aphasia Examination.* Lea & Febiger, Philadelphia, 1983.

121. deAjuriaguerra J, Tissot R: Some aspects of language in various forms of senile dementia: Comparisons with language in childhood. In Lenneberg EH, Lenneberg E, eds., *Foundations of language development,* Vol. 1, pp 325–339. Academic Press, New York, 1975.

122. Ernest B, Dalby M, Dalby A: Aphasic disturbances in presenile dementia. *Acta Neurol Scand* 1970; 46:99–100.

123. Bayles KA, Tomoeda CK: Confrontation and generative naming abilities of dementia patients. In Brookshire RH, ed., *Clinical Aphasiology Conference Proceedings,* pp 304–315. BRK, Minneapolis, 1983.

124. Huff FJ, Corkin S, Growdon JH: Semantic impairment and anomia in Alzheimer's disease. *Brain Lang* 1986; 28:235–249.

125. Kaszniak AW, Wilson RS: Longitudinal deterioration of language and cognition in dementia of the Alzheimer's type. Symposium: Communication and Cognition in Dementia: Longitudinal Perspectives. International Neuropsychological Association, San Diego, 1985.

126. Neils J, Boller F, Cole M, et al: Naming ability in mild Alzheimer's disease subjects. Paper presented at the annual convention of the American Speech–Language-Hearing Association, New Orleans, LA, 1987.

127. Allison RS: *The senile brain.* Edward Arnold, London, 1962.

128. Grossman M: The game of the name: An examination of linguistic reference after brain damage. *Brain Lang* 1978; 6:112–119.

129. Irigaray L: Approche psycholinguistique de langage des dements. *Neuropsychologia* 1967; 5:25–52.

130. Obler LK: Review of *Le langage des dements. Brain Lang* 1981; 12:375–386.

131. Warrington EK: The selective impairment of semantic memory. *Q J Exp Psychol* 1975; 27:635–637.

132. Bayles KA, Boone DR: The potential of language tasks for identifying senile dementia. *J Speech Hear Disord* 1982; 47:210–217.

133. Skelton-Robinson M, Jones S: Nominal dysphasia and the severity of senile dementia. *Br J Psych* 1984; 145:168–171.

134. Hart S: Language and dementia: A review. *Psychol Med* 1988; 18:99–112.

135. Grober H, Buschke H, Kawas C, et al: Impaired ranking of semantic attributes in dementia. *Brain Lang* 1985; 26:276–286.

136. Constantinidis J: Is Alzheimer's disease a major form of senile dementia? Clinical, anatomical, and genetic data. In Katzman R, Terry RD, Bick KL, eds., *Alzheimer's disease: Senile dementia and related disorders,* pp 15–25. Raven Press, New York, 1978.

137. Emery OB: Language and memory processing in senile dementia of the Alzheimer's type. In Light LL, Burke DM, eds., *Language, memory, and aging,* pp 221–243. Cambridge University Press, New York, 1988.

138. Linebarger M, Schwartz M, Saffran E. Sensitivity to grammatical structure in so-called agrammatic aphasics. *Cognition* 1983; 13:361–392.

139. Kempler D, Curtiss S, Jackson C: Syntactic preservation in Alzheimer's disease. *J Speech Hear Res* 1987; 30:343–350.

140. Sohlberg MM, Mateer CA: *Introduction to cognitive rehabilitation: Theory and practice.* Guilford Press, New York, 1989.

141. Breitner JC, Folstein M: A prevalent disorder with specific clinical features. *Psychol Med* 1984; 14:63–80.

142. Chapey R, ed., *Language intervention strategies in adult aphasia.* Williams & Wilkins, Baltimore, 1994.

143. National Institute on Aging Task Force: Senility reconsidered: Treatment possibilities for mental impairment in the elderly. *JAMA* 1980; 244:259–263.

144. National Institute of Health Consensus Conference. *JAMA* 1987; 258:3411–3416.

145. Schear JM, Skenses LL. The interface between clinical neuropsychology and speech–language pathology in the assessment of the geriatric patient. In Ripich D, ed., *The handbook of geriatric communication disorders,* pp 59–80. Pro-Ed, Austin, TX, 1991.

146. Danks J, Glucksberg S: Experimental psycholinguistics. *Ann Rev Psychol* 1979; 313–339.

147. Lemme M, Danes N: Models of auditory linguistic processing. In Lass N, McReynolds L, Northern J, Yoder D, eds., *Speech, language, and hearing:* Vol. 1. *Normal Processes.* Saunders, Philadephia, 1982.

148. Kertez A: *Western aphasia battery.* Grune & Stratton, New York, 1982.

149. Porch BE: *Porch index of communicative abilities.* Consulting Psychologists Press, Palo Alto, 1967.

150. Bayles KA, Tomoeda CK: *Arizona battery for communication disorders of dementia* (ABCD). Canyonlands Publishing Company, Tucson, 1991.

151. Shadden BB: The use of discourse analyses and procedures for communication programming in long-term care facilities. *Lang Dis* 1995; 15:75–86.

152. Dunn LM, Dunn LM: *Peabody picture vocabulary test—revised.* American Guidance Service, Circle Pines, 1981.

153. Smith SR, Murdoch BE, Chenery HJ: Semantic abilities in dementia of the Alzheimer type. *Brain Lang* 1989; 36:314–324.

154. Borkowski JG, Benton AL, Spreen O: Word fluency and brain damage. *Neuropsychologia* 1967; 5: 135–140.

155. Butters N, Granholm E, Salmon DP, et al: Episodic and semantic memory: A comparison of amnesic and demented patients. *J Clin Exp Neuropsychol* 1987; 9:479–497.

156. Monsch AU, Bondi MW, Butters N, et al: Comparison of verbal fluency tasks in the detection of dementia of the Alzheimer type. *Arch Neurol* 1992; 49:1253–1258.

157. Shewan CM: *Auditory comprehension test for sentences.* Linguistics Clinical Institutes, Chicago, 1979.

158. DeRenzi E, Faglioni P: Normative data and screening power of a shortened version of the token test. *Cortex* 1978; 14:41–49.

159. Spellacy FJ, Spreen O: A short form of the token test. *Cortex* 1969; 5:390–397.

160. DeRenzi E, Ferrari C: The reporter's test: A sensitive test to detect expressive disturbances in aphasics. *Cortex* 1978; 14:279–293.

161. Rey A: *L'examen clinique en psychologie.* Presses Universitaires de France, Paris, 1964.

162. Wechsler D: *Wechsler memory scale revised.* The Psychological Corporation, New York, 1987.

163. Ross-Swain D, Fogle P: *Ross information processing assessment—Geriatric (RIPA-G).* Pro-Ed, Austin, TX, 1996.

164. Golding E: *The Middlesex elderly assessment of mental state (MEAMS).* Thames Valley Test Company, Fareham, 1988.

165. Whitehouse PJ, Rabins PV: Quality of life and dementia. *Alzheimer Dis Assoc Disord* 1992; 6:135–137.

166. Larson R: Thirty years of research on the subjective well-being of older americans. *J Gerontol* 1978; 33:109–125.

167. Mendola WF, Pelligrini RV: Quality of life and coronary artery bypass surgery patients. *Soc Sci Med* 1979; 13:457–461.

168. Ishi-Kuntz M: Social interaction and social well-being: Comparison across stages of adulthood. *Aging Hum Devel* 1990; 30:15–35.

169. Clark LW: Interventions for persons with Alzheimer's disease: Strategies for maintaining and enhancing communicative success. *Lang Dis* 1995; 15:47–65.

170. ASHA Committee on Communication Problems in Aging: The roles of speech–language pathologists and audiologists in working with older persons. *ASHA* 1988a; 30:80–84.

171. ASHA Committee on Communication Problems in Aging: Provision of audiology and speech–language pathology services to older persons in the nursing home. *ASHA* 1988b; 30:72–74.

172. Glickstein JK, Neustadt GK: *Reimbursable geriatric service delivery: A functional maintenance therapy system.* Aspen Publishers, Rockville, 1992.

173. Glickstein JK, Neustadt GK: Speech–language interventions in Alzheimer's disease: A functional communication approach. *Clin Comm Dis* 1993; 3:15–30.

174. Stephens L, ed.: *Reality orientation: A technique to rehabilitate elderly and brain-damaged patients with a moderate to severe degree of disorientation.* American Psychiatric Association, Washington DC, 1969.

175. Hussian RA: *Geriatric psychology: A behavioral perspective.* Van Nostrand Reinhold, New York, 1981.

176. Reisberg B: *Brain failure: An introduction to current concepts of senility.* Free Press/Macmillan, New York, 1981.

177. Burton M: Reality orientation for the elderly: A critique. *J Adv Nurs* 1982; 7:427–433.

178. MacDonald ML, Settin JM: Reality orientation vs. sheltered workshops as treatment for the institutionalized aging. *J Gerontol* 1978; 33:416–421.

179. Hanley IG: Reality orientation in the care of the elderly patient with dementia—Three case studies. In Hanley I, Gilhooly M, eds., *Psychological therapies for the elderly.* New York University Press, New York, 1986.

180. Hanley IG: *Individualized reality orientation: Creative therapy with confused elderly people.* Winslow Press, Bicester, 1988.

181. Lam DH, Woods RT: Ward orientation training in dementia: A single case study. *Inter J Geriat Psych* 1986; 1:145–147.

182. Baines S, Saxby P, Ehlert K: Reality orientation and reminiscence therapy: A controlled cross-over study of confused elderly people. *Br J Psych* 1987; 151:222–231.

183. Wallis GG, Baldwin M, Higgenbotham P: Reality orientation therapy: A controlled trial. *Br J Med Psychol* 1983; 56:271–278.

184. Woods RT: Reality orientation and staff attention: A controlled study. *Br J Psych* 1979; 134:502–507.

185. Greene JG, Timbury GC, Smith R, et al: Reality orientation with elderly patients in the community: An empirical evaluation. *Age & Aging* 1983; 12:38–43.

186. Holden UP, Woods RT: *Reality orientation psychological approaches to the 'confused' elderly,* 2nd ed. Churchill Livingstone, Edinburgh, 1988.

187. Miller E, Morris R: Management of dementia. In Miller E, Morris R: *The psychology of dementia.* John Wiley & Sons, Chichester, 1993.

188. Zgola JM, Coulter LG: I can tell you about that: A therapeutic group program for congnitively impaired persons. *Amer J Alzheimer Care Rel Dis* 1988; July/August: 17–22.

189. Anderson JR: A spreading activation theory of memory. *J Verb Learn Behav* 1983; 22:261–295.

190. Kiernat J: The use of life review activity with confused nursing home residents. *Am J Occup Ther* 1979; 33:306–310.

191. Osborne C: Reminiscence: When the past eases the present. *J Gerontol Nurs* 1989; 15:6–12.

192. Mateer C, Sohlberg M: A paradigm shift in memory rehabilitation. In H. Whitaker, ed., *Neuropsychological studies of non-focal brain injury: Dementia and closed head injury,* pp 180–210. Springer-Verlag, New York, 1988.

193. Bourgeois MS: Evaluating memory wallets in conversations with persons with dementia. *J Speech Hear Res* 1992; 35:1344–1357.

194. Hughston GA, Merriam SB: Reminiscence: A nonformal technique for improving cognitive functioning in the aged. *Int J Aging Hum Dev* 1982; 15:139–149.

195. Ziol E, Dobres R, White, L: *Communicative interaction: Group activities for cognitively impaired elderly.* Imaginart International, Inc., Bisbee AZ, 1996.

196. Rabins P: Management of irreversible dementia. *Psychosometics* 1982; 22:591–597.

197. Zarit JM: Predictors of burden and stress for caregivers of senile dementia patients. Unpublished doctoral dissertation. University of Southern California, San Diego, 1982.

198. Kinney JM, Stephens MAP: Caregiving hassles scale: Assessing the daily hassles of caring for a family member with dementia. *Gerontologist* 1989; 29:328–332.

199. Santo Pietro MJ, Decotiis E, McCarthy J, et al: Conversation in Alzheimer's disease: Implication of semantic and pragmatic breakdowns. Paper presented at American Speech–Language-Hearing Association, Seattle, 1990.

200. Bayles KA, Tomoeda CK: Caregiver report of prevalence and appearance order of linguistic symptoms in Alzheimer's patients. *Gerontologist* 1991; 210–216.

201. Orange, JB: Perspectives of family members regarding communication changes. In Lubinski R, ed., *Dementia and communication.* Mosby-Year Book, Philadelphia, 1991.

202. Feil N: Validation therapy. *Geriat Nurs* 1992; 13: 129–133.

203. Morton I, Bleathman C: The effectiveness of validation therapy in dementia: A pilot study. *Int J Geriat Psych* 1991; 6:327–330.

204. Feil N: V/F *Validation: The Feil method.* Edward Feil Productions, Cleveland, 1982.

205. Alprin SI: Unpublished study of staff attitudes after validation. Cleveland State University, Cleveland, 1980.

206. Dietch JT, Hewett LJ, Jones S: Adverse effects of reality orientation. *J Am Geriatr Soc* 1989; 37:974–976.

207. Fritz A: *The language of resolution among the old-old: The effect of validation therapy on two levels of cognitive confusion.* Unpublished paper, Chicago, 1986.

208. Peoples N: Validation therapy versus reality orientation as treatment for disoriented institutionalized elderly. Unpublished Master's Thesis, University of Akron, 1982.

209. Benjamin BJ: Validation therapy: An intervention for disoriented patients with Alzheimer's disease. *Lang Dis* 1995; 15:66–74.

210. Ripich D, Wykle M: A program for nursing assistants with Alzheimer's patients. Paper presented at the American Gerontology in Higher Education Conference, Kansas City, 1990a.

211. Ripich D, Wykle M: Developing healthcare professionals' communication skills with Alzheimer's disease patients. Paper presented at the Annual Meeting of the American Society on Aging, San Francisco, 1990b.

212. Ripich DN: *Alzheimer's disease communication guide: The FOCUSED Program for Caregivers.* The Psychological Corporation, San Antonio, 1996.

213. Clark LW, Witte K: Dealing with dementia in long-term care. Miniseminar Presentation for annual convention on New York State Speech, Language, and Hearing Association, Kiamesha Lake, 1989.

214. Clark LW: Caregiver stress and communication management in Alzheimer's disease. In Ripich D, ed., *Handbook of geriatric communication disorders,* pp 127–142. Pro-Ed, Austin, TX, 1991.

215. Ripich DN: Language and communication in dementia. In Ripich DN, ed., *Handbook of geriatric communication disorders,* pp 255–284. Pro-Ed, Austin, TX, 1991.

216. Poulshock SW, Deimling GT: Families caring for elders in residence: Issues in the measurement of burden. *J Gerontol* 1984; 39:230–239.

217. Carroll D: *When your loved one has Alzheimer's disease.* Harper and Row, New York, 1989.

Otolaryngology and the Speech–Language Pathologist

20

Medical and Surgical Management in Otolaryngology

MICHAEL S. BENNINGER AND GLENDON M. GARDNER

CHAPTER OUTLINE

History and Physical Examination

Oral Cavity, Oropharynx, Nasopharynx

Nasal and Sinus Disorders

Anatomy of the Larynx

Physiology of the Larynx

Gastroesophageal and Pharyngeal Reflux Disease

AIDS and Otolaryngology

Otolaryngologists and speech–language pathologists work closely together to provide comprehensive services to patients with disorders and diseases of the head and neck because of the impact of these structures on communication and swallowing. While not all otolaryngologic patients require intervention by a speech–language pathologist, a knowledge of the more commonly encountered disorders and their effect on speech and swallowing functions is crucial. Medical treatment and surgical repair and resection can result in post-treatment effects that require management by a speech–language pathologist.

In this chapter, we will discuss the process by which the otolaryngologist diagnoses head and neck disorders, diseases and disorders of the oral cavity, oropharynx and nasopharynx, nasal-sinus disorders, laryngeal anatomy and physiology, laryngeal disorders, trauma, and tracheostomy, special medical issues in professional voice, gastroesophageal

reflux disease, and head and neck manifestations in AIDS.

HISTORY AND PHYSICAL EXAMINATION

When a patient presents to an otolaryngologist with a complaint involving the upper airway or head and neck, the first and perhaps most critical part of the assessment is obtaining a thorough history. It is during the history that the otolaryngologist establishes a relationship with the patient and begins the mutual exchange of information in a manner that breeds trust. Traditionally, the history begins with a clarification of the chief complaint in an attempt to identify factors that will be pertinent to the subsequent evaluation and treatment. The time from onset, the severity of the symptoms, whether or not the symptoms vary by time of day or exposure to certain environments or conditions, and any previous treatment for this condition should be obtained. It is important, however, to not become so focused on the main complaint that important peripheral information pertinent to the disorder or other conditions that may require assessment is ignored. A general review of other head and neck symptoms follows and then questions are asked regarding general medical health and other medical problems. A list of medications and a history of previous diseases or surgeries should be obtained. Any habits that might influence health should be considered, particularly eating habits, or whether or not the individual uses tobacco or alcohol. One cannot underestimate the power of the history, because often the physician can come to a tentative diagnosis prior to any physical contact with the patient.

The head and neck physical examination usually begins during the history. At that time, the physician tests speech and voice, assesses gross hearing, and observes any abnormalities of facial movement or skin conditions or masses. It is important during the head and neck exam to thoroughly examine all structures. To overcome this potential pitfall, it is reasonable to follow a sequence of evaluation despite the presenting disorder. The skin and scalp are usually evaluated first followed by an examination of the ears. The external ear and ear canal are assessed with an otoscope to identify inflammation or skin conditions. The middle ear is visualized for normal landmarks and absence of infection, masses, fluid or retraction of the ear drum. Air insufflation (pneumatic otoscopy) is particularly useful in evaluating middle ear function, negative pressure, or fluid. If any concerns are raised during otoscopy, a microscope can be used to better delineate any potential abnormalities. Hearing can be assessed with the use of tuning forks although if any concerns are raised related to the hearing, then a formal audiogram should be recommended.

A nasal examination is generally obtained with a head mirror, indirect light, and a nasal speculum. Decongesting the nose will allow for improved visualization into its more posterior aspects. If concerns are raised, if visualization is difficult, or if a diagnosis needs confirmation, nasal endoscopes can be used.[1] The oral cavity should be examined with mirror indirected light so that two hands can be used to manipulate the tongue and other mucosal surfaces. All areas should be seen. The tongue blades can then depress the tongue to see the oropharynx, tonsils, and tongue base. Keeping the tongue blades just anterior to the junction of the anterior two-thirds and posterior

one-third of the tongue and having the patient gently breathe will minimize the gagging sensation. With the tongue compressed, a nasopharyngeal mirror can be used to assess the nasopharynx.

The larynx should be initially visualized with a laryngeal mirror. The tongue is grasped and gently pulled forward. The mirror is inserted to a point just anterior to the palate, and light is directed to allow visualization of the pharynx and larynx. Avoidance of touching the palate or having the patient phonate prior to placing the mirror will minimize the gag reflex. Almost all patients can be visualized well with a mirror. It is important to focus not just on the vocal folds because other important findings related to the base of tongue, posterior pharyngeal walls, pyriform sinus, epiglottis, and valleculae may be missed. Different vowel sounds will allow different angles to the larynx. Indirect laryngoscopy allows for a global view of the larynx and should be performed prior to any further techniques to visualize the larynx although it is limited in that it cannot see the larynx during running speech or singing. To supplement the mirror view and visualize the larynx during running speech, or if visualization is limited, a flexible laryngoscope can be passed. Usually this is passed through the nose after decongestion and occasionally after application of a topical anaesthetic. Not only is this instrument valuable in larynx assessment, it can be used to better visualize the nasopharynx and for functional assessment of swallowing (FEES)[2] or even for voice modification or biofeedback training. Video images can be obtained for following the progress of treatment, documentation, and discussions with the patient, family, or referring physician.[3] To further augment the examination of the larynx, videostroboscopy of the larynx can be performed to assess vocal fold vibration.

The neck should be palpated for any masses, neck muscular problems, or asymmetry. The thyroid is then palpated at rest and during swallowing. Pulsating masses can be auscultated to help identify a vascular lesion. Fine needle aspiration is a useful tool in obtaining a pathologic diagnosis and has obviated the need in many cases for open biopsy. A neurologic assessment of the cranial nerves is part of the routine examination while selective assessments of balance function should be performed if such a disorder is suggested by the preceding evaluation. A general physical examination is usually not performed on a routine basis by an otolaryngologist, although selected exams, such as of the lungs or heart, may be performed if prompted by the H and P.

Other tests will be determined by the findings of the history and physical examination. CT and MRI scanning are very useful in assessing head and neck masses or tumors and ruling out intracranial or skull base disease. CT scans are particularly useful in evaluating sinus disease. A chest X-ray is helpful in patients with head and neck tumors, cough, or hemoptysis. Swallowing and gastroesophageal reflux assessment may be considered in patients with swallowing complaints. Other medical evaluations will be determined by the suspicions of disease. On occasion, an evaluation under anaesthesia may be necessary to stage cancer, obtain biopsies, or clarify diagnosis.

ORAL CAVITY, OROPHARYNX, NASOPHARYNX

Anatomy

The boundaries of the oral cavity are the lips anteriorly, the buccal (cheek) mucosa laterally, the anterior tonsillar pillars posteriorly, the hard palate superiorly, and the floor of mouth inferiorly (Figure 20–1). The oral cavity contains the teeth and alveolar ridges of the mandible and maxilla, the anterior two-thirds of the tongue, and the hard palate. It is also the site of the orifices of the ducts of the major salivary glands.

The oropharynx begins at the anterior tonsillar pillars and extends to the hyoid bone inferiorly and to the level of the soft palate superiorly where the nasopharynx begins (Figure 20–2). The tonsils, soft palate, posterior one-third of the tongue (base of tongue), and suprahyoid epiglottis are located in the oropharynx. The nasopharynx is bounded anteriorly by the choana and contains the tori tubarious and the adenoids.

Function and Congenital Anomalies

The oral cavity, pharynx, and nasal cavities serve many functions. The oral cavity, oropharynx, and hypopharynx are the entrance to the digestive tract. The pharynx, nasal cavities, and oral cavity form the resonator of the voice. Abnormalities of these structures may affect speech or swallowing.

Choanal Atresia

In general, congenital problems are a result of either failure of a closed structure to open (e.g., choanal atresia) or the failure of a structure to close properly (e.g., cleft palate). The nasal placode is a thickening of the ectoderm (outer surface) of the face that develops during the third or fourth weeks of gestation and invaginates, creating two nasal pits a week later.[4] The forming nasal cavity remains

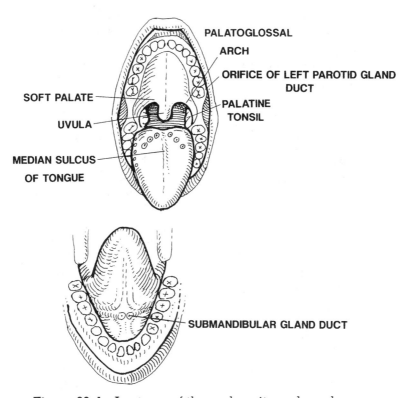

Figure 20–1. Anatomy of the oral cavity and oropharynx.

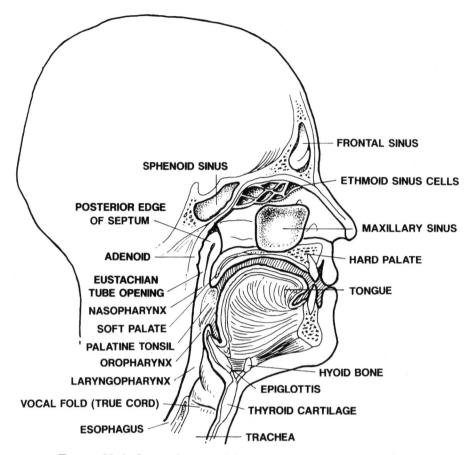

Figure 20–2. Lateral view of the upper aerodigestive tract.

separate from the pharynx at the bucconasal membrane. This membrane usually ruptures at about the eighth week of gestation. Failure to rupture leads to choanal atresia, which can be uni- or bilateral. (The choana is the junction between the nasal cavity and nasopharynx.)

Infants are obligate nasal breathers—they must breathe through their noses. The high position of the infant's larynx that causes them to breathe through the nose also enables them to eat and breathe simultaneously. Bilateral choanal atresia presents at birth with symptoms of choking, inability to nurse, and cyanosis. The diagnosis is made by unsuccessfully attempting to pass red rubber catheters through the nose to the pharynx. Various devices, the simplest of which is a baby bottle nipple with the end cut off, are used to allow the infant to breathe through the mouth. Feeding tubes are sometimes necessary initially. Tracheotomy rarely is needed. By two or three weeks of age, the infant has often learned to breathe orally.

Surgical opening of the atresia is often done at 10 weeks. There are several different techniques for repairing choanal atresia including transnasal and transoral/transpalatal approaches.

Unilateral choanal atresia is less obvious and is often not diagnosed for months to years. Unilateral chronic nasal discharge is often the only symptom. Hyponasal speech is also not uncommon. Choanal atresia may be associated with other congenital anomalies.

Cleft Lip and Palate

The palate is formed by the fusion of several structures including the frontal nasal process and the palatal shelves of the maxilla, while the upper lip is a fusion of the lateral and medial nasal processes. This process takes place around the tenth week of gestation. Failure of proper fusion or improper breakdown of epithelial bridges may result in a variety of abnormalities of the upper lip, nose, and/ or palate.

The least severe deformity is diastasis of the musculature of the soft palate or a submucosa cleft palate. These patients may present with velopharyngeal insufficiency with hypernasal speech and nasal regurgitation of fluids. Speech therapy often benefits patients with mild cases. For more severe cases, surgical procedures are available to reestablish the muscular integrity of the soft palate, augment the posterior pharyngeal wall, or partially close the nasopharynx with flaps.

The most severe clefting is bilateral cleft lip and complete clefting of the hard and soft palates. Various combinations of cleft lip and palate can exist, resulting in different types of feeding, speech, and cosmetic problems. Feeding difficulties in cleft palate are first due to the infant's inability to generate negative pressure to suck as air leaks through the cleft. Food in the oral cavity and oropharynx also refluxes freely into the nasopharynx and nasal cavity. Unrepaired cleft palate also results in a severely hypernasal voice which may cause unintelligible speech. Repair of the lip is usually done when the child has fulfilled the "rule of tens"—i.e., 10 weeks old, 10 pounds, hemoglobin of 10 gm.[5] The palate is repaired somewhat later between 12 and 24 months of age.[5]

Abnormalities of the musculature of the soft palate will often lead to eustachian tube dysfunction due to the relationship of the tensor veli palatini and levator palatini muscles to the tori tubarius, the openings of the eustachian tubes. Middle ear effusions and sometimes more extensive ear disease are often seen in cleft palate patients. Placement of tympanostomy tubes to prevent problems from developing is advisable.

Velopharyngeal insufficiency can also be the result of lack of innervation to the soft palate via the vagus nerve. This may be seen in cerebral palsy or following polio myelitis. A prosthesis that lifts the soft palate is often very effective. Bilateral lesions of the vagus nerves are extremely unlikely, whereas resection of a skull base tumor can often result in a unilateral vagal palsy with unilateral weakness of the soft palate. Surgical attachment of the paralyzed side to the posterior nasopharyngeal wall relieves these patients of their symptoms quite well.[6]

Adenotonsillar Hypertrophy

The adenoids and palatine tonsils (commonly known just as the tonsils) are part of the ring of lymphatic tissue in the pharynx that, with the lingual tonsils, make up Waldeyer's ring. This ring of tissue is the first part of the lymphatic system to encounter foreign substances that enter the body through the nose or mouth and is thought to sensitize the immune system to these invaders. Problems with the tonsils and adenoids can occur when they hypertrophy and obstruct the naso- and oropharynx or become chronically infected with bacteria, often group A, β-hemolytic streptococ-

cus. Hypertrophy causes hyponasal voice, nasal obstruction, snoring, chronic mouth breathing, and occasionally obstructive sleep apnea syndrome. Chronic tonsillitis causes chronic sore throat, odynophagia, and often, halitosis. If the tonsils and adenoids do not shrink with age or remain symptomatic despite medical intervention, surgical excision of the tonsils and/or adenoids usually resolves these problems. Removal of the adenoids, however, can lead to velopharyngeal insufficiency and associated symptoms of nasal regurgitation and hypernasal voice. This usually occurs only transiently, lasting days to a few weeks, in a small number of patients (less than 5%) and is very rarely permanent (less than 1%). The permanent cases are usually seen only in children with a short palate or unrecognized submucous cleft palate. Treatment includes palatal lift prostheses or surgery to lengthen the palate or adhere it to the posterior pharyngeal wall.

Tongue Disorders

Most disorders affecting the tongue are related to changes of the mucosa, changes that can occur in any of the oral mucosa. These include hyperkeratosis, dysplasia, and atrophy. Most mucosal abnormalities seen are very nonspecific and of little clinical significance. Many need to be biopsied to rule out carcinoma, but otherwise require no therapy.

Lack of sense of taste is usually due to a loss of sense of smell with no actual abnormality of the taste apparatus. However, various systemic illnesses and medications can diminish the overall sense of taste. Decreased taste and/or numbness in a specific part of the tongue should alert the clinician to the possibility of a lesion of the nerve supplying sensation to that portion of the tongue.

Motor function of the tongue is integral in chewing, manipulating a food bolus, swallowing, and articulating speech. Interruption of the motor innervation to the tongue is usually the result of stroke or other significant intracranial event or surgical trauma in the neck or floor of mouth. A malignant neoplasm of the base of skull or submandibular gland will rarely present with a unilateral tongue palsy. Fortunately, the tongue is able to accommodate a unilateral hypoglossal nerve palsy well, with very little long-term dysarthria or dysphagia, provided there are no other cranial nerve palsies.

Salivary Gland Disorders

The oral cavity is the site of the openings of the ducts of the major salivary glands and the site of many minor salivary glands. The three pairs of major salivary glands include: the parotid glands, located anterior to the ear and superficial to the angle of the mandible; the submandibular glands, just inferior and medial to the body of the mandible; and the sublingual glands, inferior to the anterior tongue. Each gland produces saliva of slightly different composition when stimulated by the autonomic nervous system. Saliva lubricates the mouth and enzymes within saliva initiate digestion of food. Dry mouth (xerostomia) results when the salivary glands cease to function properly. A chronically dry mouth is very uncomfortable, makes eating more difficult, and can lead to dental disease. Xerostomia can be due to simple problems, such as inadequate water intake and dehydration, or to more complex autoimmune diseases, such as Sjögren's syndrome in which the tissue ceases to function. A common cause of xerostomia is medication that alters the autonomic input to the glands including antihistamines and antipsychotic and antidepressant drugs. Xerostomia is also a common side effect of radiation therapy to the oral cavity and/or oropharynx. Treatment first involves identifying and treating the etiology followed by the use of oral lubricants and medications that directly stimulate the salivary glands.

Infections of the Oral Cavity, Oropharynx, Nasopharynx, and Salivary Glands

Infections can occur in many different structures within and around the oral cavity and oropharynx. They can be viral, bacterial, fungal, or due to mycobacteria, some of which cause tuberculosis. The most common infection is viral pharyngitis that causes sore throat and odynophagia (painful swallowing). The tonsils may be involved and swell enough to threaten the airway. Less common viruses, such as the herpes virus, may cause painful and infectious vesicular sores on the lips and in the mouth. Aphthous ulcers, commonly known as canker sores, are thought to be due to local trauma and possibly a nonherpetic viral infection. They are very painful, usually last about seven days, but are not contagious. Pharyngitis and tonsillitis may also be caused by bacteria. Infection by group A β-hemolytic streptococcus (strep throat) is the most feared because of its potential systemic effects such as rheumatic fever, rheumatic heart disease, and kidney disease (acute glomerulonephritis).

The salivary glands are also prone to infection. This can be viral, as in mumps, which affects the parotid glands, or suppurative sialoadenitis, in which bacteria, usually staphylococcus aureaus, may infect any of the salivary glands. Stones within the ducts or glands themselves (sialolithiasis) will make bacterial sialoadenitis more likely as will dehydration and other causes of xerostomia as discussed above.

Treatment of these various infectious processes varies according to the etiology and structure involved. Hydration, analgesics, and antipyretics relieve most symptoms. Some viruses may be treated with specific antiviral agents (e.g., acyclovir is effective against herpes simplex), while most other viruses are not deterred by antiviral agents. Bacterial infections are treated with antibiotics. Occasionally a bacterial infection will progress into an abscess that does not respond to antibiotic therapy. Surgical drainage is then required. This can be done either through the mouth or the neck. Rather severe, life-threatening infections can develop if the abscess extends into the neck where it can involve the great vessels or cause enough swelling to obstruct the airway. Incision and drainage of a deep neck abscess and sometimes tracheotomy are performed emergently in those cases.

Neoplasms of the Oral Cavity, Oropharynx, and Salivary Glands

The most common malignant tumor of the oral cavity and oropharynx is squamous cell carcinoma that is usually caused by tobacco use and, to a lesser extent, alcohol abuse. This is covered in detail in Chapter 23.

Tumors may also develop within the salivary glands. If these are benign or malignant but diagnosed early, excision of the gland may effect a cure. Although relatively straightforward for the submandibular glands, it is much more complex for the parotid glands. The facial nerve leaves the skull base just inferior to the ear and courses through the substance of the parotid gland to the muscles of the face that it innervates. Any surgery of the parotid gland must begin with identification and careful dissection of the facial nerve to avoid inadvertent injury that could result in unilateral complete facial paralysis with inability to close the eye, the lips, and obvious cosmetic deformity.

Trauma of the Oral Cavity

Trauma to the oral cavity may be blunt or penetrating with the former more common. Motor vehicle accidents and assaults are responsible for most blunt injuries that result in mandible fractures. Treating these fractures to re–establish normal occlusion may be achieved with a variety of techniques, including long-term (6 weeks) maxillomandibular fixation (MMF, wiring the jaws together) alone, MMF and wiring or plating of the fractures, or screwing and compression plating of the fractures with immediate release of MMF. The technique chosen depends on the site and direction of the fracture, as well as the surgeon's experience. When a mandible fracture is combined with other facial injuries, the repair becomes more complex and reestablishment of the normal occlusion less certain.

Penetrating injuries to the oral cavity and pharynx range from hard and soft palate lacerations that result from children falling down on objects in their mouths, such as toy trumpets or popsicle sticks, to devastating shotgun injuries sustained in unsuccessful suicide attempts. The childhood injuries deserve evaluation due to the proximity of the carotid artery to the lateral pharyngeal wall and possible damage to that structure. The injury from suicide attempts will require many procedures first to salvage as much tissue as possible and then to reconstruct the face.

Sleep Disorders

Many conditions can affect sleep. Probably the most common problem with sleep is snoring that represents turbulent airflow during sleep and affects approximately 50% of males and 30% of females. It is more common as people age and is more prevalent in people who are overweight. Snoring tends to worsen after alcohol intake and when lying flat on the back. Since snoring is a sign of obstruction, it may affect one's ability to sleep.

Although snoring is often perceived as only a problem for the snorer's bed partner, it may be a sign of the more serious condition known as obstructive sleep apnea syndrome (OSAS) in which breathing stops for periods of time during sleep (apnea). Patients with OSAS commonly complain of excessive daytime sleepiness, headaches, and chronic fatigue. The condition can lead to high blood pressure, heart rhythm problems, heart failure, sudden death, and automobile accidents due to falling asleep while driving.[7]

Apnea may be due to the central nervous system's not initiating a breath, or, more commonly, a blockage developing somewhere in the throat or nasal passages, stopping the flow of air. Various abnormalities of the facial structures and throat can promote sleep apnea by blocking breathing through the nose or throat or causing the tongue to fall back into the throat. Large tonsils, a long floppy soft palate, or a large tongue may promote this condition.[8] If sleep apnea is suspected, the patient will undergo a polysomnogram, or sleep study, which involves spending a night in the sleep laboratory, or use of home-based, mobile sleep study equipment and services. While the subject sleeps, many measurements are taken of eye movements, brain wave activity (electroencephalography, EEG), heart activity, breathing activity, and oxygen saturation (level of oxygen in blood). Based on the finding of this examination, the patient is diagnosed with either a snoring disorder only, or mild, moderate, or severe sleep apnea.

There are various treatments for sleep apnea. In those patients who are overweight, weight loss is extremely important and occasionally enough to relieve the patient of these symptoms.[8] Exercise and regimented sleep-wake cycles are also helpful.

The goal of the remainder of treatment is to keep the airway open while the patient is sleeping. This can be done with a nasal constant positive airway pressure device (nasal CPAP) in which the subject is fitted with a mask over the nose providing a constant flow of air through the nose to prevent collapse of the throat while inhaling. While particularly effective, CPAP is sometimes poorly tolerated. Other options include oral airways—devices placed in the mouth that hold the tongue and jaw forward to keep the tongue from falling back and obstructing the airway. Nasal airway devices may be helpful in some patients. The oral and nasal airways are not particularly comfortable or well tolerated. Therefore, these treatments are often abandoned by the patient who continues to suffer from the effects of sleep apnea.

Surgical procedures may permanently open the breathing passageways without the use of devices. For extremely severe sleep apnea, a tracheotomy is often done. This is the ultimate surgical procedure for this disease and works 100% of the time, but it does require long-term care of the tracheostomy tube. Most patients do not require this procedure.

Other surgical procedures are aimed at improving the airway in the nose. Several operations have been developed to open the airway at the level of the throat, the most common area that obstructs. The most popular of these is known as uvulopalatopharyngoplasty (UPPP). Here the surgeon removes the tonsils, which are usually contributing to the problem, and excess tissue from the soft palate and pharyngeal walls. UPPP creates more room in the throat and prevents collapse of the tissues while the person is sleeping. A staged, laser-assisted version of this surgery can now be performed as an outpatient procedure without general anesthesia. Procedures have also been developed to pull the jaw forward, primarily to pull the tongue forward, preventing it from falling back and blocking the airway.[7]

These procedures alter the shape and function of the pharynx and can potentially affect the voice. In most cases, if there is a change, it is a positive one with less hyponasality in the patient who has had adenoids removed or a deviated nasal septum straightened or a less muffled voice after UPPP in one with large tonsils. A potential complication of UPPP, however, is velopharyngeal insufficiency. This occurs transiently in up to 15% of patients and permanently in less than 1% of cases.

NASAL AND SINUS DISORDERS

Functions and Disorders of the Nasal Cavities and Paranasal Sinuses

The nasal cavities humidify inspired air, filter out foreign matter, provide passage of outside air to the olfactory nerves (smell), and act as a resonator for the voice. The nose is the preferred route of breathing during most activity except during strenuous exercise when the mouth is usually open. The function of the paranasal sinuses is unclear. One theory is that the sinuses serve as buffers/bumpers for trauma to the head and eyes. Another is that

hollow sinuses make the head lighter (Figures 20–2 and 20–3).

The most common nasal complaint is obstruction. Congenital problems such as choanal atresia and nasopharyngeal disease such as adenoid hypertrophy can cause obstruction. So can acquired obstructing lesions of the nasal cavities themselves. The nasal septum should be a straight, relatively thin, flat, midline structure, but it can become deviated as a person ages and obstruct (partially or completely) either one or both sides of the nose. Trauma to the nose can also cause deflection of the nasal septum and/or nasal bones. Benign masses, such as polyps or papillomas, and malignancies often also present with nasal obstruction, usually unilateral. Besides the obvious symptom of impaired nasal breathing, these patients often complain of decreased sense of smell, hyponasal speech, dry throat (especially in the morning), and snoring. Tumors may also cause pain and bleeding and more advanced cases can cause anesthesia of the face or eye symptoms.

Nasal obstruction may improve with medical therapy aimed at reducing swelling of the mucosal lining of the nose with oral decongestants, antihistamines (if allergy is a cause), steroid sprays, and humidification. When medical treatment fails, surgery is often curative. Straightening of the septum (septoplasty) and reconstruction of the entire nose (septorhinoplasty) are very effective proce-

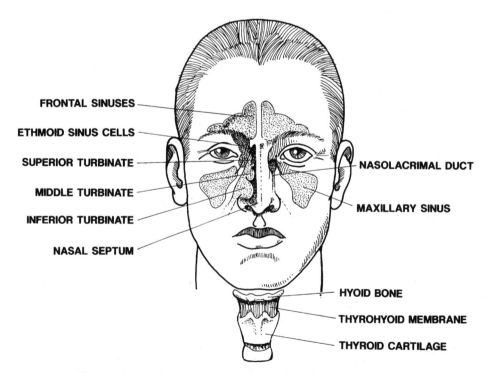

Figure 20–3. Coronal view of nasal and sinus cavities.

dures with few complications. Removal of benign lesions such as polypectomy is also relatively straightforward, although the polyps have a tendency to recur.

Epistaxis

Bleeding from the nose (epistaxis) is another fairly common problem. Most episodes of epistaxis originates from small vessels located on the anterior septum. This results in brief relatively mild, easy-to-control bleeding. Occasionally epistaxis originates from the posterior nasal cavity or nasopharynx, is much harder to control, and may possibly be life-threatening. Nasal packing or cauterizing or ligating the bleeding vessels will usually control the bleeding. Epistaxis may also be a sign of a nasal or sinus neoplasm.

Rhinitis

Allergic rhinitis is a common intermittent cause of nasal obstruction. Other symptoms include clear watery rhinorrhea, sneezing, and itchy nose and eyes. These symptoms occur in the presence of specific allergens that may be present during certain seasons (e.g., pollens, fungi) or in certain locations (e.g., dust mite, animal dander). Avoidance or elimination of the allergens provides definitive treatment although this is frequently difficult. Few patients will part with their pets, for example. Antihistamines, steroid nasal sprays, and cromolyn nasal sprays (cromolyn prevents the mast cell from releasing histamine) may be necessary. Usually only one of these classes of medications is necessary at any one time. Antihistamines have the disadvantage of sometimes causing sedation and excessively drying the mouth and pharynx, which can be a problem for professional voice users. Desensitization injections, commonly known as "allergy shots," frequently succeed in making the person less sensitive to the allergens.

Sinusitis

Sinusitis is an infection of one or more of the eight paranasal sinus cavities. It usually follows a viral upper respiratory infection or an exacerbation of allergic rhinitis. These conditions cause swelling of the nasal mucosa including the mucosa at the naturally small openings of the sinuses. Anatomic abnormalities and polyps may also block the sinus ostia. Blockage of these openings creates a closed cavity that is an excellent environment for the colonization and growth of bacteria, the most common pathogens in sinusitis. Symptoms of an acute sinusitis include purulent nasal discharge, nasal obstruction, facial pain and pressure, fever, and occasionally headache. Treatment is aimed at opening the closed sinus cavities and eradicating the bacteria. Oral and topical nasal spray decongestants, saline nasal rinses, analgesics, rest, and antibiotics are crucial. Most acute episodes of sinusitis in immunocompetent individuals clear with one course of medical therapy.

Potential, but rare, complications of acute sinusitis include spread of the infection to the orbit, with possible injury to the eye, or intracranially, with possible meningitis, brain abscess, or cavernous sinus thrombosis. These complications usually require surgical intervention to open up and drain the affected sinus and adjacent infected area, such as the orbit.

Chronic sinusitis is quite different from the acute disease, although acute exacerbations may occur in a patient with chronic disease. The common symptoms of chronic sinusitis include chronic nasal and post-nasal discharge, which is usually thick mucoid material, varying degrees of nasal obstruction, pressure, or a heavy feeling in the face and head. Facial pain and headaches are rarely seen in chronic sinusitis and fever is also uncommon. Patients are treated in a similar manner to those with acute sinusitis, but the duration of therapy is longer: antibiotics are prescribed for three or more weeks; nasal steroid sprays and oral decongestants or antihistamines (if allergy is present) are taken indefinitely. Nasal endoscopy helps to determine whether small polyps or other lesions are obstructing the sinus ostia. A CT scan is the test of choice for assessing location and extent of disease. It will often show obstruction of the ostiomeatal complex, which is the common path of drainage for the frontal, anterior ethmoid, and maxillary sinuses. It may also show thickening of the mucosal lining of the sinuses, a sign of chronic sinusitis. A patient who has severe enough symptoms and fails medical therapy is a candidate for surgery. A relatively new technique known as endoscopic sinus surgery (ESS) has greatly decreased the morbidity associated with sinus surgery and is the preferred technique.[8] With the increased ability to see the anatomy during surgery, more precise and more thorough removal of diseased tissue can be performed without the need for external incisions. Success rates are approximately 85%.[9] Nasal polyps are often seen in patients with chronic sinusitis. They are removed during ESS and are thought to recur less often after this procedure than after a simple polypectomy.

Nasal Masses

The most common benign nasal mass is the inflammatory polyp, although it is not considered a true neoplasm (Figure 20–4). As discussed above, these masses usually cause nasal obstruction and are frequently associated with allergic rhinitis or chronic sinusitis. In children, the presence of nasal polyps suggests the possibility of cystic fibrosis, which may be undiagnosed. Removal of nasal polyps involves simple polypectomy or more extensive sinus surgery, depending on symptoms and other findings. Squamous papillomas are the most common true neoplasms in the nose. They are benign and usually cured with simple excision.

Inverted papilloma is less common and also benign. It can, however, be very aggressive and is capable of eroding through adjacent bony structures into the orbit or intracranially. Removal of these lesions requires excision of the tumor with a wide margin of normal tissue. Since these are found most commonly on the lateral nasal wall, they are usually treated with a medial maxillectomy, which removes the entire lateral nasal wall, ethmoid sinus and medial wall of the maxilla. With a lesser operation, recurrence is common. The treatment of nasal-sinus malignancies is discussed in Chapter 23.

Facial Pain

Pain is a symptom that can result from many different disease processes. The most common causes of facial pain include trauma, sinusitis, and dental disease. The history will provide the diagnosis, which is usually confirmed with the physical findings. With appropriate treatment and resolution of

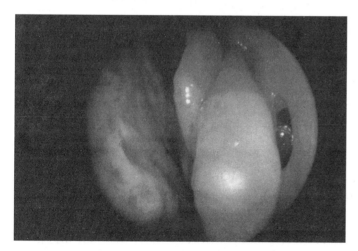

Figure 20–4. Large polyp extending from the left middle meatus into the nose. The polyps caused nasal obstruction and chronic rhinosinusitis. The patient had complete obstruction of the right nostril with polyps.

the disease, the pain also abates. Sometimes the etiology behind the pain is not apparent or the pain does not resolve with the other symptoms.

As discussed above, acute (not chronic) sinusitis is often painful. Tenderness is elicited over the maxillary or frontal sinuses if those are involved. Inflammation of the ethmoid and sphenoid sinuses can cause pain at the top of the head and occiput, respectively. The pain, however is usually not an isolated symptom, but is associated with other signs of sinusitis.

The trigeminal nerve (cranial nerve V) supplies sensation to the face. The first division (ophthalmic) supplies the forehead, eyebrows, and eyes. The second division (infraorbital) supplies the cheek, nose and upper lip and gums. The third division (mandibular) supplies the ear, mouth, jaw, tongue, lower lip, and submandibular region. When pain is located in a very specific nerve distribution area, lesions involving that nerve must be considered. Tumors involving the nerve usually cause other symptoms, but pain may be the only complaint and presence of a tumor at the base of the skull or in the face must be ruled out. When the work-up is negative, the diagnosis may be one of many types of neuralgia, which is a pain originating within the sensory nerve itself. Treatment is medical and in some cases surgical.

Otalgia (ear pain) can be caused by many different conditions of the ear itself, including trauma, infection, foreign body, tumor, and even cerumen impaction, or it can be a referred pain. The external ear canal and auricle receive sensory innervation from branches of four different nerves—the fifth (trigeminal), seventh (facial), ninth (glossopharyngeal), and tenth (vagus) cranial nerves. These nerves also supply various other parts of the head and neck and even thorax and abdomen in the case of the tenth nerve. Inflammation of another part of these nerves (e.g., the vagus nerve from a tumor of the larynx or hypopharynx) will often cause otalgia along with the local symptoms. More common conditions such as tonsillitis or an aphthous ulcer of the soft palate also commonly cause referred otalgia.

There are many craniomandibular disorders that include pain in the head and neck among many different and varied symptoms. Many of these conditions relate to the temporomandibular joint (TMJ) and surrounding structures. Internal abnormalities of the TMJ may cause local pain, otalgia, trismus, sounds within the joint during mandibular movement, and change in occlusion.[10] Extracapsular craniomandibular disorders are also known as myofacial pain dysfunction syndrome[10] and are thought to be due to an abnormal relationship of the dental apparatus, the TMJs, and the neuromuscular system. Symptoms include pains that do not seem related to the TMJ, headaches, "muffled" ears and other otologic symptoms, and various other vague facial, dental, and neck symptoms. The work-up is first aimed at finding and correcting the underlying cause of the symptoms, such as an intracapsular lesion of the TMJ or dental malocclusion. This may require simple measures such as bite blocks to align the occlusion at night and prevent bruxism, or may require surgery of the TMJ itself. Other treatments include transcutaneous electrical neural stimulation (TENS) to control muscle spasms and relieve pain.

ANATOMY OF THE LARYNX

To understand the anatomy of the larynx, it is imperative to realize that the larynx is not an anatomic site unto itself. Much of the function of the larynx is dependent on the structures that are attached and integrated with the larynx. These include the muscles and soft tissues of the neck, the trachea and the esophagus, the hyoid and mandibular bones, and the muscles of the tongue. Functionally, the larynx depends on the integration of activities with the nervous system, both afferent and efferent impulses, and coordination of activities via the central nervous system and the spinal cord. It is often simplest to think of the larynx in relationship to its four major tissue types: cartilages, muscles, nerves, and blood vessels.

There are five primary laryngeal cartilages: the thyroid cartilage, cricoid cartilage, epiglottis, and a pair of arytenoid cartilages (Figures 20–5 through 20–7). In addition, there are smaller cartilages whose function is not perfectly clear. These are the paired cuneiform and corniculate cartilages that lie in the aryepiglottic folds superior to the arytenoid cartilages. The thyroid cartilage, whose name is derived from the Greek word for "shield," is the largest cartilage in the larynx and encompasses the anterior and lateral skeletal structure of the larynx. The cartilage has a greater and lesser cornua to which are attached the thyrohyoid ligament and the cricothyroid ligament, respectively, and bilateral ala. The cartilage also has an oblique line on the ala to which is attached the inferior constrictor muscle. This attachment is important for the superior movement of the larynx with swallowing. The anterior thyroid cartilage extends from the thyroid notch to the anterior-inferior cartilage. The angle of the anterior cartilage tends to

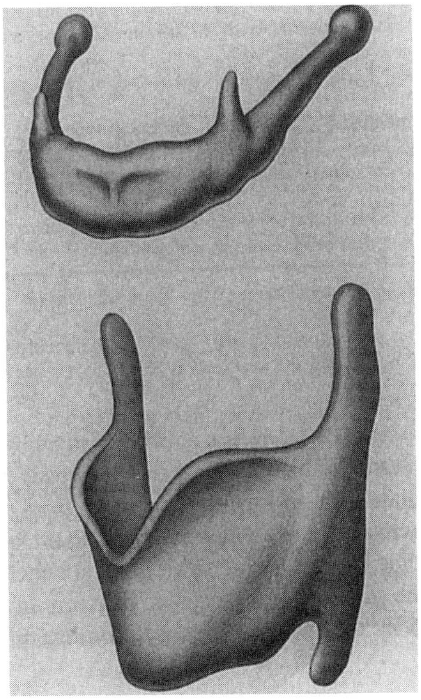

Figure 20–5. Hyoid bone and thyroid cartilage. *Source:* From Tucker HM: *The Larynx,* 2nd Ed., 1993; New York, Thieme. Reprinted with permission.

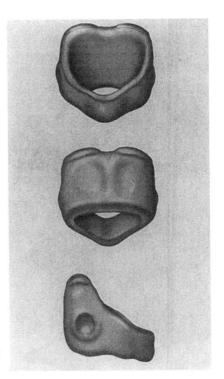

Figure 20–6. Cricoid cartilage. *Top,* anterior view. *Middle,* posterior view. *Bottom,* lateral view. *Source:* From Tucker HM: *The Larynx,* 2nd Ed., 1993; New York, Thieme. Reprinted with permission.

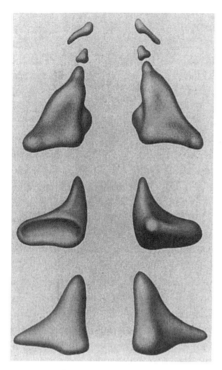

Figure 20–7. Arytenoid cartilages. *Top,* posterior view with cuneiform and corniculate cartilages above. *Middle,* inferior view. *Bottom,* anterior view. *Source:* From Tucker HM: *The Larynx,* 2nd Ed., 1993; New York, Thieme. Reprinted with permission.

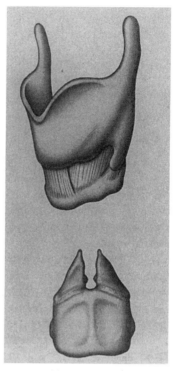

Figure 20–8. Cricothyroid joint, membrane, and ligament, above; cricoarytenoid joints, posterior view, below. *Source:* From Tucker HM: *The Larynx,* 2nd Ed., 1993; New York, Thieme. Reprinted with permission.

be more acute in men (90°) than in women (120°), which makes it more prominent in the neck—hence the term "Adam's apple."

The cricoid cartilage lies just below the thyroid cartilage and is joined to the thyroid cartilage at the cricothyroid joint between the inferior cornua of the thyroid and the lateral joint capsule of the cricoid (Figure 20–8). This joint allows for rotation of the cricoid in relationship to the thyroid cartilages. The cricothyroid membrane attaches the anterior-lateral aspects of the inferior thyroid to the superior cricoid. The cricoid cartilage is the only complete ring in the upper airway with the thyroid cartilage and the tracheal rings being open posteriorly. In neonates and infants, this is the narrowest part of the upper airway and is the most common site for upper airway obstruction. Swelling of the tissues of the subglottic region surrounded by the complete ring, fixed cricoid cartilage accounts for the airway obstruction in croup. In older children and adults, the narrowest area is the rima glottis or space between the free margins of the true vocal folds. The cricoid cartilage is shaped like a signet ring with the larger face pos-

terior. On the upper surface of the signet portion is the cricoarytenoid joint. This joint is unique in that it allows for both rotation of the arytenoids and also anterior-posterior sliding.

The arytenoid cartilages are paired cartilages that lie on top of the cricoid cartilage at the cricoarytenoid joint. In addition to the joint, there are three main surfaces (processes) of the arytenoids: the muscular process to which is attached the interarytenoid muscles, the posterior cricoarytenoid muscle, and a portion of the thyroarytenoid muscle, the vocal process with the attachment of the vocalis ligament anteriorly and the lateral process which attaches the lateral cricoarytenoid muscle.

The epiglottis is different from the other cartilages of the larynx in that it is primarily hyalin cartilage (Figure 20–9). This cartilage does not ossify, while the other cartilages do ossify with age. The epiglottis is attached to the upper, mid-posterior surface of the thyroid cartilage at the petiole, and laterally with the arytenoids by the aryepiglottic folds. There is an upper (lingual) and a lower (laryngeal) surface of the epiglottis. The vallecula is

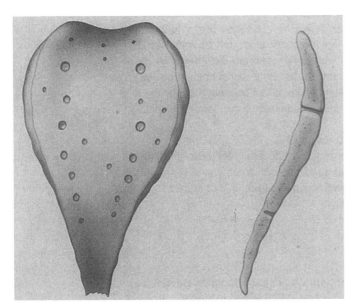

Figure 20–9. Epiglottic cartilage. Note perforations. *Source:* From Tucker HM: *The Larynx,* 2nd Ed., 1993; New York, Thieme. Reprinted with permission.

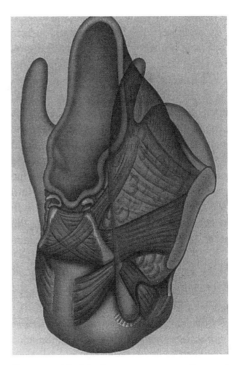

Figure 20–10. Intrinsic muscles of the larynx. *Source:* From Tucker HM: *The Larynx,* 2nd Ed., 1993; New York, Thieme. Reprinted with permission.

the area where the epiglottis meets the base of the tongue.

There are both intrinsic and extrinsic muscles of the larynx. The intrinsic muscles of the larynx are the thyroarytenoid, interarytenoid, posterior cricoarytenoid, and the lateral cricoarytenoid muscles while the extrinsic muscles are the cricothyroid muscles (Figure 20–10). The intrinsic muscles receive their motor innervation primarily from the recurrent laryngeal nerves (RLN) with a small portion coming from the superior laryngeal nerve (SLN)[11] while the cricothyroid receives its motor innervation from the superior laryngeal nerves (Figure 20–11).

The lateral cricoarytenoid muscles result in rotation of the vocal process of the arytenoids toward the midline, thereby tightening the vocal folds and slightly elongating them (Figure 20–12). The thyroarytenoid (TA) muscles tense the vocal folds by shortening the arytenoids in relationship to the thyroid cartilage. The TA muscles along with the overlying vocalis ligament and mucosa are the structures that form the true vocal fold. The interarytenoids pull the muscular processes of the arytenoids together resulting in adduction and the cricothyroid muscles rotate the thyroid on the cricoid cartilages thereby elongating and tensing the vocal folds. These muscles work in delicate concert to adduct the vocal folds and adjust pitch. The only pure abductor of the larynx is the posterior cricoarytenoid muscles that rotate the vocal processes of the arytenoids laterally as they pull

the muscular processes medially. Although there is some debate, the cricothyroid muscles may also play a role in abduction with deep inspiration or with hypercapnia.

The major nerve supply to the larynx is from the superior and recurrent laryngeal nerves that are branches of the vagus (X) nerve. The SLN leaves the vagus just after it exits the skull base and splits into internal and external branches. The internal branch passes through the thyrohyoid membrane to supply sensory innervation to the epiglottis and the larynx down to the level of the true vocal folds. If this sensory input is lost, there can be a significant effect on swallowing and patients may be prone to aspiration. The external branch stays external to the larynx and supplies motor innervation to the cricothyroid muscles. The RLNs receive their names because they leave the vagus nerve low in the neck and loop (recur) in the chest prior to ascending in the tracheo-esophageal groove to innervate the intrinsic muscles of the larynx and provide sensation to the lower edge of the vocal folds and the subglottic region. The right RLN loops under the subclavian artery that is higher in the neck than the left RLN, which loops under the arch of the aorta. The nerve impulses in the left RLN are slightly faster than in the right; this allows them to reach the respective

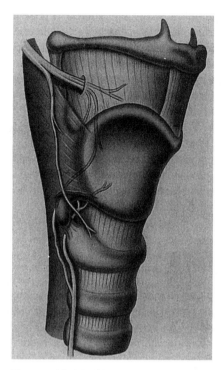

Figure 20–11. Nerve supply of the larynx. Superior laryngeal nerve course from above and recurrent laryngeal nerve approaches from below. Also note inferior constrictor muscle. *Source:* From Tucker HM: *The Larynx,* 2nd Ed., 1993; New York, Thieme. Reprinted with permission.

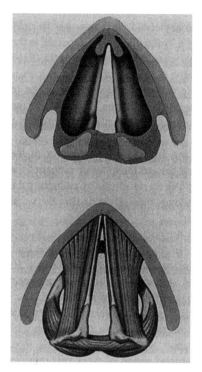

Figure 20–12. Horizontal section of larynx through the ventricles. Mucosa intact, above; mucosa removed to show intrinsic muscles of vocal folds, below. *Source:* From Tucker HM: *The Larynx,* 2nd Ed., 1993; New York, Thieme. Reprinted with permission.

muscles of the larynx at the same time.[12] The longer loop of the left RLN into the chest results in a higher likelihood that the left RLN will be injured by pathology in the chest.[13]

The microanatomy of the vocal folds has been well described[14] and is crucial for an understanding of the pathology and physiology of the larynx and necessary for planning treatment (Figure 20–13). The vocal folds are composed of sequential layers. The most superficial layer is the mucosa, which is stratified squamous epithelium primarily without glandular structures. Deep to the mucosa are three layers of lamina propria: a superficial layer of loose connective tissue (Reinke's space), a middle transitional layer, and a deep layer of dense connective tissue and collagen (thyroid ligament). Deep to the thyroid ligament is the medial belly of the vocalis (TA) muscle. It is believed that with lower pitch and tension these distinct layers move independently from one another, but with elevated pitch and greater tension they tend to move more as a single unit.

PHYSIOLOGY OF THE LARYNX

The larynx has three major functions: protection, respiration, and phonation. Protection of the lungs reveals the critical role of the larynx in swallowing. Laryngeal physiology is based on a complex interaction of concerted muscular activity, sensory and motor nerve input, reflexes, and glandular secretions. It is difficult to summarize all these activities, although some general physiological principles apply.

Phonation, or the production of voice, is the result of the action of the lungs, the larynx, and the resonating cavities of the lower and upper airways. As the vocal folds are brought together through the actions of the intrinsic and extrinsic muscles of the larynx, and as passive or forced-active exhalation occurs, subglottic pressure increases until it overcomes the pressure of the vocal folds held in position. The vocal folds will then part for a short period of time depending on the level of subglottic pressure and the tightness of the apposition of the

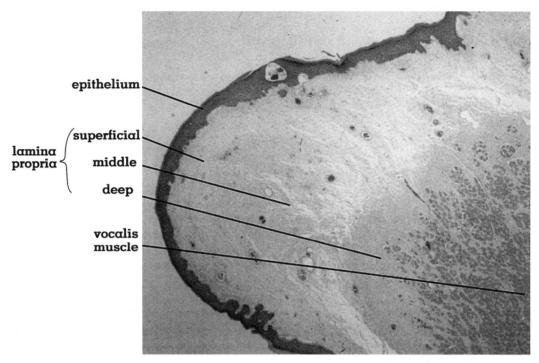

Figure 20–13. Histologic coronal section of the vocal fold.

vocal folds. As the vocal folds separate to allow passage of the air, two events occur that tend to bring the vocal folds back to the midline: (1) The natural tension and pressure of the vocal folds becomes greater than the decreasing subglottic pressure and (2) the Bernoulli effect occurs, which pulls the vocal folds back to the midline. As the subglottic pressure rapidly increases, the cycle is repeated. This repetitive cycle of vocal fold closing and opening is called the myoelastic-aerodynamic theory of phonation.[14] Factors that would allow this to occur more quickly would be associated with an increase in vocal fold frequency and an elevated pitch. These would be increasing subglottic pressure, decreasing the mass of the vocal folds, or increasing the tension on the vocal folds. Similarly, decreased subglottic pressure, increased mass, or decreased tension would result in lowering the pitch. A mass lesion, poor pulmonary support, a thicker vocal fold (as in a male), or lesser tension would all be associated with decreased pitch.

Loudness is determined by the amplitude of the vibration. Loudness can be increased or decreased without changing pitch. Other factors instrumental in voice production involve the resonating cavities of the upper airway, particularly the pharynx and oral cavity. Speech is dependent on voice production, resonation, and articulation. Although subtle refinements in the voice are produced at the level of the larynx, the vocal folds are not necessary for voice production. Some individuals use their false vocal folds for voice production while laryngectomees can produce voice through vibration of the cricopharyngeus. Quality of voice is dependent on culture, age, sex, and many other factors such as individual taste and preference.

Benign Laryngeal Disorders

As described above, the larynx serves to protect the airway from aspiration, provides a valve for generating an effective cough, and is the source of the sound that is shaped by the rest of the vocal tract to produce the voice. Benign laryngeal disorders can affect any or all of these functions.

Most benign laryngeal disorders cause a change in voice, usually referred to as "hoarseness." This term, among otolaryngologists and voice pathologists, is interpreted as a rough, raspy voice often with lowering of the pitch. Unfortunately, it is not quite as well defined among other physicians and the general public, and a careful history must be obtained to determine the exact nature of the voice change.[15] Pain in the region of the larynx, shortness of breath, and dysphagia may also be complaints associated with benign laryngeal disorders.

Epiglottitis

Epiglottitis, also known as supraglottitis, is an acute infection of the epiglottis and aryepiglottic folds usually caused by *Haemophilus influenza* type B (Hib). It has historically been most common in children, aged 2 to 4 years, but since the introduction of a Hib vaccine, the incidence in children has declined, while in adults it has remained stable.[16] Symptoms include rapid onset of fever, sore throat, odynophagia, and sometimes shortness of breath. Patients usually sit upright with the head extended, drooling. The severe swelling of the supraglottic structures may lead to obstruction of the airway and death by asphyxiation. Management in children involves rapidly, but calmly, controlling the airway, usually with intubation in the operating room, and then administering antibiotics. The child remains intubated until the inflammation has resolved, usually after 2 to 3 days. Adults, who are more easily examined and have a larger airway to start with, may be managed more conservatively in less severe cases. Tracheotomy is rarely needed.

Laryngomalacia

Laryngomalacia is abnormal flaccidity of the laryngeal tissues that collapse during inspiration, causing inspiratory stridor. This may occur shortly after birth and usually resolves spontaneously in 6 to 18 months if, as in most cases, the child is otherwise normal. The stridor fluctuates in intensity and is worse with increased inspiratory effort, such as during crying or feeding. Rarely is intervention required.[17]

Laryngitis

The most common disease of the larynx is laryngitis, which is an inflammatory condition with several different etiologies. The most common form of laryngitis is a viral infection and is usually associated with an upper respiratory tract infection. Physical findings include erythema of the vocal folds and arytenoid mucosa, excess mucus, and sometimes edema of the vocal folds. Hydration, humidification, analgesic/anti-inflammatory medications, mucolytics, modified voice use, and avoidance of irritants such as cigarette smoke, are the mainstays of treatment while the viral illness runs its course. In fact, these treatments will help in any laryngeal disorder. Croup, which is a viral infection of the proximal trachea and subglottic region seen more commonly in young children, causes a barking cough, hoarseness, and often inspiratory stridor. Most cases respond to humidification and/or cool air while more severe cases require systemic steroids and occasionally even intubation for airway protection.

Laryngitis is also caused by gastropharyngeal reflux disease (GPRD) and by exposure to inhaled irritants such as smoke, steam, caustic gases, and other noxious substances.[18]

Chronic cough due to pulmonary disease may also lead to inflammation of the glottis, frequently in the region of the vocal processes of the arytenoids that make rather violent contact with throat clearing and uncontrolled coughing fits. Some medications used to treat asthma, such as inhaled steroids, may also cause edema and erythema of the vocal folds.

Benign Laryngeal Masses, Nodules, Polyps and Cysts

Any lesion that changes the mass of one or both vocal folds or prevents the vocal folds from closing completely during the glottic cycle will cause dysphonia. The common benign lesions of the vocal folds include vocal fold nodules, polyps, and cysts. A less common lesion is sulcus vocalis. Each of these has a different etiology and treatment. Often, the diagnosis of a vocal fold lesion is obvious on indirect or fiberoptic laryngoscopy. Videostroboscopy is of help in differentiating between the different masses in one-fourth to one-third of cases.[19,20]

Nodules are the result of vocal abuse and are usually bilateral symmetric lesions that involve the mucosa and submucosal space (Figure 20–14). Repeated contact at the mid-portion of the membranous vocal folds causes thickening and often

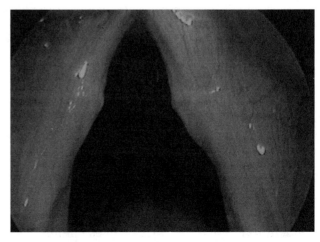

Figure 20–14. Bilateral vocal fold nodules.

incomplete keratinization of the mucosa.[21] The junction between the epithelium and submucosa, the basement membrane zone (BMZ), is often damaged.[21] Often, what appears to be a nodule is actually transient localized edema sometimes referred to as "physiologic swelling" that usually resolves 1 to 2 days following heavy voice use.[22] For longer lasting lesions, voice therapy is the primary treatment. Surgery is reserved for those patients whose dysphonia persists after 3 to 6 months of intense therapy.[22,23] When surgery is necessary, very conservative excision of only the abnormal tissue is performed. All normal mucosa should be preserved and extreme care taken to avoid trauma to the vocal ligament that is not typically abnormal with vocal nodules. This may be done with either very fine microsurgical instruments or with the CO_2 laser, although controversy exists regarding the use of the laser for vocal nodules.[22–26]

Intracordal cysts may be epidermoid cysts, which are most likely congenital, or mucus retention cysts resulting from obstruction of mucous gland ducts that in turn may be due to inflammatory and/or traumatic processes.[27] (Figure 20–15). Frequently, there is no apparent predisposing cause. Only the epidermoid cyst is a true cyst; it is located in the submucosa, often with surrounding fibrous reaction.[21] Such a cyst is usually unilateral although a contralateral reactive nodule may be present making the misdiagnosis of classic vocal fold nodules somewhat common. Videostroboscopy is especially helpful in differentiating between these two entities.[20] While voice therapy may improve the voice despite the presence of the cyst, excision is usually required to achieve the best voice result. Preoperative voice therapy does improve the likelihood of a good result.[28] Excision of cysts is usually carried out using microdissection with "cold" instruments (i.e., no laser). An incision is made through the mucosa into Reinke's space (superficial layer of the lamina propria) and the mucosa elevated off of the cyst. The cyst is then dissected from the vocal ligament (middle and deep layers of lamina propria) with great care to avoid trauma to that structure and prevent rupturing the cyst.[22–25,29] Excising the cyst intact is the only way of ensuring that the entire cyst has been removed, lessening the likelihood of recurrence.[25] The often encountered contralateral reactive nodule is assessed intraoperatively as to consistency. If it is soft, it will often resolve after excision of the cyst; but if it is hard and fibrotic, the nodule should be excised as discussed above for vocal nodules.

Vocal fold polyp is a term that includes any non-neoplastic-appearing lesion that is not a nod-

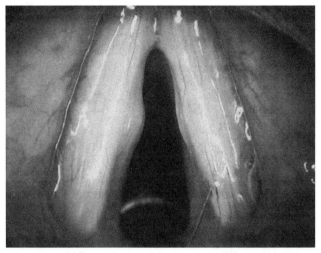

A

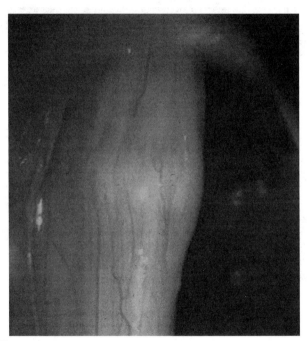

B

Figure 20–15. (**A**) Left vocal fold cyst with small reactive right vocal fold nodule. (**B**) Close up of left vocal fold cyst (different patient than 2A). See Color Plate 9.

ule or granuloma (Figure 20–16). Polyps may be broad based or pedunculated, unilateral or bilateral, firm or extremely soft, very small (2 mm) or huge, appearing to obstruct the airway, although they rarely do as they flop in and out of the lumen. They may be the result of a submucosal hemorrhage, vocal abuse, or smoking. The onset of dysphonia associated with a hemorrhagic polyp is usually sudden with a history of severe coughing or screaming immediately prior to onset of the disorder not uncommon. With pedunculated polyps, the result after excision is excellent. The procedure

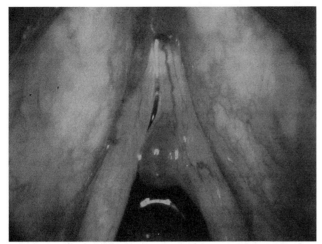

A

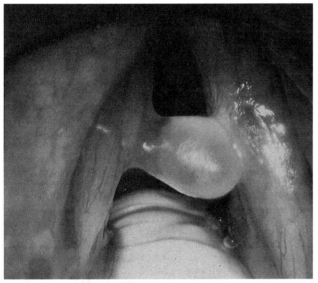

B

Figure 20–16. (A) Hemorrhagic polyp of right vocal fold with obvious enlarged feeding vessel. Also noted are polypoid changes of left anterior false vocal fold. **(B)** Pedunculated polyp of left vocal fold with reactive changes of right vocal fold (partially seen at anterior aspect of polyp on left vocal fold). See Color Plates 10 and 11.

involves making an incision at the base of the lesion, again taking care to avoid trauma to the surrounding normal mucosa and the underlying vocal ligament. Broad-based sessile polyps are excised with the same techniques, but the resulting mucosal defect is naturally larger, and the results, while still usually excellent, are less predictable. Excision may be done with microsurgical instruments or with the CO_2 laser.[22,24,26]

Diffuse, chronic edema of the true vocal fold may be referred to as Reinke's edema, polypoid corditis, or polypoid degeneration[21] (Figure 20–17).

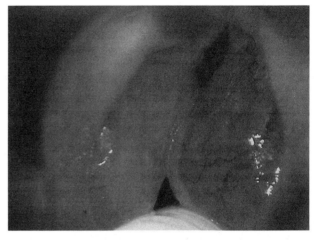

Figure 20–17. Severe polypoid degeneration of both true vocal folds in a long-time smoker. See Color Plate 12.

There is a generalized accumulation of fluid within the matrix of the superficial layer of the lamina propria, or Reinke's space.[23] This is usually due to smoking and other sources of chronic irritation, such as chronic coughing and throat clearing and may be related to GPRD as well. It may also represent myxedema of hypothyroidism. With mild or early polypoid corditis, an improvement may be seen with a cessation of the inciting irritation, such as smoking. Long-standing cases will require surgical intervention for improvement of the voice. It is crucial that smokers quit prior to or at least at the time of surgery to avoid a recurrence of the condition.[30,31] Surgery involves making an incision on the superior surface of the true vocal fold through the mucosa into Reinke's space and elevating the mucosa. The edematous matrix is then removed, taking care to avoid trauma to the vocal ligament, and the mucosa redraped and trimmed.[29] If the mucosa is relatively normal, its preservation will yield a better result than simply stripping it all away.[30] If, however, there are changes, such as leukoplakia, suggestive of a neoplastic process, the abnormal mucosa must be removed for histologic examination.

Sulcus vocalis is an extremely rare condition in which there is a furrow, or sulcus, of mucosa along the rima glottis that is adherent to the underlying vocal ligament (Figure 20–18). There are several types of sulcus vocalis including physiologic sulcus, type 2 sulcus (vergeture), and type 3 sulcus vocalis. Different theories explain the etiology of each of these types including rupture of a previously present intracordal cyst for the third type. Treatment depends first on identifying the pathology correctly. Type 2 sulcus (vergeture) is treated with microdissection and type 3 with excision.[32]

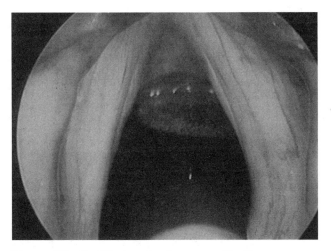

Figure 20–18. Bilateral sulcus vocalis. Furrows are seen on the medial aspect of both true vocal folds.

Benign Neoplasms

The most common benign neoplasm of the vocal fold, by far, is the squamous papilloma.[33] (Figure 20–19) Laryngeal papillomatosis is more common in children, but can occur at any age. Dysphonia is the first symptom, but neglected or aggressive disease can progress to airway obstruction and even death. The etiology seems to be human papilloma virus (HPV) infection, but an infecting source is usually not apparent. Treatment is microdissection or CO_2 laser ablation of the papillomata to restore the airway and normal contours of the vocal folds improve voice. The disease is extremely unpredictable and may recur within one month or disappear forever after only one treatment. Because of this uncertain prognosis, surgical excision must be conservative and preserve all normal

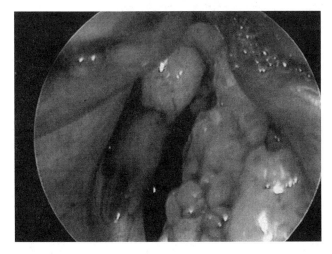

Figure 20–19. Extensive papillomatosis of the larynx in an adult. The entire right true vocal fold and the anterior left true vocal fold are involved. See Color Plate 13.

anatomy despite often very extensive disease that obscures all normal landmarks. Overaggressive surgery can lead to scarring of the vocal folds and formation of glottic webs that impair both voice and airway.[34] When the papillomatosis goes into remission, which in children often happens at puberty, the remaining laryngeal abnormalities are often the result of the surgery, not the disease process itself. Avoiding surgical trauma to the larynx can be difficult since these patients, especially children, commonly undergo many procedures. In more severe cases, the papillomatosis may spread down the trachea and even reach the carina and mainstem bronchi.

Benign neoplasms of the vocal folds, other than papillomata, are extremely rare. Other tumors include oncocytic tumors, granular cell tumors, hemangiomas, adenomas, rhabdomyomas, and neurofibromas.[33] Treatment usually involves excision with a minimal amount of normal tissue.

Granulomata are lesions that are not considered true neoplasms and consist of masses of granulation tissue. They commonly occur on the vocal process of the arytenoid cartilage as a result of some irritation such as endotracheal intubation, frequent coughing and throat clearing, vocal abuse with a hard glottal attack or gastropharyngeal reflux disease (GPRD).[35] (Figure 20–20) Ossification of the arytenoid cartilage as determined by CT scan suggests that perichondritis may play a role.[36] Treatment options include anti-reflux measures, voice therapy, steroids, surgical excision, and Botox injection (to decrease the force of arytenoid contact).[37] Granulomas have a tendency to recur after excision if the inciting etiology, such as GPRD, is not eliminated; this is best addressed before surgery.[18,22,23,36]

Functional Voice Disorders

Not all dysphonia is attributable to vocal fold masses or neurologic disorders. Occasionally, a patient will describe onset of a rough raspy voice, a weak breathy voice, or a whisper voice following an episode of laryngitis. With resolution of the other symptoms of laryngitis (pain, dysphagia, cough) the dysphonia persists. The history often includes periods of normal voice followed by sudden unexplained onset of the dysphonic voice, although the dysphonia can be constant for long periods of time. The patient often attributes the sudden changes to some real phenomenon such as cold air, change in weather, or perceived allergies and sinus-related disease. Onset may also be slow and gradual. Laryngeal examination may reveal many different findings including an open posterior glottis with rotated arytenoids, an open glottis

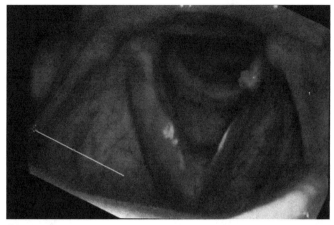

A

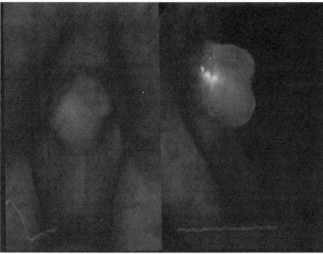

B

Figure 20–20. (A) Small granuloma of the left vocal process of the arytenoid cartilage. Also note thickening of the mucosa overlying the right vocal process and tenacious mucus on the membranous true vocal folds bilaterally. **(B)** A larger right-sided granuloma at the superior aspect of the vocal process. In this patient, the lesion does not impair glottic closure, and the voice was normal. See Color Plates 14 and 15.

along the entire length of the vocal folds with normal motion, and various configurations of supraglottic hyper function. While there is generally no organic disease to be found, continued abnormal laryngeal behavior may lead to the development of a secondary lesion such as vocal nodules.

The abnormal voice in the patients with rapid onset of dysphonia described above is due to improper vocalization technique, although it is usually done unconsciously. It is thought that during an acute laryngeal illness, when changes in the vocal folds alter the voice, some patients will alter their speaking technique, sometimes in improper ways,

to overcome the laryngeal pathology. When the acute inflammation resolves, most people naturally resume their normal speaking technique, but a minority will continue their maladaptive behavior unaware of what they are doing. Many of these patients have been told by other physicians that there is nothing wrong with them and that "it's all in your head." Many are quite frustrated by the time they meet an otolaryngologist or speech–language pathologist who understands their problem. Fortunately, these patients usually respond quickly to voice therapy when properly applied.

Excessive muscular tension within the larynx will also cause dysphonia with the only abnormal finding that of various patterns of constriction of the supraglottis. This group of nonorganic voice disorders are referred to as muscle tension dysphonia, which is a subclass of functional voice disorders.[38] When such a diagnosis is entertained, any suggestion of organic disease should be worked up while voice therapy is commenced. Often supraglottic hyperfunction is compensating for organic glottic insufficiency due to vocal fold immobility, a defect in the vocal fold, or a mass that impairs closure.

In some cases, a functional voice disorder is conscious and the patient is looking for gain from his or her problem. This gain may be in the form of increased attention or sympathy from friends and family or monetary in the form of disability claims. The clinician must be alert to this possibility because these patients are often quite resistant to therapy. Premature surgical intervention must be avoided to prevent creation of real iatrogenic laryngeal abnormalities.

Conversion aphonia or dysphonia usually has sudden onset and is associated with a predisposing event that may have nothing to do with the voice at all.

Neurolaryngology

Neuroanatomy and Reflexes

The gross neuroanatomy of the larynx was described in some detail in the preceding sections. However, much of laryngeal function depends on fine coordination of proprioception, chemical and temperature receptors, and efferent muscular innervation. This fine balance can be upset with injuries to the laryngeal nerves, mucosal injury, or neurologic disorders or diseases.

Vocal Fold Paralysis

The innervation of the laryngeal muscles can be disrupted anywhere from the nucleus ambiguous to the neuromuscular junction. If this injury is partial and some muscular activity occurs, then such an injury is called a paresis. If complete, then the injury is termed a paralysis. Vocal fold paralysis can be temporary or permanent. One problem with evaluating an immobile vocal fold is that when a vocal fold is immobile it can be due to loss of innervation (paralysis) or joint fixation. For the sake of this discussion, a distinction is made when relevant but otherwise lack of movement of the vocal fold is termed vocal fold immobility, either unilateral (UVFI) or bilateral (BVFI). The most common etiologies for VFI determined by recent review at Henry Ford Hospital are noted in Table 20–1. Although iatrogenic injury, primarily during thyroid surgery, has traditionally been the most common causes of both UVFL and BVFI, nonlaryngeal neoplasms have recently become the most common identifiable cause.[39-41] (Figure 20–21) Because of this, unless a cause is clearly identified, some evaluation of the neck and chest is recommended to rule out a neoplasm. At present, we recommend a chest X-ray and a CT or MRI scan of the neck from the skull base to the thoracic inlet, essentially following the entire course of the superior and recurrent laryngeal nerves.[42] It is likely that idiopathic paralysis is the most common cause, but since many of these are felt to recover spontaneously, the temporary dysphonia may be overlooked or disregarded as anything more than "laryngitis."

UVFI is most commonly caused by injury to the laryngeal nerves, although joint disruption or fixation from intubation, neck trauma, or rheumatoid arthritis should be considered. Once the etiology of the immobility is ascertained, or once a neoplastic cause is ruled out for idiopathic immobility, then treatment is determined by the cause and the like-

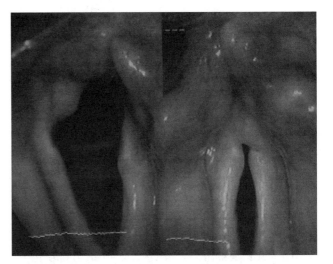

Figure 20–21. Left unilateral vocal fold paralysis: (left) during inspiration with normal abduction of the right vocal fold and (right) during phonation with incomplete glottic closure and a resultant weak breathy voice. The etiology was metastatic carcinoma from the bladder to the mediastinum with involvement of the left recurrent laryngeal nerve. See Color Plate 16.

lihood of recovery. A dislocated arytenoid should be reduced, a transected nerve reanastamosed and rheumatoid arthritis appropriately treated. Electromyography of the larynx can be performed to clarify whether the immobility is caused by joint fixation or paralysis or to help determine if recovery is likely in a paralyzed fold.

If a paralysis is confirmed, then the clinician has an opportunity to observe the patient or recommend a course of voice therapy. Some patients will regain a satisfactory voice with voice therapy alone, obviating the need for more aggressive management.[39] Many recommend a period of observation and a short course of voice therapy for up to a year prior to surgical treatment to allow adequate time for accommodation or wait for nerve recovery, which can take up to a year. With the availability of EMG, some of the guesswork has been eliminated. Even if denervated, vocal fold recovery can return. However, if there is no evidence of regeneration at six months, or if there is no recruitment even if some reinnervation has occurred, our experience has been that it is very unlikely that function will return.[39] If by that time the voice is inadequate for the patient's social and occupational needs despite a course of voice therapy, then surgical management should be considered. Some patients may require earlier intervention, particularly if they have significant problems with aspiration or a voice that significantly limits the patient's ability to fulfill occupational needs.

Table 20–1. Common Etiologies of Vocal Fold Immobility at Henry Ford Hospital (1985–1991).

Etiology	Number of Patients (%)
Miscellaneous (including idiopathic)	54 (33.9)
Malignancy (not including larynx)	39 (24.5)
Trauma/iatrogenic (not including thyroidectomy)	36 (22.7)
Thryroidectomy	16 (10.1)
Neurologic	14 (8.8)
Total	159 (100)

The type of surgical correction considered depends on a number of factors including the patient's need or desire for improvement of voice, the available techniques, the surgeon's experience, the degree of glottal insufficiency, and the urgency or need for permanency of the procedure. Many techniques are available and combinations of techniques are occasionally needed. Vocal fold injections have been used for many years and a variety of substances have been found to be of value. If a temporary improvement is needed, then gelfoam can be injected into the vocal fold. This usually lasts anywhere from 4 to 8 weeks and then resorbs. It is also a good technique for predicting the results of more permanent therapy or while waiting for possible recovery. Teflon paste injection is a generally reliable and predictable method of medializing the paralyzed vocal fold. In recent years, it has lost favor because of delayed granuloma formation and the irreversibility of the procedure. At present, we recommend Teflon in patients who have a paralyzed fold and whose life expectancy is short or in patients whose general health makes them a poor operative risk. Collagen has been found to be a good method of closing small glottic defects but large defects have not responded well. Similarly, implantation or injection of autologous adipose has been recommended for small defects or to fine tune the results of other procedures. Both collagen and fat have the disadvantages of resorption and loss of effect, although some partial long-term persistence of fat has been identified. These may become more useful as more experience is gained.

The preferred method of surgically managing UVFP by most otolaryngologists at this time is by surgically medializing the vocal folds. Since initially described by Isshiki et al., vocal fold medialization, initially with cartilage, and now primarily with silastic, has become the mainstay of treatment.[43] The objective is to implant silastic through a small window in the thyroid cartilage and push the immobile fold toward the midline to allow approximation from the opposite fold on phonation. Excellent results can be obtained, particularly in young patients or those in whom the superior laryngeal nerve innervation to the cricothyroid muscle remains intact.[39,44,45] Recently, other substances such as hydroxyapatite have been used in place of silastic,[46] although silastic is readily available and used by most laryngeal surgeons. The advantages of silastic medialization in vocal fold injection is that it allows for predictable results; the implant can be removed and revised if the results are suboptimal. The major disadvantage is that medialization may not adequately close a large posterior glottal chink, particularly in patients with combined SLN and RLN paralysis.

Arytenoid adduction (AA) is a procedure in which the arytenoid is rotated in a direction simulating the action of the lateral cricoarytenoid muscle, thereby adducting the vocal process to the midline. This procedure has become the preferred method of closing large posterior glottic gaps and can be performed alone or more commonly in conjunction with silastic medialization.[45] The disadvantages of AA are primarily related to some technical difficulties associated with the procedure, although in experienced hands it has been an excellent addition to the capabilities in managing UVFI.

One disadvantage of vocal fold injection, silastic medialization, and AA is that they are static procedures directed at pushing or pulling the immobile vocal fold to the midline for approximation from the opposite fold and therefore do not return innervation to the vocal folds. Vocal fold reinnervation can potentially resume some vocal fold motion. Originally, nerve-muscle pedicle reinnervation was recommended and although there was some evidence of clinical success and prevention of vocal fold atrophy would occur,[47] an inability to reliably produce vocal fold motion resulted in an interest to develop other methods of reinnervation. Subsequently, phrenic nerve and ansa cervicalis anastomosis to the recurrent laryngeal nerve or implantation directly into the laryngeal muscles have been described with some success.[48] The ease and predictability of silastic medialization and AA have prevented more widespread use of reinnervation, but with ongoing investigation it is likely that this will become a more important method.

The management of bilateral vocal fold immobility is also dependent on identification of the etiology that will guide early management. In many cases, particularly in neonates and infants, tracheostomy may be necessary to manage the airway obstruction. Long-term management will depend on the likelihood or timing of potential recovery. In those cases where recovery is unlikely, surgical management is usually necessary, although an occasional patient will function surprising well with no treatment. Such patients will have a satisfactory voice, but are usually limited in their activity levels by airway inadequacy.

When considering surgical treatment of BVFI, it is important to realize the delicate balance between good voice quality and a satisfactory airway. In general, efforts to dramatically improve the airway will result in a poorer voice and, conversely, attempts to retain normal voice will result in some compromise in airway, particularly with exercise or exertion, although a satisfactory balance is commonly attained. A number of options have been advocated for lateralization of one or both vocal folds in BVFI. The first was an external direct lateralization as described by Woodman.[49] With the advent of more sophisticated endoscopic microlaryngeal techniques and particularly advances in laser technology, the Woodman procedure has been largely abandoned except in very complicated or scarred larynges. The principles of microscopic or laser surgery rely on reduction of the bulk of one or both vocal folds. This can include an arytenoidectomy, partial arytenoidectomy, or partial cordectomy with each having distinct advantages.[50,51] Usually, the technique used is predominantly determined by the experience of the surgeon with one or more techniques.

Spasmodic Dysphonia

Spasmodic dysphonia (SD) is a neurologic disorder of the larynx of unknown cause that is manifested by two different characteristic voice abnormalities: adductor SD characterized by a strained or strangled voice with effortful speech and abductor SD characterized by episodes of breathiness and rapid air loss as the vocal folds spasm in an abducted position.[52] Adductor SD is much more common that abductor SD. A rare patient will have a combined adductor-abductor SD. Although the cause of SD is unknown, onset may occur after a traumatic event such as head trauma or a neurologic event. In some cases there may be a family history or genetic predisposition. SD is a focal dystonia of the larynx and although it usually occurs in isolation, there is an associated tremor or other dystonia in about one-fourth of patients. In most cases the onset is somewhat insidious with gradually worsening symptoms that tend to be progressive. Many patients give a history of many years of worsening symptoms at first overlooked and then attributed to a functional or psychogenic cause until a diagnosis of SD is made. With better recognition of this disorder and the development of a national network of SD support groups, SD diagnosis at an early stage is becoming much more common.

The diagnosis of SD is made by the recognition of the characteristic voice and confirmed by flexible laryngoscopy where the episodes of spasm can be observed during conversational speech or when prompted by passages that precipitate spasm. At times, the diagnosis is difficult because of an associated tremor or other neurologic or neuromuscular disorder. The treatment of SD begins with a course of voice therapy. In some cases, particularly in patients with early disease, voice therapy may be adequate to keep the individual functioning well and may minimize other procedures in those who require further treatment.

Unfortunately, the natural history of SD is for progression so that treatment other than voice therapy is ultimately needed. The first described successful surgical treatment for SD was unilateral recurrent laryngeal nerve section. This procedure was successful in most patients but with long follow-up as many as 50% of patients had recurrence of their symptoms and some had worse voices because of loss of unilateral innervation. Because of these problems, other techniques were explored. Thyroplasty with retrusion of the anterior commissure similarly had good initial results but long-term success was only achievable in about 50% of patients while most had significant deepening of the voice. Selective denervation has been described more recently, but there is not enough experience to predict long-term efficacy.

The treatment of choice for most laryngologists who treat patients with SD is botulinum toxin type A injections.[52] BOTOX blocks the chemical interaction at the neuromuscular junction. It has been used successfully in both adductor SD, where it is almost universally effective, and in abductor SD, where results have been good but somewhat more unpredictable. The disadvantage of BOTOX is that results are temporary and patients require repeat injections every 3 to 6 months. Overall, the high success rate and the minimal morbidity associated with the procedure have resulted in BOTOX becoming the treatment of choice for most cases of SD at this time. Continuation of voice therapy between injections has been found to prolong the time between injections.

Neurologic Disorders Affecting Voice

The nervous system is critical to the production of voice in coordinating the activities of the lungs, larynx, and resonating cavities. Kinesthetic and proprioreceptive feedback is necessary for the control of phonation both through voluntary control and reflex action.[52,53] Alterations in the sensory or motor function of any of the components necessary to the production in the voice or speech may dramatically impact function. Although most neurologic disorders have some effect on voice, a few stand out either because of their selectivity to voice dysfunction or their frequency in the population. These are discussed in more detail.

Tremor can cause significant problems in voice production. The tremor may occur because of a global disorder such as Parkinson's disease or may only occur with phonation, or an essential voice tremor. At times, the tremor may worsen with stress or illness. Physical examination will usually identify the tremor, although tremor may be confused with other neurologic voice disorders such as spasmodic dysphonia. Once identified, mild tremor can usually be managed with voice therapy or beta-adrenergic blockers, although more significant tremors may be difficult to control even with substantive pharmacologic therapy.

Multiple sclerosis (MS) is a disease of undetermined cause characterized by demyelination of the white matter of the brainstem, spinal cord, cerebellum, and periventricular region. MS classically presents with Charcot's triad of nystagmus, dysarthric speech, and intention tremor, although this triad may not be present in many patients. MS often involves a number of motor and sensory functions of the head and neck including smell, vision, facial weakness, alterations in balance and hearing, and dysarthric speech. The prevalence of MS is greater in the higher latitudes of both the southern and northern hemispheres and can affect as many as 80 per 100,000 persons in some places in the United States. Most patients present between the ages of 20 and 40 with a slight male predominance.[52,54] The hallmark of MS is recurring episodes of focal neurologic deficits that remit and recur, sometimes over relatively long periods. Over time, unfortunately, the disease does progress with resultant permanent neurologic deficits. The diagnosis is made in an individual with suspicious symptoms by MRI scanning which shows evidence of demyelination or by spinal tap. The treatment of MS is symptomatic. Speech, voice, swallowing, balance therapy, and hearing augmentation can be of great value in treating the patient with MS. Adrenocorticosteroid may be of value during the active phase of the disease.

Myasthenia gravis is a disease characterized by fatiguability of muscles with gradual return of muscle strength after use. Although it can affect any striated muscle, there is an increased susceptibility of the muscles innervated by cranial nerves, particularly those innervated by the facial, vagus, and oculomotor nerves. Myasthenia has a male predominance of 2:1 and occurs in approximately 10 per 100,000 people.[52,54] The peak onset is in the sixth to seventh decades for men and third decade for women. Dysphonia or dysarthria occur in 6 to 25% of individuals, with the most common symptom being ptosis. Vocal fatigue with use or fatigue of the lips, tongue, and mouth while speaking or chewing are common complaints. Laryngeal dysfunction has been found to be abnormal in 60% of affected individuals. The diagnosis is made by a history of muscle fatigue with use and confirmed by a tensilon test. Electromyography will show fatigue on repeat electrical stimulation. The treatment of myasthenia is with acetyl cholinesterase inhibitors, steroids, and in some cases thymectomy.

Laryngeal Trauma

Laryngeal trauma is often fatal and the total number of cases is difficult to measure because many victims do not reach health care facilities. Significant laryngeal injury may be the result of either blunt or penetrating trauma with motor vehicle accidents the most common cause of blunt injuries. The importance of correctly identifying an injury to the larynx or trachea is reflected in the ABCs of trauma evaluation: Airway, Breathing, Circulation.

If the airway is obstructed or becoming obstructed, it must be reestablished immediately. With significant laryngeal trauma, transoral endotracheal intubation is often impossible or even dangerous because it can convert a partial obstruction to a complete one.[58] Therefore, a surgical airway, usually a tracheotomy, is performed to bypass the obstructed segment. Once the airway has been secured, other injuries have been assessed, and the patient stabilized, the nature of the laryngeal injury is determined. If the patient is stable from the start, the larynx can be evaluated before any intervention. Preoperative evaluation includes indirect or fiberoptic laryngoscopy and CT scan of the larynx.[59]

While acute obstruction of the airway is the most dangerous aspect of laryngeal trauma, the long-term complications of laryngeal trauma can be devastating. Loss of the normal dimensions of the cartilaginous framework of the larynx and trachea or scarring within the lumen can cause chronic obstruction requiring long-term tracheotomy. Loss of innervation to the larynx can cause both airway and voice problems. Disruption and scarring of the vocal folds will cause varying degrees of voice problems. Occasionally, the larynx becomes incompetent, resulting in aspiration and dysphagia.

The surgeon's goal when repairing the injured larynx is to avoid these chronic complications. This is achieved by trying to restore the original anatomy. Disrupted mucosa is sewn or grafted if there has been tissue loss. Internal laryngeal ligaments must be reattached to the cartilaginous framework, especially the anterior commissure. The laryngeal framework is restored to its original shape with use of wires, sutures, or microplates.[60] (Figure 20–22) Stents are sometimes necessary to maintain a lumen during the healing process, al-

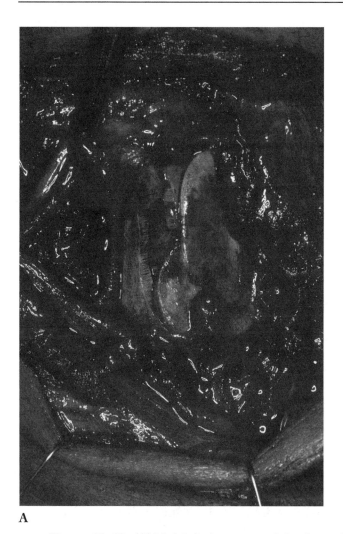

A   B

Figure 20–22. (**A**) Multiple fractures of the thyroid cartilage after a motor vehicle accident. The mucosa of the true and false vocal folds was also disrupted (not seen). (**B**) After repair of the mucosal injuries and reconstruction of the cartilagenous framework with microplates. See Color Plates 17 and 18.

though the stents themselves can cause tissue reaction and scarring.

After the initial repair of the laryngeal injury, more surgery may be necessary if problems persist with airway, voice, or swallowing. These revision procedures may be done either endoscopically or through an open approach, depending on the particular problem being addressed. Once healing is complete, most patients can be decannulated. Voice results are more difficult to predict and after severe trauma, a "normal" voice is sometimes impossible to obtain. A functional voice is sometimes the most realistic goal.[58] Dysphagia is not usually a severe long-term problem following laryngeal trauma.

Tracheo(s)tomy

Tracheotomy is the surgical opening of the trachea to achieve an airway directly from the anterior neck to the trachea, bypassing the oral and nasal cavities, pharynx, and larynx. Tracheostomy, as opposed to tracheotomy, implies a permanent opening, although the two terms are commonly used interchangeably. Tracheotomy is performed for two basic reasons: to bypass an obstruction of the airway above the proximal trachea or to provide stable, long-term easy access to the airway, usually for mechanical ventilation or pulmonary toilet.

Upper airway obstruction is caused by many different processes. Tumors of the upper aerodigestive tract may block the breathing passages. Surgery to remove these lesions can also result in enough swelling, usually short term, to obstruct breathing. Tracheotomy bypasses the region of obstruction in the pharynx in patients with severe obstructive sleep apnea. Facial trauma or deep neck abscesses may cause enough swelling to require tracheotomy until that problem has resolved. Bilateral vocal fold paralysis, laryngeal and subglottic stenosis, and tracheal stenosis often lead to tracheotomy either as a permanent treatment or for securing the airway while surgical procedures are performed on the larynx or trachea to relieve the constriction. Patients with chronic lung disease and other systemic illnesses that require long term (greater than seven days) mechanical ventilation will benefit from tracheotomy by removing the endotracheal tube from the larynx and subglottis where it can cause injuries that may result in dysphonia or stenosis. The tracheotomy tube is also more comfortable, better tolerated,[61] and easier to care for than an endotracheal tube, which passes through the nasal or oral cavities on its way to the larynx. The shorter tracheotomy tube also decreases ventilatory dead space, thereby easing the process of weaning from the ventilator.

Tracheotomy involves making an incision through the anterior skin of the neck, dissecting between the strap muscles, avoiding or dividing the isthmus of the thyroid gland, and entering the trachea through its anterior wall in the region of the second or third tracheal rings. Fortunately, these structures, in a thin person, are relatively close to the skin, making the procedure fairly straightforward. It is much more difficult in a person with a deep neck abscess, a neck tumor, severe scarring of the trachea itself, or in an obese person, which is often the case in patients with severe obstructive sleep apnea.

An emergency tracheotomy, in a patient with a rapidly deteriorating airway such as a trauma patient, can be a very stressful procedure and the need for speed as well as the often altered anatomy make this somewhat more difficult than an elective procedure. A tracheotomy done for obstruction provides an airway for the patient to breathe, but does not limit the ability to speak if the obstructing lesion does not impair laryngeal function. Once air is inspired through the tube into the lungs, the air can be exhaled past the tube or through a hole in the superior aspect of the tube (fenestrated tube) by plugging the external hole of the tube to redirect the air through the larynx. This can be done with a finger or a one-way valve placed on the end of the tube such as the Passy-Muir valve. If the tube is needed for long-term ventilation, a cuff around the end of the tube will stop air from passing around the tube since all the air must flow from the ventilator to the lungs without leaking. This prevents speaking. There are some devices that provide an external airflow above the tracheotomy tube and through the larynx for speaking while on a ventilator.

Swallowing is sometimes affected by placement of a tracheotomy by limiting the elevation of the larynx and trachea during the swallow. In most cases, however, the patient will be able to take an oral diet soon after the tracheotomy, providing that other medical conditions do not preclude it. A cuffed tube may impair swallowing by compressing the esophagus.

Aspiration is sometimes cited as an indication for tracheotomy in the hopes that a cuffed tube will prevent passage of food and saliva into the distal trachea. This is not a dependable method for preventing aspiration, however, so other indications for the tracheotomy should be present. Swallowing therapy should also be undertaken before the surgical procedure is performed.

Tracheotomy is a temporary condition. The tract through which the tube is placed is skin-lined only on those rare occasions when a permanent stoma is created. In most cases, when the tube is no longer needed, it can be removed and the hole will heal within days or weeks. The resulting scar is usually mild if the tube has been in place for only a short time. The longer it has been in place, the more noticeable the scar. Revision of the scar for a better cosmetic appearance is possible at a later date. Even a temporary tracheotomy wound will rarely require surgical closure. Long-term side effects of tracheotomy, which are not common, include stenosis of the trachea at the site of the stoma, voice disorders, and, rarely, dysphagia.

Professional Voice Disorders

Performing or professional vocalists may experience unique and difficult-to-manage problems related to voice. Since their lifestyle and often livelihood depend on the quality of their voices, even minor alterations can have significant consequences. Furthermore, the drive necessary to be successful and the personality required to be visible may result in voice overuse at a time when voice moderation would be preferred. The lifestyle of performers is often not conducive to preferred voice behaviors. The professional often has an aggressive travel or recording schedule intermixed with interviews. They usually perform at night and eat after performances predisposing them to GPRD. They have poor control over such environmental issues as dryness and dust, particularly when on the road. The avocational singer frequently performs after a full day's work or family commitments and often requires substantial voice use.

The most critical part of the evaluation of the singer or professional speaker is the history. Not only should clinicians question the severity, timing, and onset of the dysphonia, they should assess the performer's experience, training, and lifestyle. The time of the next performance and any important career performances that are upcoming should be determined. The choir singer who does not solo and does not have to sing for two weeks would be approached very differently from the star opera or pop singer who has a key performance in three hours. Lifestyle behaviors that could be detrimental to voice use such as substance abuse or eating disorders such as bulimia should be identified. Environmental factors such as allergies, dryness, dust, or frequent travel may all impact the voice. A list of medications should be obtained. Certain medications such as diuretics or antihistamines may be used by performers without their realizing the potential drying effect, and these and all other medications should be identified.

The physical examination should be complete and include any areas identified as possible problems through the history. The oral cavity and pharyngeal examinations should look for signs of inflammation, dryness, or evidence of reflux or allergies. Palpation of the neck may reveal neck tightness or tenderness and scalloping of the tongue may be a sign of tension. The larynx should first be viewed with a mirror to give a global view of the pharynx and larynx. Most diagnoses will be made through history, and mirror laryngoscopy (although videostroboscopy may give additional information) is helpful in patient education and very useful in following progression of the disorder or the response to treatment. Objective voice evaluations are especially important in the evaluation of the singer to allow for assessment of minor changes in voice or progress in treatment that might not be assessed by visualization of the larynx.

The treatment of dysphonia in the performer usually involves the multidisciplinary input of the otolaryngologist and speech–language pathologist and often requires the aid of a trained teacher of music and singing. Simple conservative measures are helpful in most individuals regardless of their specific pathology. These would include education regarding diet and lifestyle, hydration, humidification, anti-reflux measures, and caution regarding excessive, prolonged, or abusive vocalization. Assessment of the singing range may identify whether or not the material is "right" for the singer. In many cases, particularly in amateur singers, technical problems with voice production would require professional voice instruction. Voice training from a speech–language pathologist will minimize the negative effects of improper speaking voice use and may carry over to the singing voice.

On occasion, acute disorders, such a virus or upper respiratory tract infection, may occur at a time where performances cannot be canceled or changed. In such cases, it is critical for the voice treatment team to determine whether or not proceeding has the potential for long-term or even permanent injury to the voice. If this is likely, then the performance should be canceled.

Fortunately, these are rare circumstances. Usually the singer can be managed with symptomatic treatment such as humidification, hydration, decongestants, and mucolytics. Antihistamines should be avoided, if possible, because of their potential drying side effects and inhalant steroids are not of value and may even be contraindicated in acute laryngeal inflammation. If evidence of an infection exists, antibiotics should be started with the type of antibiotic being determined by the likely pathogens or by culture. On rare occasions such symptomatic treatment is not sufficient and a short course of systemic steroids may be considered.

Chronic voice disorders are not uncommon in performers. The most common significant disorders are focal edema (Reinke's) or vocal nodules. With proper voice training and modifications along with lifestyle measures, these resolve in almost all patients. Fortunately, surgery in performers is rarely indicated. If, however, this becomes necessary, then it should be performed by an experienced laryngologist utilizing microscopic surgical techniques. Postoperative care should be aggressive and multidisciplinary. The recovery should be graduated and the performer should only return to singing when there is evidence of complete recovery.

GASTROESOPHAGEAL AND PHARYNGEAL REFLUX DISEASE

Gastroesophageal (GERD) and gastropharyngeal (GPRD) reflux have been recently identified to either be causative or a cofactor in many diseases and disorders of the esophagus, pharynx, larynx, and upper respiratory tract. Recent studies have shown that reflux is a likely cause of unexplained cough, globus sensation, hoarseness, and chronic throat clearing.[55] Furthermore, GPRD is often confused with sinus disease in that patients complain of thick mucus sticking in the throat and attribute such symptoms to posterior nasal drainage from sinus disease, even if they have no other nasal or sinus symptoms. The throat clearing can become habitual, and the symptoms perpetuate.

There are four major mechanisms for the prevention of GERD or GPRD: (1) the upper esophageal sphincter (UES), which is primarily the cricopharyngeus muscle that has resting tone and relaxes with swallowing; (2) esophageal motility; (3) the lower esophageal sphincter (LES), which is a pseudo sphincter created by a pressure differential between the thorax and abdominal cavities; (4) gastric motility and emptying. The three major causes of reflux disease are decreased esophageal motility, decreased LES tone, and delayed gastric emptying.[56] There is some debate related to the role of the UES in reflux disease, but given that pharyngeal reflux occurs, this would suggest an important role. Most reflux disease is the result of lifestyle and diet. High fat foods, alcohol, caffeine, and large meals all predispose to reflux. Furthermore, late night eating, just prior to bedtime prompts acid/pepsin production to digest the food while recumbency prevents the gravitational aid in prevention of reflux. Overweight individuals are more likely to reflux, and age can result in changes in LES tone. Finally, hiatal hernias can result in loss of LES prevention of reflux.

The typical patient with GPRD often presents with a different constellation of symptoms from those with GERD. Where GERD patients often complain of dyspepsia and heartburn, those with GPRD will usually have nonspecific symptoms such as mild hoarseness usually worse in the morning, a foreign body or "globus" sensation, nocturnal cough, or the need to chronically clear the throat. The diagnosis in such patients is usually made by history suggestive of reflux. The physical examination may reveal some thickening or edema of the posterior commissure or arytenoids, and occasionally will reveal erythema or cherry-red arytenoids. With advanced or prolonged reflux, contact ulcers, granulomas, leukoplakia, evidence of chronic inflammation, or diffuse edema can be seen. There has been some suggestion that reflux may even be a factor or cofactor in the development of laryngeal cancer. Evidence is growing that in some patients reflux may precipitate laryngospasm or exacerbate asthma. Finally, a relationship has been established between reflux and sudden infant death syndrome (SIDS).[57]

The treatment of GPRD depends on the severity of symptoms and the certainty of the diagnosis. In most cases diet and lifestyle are the major causes of GERD and GPRD, and dietary and lifestyle modifications will be adequate to alleviate the symptoms. Smaller meals; a low fat diet; avoidance of alcohol, tobacco and caffeine; not eating for three to four hours to bedtime; weight control; and elevation of the head of bed will control the symptoms in most patients. With severe reflux and hiatal hernia, avoidance of heavy lifting, stooping, or tight clothing may be recommended. If these conservative measures are unsuccessful, a trial of antacids, especially at bedtime, may be suggested. If unsuccessful, a trial of a more aggressive pharmacological treatment can be considered or objective testing if the diagnosis is uncertain.

A number of tests have been advocated for the diagnosis of GERD and GPRD. A barium cine swallow may make the diagnosis or identify a hiatal hernia, but has a relatively high false negative rate. Acid perfusion tests, pH probing, esophageal manometry, and endoscopy can be considered. The gold standard for evaluation of reflux, particularly GPRD, is 24-hour double pH probe testing that allows measurement in the lower esophagus and pharynx simultaneously and during the day and night. These tests may be cumbersome for the patient and are expensive. An alternative to testing is by a trial of medication. A proton-pump inhibitor, Prilosec, results in acid suppression in most patients and therefore should eliminate symptoms if reflux is the cause. Occasionally, doubling of the recommended dosage is necessary. If this is successful in disease control, then a dietary-lifestyle modification should be implemented. The Prilosec can be continued, although most patients can be converted to a less expensive medication such as an H-2 blocker. Since decreased esophageal and gastric motility and decreased LES pressure are the major causes of reflux, a motility agent such as Propulcid may be more physiologic and would be an excellent alternative to acid suppression.

AIDS AND OTOLARYNGOLOGY

Acquired immunodeficiency syndrome (AIDS) is caused by the human immunodeficiency virus (HIV). This disease has had a profound impact on otolaryngology as with all areas of medicine. Many patients will experience their first symptoms of AIDS in the head and neck. Otolaryngologists must be alert to the signs of AIDS and prepared to make the diagnosis when these patients present.

While there are certain infectious processes that are much more common in AIDS patients, all common infections may occur in the AIDS population including sinusitis, pharyngitis, tonsillitis, otitis media, and externa. These frequently seen conditions, however, will often fail to respond to the usual course of treatment, requiring repeated courses of antibiotics and perhaps surgery when complications occur. This resistance to treatment should alert the clinician to a possible immunodeficiency.

Candida infections of the oral cavity, pharynx, larynx, and esophagus are more common in patients with AIDS. Herpes simplex and zoster infections[62] are also more frequent and more severe in AIDS patients. Giant herpetic ulcers may affect the mouth, nose, or face.[63] Other ulcers of the oral cavity, specifically aphthous ulcers, may also develop into giant ulcers and are extremely painful and difficult to treat. Hairy leukoplakia is a benign and painless condition that is also associated with HIV infection.

Nasopharyngeal lymphoid proliferation may present with nasal obstruction, snoring, and serous otitis media with hearing loss. The findings of apparent adenoid hypertrophy in an adult with HIV infection risk factors should prompt the appropriate tests.

Kaposi's sarcoma is a previously rare neoplasm that is the most common neoplastic process in AIDS patients.[64] These lesions may be in the skin, lymph nodes, or any mucosal surface of the head and neck. Treatment is symptomatic.

The most common neck mass in patients infected with HIV is the enlarged lymph node. If one of these enlarged node becomes significantly larger than the rest, a diagnosis of lymphoma, which is associated with AIDS, must be considered. Benign lymphoepithelial lesions of the parotid glands have also been noted in patients who are HIV seropositive.[65] These lesions are typically cystic, bilateral, and can grow quite large. Diagnosis is based on the clinical presentation and fine needle biopsy to rule out other neoplasms. Excision, which involves superficial or total parotidectomy with facial nerve dissection, is reserved for neoplasms; benign lymphoepithelial lesions of the parotid glands should be followed for repeated aspirations of fluid as needed for comfort or sudden changes in size that may indicate the development of a lymphoma.

Fifty percent of AIDS patients will present with an opportunistic pulmonary infection such as *pneumocystis carinii* pneumonia. Cough is the most common symptom of these infectious processes.

SUMMARY

Otolaryngologic patients can present with disorders that affect speech functions (phonation, resonance, and articulation) and swallowing. Communication between the disciplines of otolaryngology and speech–language pathology can be fostered by familiarity with the process of diagnosis and treatment in each area. This chapter provides an introduction to those areas in the field of otolaryngology that are of the most significance to the speech–language pathologist.

CASE ONE

A 43-year-old woman experiences blunt trauma to the left neck secondary to a snowmobile accident. She immediately noticed a change in voice and mild dysphagia. On presentation, she was noted to have ecchymosis of the left neck and an immobile vocal fold in a paramedian position with incomplete approximation from the other fold. She had no shortness of breath or problem swallowing. She was discharged to be reevaluated in three to four weeks. On repeat evaluation, the vocal fold was still found in a paramedial position with improved, but incomplete approximation from the other side. Her voice remained breathy with poor glottic stops. A videostroboscopic analysis revealed asymmetrical vertical plane and asymmetrical vibration with a large glottic chink. The patient was referred for voice therapy. Following six weeks of intensive voice therapy, the patient had improvement of her voice with longer maximum phonatory times and decreased air wasting. Nonetheless, her voice was inadequate for her occupational needs. She is in sales for a major manufacturing corporation.

Electromyography of the larynx was performed and showed fibrillation potentials from the thyroarytenoid muscle and normal innervation of the cricothyroid muscle. To temporize her voice, vocal fold injection of gelfoam was performed with near normalization of the voice. On six-week evaluation, the vocal fold was again found to be lateralized. However, there was good approximation from the opposite side and, although mildly dysphonic, the patient has satisfactory voice for her occupational need. It was elected to have her continue her voice therapy and follow-up in six months. On repeat evaluation, her voice had returned completely to normal, and physical examination revealed a normally mobile left vocal fold, good approximation of the midline, and return of normal vocal fold waveform vibration on videostroboscopy.

This case has value to the speech–language pathologist because it shows the somewhat elongated course of patients with vocal fold paralysis. It verifies the critical role of voice therapy in the early stages of the disease with the potential of vocal fold normalization through accommodation. It also confirms the important roles of diagnostic testing, including videostroboscopy, airflow analysis, and electromyography in the evaluation and treatment of patients with unilateral vocal fold immobility.

CASE TWO

A 5-year-old boy was referred from his pediatrician to an otolaryngologist for chronic mouth breathing, snoring, hyponasal speech, periods of apnea at nighttime, and enuresis. Physical examination revealed 3+/4 tonsil hypertrophy and diffuse adenoid hypertrophy. Given the child's history of obstructive sleep apnea symptoms enuresis, and tonsilar and adenoid hypertrophy, a tonsillectomy and adenoidectomy were performed. Although the child immediately experienced improvement in his sleep, elimination of his snoring, enuresis, and chronic mouth breathing, the parents noted that the child's voice had changed from being hyponasal to very hypernasal with a loss of air with production of certain oral sounds, persisting for two weeks following the procedure. Examination of the pharynx revealed good healing in the tonsilar and adenoid sites and normal movement of the palate. The otolaryngologist recommended observation, and six weeks following the surgery the hypernasal speech had stopped.

The tonsils and adenoids play a critical role in obstructive symptoms and hyponasal speech in children. On surgical removal of the tonsils and adenoids, the obstructive symptoms usually completely resolve. However, in children with very large adenoids, there may be a temporary inability of the palate to accommodate for the loss of adenoid tissue. This results in temporary hypernasal speech, which will almost always cease spontaneously. In the rare occasions where hypernasal speech persists, assessment and treatment by a speech–language pathologist will result in normalization of the nasal speech. Because of this potential sequelae, adenoidectomy is recommended for children with Down's syndrome, cleft, or submucous cleft palate only under rare circumstances.

STUDY QUESTIONS

1. What are the anatomic boundaries of the oral cavity?

2. What are the symptoms of bilateral choanal atresia in a newborn infant? Why do they occur?

3. Identify common causes of velopharyngeal insufficiency in children.

4. What are common causes of xerostomia?

5. Describe the sensory innervation to the face.

6. How do the cricothyroid muscles act to aid in adduction of the vocal fold? What is the innervation of this muscle?

7. Explain the myoelastic aerodynamic theory of phonation.

8. Name three causes for Reinke's space edema.

9. What are the two most common causes of unilateral vocal fold paralysis?

10. How does botulinum toxin act to eliminate the symptoms of spasmodic dysphonia? Is this effect permanent? Why?

11. What is the most important part of the clinical evaluation of a voice disorder in a performer?

12. Describe three common head and neck manifestations of AIDS.

REFERENCES

1. Benninger MS: Nasal endoscopy: Its role in office diagnosis. *Am J Rhinol* (in press).

2. Bastian RW: Videoendoscopic evaluation of patients with dysphagia: An adjunct to the modified barium swallow. *Otolaryngol Head Neck Surg* 1991; 104: 339–350.

3. Benninger MS: The medical examination. In Benninger MS, Jacobson B, Johnson A, eds., *Performing arts medicine: The care and prevention of professional voice disorders,* pp 86–96. Thieme, New York, 1994.

4. Moore KL: *The developing human,* 2nd ed. W. B. Saunders, Philadelphia, 1977.

5. Bumsted RM: Cleft lip and palate. In Cummings CW, Frederickson JM, Harker LA et al., eds., *Otolaryngology—Head and neck surgery,* pp 1129–1168. C. V. Mosby, St. Louis, 1986.

6. Netterville JL, Vrabec JT: Unilateral palatal adhesion for paralysis after high vagal injury. *Arch Otolaryngol Head Neck Surg* 1994; 120:218–21.

7. Goode, RL: Sleep disorders. In Cummings CW, *Otolaryngology—Head and neck surgery,* ed. 1449–1457. Mosby-Year Book, St. Louis, 1986.

8. Redline S, Young T: Epidemiology and natural history of obstructive sleep apnea. *ENT J* 1993; 72:20–26.

9. Benninger MS, Mickelson SA, Yaremchuk K: Functional endoscopic sinus surgery. Morbidity and early results. *Henry Ford Hospital Med J* 1990; 38:5–8.

10. Cooper BC: Craniomandibular disorders. In Cooper BC, Lucente FE, eds., *Management of facial, head and neck pain,* pp 153–255. W.B. Saunders, Philadelphia, 1989.

11. Sanders I, Wu B, Liancai M, et al: Innervation of the human larynx. *Arch Otolaryngol Head Neck Surg* 1993; 119:934–939.

12. Harrison DFN: Fibre size frequency in the recurrent laryngeal nerves of man and giraffe. *Acta Otolaryngol* 1981; 91:383–389.

13. Benninger MS, Schwimmer C: Functional neurophysiology and vocal fold paralysis. In Gould J, Rubin, eds., *Diagnosis and care of voice disorders,* pp 105–121. Igaku-Shoin Publishers, Tokyo, 1995.

14. Colton RH: Physiology of phonation. In Benninger MS, Jacobson B, Johnson A, *Vocal arts medicine: The care and prevention of professional voice disorders,* pp 30–60. Thieme, New York, 1993.

15. Gardner GM, Benninger MS: The definition and measurement of hoarseness. *Curr Opin Oto-Head Neck Surg* 1996; 4:113–120.

16. Frantz TD, Rasgon BM: Acute epiglottitis: Changing epidemiologic patterns. *Otolaryngol Head Neck Surg* 1993; 109:457–460.

17. Frantz TD, Rasgon BM, Quesenberry Jr. CP: Acute epiglottitis in adults. *JAMA* 1994; 272:1358–1960.

18. Koufman JA, Wiener GJ, Wu WC, Castell DO: Reflux laryngitis and its sequelae: The diagnostic role of ambulatory 24–hour pH monitoring. *J Voice* 1988; 2:78–89.

19. Woo P, Colton R, Casper J, Brewer D: Diagnostic value of stroboscopic examination in hoarse patients. *J Voice* 1991; 5:231–238.

20. Sataloff RT, Spiegel JR, Hawkshaw MJ: Strobovideolaryngoscopy: Results and clinical value. *Ann Oto, Rhin Laryngol* 1991; 100:725–727.

21. Loire R, Bouchayer M, Cornut G, Bastian RW: Pathology of benign vocal fold lesions. *ENT J* 1988; 67: 357–362.

22. Sataloff RT: Structural and neurological disorders and surgery of the voice. In Sataloff R, ed., *Professional voice: The science and art of clinical care,* pp 267–299. Raven Press, New York, 1991.

23. Werkhaven J, Ossoff RH: Surgery for benign lesions of the glottis. *Otolaryngol Clin North Am* 24: 1991; 1178–1201.

24. Ford CN: Phonosurgery. In Benninger MS, Jacobson BH, Johnson AF, eds., *Vocal arts medicine,* pp 344–355. Thieme, New York, 1994.

25. Bouchayer M, Cornut G: Microsurgical treatment of benign vocal fold lesions: Indications, technique, results. *Folia Phoniatr* 1992; 44:155–184.

26. Shapshay SM, Rebeiz EE, Bohigian RK, Hybels RL: Benign lesions of the larynx: Should the laser be used? *Laryngoscope* 1990; 100:953–957.

27. Milutinovic Z, Vasiljevic J: Contribution to the understanding of vocal fold cysts: A functional and histologic study. *Laryngoscope* 1992; 102:568–571.

28. Koufman JA, Blalock PD: Is voice rest never indicated? *J Voice* 1989; 3:87–91.

29. Courey MS, Gardner GM, Stone RE, Ossoff RH: Endoscopic vocal fold microflap: A three-year experience. *Ann Otol Rhinol Laryngol* 1995; 104:267–273.

30. Lumpkin SMM, Bennet S, Bishop SG: Postsurgical follow-up study of patients with severe polypoid degeneration. *Laryngoscope* 1990; 100:399–402.

31. Hojslet PE, Moesgaard-Nielson V, Karlsmore M: Smoking cessation in chronic Reinke's oedema. *J Laryngol Otol* 1990; 104:626–628.

32. Ford CN, Inagi K, Bless DM, et al: Sulcus vocalis: A rational analytical approach to diagnosis and management. *Ann Otol Rhinol Laryngol* 1996; 105:189–200.

33. Jones SR, Myers EN, Barnes L: Benign neoplasms of the larynx. *Otolaryngol Clin N Amer* 1984; 17:151–178.

34. Ossoff RH, Werkhaven JA, Dere H: Soft-tissue complications of laser surgery for recurrent respiratory papillomatosis. *Laryngoscope* 1991; 101:1162–1166.

35. Olson NR: Laryngopharyngeal manifestations of gastroesophageal reflux disease. *Otolaryngol Clin N Amer* 1991; 24:1201–1213.

36. McFerran DJ, Abdullah V, Gallimore AP, Pringle MB, Croft CB: Vocal process granulomata. *J Laryngol Otol* 1994; 108:216–220.

37. Nasri S, Sercarz J, McAlpin T, Berke G: Treatment of vocal fold granuloma using botulinum toxin type A. *Laryngoscope* 1995; 105:585–588.

38. Koufman JA, Blalock PD: Functional voice disorders. *Otolaryngol Clin N Amer* 1991; 24:1059–1073.

39. Benninger MS, Crumley RL, Ford CN, et al: Evaluation and treatment of the unilateralparalyzed vocal fold. *Otolaryngol Head Neck Surg* 1994; 111:497–508.

40. Terris DJ, Arnstein DP, Nguyen HH: Contemporary evaluation of unilateral vocal cord paralysis. 1992; 107:84–89.

41. Tucker H. Vocal cord paralysis 1979: Etiology and management. *Laryngoscope* 1979; 90:585–590.

42. Altman J, Benninger MS: The evaluation of unilateral vocal fold immobility; Is chest x-ray enough? *J Voice* (in press).

43. Isshiki N, Morita H, Okamura H, et al: Thyroplasty as a new phonosurgical technique. *Acta Otolaryngol* 1974; 78:451–456.

44. Koufman JA: Laryngoplasty for vocal fold medialization; an alternative to Teflon. *Laryngoscope* 1987; 96: 726–731.

45. Netterville JL, Stone RE, Tucker ES, et al: Silastic medialization and arytenoid adduction: The Vanderbilt experience. A review of 116 phonosurgical procedures. *Ann Otol Rhinol Laryngol* 1993; 102:413–424.

46. Cummings CW, Purcell LL, Flint PW: Hydrorylapatite laryngeal implants for medialization: Preliminary report. *Ann Otol Rhinol Laryngol* 1993; 102: 843–851.

47. Tucker HM: Nerve-muscle pedicle reinnervation of the larynx: Avoiding the pitfalls and complications. *Ann Otol Rhinol Laryngol* 1984; 91:440–444.

48. Crumley RL: Update: Ansa cervicalis to recurrent laryngeal nerve anastomosis for unilateral laryngeal paralysis. *Laryngoscope* 1991; 101:384–387.

49. Woodman D: A modification of the extralaryngeal approach to arytenoidectomy for bilateral abductor paralysis. *Arch Otolaryngol* 1946; 43:63–65.

50. Ossoff RH, Duncavage JA, Shapshay SM, Krespi YP, Session GA: Endoscopic laser arytenoidectomy revisited. *Ann Otol Rhinol Laryngol* 1990; 99:764–771.

51. Dennis DP, Kashima H: Carbon dioxide laser posterior cordectomy for treatment of bilateral vocal cord paralysis. *Ann Otol Rhinol Laryngol* 1989; 98:930–934.

52. Benninger MS: Dysphonias secondary to neurologic disorders. *J Singing* 1996; May/June: 29–32.

53. Kirchner JA: Laryngeal afferent systems in phonatory control. *ASHA Rep* 1981; 11:31–35.

54. Garfinkle TJ, Kimmelman CP: Neurologic disorders: Amyotrophic lateral sclerosis, myasthenia gravis, multiple sclerosis, and poliomyelitis. *Am J Otolaryngol* 1982; 3:204–212.

55. Koufman JA: The otolaryngologic manifestations of gastroesophageal reflux (GERD): A clinical investigation of 225 patients using ambulatory pH monitoring and an experimental investigation of the role of acid and pepsin in the development of laryngeal injury. *Laryngoscope* (Suppl) 1991; 53:71–78.

56. Benninger MS: Treatment of dysphonias secondary to gastroesophageal reflux. In Clemente P, ed., *Voice update.* Elsevier Science, Amsterdam, 1996.

57. Kelly DH, Shannon DC: Sudden infant death syndrome and near sudden infant death syndrome: A review of the literature 1964–1982. *Pediatric Clin North Am* 1982; 19:1241–1261.

58. Schaefer SD: The acute management of external laryngeal trauma. A 27-year experience. *Arch Otolaryngol Head Neck Surg* 1992; 118:598–604.

59. Schaefer SD. Use of CT scanning in the management of the acutely injured larynx. *Otolaryngol Clin N Am* 1991; 24:31–36.

60. Woo P: Laryngeal framework reconstruction with miniplates. *Ann Otol Rhinol Laryngol* 1990; 99: 772–777.

61. Astrachan DI, Kirchner JC, Goodwin WJ Jr: Prolonged intubation vs. tracheotomy: Complications, practical and psychological considerations. *Laryngoscope* 1988; 98(11):1165–1169.

62. Marcusen DC, Sooy CD: Otolaryngologic and head and neck manifestation of acquired immunodeficiency syndrome (AIDS). *Laryngoscope* 1985; 95: 40105.

63. Lucente FE: Impact of the acquired immunodeficiency syndrome epidemic on the practice of laryngology. *Ann Otol Rhinol Laryngol* 1993; 102:1–23.

64. Singh B, Har-El G, Lucente FE: Kaposi's sarcoma of the head and neck in patients with acquired immunodeficiency syndrome. *Otolaryngol Head Neck Surg* 1994; 111:618–624.

65. Tunkle DE, Loury MC, Fox CH, et al: Bilateral parotid enlargement in HIV-seropositive patients. *Laryngoscope* 1989; 99:590–595.

21

Assessment and Management of Voice Disorders in Adults

Barbara H. Jacobson, Joseph C. Stemple, Leslie E. Glaze, and Bernice K. Gerdeman

---

CHAPTER OUTLINE

Principles of Diagnosis and Management

Diagnostic and Management Issues for Specific Voice Disorders

Intraoperative Monitoring

Competencies for Voice Pathologists

A knowledge of laryngeal anatomy and physiology is critical to the practice of medical speech–language pathology. Diseases and disorders that affect communication and swallowing in general often impact laryngeal functioning. In addition, surgical and medical procedures (e.g., thyroidectomy, intubation for respiratory failure) can result in detrimental effects on voice production through direct injury to laryngeal structures or through damage to peripheral nerves. The diagnosis and management of voice disorders rely heavily on a familiarity with the fields of otolaryngology, neurology, pulmonary medicine, gastroenterology, and surgical specialties (thoracic surgery, general surgery, neurosurgery). Physicians in these specialties refer patients to speech–language pathologists with questions regarding confirmation of the voice disorder, description of the dysphonia, prognosis for improvement with voice therapy (either alone or combined with other treatment modalities), subsequent coordinated management, and, finally, behavioral therapy for the disorder. Practice guidelines in speech–language pathology state that patients with suspected voice disorders cannot be treated without an otolaryngologic examination.[1]

Laryngeal cancer and airway compromise may present as hoarseness. Due to the life-threatening nature of these conditions, a laryngoscopic exam must be performed by an otolaryngologist before beginning any treatment program for a patient with a voice disorder.

In this chapter, we present a broad overview of voice pathology practice in the medical setting. We discuss general principles relating to the diagnosis and management of voice disorders, specific diagnostic and treatment issues for various classes of voice disorders, and intraoperative monitoring in phonosurgery. For more information about the diagnosis and management of voice disorders, several texts provide excellent coverage of this topic.[2–7] Within this book, the reader is referred to Chapters 20, 22, 24, and 26 for other relevant discussion.

PRINCIPLES OF DIAGNOSIS AND MANAGEMENT

In this section we will discuss general issues related to the diagnosis and management of voice disorders. Until the early 1980s, the practice of voice pathology relied heavily on auditory perceptual judgments of voice production for the differential diagnosis of dysphonias. However, in the last 15 years, clinical voice laboratories have emerged, and current practice in voice pathology relies on the "objective" analysis of voice production to complement perceptual analysis. This shift to more technology-based practice has placed increased demands on voice pathologists to be knowledgeable about instrumental measures and their application to diagnosis and treatment. Many clinicians use endoscopy and computer-based programs as treatment modalities to supplement traditional voice therapy. It is expected that this trend will continue, and competencies developed by ASHA reflect this.

Diagnosis

The aims of the diagnostic process for voice disorders are not so very different from those in other areas of specialization in speech–language pathology. Ultimately, the goal of assessment in medical speech–language pathology is to answer the question proposed by the referring physician. Steps in this process include: establishing an etiology, identifying factors contributing to the disorder, creating a hierarchy of those factors in order of significance, estimating the severity of the disorder (from the clinician and patient perspectives), determining a treatment approach, identifying outcomes measures that will support treatment effectiveness, establishing prognosis, and determining other appropriate referrals. The tools that a speech–language pathologist uses for the diagnosis of voice disorders are the history of the disorder, auditory perceptual analysis, instrumental measures, and descriptive scales of severity. Table 21–1 lists types of voice disorders and the etiologies that are associated with them.

Obtaining the History

Obtaining the history is one of the most important steps in the evaluation process for voice disorders. In neurogenic communication disorders, testing determines the nature of the disorder; in voice disorders, the history may provide most of the facts necessary to diagnosis the dysphonia and determine the etiology. Information gathered during history taking often drives the remainder of the assessment and determines what direction it takes. Appendix A is an example of a form that can be used to collect pertinent information. Certain elements of the history are significant for establishing

the etiology of the voice disorder. Factors that are important in differential diagnosis are: the patient's description of the problem; onset (sudden vs. gradual); character of the dysphonia (consistent vs. variable); voice use patterns (at work, during leisure, at school); other associated events and/or co-occurring illnesses at the time of the onset of the dysphonia; and occurrence of the dysphonia (lifelong vs. isolated event). Information regarding medical and surgical history, medications (including over-the-counter and illicit drugs), hydration, caffeine intake, smoking and alcohol use, and history of psychological intervention are important. A review of the medical history with attention to the types of prior illnesses (e.g., back pain, chronic headaches) may be helpful in establishing a history of somatization. Finally, work and social histories help to establish the patient's personality style and his or her manner of coping with daily stresses.

Auditory Perceptual Analysis

Ear judgments of voice quality have been used for many years in the diagnosis of voice disorders. Clinicians rely on auditory perceptual assessments of voice production for the monitoring of voice disorders. The experienced clinician has developed the listening skills required to discriminate voice characteristics. However, as studies have shown, a great deal of intrajudge and interjudge variability may preclude development of a reasonable listening instrument for the perceptual judgment of voice.[8–10] The presence of such variability means that a group of clinicians in a particular hospital or clinic setting should train themselves to judge auditory perceptual parameters of voice (and speech production and visual perceptual parameters, for that matter) similarly. This is accomplished through listening to anchoring tapes that are periodically reviewed by the clinician to realign internal listening standards and through reliability sessions in which a group of clinicians reaches consensus on judging vocal parameters.

The collection of information for perceptual analysis usually consists of two portions: a controlled elicited task section and free conversation. The tasks are designed for the analysis of: voice quality (hoarse/rough, hoarse/breathy, strained/strangled, breathiness, aphonia, pitch breaks), pitch appropriateness and range, and loudness appropriateness and range. An s/z ratio (for an estimation of the relationship between lung volumes available for speech and glottic competence) is calculated. To identify specific abusive voice produc-

Table 21–1. Etiologies Associated with Various Types of Voice Disorders

Type of Voice Disorder	Possible Etiologies
Functional (nodules, polyps, cysts, edema, musculo-skeletal tension, Reinke's edema, contact ulcer, granuloma)	Voice production techniques (misuse) Voice use/hygiene (abuse, overuse)
Atypical (psychogenic) (dysphonia/aphonia in presence of normal-appearing larynx, musculoskeletal tension)	Conversion event Psychiatric illness Nonspecific
Neurogenic (paresis, paralysis, myoclonus, spasmodic dysphonia, tremor, apraxia)	Upper motor neuron—amyotrophic lateral sclerosis (ALS), cortical/subcortical stroke, multiple sclerosis (MS), Lower motor neuron—direct damage to recurrent laryngeal nerve/superior laryngeal nerve, idiopathic (unknown etiology); brainstem stroke, MS, ALS, neurofibromatosis Extrapyramidal—Parkinson's disease (PD) Huntington's chorea (HC), MS Cerebellar—stroke, MS, degeneration Myoneural junction/muscle—myasthenia gravis, polymyositis, muscular dystrophy TBI (multiple neurologic sites)
Local irritation/systematic effects (edema, Reinke's edema, granuloma)	Gastroesophageal reflux Drugs (corticosteroid inhalers, antihistamines) Irritative inhaled substance (cigarettes, environmental) Allergies Lupus, Rheumatoid arthritis URI Menopause Sarcoidosis Intubation
Neoplastic (benign—papilloma, amyloid deposit; malignant)	Carcinoma (usually squamous cell) Papillomatosis Leukoplakia/Dysplasia Amyloidosis

tion behaviors, spasm, and tremor, the patient may repeat target words or sentences (e.g., tasks such as vowel-initial sentences and voiced/voiceless contrast sentences). Table 21–2 lists some tasks that can be used in a protocol for perceptual analysis.

The information obtained during the history and auditory perceptual analysis prepares the clinician for expected findings during instrumental voice analysis. Hypotheses formed during this initial phase can be tested and compared with acoustic, aerodynamic, and videostroboscopic findings.

The Clinical Voice Laboratory

The data generated by instrumental measures of voice constitute the first step toward objective description of voice quality. Knowledge of anatomy and physiology of the larynx and the mechanics of

voice production can be examined indirectly through the use of instrumental vocal function measures, including acoustic analysis, aerodynamic measurement, movement tracings, and laryngeal imaging (see Chapter 22). Today, the clinical voice pathologist has the opportunity to employ a number of instrumental tools for assessment, treatment monitoring, and direct biofeedback of voice production (Table 21–3). This complementary information improves understanding of the capabilities in normal and professional speakers and the voice production limits of disordered patients.

The clinical applications of these instruments can be directed at a number of purposes, including pathology detection, assessment of severity, differential diagnosis of a voice problem, and as a primary treatment tool. Objective measures of both vocal function and observation of the laryngeal

Table 21–2. Tasks that Can Be Used for Auditory Perceptual Analysis

Task	Objective	Expected Behavior
Sustained vowel	Judge voice quality, glottic competence	Duration—18–20 secs
Sustained /s/ and /z/	s/z ratio—estimate glottic competence	≤1.4
Singing up musical scale	Estimate pitch range	16 notes (2 octaves)
Soft—loud voice production	Assess ability to vary loudness and to produce a shout	Appropriate shout; adequate variation from soft to loud voice
Oral reading—standard passage	Compare to sustained vowel/ free conversation	Variations in pitch/loudness; adequate replenishing breaths
Free conversation	Compare to sustained vowel/oral reading; assess effects of emotion on voice	As above for oral reading (with more inflection); voice production is consistent
Coughing, throat clearing, laughter	Assess non-speech vocal fold behavior	Sharp glottal coup
Specific words/sentences; varying loudness and pitch	Elicit hard glottal attack, adductor/abductor spasm, tremor, seek variations in voice disorder	Absence of symptoms

Table 21–3. Instrumental Measures in the Voice Laboratory

Technique	Information	Equipment and Function
Acoustic recording and analysis	Fundamental frequency Intensity Signal/harmonics-to-noise ratio Perturbation measures Spectral features Voice Range Profile	Microphone, playback speakers High-quality audio recording system Computer capabilities: recording, filtering, analog/digital/analog conversion Data storage, and retrieval Acoustic analysis software Sound Spectogram
Aerodynamic measurement	Airflow rate and volume Subglottal (intraoral) pressure Laryngeal resistance Phonation threshold pressure	Oral-nasal airflow mask Oral sensing tube Pneumotachometer or warm wire anemometer
Stroboscopic imaging of the larynx (see Chapter 22 for full description)	Gross structure Gross movements Vibratory characteristics	Endoscopes (rigid, flexible) Stroboscopic light generator, audio and contact microphones Camera pack, lens, coupling devices SVHS recorder, monitor, color video printer
Electroglottography (EGG)	Vocal fold contact area	Electroglottograph
Electromyography (EMG)	Muscle activity	Electromyography recorder

image can be used by the voice pathologist to display, instruct, motivate, and justify treatment needs. Instrumental feedback may assist with achieving target behaviors. Repeated pre- and post-test measurements may reinforce the patient's progress. Finally, information about the vocal pathology offers an illustration or documentation of the pathology that may be more convincing than perceptual judgments of voice quality alone.

The user must always recognize that all non-invasive voice laboratory measurements are *indirect* estimates of vocal function from which one might make inferences about voice quality or laryngeal status. (Note that the only direct measure of vocal function is percutaneous electromyography, which is invasive and requires collaboration with an otolaryngologist or neurologist in the clinical setting.) Thus, the levels of observation that are represented by various measurement tools also dictate the limits to interpretation of data.[11]

Acoustic Measurements

Acoustic measures of voice production provide objective and noninvasive measures of vocal function. Increasingly, these measures are available at an affordable cost and voice pathologists find them a convenient indirect measure to document voice status across time. Figure 21–1 shows an acoustic analysis system for recording, storing, and analyzing the speech signal. Acoustic analysis routines are written based on assumptions of a nearly periodic, stable sound source, and recording protocols must accommodate this underlying principle. A sustained or extracted vowel portion must be of sufficient length to preserve the validity of acoustic measurement.[12] If the pathologic sound source is aphonic or so irregular (e.g., spasmodic dysphonia) that the patient cannot produce a sustained vowel, then acoustic analysis cannot be used with confidence for that speaker.

Recently, progress has been made toward recommendations on agreed guidelines for valid acoustic analysis. Acoustic signals may be classified into three types, according to the periodicity and stability of the sound source. Table 21–4 summarizes the three signal types and the recommended analysis schemes. A full description of the summary recommendations is available from the National Center for Voice and Speech (NCVS).[13]

Variations in fundamental frequency, intensity, and vowel selection will affect the resulting acoustic measures.[14–16] The number of trials must be adequate to represent the speech behavior. The voice pathologist must observe the patient's production carefully to elicit the most representative production. Test-retest reliability has also been a concern for users of acoustic analysis data. There is an inherent amount of intrasubject variability in all speech and voice productions. To use acoustic measures for pre- and post-treatment comparison, it is critical to exact a stable baseline measure. Table 21–5 displays a sample recording protocol for acoustic measures.

Fundamental Frequency

Once the pitch period (T) is detected, then fundamental frequency (Fo) can be calculated from the reciprocal ($Fo = 1/T$). Fundamental frequency is the rate of vibration of the vocal folds, and is expressed in Hertz (Hz), or cycles per second. Fundamental frequency is the acoustic measure of an audioperceptual correlate, pitch. The mean fundamental frequency can be measured during sustained vowels or extracted from connected speech.

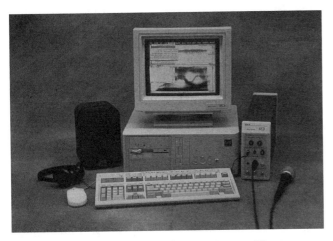

Figure 21–1. Acoustic analysis system. Photo courtesy of Kay Elemetrics.

Table 21–4. NCVS Classification of Voice Signals

	Signal Quality	Acoustic/Perceptual Measure
Type 1	Nearly periodic	Perturbation analysis
Type 2	Strong modulations (vibrato, tremor) intermittency (glottal fry, voice breaks)	Visual display (e.g., spectrogram); perturbation unreliable
Type 3	Chaotic or random	Perceptual judgments of voice quality; acoustic analysis unreliable

Table 21–5. Suggested Protocol for Acoustic Analysis

Task	Measure

Sustained vowel (3 trials each)
    comfort pitch
    high pitch (excluding falsetto)
    low pitch (excluding glottal fry)
	Fundamental frequency (Hz)
	Jitter (%, msec)
	Shimmer (dB)
	Harmonics-to-noise ratio

Glissando (vowel glide from lowest point [f_1] in pitch range to highest point [f_2]	Semitone range {formula = [log (f2/f1) × 39.86]}
Soft to loud voice (count from 1 to 5)	Lowest intensity (dB) Highest intensity (dB)
Read passage	Speaking fundamental frequency Habitual intensity (dB)
Conversation	Speaking fundamental frequency

Variation in fundamental frequency during connected speech can be used to reflect changes in intonation. Fundamental frequency range, also called *phonational range,* measures the highest and lowest pitch a patient can produce. The numerical values of fundamental frequency are nonlinear. For example, the pitch difference between 200 and 400 Hz is far greater than the perceptual difference between 600 and 800 Hz. Therefore, the top and bottom frequencies measured in phonational range can be "normalized" on the musical scale and expressed as a number of notes, or *semitones.*[17]

Perturbation Measures

There are many fine waveform analysis routines, but most acoustic analysis programs offer measures of voice perturbation. Perturbation is defined as the cycle-to-cycle variability in a signal, and two common expressions of this term are *jitter* (frequency perturbation) and *shimmer* (amplitude perturbation). There is a range of mathematical calculations for these terms, which may vary based on three general parameters:[18,19]

1. Length of the analysis window: short versus long-term averages
2. Absolute or relative measurement units: ratio or percentage
3. Statistical expression: central tendency (e.g., mean jitter) or variability (e.g., coefficient of variation of frequency)

Technical capabilities continue to improve, and optimal recording standards and equipment specifications may lead to increased stability and validity of acoustic measures.[20–22]

Harmonics-to-Noise Ratio

Acoustic analysis programs often produce a ratio measure of the energy in the voice signal over the noise energy in the voice signal. Greater signal or harmonic energy in the voice is thought to reflect better voice quality. Large noise energy (random aperiodicity in the voice signal) represents more abnormal vocal function.[3,23]

Intensity

Vocal intensity (Io) is the acoustic correlate of another perceptual attribute, loudness. It is referenced to sound pressure level (SPL) and measured on the logarithmic decibel (dB) scale. Both mean intensity and intensity range (maximum and minimum) are useful measures of vocal function. Intensity measurements can be made with a number of different instruments, including sound level meters, acoustic analysis programs, and some aerodynamic measurement devices. However, intensity measures are subject to several artifacts, including influence of ambient or background noise, inconsistencies in mouth to microphone distance, and variations with changes in speech task, vowel production, or fundamental frequency. A standard, well-monitored elicitation protocol will help minimize the potential sources of error in intensity measures.

Phonetogram

The phonetogram, also known as the voice range profile (VRP) or the physiological frequency range of phonation (PFRP) has been used by teachers of voice and phoniatricians (a term used outside the

United States for physicians who treat voice disorders) for many years and has gained attention for its wide application to functional changes in voice production. In a systematic progression from lowest to highest pitch, the patient produces a frequency range at lowest and highest intensity levels. The resulting plot is an ellipse-shaped frequency/intensity profile, and its dimensions are expressed in semitones. This comprehensive assessment is a useful measures for before and after treatment and for long-term monitor of vocal range development in professional voice users.[24,25]

Spectral Analysis

The sound spectrogram displays the glottal sound source and filtering characteristics of the speech signal across time. Both formant frequency energy (vocal tract resonation) and noise components (aperiodicity, transient or turbulent noise) of speech production are presented in a three-dimensional scale. The horizontal axis is time. The vertical axis is frequency, with the lowest energy band representing the fundamental, and formant trajectories above. A third scale is the darkness or "gray" scale (or color difference) that represents intensity change. Spectrogram analysis can provide an estimate of the harmonic to noise ratio of a speech production. Another form of spectral analysis is the line spectrum, which plots all harmonic energies at a single time point. Frequencies are plotted on the horizontal axis; amplitude on the vertical axis. Advanced mathematical routines, such as fast Fourier transform (FFT) and linear predictive coding (LPC), have been applied to spectral analysis to identify formant characteristics.[18,26] For voice pathologists, spectral analysis is useful in assessing the interaction between the sound source and vocal tract (supraglottic) influences.

Aerodynamic Measurements

Aerodynamic measurements are interpreted as a reflection of the valving activity of the larynx, representing both vocal fold configuration and movement, structure, and function.[27] Figure 21–2 displays an aerodynamic recording system for measurement of airflow and pressure during speech production. Air flow and pressure can be measured under stable and transient speech productions. Average airflow rate or flow volume during sustained productions would reflect long-term or average aerodynamic measures. Momentary changes in oral pressure measured during production of plo-

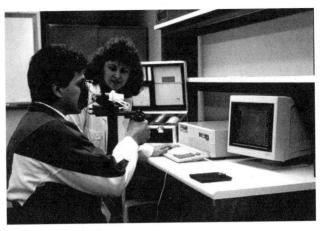

Figure 21–2. Aerodynamic analysis system. Photo courtesy of Kay Elemetrics.

sive or fricative consonants are examples of transient or short-term aerodynamic measures.[28,29] Derived measures, such as laryngeal resistance or glottal power, integrate pressure and flow in a single measure.[17,30,31]

Like all instrumental measures, aerodynamic assessment must be observed carefully to avoid equipment or task artifact. Airflow masks, oral pressure sensing tubes, and oral coupling tubes require an airtight seal with the face or lips. The examiner must attempt to ensure patient compliance and comfort to elicit as natural a speech production as possible. Multiple trials are always useful for securing a stable baseline. Finally, the validity of aerodynamic measures should be verified by conducting a standard calibration routine prior to each examination session. Table 21–6 displays a sample aerodynamic recording protocol.

Flow Measurement

There are two basic measurements of airflow used in speech production: flow volume and flow rate. Volume is the total amount of flow used during a certain production, such as a maximum phonation time. Volume is generally measured in liter or milliliter units. The spirometer is a respiratory measurement device that records volume measures. Two forms of this instrument are available: wet and dry spirometers. The wet spirometer has two chambers with known volumes of air and water contained within. As the patient blows air into the upper chamber, the volume of water displaced by the flow is measured directly. The dry spirometer utilizes a turbine mechanism. As air passes across the turbine, the number of rotations is calibrated with specific volume amount.[3,18]

Table 21–6. Suggested Protocol for Aerodynamic Analysis

Task	Measure
Deep inhalation/slow exhalation (2 trials)	Estimated vital capacity/flow volume
Deep inhalation/fast exhalation (2 trials)	Forced vital capacity
Sustained vowel (3 trials each) comfort pitch highest sustainable pitch (excluding falsetto) lowest sustainable pitch (excluding glottal fry)	Phonation volume Airflow rate Peak flow rate Phonation time
/ipipipipi/ (on one exhalation)	Subglottal pressure Glottal resistance Glottal efficiency Glottal power

The measurement of airflow rate is somewhat less direct, and a range of devices and techniques are available. The most common airflow device is the pneumotachograph, which uses the principle of differential pressure across a known resistance to estimate flow rate. A pneumotachograph is essentially a metal tube, with a mechanical resistance (usually a wire mesh screen or a series of small tubes) inside. As airflow is blown through the tube and its resistance, differential pressures are measured at sites directly upstream and downstream to the resistance and flow is calculated using the differential pressure divided by the resistance. The amount of flow divided over the amount of time equals flow rate. A second device used to measure airflow is the warm wire anemometer. When flow passes over a warm wire within this instrument, the wire is cooled, changing the electrical resistance of the wire with the change in temperature. The change in resistance in the wire is proportional to the flow, and flow rate can be calculated from that change.[18,28]

Subglottal Air Pressure Measurement

Pressure is defined as the force per unit area, acting perpendicular to the area. In voice production, respiratory (subglottal) pressure acts as a force building up below the adducted vocal folds, rising until the folds open and are set into oscillation. Subglottal air pressure is essentially the power supply, and variables such as vocal fold stiffness, hyperfunctional compression, and incomplete glottic closure will influence the amount of subglottal effort needed to initiate phonation. Thus, voice pathologists use measures of subglottal pressure as an indicator of the valving characteristics of the vocal folds.

Estimating Subglottal Pressure: Subglottal pressure can only be measured directly through an invasive procedure that requires a needle puncture into the tracheal space directly below the vocal folds. A noninvasive, indirect estimate of subglottal pressure has been used clinically by measuring the intraoral pressure during production of an unvoiced plosive consonant. This pressure is an accurate estimate of the subglottal pressure only under the following assumptions:

1. The oral plosive constriction creates a momentary airtight seal, which provides a continuous opening from the lungs to the lips (assuming the velum is closed, or nares are pinched to avoid nasal leak).
2. The vocal folds are open so that the oral pressure produced in the plosive production is analogous with the respiratory effort that would be available as driving pressure to set the vocal folds in oscillation.[32]

Subglottic pressure is estimated from repeated production of an unvoiced plosive + vowel syllable (e.g., /pi/). An oral tube is placed between the closed lips and connected to a pressure transducer. The oral catheter must be placed carefully in the mouth, sealed by the lips, and not occluded by the tongue. The length, diameter, and angle of the tube can influence the pressure measurement.[18] The peak intraoral pressure recorded during the plosive production is considered to equal the tracheal pressure.

Phonation Threshold Pressure

Titze[33,34] defines phonation threshold pressure as the minimal pressure required to set the vocal folds into oscillation. The measure has been estimated indirectly using intraoral pressures described above, measured at the exact moment of voice onset for barely audible phonation.[35] In general terms, phonation threshold pressure can be interpreted as a measure of the effort needed to begin phonation. Because speakers with vocal pathologies frequently report greater effort in "turning the voice on," this new measure may prove highly useful for assessing effects of treatment or phonosurgical results.

Laryngeal Resistance

Derived measures utilize measures of pressure and flow in a ratio or product. Laryngeal resistance is the quotient of peak intraoral pressure (estimated from production of an unvoiced plosive) divided by the peak flow rate (measured from production of a vowel) as produced in a repeated train of a consonant + vowel syllable.[36] This measurement is intended to reflect the overall resistance of the glottis and, by extension, serve as an estimate of the valving characteristic, whether too tight (hyperfunctional), too loose (hypofunctional), or normal.[30,31] Unfortunately, derived measures pose some limits to interpretability. The magnitude of the derived value (e.g., high laryngeal resistance) is not meaningful without examining the separate contributions of pressure and flow. For example, a measure of increased laryngeal resistance values might be attributable to excessive subglottal pressure, insufficient transglottal flow, or both.

Other Physiological Measures of Function

Inverse Filter

Any signal measured at the mouth is a product of two components, the glottal sound source and the resonance characteristic from the vocal tract. Inverse filtering is a technique that theoretically isolates these two components; the supraglottic or vocal tract influence is removed, leaving intact the glottal waveform only. Inverse filtering has been applied to both acoustic waveforms and airflow measurements. The pattern of the inverse filtered waveform can be described in terms of opening and closing slopes, speed and open quotients, and waveform minima and peaks.[3,37] One limit to the inverse filter process is the imprecise estimation of vowel format frequencies and vocal tract area functions for the individual speaker.[34]

Electroglottography (EGG)

Electroglottography is a noninvasive technique that uses electrical current passing through the neck to measure vocal fold contact across time. Figure 21–3 shows a typical electroglottograph. Two electrodes are placed on either side of the thyroid alae, with a small electrical current passing through as the vocal folds vibrate. Tissue conducts the current better than air, so the resistance will increase when the vocal folds are opening and decrease during the closing phase. The EGG waveform displays this variable resistance and serves as an analog of vocal fold opening and closing gestures during vibration, with peaks and troughs representing maximum points of ab- and adduction.[38] The technique is not without artifact, however, because variations in tissue thickness, electrode placement, mucous interference, and laryngeal movements can produce error in this measure.[39] Nonetheless, EGG has been used in combination with other physiological measures of vocal function for cross-validation through simultaneous measurement. A most useful application was suggested by Karnell,[40] who synchronized an EGG signal with stroboscopy flash pulses to offer a real-time monitor of the vibratory phase points across the stroboscopic image.

Electromyography (EMG)

Electromyography is a direct measure of laryngeal function and, as an invasive procedure, must be performed clinically by a neurologist or otolaryngologist. Electrodes are inserted percutaneously (through the neck) into specific laryngeal muscles, and the pattern of electrical activity is studied. The

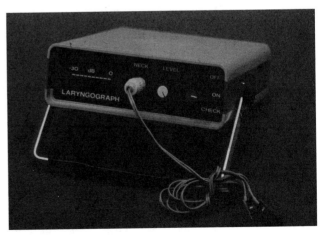

Figure 21–3. Electroglottograph. Photo courtesy of Kay Elemetrics.

electrical signals recorded from the muscles are interpreted as normal or pathologic based on four basic features: timing (onset and offset) of muscle activity, and the pattern, number, and amplitude of muscle action potentials. The widest application of laryngeal EMG is for diagnosis and prognosis in vocal fold neuropathy, including paralysis, dystonia, and other neuromuscular disorders, and for discriminating vocal fold paralysis from mechanical fixation of the cricoarytenoid joint. A more recent clinical application of percutaneous EMG is to identify the correct site of BOTOX injection for treatment of spasmodic dysphonia.[24,40–43]

Normative Data

The number of instrumental measures of voice has expanded greatly over the past decades. Acoustic, aerodynamic, imaging, and physiologic measures of vocal function have been enhanced by better recording devices, signal processing techniques, and analysis routines. Voice pathologists have recognized the clinical applications of these measurement tools to integrate instrumental measurements in the diagnosis and treatment of voice-disordered patients. Yet, interpretation must be done with care and users must be knowledgeable about the risks of artifact and error to ensure valid application of these measures. Some normative data is available for acoustic and aerodynamic analysis.[3,14,44–47] Clinicians who use instrumental analysis in their practice are encouraged to collect data on normal voice production with their equipment using their standardized protocols. As investigation into valid, reliable, and meaningful instrumental measures evolves, progress will continue in determining the markers of normal voice production.

Assessing Severity

The severity of a voice disorder is relative to the perspective of the speech–language pathologist and the patient. Studies comparing clinicians' and patients' ratings of voice disorder severity and impact on daily functioning typically demonstrate a disparity in the perceptions of these two groups.[48,49] Intuitively, this makes sense. Many factors contribute to how patients evaluate the effects of dysphonia on their lives. A person who is retired, lives alone, and has few social contacts may feel less handicapped by vocal fold immobility than another individual who has a more active social life and increased speaking demands. Perceptions of severity may even change as a patient moves through the continuum of care. For example,

a patient who developed granulomas secondary to prolonged intubation for respiratory failure may report less handicap from dysphonia immediately after extubation due to pressing concerns regarding her unstable medical status. However, as her condition improves and she moves from the ICU to a step-down unit to a regular medical floor, she may perceive her voice disorder as more severe as she attempts to communicate with family, friends, and medical staff.

Judgments of severity can be made in several different ways. Commonly, clinicians rate the severity of a dysphonia along a "mild" to "profound" continuum. Patients may be asked to provide a similar rating. However, this may not provide the necessary sensitivity for demonstrating changes in dysphonia subsequent to treatment. Tools are available that can be used for assessing treatment outcomes. ASHA has developed a series of functional communication measures (FCMs) for a variety of communication and swallowing disorders. The FCM for voice disorders (FCMVD) is a scale of severity that assigns numbers from 0 to 7 to describe the range of functional impairment. This scale may not be sensitive enough to reflect change for patients with relatively mild voice disorders. The Special Interest Division 3 has developed a treatment outcomes for voice instrument to be used to gather severity information for patients with voice disorders.

Measures of quality of life have gained recent prominence in the drive to collect relevant data for assessing treatment outcomes. Some standardized and nonstandardized tools are available for voice disorders. Llewellyn-Thomas et al.[49] developed a series of scales for the assessment of the effects of radiation therapy on voice and daily functioning in laryngeal cancer patients. Patients judged their ability to use their voices in work and social situations as well as the quality of their voices. Smith et al.[50] developed a questionnaire that collected information from patients regarding the functional impact of voice disorder on aspects of their lives. Information on employment, symptoms, risk factors, and family history was also elicited. In this study, significant effects were reported for work activities and social interaction for older patients. Jacobson et al. developed the Voice Handicap Index (VHI) which is an instrument for assessing patient self-perceived handicap.[51] It is a 30-item scale with 3 subscales (physical, emotional, and functional subscales). A patient's total scale score must change by 18 points (in either direction) to demonstrate a change in self-perceived handicap that is not related to random variation. The further development of sensitive, reliable, and valid tools for assessing quality of life and the effects of medical, surgical, and behavioral interventions is required not only to understand the patient's perception of his or her voice disorder, but also to respond to third-party payor demands for demonstrated treatment effectiveness.

Other Assessment Components

An oral-peripheral examination should always be a part of a voice evaluation. A thorough assessment includes observation of structures at rest and during speech and non-speech movements. An evaluation of laryngeal area muscle tension is an integral part of the evaluation. Using Aronson's technique for palpating suprathyroid, thyroid, and infrathyroid structures (especially thyrohyoid space), judgments about resting muscle tension and extent of movement on contraction when phonating can be made.[7]

Other important elements include informal assessments of speech and language, hearing screening, and informal screening for dysphagia. Some patients with vocal fold paralysis, laryngeal cancer, and neuromuscular disease are at risk for dysphagia and any symptoms should be noted. In addition, patients with musculoskeletal tension dysphonia can report a globus (lump in the throat) sensation that may affect their swallowing function.

Principles of Treatment

The treatment of voice disorders has traveled the historical path from elocution-based treatments and public speaking applications to more specific physiological approaches to voice therapy. The earliest speech–language pathology texts that discussed therapy for voice disorders described behavioral voice use changes that were meant to develop improved vocal habits as well as some specific methods of modifying improper vocal components such as breathing, posture, pitch, and loudness.[52,53]

Boone[54] was perhaps the first to compile a collection of voice care ideas and formulate a philosophy or orientation of voice treatment that was called symptomatic voice therapy. The focus of symptomatic voice therapy was and remains the modification of deviant vocal symptoms identified by the voice pathologist during the diagnostic voice evaluation. These symptoms may be breathiness, low pitch, glottal fry phonation, the use of hard glottal attacks, and so on. Symptomatic voice therapy is based on the premise that most voice disorders are caused by the functional misuse or abuse of the voice components including pitch, loudness, respiration, phonation, and rate. When identified through the diagnostic process, the misuses are eliminated or reduced through various voice therapy techniques. To this end, Boone[54] described 20 therapy techniques that he named "voice facilitating techniques." These techniques were developed to modify the inappropriate vocal symptoms—thus the term symptomatic voice therapy. The symptomatic approach to voice care continues today as described in detail by Boone and McFarlane.[55]

Aronson[56] suggested that voice therapy often focuses on identification and modification of the emotional and psychosocial disturbances associated with the onset and maintenance of the voice problem. This psychogenic voice therapy orientation is based on the assumption of underlying emotional causes for the voice disturbance. When these causes are resolved, a resolution of the voice disorder will also occur. Aronson,[7] Case,[6] Colton and Casper,[3] and Stemple, Glaze, and Gerdeman[2] further discussed the need for determining the emotional dynamics of the voice disturbance from the perspectives of emotions as a cause for voice disorders and voice disorders being the cause of emotional disequilibrium.

Stemple[57] suggested an etiologic voice therapy orientation based on the reasonable assumption that there is always a cause for the presence of the voice disorder. If that cause (or causes) can be identified, then appropriate treatments can be devised for modifying or eliminating those causes. Once modified, the voice production has the opportunity to improve or return to normal. During the diagnostic evaluation, much effort is focused on identifying the direct and indirect causes of the voice disorder. Once the etiologic factors are treated, the vocal symptoms often improve without direct manipulation of the voice components. Direct symptom modification (i.e., raising the pitch, reducing breathiness, and so on) is reserved for situations where the inappropriate use of a voice component is found to be the primary etiologic factor. Etiologic voice therapy presumes that, once identified, the cause of the voice disorder can be modified or eliminated leading to improved voice production.

A physiologic voice therapy orientation is composed of holistic voice therapies devised to alter or modify the physiology of the vocal mechanism.[2] Normal voice production depends on a balance among respiratory airflow; laryngeal muscular strength, tone, balance, coordination, and stamina; and coordination among these and the supraglottic resonatory structures. Any disturbance in the physiologic balance of these three vocal subsystems may lead to a voice disturbance. Physiologic voice therapy strives to balance the physiology of voice production through direct physical exercise and manipulations of the laryngeal, respiratory, and resonatory systems. Examples of these physiologic therapies include the holistic approaches known as vocal function exercises,[58] resonant voice therapy,[59] and the accent method.[60] In addition, special care is taken to account for the health of the vocal fold cover. This care may be related to proper mucosal hydration, attention to voice abuse reduction, or anti-reflux regimens as examples.

An eclectic voice therapy orientation is the combination of any and all of the other orientations of voice therapy. Successful voice therapy is dependent on the voice pathologist using all of the therapy techniques that seem appropriate for individual patients. Many patients may share the same diagnosis; however, the etiologies and personalities, vocal needs, and emotional reactions to their voice problems may be very different. Because of these differences, the same pathologies may require very different management approaches.[2] Utilizing a case study, let us examine a typical patient with a voice disorder from the perspective of each voice therapy orientation.

CASE ONE

The patient was a 32-year-old woman who was diagnosed by the laryngologist as having small bilateral vocal fold nodules. The patient was referred for a voice evaluation and a voice therapy program.

History of the Problem

The patient was referred to the otolaryngologist by her internist when, during a regular physical examination, the patient complained of intermittent hoarseness, voice fatigue, loss of the upper part of her singing voice, and occasional aching in her throat. She reported that her voice quality was a little worse in the morning, cleared some as the day progressed, and then worsened again by evening. The overall frequency and severity of the problem had increased over the past six months.

Medical History

The patient reported undergoing a tonsillectomy and appendectomy as a teenager. In addition to the surgeries, she was hospitalized for anorexia and bulimia on two different occasions. The last hospitalization lasted for three weeks and occurred 18 months prior to the evaluation. The patient continues to be treated for the eating disorder with bimonthly counseling and for mild depression with medication.

Chronic medical conditions included asthma and frequent bronchitis, as well as air-borne allergies. The patient also complained of heartburn. Daily medications were taken for depression, inhalers and steroids for asthma, antihistamines for allergies, and over-the-counter antacids. The patient also admitted to smoking approximately 10 cigarettes per day for the past 10 years. Her liquid intake was poor, consisting of approximately three cups of caffeinated coffee and four cans of caffeinated soda per day. Chronic throat clearing was noted throughout the evaluation. The patient indicated that on a day to day basis she felt only "fair" due to stress, fatigue, and frequent headaches caused by her allergies.

Social History

The patient was married for 10 years, but had presently been separated from her husband for 3 months, causing much stress and tension. She had three daughters ages 9, 7, and 4. The middle child was suspected of having a significant learning and behavioral disorder that contributed to the daily stress. The patient was not reticent to talk about her depression and indicated that her unhappy marriage, the problem with her child, and her own poor self-concept were the major contributors to her emotional problems. The problems were now compounded by the pending divorce.

The patient had been employed for 6 years by an automobile factory that made plastic dashboards. She indicated that her specific job was in the "molding room" where the plastic was heated and molded in large machines. The molding process created fumes and vapors that apparently caused the patient much coughing during the day. In addition, the machines were noisy, requiring the workers to talk loudly to be heard. Most talking on the job was social among eight people who worked in a large, well-ventilated room.

Nonwork activities included mothering her children with associated harsh voice use, talking on the telephone with her sister, and singing soprano in the church choir. Her singing was presently curtailed because of the voice problem.

Oral-Peripheral Examination

The structure and function of the oral mechanism appeared to be well within normal limits for speech and voice production. The laryngeal sensations of dryness and occasional thickness were reported by the patient. Laryngeal area muscle tension and neck tension were demonstrated by the patient.

Voice Evaluation

The patient's voice quality was described as mild to moderately dysphonic, characterized by low pitch, inappropriate loudness, and husky dry hoarseness.

Respiration: s/z = 25 sec/10 sec; Patient demonstrated a thoracic, supportive breathing pattern. She tended to speak on residual air, especially toward the end of phrases.

Phonation: Breathiness and glottal attacks were noted during conversational voice. Occasional glottal fry was noted toward the end of phrases.

Resonation: Voice was produced with an elevated larynx and retracted tongue.

Pitch: Patient demonstrated an unusually low pitch conversationally.

Loudness: Patient spoke unusually loud for the speaking situation.

Rate: Normal

Acoustic measures and aerodynamic analysis revealed the following:

Fundamental frequency = 165 Hz
Frequency range = 140 to 480 Hz (21.3 semitones)
Jitter percent: sustained vowels = .56
Shimmer dB: sustained vowels = .67
Intensity (habitual) = 76 dB
Airflow volume = 3,200 ml
Airflow rate = 252 ml/sec, modal pitch
Phonation time = 12.7 sec
Subglottic air pressure = 8.6 cm/H_2O

Laryngeal videostroboscopic observation revealed moderate-sized bilateral vocal fold nodules. Glottic closure was hourglass with a mild ventricular fold compression. The amplitude of vibration and the mucosal wave were moderately decreased bilaterally. The open phase of the vibratory cycle was mild to moderately dominant, while the symmetry of vibration was irregular by 50%. In short, the patient demonstrated a stiff, out-of-phase vocal fold vibration.

Impressions

The patient presented with a voice disorder secondary to these possible etiologic factors:

- Long-term cigarette smoking
- Harsh employment environment in terms of fumes and talking over noise

- Poor hydration and large caffeine intake
- Frequent regurgitation
- Possible gastroesophageal reflux disease
- Asthma and frequent bronchitis
- Air-borne allergies
- Prescription medications causing mucosal drying
- Frequent coughing and throat clearing
- Emotional instability
- Shouting at her children
- Talking too loudly in general conversation
- Using a low pitch
- Laryngeal area muscle tension

Recommendations

Symptomatic Voice Therapy. General focus would use facilitating techniques to:

1. Raise pitch
2. Reduce loudness
3. Reduce laryngeal area tension and effort

This direct symptom modification would follow an explanation of the problem and would run concurrently with modification of the vocally abusive behaviors including:

1. Smoking
2. Caffeine intake
3. Coughing and throat clearing
4. Shouting at her children

Psychogenic Voice Therapy. General focus would explore the psychodynamics of the voice disorder. This exploration would include:

1. Detailed patient interview to determine the cause and effects of stress, tension, and depression
2. Determination of the exact relationship of emotional problems and voice problem
3. Counseling the patient about the effects of emotions on voice problems
4. Reduction of musculoskeletal tension caused by emotional upheaval
5. Support of ongoing psychological counseling.

Secondary focus would deal with modification/elimination of the abusive behaviors including:

1. Smoking
2. Caffeine
3. Coughing and throat clearing

Inappropriate use of pitch and loudness would most likely be viewed as obvious symptoms of the voice problem. As the psychodynamics improve, the voice symptoms would be expected to improve.

Etiologic Voice Therapy. General focus would be to identify the primary and secondary causes of the voice disorder and then to modify or eliminate these causes. The primary causes would include:

1. Smoking
2. Laryngeal dehydration from poor hydration, caffeine intake, and drugs
3. Voice abuse such as talking loudly over noise at work, shouting at her children, coughing, and throat clearing
4. Inhalation of plastic fumes

Secondary causes that may be more the result of the problem as opposed to a cause would be:

1. Laryngeal area muscle tension due to increased mass and stiffness
2. Low pitch due to increased mass
3. Increased loudness due to effort to force stiff, heavy folds to vibrate

Therapy would focus on modification or elimination of the primary etiologic factors. The patient would be supported in her effort to stop smoking, encouraged to begin a hydration program and reduce caffeine intake, given vocal hygiene counseling in an effort to reduce the vocally abusive habits, and encouraged to wear a mask to filter her breathing at work. The secondary causes of tension—low pitch and increased loudness—would be expected to spontaneously improve as the primary causes were modified and the vocal fold condition improved.

Physiologic Voice Therapy. General focus would be to evaluate the present physiologic condition of the patient's voice production and develop direct physical exercises or manipulations to improve that condition. This patient demonstrated increased mass and stiffness of the vocal folds that changed the physical dynamics of vocal fold vibration. Indeed, she was required to build greater subglottic air pressure to initiate and maintain vibration that required a high airflow rate. This increased pressure caused her to speak too loudly in conversation. She also attempted to overcome these problems by making physical adjustments such as increasing supraglottic tension in an effort to maintain her voice. When added to the mucosal and muscular stiffness, vocal hyperfunction was the result. The management program would therefore include:

1. Vocal function exercises designed to restrengthen and balance the laryngeal musculature and balance airflow to muscular activity and improve supraglottic placement of the tone

2. Hydration program and decrease in caffeinated products to improve the mucous membrane of the vocal folds
3. Discussion of medications with the patient's physician
4. Elimination of habit coughing and throat clearing
5. Vocal hygiene counseling for elimination of direct voice abuse

Eclectic Voice Therapy. In the review of these orientations it is obvious that each management approach has certain strengths as well as inherent weaknesses. Patients may best be treated with the understanding and use of all these orientations. Therefore, eclectic voice therapy is obviously the treatment of choice with any voice disordered patient. This patient would best be served when the management plan included

1. Symptom modification
2. Elimination/modification of the causes
3. Attention to the psychodynamics of the problem
4. Direct physiologic exercise and attention to the mucosal covering of the vocal folds.

DIAGNOSTIC AND MANAGEMENT ISSUES FOR SPECIFIC VOICE DISORDERS

Functional Voice Disorders

This classification of voice disorders includes those that result from abuse, misuse, or overuse of the voice. Inappropriate use of the voice can cause vocal nodules, vocal polyps, Reinke's edema, vocal cysts, contact ulcers, and granulomas. (See Chapter 20 for a discussion of the pathophysiology of the these lesions.) In clinical practice, these are the most common pathologies seen.[61] In the past, speech–language pathologists and otolaryngologists have used the term "functional" to refer to disorders that were psychogenic in nature. For the purposes of this chapter, we will use the term to refer to voice disorders that result when patients (1) generate voice in a way that disrupts the balance between respiration, phonation, and resonation necessary for efficient voice production (including increased musculoskeletal tension) and (2) use abusive voice behaviors (yelling, throat clearing, etc.).

Vocal Nodules

Vocal nodules are the most common of the structural lesions causing dysphonia. They may be separated into "acute" and "chronic" categories.

Videostroboscopy is often required to distinguish between these two types. Prognosis is excellent for elimination of nodules with voice therapy for nodules that are "acute" in nature (i.e., softened, more pliant). For hardened, chronic nodules, the outcome with voice therapy alone is somewhat uncertain. Murry and Woodson[62] compared various management paradigms for patients with vocal nodules (voice therapy alone, surgery alone, and surgery and voice therapy) and found that improvements in voice were achieved with all three models. The type of nodule (chronic vs. acute) was not a variable in this study. They discussed the need to consider the potential risks of surgery (disturbance of the cover of the vocal fold) and its cost balanced with its benefits when compared to voice therapy.

Vocal Polyps

A polyp generally presents as a unilateral lesion. This mass can be quite large and when it involves the entire extent of the vocal fold, it is considered to be Reinke's space edema or polypoid degeneration. The lesion can also be supra- or infraglottic. On occasion, a reactive nodule will be present at the corresponding area on the opposite vocal fold. Polyps are most often treated surgically with postoperative voice therapy.[3] However, there may be a place for preoperative voice therapy in eliminating reactionary edema around the site of the polyp, thereby clearing the surgical field for the surgeon. While polyps can result from a single event of yelling or shouting, rather than from chronic voice abuse, voice therapy may still be required to return voice production to its premorbid state. Smoking is a significant etiology for polypoid degeneration and patients must be counseled regarding the probable return of polyps if they continue to smoke.

Vocal Fold Cysts

Cysts also usually appear as a unilateral lesion. As with polyps, there may be a reactive nodule on the vocal fold opposite the cyst. Often these masses are long-standing and in some cases asymptomatic. Videostroboscopy plays an important role in differentiating cysts from nodules (when there is a reactive nodule to the cyst). Elimination of vocal cysts is best achieved with surgery. Voice therapy is indicated preoperatively to reduce edema, if necessary. Postoperatively, voice therapy can lessen the effects of any voice use behaviors that may have contributed to the development of the cyst and restore the voice to its premorbid state.

Contact Ulcers and Granulomas

Contact ulcers and granulomas occur at the posterior commissure and vocal processes. Both lesions have been considered to occur from "aggressive" speaking styles that cause increased pressure and irritation at the vocal processes.[54] They are often seen as result of intubation. However, while manner of voice production may be implicated in the development of either type of lesion, gastroesophageal reflux disease (GERD) appears to be the likely culprit in patients without intubation.[63] Granulomas frequently recur and a partnership between the speech–language pathologist and otolaryngologist is crucial in their treatment.

Musculoskeletal Tension Dysphonia

Musculoskeletal tension dysphonia (MSTD), also referred to as muscular tension dysphonia, arises from the misuse of extrinsic and intrinsic laryngeal muscles to produce voice. Often the larynx is virtually immobile in the neck and patients can withdraw in pain when the thyroid cartilage and thyrohyoid space are palpated. Patients with MSTD may also complain of a globus sensation at rest and/or during swallowing. Characteristic vocal fold appearances are associated with MSTD. Morrison and Rammage[4] offered a discussion of the typical presentations of this disorder. They felt that MSTD can occur as either a primary (as a result of psychological stressors) or secondary (as the result of organic disease) disorder. Management of laryngeal area muscle tension is indicated for all patients who present with significant tension and pain at the larynx. Roy and Leeper[64] presented results of a study in which manual tension reduction[7] was used to reduce dysphonia. Seventeen patients with MSTD (and normal-appearing vocal folds) who underwent therapy demonstrated improvement in auditory perceptual and acoustic measures after therapy. Therapeutic massage (by a licensed or certified massage therapist) may be help reduce overall body tension.

Atypical (Psychogenic) Voice Disorders

While the majority of voice disorders seen by the voice pathologist involve some form of voice misuse or abuse, challenging, atypical disorders associated with personality and/or emotional disorders also exist. The major types of laryngeal pathologies caused by personality conflicts are conversion aphonia, conversion dysphonia, and mutational falsetto. The management plans for these pathologies include four major stages. The first stage is the medical evaluation. As with all voice disorders, it is essential that the presence of organic pathology be ruled out prior to the initiation of therapy. The report of normal laryngeal structures will also confirm the diagnosis of a personality related disorder in the presence of inappropriate and often unusual vocal symptoms.

The second treatment stage is the diagnostic voice evaluation. During the evaluation, the voice pathologist, through a detailed psychosocial interview, will develop the history of the pathology and learn how the patient functions socially and physically within the environment. An impression of the patient's personality will evolve. The diagnostic time is also used to prepare the patient for vocal change. This is accomplished by explaining to the patient how the vocal mechanism works and by describing what is happening physiologically within the larynx to create the present voice. Although no attempt is yet made to explain why this is occurring, the physiological description provides the patient with a rationale for the vocal problems.

The third stage of vocal treatment is the direct manipulation of the voice. The type of manipulation will vary, depending on the phonation abilities demonstrated by the patient. Vocal manipulation most often begins during the diagnostic evaluation. The expected result is a dramatic change in the voice toward normal phonation. Greene[65] and Boone[54] both reported that these patients often attain normal voicing during the first treatment session. This has also been our experience.

The final stage of treatment involves counseling to determine why the disorder was present. The conversion voice disorders occur in patients who have undergone some physical or emotional trauma. It is the patient's subconscious effort to escape the unpleasant situation or the memory of the situation that promotes the reaction. Once normal voicing has been achieved, it is a natural transition to begin examining why the problem existed. By this time the voice pathologist has gained an excellent trust and rapport with the patient. With interview questions that are structured in a nonthreatening manner, the voice pathologist can usually determine the cause of the problem. Patients frequently volunteer the necessary information, which often opens a floodgate of emotion.

Once the cause or causes have been identified and discussed, the voice pathologist needs to determine if further professional counseling is advisable. If so, the appropriate referral should be discussed with the patient and made with the patient's consent. Let us now examine each personality-related laryngeal pathology.

Conversion Aphonia

Conversion voice disorders, called hysteric, hysterical, nervous, functional, and psychosomatic aphonia, have been discussed in medical journals for scores of years. Many treatments have been advocated in the literature. Russel[66] suggested that hysteric aphonia was a mental or moral ailment that required moral treatment. The method of cure was "to rouse the will, and thus rid the body of its thousand morbid things." Ward[67] advocated the application of an astringent to the vocal folds along with simultaneous electric shock. The pain of both procedures would influence the patient to talk. Goss,[68] Ingals,[69] and Bach[70] also utilized painful "remedies" such as bitter tonics, iron, quinine, arsenic, and strychnine. Techniques advocated today are certainly less radical but no less imaginative. Let us examine three of these strategies.

Strategy 1: By the time patients with conversion aphonia are referred to the voice pathologist, they are often truly seeking relief from the disorder and are subconsciously ready for change. Often, the event that precipitated the need for the conversion reaction has passed. Some patients may continue to receive secondary gains from the disorder and resist all therapeutic modifications, but the majority will respond quickly to direct voice therapy.

Following the interview period of the diagnostic evaluation, the voice pathologist will present a physiological description of the vocal mechanism, utilizing simple line drawings, video prints, or actual video of the vocal folds. This will demonstrate how the adductor muscles are not pulling the vocal folds together, causing the voice to be whispered. With this visual approach, the voice pathologist has given the patient a nonthreatening, reasonable explanation as to why phonation is not occurring. No comment is yet made regarding the patient's inherent ability to phonate. In fact, the "blame" for lack of phonation has been removed from the patient and placed squarely on the faulty laryngeal mechanism.

Traditional therapy approaches then examine the patient's ability to phonate during non-speech phonatory behaviors such as coughing, throat clearing, laughing, crying, sighing, and gargling. When phonation is identified in one of these behaviors, it is then shaped into vowel sounds, nonsense syllables, words, and short phrases. The voice pathologist must demonstrate much patience at this time. Most patients have not phonated for several weeks. The possibility of proceeding too quickly and frightening the patient away from phonation is present. Once good, consistent phonation is established under practice conditions, the voice pathologist begins to gently insist that it be used during the therapy conversations.

Strategy 2: Another therapy technique utilizes the falsetto voice. The patient again is instructed in the physiology of the laryngeal mechanism and how it relates to the vocal difficulties. It is explained that we are going to manipulate the vocal mechanism in a manner that will force the muscles to pull the vocal folds together. The voice pathologist then produces the falsetto tone on the sound /aI/. The patient is told in a matter-of-fact manner that everyone can produce this tone, even those who are having vocal difficulties. The falsetto is again demonstrated by the voice pathologist, and the patient is instructed to produce the same sound. Some patients initially resist the falsetto production, but in our experience, with a little coaching, the majority of patients will eventually produce the tone. The falsetto is then stabilized briefly on vowels.

It is explained to the patient that we are going to use the muscle tension created by producing the falsetto tone to force the vocal folds to pull together normally. The patient is then given a list of two-syllable phrases and asked to read them in the falsetto voice. During this exercise, the patient is constantly encouraged to read swiftly and loudly. After the voice stabilizes in a relatively strong falsetto, the patient is halted and asked to match the clinician singing down the scale about three to four notes from the original falsetto tone. The patient is then asked to continue reading the phrases at this new pitch level. The same procedure is repeated two or three more times until the patient is fairly closely approximating a normal pitch level. The patient is continually encouraged to produce these phrases louder and faster until eventually the voice "breaks" into normal phonation.

Occasionally, the patient will approximate normal phonation but then hesitate as if somewhat reluctant to produce normal voice. When this occurs, the patient is instructed to "drop way down" and produce a guttural voice quality while reading the phrases. This will "produce more tension." After a few minutes, the patient is taken back to the falsetto voice with the break into normal phonation usually occurring soon after.

Strategy 3: Another technique that we have found useful is the use of direct visual feedback using laryngeal videoendoscopy. While the patient is being scoped, either with rigid or flexible endoscopes, an explanation is given related to the positioning of the vocal folds and how that positioning relates to the present vocal problem. The patient is able to monitor the video over the voice pathologist's shoulder. The patient is then instructed in various manipulations of the vocal folds such as deep breathing, light throat clearing, and attempts to produce tones of various loudness levels and pitches. We have had surprising success in the quick return of normal voicing using this procedure.

It is extremely important that the voice pathologist be patient when utilizing any of these techniques. The normal time frame from aphonia to normal voice is approximately 30 to 45 minutes. Why do these techniques work?

1. The patient is ready for change.
2. The voice pathologist has given a reasonable explanation for why the voice is gone.
3. The voice pathologist has demonstrated confidence in the therapeutic techniques.

Following return of voice, it is necessary to explore the actual cause for the conversion reaction. It is desirable to do this in a direct manner by suggesting to the patient that stress may very often contribute to this lack of vocal fold closure. By this time the patient has developed strong confidence in the voice pathologist and often freely provides information related to psychosocial problems that may be related to the development of the conversion reaction. Appropriate counseling or referrals may then be accomplished.

Conversion Dysphonia

Aphonia is the most common conversion voice disorder, but many other vocal symptoms with varying degrees of dysphonia may occur as conversion voice disorders. The voice pathologist recognizes these vocal symptoms as a conversion disorder when the medical exam yields normal appearing vocal folds; when the history of the problem yields limited reason for the occurrence of a voice disorder; with the recognition of an atypical voice quality when compared to "normal" dysphonias; and in the patient's ability to produce normal phonation while producing non-speech vocal behaviors.

Treatment for conversion dysphonia follows the same approach as that suggested for the aphonic patient. It is important to note that some very bizarre sounding dysphonias can occur. Seldom, however, can a conversion voice disorder patient create a vocalization that the voice pathologist cannot also produce. True hoarseness is difficult to imitate. A helpful aid in determining exactly how the patient is producing voice and for confirming the conversion disorder diagnosis is to imitate the vocal behavior.

Functional Falsetto

Functional falsetto is the production of the preadolescent voice in the post-adolescent male. The falsetto voice often draws unwanted attention to the post-pubescent, physically mature patient. Whatever the reason for the development of this voicing behavior, most patients are ready and willing to modify the voice with direct therapy.

Treatment Strategies

Several therapy techniques are used to modify mutational falsetto voices. The first step of any technique is to offer the patient a reasonable explanation for the vocal difficulty. We often describe to patients how the vocal folds rapidly grow during puberty causing an awkwardness in how the vocal muscles work. This awkwardness causes the muscles to "pull" inappropriately, not permitting a deeper voice to be produced. The exercises used are designed to encourage the appropriate "pull." The second step is to utilize direct vocal manipulation. The following procedure is recommended:

1. Ask the patient to produce a hard glottal attack (HGA) on a vowel. Demonstrate how the vowel should be produced with effort closure. When the glottal attack is produced correctly, the pitch will break into the normal lower register as the falsetto positioning for the HGA cannot initiate this form of effort closure. If the pitch does not break, grasp the larynx with your thumb and index finger and hold it in a lowered position in the neck as the vowel is being produced. If, after several trials, this fails to elicit the desired sound, depress the tongue with a tongue depressor, again as the patient produces the glottal attack.
2. When the lower pitch is produced, identify it immediately as the appropriate voice

sound. Have the patient repeat it several times using the glottal attack. Then produce several different vowel sounds while attempting to reduce and then extinguish the effort of the glottal attack. Stabilize the normal voice on vowel prolongations.
3. Immediately move from vowels into words and phrases while maintaining the lower voice register. Attempt to expand the phrases through paragraph reading and into conversational speech during the initial therapy session.

Using this approach, the voice change is expected to be sudden and the progress of therapy rapid. The best way of accomplishing this sudden improvement is for the voice pathologist to be aggressive with the therapy approach. It must be remembered that the voice is new to the patient. His auditory feedback system does not yet identify the new voice as belonging to him. Initially, the voice may want to shift back into the falsetto. Positive encouragement may be necessary. Follow-up sessions may be utilized to stabilize the new voice.

Most patients are somewhat excited by and proud of the new voice while some are embarrassed by the sudden voice quality change. When the latter is the case, the patient may require a gradual desensitization program as a part of the stabilization process. A desensitization program involves establishing with the patient a personal hierarchy of communication experiences from the least difficult to the most difficult speaking situation. A typical hierarchy may include:

1. Talking to strangers in a fast food restaurant or a store
2. Talking to family members
3. Talking to selected friends
4. Talking in the classroom.

Neurogenic Voice Disorders

Voice production is affected in many neurologic diseases and disorders. In this section, we will describe the salient features of voice in these disorders and briefly review treatment approaches. When discussing the differential diagnosis of neurogenic voice disorders, it is helpful to categorize them in terms of upper motor neuron, lower motor neuron (including peripheral nerve), extrapyramidal, cerebellar, and myoneural junction and muscle disorder etiologies. The diagnosis of these voice disorders relies on a careful examination of the patient's medical history (including radiological exams), family history, and extent and course of symptoms. Some neurologic disease (e.g., ALS) may present initially as change in voice and the speech–language pathologist can provide important information for eventual diagnosis. A referral to a neurologist may be indicated when you observe (or patients describe) any weakness in their extremities, fasciculations (twitching) in muscles, loss of sensation, and/or gait disturbances that are not explained by previous medical history.

Upper Motor Neuron Disorders

Relevant neurologic disorders that result from upper motor neuron (UMN) disturbance are cortical and subcortical strokes, pseudobulbar/supranuclear palsy, and some presentations of amyotrophic lateral sclerosis (ALS) and multiple sclerosis (MS). The most obvious vocal characteristic is harshness and/or hoarseness with a spastic component. Patients with dominant hemisphere strokes (in Broca's area) can exhibit phonatory apraxia. They are unable to initiate phonation or other non-speech laryngeal behavior (coughing, clearing throat) volitionally. Occasionally, patients will complain of a gradual onset of hoarseness that, on careful listening, appears to be spastic and strained in nature. This may be the first sign of a bulbar presentation of ALS. In addition, Silbergleit[71] has shown that ALS patients with perceptually normal voices demonstrate abnormal acoustic measures when compared to normal age- and sex-matched subjects.

Treatment for patients with voice disorders related to UMN disorders is directed toward improving the functioning of all systems involved in voice production. For patients with ALS, exercise is *not* indicated. These patients will eventually require augmentative communication systems. Amplification systems may be of use for patients who have relatively intact speech, but are unable to produce adequate loudness.

Lower Motor Neuron Disorders

For our purposes, this category of voice disorders includes those that result from damage or disorders in the brainstem and peripheral nerves. Dysphonia may be absent or minimal if the vocal fold is paretic and there is good compensation from the intact vocal fold. The salient auditory perceptual characteristics of vocal fold immobility are breathiness, hoarse/breathy quality, and diplophonia. Inspiratory stridor can signal the possibility of bilateral recurrent laryngeal nerve damage. In unilateral vocal fold immobility due to recur-

rent laryngeal nerve damage, patients will often use a higher than normal habitual pitch. This occurs because the cricothyroid muscle is still intact on that side and can still assist in vocal fold adduction. When either one or both vocal folds are paralyzed in the abducted position (adductor paralysis), then the risk of dysphagia exists. Patients with ALS can have lower motor neuron damage as can patients with MS. Vocal fold appearance can assist in the determination of the site of the lesion (Table 21–7).

Otolaryngologists usually delay any surgical intervention (vocal fold augmentation or medialization) until six months to one year after the onset of vocal fold immobility. Voice therapy is indicated to speed the development of overadduction by the normal vocal fold and to minimize maladaptive phonatory behaviors (muscular tension, ventricular fold adduction).

Extrapyramidal Disorders

Disorders considered extrapyramidal in nature include Parkinson's disease (PD) and Huntington's chorea (HC), among others. Essential voice tremor is generally thought to be caused by extrapyramidal damage. PD is the most common disorder in this group. Patients with PD have "hypokinetic" dysarthria and voice production is characterized by monopitch, reduced loudness, and low pitch.[72] Patients with HC have "hyperkinetic" dysarthria and voice is strained and monopitch in quality.[7]

Ramig et al.[73] have developed a treatment program for patients with PD. This approach capitalizes on the ability of patients to use voluntary control of loudness and pitch to improve overall speech production. Studies have demonstrated direct effects on instrumental measures.[74,75]

Cerebellar Disorders

Damage to the cerebellum through degeneration or stroke results in voice that may be hoarse with fluctuations in loudness and pitch. Movements of the vocal folds and respiratory system are incoordinate. Treatment is designed to improve the timing of the onset of phonation with respiratory support.

Spasmodic Dysphonia

Spasmodic dysphonia (SD), as described in Chapter 20, is considered a neurogenic voice disorder of uncertain etiology. Spasmodic dysphonia is not a disease, nor is it associated with one specific neurologic disease. Blitzer et al.[76] describe SD as a

Table 21–7. Vocal Fold and Palatal Appearance as a Result of Brainstem or Peripheral Nerve Damage

Site of Lesion	Unilateral Damage	Bilateral Damage
Above the level of origins of pharyngeal, superior laryngeal, and recurrent laryngeal branches of the vagus	Ipsilesional vocal fold remains in abducted position on phonation; decreased palatal elevation on the same side	Both vocal folds are fixed in abducted position on phonation; decreased palatal elevation bilaterally
Below the origin of the pharyngeal branch and above origins of superior laryngeal and recurrent laryngeal branches	Vocal folds appear as above; palatal elevation is normal	Vocal folds appear as above; no effect on palatal elevation
Superior laryngeal nerve	Vocal fold adduction occurs, but there is tilt of anterior commissure and epiglottis away from the side of the lesion; palatal elevation is normal	Bowed vocal folds with overhanging epiglottis; no effect on palatal elevation
Recurrent laryngeal nerve	Ipsilesional vocal fold fixed in paramedian position; palatal elevation is normal	Both vocal folds fixed in paramedian position; no effect on palatal elevation

Source: From Aronson A: *Clinical voice disorders,* 3d ed. Thieme, New York, 1990.

dystonia (an excess of normal movement); this argues for its inclusion as an extrapyramidal disorder. SD is classified into adductor (AD), abductor (AB), and mixed types. In some patients, there is a familial history of other dystonias (e.g., blepharospasm, stuttering). Flexible fiberoptic laryngoscopy is the preferred imaging technique for diagnosis because AD and AB spasms may disappear during the sustained phonation required for visualization under rigid endoscopy. Tremor may also be perceived at high sustained pitch. Atypical (psychogenic) voice disorders can present as SD and discriminating the two can be difficult.

Many patients obtain symptomatic relief with BOTOX injections. However, not all choose to undergo this treatment, and voice therapy may help them to reduce some behaviors they have developed as a result of the muscular effort necessary to produce voice. Murry and Woodson found that voice therapy that occurred after injections of BOTOX was effective in prolonging the amount of time between injections for patients with AD SD.[77]

Myoneural Junction and Muscle Disorders

Myasthenia gravis (MG), polymyositis, and oculopharyngeal dystrophy are examples of diseases characterized by disturbances of the myoneural junction (e.g., MG) or muscle (e.g., polymyositis). Voice symptoms are related to the site of damage. For patients with MG, progressive hypophonia occurs with use. Patients with a description of rapid vocal fatigue are assessed by using a counting task (up to 100 and beyond). Gradual deterioration of the voice is apparent with increased duration of counting. Treatment is usually symptomatic.

CASE TWO

L.W. was a 62-year-old man who was referred by an otolaryngologist for assessment of voice. His primary complaint was hoarseness for the past six months. The otolaryngologist indicated that laryngoscopic exam was normal.

History of the Problem

The patient noticed the onset of hoarseness approximately six months ago. It was not associated with an upper respiratory infection or surgery. He had not noticed any worsening of his hoarseness, but his daughter, who lived out of state, had told him that she felt it was worse. His voice was bad in the morning, better throughout the day, but worsened at night, especially with fatigue. The patient described some difficulty in producing sufficient loudness in noise (e.g., restaurants, noisy parties).

He noted that he had occasional difficulty swallowing dry foods (e.g., crackers, bread).

The patient drank 6 glasses of water daily. Alcohol intake was rare (less than 1 time/month). He drank decaffeinated coffee and noncaffeinated soda.

Medical History

There was no recent history of surgery. The patient had a history of hypertension, osteoarthritis, and seasonal allergies. There were no complaints associated with GERD. Current medications included Cardizem, an over-the-counter antihistamine, and ibuprofen. There was no prior smoking history.

Social History

The patient was married and lived with his wife. He was a retired auto factory worker. Leisure activities included gardening, reading, and a monthly social club. He described his speaking demands in these activities as moderate.

Oral-Peripheral Exam

Facial symmetry was present. Strength and force against resistance was WNL for jaw, lips, and tongue. There were questionable fasciculations in the tongue. Gag reflex was present bilaterally. Palatal elevation was symmetric, but appeared slow. The patient noted occasional thick secretions. There was no laryngeal area muscle tension.

Voice Evaluation

Voice quality was mildly dysphonic and was characterized by low pitch and hoarse/rough quality.

  Respiration: s/z ratio = 20/18 sec (1.11). Breathing pattern was thoracic. The patient used adequate replenishing breaths during conversation.
  Phonation: Occasional strained voice was heard throughout the assessment, especially at the end of a phrase.
  Resonation: WNL.
  Pitch: Habitual pitch was low. Pitch variability during conversation was somewhat reduced.
  Loudness: WNL in conversation. Vocal fold compression was reduced on the shout.
  Rate: WNL.

Abuses

No hard glottal attacks were apparent during this assessment. The patient reported no chronic throat clearing, coughing, or yelling and shouting. Acoustic and aerodynamic measures were as follows:

  Fundamental frequency = 100 Hz
  Frequency range = 90 to 225 Hz (15.8 semitones)
  Jitter = .33 msec

Shimmer = 5.67 %
Intensity (habitual) = 68 dB
Airflow volume = 3000 ml
Airflow rate = 196 ml/sec, habitual pitch
Phonation time = 14 sec
Subglottic air pressure = 6 cm H_2O

Laryngeal videostroboscopy revealed no obvious laryngeal pathology. Glottic closure pattern was complete. Vocal fold adduction and abduction appeared symmetric but slightly sluggish, especially during repetitive /i/ production. Vibratory amplitude of both vocal folds was diminished. Vibratory symmetry was irregular by 25%.

Impressions

The patient presented with a mild dysphonia of an uncertain etiology. Vocal hygiene and voice production appeared to be WNL. There was no history of a precipitating respiratory infection or surgery. The presence of questionable tongue fasciculations combined with diminished speed and briskness of movement of both vocal folds pointed toward a possible neurologic etiology.

Recommendations

  1. Referral to neurology for assessment.
  2. Postpone voice therapy until definitive diagnosis.
  3. Consider videofluoroscopic swallowing evaluation.

Full neurological examination revealed that the patient was in the early stages of ALS, with a bulbar presentation. The patient was followed in an interdisciplinary ALS clinic and appropriate speech pathology interventions occurred as needed (education, swallowing assessment, augmentative communication). No voice therapy was recommended for this patient after diagnosis, but education regarding optimal voice use helped him to preserve his voice and speech as long as possible.

Neoplastic Lesions

Vocal fold masses that fall into this category are differentiated from functional voice disorders because they arise from disease processes. Patients may develop secondary poor voice production behaviors as a means of compensating for lesions. Otolaryngologists provide the primary management for these patients. The most common malignant tumor is carcinoma (usually squamous cell). Leukoplakia and dysplasia are considered precancerous conditions and patients will be closely monitored by the otolaryngologist. Benign lesions included in this group are papillomas and amyloid masses. Voice therapy is generally secondary to surgical or medical management. Intervention occurs after medical or surgical procedures.

Papilloma is commonly treated by surgical removal of the lesions. Within the last several years, another treatment has been proposed for papilloma. Photodynamic therapy (PDT) has been approved, as of this writing, for qualified individual researchers to treat papilloma. PDT has FDA approval for patients with esophageal cancer. In PDT, patients receive an injection of a photosensitive drug. This drug is eventually shed from the body but retained longer in abnormal cells and in the skin. A laser light source is directed toward the abnormal cells (tumor or papilloma). In essence, the drug enhances the sensitivity of the mass to light and the tumor begins to reduce in size. Patients who undergo this therapy are extremely light-sensitive for approximately 30 days after receiving the drug and are counseled to stay out of the sun. Patients with papilloma who are undergoing this procedure have removal or debulking of the papilloma at the time of the drug injection and light exposure. There are no large-scale clinical studies documenting the effectiveness of this treatment; however, our anecdotal experience has been that PDT reduces the frequency of surgery for papilloma removal, resulting in less potential for dysphonia secondary to vocal fold scarring. Post-surgically, voice therapy is useful for helping patients to achieve the best voice possible with their existing laryngeal condition.

Paradoxical Vocal Fold Movement

Paradoxical vocal fold movement is characterized by wheezing or inspiratory stridor due to inappropriate closure of the true vocal folds throughout the respiratory cycle. This adductory vocal fold movement produces respiratory airway obstruction that may be intermittent or continuous, ranging from mild to severe "episodes" depending on the degree of uncontrolled glottal closure during inhalation. Individuals with this disorder demonstrate normal vocal fold movement during sustained phonation and speech. During an episode, they may often have normal inhalations between phrases while speaking. During a normal respiration cycle, the true vocal folds abduct (Figure 21–4) with inhalation and partially adduct with exhalation. This

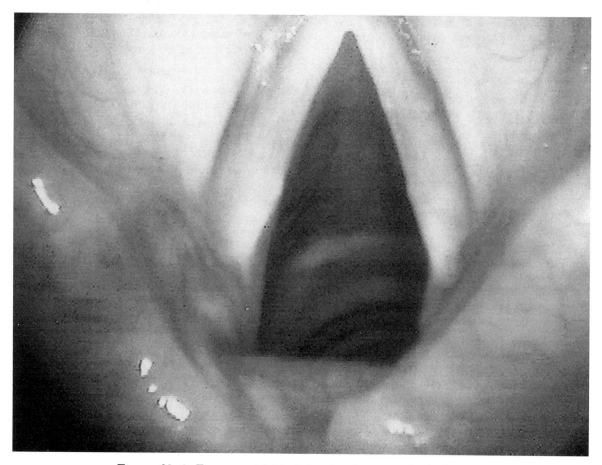

Figure 21–4. True vocal fold abduction in normal inhalation.

physiological cycle allows unimpeded movement of air into the lungs during inspiration and helps maintain alveolar patency by providing positive airway pressure during expiration.

There are many synonyms in the medical literature used to reference paradoxical vocal fold movement (Table 21–8).

The nature of the onset of paradoxical vocal fold movement is not well understood and the incidence is unknown. Onset has been reported in individuals from ages 3 to 82 with greater frequency in the adult population between the second and fourth decades. A female predominance is also suggested among the adult cases. Participation in competitive sports or strenuous physical activity or family/individual expectations toward high achievement is also reported with younger individuals.

Predisposing and precipitating factors of paradoxical vocal fold movement have been reported to occur in several different categories: (1) associated with or masquerading as asthma;[78–83] (2) exercise-induced stridor or wheezing;[84–86] (3) as a focal laryngeal dystonia, or part of Gerhardt's syndrome;[87] (4) psychogenic;[88–93] (5) drug-induced laryngeal dystonic reactions;[94] and (6) associated with gastro-esophageal reflux.[95,96]

The diagnosis of paradoxical vocal fold movement is one of exclusion. Individuals with paradoxical vocal fold movement often present with acute respiratory distress requiring emergency medical treatment. The differential diagnosis of an acute episode of airway obstruction in an adult includes allergic reaction, foreign-body obstruction, infection, aspiration, vocal fold paresis or paralysis, laryngeal trauma or abnormality, and mass lesion. Although each case is managed individually, a trained multidisciplinary team consisting of specialists from pulmonary, otolaryngology, psychiatry, gastroenterology, and speech–language pathology can accurately diagnosis and facilitate the cessation of the paradoxical vocal fold episodes.

Medical testing may include assessment of pulmonary flow volume loops, arterial blood gases, bronchial challenge testing (methacholine/histamine challenge), and chest X-rays. Brugman and Newman[97] have stated that the gold standard for paradoxical vocal fold movement diagnosis is transnasal fiberoptic laryngoscopy during an acute attack. During a paradoxical episode of inspiratory stridor, a diamond-shaped posterior glottal chink or ventricular fold compression with vocal fold adduction is observed (Figure 21–5). With direct observation of the true vocal folds, Koufman[95] reported certain tasks such as phonating the vowel /i/ and sniffing, in rapid alternating succession, counting rapidly and loudly, and non-speech tasks of coughing, panting, and throat clearing may reveal a pattern of vocal fold adductory and abductory movement consistent with paradoxical movement.

Treatment intervention to reduce or eliminate episodes includes psychiatric, pharmacologic, and behavioral approaches. Over the years, a number of therapeutic interventions have been prescribed in an attempt to treat this disorder (Table 21–9). These fall into the categories of psychiatric, pharmacologic, and behavioral management. Psychiatric intervention in the form of psychotherapy using methods of relaxation and supportive therapy[90,91,98] has been effective when emotional or psychological issues and family dynamics have been involved. Pharmacologic interventions including bronchodilators have been used in an attempt to relieve symptoms[88,99]; however, success depends on the etiology of the disorder. Loughlin and Koufman[96] reported on 12 adult patients who presented with episodic stridor or laryngospasms related to eating or in some cases, awakened from

Table 21–8. Medical Descriptors for Paradoxical Vocal Fold Movement

Atypical asthma	Laryngeal stridor
Emotional laryngeal wheezing	Munchausen's stridor
Emotional laryngospasms	Non-organic airway obstruction
Episodic laryngeal dyskinesia	Paradoxical vocal cord dysfunction
Factitious asthma	
Functional laryngeal obstruction	Pseudoasthma
Functional upper airway obstruction	Psychogenic stridor
Hysterical stridor	Psychosomatic stridor
Laryngeal asthma	Variable vocal cord dysfunction
Laryngeal dyskinesia	Vocal cord dysfunction
Laryngeal spasm	Upper airway obstruction

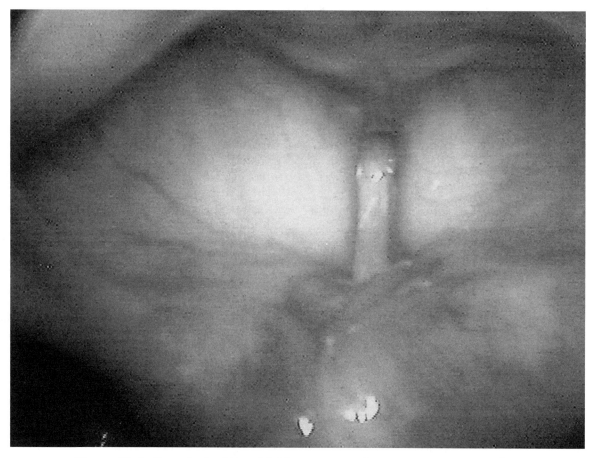

Figure 21–5. Paradoxical vocal fold movement during inspiratory stridor.

a sound sleep. Laryngeal examinations revealed signs of gastroesophageal reflux that included laryngeal erythema, arytenoid and interarytenoid edema and erythema, and Reinke's edema. Abnormal results from a 24-hour, double-probe pH monitoring were found in 10 of the 12 patients. It was reported that all patients had cessation of the laryngospasms within 1 to 4 months following an antireflux regimen consisting of dietary and lifestyle modifications and the administration of oral omeprazole. Symptoms are not routinely controlled with pharmacologic agents when the episodes are functional or psychogenic in origin.[100,101]

Speech therapy alone or in combination with other treatment intervention has proven to be successful in the reduction or elimination of paroxysms of wheezing, stridor, and dyspnea. Martin, Blager, and Gay, et al.[81] have presented a nonthreatening treatment approach that facilitates laryngeal relaxation by maintaining continuous airflow through the glottis utilizing diaphragmatic breathing. Through therapy focusing on self-awareness, the individual is encouraged to become aware of

sensations of heightened laryngeal and respiratory tension during an episode in comparison to laryngeal sensations when voluntary control is exercised. Therapy techniques include relaxation exercises to relax the oropharyngeal and upper body musculature, utilizing diaphragmatic breathing without laryngeal constriction or tension, and focusing on prolonged exhalation. Individuals are encouraged to practice therapy techniques daily and to use the techniques at the first sign of laryngeal tightness or stridor.

CASE THREE

This patient was an 18-year-old female college athlete who had received a full scholarship to play basketball. She was diagnosed by a pulmonologist as having inspiratory stridor during exercise. Her symptoms of noisy, labored breathing occurred during rigorous exercise workouts especially when doing consecutive sprints and playing in the basketball games.

Table 21–9. Therapeutic Interventions for Paradoxical Vocal Fold Movement

Adrenal corticosteroids
  Hydrocortisone
  Beclomethasone
Anti-anxiety agents
  Diazepam
Anticholinesterase agents
  Edrophonium
Antihistamines
  Diphenhydramine
  Hydroxyzine
Antipsychotic agents
  Chlorpromazine
B_2-agonists
Calcium antagonists
  Nifedipine
H_1 receptor antagonists
  Cromolyn sodium
H_2 receptor antagonists
  Cimetidine
  Ranitidine
Nebulized B-adrenergic agents
Nonnarcotic analgesics
  Acetaminophen
Orphan drug
  Botulinum toxin
Parasympathetic antagonists
  Atropine
Proton pump inhibitor
  Omeprazole
Sympathomimetic (adrenergic) agents
  Ephedrine
  Epinephrine
  Inhaled albuterol
  Isoproteronol
Tricyclic antidepressants
  Amitriptyline
  Desipramine
Xanthine derivatives
  Aminophylline
  Theophylline

Biofeedback techniques
Breathing exercises
Bilateral laryngeal nerve block
Continuous positive airway pressure (CPAP)
Helium-oxygen mixture
  Humidified air
  Intubation
Intermittent positive pressure ventilation
Oxygen
Placebo therapy
Psychotherapy
Relaxation techniques
Right phrenic nerve transplant
Speech therapy
Self-hypnosis
Tracheostomy
Visual feedback

History

Past medical history was positive for mild tuberculosis when she was eight years old that was treated successfully without sequelae. She was never restricted in any physical activities on the basis of her heart or lungs. While in high school she played basketball as a forward/center and graduated as one of the highest average rebounders per game in the state. She also ran track and competed in the district finals in hurdles. During her freshman year in college and approximately four months into basketball season, she reported dyspnea after wind sprints and during basketball practice. She was evaluated by a pulmonologist and diagnosed with exercise-induced asthma. Her symptoms continued throughout the basketball season. She was only able to exert herself maximally for approximately 5 minutes before she would experience dyspnea. During her freshman season, a number of different medications were tried including, Azmacort, Albuterol, Serevent, Ventolin, Aerobid, Proventil, Medrol dose pack, and Pepcid. Minimal improvement of her symptoms was noted. After the season was completed, the respiratory symptoms disappeared.

When practice resumed in the fall of her sophomore year, the symptoms resumed and were exacerbated with almost any form of exercise. The athletic trainer stated that her noisy breathing was so loud that it echoed in the gymnasium. After running just one sprint, the trainer reported that her breathing would get progressively louder, with wheezing and air hunger, forcing her to stop and bend over. The wheezing would last up to several minutes before subsiding. The patient reported no relief from the bronchial dilators. She subsequently was evaluated by another pulmonologist who prescribed a thallium stress test. The results of this examination and spirometry were normal. The pulmonologist, on listening to a recorded sample of an episode, suspected a vocal cord dysfunction syndrome. The patient was then referred to an otolaryngologist who then referred her to our voice clinic.

Evaluation

A thorough case history was taken and a videolaryngoscopy examination was completed. This patient was unable to spontaneously reproduce the sound that was made during the acute episodes. She described the acute attack as not being able to get enough air, shortness of breath, tightness in the throat and upper chest, and a feeling of her throat closing. During the videolaryngoscopy examination the patient was able to view her own exam on a monitor. She was requested to adduct the true vocal folds while inhaling and produce inspiratory

stridor. She reported that this was the exact sensation of "not being able to breath in, to get air" that she felt during an episode.

During the case history, the patient reported that she felt an extreme amount of pressure from her father and coach to play basketball. These episodes were emotionally upsetting to her and she was scared that she would be red shirted for the season. She stated that she just didn't know what else to do since the bronchodilators were not effective.

Treatment

Therapy was initiated utilizing the treatment approach suggested by Martin et al.[81] This patient was taught to inhale or sniff in through the nose and gently exhale through the mouth. It was also recommended to prolong exhalation through pursed lips or by saying a soft /s/ or /f/. Attention was given to abdominal expansion during inhalation and relaxation during exhalation by placing her hand on the abdomen. In addition, visual imaging techniques were taught as a method of keeping the glottis open during rapid breathing. These included visualizing the throat being as wide open as a baseball during inhalation and picturing her vocal folds in complete abduction during inhalation as was seen on the videolaryngoscopy examination. Other techniques were used to help her gain control over fast breathing. She was taught to inhale and exhale with an open jaw and relaxed tongue using diaphragmatic breathing. During an episode she was coached to sniff in through the nose and count aloud on exhalation. She was encouraged to remain upright, walking around instead of bending over, and stopping all activity.

The patient's athletic trainer was present for all therapy sessions. He then served as her coach outside the therapy setting especially during basketball practices. Eleven basketball drills were identified that presented difficulty for this patient. For each practice, the trainer was asked to keep a log of her respiratory episodes with each drill. At the end of each practice, the patient was able to review the number of drills partially or totally completed, total number of seconds/minutes spent in recovering from the episodes, number of seconds/ minutes each episode lasted, and total number of minutes of actual practice. Videotapes of her practices were also reviewed with the athletic trainer, speech–language pathologist, and patient. The speech–language pathologist also observed the patient during selected basketball practices and games. This patient was followed over a four-month period. During that time the bronchodilators were gradually reduced and then eliminated. Toward the end of the basketball season, this patient was able to complete all practice drills and played in competitive games without incident.

INTRAOPERATIVE MONITORING

The team approach to voice care is further emphasized by the voice pathologist's role in intraoperative monitoring. The expanded role of the medical speech–language pathologist was never more evident then by the role now played in surgery. Speech–language pathologists and audiologists who have been in the field for more than ten to fifteen years well remember a time when we were restricted to evaluations and treatments that involved only external contact with our patients. Audiologists did not look in ears. Speech–language pathologists did not study vocal function. As a profession, however, we gradually demonstrated the value of our education and knowledge and earned the right to be full team members in the care of patients with communication disorders.

Developing the expertise to fit voice prostheses in the laryngectomized patient was one of the first direct team relationships between the voice pathologist and the otolaryngologist. Soon after, speech–language pathologists became the caregivers for individuals with swallowing disorders. The expertise developed in this area expanded to the dysphagia diagnostic setting including working as a team member with radiologists during the modified barium swallow radiographic examination. With the advent of BOTOX injections for the treatment of spasmodic dysphonia, again, voice pathologists have teamed with otolaryngologists and, in some cases, neurologists. This teamwork includes monitoring actual injections and then the injection's effects on voice to determine future dosage requirements.

More recently, voice pathologists have teamed with their surgical colleagues to directly monitor vocal fold position and voice quality during Type 1 thyroplasty for patients with vocal fold paralysis.[102] The voice pathologist's role with these patients begins soon after the diagnosis of unilateral vocal fold paralysis is made by the otolaryngologist. Once the etiology is known, or other disease processes have been ruled out, the voice pathologist will often study the patients vocal function and voice capabilities through stroboscopy and acoustic and aerodynamic measures. Often, a short-term direct therapy program designed to enhance glottic closure will be administered. When the appropriate waiting period for recovery has passed, and if voice quality remains inadequate, then the patient may be scheduled for a vocal fold medialization procedure. The patient's vocal function will again be studied by both the voice pathologist and the otolaryngologist just prior to the surgery. The stroboscopic study will provide a visual display of the current closure pattern permitting the surgeon a presurgical idea of the size of the glottal gap as well as the anterior-posterior closure relationships. This information enables the surgeon to preplan the size and shape of the silastic implant.

On the day of surgery, the voice pathologist enters the surgical suite with the appropriate instrumentation as the room is being prepared for the procedure. The instrumentation may include just flexible videoendoscopy, or endoscopy with videostroboscopy capabilities. The room is situated so that the instrumentation is located at the patient's head and the endoscope will easily reach the patient and the monitor may be easily viewed by the voice pathologist and the surgeon. The endoscope may be suspended from an IV pole or may access the patient from a custom scope holder as described by Kelly and Wilson.[103] When the patient is situated on the surgical table, a drape is placed over the head from the chin and attached to IV poles at each side and above the patient's head. This drape allows the voice pathologist to have access to the nose with the flexible endoscope without breaking the sterile field.

Once the surgeon has exposed the thyroid cartilage and excised the window through which the silastic implant will be inserted, the voice pathologist introduces the flexible fiberoptic scope through the patient's nose. The vocal folds are visualized and the patient is asked to phonate. The relative positions of the folds are noted as well as the current voice quality. The surgeon then creates a custom implant from the silastic block. The exact size and placement of the implant is critical; if positioned too high or low, a vertical level mismatch will result, and voice quality will be suboptimal. If the implant is too large, it may cause the glottal compensation to be too great, resulting in a strained voice; if too small, the voice will remain breathy.

As the surgeon inserts the implant through the window of the thyroid cartilage and locks it in place, the voice pathologist asks the patient to phonate. The position of the vocal folds is monitored as well as the patient's voice quality. The voice pathologist may have a running commentary with the surgeon relative to the positioning such as, "too high, too low, not enough posterior closure, over-compressed, under-compressed, just right." At the same time, the patient's voice quality is monitored and the relationship between what is visualized and the voice quality is studied. The goal is to establish the optimal voice quality through the excellent positioning of the silastic implant.

Intraoperative monitoring by the voice pathologist for Type 1 thyroplasty has enhanced the results of this surgical treatment of unilateral vocal fold paralysis. This technique is yet another example of the teamwork between the otolaryngologist and the voice pathologist that has improved the care of voice disordered patients.

SUMMARY

In the field of medical speech–language pathology, laryngeal function is heavily integrated into considerations of diagnosis and treatment for a variety of communication and swallowing disorders. Disturbances in phonation can occur in many neurologic diseases and disorders. Medical and surgical management places patients at risk for the development of iatrogenic laryngeal pathologies such as granuloma (from intubation) and edema (drug-induced effects). The speech–language pathologist must be alert to these possible etiologies for dysphonia and aphonia. In addition, atypical voice disorders (including paradoxical vocal fold movement) may occur as reactions to illness or medical treatment as well as to life events.

While speech–language pathologists continue to rely on auditory perceptual analysis for a portion of diagnosis and treatment monitoring, the availability of instrumentation and technology for laryngeal imaging and analysis has altered the scope of practice. The competencies required for providing service to patients have expanded and have shifted this subspecialty to a more medical focus than in the past. The topics covered in this chapter outline the extent of knowledge needed to function as a consultant to physicians and as a provider of voice therapy based on a solid foundation of laryngeal physiology.

COMPETENCIES FOR VOICE PATHOLOGISTS

The following list of competencies is an adaptation of those proposed by Special Interest Division 3. These are in draft form. (Division 3 Newsletter: Competencies for Voice Pathologists. pp. 5–7. ASHA, Rockville, MD, June 1996)

Academic Competencies

1. Understand normal anatomy and physiology of speech production. Apply knowledge of central and peripheral nervous system control to physiology of speech and singing. Understand the influence of age and gender.
2. Understand how deviations in anatomy and physiology of the laryngeal mechanism produce abnormal voice.
3. Apply knowledge of medical conditions to understand the potential influence on laryngeal health or voice production.
4. Apply knowledge of the etiology and clinical course of head and neck cancer to understand the anatomical, physiological, acoustical, and psychosocial consequences of the disease.
5. Know the clinical methods of voice assessment, including auditory-perceptual judgments, acoustic analysis, physiological measurements, and visualization/imaging techniques, and their risks and limitations.
6. Apply knowledge of the benefits, limits, physiological consequences, and potential side effects of medical, surgical, and behavioral interventions to improve voice function.
7. Know basic principles of electronics applicable to the use of voice laboratory instrumentation. Adhere to standards for electrical safety and universal precautions.

Clinical Competencies: Assessment, Diagnosis, and Management

8. Demonstrate ability to conduct thorough, but succinct clinical case history interviews.
9. Demonstrate ability to obtain a representative sample of voice production and describe it accurately and reliably.
10. Demonstrate ability to collect appropriate and reliable acoustic and physiologic measures of voice and to interpret the data.
11. Demonstrate competency in one or more imaging techniques used to visualize the larynx, vocal tract, and nasopharynx.
12. Synthesize and evaluate case history, perceptual, and instrumental data to diagnose voice disorders.
13. Demonstrate ability to develop clinical care paths and to evaluate and modify treatment plans as needed.

14. Demonstrate ability to write succinct reports.

15. Apply principles of behavioral modification to voice rehabilitation treatment plans.

16. Select and implement appropriate rehabilitation therapies for patients with congenital or acquired structural changes in the phonatory mechanism.

17. Demonstrate ability to inform patients of the goals, procedures, respective responsibilities, and likely outcomes of treatment. Demonstrate appropriate ability to counsel patients as needed.

18. Demonstrate ability to assess and respond to interdisciplinary effects of voice disorders or vocal pathology on communication, swallowing, emotional health, and vocational status. Make appropriate referrals as needed. Function effectively on a team.

19. Collect, analyze, and interpret treatment outcomes and patient satisfaction data to assess efficacy of therapies, clinical care paths, and provide justification of service delivery.

STUDY QUESTIONS

1. Describe the physiology of paradoxical vocal fold movement.

2. Explain the various symptoms of atypical voice disorders.

3. Discuss the basic instruments and their function as they are used in the evaluation of voice.

4. What are the limitations of instrumental voice assessment?

5. What are the steps in the diagnostic process in voice disorders?

6. Specify the vocal pathologies in which voice therapy is a primary treatment option.

7. Prepare a checklist that a speech–language pathologist might use for educating a patient who has a voice disorder.

8. Discuss the various emphases in the following approaches to voice disorders:
   Symptomatic therapy   Etiologic therapy
   Physiologic therapy   Eclectic therapy
   Psychogenic therapy

9. What is the role of the SLP in intraoperative monitoring of phonosurgery?

10. Describe the voice symptoms in the following neurological diseases:
    Amyotrophic lateral   Multiple sclerosis (MS)
    sclerosis(ALS)
    Parkinson's disease   Myasthenia gravis (MG)
    (PD)
    Pseudobulbar palsy   Brainstem stroke
    Neurofibromatosis   Cerebellar degeneration

REFERENCES

1. Task Force on Clinical Standards: Voice assessment. In: *Preferred practice patterns for the professions of speech–language pathology and audiology.* American Speech–Language-Hearing Association, November, 1992.

2. Stemple J, Glaze L, Gerdeman B: *Clinical voice pathology: Theory and management,* 2nd ed. Singular Publishing, San Diego, 1995.

3. Colton R, Casper J: *Understanding voice problems: A physiological perspective for diagnosis and treatment,* 2nd ed. Williams and Wilkins, Baltimore, 1996.

4. Morrison M, Rammage L: *The management of voice disorders.* Singular Publishing, San Diego, 1994.

5. Andrews ML: *Manual of voice treatment: Pediatrics through geriatrics.* Singular Publishing, San Diego, 1995.

6. Case J: *Clinical management of voice disorders,* 2nd ed. Pro-Ed, Austin, TX, 1996.

7. Aronson A: *Clinical voice disorders: An interdisciplinary approach,* 2nd ed. Thieme, New York, 1990.

8. Kreiman J, Gerratt BR, Kempster GB, et al: Perceptual evaluation of voice quality: Review, tutorial, and a framework for future research. *J Speech Hear Res* 1993; 36:21–40.

9. Gerratt B, Kreiman J, Barroso N, et al: Comparing internal and external standards in voice quality judgments. *J Speech Hear Res* 1993; 36:14–20.

10. Bassich CJ, Ludlow CL: The use of perceptual methods by new clinicians for assessing voice quality. *J Speech Hear Disorders* 1986; 51:125–133.

11. Titze IR: Measurements for assessment of voice disorders. In *Assessment of speech and voice production: Research and clinical applications,* pp 42–49. National Institute on Deafness and Other Communicative Disorders, Bethesda, MD, 1991.

12. Karnell MP: Laryngeal perturbation analysis: Minimum length of analysis window. *J Speech Hear Res* 1991; 34:544–548.

13. Titze IR: *Summary statement of the workshop on acoustic voice analysis.* National Center for Voice and Speech, Iowa City, IA, 1995.

14. Glaze LE, Bless DM, Susser RD: Acoustic analysis of vowel and loudness differences in children's voice. *J Voice* 1990; 4:37–44.

15. Horii Y: Jitter and shimmer differences among sustained vowel phonations. *J Speech Hear Res* 1982; 25:12–14.

16. Orlikoff RF, Kahane JC: Influence of mean sound pressure level on jitter and shimmer measures. *J Voice* 1991; 5:113–119.

17. Hirano M: *Clinical examination of voice.* Springer-Verlag, New York, 1981.

18. Baken RJ: *Clinical measurement of speech and voice.* College-Hill Press, Boston, 1987.

19. Orlikoff RF, Baken RJ: *Clinical voice and speech measurement.* Singular Publishing, San Diego, 1993.

20. Titze IR: Towards standards in acoustic analysis of voice. In I. R. Titze, ed., *Progress Report 4,* pp 271–280. National Center for Voice and Speech, Iowa City, IA, 1993.

21. Titze IR, Horii Y, Scherer RC: Some technical considerations in voice perturbation measurements. *J Speech Hear Res* 1987; 30:252–260.

22. Titze IR, Winholtz WS: Effect of microphone type and placement on voice perturbation measurements. *J Speech Hear Res* 1993; 36:1177–1190.

23. Milenkovic PH: Least mean squares of waveform perturbation. *J Speech Hear Res* 1987; 29:529–538.

24. Bless DM: Assessment of laryngeal function. In CN Ford, DM Bless, eds., *Phonosurgery,* pp 91–122. Raven Press, New York, 1991.

25. Titze IR: Acoustic interpretation of the voice-range profile (phonetogram). *J Speech Hear Res* 1992; 34:21–35.

26. Kent RD, Read C: *The acoustic analysis of speech.* Singular Publishing, San Diego, 1992.

27. Schutte HK: Integrated aerodynamic measurements. *J Voice* 1992; 6:127–134.

28. Miller CJ, Daniloff R: Airflow measurements: Theory and utility of findings. *J Voice* 1993; 7:38–46.

29. Scherer RC: Aerodynamic assessment in voice production. In *Assessment of speech and voice production: Research and clinical applications* pp 42–49. National Institute on Deafness and Other Communicative Disorders, Bethesda, MD, 1991.

30. Hoit JD, Hixon TJ: Age and laryngeal airway resistance during vowel production in women. *J Speech Hear Res* 1992; 35:309–313.

31. Melcon M, Hoit JD, Hixon TJ: Age and laryngeal airway resistance during vowel production. *J Speech Hear Dis* 1989; 54:282–286.

32. Netsell R: Subglottal and intraoral air pressures during intervocalic contrast of /t/ and /d/. *Phonetica* 1969; 20:68–73.

33. Titze IR: Phonation threshold pressure: A missing link for glottal aerodynamics. In IR Titze, ed., *Progress Report* 1, pp 1–14. National Center for Voice and Speech, Iowa City, IA, 1991.

34. Titze IR: *Principles of voice production.* Prentice-Hall, Englewood Cliffs, NJ, 1994.

35. Verdolini-Marston K, Titze IR, Drucker DG: Changes in phonation threshold pressure with induced conditions of hydration. *J Voice* 1990; 4:141–151.

36. Smitheran J, Hixon TJ: A clinical method for estimating laryngeal airway resistance during vowel production. *J Speech Hear Dis* 1981; 46:138–146.

37. Fritzell B: Inverse filtering. *J Voice* 1992; 6:111–114.

38. Childers DG, Alsaka YA, Hicks DM, et al: Vocal fold vibrations: An EGG model. In T Baer, C Sasaki, K Harris, eds., *Laryngeal function in phonation and respiration,* pp 11–202. College-Hill Press, Boston, 1987.

39. Colton RH, Contour EG: Problems and pitfalls of electroglottography. *J Voice* 1990; 4:10–24.

40. Karnell MP: Synchronized videostroboscopy and electroglottography. *J Voice* 1989; 3:68–75.

41. Harris K: *Electromyography as a technique for laryngeal investigation.* ASHA Reports 1981; 11:70–87.

42. Hirose H: Electromyography of the Laryngeal and Pharyngeal Muscles. In CW Cummings, JM Frederickson, LA Harker, et al., eds., *Otolaryngology-head and neck surgery,* pp 1823–1828. Mosby, St. Louis, 1986.

43. Ludlow CL: Neurophysiological assessment of patients with vocal motor control disorders. In *Assessment of speech and voice production: Research and clinical applications,* pp. 161–171. National Institute on Deafness and Other Communicative Disorders, Bethesda, MD, 1991.

44. Holmberg EB, Hillman RE, Perkell JS: Glottal airflow and transglottal air pressure measurements for male and female speakers in soft, normal, and loud voice. *J Acous Soc Am* 1988; 84:511–529.

45. Holmberg EB, Hillman RE, Perkell JS: Glottal airflow and transglottal air pressure measurements for male and female speakers in low, normal and high pitch. *J Voice* 1989; 3:294–305.

46. Glaze LE, Bless DM, Milenkovic PH, et al: Acoustic characteristics of children's voice. *J Voice* 1988; 2:312–319.

47. Bless DM, Glaze LE, Biever-Lowery DM, et al: Stroboscopic, acoustic, aerodynamic, and perceptual attributes of voice production in normal speaking adults. In IR Titze, ed., *Progress Report 4,* pp 121–134. National Center for Voice and Speech, Iowa City, IA, 1993.

48. Jacobson B, Bush C, Grywalski C: Voice handicap index (VHI) and clinicians' perceptual judgments: A comparison. Presented at ASHA Convention, Seattle, 1996.

49. Llewellyn-Thomas HA, Sutherland HJ, Hogg SA, et al: Linear analogue self-assessment of voice quality in laryngeal cancer. *J Chronic Dis* 1984; 37:917–924.

50. Smith E, Verdolini K, Gray S, et al: Effects of voice disorders on quality of life. *NCVS Status Prog Rep* 1994; 7:1–17.

51. Jacobson BH, Johnson A, Grywalski C, et al: The voice handicap index (VHI): Development and validation. *Am J Speech–Lang Path* 1997; 6:66–70.

52. West R, Kennedy L, Carr A: *The rehabilitation of speech.* Harper and Brothers, New York, 1937.

53. Van Riper C: *Speech correction principles and methods.* Prentice-Hall, Englewood Cliffs, NJ, 1939.

54. Boone D: *The voice and voice therapy.* Prentice-Hall, Englewood Cliffs, NJ, 1971.

55. Boone D, McFarlane S: *The voice and voice therapy,* 4th ed. Prentice-Hall, Englewood Cliffs, NJ, 1993.

56. Aronson A: *Clinical voice disorders: An interdisciplinary approach.* Thieme, New York, 1980.

57. Stemple J: *Clinical voice pathology: Theory and management.* Charles E. Merrill, Columbus, OH, 1984.

58. Stemple J: *Voice therapy: Clinical studies.* Mosby Year Book, St. Louis, 1993.

59. Verdolini-Marston K, Burke M, Lessac A, et al: A preliminary study on two methods of treatment for laryngeal nodules. *J Voice* 1995; 9:74–85.

60. Smith S, Thyme K: *Accent Metoden: Special Paedagogisk Forlag A-S.* Herning, Denmark, 1978.

61. Herrington-Hall B, Lee L, Stemple J, et al: Description of laryngeal pathologies by age, sex, occupation in a treatment seeking sample. *J Speech Hear Dis* 1988; 53:57–65.

62. Murry T, Woodson GE: A comparison of three methods for the management of vocal fold nodules. *J Voice* 1992; 3:271–276.

63. Koufman JA: The otolaryngologic manifestations of gastroesophageal reflux disease (GERD): A clinical investigation of 225 patients using ambulatory 24-Hour pH monitoring and an experimental investigation of the role of acid and pepsin in the development of laryngeal injury. *Laryngoscope* 1991; 101:1–78.

64. Roy N, Leeper HA: Effects of the manual laryngeal musculoskeletal tension reduction technique as a treatment for functional voice disorders: Perceptual and acoustic measures. *J Voice* 1993; 3:242–249.

65. Greene M: *The voice and its disorders,* 3rd ed. J.P. Lippincott, Philadelphia, 1972.

66. Russell J: A case of hysterical aphonia. *Br Med J* 1864; 8:619–621.

67. Ward W: Hysterical aphonia. *Chicago Med J Examiner* 1877; 34:495–505.

68. Goss F: Hysterical aphonia. *Boston Med Surg J* 1878; 99:215–222.

69. Ingals, E: Hysterical aphonia, or paralysis of the lateral crico-arytenoid muscles. *JAMA* 1890; 15:92–95.

70. Bach J: Hysterical aphonia. *Med News-Phil* 1890; 57:263–264.

71. Silbergleit AK: Acoustic analysis of voice in amyotrophic lateral sclerosis. Unpublished doctoral dissertation, Wayne State University, 1993.

72. Darley FL, Aronson AE, Brown JR: Motor speech disorders. W.B. Saunders, Philadelphia, 1975.

73. Ramig L, Pawlas A, Countryman S: The Lee Silverman voice treatment (LSVT): A practical guide to treating the voice and speech disorders in Parkinson disease. National Center for Voice and Speech, Iowa City, IA, 1995.

74. Ramig LO, Dromey C: Aerodynamic mechanisms underlying treatment related changes in SPL in patients with Parkinson disease. *J Speech Hear Res* 1996; 39:798–807.

75. Smith ME, Ramig LO, Dromey C, et al: Intensive voice treatment in Parkinson's disease: Laryngostroboscopic findings. *J Voice* 1995; 9:453–459.

76. Blitzer A, Lovelace RE, Brin MF, et al: Electromyographic findings in focal laryngeal dystonia (spastic dysphonia). *Ann Otol Rhino Laryngol* 1985; 94:591–594.

77. Murry T, Woodson GE: Combined-modality treatment of adductor spasmodic dysphonia with botulinum toxin and voice therapy. *J Voice* 1995; 9:460–465.

78. Christopher K, Wood R, Eckert R, Blager F, Raney R, Souhrada J: Vocal-cord dysfunction presenting as asthma. *N Engl J Med* 1983; 308:1566–1570.

79. Brown T, Merritt W, Evans D: Psychogenic vocal cord dysfunction masquerading as asthma. *J Nerv Ment Dis* 1988; 176:308–310.

80. Hayes J, Nolan M, Brennan N, FitzGerald M: Three cases of paradoxical vocal cord adduction followed up over a 10-year period. *Chest* 1993; 104:678–680.

81. Martin R, Blager F, Gay M, et al: Paradoxic vocal cord motion in presumed asthmatics. *Sem Resp Med* 1987; 8:332–337.

82. Newman K, Dubester S: Vocal cord dysfunction: Masquerader of asthma. *Sem Resp Crit Care Med* 1994; 15:161–167.

83. Sette L, Pajno-Ferrara F, Mocella S, et al: Vocal cord dysfunction in an asthmatic child: Case report. *J Asthma* 1993; 30:407–412.

84. Hurbis C, Schild J: Laryngeal changes during exercise and exercise-induced asthma. *Ann Otol Rhinol Laryngol* 1991; 100:34–37.

85. Kivity S, Bibi H, Schwarz Y, et al: Variable vocal cord dysfunction presenting as wheezing and exercise-induced asthma. *J Asthma* 1986; 23:241–244.

86. Lakin R, Metzger W, Haughey B: Upper airway obstruction presenting as exercise induced asthma. *Chest* 1984; 86:499–501.

87. Marion MH, Klap P, Perrin A, et al: Stridor and focal laryngeal dystonia. *Lancet* 1992; 339:457–458.

88. Barnes S, Grob C, Lachman B, Marsh B, Loughlin G: Psychogenic upper airway obstruction presenting as refectory wheezing. *J Ped* 1986; 109:1067–1070.

89. Cormier Y, Camus P, Desmeules M: Non-organic acute upper airway obstruction: Description and a diagnostic approach. *Amer Rev Resp Dis* 1980; 121:147–150.

90. Kissoon N, Kronick J, Frewen T: Psychogenic upper airway obstruction. *Pediatrics* 1988; 81:714–717.

91. Selner J, Staudenmayer H, Koepke J, et al: Vocal cord dysfunction: The importance of psychologic factors and provocation challenge testing. *J Allergy Clin Immunol* 1987; 79:726–733.

92. Sim T, McClean S, Lee J, et al: Functional laryngeal obstruction: A somatization disorder. *Am J Med* 1990; 88:293–295.

93. Skinner D, Bradley P: Psychogenic stridor. *J Laryngol Otol* 1989; 103:383–385.

94. Koek R, Pi E: Acute laryngeal dystonic reactions to neuroleptics. *Psychosomatics* 1989; 30:359–364.

95. Koufman J: Paradoxical vocal cord movement. *Visible Voice* 1994; 3:49–53,70–71.

96. Loughlin C, Koufman J: Paroxysmal laryngospasm secondary to gastroesophageal reflux. *Laryngoscope* 1996; 106:1502–1505.

97. Brugman S, Newman, K: Vocal cord dysfunction. *Med/Sci Update* 1993; 11:1–5.

98. Caraon P, O'Toole C: Vocal cord dysfunction presenting as asthma. *Irish Med J* 1991; 84:98–99.

99. Corren J, Newman K: Vocal cord dysfunction mimicking bronchial asthma. *Postgrad Med* 1992; 92:153–156.

100. Ophir D, Katz Y, Tavori I, et al: Functional upper airway obstruction in adolescents. *Arch Otolaryn Head Neck Surg* 1990; 116:1208–1209.

101. Patterson R, Schatz M, Horton M: Munchausen's stridor: Non-organic laryngeal obstruction. *Clin Allergy* 1974; 4:307–310.

102. Isshiki N: Laryngeal framework surgery. *Adv Otolaryng-Head Neck Surg* 1991; 5:37–56.

103. Kelly D, Wilson K: Improving thyroplasty outcome by intraoperative monitoring. Presented at the Pacific Voice Conference, San Francisco, 1996.

Appendix A
Henry Ford Hospital
Division of Speech–Language Sciences & Disorders
Patient History Form

Name _____   Date _____

Age _____   Occupation _____

Referring Physician _____

Physician Diagnosis _____

Description of the Problem

1. Please describe your voice problem: _____
_____
_____

2. When did you first notice the problem: _____
_____

3. How did the problem begin? Suddenly _____   Gradually _____
   Intermittently _____

4. How has the voice problem changed since the onset? Improved_____
   Worsened _____   No change _____   Fluctuates _____

Voice Symptoms

5. Have you had any of the following symptoms?

   _____ hoarseness lasting more than 1 week   _____ loss of voice
   _____ tired voice after lengthy talk   _____ change in pitch
   _____ tension in neck muscles   _____ difficulty maintaining a loud voice
   _____ pain in neck muscles   _____ sore throat
   _____ need to clear throat   _____ fullness in nose and throat
   _____ excessive coughing   _____ tightness in nose and throat
   _____ dry throat and/or mouth   _____ shortness of breath while speaking or singing
   _____ feeling of lump in the throat   _____ scratchy throat

6. Have your seen a physician for your voice? Yes _____   No _____
   If yes, for what reason? _____

7. Have you ever seen a speech–language pathologist? Yes _____   No _____
   If yes, for what reason? _____

8. If you have received advice or treatment for a voice problem, what were the recommendations given?
   _____ voice rest   _____ medications
   _____ humidification   _____ anti-reflux program
   _____ surgery   _____ voice instruction
   _____ voice therapy   _____ vocal hygiene instructions (e.g. reduce throat clearing, reduce loud talking)

9. When is your voice best? Early morning _____   Afternoon _____
   Evening _____   Night_____

10. When is your voice the worst? Early morning _____   Afternoon _____
    Evening _____   Night _____
11. What do you think caused your voice problem? _____

Past Medical History
12. Have you had or do you have any major illnesses (dates)? _____
    _____

13. Have you had any major surgeries (dates)? _____
    _____

14. Do you have allergies? Yes _____   No _____
    If yes, please describe. _____
15. What medications are you currently taking (prescribed and over-the-counter)?
    _____
    _____

Personal/Lifestyle
16. Do you currently smoke? Yes _____   No _____
17. Did you ever smoke? Yes _____   No _____
18. If you answered "yes" to either item 16 or 17:
    a. How many packs per day? _____
    b. How may years of smoking? _____
    c. If you used to smoke, when did you stop? _____
19. Indicate your consumption of the following beverages:
    a. alcohol   Yes_____   No_____   If yes, how much per week _____
    b. caffeinated coffee or tea   Yes_____   No_____   If yes, how much per day _____.
    c. caffeinated soda   Yes _____   No _____   If yes, how much per day _____
20. What is your current job? _____
21. Are you exposed to fumes/dust/particulates at home or on the job or at home?
    Yes _____   No _____
22. In what types of physical activities (e.g., exercise) do you participate regularly?
    _____
23. At what time do you usually eat your last meal or snack? _____
24. Do you play any musical instruments? Yes _____   No _____   If so, what instrument?
    _____

Voice Use
25. Does your occupation require you to use your voice frequently? Yes_____   No_____
26. Are you involved in any of the following activities?

Long telephone conversations	Never _____	Occasionally _____	Frequently _____
Teaching to groups of people	Never _____	Occasionally _____	Frequently _____
Speaking in large rooms	Never _____	Occasionally _____	Frequently _____
Singing before a group	Never _____	Occasionally _____	Frequently _____
Choral singing	Never _____	Occasionally _____	Frequently _____
Teaching instrumental or vocal music	Never _____	Occasionally _____	Frequently _____
Preaching	Never _____	Occasionally _____	Frequently _____
Taking voice instruction	Never _____	Occasionally _____	Frequently _____
Taking acting instruction	Never _____	Occasionally _____	Frequently _____
Speaking on television or radio	Never _____	Occasionally _____	Frequently _____
Acting in plays	Never _____	Occasionally _____	Frequently _____
Coaching a sport	Never _____	Occasionally_____	Frequently_____
Public speaking	Never _____	Occasionally_____	Frequently_____
Aerobics or gymnastics instruction	Never _____	Occasionally_____	Frequently_____
Excessively long conversations	Never _____	Occasionally_____	Frequently_____
Cheerleading	Never _____	Occasionally_____	Frequently_____
Leading meetings	Never _____	Occasionally_____	Frequently_____

27. Do you currently take voice or acting instruction? Yes____No____
28. If you sing, what is your repertoire? _____
29. If you sing, what is your range? Bass____ Baritone____ Tenor____
    Alto____Soprano____
30. Do you warm up before performing? Yes____ No____
31. Do you cool down after performing? Yes____ No____
32. If you sing, how long are your practice sessions/rehearsals?_____
33. Please complete the following chart, indicating your use of voice in speaking activities. For each day of the week and time of day, indicate the "average" amount of time (i.e., hours) you spend talking in one of the activities above (or in another vocally demanding activity).

	Sunday	Monday	Tuesday	Wednesday	Thursday	Friday	Saturday
morning							
afternoon							
evening							
night							

34. Please complete the following chart, indicating your use of voice in *singing* activities. For each day of the week and time of day, indicate the "average" amount of time (i.e. hours) you spend singing.

	Sunday	Monday	Tuesday	Wednesday	Thursday	Friday	Saturday
morning							
afternoon							
evening							
night							

22

Videoendoscopy in Speech and Swallowing for the Speech–Language Pathologist

Michael P. Karnell and Susan Langmore

CHAPTER OUTLINE

Indications for Videoendoscopy

Videoendoscopy for Disorders of Resonance

Videoendoscopy for Disorders of Voice

Videoendoscopy for Swallowing Disorders

Risks Associated with Videoendoscopy

Endoscopy has been used by physicians and speech–language pathologists for related yet very different purposes. Physicians employ the procedure to help them arrive at medical diagnoses that may subsequently lead to medical or surgical intervention. They attempt to uncover the underlying causes of structural abnormality (e.g., benign or malignant tissue changes or structural abnormalities in response to trauma or congenital abnormality), neuromotor abnormality (e.g., recurrent laryngeal nerve paralysis), or neurosensory deficit (e.g., superior laryngeal nerve dysfunction) observed endoscopically. Depending on the diagnosis, the physician may suggest treatment options to either eliminate the cause of the disorder or, when that is not possible, treat the symptoms associated with it.

Speech–language pathologists do not use endoscopy to make medical or surgical diagnoses.

Speech–language pathology is an applied behavioral discipline. Therefore, speech–language pathologists use endoscopy to observe, understand, and document the anatomical and physiological correlates of resonance, voice, and swallowing behavior. Such observations, in the context of the complete functional assessment, may then become the basis for making decisions about whether and what type of behavioral management may be indicated in the overall treatment plan for the patient. Many disorders requiring behavioral management also may necessitate medical/surgical diagnosis and treatment. Consequently, it is standard practice in speech–language pathology to require patients who have a suspected anatomical or physiological disorder affecting resonance, voice, or swallowing to have a medical/surgical evaluation *before* behavioral management is considered. We believe the patient

563

undergoing the diagnostic process is usually best served when the speech–language pathologist and medical professional consider endoscopic data as a team. Subsequently, speech–language pathologists may further employ videoendoscopy as a behavioral management tool.

The purpose of this chapter is to *briefly* outline how speech–language pathologists incorporate videoendoscopy into the behavioral assessment process. Complete consideration of the many theoretical, technical, and practical issues involved is not possible and interested readers are encouraged to consider other works for additional detail regarding anatomy and physiology, instrumentation, technique, interpretation, and data management.[1–3] We assume that readers will already have a firm foundation in non-endoscopic assessment and management of speech, resonance, and swallowing disorders in adults and children.

INDICATIONS FOR VIDEOENDOSCOPY

Speech–language pathologists use endoscopy to evaluate patients with any of three general disorder types. These include patients with (1) resonance disorders (hypernasality or hyponasality) due to suspected innappropriate oral/nasal coupling during speech, (2) voice disorders resulting from suspected abnormalities in the vibratory characteristics of the vocal folds, and (3) swallowing disorders due to suspected abnormalities in the patient's ability to move food safely from the mouth into the esophagus. Some other special cases arise from time to time that do not fit well into these three general groups, but the vast majority are focussed on velopharyngeal (VP) function for resonance, laryngeal function for voice, or pharyngeal/laryngeal functioning for swallowing. Additional detailed indications for videoendoscopic evaluation of swallowing are provided later in this chapter.

VIDEOENDOSCOPY FOR DISORDERS OF RESONANCE

Patients with hypernasal speech usually have some degree of velopharyngeal insufficiency (VPI) secondary to cleft lip and palate, neuromotor deficit, or surgical resection of palatopharyngeal tumor. Hypernasality may also be the result of oral/nasal fistula in patients with adequate functioning velopharyngeal mechanisms. When these problems are identified, treatment usually involves sur-

gical or dental prosthetic management. Phoneme specific VPI, which affects only one or two phonemes, is a rare phenomenon that appears to be due to incorrect speech learning. It is successfully treated with speech therapy.

Normal oral/nasal resonance for speech requires rapid, finely coordinated alterations in velopharyngeal movements to achieve (1) velopharyngeal closure for oral speech sounds and (2) velopharyngeal opening for nasal speech sounds and respiration. Velopharygeal assessment requires a thorough understanding of the anatomical and physiologic bases of normal velopharyngeal movements during oral and nasal speech. When VPI is suspected, velopharyngeal physiology must be carefully observed as the patient is led through a well planned sequence of speech samples that place varying demands on the velopharyngeal mechanism. Videoendoscopy is useful to determine whether the patient has the potential to overcome VPI by behavioral means or, more commonly, whether physical management (surgery or prosthetics) is likely to help.

Videoendoscopy to assess velopharyngeal closure is indicated only if the patient has perceptible, audible, clinically significant hypernasality and/or audible nasal emission of air during speech production. Therefore, a careful assessment of the patient's resonance capabilities by a certified speech–language pathologist with experience examining individuals with VPI is imperative before videoendoscopy is planned or carried out.

Procedures for Examining Hypernasality due to VPI

Videoendoscopy for assessment of VPI is most commonly accomplished using a flexible endoscope positioned in the nasopharynx so that the entire velopharyngeal mechanism is in view (Figure 22–1). Positioning the endoscope in this manner may be accomplished by inserting the scope either through the inferior or middle nasal meatus.[1] If the velopharyngeal mechanism cannot be observed entirely within a single view, the endoscope may be rotated from one location to another within the nasopharynx so that all aspects of the velopharyngeal mechanism may be carefully assessed.

The speech samples used during videoendoscopy should be designed to control for the frequency of occurrence of normal oral/nasal coupling that occurs during nasal consonant productions (Table 22–1). If hypernasality is suspected, speech samples that contain no nasal consonants are required so that if oral/nasal coupling occurs, it is

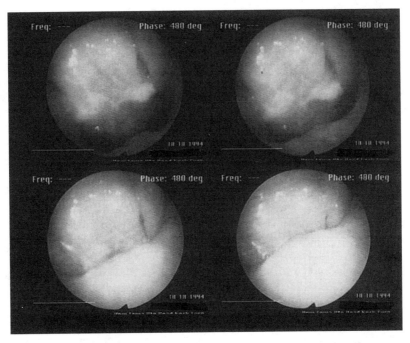

Figure 22–1. Normal velopharyngeal closure. At rest (*top left*), all margins of the velopharyngeal port are in view. As closure begins (*top right*), the velum moves posteriorly and the lateral walls move medially. At the moment of velopharyngeal closure (*bottom left*), a complete seal is achieved. Additional velar movement occurs (*bottom right*) beyond that needed for closure when pressure consonants are produced. See Color Plate 19.

clear to the observer that such coupling is inappropriate and not due to the coarticulatory effects of nasal consonant contexts. These samples should be brief and include a variety of oral pressure consonants, vowels, and semivowels to vary the demands on the velopharyngeal mechanism and determine the consistency and severity of VPI. Samples that include a mix of nasal and non-nasal consonants should also be tested to determine how well the patient makes transitions between sounds that require oral/nasal coupling and sounds that do not.

Findings and Treatment

Videoendoscopic assessment of velopharyngeal movement should be considered in terms of the relative contributions of the velum, right and left lateral pharyngeal walls, and the posterior pharyngeal wall to velopharyngeal closure. The occurrence,

Table 22–1. Examples of Speech Samples for Use During Velopharyngeal Videoendoscopy

All Oral Samples with Pressure Consonants	All Oral Samples without Pressure Consonants	Mixed Oral/Nasal Samples
Ride the bus.	You were away.	Mama made some lemon jam.
Go to school.	Where were you?	Ten men came in when Jane rang.
Did Dad do it?	We were away earlier.	Benny's nose was on the window.
Forty-four fat fish	Roll a yellow wheel.	Come to my house tonight.

consistency, and timing of closure should be considered within the context of the phonetic makeup of the utterance spoken. Detailed observations and measurements of each component have been suggested by Golding-Kushner et al.[4] Typical videoendoscopic observations of velopharyngeal function are listed in Table 22–2.

Endoscopic findings may indicate that the patient has either consistent or inconsistent VPI. Patients with consistent severe VPI (Figure 22–2) appear unable to achieve velopharyngeal closure at any time during speech production and have a clearly observable open VP port regardless of the phonetic makeup of the speech sample performed. Such individuals usually demonstrate complete velopharyngeal closure during swallowing. Such capability *should not* be considered evidence of potential for function during speech, however, since the neuromotor control mechanisms for speech and swallowing are distinctly different.[5]

Consistent VPI

Individuals with consistent VPI require physical management. If the velum appears physically short relative to the depth of the VP port and if the movements of the lateral and posterior pharyngeal walls cannot compensate for the velar deficit, either surgical management (pharyngeal flap, sphincter pharyngoplasty, or palatal lengthening) or prosthetic management (obturator or "speech bulb") will be necessary to treat the patient. If the velum appears to have adequate length but does not move due to paralysis, prosthetic management (palatal lift) is indicated. The selection of the treatment approach also depends on the specific details of each

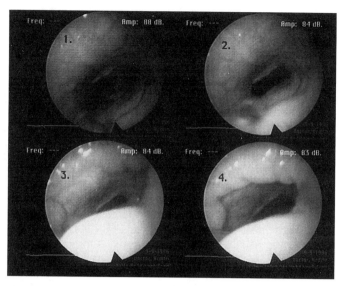

Figure 22–2. Severe consistent velopharyngeal insufficiency. At rest (*top left*), maximum velopharyngeal opening is visible. As movement toward closure begins (*top right*), the posterior margin of the velum moves posteriorly. Movement toward closure proceeds with additional posterior velar movement (*bottom right*). At maximum closure (*bottom right*), medial movement of the lateral walls and anterior movement of the posterior wall fail to compensate for inadequate velar movement.

individual patient's needs and takes into consideration overall patient health, hygiene, and patient or family preferences.

Inconsistent VPI

Patients whose severity of VPI is mild to moderate generally appear to have adequate or nearly ade-

Table 22–2. Typical Observations Made During Videoendoscopic Examination of Velopharyngeal Closure

Videoendoscopic Observations	Possible Findings
Movement of the velum, left and right pharyngeal walls, and posterior pharyngeal wall	Rate each component as no movement, moderate movement, or marked movement.
Consistency of velopharyngeal closure	Rate as consistently complete, inconsistent, consistently incomplete.
If incomplete or inconsistent describe severity.	Mild (inappropriate opening appears less than 10% of at rest port size), Moderate (10–20%), or Severe (>20%)
If inconsistent, describe nature of inconsistency.	Phoneme specific VPI, opening during vowels/semivowels only, leakage during pressure consonants only, etc.
Location of opening	Left side only, midline, right side only.

quate velar length and achieve considerable movement of the velopharyngeal mechanism toward closure. Some marginal patients may appear to achieve complete velopharyngeal closure at least momentarily during non-nasal speech production (Figure 22–3). Morris[6] described this phenomenon as "Sometimes But Not Always" closure or SBNA. Others may appear to come very close to achieving velopharyngeal closure without completely reaching closure (Figure 22–4). Morris[6] described these patients as having "Almost But Not Quite" closure. In our experience, however, most of these patients actually achieve at least momentary closure during some non-nasal consonant sounds. Other types of inconsistent or marginal VPI likely exist. Most marginal patients who require treatment receive the same forms of physical management described above for consistent VPI cases. Various approaches to posterior pharyngeal wall augmentation have been used at some centers. One of these is described in Case One. However, some patients may be suitable for behavioral management.

Except for patients with phoneme-specific VPI, there is no simple means of determining how to identify which patients who inconsistently achieve closure are most likely to adequately benefit from behavioral management. Several factors are taken into consideration. These include (1) the frequency of occurrence of adequate closure, (2) the phonetic

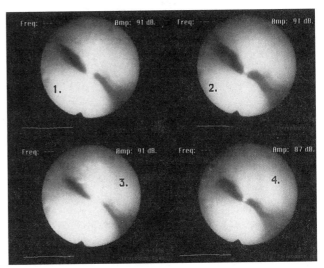

Figure 22–4. Marginal VPI: Almost But Not Quite. Maximum movement (*top left*) associated with initial [tʃ] in "Chop the wood." fails to achieve closure. During the subsequent vowel [c], a slight increase in velopharyngeal area is visible (*top right*). Near closure is achieved during production of initial [th] in "the" (*bottom left*) followed by an slight increase in opening during the subsequent vowel [a] in "the."

patterns associated with the occurrence of adequate closure, and (3) the patient's ability to modify either the frequency or phonetic patterns in response to clinical stimulation or biofeedback. A well-designed videoendoscopic evaluation with a cooperative patient should go a long way toward determining whether the patient is a candidate for speech therapy on the basis of these three observations.

CASE ONE

A 15-year-old female was evaluated as part of a general cleft palate-craniofacial clinic visit for possible VPI. She had a repaired bilateral complete cleft lip and palate. Nasal resonance was judged as a 3 on a scale where 1 = normal oral/nasal resonance and 10 = severe consistent hypernasality. She demonstrated no audible nasal emission of air, no articulation errors, no denasality, and no hoarseness. Nasalance measures were 32% during production of the Zoo passage, 40% during production of low pressure sentences,[7] and 65% during nasal sentences. Normal nasalance during the Zoo and low pressure sentences at our clinic is estimated as less than 30%.

On videoendoscopic examination, marked velar movement and moderate left and right lateral wall movement toward closure were observed. No

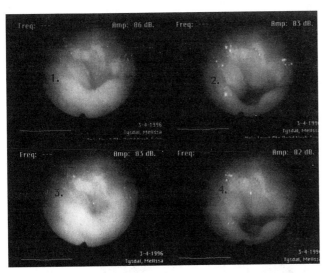

Figure 22–3. Marginal VPI: Sometimes But Not Always. Complete closure (*top left*) is achieved with oral closure for the initial [p] in "Popeye plays baseball." Closure fails (*top right*) as oral pressure for initial [p] is released and the following vowel is produced. Closure is reestablished (*bottom left*) for the medial [p] in "Popeye" followed again by opening (bottom right) for the final diphthong [aI].

posterior wall movement was visible. A small (approximately 5% of at rest velopharyngeal opening area) was consistently visible at the midline of the posterior pharyngeal wall where an indentation existed in the adenoid pad (Figure 22–5). Because of the relatively minor severity of the symptoms, no treatment was recommended.

The patient reported she was not interested in pursuing treatment at the time of her clinic visit. However, eight months later she requested treatment and surgical injection of autologous fat was performed at the site of the midline notch in the adenoid pad.

The patient was examined again five months post-surgery. The patient nasality was judged a 2, a slight improvement from the preoperative rating of 3. Consistent with her preoperative status, no articulation errors, audible nasal emission of air, or denasality were observed. Nasalance measures were substantially improved, however. During production of the Zoo passage, nasalance was 18%, down 14 percentage points compared to preoperative measurement. Nasalance during production of the low pressure sentences was 29%, down 11 percentage points. Nasalance during the nasal sentences was also reduced compared to preoperative status to 53%.

During videoendoscopy, she demonstrated ability to achieve complete velopharyngeal closure during most speech sounds. However, some inconsistent breaches in closure were observed at the left

lateral port and appeared to result from a physiological relaxation of velar elevation during some vowels and semivowels rather than from anatomical defect. The midline deficit in the adenoid pad was no longer visible and no oral/nasal coupling was observed at that site (Figure 22–6). The patient reported satisfaction with her speech. She has not requested additional treatment since that time.

VIDEOENDOSCOPY FOR DISORDERS OF VOICE

Patients with voice disorders may have impaired vocal fold vibration due to a variety of disorders affecting the larynx. These include laryngeal trauma, laryngeal tissue pathology, laryngeal nerve paralysis, or vocal misuse. Consequently, some patients may have difficulty adducting their vocal folds adequately for phonation or abducting them adequately for respiration. Others may have difficulty initiating, maintaining, or controlling the vibratory movements of the vocal folds necessary for acceptable, functional phonation. Some patients have complex combinations of laryngeal problems.

Video*stroboscopy* (videoendoscopy using illumination from a controlled stroboscopic light source) enables assessment of the two major types of laryngeal movements necessary for adequate voice production and respiration.[1,2] The first major type involves vocal fold adductor/abductor movements. Glottal adduction is observed as the lateral

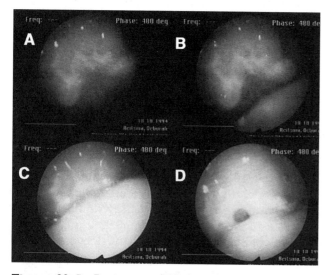

Figure 22–5. An inverted V-shaped notch appears in the adenoid pad at rest (*top left*) and as the velum approaches during a closing gesture (*top right*). Complete closure is achieved temporarily (*bottom left*) followed by a small leak at the location of the notch (*bottom right*).

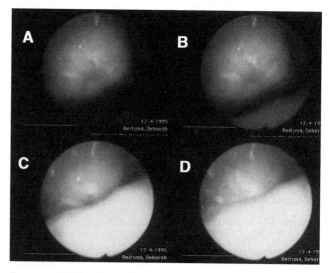

Figure 22–6. After fat injection at midline of the posterior wall, the notch visible in Figure 22–5 was reduced and the nasal escape at that location was eliminated.

cricoarytenoid muscles contract to bring the vocal folds toward the glottal midline (adduction) for voiced speech sounds. Glottal abduction occurs as the posterior cricoarytenoid muscles contract to move the vocal folds away from the glottal midline (abduction) for voiceless speech sounds and respiration. The second major type of laryngeal movement involves the vibratory movements of the vocal folds themselves observable during voiced phonation. Videoendoscopy without a stroboscopic light enables assessment of only adductor/abductor movements. A stroboscopic light source is necessary for clinical assessment of vocal fold vibration. Stroboscopy provides a *simulated* slow motion image of the vocal folds. The view of the vibratory cycle on videotape is a composite of many cycles. This discussion will focus on videostroboscopy as the preferred method of clinical observation of laryngeal movements for voice and respiration.

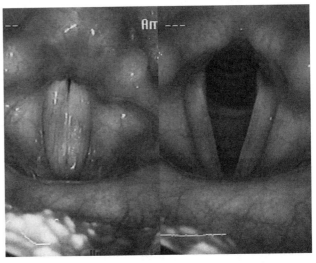

Figure 22–7. Typical view through a rigid endoscope of vocal folds during adduction (*left*) and abduction (*right*). See Color Plate 20.

Procedures for Examining Laryngeal Function for Voice

Videostroboscopy should be performed using a rigid oral endoscope whenever possible for maximum image quality. Flexible nasal endoscopes may be used when the rigid oral scopes cannot be tolerated by the patient or when there is interest in obtaining laryngeal function information during unencumbered speech production. It is wise, therefore, to have both a rigid and a flexible endoscope available.

The videostroboscopic view should include all the structures from the arytenoids to the glottal anterior commissure during glottal adduction and abduction (Figure 22–7). Whenever possible, it is useful to obtain views of the left and right pyriform sinuses as well as the epiglottis and valeculae. When the rigid oral endoscope is used to observe vocal fold vibratory movements (Figure 22–8), laryngeal maneuvers are generally limited to voiced sustained [i] productions while the patient attempts low pitch, high pitch, comfortable pitch, low loudness, moderate loudness, and increased loudness. Abducted views of the folds are obtained during inspiration.

The flexible endoscope may be used to obtain vocal fold vibratory information when the rigid scope cannot be used. The flexible scope must be advanced into the laryngeal vestibule while the patient sustains [i] or [u] phonation. This technique requires experience and a steady hand (see Karnell[1] for a more detailed description of technique). The clinician should withdraw the endoscope

back to oropharynx when the patient stops phonating so the endoscope will not come in contact with the epiglottis during swallowing or spontaneous speech. Close inspection of the vocal folds during quiet respiration is typically possible if the patient is instructed to neither speak nor swallow as the flexible endoscope is carefully advanced into the laryngeal vestibule. Care must be taken, however, to prevent contact with structures in the laryngeal vestibule so as to avoid stimulating a cough response. When the flexible nasal endoscope is used to observe ongoing speech production, the lens

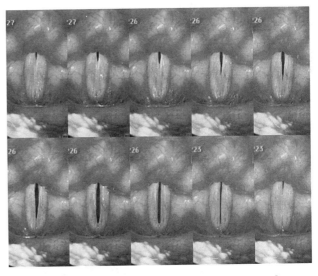

Figure 22–8. Sequence of vocal fold images during a complete stroboscopic vibratory cycle. The sequence progresses left to right across the top then across the bottom left to right.

should be positioned above the tip of the epiglottis while the patient speaks so that epiglottic contact with the endoscope may be avoided.

Findings and Treatment

The absence or reduction of abductor/adductor movement of one or both vocal folds is indicative of a recurrent laryngeal nerve paralysis or paresis (Figure 22–9). The effects of arytenoid fixation appear similar to recurrent laryngeal nerve paralysis in some cases. Laryngeal EMG is useful for confirming the presence or absence of laryngeal motor nerve activity.

Laryngeal vibratory activity is typically described in terms of the characteristics listed in Table 22–3. Vibratory amplitude of the two folds and phase symmetry are useful for identifying unilateral or asymmetrical effects of pathology. Unilateral laryngeal paralysis or unilateral growths may cause the affected vocal fold to vibrate with less amplitude and/or out of phase relative to the unaffected vocal fold (Figures 22–10 and 22–11). The presence of adynamic segments suggests excessive stiffness in the affected portion of the vocal fold. The quality of the vocal fold mucosal wave is often considered an index of vocal fold tissue stiffness. Excessively stiff vocal folds do not show a well-defined mucosal wave (Figure 22–10). Adequacy of glottal closure is an indication of glottal valving efficiency (Figure 22–12).

Additional observations are frequently useful for their descriptive value. The quality of the edges

Table 22–3. Typical Observations Made During Videostroboscopic Examinations of Vocal Vibratory Function[8]

Observation	Finding
Vibratory amplitude	Indicate reduced, adequate, great amplitude for right and left folds.
Phase symmetry	Always in phase, inconsistently in phase, always out of phase.
Mucosal wave	Reduced, normal, or great for right and left folds.
Glottal closure	Complete, incomplete at the time of maximum vocal fold contact.
Open quotient	Time during vibratory cycle when folds are *not* in contact divided by total duration of the cycle (Normal is approximately .50).

of the vocal folds reflects the integrity of the medial surfaces of the folds that contact one another during phonation (Figure 22–13). The presence of supraglottic compression (Figure 22–14), either as medial displacement of the ventricular folds or as anterior displacement of the arytenoids toward a posteriorly displace epiglottis, is usually indicative of excessive vocal strain. Supraglottic com-

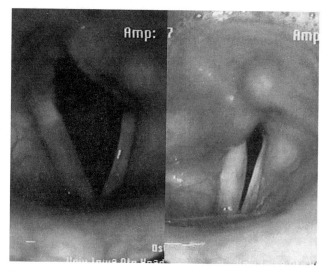

Figure 22–9. Abducted (*left*) and adducted (*right*) view of larynx with left laryngeal paralysis. Note the bowing of the affected left vocal fold visible in the abducted view. See Color Plate 21.

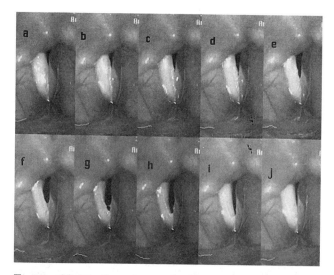

Figure 22–10. Sequence demonstrating vibratory amplitude asymmetry. Note the normal vibratory displacement of the right true vocal fold compared to the relative immobility of the left fold. Also, the mucosal wave visible on the right vocal fold is absent from the left.

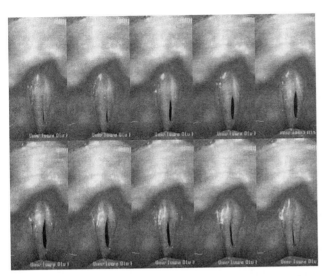

Figure 22–11. Sequence demonstrating vibratory phase asymmetry.

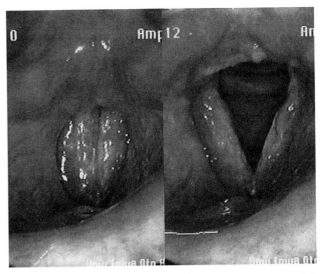

Figure 22–13. Adducted (*left*) and abducted (*right*) views of rough/irregular vocal folds. See Color Plate 22.

pression in the presence of incomplete glottal closure may be compensatory in nature. The presence of vocal fold abnormalities may be described or provisionally named provided it is clear to the speech–language pathologist, the patient, and the physician that the specific nature of tissue abnormalities is for the physician to diagnose. Physician review of the videostroboscopic records is frequently helpful for medical diagnosis of many types of neurogenic laryngeal disorders and common tissue pathologies such as nodules, polyps, edema, erythema, and so on. Some tissue abnormalities require direct laryngocopy and biopsy for adequate diagnosis. Severe dysphonia in the ab-

sence of tissue abnormalities or movement disorders is usually indicative of a functional disorder.

CASE TWO

A 37-year-old female reported a history of hoarse, breathy, weak voice since the age of 19. No diagnosis had previously been made and no treatment had been performed. Her voice quality was clinically judged as G2 R2 B2 A1 S0 on the GRBAS scale.[8] The patient judged her own voice quality as a 4 on a scale where 0 was perfectly normal voice and 6 was the worst voice she could imagine for herself.

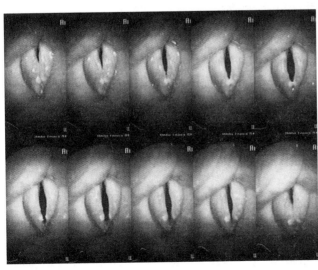

Figure 22–12. Sequence demonstrating incomplete posterior glottal closure.

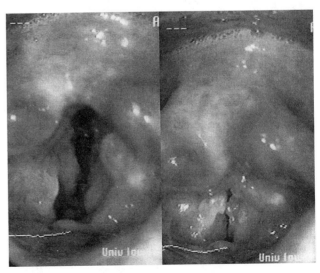

Figure 22–14. Abducted (*left*) and adducted (*right*) views of rough/irregular vocal folds with supraglottic compression during adduction. See Color Plate 23.

Videostroboscopy demonstrated the patient had a left unilateral laryngeal paralysis. On abduction, the right true vocal fold appeared smooth and straight but the left fold appeared somewhat bowed (Figure 22–9). During voice production, glottal closure was incomplete throughout the vibratory cycle, vibratory amplitude was asymmetrical (R > L), and no mucosal wave was visible on the affected vocal fold (Figure 22–15). No supraglottic compression or vibratory phase asymmetry was observed. No adynamic segments were observed.

Left vocal fold medialization was surgically accomplished using a Gortex implant eight months after our initial evaluation. A follow-up evaluation was completed six weeks after surgery. At that time the patient's voice was judged G1 R1 BO AO SO. The patient's self-evaluation of voice quality improved from the preoperative rating of 4 to a postoperative rating of 0 (normal).

Adequate vocal fold contact was observed via videostroboscopy along the anterior two-thirds of the vocal folds (Figure 22–16). A small posterior glottal chink persisted but was considered within normal limits for an adult female. Vibratory amplitude and phase were symmetrical. Mucosal wave was visible bilaterally, but more clearly demonstrated on the unaffected fold. The patient reported satisfaction with her voice quality and no additional treatment was planned.

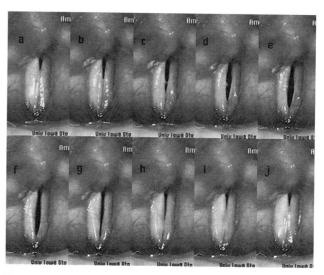

Figure 22–16. Postoperative vibratory sequence in the same patient demonstrated in Figure 22–15 showing improved vocal fold contact and normal vibratory amplitude and phase symmetry.

VIDEOENDOSCOPY FOR SWALLOWING DISORDERS

Oropharyngeal dysphagia can occur for a variety of reasons. The most frequent medical etiologies of dysphagia are neurological damage, most commonly stroke, structural damage due to surgical excision of diseases of the base of skull or head and neck structures, and repeated translaryngeal intubations or placement of a tracheostomy tube. Patients with severe pulmonary disease may also experience dysphagia, as well as those who are extremely debilitated or obtunded. In children, dysphagia can be a component of several congenital, developmental, or acquired medical problems. Speech–language pathologists may screen for dysphagia that involves the oral, pharyngeal, and/or esophageal stages, but they usually have expertise only in the oral and pharyngeal stages, and refer esophageal stage problems to gastroenterology.

The first steps in evaluation of dysphagia should include a review of the medical history, an interview, and a clinical examination of oral, laryngeal, and respiratory function. Following this, an instrumental examination is often performed.

Endoscopy and Fluoroscopy: Two Procedures for Evaluating Oropharyngeal Dysphagia

While fluoroscopy has become a standard examination for oropharyngeal dysphagia, nasendoscopy is an excellent alternative procedure, and

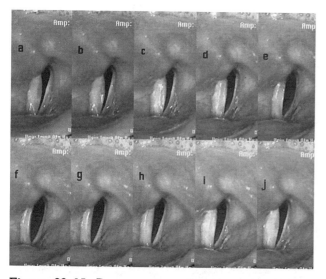

Figure 22–15. Preoperative vibratory sequence in a patient with left TVF paralysis demonstrating incomplete glottal closure, vibratory asymmetry, and phase asymmetry.

in some cases will provide more meaningful information. Indications for performing an endoscopic examination versus a fluoroscopic examination are listed in Table 22–4. Indications for the two examinations have been debated in the literature, and continue to be the subject of much discussion.[9,10]

There are practical reasons for choosing endoscopy over videofluoroscopy. For example, when the patient is critically ill, intubated, or requires continuous monitoring, videoendoscopy may be safer and easier for the patient to tolerate than videofluoroscopy. The portability of the endoscopic exam allows it to be brought to the patient's bedside where the exam can be done in a safer and more comfortable environment than the fluoroscopy suite.

Table 22–4. Indications for a FEES[SM] or Fluoroscopy Examination

Indications for a FEES Exam (practical and clinical indications)

Need exam that day—can do it anywhere, anytime

Positioning in fluoroscopy problematic—e.g., patient bedridden, weak, has contractures, in pain, has decubitis ulcers, quadriplegic, wearing neck halo, obese, on ventilator.

Transportation to fluoroscopy problematic—medically fragile/unstable patient (in ICU; cardiac or other monitoring in place; on ventilator; nursing/medical care must be with patient)

Transportation to hospital problematic—nursing home issues, including cost of transportation, resources needed to accompany patient, strain on patient, patient fearful of leaving familiar surroundings, etc.

Concern about excess radiation exposure

Concern about aspiration of barium, food, and/or liquid in patient with potentially severe dysphagia or very limited ability to tolerate any aspiration; e.g., brainstem CVA with suspected absent swallow reflex; patient tube fed for prolonged period; poor pulmonary status; poor immunologic status. FEES can give you a more conservative examination.

Post-intubation or post-surgery—esp. CABG, carotid endarterectomy, or any surgery where RLN was vulnerable). Endoscopy an visualize larynx directly for signs of trauma or neurologic damage and assess laryngeal competence.

Current or recent tracheostomy—suspect laryngeal competence is compromised

Need to assess status of secretions—ability of patient to manage secretions

Want time to assess fatigue or swallow status over a meal

Want therapeutic exam

Want enough time to try out several maneuvers, several consistencies, etc.; you want to try real foods; you want caregiver to hold baby in several positions, etc.

Need repeat exam to assess change; to assess effectiveness of maneuver

Want to try biofeedback

When these symptoms are present:

    Hypernasal voice

    Hoarse, breathy voice

    Wet voice quality

    Rapid respiratory rate; effortful breathing

Indications for Fluoroscopy (practical and clinical indications)

Patient will not accept/tolerate endoscopy

Oral stage problem needs to be imaged

Esophageal stage problem or gastroesophageal reflux (GER) suspected; want to visualize esophageal motility and GE reflux

Globus complaints; possible cricopharyngeal (CP) dysfunction

Possible cervical osteophytes

Vague symptomotology from patient; need comprehensive view

Need to identify which bolus propulsion force/ structural movement is weak (e.g., tongue, vs. laryngeal elevation)

Need to verify aspiration of thin liquids during the swallow

Need to get better impression of amount of aspiration

There are also clinical indications for choosing an endoscopic exam as opposed to fluoroscopy. A common example is the patient who has a breathy or hoarse voice quality and for whom a direct look at the larynx would be beneficial. Intubation can easily cause laryngeal trauma and surgery can result in damage to the laryngeal nerve as an unexpected complication. The resultant structural and physiologic changes to the larynx that directly affect swallowing are best revealed by endoscopy.

Children with dysphagia as well as adults benefit from endoscopy. Some advantages for infants or children are the ability to be tested in a natural seating position (even held in the parent's arms), with typical liquids or foods, and the absence of radiation exposure. Voluntary compliance and cooperation from children are not always assured, however.

The views provided by videoendoscopy and videofluoroscopy are distinctly different. Fluoroscopy provides an image of the *shadow* of oral, pharyngeal, and esophageal structures and reveals the movements of these structures in relation to bolus flow. Endoscopy offers a detailed and semidirect view of the hypopharynx and larynx as the bolus flows past. The endoscopic view is usually obliterated for about .5 second during the height of each swallow, except in cases where pharyngeal compression and/or laryngeal elevation is significantly reduced. The fluoroscopic view is limited in time by radiation exposure constraints so that the fluoroscopy unit is generally turned off between every swallow and total viewing time is limited to 3 to 5 minutes. Endoscopy can provide a constant view over a prolonged period of time. It can reveal problems that occur over time. Fluoroscopy can provide a clearer representation of subglottic aspiration.

While there are significant differences between the two procedures, they have similar purposes and outcomes. Both fluoroscopic and endoscopic procedures can be used to detect the presence of dysphagia, both can reveal the nature of the problem, and both will allow the examiner to make the recommendations needed for adequate management of the problem.

Endoscopic Procedure for Examining Swallowing Function

Langmore, Schatz, and Olson published the first description of a procedure for evaluating swallowing with endoscopy.[11,12] It is known as the FEES^{SM}* procedure, and we will briefly describe it here. A standard flexible laryngoscope is attached to a videocamera, light source, videotape recorder, and monitor and is then passed transnasally to a point just above the epiglottis where the hypopharynx and larynx can be optimally viewed (Figure 22–17). For most of the exam this is the position of choice; however, after each swallow, the scope is briefly passed into the laryngeal vestibule so that the true vocal folds and the subglottic shelf (membranous portion of the thyroid and cricoid cartilage positioned just below the true vocal folds) can be examined more closely for evidence of penetration or aspiration (Figure 22–18).

Patient comfort is paramount for this examination because the objective is to assess habitual swallowing function and be able to keep the endoscope in place for as long as 30 minutes. If the patient requests a topical anesthesia to help dull the sensation inside the nose, the examiner places a small amount (about 1 ml) of viscous Lidocaine 2% in the nares that will be used to pass the endoscope. An oral spray is never used since this would depress sensation in the pharynx or larynx and might affect swallowing function.

The FEES^{SM} protocol is shown in Table 22–5. There are two major parts to a complete FEES^{SM} examination. Part I consists of a sensorimotor examination of pharyngeal and laryngeal function to assess such parameters as strength, range, symmetry, and briskness of movement. Anatomy is also viewed for its effect on swallowing function. The second part of the FEES^{SM} exam involves delivery of food and liquid to directly assess swallowing of these materials.

Part I of the FEES^{SM} exam is necessary for understanding the underlying anatomical or physiological cause of the dysphagia. The appearance of all the pharyngeal and laryngeal structures are observed for their effect on swallowing function. Edema is a common finding after intubation that can account for a temporary dysphagia due to reduced sensation and mobility of the affected

---

* FEES^{SM} is a service mark of Susan E. Langmore, Ph.D. Use of this service mark indicates that the endoscopic examination of pharyngeal swallowing herein performed or reported on was consistent with the procedure developed by Susan E. Langmore, Ph.D., and described in this chapter. It implies that the examination was a complete assessment of pharyngeal swallowing, including an examination of sensorimotor function of the pharyngeal and laryngeal structures, evaluation of ability to swallow all appropriate consistencies of food and liquid, and use of trial therapy, when appropriate, to determine what alterations or maneuvers helped to alleviate the problem.

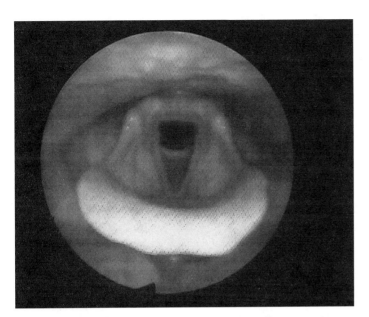

Figure 22–17. View of the hypopharynx with the tip of the endoscope positioned just superior to the epiglottis so that the laryngeal vestibule and structures surrounding it can be viewed. The typical position for the endoscope just prior to the swallow.

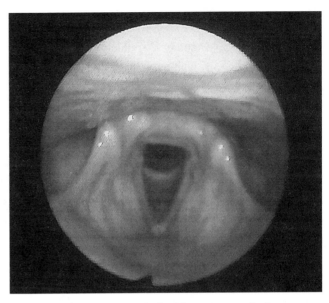

Figure 22–18. View of the larynx, including arytenoids, true vocal folds, and sub-glottic shelf. This view should be obtained between swallows for a brief period to inspect for signs of aspiration.

structures. Any suspicious growths or unusual appearance of the mucosal surface would alert the speech pathologist to a possible medical pathology and would warrant referral to otolaryngology.

Following the FEES[SM] protocol, pharyngeal and laryngeal function are then assessed via a series of tasks such as asking the patient to repeat "kuh-kuh-kuh" (for back of tongue movement), dry swallow (velopharyngeal closure), hold the breath (true vocal fold adduction), hold the breath tightly (true and false vocal fold adduction and complete arytenoid medial contact), sustain breath holding for several seconds, and sniff (laryngeal abduction). Airway protection is tested in detail since this function is so critical for prevention of aspiration.

Over the first few minutes of the examination, the examiner observes the status of any standing secretions, the ability of the patient to swallow or clear these secretions, and the frequency of spontaneous dry swallows. The presence of excess, standing secretions is an important clue to a dysphagia and has been shown to be an excellent predictor of aspiration of food and liquid.[13] It is therefore an important part of the FEES[SM] examination.

Laryngeal and pharyngeal sensation are then assessed. An indication of sensation is revealed by the patient's response to the presence of the endoscope, but, if this is in question, it can be directly tested by lightly touching the back of tongue, lateral pharyngeal walls, base of tongue, and finally,

if necessary, the tip of epiglottis. By leaving the laryngeal structure (epiglottis) to the end, and only touching it if the patient is insensate to the touch of other structures, an adverse reaction will be avoided. Recently, a special endoscope has been developed (Pentax Precision Instrument Corporation, Orangeburg, NY) to directly test and quantify sensory threshold. It has a second channel that can deliver a calibrated pulse of air to the structures of interest. Preliminary research with this instrument suggests that it may have great clinical utility.[14,15]

After the anatomical and physiological function of the pharynx and larynx have been evaluated, the FEES exam progresses to the delivery of food and liquid so that actual swallowing of these materials can be evaluated. Every bolus is dyed green or blue so that it is more visible and distinct from surrounding mucosal surfaces. A variety of bolus amounts and consistencies are given to the patient and his or her ability to swallow them safely and adequately are noted. Abnormal function is identified by signs such as residue, spillage, laryngeal penetration, and aspiration of material below the true vocal folds. Pharyngeal delay time is calculated and reduced or delayed epiglottic retroflexion is noted. Timing of airway closure with bolus flow is also noted.

As soon as a problem is identified, the examiner intervenes with appropriate therapeutic alterations to observe their effect on swallowing. These alterations might include instructing the patient to

Table 22–5. FEES^{SM} Examination Protocol

Anatomic-Physiologic Assessment

A. Velopharyngeal Closure

At juncture of velum and nasopharynx, view sphincteric closure as the patient swallows and phonates oral and nasal sounds and sentences. Administer liquid while scope is in nose if nasal reflux is to be assessed.

B. Appearance of Hypopharynx and Larynx at Rest

Scan around entire HP to note appearance, symmetry, and abnormalities that warrant an ENT referral for suspected pathology.

C. Handling of Secretions and Swallow Frequency

Observe amount and location of secretions in lateral channels, laryngeal vestibule, and/or subglottally. Note this over a 2 to 5 minute segment, as you proceed with the exam. Also note frequency of dry swallows over a period of at least 2 minutes. Optional: Drop green food color on tongue to mix with saliva if you need a better view.

D. Base of Tongue

Task: Say "kuh-kuh-kuh " several times.
Observe extent of movement and symmetry.

E. Respiration

Observe laryngeal structures for rest breathing. Note extent, symmetry, and rate of movement.
Task: Sniff or deep inhalation (note abduction)

F. Airway Protection

Task: Cough
Task: Hold your breath—at the level of the throat
Task: Hold your breath very tightly
Task: Hold your breath to the count of 7

G. Phonation

Task: Hold "ee"
Task: Repeat "hee-hee-hee" 5 to 7 times
Task: Count from 1 to 10.
Task: Glide upward in pitch.

H. Pharyngeal musculature

Task: Hold your breath and blow out cheeks forcefully.
Observe the depth and symmetry of pyriform sinuses.
Task: Strain your voice and grunt or say "ee" in a very loud, high voice.
Observe and middle and inferior constrictors- extent and symmetry of contraction.

Swallowing Food and Liquid

All foods/liquids are dyed green with food coloring.

Guidelines

Increase amount with each presentation unless aspiration occurs.
Repeat any amount that results in aspiration—unless severe aspiration.
Discontinue that amount if aspiration occurs twice.
Try less than 5 cc *only* if patient at very high risk for aspirating.
Give measured amounts if exact bolus size needs to be known; otherwise give functional amounts such as teaspoons, tablespoons, drinks from cup, straw.
Give instructions to swallow on command only to sort out the specific nature of an observed problem with spillage; otherwise let patient swallow at his or her own rate.
Give material that is light in color so that it will be visible.

Table 22–5. (continued)

Anatomic-Physiologic Assessment

Order of Consistencies will vary, depending on patient needs and the problems observed. Suggested consistencies to try include the following:

Ice chips—½ tsp. of ice chips (dyed green!)
  Begin with this consistency if patient is NPO at present and/or appears to be at high risk for aspiration (e.g., has standing secretions in HP).
  Repeat this several times. Note the effect on clearance of secretions, ability of patient to swallow the ice chips, and sensitivity of patient to any aspiration of ice chips.

Pureed food—5 cc, 10 cc, 15 cc of applesauce, pudding, etc.

Soft solid food—e.g., cheese sandwich.
  Allow the patient to take a bite sized portion.

Hard, chewy, crunchy food
  Give this consistency if regular diet is being considered

Thin Liquid—5 cc, 10 cc, 15 cc, 20 cc, 5 consecutive swallows.
  Milk or other translucent thin liquid (white in color) is good for visibility.

Thick Liquid—5 cc, 10 cc, 15 cc, 20 cc, 5 consecutive swallows.
  Give this consistency if indicated (from performance on thin liquids or pureed).
  Give nectar and honey consistencies for more precise information.

Therapeutic Positions, Maneuvers and Other Alterations in Bolus Delivery

Apply these at all appropriate points in the exam—generally as soon as the problem is observed. Use the strategy appropriate for the observed problem, including head turn, chin tuck, effortful swallow, supraglottic swallow or modification of this, Mendelsohn maneuver, dry swallows, and delivery by spoon, straw, or cup.

Hypopharyngeal/Laryngeal Sensory Testing

Can be directly tested by lightly touching the pharyngeal mucosal wall with the tip of the scope, then the base of tongue, and, if no response, the tip of epiglottis. If quantitative measure of sensory threshold can be obtained, this is preferable.

---

assume another posture such as chin-tuck, teaching the patient a swallow maneuver such as the controlled breath-hold prior to swallowing, or adjusting the bolus consistency, size, or method of delivery. The examination ends when the examiner understands the nature of the problem, has determined which bolus amounts and consistencies can be swallowed effectively and safely, and noted what therapeutic alterations facilitate swallowing.

Whenever possible, the patient, the family, and nursing staff that feed the patient are involved in the examination and participate in decision making regarding possible treatment for the swallowing problems that are observed. It has been our clinical experience that education of and collaboration with these significant persons are the most effective means of developing realistic and meaningful treatment goals and ensuring compliance with the treatment plan.

Findings

When swallows are observed endoscopically, there is a brief period during the height of the swallow, lasting about .5 second, where the view is obscured. This period, known as "white-out," is not usually a problem for the experienced examiner who is able to deduce what happened during this brief time. The risk of excessive radiation to the patient limits total viewing time to a period of 3 to 5 minutes for the complete examination. Endoscopy has the advantage of being able to maintain a view for a prolonged period of time, often up to 30 minutes if the patient is comfortable. Much information if gained by maintaining a prolonged and constant view, as, for example, when the patient refluxes material into the pharynx after several minutes of eating. It is also possible to make more naturalistic observations of how the patient really eats and how he or she spontaneously reacts to observed problems such as residue buildup or laryngeal penetration of material. When scoring and reporting on a FEES^SM exam, it is often most useful to describe the abnormal findings that occur over time with each consistency—for example, to describe how the patient handled pureed food, solid food, and liquids.

Scoring a FEES^SM exam can be done by simply noting the abnormal findings as they occur.

Possible observations might include spillage of pureed material to the level of pyriforms before the swallow, residue left in right lateral channel, aspiration of liquid before the swallow, and so on. After the exam is scored, the more difficult task is to interpret these findings. Interpretation requires the examiner to relate the individual findings to the underlying anatomy and pathophysiology that created the particular pattern observed. This not only explains the dysphagia, but provides the rationale for the treatment plan. There are five major types of underlying anatomical or physiological causes of dysphagia: (1) incomplete bolus clearance; (2) inadequate airway protection; (3) mistiming of bolus propulsion and airway protection; (4) inadequate sensation; and (5) abnormal anatomy. These five problems can all be revealed from a FEES[SM] examination.

Incomplete Bolus Clearance

The first major problem causing dysphagia is incomplete or inadequate bolus propulsion, evidenced by residue of bolus left behind after the swallow (Figure 22–19). If residue falls into the laryngeal vestibule after the swallow, it will continue to fall by gravity or inhalation as the airway opens and eventually can be aspirated. The underlying pathophysiology causing the residue may be weakness of the lingual, pharyngeal, or laryngeal structures, or presence of an obstruction in the bolus

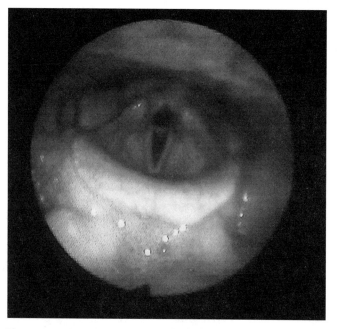

Figure 22–19. Residue of pureed material left in the vallecule and lateral channels after the swallow. See Color Plate 24.

path. While residue, the patient's reaction to the residue, and the path it eventually takes are clearly seen by endoscopy, identifying the specific source of a possible weakness is more difficult and fluoroscopy may be needed to help sort this out if this information is critical for treatment. On the other hand, if there was an obstruction to bolus flow, this problem is apparent from the endoscopic view. This large feeding tube can restrict movement of the arytenoids and epiglottis, and serve as a conduit for collecting food along its surface.

Mistiming of Bolus Propulsion and Airway Protection

A second major cause for dysphagia is inadequate airway protection, resulting in aspiration of material during the swallow. As with inadequate bolus propulsion, the underlying pathophysiology is often thought to be weakness or incomplete valving of the laryngeal structures (epiglottic retroversion, arytenoid adduction and tilt forward, true and false vocal fold adduction). While fluoroscopy is better for viewing aspiration of the bolus as it occurs during the swallow, endoscopy is the superior tool for judging the source of the weakness, or laryngeal incompetence. The tasks requested of the patient in the first part of the FEES[SM] examination (hold your breath, etc.) assess the ability of the larynx to protect the airway and general mobility, symmetry, and briskness of laryngeal movment. If aspiration does occur during the swallow, it is usually apparent on endoscopy from residue of the bolus left in the laryngeal vestibule (Figure 22–17) or on the subglottic shelf. If it occurs just as the swallow begins, the view is still available to the endoscopist and it can be seen directly. If unsure, the endoscopist can ask the patient to cough and see if any material is expelled. Some researchers, comparing endoscopy to fluoroscopy, have verified that endoscopy is sensitive to aspiration, in spite of losing the view for .5 second.[12,16]

Inadequate Airway Protection

A third major cause for dysphagia is mistiming of bolus propulsion and airway protection. This problem of mistiming, often described as a problem in delaying the pharyngeal response, is the most common abnormal pattern reported for patients with neurogenic dysphagia and is responsible for the most frequent occurrence of aspiration.[17–19] The observed event that signals this problem is spillage of material into the hypopharynx prior to the initiation of the swallow (Figure 22–20).

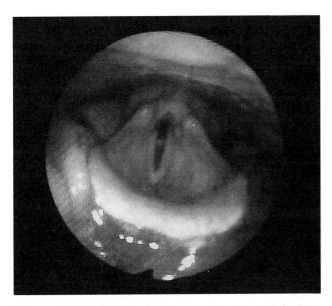

Figure 22–20. Spillage of pureed material before the swallow has begun. The material has spilled nearly to the pyriform recesses without any indication of the swallow initiation, indicating a pharyngeal delay. See Color Plate 25.

Spillage has been attributed to several underlying problems, including (1) poor oral control or sensation, allowing the bolus to fall into the pharynx during the oral stage; (2) delay initiating the swallow because of reduced sensation, slow or incomplete transmission or processing of sensory information, or slow, incomplete transmission of the final motor command to swallow; and/or (3) difficulty coordinating the many different structural movements that must occur nearly simultaneously at the onset of the swallow. Pharyngeal delay time, or a temporal measure of how long the bolus was in the pharynx before the swallow began, is a very useful and quantitative measure of the problem and can be readily calculated from endoscopy as well as fluoroscopy. If the spillage is excessive, the bolus can overflow the lateral channels or the pyriforms and enter the laryngeal vestibule. Because the swallow has not yet begun, the airway will probably be open, and thus the bolus can enter the glottis and be aspirated. All these events are directly viewed with endoscopy because the swallow has not yet begun.

Inadequate Sensation

Reduced sensation, the fourth underlying problem, can be directly assessed with a FEES^SM examination. It is possible that reduced sensitivity is a major cause for a delayed initation of the swallow.

Impaired sensation also reduces a patient's awareness and response to residue, penetration, or aspiration. Further research is needed to determine which patients with dysphagia have a measurable reduction in peripheral sensitivity and how that impairment is associated with other observed swallowing problems. As we understand this problem better, more effective treatment paradigms may emerge for dealing with this loss.

Abnormal Anatomy

Abnormal anatomy has been observed to directly impair swallowing function in many ways. It can prevent effective bolus clearance or airway closure because it creates an obstruction or diverts the bolus in an unfavorable direction. Even normal variations in anatomy will affect the path taken by the bolus. For example, some persons have an epiglottis with a curled tip that rests against the base of the tongue. Even a small amount of spillage cannot be tolerated by these individuals, since the bolus will be directed into the vestibule rather than into an open vallecular recess. Endoscopy can clearly image the anatomy of the pharynx or larynx.

Treatment

Endoscopy is a useful tool to guide the treatment or management of a dysphagia. Because it is portable, the examination can be brought to many patients who would otherwise not have the advantage of an instrumental examination. After an endoscopic exam, the clinician should have a better understanding of the problem and can plan more effective treatment.

Another advantage of endoscopy as a managment tool is that the FEES^SM exam can be done in the presence of, and with the cooperation of the patient, family, nursing staff, and anyone else involved in the patient's world of eating. The visual image can be discussed, the abnormal findings can be explained, and the entire 'team' can be involved in making decisions about what should be done. Compliance is greatly improved in such an environment.

The FEES^SM examination may be best thought of as a *therapeutic* examination. As soon as the patient experiences difficulty with a bolus, the examiner may alter conditions to find a safe and effective way for the patient to swallow. This may involve increasing or decreasing the bolus size, changing the consistency of the bolus, altering the method of food delivery, teaching the patient a swallow maneuver, or altering posture. All therapeutic applications can be tried without the time constraints of fluorscopy and their effect can be shown directly to the patient and caregivers for their understanding and input. If fatigue is a mitigating factor, there is ample time to observe the effects of fatigue on swallowing performance. Recommendations regarding diet, treatment, and management follow directly from "testing" therapeutic interventions during the initial assessment. Follow-up FEES examinations may be done with the sole purpose of testing the effectiveness or continued need for a therapeutic alteration.

Finally, endoscopy can be used directly as a feedback tool. By turning the patient to face the monitor, it can provide visual biofeedback. We have employed endoscopy to teach a more protective and consistent pattern of airway closure, emphasize the effects of a different posture, and increase a patient's awareness of spillage, residue, penetration, or aspiration. Most patients don't want an endoscope placed in their nose daily, but one or two sessions is tolerated well by most.

CASE THREE

A patient in the Intensive Care Unit had coronary artery bypass graft surgery (CABG), which was reported to be uneventful. The day following surgery, he was offered some thin liquids, and on the second day, began receiving meal trays of liquids and soft foods. He coughed regularly while eating and complained of difficulty swallowing. A FEES examination was done at bedside in the Intensive Care Unit.

Findings
Before delivery of food and liquid, the larynx and hypopharynx were viewed. Reduced movement of the left vocal fold and arytenoid were noted at rest, for breath holding, and phonation. Complete closure of the airway was only achieved with great effort. In addition, left lateral pharyngeal wall contraction appeared to be reduced at the onset of dry swallows. Secretions were visible throughout the hypopharynx and in the laryngeal vestibule and were actively aspirated, although the patient inconsistently and ineffectively attempted to clear them with throat clearing and coughing. The entire laryngeal vestibule was edematous.

Ice chips (½ tsp. × 5) were first delivered to the patient and were swallowed fairly successfully (only ⅕ with some aspiration). Therefore, food and liquids were delivered to assess swallowing function. There was a consistent slight delay initiating the swallow of about 1 second, with pureed boluses falling mid-way down the lateral channels but liq-

uid boluses falling to the pyriforms and sometimes (2 to 5 times) flowing into the laryngeal vestibule before the swallow was initiated. The swallow itself was weak, with reduced pharyngeal wall medial wall movement on the left side and with more residue on the weakened left side. Although the patient attempted to clear this residue spontaneously with as many as 7 or 8 dry swallows, he was ineffective in clearing the bolus. On 2 to 5 swallows of thin liquid, aspiration occurred before the swallow was initiated, and on 1 to 3 swallows of pureed, aspiration during the swallow was evidenced by residue of material on the subglottic shelf. Head turning to the patient's affected left side did appear to reduce the residue, but significant residue still remained on the right side. More food was not given, but if it had been, the buildup of residue would have resulted in aspiration of the residue at some point.

Impressions
Severe dysphagia, characterized by the following: (1) weakened laryngeal, pharyngeal (and possibly lingual) movement, especially on the left side, causing incomplete bolus clearance and airway protection and allowing aspiration to occur during and after the swallow; (2) mild delay initiating the swallow, causing some spillage of material into the hypopharynx prior to the swallow and aspiration before the swallow; (3) anatomy was altered by edema of laryngeal structures; and (4) sensation was suspected to be mildly reduced, especially for those structures that were edematous and possibly more on the affected left side. The changes in anatomy and sensation may be largely related to the intubation during and postsurgery, while the weakness on the left side suggests possible neurologic damage to the recurrent laryngeal nerve. The delay initiating the swallow may be related to reduced sensation or may be a temporary condition related to the recent trauma and fatigue of undergoing major surgery.

Recommendations
The patient is not able to take food or liquid safely by mouth at this time. Ice chips are recommended as tolerated by the patient to help dilute and clear secretions that might otherwise accumulate in the hypopharynx and be aspirated. Reevaluation (FEES) in 3 days to determine if there has been a change in swallowing function. Direct therapy is not recommended at this time because of his weakened state and anticipated spontaneous improvement in function. Consider alternative means of nutrition at this time.

Comment

Several key findings that accounted for the dysphagia were apparent from the endoscopic exam: altered anatomy, reduced movement/weakness of the left side of the larynx (innervated by the recurrent laryngeal nerve) and pharynx (CNs IX and X), mild delay initiating the swallow with spillage and aspiration of liquids before the swallow. Although the event of aspiration of pureed foods was not directly observed, it was evidenced from residue after the swallow. Further information that might be gained from a fluoroscopy study was not felt to be necessary or even useful at this time. A repeat FEES exam was believed to be indicated in a few days to determine whether the edema had subsided, whether the patient was swallowing his secretions successfully, and whether the reduced movement of the left side of the larynx and pharynx was still present. An improvement in any of these conditions would signal a possible readiness for food or liquid.

RISKS ASSOCIATED WITH VIDEOENDOSCOPY

The risks are negligible when performing rigid oral endoscopy for evaluating laryngeal function for voice production, provided the clinician has received adequate training and no topical anesthetic is applied. The potential for stimulating a cough or gag response is always present but usually can be minimized with appropriate technique. However, if the patient's gag reflex is sufficiently sensitive that an adequate view of the larynx is not possible, application of oral anesthetic or use of nasal videoendoscopy may be necessary.

When topical anesthetic is applied, there is a small risk of allergic reaction to the anesthesia. Medical clearance to apply topical anesthesia should be obtained prior to using such agents for clinical purposes and application should be limited to institutions that provide medical support should an unexpected reaction occur. Also, when applying anesthesia for FEES, only a very small amount (about 1 ml) of viscous lidocaine is inserted partly into one of the nares so that only the most narrow part of the nose (usually between the median septal wall and the inferior turbinate) is numbed. By using viscous lidocaine rather than a spray, sensitivity in the pharynx and larynx for intact swallowing function is preserved, and any risks from using an anesthetic that might pass into the lungs is eliminated. A FEES[SM] protocol requires that the anesthetic, if used, be lidocaine 2% hydrocloride gel, which is one of the safest anesthetics available. If any reaction should occur, it will likely be a localized reaction within the nose itself.[20]

Three other possible risks from nasal endoscopy are nose bleed, vasovagal response, and laryngospasm. All these are largely preventable because of the nature of the examination. Well-trained clinicians carefully monitor passage of the endoscope through the nasal lumen using visual and tactile feedback to assure there is minimal contact pressure between the endoscope insertion tube and the nasal mucosa. Visual feedback occurs as the clinician views the nasal passage through the endoscope or on the television monitor. Tactile feedback occurs as the clinician senses resistance to passage of the endoscope as the clinician's thumb and forefinger gently guide the insertion tube forward. Resistance to insertion can be felt as it occurs, and the scope position can be adjusted to avoid discomfort or nosebleed.

Risk of laryngospasm is minimized by avoiding direct contact between the endoscope and the true vocal folds, arytenoids, and epiglottis during laryngeal and swallowing examinations. The epiglottis is only intentionally touched during a FEES if laryngeal sensitivity is highly suspect. Laryngospasm has been reported in the literature only when the stimulus is perceived by the patient as extremely noxious, as may occur during a sudden gastroesophageal reflux event.[21] It is most commonly reported in patients who have undergone general anesthesia and are being extubated.[22] If laryngospasm should occur, it will most likely break spontaneously. The endoscope should be withdrawn and the patient instructed to try to relax. If this does not work, the Heimlich maneuver or oxygen can be applied intra-orally to break the laryngospasm.

Vasovagal response, or fainting, is usually due to patient anxiety.[23,24] This complication is preventable as long as the examiner monitors the patient carefully and conveys an air of calm reassurance. Heart rate can be monitored during the exam and if the pulse quickens dramatically, signaling a possible vasovagal response, the exam should be terminated. If the patient does faint, he or she should be laid supine with the feet above the head. Smelling salts can be applied and medical assistance should always be sought. Vasovagal response can be dangerous in the patient who has an acute cardiac condition with predisposition to bradycardia or cardiac dysrhythmia.[25,26] The authors would recommend that a physician be available for procedures done on patients with complex health problems.

Aspiration is a potential complication that accompanies all dysphagia examinations. The FEES[SM] protocol calls for a conservative approach to this problem. If the patient has not eaten by mouth for awhile or if a swallow reflex is suspected to be absent, the protocol calls for delivery of 2 ml ice chips as the first external bolus to be swallowed. Only after several successful swallows of ice chips would the patient be given food or liquid that, if aspirated, would be potentially much more harmful to the lungs. This stands in contrast to the fluoroscopy procedure, where barium or barium-laced food and liquid must be delivered to the patient to assess swallowing potential. It is probably worth emphasizing that the unlikely but possible risks associated with either endoscopy or fluoroscopy are far less serious than the well-known risks of aspiration, which are likely to continue if the speech–language pathologist is unable to assess the problem and intervene in a meaningful way.

Risks associated with nasal endoscopy are somewhat more complex than those associated with oral endoscopy. We maintain that flexible nasal endoscopy should be performed only in environments that provide medical support.

Transmission of infectious disease is always a concern when performing endoscopy. Endoscopes must be cleaned according to guidelines such as those developed by the Association of Professionals in Infection Control and Epidemiology and the Association for the Advancement of Medical Instrumentation.[27,28] These guidelines change from time to time so it is important to stay current with recent developments. Use of Universal Precautions[29] is advised to protection both patient and clinician.

SUMMARY

There are many reasons why the speech–language pathologist should be involved in performing videoendoscopic assessment of resonance, voice, and swallowing. The speech–language pathologist who performs endoscopy has extensive training in normal anatomy and physiology of speech production and swallowing and behavioral manipulation of speech behavior. The speech–language pathologist is also acutely aware of the *variability* of normal anatomical and physiological requirements for voice, speech, and swallowing function. Knowing the difference between normal variability and abnormal function is often the key in interpreting videoendoscopic recordings.

Videoendoscopy requires a degree of tolerance, cooperation, and stimulability on the part of the patient given the presence of the scope. It is critical that the patient be as comfortable as possible so the speech and voice tasks and foods and liquids provided evoke natural resonance, voice, or swallowing function. Speech–language pathologists skilled in behavioral manipulation have special competencies that lend themselves to successful, high-quality videoendoscopic assessments of voice, speech, and swallowing. The speech–language pathologist has training in principles of behavioral modification and motor learning that is critical to conducting the videoendoscopic examination in a manner that lends itself to assessing the extent to which behavioral intervention (therapy) may be useful as part of the overall treatment plan. The involvement of the speech–language pathologist is warranted in maximizing the value of the videoendoscopic assessment of voice, resonance, and swallowing.

STUDY QUESTIONS

1. What are some indications for speech–language pathologists to use endoscopy?

2. When is videoendoscopy used to assess velopharyngeal closure?

3. What speech samples should be included in the videoendoscopic examination of velopharyngeal closure for speech?

4. What are the two major types of laryngeal movements observed during the videoendoscopic examination of voice.

5. When is flexible endoscopy is used during the videoendoscopic examination of voice?

6. What parameters of vocal fold appearance and motion are usually observed during videostroboscopy?

7. What elements of anatomy and physiology of the swallow may be seen using videoendoscopy?

8. What are the indications for a FEES examination?

9. What pathophysiology does spillage of material into the hypopharynx before the swallow is initiated?

REFERENCES

1. Karnell MP: *Videoendoscopy—From velopharynx to larynx.* Singular Publishing, San Diego, 1994.
2. Hirano M, Bless DM: *Videostroboscopic examination of the larynx.* Singular Publishing, San Diego, 1993.
3. Langmore SE, McCulloch TM: Examination of the pharynx and larynx and endoscopic examination of

pharyngeal swallowing. In Perlman AL, Schulze-Delrieu K, eds., *Deglutition and Its Disorders,* pp 201–226. Singular Publishing, San Diego, 1997.

4. Golding-Kushner KJ, Argamaso RV, Cotton RT, Grames LM, Henningsson G, Jones DL, Karnell MP, Klaiman PG, Lewin ML, Marsh JL, McCall GN, McGrath CO, Muntz HR, Nevdahl MT, Rakoff SJ, Shprintzen RJ, Sidoti EJ, Vallino LD, Volk M, Williams WN, Witzel MA, Dixon-Wood VL, Ysunza A, D'Antonio L, Isberg A, Pigott RW, Skolnick L: Standardization for the reporting of nasopharyngoscopy and multiview videofluoroscopy: A report from an international working group. *Cleft Palate J* 1990; 27:337–347.

5. Shprintzen RJ, Lencione RM, McCall GN, Skolnick ML: A three dimensional cinefluoroscopic analysis of velopharyngeal closure during speech and nonspeech activities in normals. *Cleft Palate J* 1974; 11:412–428.

6. Morris HL: Types of velopharyngeal incompetence. In Winitz H, ed., *Treating articulation disorders: For clinicians by clinicians.* University Park Press, Baltimore, 1984.

7. Karnell MP: Nasometric discrimination of hypernasality and turbulent nasal airflow. *Cleft Palate J* 1995; 32:145–148.

8. Hirano M: *Clinical examination of voice.* Springer-Verlag, New York, 1991.

9. Kidder TM, Langmore SE, Martin BJW: Indications and techniques of endoscopy in evaluation of cervical dysphagia: Comparison with radiographic techniques. *Dysphagia* 1994; 9:256–261.

10. Langmore SE, Logemann JA: After the clinical bedside swallowing examination: What next? *Am J Speech–Lang Path* 1991; 1:13–20.

11. Langmore SE, Schatz K, Olsen N: Fiberoptic endoscopic examination of swallowing safety: A new procedure. *Dysphagia* 1988; 2:216–219.

12. Langmore SE, Schatz K, Olsen N: Endoscopic and videofluoroscopic evaluations of swallowing and aspiration. *Ann Otorhinolaryn* 1991; 100:678–681.

13. Murray J, Langmore SE, Ginsberg S, Dostie A: The significance of accumulated oropharyngeal secretions and swallowing frequency in predicting aspiration. *Dysphagia* 1996; 11:99–103.

14. Aviv JE, Martin JH, Keen MS, Debell M, Blitzer A: Air pulse quantification of supraglottic and pharyngeal sensation: A new technique. *Ann Otorhinolaryn* 1993; 102:777–780.

15. Aviv JE, Martin JH, Sacco RL, Zagar D, Diamond B, Keen MS, Blitzer A: Supraglottic and pharyngeal sensory abnormalities in stroke patients with dysphagia. *Ann Otorhinolaryn* 1996; 105:92–97.

16. Miller CK, Willging JP, Strife JL, Rudolph CD: Fiberoptic endoscopic examination of swallowing infants and children with feeding disorders. *Dysphagia* 1994; 9:266.

17. Horner J, Buoyer FG, Alberts MJ, & Helms MJ: Dysphagia following brain-stem stroke: Clinical correlates and outcome. *Arch Neurol* 1991; 48:1170–1173.

18. Horner J, Massey EW, Riski JE, Lathrop DL, Chase KN: Aspiration following stroke: Clinical correlates and outcome. *Neurol* 1988; 38:1359–1362.

19. Veis SJ, Logemann JA: Swallowing disorders in persons with cerebrovascular accidents. *Arch Phys Med Rehab* 1985; 66:372–375.

20. Eyre J, Nally FF: Nasal test for hypersensitivity including a positive reaction to lignocaine. *Lancet* 1971; 1:264–265.

21. Bortolotti M: Laryngospasm and reflex central apnea caused by aspiration of refluxed gastric contents in adults. *Gut* 1989; 30:233–238.

22. Staffel GJ: The prevention of postoperative stridor and laryngospasm with topical lidocaine. *Arch Otolaryng Head Neck Surg* 1991; 117:1123–1128.

23. Kelly TJ: Mechanics and treatment of vasovagal syncope. *Patient Care* 1991; 62:216–218.

24. Kleinknecht RA, Lenz J, Ford G, DeBerard S: Types and correlates of blood injury-related vasovagal syncope. *Behav Res Therapy* 1990; 28:289–295.

25. Fitzpatrick A, Theodrakis G, Vardas P, Kenny RA, Travill CM, Ingram A, Sutton R: The incidence of malignant vasovagal syndrome in patients with recurrent syncope. *Eur Heart J* 1991; 12:389–394.

26. Van Lieshout JJ, Weiling W, Karemaker JM, Eckberg DL: The vasovagal response. *Clin Sci* 1991; 81:575–586.

27. Rutala WA: APIC Guideline for selection and use of disinfectants. *Am J Infect Control* 1996; 24:313–342.

28. American National Standard: *Safe use and handling of glutaraldehyde-based products in health care facilities.* ANSI/AAMI ST58, 1996.

29. Center for Disease Control: Recommendations for prevention of HIV Transmission in Health-Care Settings. *MMWR* 1987; 36 Suppl. No. 25.

Appendix A
Competencies

Successful, safe performance of videoendoscopy requires the skills of a competent clinician. The following list of competencies have been adapted from those proposed by the American Speech–Language-Hearing Association Special Interest Division (SID 3) for Voice and Voice Disorders Subcommittee for Training Guidelines for Laryngeal Videoendoscopy/Stroboscopy. While these preliminary guidelines do not represent official ASHA policy and are likely to be revised, we feel they are worth presenting here for consideration and discussion.

1. Familiarity with the various roles of medical doctors, speech–language pathologists, nurses, and support staff involved in the provision of videoendoscopy.
2. Ability to communicate well with medical doctors, nurses, and patients in an interdisciplinary patient-care environment.
3. Familiarity with normal and pathological velopharyngeal, laryngeal, and pharyngeal anatomy and physiology, medical terminology as it pertains to velopharyngeal, laryngeal, and swallowing disorders, and principles and techniques of speech, voice, and swallowing therapy.
4. Familiarity with the various approaches to becoming trained to perform videoendoscopy.
5. Ability to identify, select, assemble, operate, and maintain the equipment necessary to perform videoendoscopy.
6. Ability to recognize ad identify patients who are appropriate for videoendoscopy.
7. Ability to technically perform videoendoscopy using oral and flexible endo-

scopes in a manner that yields maximum quality recordings.
8. Ability to interpret effects of behavior and anatomy on physiology in coordination and cooperation with medical colleagues.
9. Ability to concisely describe videoendoscopy findings and interpretations for professional communication purposes.
10. Ability to organize, store and retrieve LVES data for quality assurance and treatment efficacy purposes.

Becoming competent requires a mix of training and experience. Competence also requires interest, ability, and motivation on the part of the clinician. Not all clinicians have the innate qualities necessary to perform effective videoendoscopy. Identification of the presence or absence of these attributes in prospective endoscopists is the responsibility of both teachers and students of videoendoscopy.

We support flexibility in the training process. Strict guidelines that specify numbers of procedures performed or amount of time in training should be avoided when possible. The training process should be tailored to provide efficient yet thorough preparation for each clinician who is interested in learning to perform videoendoscopy.

23

Rehabilitation of the Head and Neck Cancer Patient

MICHAEL S. BENNINGER AND CINDY GRYWALSKI

Cancer is second only to heart disease as the major cause of death in the United States, accounting for approximately 22% of all deaths.[1] Head and neck cancers account for approximately 10% of all cancers and 5% of all cancer deaths, if skin cancers are included. The American Cancer Society estimated that there were 41,090 newly diagnosed cases of oral cavity, pharyngeal, and laryngeal cancers in the United States during 1996, and an estimated 12,510 deaths resulted from these cancers.[2] Using these estimates, oral cavity, pharyngeal, and laryngeal cancers accounted for 3% of all newly diagnosed cancers and 2% of all deaths from cancer.

Although these percentages may not seem staggering, the effects of head and neck cancers are often pronounced, interfering with an individual's physical, psychological, and social well-being. Basic life functions can be drastically altered by the disease and the treatment regimen used to try to cure it. For this reason, head and neck cancer patients require management from a number of medical and nonmedical perspectives.

Head and neck cancers afflict more men than women, although incidence and mortality rates for women have increased over the last 30 years.[2] This increase has coincided with increases in the number of women who use tobacco, a known risk factor for head and neck cancers. Incidence and mortality rates for some head and neck cancers are higher for African Americans,[2] possibly related to differences in nutrition or socioeconomic factors that interfere with early detection and improved survival. Incidence rates for specific cancer sites within the head and neck vary with geography. For example, oral cavity and oropharyngeal cancers account for almost half of all cancers in the East and Far East.[3] The incidence of nasopharyngeal carcinoma in the people of Kwang Tung Province in China is 25 times higher than it is in whites.[4] Environmental, cultural, ethnic, and genetic conditions are likely explanations for the relationship between the predominance of a particular head and neck cancer site and geographic location.

Speech–language pathologists become involved in the therapeutic regimen for head and neck cancer patients because one or more of the basic speech subsystems (respiration, phonation, resonation, and articulation) and/or swallowing may be affected by the cancer treatment to varying degrees. Head and neck tumors are challenging to manage from a medical standpoint because of the complexity, compactness, and important functions of head and neck structures. Head and neck cancers may invade any of the organs or air-filled spaces that form the upper aerodigestive tract, from the base of the skull superiorly to the trachea inferiorly, and from the tip of the nose anteriorly to the pharyngeal wall posteriorly. When surgical removal of a head and neck tumor is undertaken, it can be difficult to maintain negative (noncancerous) margins because structures are close in proximity. Surgical resection of the tumor often involves removal of more than the tumor host structure. These tumors may seriously interfere with basic human functions, such as breathing, swallowing, and speaking. Treatment of these tumors may result in permanent physical alterations and drastic lifestyle changes. Speech–language pathologists must predicate their plans for rehabilitation of these patients with sound knowledge of normal head and neck anatomy and physiology. They must understand the functional consequences that result from alterations in head and neck structures. They need to maintain current knowledge of medical treatments for head and neck cancer. They must seek and exchange information with other medical specialists who care for this group of patients. Above all, they must apply the information they have gathered to effectively manage their patients' communication and swallowing problems, recognizing that each patient's

responses to the cancer, its treatment, and the subsequent rehabilitation course are unique.

This chapter presents a framework for provision of speech–language pathology services to head and neck cancer patients. We provide a general description of the anatomic subdivisions of the mucosal surfaces that line the head and neck, common tumor sites and symptoms for each anatomic subdivision, diagnostic procedures for head and neck cancers, medical treatment options, guidelines for the timing of speech and swallowing intervention, alterations in speech and swallowing following head and neck cancer treatment, and management procedures. The information in this chapter is primarily intended to assist speech–language pathologists who are preparing to work with head and neck cancer patients in a medical setting by offering basic information and practical guidelines. The framework for rehabilitation presented in this chapter emphasizes the health care team approach because treatment for head and neck cancer patients is multifaceted and requires information from many different medical and nonmedical perspectives.

ANATOMICAL REGIONS OF THE HEAD AND NECK

The most common cancer of the head and neck is squamous cell carcinoma, which may involve any of the mucosal surfaces of the upper aerodigestive tract. Tumors that form on these mucosal surfaces can have an impact on speech and swallowing. Our discussion of head and neck anatomy focuses on these internal structures, where tumors are frequently found. It is helpful to conceptualize the internal head and neck region as four distinct compartments with landmark structures and air-filled spaces that can be found in each one, keeping in mind that tumors frequently do not contain themselves inside these somewhat arbitrarily determined compartments. The following description of head and neck anatomy is general at best. Readers who want more thorough descriptions are referred to sources that devote major emphases to the anatomy of the speech and swallowing mechanisms, such as the one by Zemlin.[5]

The four major intrinsic cavities of the head and neck region are the nasal cavity, the oral cavity (including lips, cheeks, and buccal spaces), the pharyngeal cavity, and the laryngeal cavity (Figure 23–1). The framework for these cavities is bony and cartilaginous. Muscles and connective tissues attach to the framework, and all is covered with a lining of moist mucosa. The structures and air spaces located in each cavity help to define the anatomic boundaries.

The Nasal Cavity

The nasal cavity serves as a passage for air and is divided medially by the nasal septum into somewhat symmetrical chambers. The anterior nares (nostrils) connect the nasal cavity with the external environment. The posterior nares (choanae) connect the nasal cavity to the nasopharynx. Other important structures to be noted in the nasal cavity are the superior, middle, and inferior nasal turbinates. These tissue masses serve to heat, moisten, and filter nasally inhaled air. The sinuses and the lacrimal (tear) system drain into the nose by way of the meatuses of the turbinates. Cranial nerve I (olfactory) innervates the upper portion of the nose.

The Oral Cavity

The oral cavity can be thought of as the mouth. It contains a number of structures necessary for speech and swallowing. It is bounded anteriorly by the lips, laterally by the buccal (cheek) spaces, posterolaterally by the anterior faucial pillars, superiorly by the juncture of the hard and soft palates, and inferiorly by the floor of the mouth, with its mobile anterior two-thirds of the tongue. Important structures in the oral cavity are the lips, teeth, gums, buccal mucosa, upper alveolar ridge, lower alveolar ridge, retromolar gingiva (retromolar trigone), floor of the mouth, sublingual salivary gland and ducts, hard palate, and freely mobile portion (anterior and middle third portions) of the tongue.

The Pharynx

The pharynx is a tube-shaped cavity made up primarily of connective tissue superiorly and muscle tissue inferiorly. It allows the passage of air and food. In adults, the superior border of the pharynx is at the level of the base of the skull and the inferior border is at the level of the cricoid cartilage and the sixth cervical vertebra. The pharynx is divided into three sections: the nasopharynx, the oropharynx, and the hypopharynx. The nasopharynx connects superiorly with portions of the sphenoid and occipital bones of the skull. On its lateral walls are the openings to the eustachian tubes, which communicate with the tympanic cavities bilaterally. The soft palate is the inferior border of

the nasopharynx as well as the superior border of the oropharynx. The oropharynx extends inferiorly to the level of the hyoid bone, and connects with the oral cavity anteriorly at the anterior faucial pillars. The oropharynx contains the posterior third portion of the tongue, or tongue base, and the palatine tonsils. Contiguous with the oropharynx is the hypopharynx, with its superior border at the level of the hyoid bone. Its inferior border is the pharyngoesophageal segment, a sphincter of muscle that marks the bottom of the pharynx and the top of the esophagus. Laterally, the hypopharynx shares margins with the larynx at the pyriform sinuses, although the medial walls of the pyriform sinuses are considered part of the larynx.

The Larynx

The intrinsic larynx is the fourth major head and neck cavity. It is suspended superiorly from the U-shaped hyoid bone by accessory laryngeal muscles. The hyoid bone can be considered a part of the larynx because it is an important attachment site, although it is also considered a lingual bone because a number of lingual muscles attach to it.[6] The larynx extends from the epiglottis and valleculae superiorly to the lower border of the cricoid cartilage inferiorly. Valleculae are bilateral grooves formed by the tongue base and epiglottis that act as holding tanks for material about to be swallowed and channel it away from the laryngeal inlet. Like the pharynx, the larynx is divided into three distinct anatomical sections: the supraglottic larynx, the glottic larynx, and the subglottic larynx. The supraglottic larynx contains the epiglottis (lingual and laryngeal aspects), ventricular folds (false vocal folds), the superior portions of the arytenoid cartilages, and the aryepiglottic folds. The glottic larynx runs the horizontal length of the true vocal folds from the anterior commissure, where the vocal folds have a common attachment to the inner angle of the thyroid cartilage, to the posterior commissure, where each fold attaches to its respective arytenoid cartilage at the vocal process. The superior border of the glottic larynx is the laryngeal ventricle, which is the space that separates the false and true vocal folds. The inferior border of the glottic larynx, marked at 1 cm below the free medial margins of the true vocal folds, is the superior border of the subglottic larynx. The lower margin of the cricoid cartilage is the inferior boundary of the subglottic larynx, where the trachea begins. The four major internal cavities of the head and neck are shown in Figure 23–1.

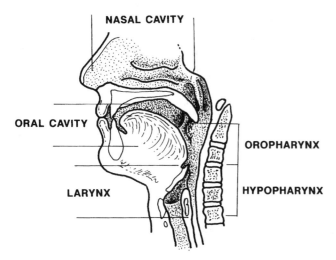

Figure 23–1. The four internal compartments of the head and neck.

Neural, Vascular, and Lymphatic Systems

It is important to keep in mind that the head and neck region contains bone, cartilage, and neural, vascular, and lymphatic networks that can become involved directly or indirectly in the neoplastic disease process. Cranial nerves V (trigeminal), VII (facial), IX (glossopharyngeal), X (vagus), XI (spinal accessory), and XII (hypoglossal) have sensory and motor branches coursing through the head and neck that could be disturbed by perineural invasion of the tumor or its treatment.

The function of lymphatics is to return water and protein to the blood from interstitial fluid.[7] Lymphatic vessels and nodes are well represented in the head and neck. Regional lymph node status is one of the components of head and neck tumor classification and staging (the "N" in the TNM classification system). Lymph is a clear, watery fluid that flows through lymphatic vessels and one or more lymph nodes before leaving the neck by way of the thoracic duct or the right lymphatic ducts. Passage of lymph through more than one lymph node may explain tumor spread in this region, as lymph from an area of tumor travels through a number of head and neck lymph nodes before leaving the area. The system of lymphatic drainage in the head and neck is relatively closed off from the rest of the body, and provides probable explanations for the local containment of tumor spread frequently seen in his region.[8] Lymphatic representation is much more limited and confined in the intrinsic structures of the larynx than it is in external laryngeal structures, resulting in mechanisms of metastasis that are more limited and confined as well.[9] More extensive nodal involvement indicates less favorable prognosis.[10,11]

TISSUE CHANGES IN HEAD AND NECK CANCER

The four major internal cavities of the head and neck form a contiguous tract for air and food, called the upper aerodigestive tract. A mucous membrane consisting of stratified squamous epithelium lines the oral cavity, oropharynx, hypopharynx, and glottic larynx; the nasal cavity, supraglottic larynx, and subglottic larynx have ciliated columnar epithelium; and the nasopharynx has mixed mucosa.[8] There are a number of histological changes that can occur in these membranous linings. Some of these changes result in benign growths, such as nodules, polyps, and cysts. Some cellular changes indicate a precancerous state. Leukoplakia is a term that describes a "white patch" of abnormal growth and signifies changes in the normal mucosa, some which may be premalignant. Atypia, metaplasia, dysplasia, and hyperplasia are other terms used to describe cellular changes in normal mucosa that may be precancerous. In the head and neck, squamous cell carcinoma is by far the most common type of malignancy, and the one discussed in this chapter. It is found in 90% of all laryngeal cancers.[12] Adenocarcinomas (malignant tumors originating in accessory salivary and mucous gland epithelium) and sarcomas (malignant tumors originating in bone, cartilage, muscle, or connective tissue) occur much less frequently in the head and neck. The earliest detectable malignant change in the squamous epithelium is called carcinoma in situ. The cellular changes associated with carcinoma in situ are restricted to the thickness of the epithelium, and do not invade the basement membrane or other tissue layers.[13] More invasive cellular changes are systematically classified and staged, as explained below.

Almost all malignant cellular changes in the head and neck are reactions to chronic irritation, and most of this irritation is associated with common carcinogenic agents, principally tobacco (including smokeless) and alcohol. Gastroesophageal reflux has been studied as a comorbid condition for some cancers, particularly cancer of the larynx.[14] Poor oral hygiene has also been studied for its role in oral cavity cancers.[4] There has been research interest in the area of cancer genetics that may help to identify individuals who are more likely to develop head and neck cancers or have a worse prognosis. Loss or inactivation of certain tumor supressor genes has been found in patients with squamous cell carcinoma of the head and neck, and this loss has been related to poor patient survival.[15]

HEAD AND NECK TUMOR SITES AND SYMPTOMS

The site and size of the tumor determine the constellation of symptoms that patients with head and neck cancer experience.[16] The universal symptoms of pain, bleeding, and a nonhealing sore or ulcer are common. Otalgia, or ear pain, is often reported, but this is more often a referred pain from tumors in the oral cavity, pharynx, larynx, or trachea than from an ear tumor. A lump or thickening on the neck or in the mouth is reported by patients, as is difficulty in chewing, swallowing, and moving the tongue or jaw.

Less than 1% of all malignancies are carcinomas of the nasal and paranasal areas.[17,18] Patients with nasal cavity tumors do not typically work with a speech–language pathologist because speech and swallowing dysfunction are atypical. Large, obstructive tumors in the nasal or nasopharyngeal cavity certainly could cause hyponasal resonance, but a more critical symptom is blockage of nasal airflow, and this requires medical management.

Common tumor sites in the oral cavity are the anterior floor of the mouth, the lateral floor of the mouth, the mobile portion of the tongue, and the hard palate. Oral cavity cancers appear as lumps in the mouth or ulcers that do not heal. They may become irritated and bleed during chewing or denture use. Patients may report that they have been eating softer diets to ease mouth pain.

The tonsil, base of tongue, and soft palate are common sites for tumors in the oropharynx. Tumors here are often asymptomatic in the early stages, and as a result they are associated with increased metastatic rates, treatment failures, and mortality rates. Sixty percent of tonsil or base of tongue tumors metastasize regionally.[19] An external neck mass may be the initial symptom from any head and neck tumor, although it is more common in nasopharyngeal, oropharyngeal, and hypopharyngeal cancers. Another common symptom with pharyngeal tumors is ear pain. This is a referred pain from the tumor site to the ear mediated by cranial nerves VII, IX, or X. Dysphagia and odynophagia are common complaints. Hoarseness is present only in fairly advanced hypopharyngeal cancers. A gradually worsening sore throat is a typical symptom of oropharyngeal tumors.

Early nasopharyngeal tumors may produce mild nasal obstruction and posterior nasal drainage, but these symptoms can often be ignored by patients because they are common occurrences in general. The two most commonly presenting symptoms of nasopharyngeal tumors are serous otitis media from eustachian tube obstruction and a neck mass. As these tumors advance, worsening nasal obstruction and epistaxis (nosebleeding) may occur.

Tumors in the supraglottic larynx are primarily found on the epiglottis, the aryepiglottic fold, or the false vocal fold. Tumors in the glottic larynx are typically on the vocal folds. These structures form the three levels of sphincteric airway protection during swallowing.[20] When supraglottic tumors are surgically excised, the supraglottic laryngectomy patient is left with only the true vocal folds for airway protection and this may cause serious swallowing problems. Fortunately, most patients can eat and swallow in a satisfactory manner following supraglottic laryngectomy with appropriate swallowing therapy. Early cancerous lesions on the true vocal folds cause persistent hoarseness or a breathy voice, and concern for the detrimental voice change usually brings patients to the otolaryngologist. Other symptoms of laryngeal cancer that are reported in the course of the disease are scratchy throat, dysphagia, odynophagia (painful swallowing), hemoptysis (spitting up blood), chronic cough, and otalgia. Dyspnea (breathing difficulty), stridor (noisy inhalation), and halitosis (foul-smelling breath) are generally late appearing symptoms, indicative of airway obstruction and tissue necrosis. Isolated subglottic tumors are rare, but the subglottis may be the site of tumor extension.

Systemic (entire body) symptoms are uncommon in patients with squamous cell carcinoma of the head and neck, except in advanced disease when weight loss and general feelings of malaise and fatigue occur. Halitosis is common in many patients with head and neck cancers, particularly in those who consume alcohol excessively. Since most of these patients have had a long history of tobacco exposure, it is not unlikely that they will have sequelae of such exposure, such as chronic obstructive pulmonary disease, emphysema, hypertension, or even lung cancer. These other medical conditions should be considered when planning treatment. For example, a supraglottic laryngectomy for removal of an epiglottic tumor may be contraindicated if the patient also has severe pulmonary disease and cannot risk compromised swallowing.

Patients with any of the symptoms discussed above may find their way to a speech–language pathologist for evaluation of speech, voice, and/or swallowing before a medical exam has taken place. Since a malignant tumor may be the cause of patients' symptoms, referral to an otorhinolaryngologist is necessary. Delays in diagnosis and treatment can be avoided by the astute clinician who recognizes the importance of the physical exam in the expedient identification and treatment of head and neck cancers.

DIAGNOSIS OF HEAD AND NECK CANCER

Obtaining the History

A patient who is experiencing physical or functional changes of head and neck structures will very frequently be referred to an otorhinolaryngologist. Clinical assessment comprises a medical history and a physical exam, which then may lead to further testing, such as roentgenographic imaging, computed tomography, magnetic resonance imaging, blood sampling, and tissue biopsy procedures. A thorough history of presenting symptoms is most essential in the evaluation of patients with head and neck cancers. Risk factors associated with development of carcinoma need to be identified, particularly remote and current exposure to tobacco and alcohol. Other important areas of questioning pertain to previous medical or surgical problems, current use of medications, and the course of symptom progression. It would be remiss if history taking did not include assessment of the patient's psychosocial status because this provides information about likely coping abilities and available support from family and friends if medical management is undertaken.

The Physical Exam

Once a complete history has been obtained, the physical exam is undertaken to palpate areas of the head and neck, including lymph node areas on the neck, and visually inspect the skin, scalp, and mucosal surfaces of the ears, nose, oral cavity, pharynx, and larynx. Indirect exams with a light, a head mirror, and a small angled laryngeal mirror placed strategically in the oropharynx are used to look at the nasopharynx, hypopharynx, and larynx. If a patient's strong gag prohibits indirect examination of the larynx, a topical anesthetic may be used to numb the oropharynx or it may be necessary to transnasally pass a flexible fiberoptic endoscope, an instrument made up of long, very thin cylinders, some of which illuminate the larynx and others that allow its viewing through an eyepiece. It may be necessary to assess the vibratory function of the vocal folds with laryngeal videostroboscopy. This exam simulates slow motion of vocal fold vibration by controlling the timing of light flashes on the larynx during phonation. With laryngeal videostroboscopy, the effects of vocal fold lesions on vibratory function can be determined. It may allow for identification of an adynamic segment of the vocal fold, such as an area of leukoplakia, that may suggest early invasion of a lesion.[21] Exams with the flexible fiberoptic endoscope and laryngeal stroboscope allow for videotaped documentation and tracking of the tumor throughout the course of treatment. Videotaped exams also make it possible to present and discuss a case at a tumor board conference. The composition and function of a multidisciplinary tumor board for head and neck cancer are discussed later in the chapter.

For optimal direct viewing of the larynx and pharynx, a direct pharyngoscopy/laryngoscopy is frequently performed. This procedure is the key to accurate diagnosis and staging of the disease. It is generally not a procedure done in the clinic, but one performed in the operating room with the patient under general anesthesia. Bastian[22] has described a clinic procedure using a flexible laryngoscope and adequate anesthesia to appropriately stage the tumor and obtain biopsies, obviating the need for general anesthesia in the operating room. At the time of the direct pharyngoscopy/laryngoscopy, a tissue biopsy is usually obtained and sent to a pathology laboratory for confirmation of malignancy. This procedure can also be used to identify a possible second primary tumor. Individuals with a tumor in the head and neck have a 7% chance of having a second tumor somewhere else in the aerodigestive tract.[23] This could be in the pharynx, larynx, lungs, or esophagus. The chance of having a second primary tumor has made some medical practitioners advocate the use of triple endoscopy (direct bronchoscopy, esophagoscopy, and pharyngoscopy/laryngoscopy) for all patients with an index squamous cell carcinoma (tumor responsible for the patient's symptoms), but this is not always necessary. Direct pharyngoscopy/laryngoscopy is the usual procedure for the evaluation and staging of most head and neck cancer patients, and bronchoscopy and esophagoscopy may be reserved for patients who report symptoms that would suggest pulmonary or esophageal involvement.[23]

Noninvasive imaging techniques are also used to gather diagnostic information, particularly in the detection of metastatic disease. The two most common techniques used with head and neck cancers are computerized tomographic (CT) scanning and magnetic resonance imaging (MRI). A CT scan provides a series of X-ray views in slices of the head and neck. MRI uses radio waves traveling through a magnetic field to make detailed images of head and neck structures. These tests have functional prediagnostic applications and provide important information about tumor features, but the clinical and operative examinations are the primary information sources used to stage the disease.

CLINICAL TUMOR CLASSIFICATION

Squamous cell carcinomas of the head and neck are clinically classified based on the findings from the physical exam and any other procedures that were administered prior to the initiation of treatment, such as endoscopy, fine needle aspiration biopsy, CT scanning, MRI, chest films, and blood chemistry tests. Clinical staging follows the American Joint Commission for Cancer Staging,[24] and is commonly referred to as the TNM system. The "T" stands for the size and/or anatomical extent of the primary tumor and is followed by either the letters "I" and "S," which abbreviate "in situ," or a number ranging from 0 to 4. A T0 classification is reported when there is no tumor; a TIS lesion is reported when the tumor is a carcinoma in situ, the earliest identifiable neoplasm; and T_1, T_2, T_3, and T_4 lesions are reported based on gradually increasing tumor size, with a T_1 lesion smaller than a T_4 lesion.

The next part of the classification system is the "N," which is used to report the number, size, and location of local lymph nodes that have become involved in the disease process by way of a number ranging from 0 to 3. An N_0 is reported when no regional lymph node involvement is found; an N_3 represents a single large node or multiple nodes on the same, opposite, or both sides of the tumor. This classification describes lymph node metastasis to the neck only, and is dependent only on the neck disease and not on the size of the primary tumor. In addition, lymph node metastasis is usually described by the location of the nodes in the neck, using the following neck divisions: submental and submaxillary triangle nodes; high, middle, and low jugular chain nodes; posterior triangle nodes; and peritracheal nodes.[25]

The final classification marker is the "M" that is used to describe metastasis (spread) of the tumor to distant body regions. Except for a classification of M_X, which is reported when distant metastasis cannot be assessed (an "X" after any of the tumor classification markers indicates an inability of that component to be assessed), this classification is basically binary, with M_0 indicating no distant metastasis and M_1 indicating that distant metastasis is present.

Table 23–1. Staging of Head and Neck Carcinoma

Stage I	$T_1N_0M_0$
Stage II	$T_2N_0M_0$
Stage III	$T_3N_0M_0$ or $T_{1-3}N_1M_0$
Stage IV	$T_4M_{0-1}M_0$ or $T_{1-4}N_{2,3}M_0$ or any T, any N, M_1

Distant metastases are uncommon in squamous cell carcinoma of the head and neck except in advanced or recurrent disease, with the lungs being a common metastatic site. Because these patients usually have a history of chronic smoking, and pulmonary compromise is often present, a chest X-ray is recommended as part of the pretreatment workup.

Once the TNM classification markers have been assigned, they may be grouped into one of four stages, ranging from the earliest cancers that fall into the Stage I category to those most advanced that are placed into the Stage IV category (Table 23–1). These stages have substantial prognostic significance because likelihood of treatment failure and worsening chance for survival are associated with each advancing stage.

MEDICAL AND SURGICAL MANAGEMENT OF HEAD AND NECK CANCERS

Surgery and radiation therapy are the most common treatment modalities for squamous cell carcinoma of the head and neck. Surgical excision may be done with microsurgical instruments or a microspot laser. Surgery and radiation therapy may be administered alone, in combination with each other, or in combination with other treatment modalities, depending on the nature, site(s), and extent of the disease, the current health status of the patient, and any previous treatment procedures. One of the side effects of radiation therapy, and perhaps chemotherapy, is significant change in glandular secretions with temporary or permanent decrease in salivation, resulting in dry mouth and throat, or xerostomia. Chemotherapy as the sole treatment for head and neck cancer has not shown an improvement over surgery and/or radiation therapy. However, in an attempt to reduce recurrence rates after standard therapy, even for early stage I and stage II tumors with recurrence in 10% to 40% of cases, chemotherapy is being used in an adjuvant manner after standard therapy for its reported survival benefits.[26] It is being studied for its combined effects with radiation therapy on survival rates. The combination of radiation therapy and chemotherapy is being offered to some patients with fairly advanced tumors, such as T_3 laryngeal cancers, as an organ-preserving alternative to surgical ablation. At this time, there is little evidence to support the use of chemotherapy as the sole treatment for squamous cell carcinoma of the head and neck other than for palliation; however, drug therapy may have promise for future cures. New directions in cancer treatment, such as biologic modifiers and immunotherapy, are being investigated and may well be used in future management of head and neck cancer.[27,28] One treatment option that may be considered in advanced, unresectable cancers is to "do nothing" from an aggressive medical standpoint, and such a decision should be made after carefully counseling the patient and family about the probable treatment outcomes. If this option is chosen, a hospice program could be considered. Photodynamic therapy (PDT) is currently being studied for its effects on some forms of cancer, including the oropharynx and larynx. It involves the use of a light-sensitive drug that is retained by cancerous cells. Application of light then destroys these marked cells. Skin sensitivity to light is the major side effect of PDT, and the results of its effectiveness in head and neck cancers are not yet conclusive. Although there is some controversy related to preferred treatment protocols based on treatment results at specific medical centers, and all the treatment approaches cannot be addressed in this chapter, a summary of reasonable treatment options for head and neck squamous cell carcinoma follows.

Nasal Cancers

Nasal cancers are predominantly squamous cell carcinomas, basal cell carcinomas, or malignancies of glandular origins, such as adenocarcinomas. Since many nasal tumors originate on the skin of the nose and invade the nasal cavities by direct extension, surgical excision is usually the preferred option. Because of the complicated anatomy of this region, identification of free margins of resection is frequently difficult. Graded resections with intraoperative pathologic marginal control (MOHS chemosurgery) have allowed for resections with improved reliability of complete tumor extirpation. Larger nasal tumors and those that involve the paranasal sinuses or palate require en bloc (whole) resections, which may significantly interfere with nasal breathing, balanced resonance, and swallowing. Vision may be affected by these tumors if orbital resection is required. Additional radiation

therapy or chemotherapy is usually recommended following surgery. The cosmetic effects of nasal cancers and their treatments may be devastating to the patient, but deformities can often be corrected with further surgery or prosthetics.

Oral Cavity Tumors

Oral cavity tumors are usually treated by surgery alone, or surgery and radiation therapy combined. Key functional decisions in oral cavity tumors revolve around potential effects on chewing, swallowing, and articulation of speech, as well as cosmesis. Small cancers, such as a T_1 tumor of the anterior tongue, are usually amenable to surgical excision with wide margins. Since the tongue has limited barriers against tumor spread, larger tumors usually require postoperative radiation therapy. Surgical closure of an area where the tumor was excised can, at times, be done with tissue surrounding the lesion, and this is known as primary closure. T_3 or T_4 tumors often result in large defects of the tongue, floor of mouth or mandible, and may require reconstruction with tissue from nearby body sites, such as regional myocutaneous flaps or skin grafts, and this is known as secondary closure. In these types of closures, the replaced tissue cannot provide the same function as the original tissue, and the patient will often have difficulty with swallowing and speech, sometimes severe and incapacitating. Free flaps from distant body parts can also be used for reconstruction, and there are certain donor sites especially well suited to repair large defects of the oral cavity, such as using the iliac bone from the pelvis and some of the surrounding muscle to patch portions of the mandible. Flaps with neuronal networks can be placed at the site of the surgical defect and anastomosed to existing neuronal structures, in an attempt to restore motor and sensory function to the reconstructed area.

Nasopharyngeal and Oropharyngeal Cancers

Nasopharyngeal cancers are usually treated with radiation therapy alone, although combining it with chemotherapy may provide better disease control. Small T_1 tumors may be amenable to surgical resection, although the difficulty with access to the nasopharynx and success of radiation has made surgery a rarely used option. However, salvage surgery is a possible option for those who have failed radiation therapy.

The management of cancers of the oropharynx is somewhat controversial. Both radiation therapy and surgery have been advocated as primary modalities. The decision to treat with one or the other depends mostly on the nature of the tumor. The advantage of radiation therapy is that it is more likely to preserve important structures and, in turn, their functions. Furthermore, oropharyngeal tumors tend to be particularly radiosensitive, resulting in initially good response rates. The outcome of primary radiation therapy, with surgical salvage for failures, is comparable to surgery followed by postoperative radiation therapy. Surgery usually requires reconstructive techniques such as flaps for repair of surgical deficits, and difficulties with swallowing and speech are common in all but early tumors treated with surgery. Despite these problems, many patients can learn to function adequately. Stage IV tumors of the base of the tongue usually require a total glossectomy, which typically results in profound compromise of speech and swallowing function in all but a few patients. Therefore, many medical practitioners have resorted to radiation therapy alone or combined radiation therapy with chemotherapy. It should be noted that multifraction radiation therapy can occasionally leave a patient with as much functional limitation as surgery.

Laryngeal Cancers

Patients with T_1 and T_2 cancers of the supraglottic larynx usually have successful disease control with either radiation therapy or surgery. Although partial supraglottic laryngectomy can be performed for some small cancers (such as a T_1 tumor of the epiglottis, larger tumors (such as a T_2 tumor of the false vocal fold) require a formal supraglottic laryngectomy. Surgery is more commonly performed for larger supraglottic tumors than use of radiation therapy. A supraglottic laryngectomy may leave an individual with serious swallowing difficulties, although voice would tend to be quite good. One of the most important contributing factors to the swallowing difficulties is the removal of the epiglottis. During normal swallowing, the larynx elevates and moves forward, and the epiglottis covers the laryngeal entroitis while directing the bolus (material to be swallowed) into lateral channels called the pyriform sinuses, providing protection from aspiration. This protection is lost following supraglottic laryngectomy. The false vocal folds play an important role in preventing the egress of air from the lungs and are necessary for creating subglottic pressure, which also helps to prevent aspiration. When they are removed, as in a standard supraglottic laryngectomy, swallowing

decompensates. Furthermore, these patients usually have temporary tracheostomies due to postsurgical swelling and airway obstruction, and the redirection of air through the tracheostomy tube also prevents adequate subglottic pressure. The tube holds the remaining laryngeal structures more tightly in the neck, limiting the upward and forward movement of the larynx during the swallow. It is sometimes difficult to swallow well until the tracheostomy tube has been plugged or preferably removed. Most patients who have had supraglottic laryngectomies can learn to swallow by mouth using strategies that maximize preserved swallowing abilities. Voice is typically good because the true vocal folds have been preserved. Some T_3 supraglottic cancers can be treated with extended supraglottic laryngectomies, although most T_3 and T_4 tumors require a total laryngectomy.

T_1 glottic cancers can be treated with radiation therapy or surgery, and there is some controversy over which modality is preferred. Survival with primary radiation therapy and surgical salvage of recurrent tumors is comparable to primary surgery and radiation salvage or further surgical salvage with either partial or total laryngectomy, and this survival rate has been reported as approximately 95%.[29] Since results for these two modalities are similar, a key factor in determining preferred treatment is voice outcome. Subjective judgments of voice quality in patients who have undergone radiation therapy have been inconsistent.[30–32] Selected objective measures of postradiation voices have been outside the range of normal.[33] Radiation therapy is used in an attempt to control the tumor while preserving the most natural voice possible, although there have been perceptual voice abnormalities detected by a skilled listener ten years after radiation therapy was used to treat patients with early glottic carcinoma.[34] Voice outcomes with T_1 tumors confined to one vocal fold and not involving the anterior commissure or the vocal process of the arytenoid were favorable whether treated with radiation or surgery.[35] Larger T_1 and any T_2 tumors are preferentially treated by radiation initially. Continuation of smoking following treatment, larger tissue biopsies taken for diagnoses, and complications of treatment are the key factors associated with poor voice outcome and recurrence following radiation therapy for T_1 and T_2 glottic cancer.[36] Larger T_2 cancers can be managed with partial laryngectomy or hemilaryngectomy, but less than optimal voice and swallowing outcomes would make this treatment modality less attractive than radiation therapy. Partial laryngectomy procedures, including hemilaryngectomy and supraglottic laryngectomy, are viable options in cases of radiation therapy failure, with high expectation of disease control and limited morbidity.[37]

T_3 glottic cancers have traditionally been treated with total laryngectomy, which is still considered the standard against which other treatments are compared. Swallowing is generally good after total laryngectomy, although problems do arise, and voice restoration with one of the alaryngeal voice modalities allows for functional communication. A combination of chemotherapy and radiation therapy has been offered to patients with T_3 glottic carcinomas, in an attempt to preserve the larynx, and the survival rate of these patients has been reported as comparable to the survival rate of patients who received only surgery.[38] It is reasonable to offer a patient with a T_3 laryngeal cancer either primary surgery with a total laryngectomy or laryngeal preservation with combined chemotherapy and radiation therapy, reserving surgical salvage for recurrence. T_4 glottic tumors are best treated with total laryngectomy followed by radiation therapy.

Metastatic Neck Disease

Metastatic disease to nearby areas is common in squamous cell carcinoma of the head and neck, particularly in advanced disease. The likelihood of neck metastases depends on the site and stage of the tumor. Cancers of the tonsil, tongue, nasopharynx, and pyriform sinuses are particularly likely to have metastasized, even at the time of initial presentation of the tumor. Many of these tumors have nonpalpable metastases or occult (concealed) disease in the neck. If there is obvious disease involvement, or if the likelihood of occult disease is greater than 25 to 30%, a neck dissection to remove cancerous lymph nodes should be considered. There are different types of neck dissections. One is a radical neck dissection, which occurs when all cervical lymph nodes are surgically removed. With this type of dissection, the sternocleidomastoid muscle and spinal accessory nerve are cut, resulting in difficulty with head turning and shoulder raising. Another type of neck dissection is a modified radical neck dissection, which is less ablative and preserves some nonlymphatic structures that are removed in a radical neck dissection. A CT scan or an MRI of the neck can elucidate metastatic neck disease, often prior to the nodes being palpable. Occult disease or a single metastasis less than 2 cm in size can be managed with radiation therapy in most circumstances, although the presence of larger single nodes or mul-

tiple nodes usually requires surgery. On occasion, a patient will present with a metastatic lymph node and an unknown primary tumor. In such cases, random biopsies of the nasopharynx, tonsil, base of tongue and pyriform sinuses may identify the index tumor.

The extent of lymph node metastases has been associated with prognosis. Larger lymph nodes, bilateral nodes, and multiple nodes result in higher nodal (N) staging and correspond to poorer prognosis, while solitary small (less than 3 cm) nodes correspond to a more favorable prognosis.

MULTIDISCIPLINARY MANAGEMENT

The Head and Neck Tumor Board

Many patients with head and neck cancer receive comprehensive care by a treatment and rehabilitation team. Although it is typically the otolaryngologist/surgeon who acts as the primary care coordinator, other medical specialists are needed to provide thorough management. A common forum for treatment planning and information exchange is a multidisciplinary head and neck tumor board meeting. Frequency of meetings and composition of attendees most likely depends on the number of patients treated for head and neck cancers at a given medical center and the medical specialists available. At a minimum, an otolaryngologist (who may also be the surgeon), a radiation oncologist, a medical oncologist, and a maxillofacial prosthodontist are needed to delineate the medical treatment plan. Histologic and imaging information, provided by a pathologist and a radiologist respectively, assists in this endeavor. However, tumor boards should encompass more than medical treatment specifications. Total rehabilitation cannot be achieved without a broader consideration of the person who has the cancer, and additional team members are beneficial.

One of the key individuals at a head and neck tumor board meeting is the cancer coordination nurse, or clinical nurse specialist. This individual assures that all tests and evaluation results are available, coordinates treatment activities and scheduling with the patient and family, and provides for continuity of care and facilitation of treatment, particularly when this involves combined modalities.[39]

The Role of the Speech–Language Pathologist

A speech–language pathologist is needed to provide information to the team about the swallowing and speech problems that are likely in a given patient, and the feasibility of voice restoration procedures. Any new approaches to voice restoration, speech and swallowing prosthetics, or swallowing rehabilitation can be presented in the context of discussing patients who might benefit from them. Patients in need of pretreatment evaluation and counseling can be identified at the tumor board meeting. It is helpful to have as thorough a description of the tumor and planned surgical resection as possible, perhaps even an illustration of tumor location and resection boundaries, to predict possible functional limitations. Figure 23–2 shows a case presentation form and Figure 23–3 is a basic diagram of head and neck structures on which the surgeon may draw the tumor and the planned resection margins. Patients and their family members may meet the speech–language pathologist for the first time soon after the tumor board meeting, an important first step in establishing a sound clinical relationship that will continue well into the future at various levels. Discussions between tumor board members and patients following the tumor board meeting can easily overwhelm the patient, who may be hearing the diagnosis of cancer and the details of the planned treatment for the first time, so information bombardment should be avoided. It is more important for the speech–language pathologist to meet the patient and informally obtain a cursory idea of ongoing speech, swallowing, and cognitive functioning. Pretreatment appointments can be rescheduled for another time prior to the initiation of the medical treatment, when patients will be more receptive to explanations about likely functional changes in speech and swallowing and what can be done about them.

There are other medical specialists who may not be directly involved with the decision-making process for medical management, but are called on to provide services during rehabilitation. Physical therapists may work with patients who have limited range of shoulder motion because the spinal accessory nerve was sacrificed in a radical neck dissection. Nutritionists, psychologists, psychiatrists, and vocational counselors are helpful referral sources, although they may not be regular members of the management team.[40]

TIMING OF SPEECH–LANGUAGE PATHOLOGY SERVICE

The speech–language pathologist may become involved in a head and neck cancer case at any stage along the continuum of patient care, from prediag-

nosis to posttreatment rehabilitation. Timing of service provision along this continuum is an important consideration in optimal management of speech and swallowing. Intervention can be divided into three periods: pretreatment, immediate posttreatment, and extended posttreatment. Although the timing of service provision usually varies from patient to patient because of the specific circumstances in each case, there are some general guidelines for management issues related to speech and swallowing as they crop up along the medical course.

Pretreatment Intervention

The speech–language pathologist is involved most extensively with surgical head and neck patients. This discussion pertains to the surgery patient. Presurgical consultation is highly preferred. During this period, intervention is focused on speech, language, and swallowing assessments, patient and family education, and counseling. It would be ideal for the speech–language pathologist to see every patient soon after the diagnosis and treatment options have been given. Information about likely speech and swallowing changes related to specific treatments could then be used by the patient and family in the decision-making process. If the initial meeting between the speech–language pathologist and the patient is at the time when the patient first hears the diagnosis and recommended treatment options, then getting a sense of the patient's reactions will assist in adjusting the timing of intervention procedures. Most individuals fear cancer. The issues paramount to patients who have just heard a diagnosis of head and neck cancer are the chance for cure and the effects treatment will have on their daily functioning and general well-being. The most opportune time to begin intervention may not be when the patient receives the diagnosis.

For some, pain management surpasses all other medical or personal considerations. Pain, either prior to or after treatment, can skew a patient's general perspective and limit receptiveness to intervention procedures that may at the time seem only remotely related. Initial provision of speech and swallowing services, even of something as seemingly tolerable as patient education, may have to wait until the patient's pain has been controlled. Family education may be a better intervention target at times when pain interferes with direct patient intervention. Postsurgical pain is usually not a lengthy interference in speech and swallowing intervention, but time is needed for surgical sutures to heal.

MULTIDISCIPLINARY HEAD AND NECK TUMOR CONFERENCE

NAME: DATE:

MRN: AGE:

REFERRED FROM: REFERRED TO:

PHMX: TOBACCO:

ALLEREGY: ETOH:

MEDS: FAMILY HX:

History:

Physical:

Pathology:

Radiological Studies:

TUMOR SITE: T   N   M   STAGE

Treatment Alternatives:

1)

2)

3)

Treatment Planned:

Follow-up Studies/Referrals:

Protocol Alternatives:

Figure 23–2. A multidisciplinary head and neck tumor board data collection form.

MULTIDISCIPLINARY HEAD AND NECK TUMOR CONFERENCE

NAME: MRN:

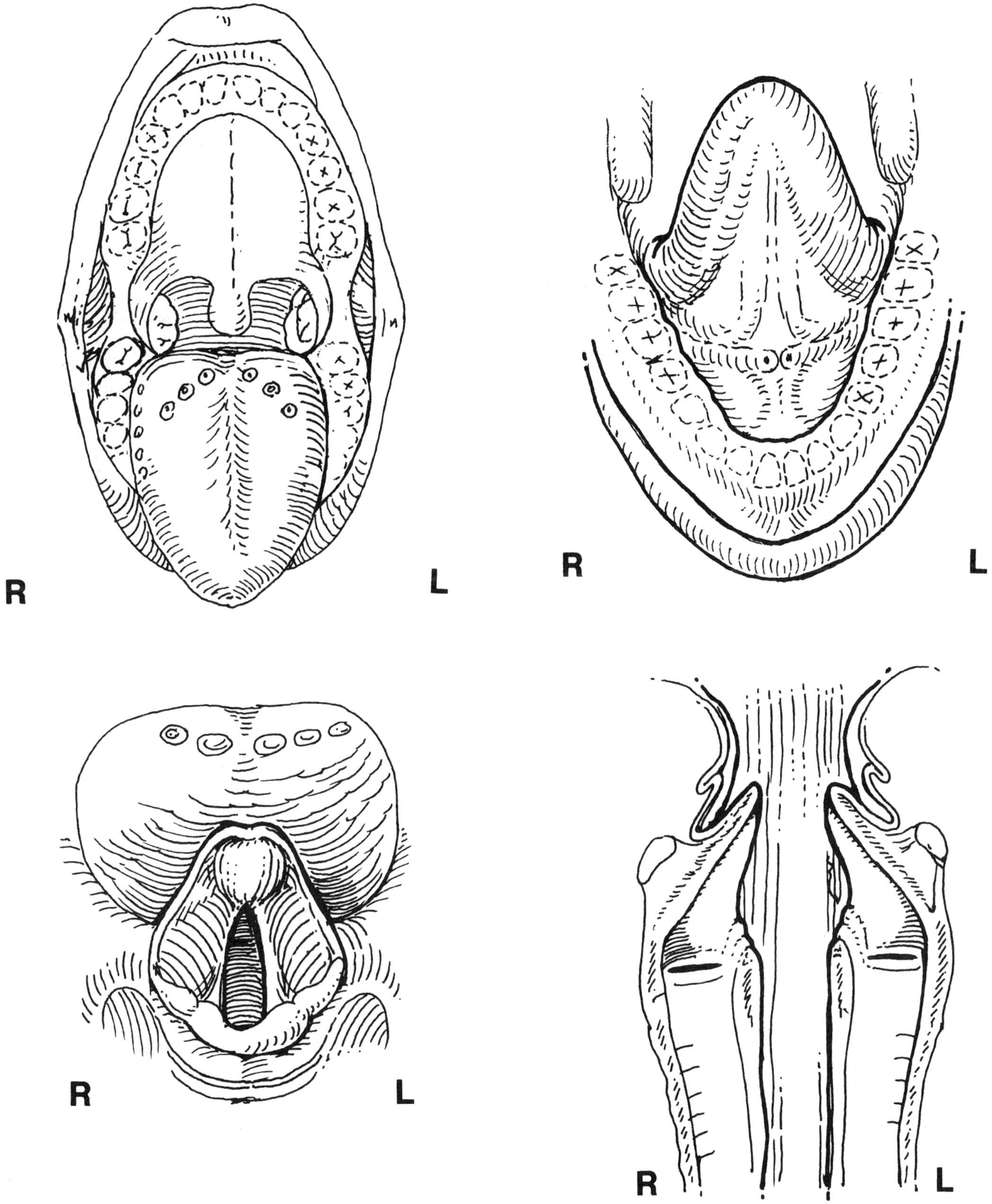

R   L   R   L

R   L   R   L

Figure 23–3. Diagram of head and neck structures for drawing surgical margins.

The speech–language pathologist should check with the surgeon for the most appropriate time to begin direct remediation procedures. Rigid adherence to guidelines for rehabilitation of speech and swallowing in head and neck cancer patients can be difficult because of the individual nature of each case. It is best to have broad goals for all patients, and step back frequently to look at the entire rehabilitation picture for each patient, making adjustments in specific speech and swallowing objectives as the patient's needs dictate. Some flexibility in the timing of information provision, communication retraining, and counseling will be necessary.

Preparation of the pretreatment session by the speech–language pathologist involves thorough review of the patient's medical record. The initial session should focus on exchange of information between the patient and the speech–language pathologist. A comfortable starting point is to have the patient tell the clinician what he or she has already been told about the diagnosis and planned treatment. This retelling can be a transition point for more specific discussion about likely changes in speech and swallowing. The course of rehabilitation should be described. Following this, the patient may list concerns about rehabilitation by order of importance. While speech–language pathologists address issues related to communication, speech, and swallowing, and these issues are often inextricably tied to the medical aspects of the patient's care, specific medical concerns should be addressed by the appropriate medical specialist. The pretreatment session should include assessment of a patient's current communication and swallowing status, physical abilities to use alaryngeal methods of communication, general cognitive function, alertness, and attentiveness. If surgery is the planned treatment and speech deficits are likely, it is a good idea to establish a reliable alternative method of communication that the patient can use during the immediate postsurgery period, such as writing, gesturing, mouthing words, or pointing to pictures on a communication board. Appendix D is a checklist of discussion topics to be covered during a preoperative or immediate postoperative counseling session.

Postsurgical Intervention

The opportunity for pretreatment intervention is not always possible. The immediate post-treatment follow-up will need to begin with the information that would have been presented during the pretreatment sessions. Even if pretreatment intervention occurred, a review of information about the effects of the surgery on speech and swallowing should provide the patient with a basis for treatment. Anatomic and physiologic changes that have altered communication and swallowing should not be skimmed over because the patient's understanding of these changes assists with further explanations about various treatment approaches. For patients who have had surgery and an uncomplicated immediate postsurgical course, speech and swallowing rehabilitation can begin within a two week period following the surgery. The surgeon should indicate that surgical sutures can withstand movement before aggressive therapy begins. Recovery complications postpone direct rehabilitation efforts, but this may be an optimal time to provide the patient and family members with necessary information and support. Immediate postsurgical speech and swallowing assessment provides a measure of the amount of impairment, which gives an indication of the length of treatment. Speech may not be a functional communication mode, and assistive or alternative methods of communication must be practiced. The immediate postsurgical period can be one of emotional upheaval because of diminished ability to communicate. In addition, patients have to deal with the physical and functional alterations as a result of the surgery. The emotional status of the patient can interfere with rehabilitation attempts. For example, total laryngectomy patients having difficulty accepting their loss of voice may be quite unmotivated during initial training of an electrolarynx. It is sometimes beneficial for patients to meet with a person who has had a similar type of surgery. Visitation should be arranged at the patient's request, however, because the amount of benefit is a function of readiness for rehabilitation. The immediate postsurgical treatment period should be the time when the patient is presented with the specific plan for speech and swallowing intervention.

Outpatient Speech–Language Pathology Services

The extended postsurgical treatment is the time when the "work" of rehabilitation gets done and the plan is put into action. Certainly patients requiring prosthetic devices, alaryngeal speech training, or specialized swallowing strategies will have extended rehabilitation courses. Patients who have been discharged from the hospital and who have returned to their typical living environment begin to experience the limitations in daily functioning that resulted from the surgery, including limitations in speaking and swallowing. The extended postsurgical period focuses on restoration of communication and swallowing to a degree that matches as closely as possible pre-morbid abilities. Motivation may wax and wane. In general, as healing proceeds and the patient begins to regain a level of lost function, motivation improves.

MANAGEMENT OF SPEECH FOLLOWING HEAD AND NECK CANCER TREATMENT

Radiation therapy and surgery are the most common treatments for head and neck cancer. These treatments are used separately, in combination, and with other forms of treatment. Radiation therapy and surgery for head and neck cancers result in relatively predictable patterns of functional deficits in speech and swallowing that can range from mild and transient to severe and chronic. These deficits are caused by tissue reactions and alterations in anatomic structures. Speech–language pathologists should have a clear understanding of likely problems in speech and swallowing following head and neck cancer treatment so that they can provide specific management techniques that restore normal function or retain functional levels as close to normal as possible. It is primarily the surgery patient who requires the most extensive speech and swallowing treatment. Resections of the tongue, mandible, palate, larynx, and pharynx result in relatively predictable speech and swallowing changes, which are the focus of this discussion.

Speech Changes and their Management

Normal speech requires sensory and motor integration of respiration, phonation, articulation, and resonation. Treatment for head and neck tumors can alter one or more of these speech systems depending on the location and size of the tumor, the planned treatments, and the patient's ability to compensate for any treatment alterations. In general, smaller tumors require less ablative treatment and result in more preserved speech function while larger tumors exact a higher functional cost. Unilateral tumors are generally not as limiting as bilateral disease. Some general predictions about alterations in speech can be given to patients prior to treatment, based on knowledge of tumor site, tumor size, and planned treatment, although each patient's specific problems will vary depending on his or her adaptability following treatment. Small tumors treated with radiation therapy alone or combined radiation therapy and surgery do not typically produce speech alterations. There are potential side effects associated with radiation therapy to the oral and oropharyngeal cavities, such as xerostomia (mucosal dryness), oral and pharyngeal mucosa inflammation, soft tissue and bone pain, and thicker consistency of saliva. These side effects usually do not interfere with speech production as much as swallowing, as will be discussed later in this chapter. Large tumors usually require extensive surgical resection, which will likely result in some degree of compromised speech.

Glossectomy

Speech deficits may occur following a glossectomy. This procedure removes part or all of the tongue. An appreciation of the tongue's function in normal articulation will assist in understanding the compromising effects that glossectomy can have on speech. Many consonants and all vowel differentiations in English require execution of precise and rapidly coordinated movements and shape alterations by the tongue.[40] The severity of the speech impairment is usually commensurate with the extent of tongue resection, the degree of limitation in tongue mobility, and the patient's ability to compensate by using intact remaining oral structures. For example, vowel differentiation in total glossectomy patients has been accomplished by widening and narrowing the pharynx.[42] Partial glossectomy patients have shown improvement in the acoustic signals for vowel distinctions by using tongue protrusion and increased jaw height.[43] Compensatory positions of the lips and jaw may become the targets of speech therapy following tongue surgery. Slower speaking rates, exaggerated articulatory movements, and sound approximations assist the glossectomy patient with clearer speech. Range of motion and strength exercises are also part of speech rehabilitation.

Although the tongue is the primary structure in the oral and oropharyngeal cavities on which clear speech depends, it is important to remember that other structures contribute to the perception of clear speech. Tumors that require surgical alteration of these structures may have deleterious effects on speech. For example, resonance may be disturbed by palatectomy or pharyngectomy.

Application of Prosthetics

Maxillofacial prosthetics are used for anatomical, functional, or cosmetic restoration for acquired surgical defects in head and neck cancer patient.[44] Intraoral prostheses restore resected portions of the oral cavity. An obturator is an intraoral prosthesis that closes an opening. For example, palatal obturators may be helpful for patients who have had a maxillectomy. An extended denture may return speech to normal for patients who have had soft palate or pharyngeal surgery with subsequent impairment of velopharyngeal closure. Glossectomy patients can benefit from a maxillary prosthesis that lowers the hard palate and facilitates improved function of a tongue with restricted movement. Since intraoral prostheses depend on the teeth or a stable denture, it is important for patients to maintain optimal oral and dental care throughout the period of medical treatment.

Rehabilitation for Laryngeal Cancer

The larynx contributes the sound source for voiced speech sounds by way of self-sustaining vocal fold vibration that valves exhaled air and converts it to acoustic output. Treatments for laryngeal tumors interfere with phonation. Small laryngeal tumors may be treated with radiation therapy alone, or a combination of radiation therapy and surgery. Radiation therapy as the sole treatment for laryngeal cancer preserves laryngeal structures, but it can irritate, dry, and inflame vocal fold mucosa and lead to a period of increased hoarseness. This, in turn, may set up hyperfunctional voice production as a compensatory reaction in a patient. Voice therapy may benefit such a patient. The speech–language pathologist provides a behavioral modification program aimed at improving voice hygiene, and an exercise program aimed at reduction of adductory forces on the vocal folds, in an attempt to prevent worsening dysphonia and optimize voice quality during and following radiation therapy.

Large laryngeal tumors usually require removal of part or all of the larynx. Conservative procedures include hemilaryngectomy and supraglottic laryngectomy. Total laryngectomy is performed when laryngeal tumors are large enough to preclude safe surgical margins with more conservative approaches. A standard hemilaryngectomy implies a resection in the superior-inferior, or vertical, plane.[9] For this reason, it is also known as a vertical partial laryngectomy. A hemilaryngectomy leaves one side of the larynx intact and some tissue bulk on the operated side. Therefore, phonation is possible, although the voice is dysphonic. A standard supraglottic laryngectomy is a horizontal resection above the level of the true vocal folds. Voice tends to be good because both vocal folds are preserved, but swallowing is often severely compromised because this procedure removes the sphincteric protection of the false vocal folds and the epiglottis with the aryepiglottic folds.[20]

Total laryngectomy removes all of the larynx. The sound source for speech is no longer coupled to respiratory function from below or articulatory and resonatory function from above. Total laryngectomy results in sudden and complete loss of voice. Patients may incorrectly assume that whispering is still possible after total laryngectomy, and the disconnection of respiratory airflow and speech articulators needs to be explained to the patient when treatment options are discussed. In addition, information about methods of alaryngeal speech must be presented in an unbiased fashion. A dependable method of communication for the period immediately following surgery needs to planned, such as writing, gestures, or picture boards. Ideally, all these concerns about communication should be brought up preoperatively so that the patients have an awareness of expected functional losses and a means of coping with them, albeit rudimentary. The types of questions patients ask about treatment-related changes in communication may indicate their level of responsiveness to rehabilitation efforts, and can be used by the speech–language pathologist to gauge the flow of information.

Postoperative speech rehabilitation for the total laryngectomy patient usually begins a few days following the surgery, while the patent is still in the hospital. Clear and concise information about the anatomical and physiological changes that resulted from the surgery and their effects on communication should be provided. There are published sources that contain essential information and helpful illustrations for new laryngectomy patients, such as the one by Keith and Thomas.[45] This source and others can be handy references for laryngectomy patient to have as reinforcement of the information provided directly by the speech–language pathologist throughout the course of rehabilitation.

Alaryngeal Speech

Alaryngeal speech options are the primary focus of rehabilitation for the total laryngectomy patient. The three most common alaryngeal speech methods are the artificial larynx (or electrolarynx), esophageal speech, and tracheoesophageal speech. It is ultimately the patient who must make the decision as to which method or methods to use. Each method has advantages and disadvantages that prospective users and their listeners will need to consider. The speech–language pathologist should present each method of alaryngeal speech in an unbiased fashion, recognizing that the best method of speech restoration for one patient may poorly suit another.

Artificial Larynges

There are many different types of artificial larynges, but each has as its primary action the deliverance of sound (usually a buzzing tone) to the oral cavity that can then be shaped into speech by the articulators. Speech–language pathologists should be familiar with these instruments and be able to provide demonstration of their use. These instruments may be grouped into four categories based on the manner of sound generation and the location on the body for sound conduction. The four categories of artificial larynges are: electronic neck-type, electronic mouth-type, electronic interdental type, and pneumatic type.[46] The electronic neck-type and electronic mouth-type artificial larynxes are the most common of these devices. The electronic neck-type artificial larynx has battery-produced sound that is conducted to the oral cavity by way of the neck tissue against which the head of the device is placed. Neck tissue should be supple and local swelling should be minimal for optimal sound conduction, making the electronic neck-type artificial larynx less functional during the immediate postoperative period. The electronic mouth-type artificial larynx conducts battery produced sound to the oral cavity by way of a mouth tube. This tube remains in the oral cavity as speech is articulated. It is preferred during the immediate postoperative period, when neck-type devices cannot be used. The electronic interdental-type artificial larynx is designed to become a part of an upper denture. The battery produced sound is activated by a handheld control. This type of artificial larynx requires coordinated efforts from the patient's physician, speech–language pathologist, and dentist. Pneumatic devices produce sound by using air from a patient's stoma to vibrate an external rubber membrane. The sound is carried to the oral cavity by a mouth tube, which remains in place while speech is articulated. Pneumatic devices are not as common as electronic devices. The various types of artificial larynges are pictured and described by Salmon.[46] An electrolarynx, battery, and battery charger are pictured in Figure 23–4.

Training in the use of an artificial larynx is part of the comprehensive speech rehabilitation pro-

gram for total laryngectomy patients. Treatment goals often include care of the device, location of body placement for optimal sound conduction, timing of sound activation with speech, reduced speaking rate, and slightly exaggerated articulatory movements. Since the artificial larynx produces continuous sound at the "push of a button," and the sound is maintained throughout the entire spoken utterance, strategies for normal phrasing and dealing with the inability to produce voice/voiceless contrasts are helpful. Advanced artificial larynx users can learn volume and pitch alterations to more closely approximate the linguistic components of normal speech, although this aspect of communication will remain severely compromised. A patient may use an artificial larynx as a primary or secondary method for communication after comparing its advantages and disadvantages with the other alaryngeal methods of communication. Demonstration by a proficient artificial larynx speaker may assist the new laryngectomy patient with the decision regarding alaryngeal speech options. Appendix E is an example of a letter of requisition for an electrolarynx, if the speech–language pathologist initiates the order.

Esophageal Speech

Esophageal speech is the second method of alaryngeal communication discussed in this chapter. It involves injection and immediate expulsion of air through a narrow sphincter of muscle fibers at the juncture of the hypopharynx and the esophagus (the pharyngoesophageal or "PE" segment), which vibrates in response to the airflow and creates sound. Thus, sound is once again powered by an air supply that vibrates an internal body structure. However, the air supply that generates sound in esophageal speech comes from air trapped within the oral and oropharyngeal cavities rather than the lungs, resulting in reduced air volumes and the need to frequently insufflate the PE segment for continuous speech. This reduced power source and the need to frequently replenish air results in salient perceptual features that distinguish esophageal speech from the other forms of alaryngeal speech.[47,48] Esophageal speech requires considerable training, and not every laryngectomy patient who tries esophageal speech will be successful at it. Major goals for communication rehabilitation with esophageal speech include optimal air intake methods, sound shaping, avoidance of stoma and air injection noise, and appropriate phrase lengths. It might be beneficial for

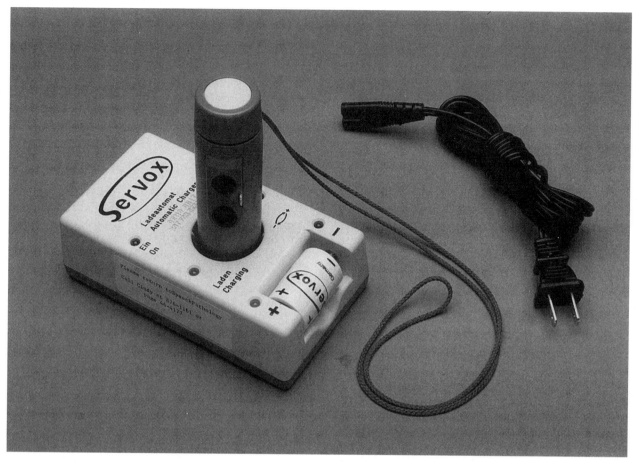

Figure 23–4. A Servox electrolarnyx, battery, and battery recharger. (Siemens Hearing Instruments, Inc., Prospect Heights, IL)

a new laryngectomy patient who is considering esophageal speech to observe and listen to a proficient esophageal speaker.

Tracheoesophageal Speech

Tracheoesophageal speech is the third alaryngeal speech option. This option requires that a fistula be surgically created in the common wall of the posterior trachea and the anterior esophagus. A voice prosthesis is housed in this fistula, with its proximal end in the stoma and its distal end in the esophageal lumen. For voice restoration, pulmonary air ready for exhalation from the stoma is redirected through the voice prosthesis by stoma occlusion. The exhaled column of air travels through the voice prosthesis, enters the esophagus, and travels superiorly to vibrate the PE segment and create sound. The tracheoesophageal (TE) puncture procedure and voice prosthesis were introduced by Singer and Blom in 1980.[49] There have been modifications in voice prostheses since then, but the original concept of sound generation by rerouting pulmonary air through a valved voice

prosthesis has remained the same. The idea of a one-way valved voice prosthesis is important because the valve allows air to enter the esophagus but prohibits secretions and food in the esophagus from entering the trachea. Occlusion of the stoma is necessary to divert pulmonary air through the voice prosthesis. Finger closure is one method of stoma occlusion. Another method involves the use of an adjustable tracheostoma valve.[50] This valve is secured over the stoma and closes with exhalation for speech, eliminating the use of a hand to speak. Doyle[9] has described tracheoesophageal speech procedures and provided photographs of various types of voice prostheses. Figure 23–5 shows three types of tracheoesophageal voice prostheses. Figure 23–6 shows an indwelling type of voice prosthesis. Appendix A lists information resources for head and neck cancer patients, including suppliers for voice restoration products.

While tracheoesophageal speech is not the preferred alaryngeal speech option for every laryngectomy patient, it has become popular and widely used. Patient candidacy should be assessed by the speech–language pathologist, preferably

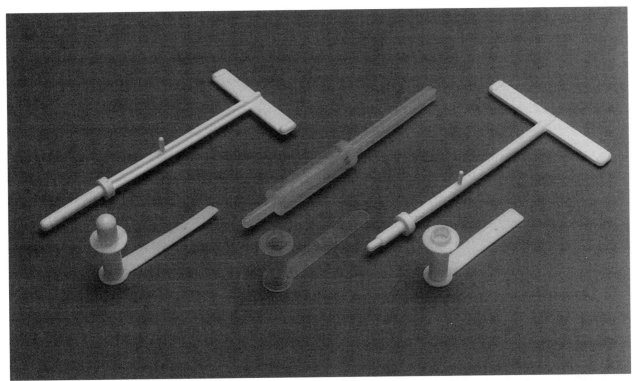

Figure 23–5. Examples of three tracheoesophageal voice prostheses. On the left is a Blom-Singer duckbill type of voice prosthesis with its inserter, in the center is a Bivona ultra low pressure voice prosthesis with its inserter, and on the right is a Blom-Singer low pressure voice prosthesis with its inserter. (Blom-Singer, Carpinteria, CA)

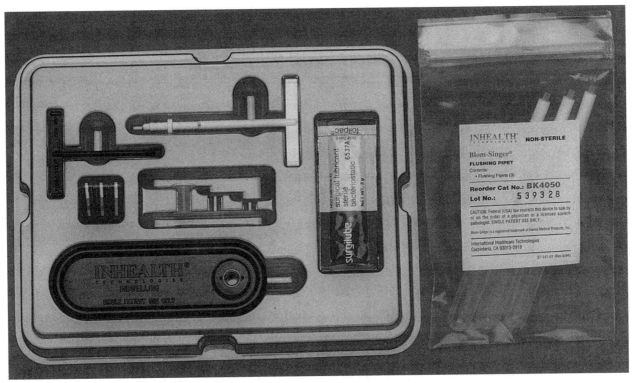

Figure 23–6. A Blom-Singer indwelling voice prosthesis kit with pipets for in situ cleaning. (Blom-Singer, Carpinteria, CA)

before any decisions regarding alaryngeal speech restoration have been solidified. Candidacy criteria include patient motivation, functional visual acuity, functional manual dexterity, adequate pulmonary support for speech, mental stability, stoma integrity, and the ability to care for and use the voice prosthesis.[51] Air insufflation of the esophagus is done by the speech–language pathologist prior to the puncture procedure to evaluate the vibratory capabilities of the PE segment. With some patients, results of esophageal air insufflation indicate that PE segment spasm, hypertonicity, or hypotonicity is interfering with sound production. Although this does not necessarily preclude a patient from acquiring tracheoesophageal speech, it indicates that further medical procedures or behavioral modifications aimed at optimizing the vibratory capabilities of the PE segment should be considered. For example, botulinum toxin injection has recently been used for relaxation of the PE segment. TE punctures may be done at the time of the total laryngectomy (primary TE puncture) or they may be done as a separate procedure after the total laryngectomy (secondary TE puncture). There is controversy surrounding the timing of the TE puncture, in part because individual patient factors that are likely to influence success with either method have not been identified.[9]

As with the other methods of alaryngeal speech restoration, the general rehabilitation goal for communication with tracheoesophageal speech is the clearest speech possible. More specific goals include prosthesis fitting, insertion, removal, and care procedures, coordination of stoma occlusion, speech onset and sound generation, appropriate effort, optimal loudness, and phrasing. Patients considering the TE puncture and voice prosthesis would benefit from a visit by tracheoesophageal speaker. In fact, it is a good idea to ask new laryngectomy patients if a laryngectomy visitor would assist them in their rehabilitation efforts at any point along the course of recovery. It should be the patient's choice whether or not to meet with a laryngectomy visitor. Patients who participate in their medical care through decision making may be more likely to adapt to functional limitations over time.

Speech–language pathologists may assist patients in choosing a method or methods of alaryngeal speech by describing the features that differentiate each of the three methods. In addition, it may be beneficial for patients to speak with and observe alaryngeal speakers who are effective communicators.

Because of the compact nature of head and neck structures, there are times when multiple structures are involved in the excision of the tumor, each with its own effect on postsurgical speech abilities. Depending on the specific site of lesion, patients may have surgical excision of both the tongue and the larynx. Serious speech deficits result in patients who have total glossectomy with total laryngectomy. The loss of the tongue interferes with articulation and the loss of the larynx interferes with phonation. These patients require lengthy and creative rehabilitative efforts for resumption of some degree of functional communication, sometimes involving augmentative or assistive communication devices.

Respiratory Changes Requiring Speech Intervention

Compromised respiration may result from a tumor in any of the internal cavities of the head and neck. Breathing difficulty may gradually worsen as the tumor grows, eventually becoming an emergency situation that could require a tracheostomy. In addition, respiration may be compromised due to lung disease from a history of smoking, which is common in head and neck cancer patients. Swelling following surgical excision of a tumor in the head and neck may necessitate the need for a tracheostomy. Respiratory compromise is a medical management problem. Once an airway has been secured, respiratory support for speech can be assessed and addressed. Succinct explanations of the normal process of respiration and the specific changes in this process resulting from the tumor and its treatment should be given to tracheostomized patients. Patients with temporary tracheostomies may be assessed for appropriateness of a speaking valve to restore voice, and then trained in its use. Certainly patients who have had permanent rerouting of oral and nasal breathing to stoma breathing with total laryngectomies have to make pronounced speech adaptations, as was previously discussed. For these patients, exhaled air from the stoma can no longer be made audible because the vocal folds have been removed, and the air cannot be shaped by articulators because it bypasses them, unless a tracheoesophageal (TE) puncture is made to restore airflow through the oral cavity. Speech–language pathologists should plan to provide laryngectomy patients with information about the respiratory changes that result from the rerouted airway, and the effects that these changes have on speech. Many of these patients would benefit from diagrams, drawings, and three-dimensional models. A discussion of common postsurgical problems related to stoma breathing might make the adjustment easier for patients. One of the most important topics for discussion should be keeping the stoma area clear of potential obstruction. Ways to deal with the increased amount and viscosity of mucous should be suggested, including adequate daily water intake, humidification of environmental air, and air filtration with stoma covers. Mucous expectoration from the stoma instead of the mouth should be discussed. Reduced ability to hold the breath at the level of the larynx may interfere with lifting heavy objects and other activities that require stabilization of the thoracic cavity, and this needs to be addressed. Reduction in smell and taste because of rerouted airflow needs to be explained. Finally, the total laryngectomy patient needs to consider some means of identification as a stoma or neck breather, since standard first aid procedures for artificial respiration (i.e., mouth-to-mouth resuscitation) would have to be modified for these patients.

SWALLOWING CHANGES AFTER HEAD AND NECK CANCER TREATMENT

Normal swallowing, like normal speech, is a well-integrated motor and sensory activity involving structures in the oral, pharyngeal, and laryngeal cavities, as well as the esophagus. In the oral cavity, the teeth, tongue, hard palate, and mandible are involved in preparation of the bolus; the tongue then collects and squeezes it posteriorly to the oropharynx. The swallow response is elicited in the oropharynx and involves closure of the velopharynx, superior and anterior movements of the hyoid bone and larynx, laryngeal closure, tongue base movement toward a bulging pharyngeal wall, peristaltic pharyngeal waves, and relaxation of the cricopharyngeal muscle.[52] After radiation therapy or surgery for head and neck tumors, difficulties at any point in the dynamic swallowing process can occur, and may range in severity from negligible and transient to severe and chronic, depending on the residual effects of the treatment and the compensatory abilities of the patient.

Effects of Radiation

Radiation therapy to the oral cavity and neck may result in inflammation and dryness of oral and pharyngeal mucosa, thickening and reduction of saliva, mouth and throat pain, changes in taste, and loss of appetite.[41] These side effects may produce dysphagia that worsens as the treatment progresses and may remain for a period of time after treatment has been completed. Radiation therapy may be used before or after surgical resection for a

head and neck tumor, producing combinations of swallowing problems related to both of the medical treatments that were used. Swallowing strategies that may benefit these patients include reduction of bolus size, modification of diet consistencies, multiple swallows for each bolus, and use of foods with strong flavors.

Effects of Surgery

Surgical resections for head and neck cancer result in predictable patterns of dysphagia related to the specific anatomic or neurologic insult produced by the resection.[53] Swallowing problems may occur following tracheostomy, glossectomy, mandibulectomy, palatal resection, pharyngectomy, and laryngectomy. A tracheostomy procedure results in dysphagia because of decreased laryngeal elevation, poorly coordinated laryngeal closure, desensitization of the reflexive cough, and pooled secretions. Cuff inflation should not be considered a protection against aspiration in patients with a tracheostomy. Oral and oropharyngeal resections cause an assortment of dysphagic symptoms, depending on the surgery site and the method of reconstruction. Restricted mobility of the lips, tongue, mandible, soft palate, and pharynx and the use of closure techniques that fill in the surgical defect with nonfunctional tissue can interfere with swallowing in the oral preparatory, oral, and pharyngeal phases of swallowing. There may be interference with chewing, diminished bolus propulsion, reduced tongue pressure, premature spillage, slow oral transit, oral cavity residue, delayed elicitation of involuntary swallowing responses, reduced pharyngeal peristalsis, pharyngeal residue, and aspiration. Subtotal laryngeal resections remove structures that act as sphincteric protection during swallowing. For example, supraglottic laryngectomy removes the false vocal folds, epiglottis, and aryepiglottic folds, which leaves only the true vocal folds to protect the airway. Dysphagia after total laryngectomy may be related to alterations in the shape and function of the pharynx, benign pharyngeal or esophageal stricture, cricopharyngeal dysfunction, and effects of radiation therapy. Of course, tumor recurrence is a suspicion when there is a change in swallowing function.

Evaluation of Swallowing

Swallowing assessment for head and neck cancer patients usually includes a clinical examination and a radiologic study. The results of assessment should pinpoint the swallowing problems, determine the effects of compensatory or facilitating strategies, and guide treatment decisions. Some common swallowing strategies used with head and neck cancer patients are: positional changes, consistency modifications, bolus size adjustments, bolus placement adjustments, effortful swallows, and double swallows. Oral prostheses and specially designed feeding utensils may improve swallowing function for these patients, depending on the specific cause for the dysphagia. Swallowing is one of those routine physiologic functions that patients may expect to resume with minimal or no effort. This is not always the case with head and neck cancer patients. The patient needs to be aware that restoration of optimal swallowing function usually requires diligent and extensive effort on his or her part and aggressive swallowing therapy on the part of the speech–language pathologist.

SUMMARY

This chapter has focused on a variety of issues surrounding the head and neck cancer patient. Speech–language pathologists who work in a medical setting need a sound understanding of head and neck anatomy and physiology and a set of specialized skills for service provision to this group of patients. Speech and swallowing problems are common and varied. Head and neck cancer patients will have optimal return of speech and swallowing function if they are provided with an intervention plan that is guided by a knowledge of the changes in normal anatomy and physiology that can occur as a result of the disease and its treatment.

CASE ONE

Case One is a 56-year-old man who smoked one pack of cigarettes daily and drank alcohol a few times each week for about 30 years. He reported a 4-month history of hoarseness at his initial otolaryngologic exam. Results of an indirect laryngeal exam showed a right vocal fold mass resembling carcinoma that extended nearly the length of the fold but did not cross at the anterior commissure. This fold was mobile. The mass was classified as T_1 N_0 M_0 and Stage I. Direct microlaryngoscopy and biopsy of the mass were done, and results of the pathology report showed squamous cell carcinoma. Radiation therapy was the recommended treatment. The patient had an initial voice evaluation prior to having radiation therapy. Voice was

moderately dysphonic at that time and there were no swallowing complaints. Laryngeal videostroboscopy showed severely reduced mucosal wave on the right fold. Voice hygiene instructions were given to the patient in an attempt to minimize voice problems during radiation therapy. These instructions included cessation of smoking, reduction of throat clearing, increased daily water consumption, and habitual use of a quiet voice with environmental adjustments to reduce the need for louder voice. Vocal quality was judged as improved when reevaluated three weeks after completion of radiation therapy. The patient was seen regularly by his otolaryngologist for the next few months. Laryngeal exams were negative during this postradiation period, but the vocal fold mucosa did not return to normal. Eight months after radiation therapy there was recurrence on the right vocal fold and extension of the tumor to the anterior portion of the left vocal fold was found. An extended hemilaryngectomy that included all of the right side of the larynx and a significant portion of the left side of the larynx was done. The hyoid bone, arytenoids, and most of the epiglottis were preserved. The epiglottis was pulled inferiorly and used to fill in the anterior portion of the thyroid cartilage that was surgically removed. Tissue from the right false vocal fold was used in place of the excised right true vocal fold. A tracheostomy was done at the time of the surgery to prevent airway compromise related to swelling. The patient was seen by the speech pathologist in the hospital three days following the surgery. An oral mechanism examination was done, but it was limited because surgical sutures could not be disturbed. Results of the oral mechanism examination showed reduced frequency of spontaneous swallow, delayed volitional swallow, pooled secretions in the oral cavity, drooling, and gurgly vocal quality. The patient was discharged from the hospital with tracheostomy and nasogastric tubes in place. He was not eating by mouth at the time of discharge, but he was handling his secretions and he had a productive cough. He had a videofluorographic study two weeks after surgery, which showed severe mechanical dysphagia with aspiration secondary to premature spillage from reduced size of valleculae and reduced constriction of reconstructed tissue at the level of the glottis. Intensive swallowing therapy was recommended. The focus of this therapy was the supraglottic swallow technique. Flexible fiberoptic endoscopy was used during therapy sessions to monitor swallowing proficiency and provide visual feedback to the patient about effortful swallow attempts. During that time, the tracheostomy tube was removed. A repeat videofluorographic study was done after four weeks of swallowing therapy, showing improved constriction of the glottis. Swallow was safe for thick and solid consistencies with the supraglottic swallowing technique. Other swallowing recommendations included an upright feeding position, small bolus size, and multiple daily feedings. The nasogastric tube was removed once nutrition was maintained with oral intake. Swallowing was reassessed during the next month in the speech pathology clinic using flexible fiberoptic endoscopy. The patient slowly started to gain weight. He reported that he had tried drinking thin liquids at home. Thin liquids were then introduced in the clinic and swallowed without clinical signs of aspiration. The patient was instructed to watch for and report any symptoms of pulmonary problems during the course of swallowing rehabilitation, but these did not occur. Swallowing rehabilitation for this extended hemilaryngectomy patient consisted of two videofluorographic studies, two bedside swallowing assessments during his hospitalization period, and two months of swallowing therapy as an outpatient with flexible fiberoptic endoscopy to monitor progress.

CASE TWO

Case Two is a 49-year-old female who had a total laryngectomy, bilateral neck dissection, and primary tracheoesophageal puncture. Radiation therapy was planned following surgery. The speech–language pathology service was consulted postoperatively. The patient was seen four days after her surgery. She used writing as her primary method of communication during the immediate postoperative period. The speech–language pathologist discussed with the patient the speech changes that resulted from anatomical and physiological changes related to the surgery. A brief explanation of voice rehabilitation methods was given. An electrolarynx was demonstrated by the clinician and tried by the patient. Sound conduction was poor with neck placement because of neck tissue swelling. Speech with cheek placement was fair. An oral adaptor was tried, but this did not improve speech intelligibility. During her seven-day stay in the hospital, the patient used a loaner electrolarynx and had daily speech therapy. Training with this device continued on an outpatient basis, after the patient's hospital discharge. She was able to use neck placement three weeks after her surgery. She had a six-week course of postoperative radiation therapy, which interfered with neck placement of the

electrolarynx and compromised speech intelligibility. During that time, she developed skin irritation around her stoma and neck swelling. A stent was kept in her stoma to prevent closure during radiation therapy. These side effects of radiation therapy interfered with swallowing and fitting of a voice prosthesis. We discussed bolus consistency modifications for her to use during the remaining portion of her radiation treatment. We postponed voice prosthesis fitting until completion of radiation therapy.

Two weeks after she completed radiation therapy, the TE puncture was sized and a voice prosthesis was inserted. Voice was quite strained and there were halts in sound production. Radiographic study of TE voice production showed hypertonicity of the upper esophageal segment, characterized by an anterior bulge of tissue at the level of the cricopharyngeal segment during voicing attempts. Treatment options included doing nothing, cricopharyngeal myotomy or injection of botulinum toxin to the hypertonic muscles. The patient did not want another surgical procedure, so she decided to have the injection. Alaryngeal voice reassessment one week after the injection showed improvement in voice and speech intelligibility without breaks in sound. In addition, tightness during swallowing lessened. The patient reported that she was able to swallow solids with less effort. Voice therapy then focused on optimizing speech by coordinating breath support with finger occlusion and adjusting lung air pressures for specific speaking situations. As she mastered TE speech, the patient became interested in an indwelling type of voice prosthesis. She had no previous trouble with yeast colonization on her voice prosthesis and she was judged to be a good candidate for an indwelling prosthesis, which was tried with success. She then became interested in trying a tracheostoma valve for hands free speech. Her speech rehabilitation resulted in good TE voice produced without the use of her hands, which allowed her to return to communication functioning that she judged to be very similar to her pre-morbid abilities.

STUDY QUESTIONS

1. Why is it important to understand normal head and neck anatomy to best serve head and neck cancer patients?

2. What are the major internal compartments of the head and neck and the important structures for speech and swallowing found in each?

3. What are the symptoms of head and neck cancer?

4. What are the diagnostic procedures frequently used for head and neck cancer?

5. What is the TNM tumor classification system.

6. How does a multidisciplinary tumor board assist in patient care?

7. What are some of the considerations in pretreatment, immediate posttreatment, and extended posttreatment intervention periods?

8. What speech changes may be anticipated after surgery of the head and neck?

9. What rehabilitative measures are used to restore speech in head and neck cancer patients?

10. What swallowing changes may be anticipated after surgery of the head and neck?

11. What rehabilitative measures are used to restore swallowing in head and neck cancer patients?

REFERENCES

1. Cancer Statistics, 1988. *CA* 1988; 38:5–22.
2. American Cancer Society: *Cancer facts and figures.* American Cancer Society, Atlanta, 1996.
3. Johns ME, Papel ID: Carcinoma of the oral cavity and pharynx. In Lee KJ, ed., *Essential otolaryngology,* 4th ed., pp 475–492. Medical Examination, New York, 1987.
4. Decker J, Goldstein JC: Risk factors in head and neck cancer. *N Eng J Med* 1982; 306:1151–1155.
5. Zemlin WR: *Speech and hearing science,* 3rd ed. Prentice-Hall, Englewood Cliffs, 1988.
6. Citardi MJ, Gracco CL, Sasaki CT: *The anatomy of the human larynx.* In Rubin JS, Sataloff RT, Korovan GS et al., eds., *Diagnosis and treatment of voice disorders,* pp 55–69. Igaku-Shoin, New York, 1995.
7. Anthony CP, Kolthoff NJ: *Textbook of anatomy and physiology,* 9th ed. C.V. Mosby, St. Louis, 1975.
8. Cachin Y: Perspectives on cancer of the head and neck. In Myers EM, Suen JY, eds., *Cancer of the head and neck,* 2nd ed., pp 1–16; Churchill Livingstone, New York, 1989.
9. Doyle PC: *Foundations of voice and speech rehabilitation following laryngeal cancer.* Singular Publishing Group, San Diego, 1994.
10. Barnes EL: Pathology of the head and neck: General considerations. In Myers EM, Suen JY, eds., *Cancer of the head and neck,* 2nd ed., pp 75–99. Churchill Livingstone, New York, 1989.
11. Richard J, Sancho-Garnier H, Micheau C: Prognostic factors in cervical lymph node metastasis in upper respiratory and digestive tract carcinomas: Study of 1,713 cases during a 15-year period. *Laryngoscope* 1987; 97:97–101.
12. Tucker HM: Malignant neoplasms. In Tucker HM: *The larynx,* 2nd ed., pp. 287–323. Thieme, New York, 1993.
13. Bauer WC: Concomitant carcinoma in situ and invasive carcinoma of the larynx. *Can J Otolary* 1974; 3: 533–542.
14. Koufman JA, Burke AJ: The causes and pathogenesis of laryngeal cancer. *Visible Voice* 1996; 5:26–46.
15. Pearlstein RP, Benninger MS, Worsham M, et al: 18Q loss of heterozygosity is a predictor of poor survival in patients with stage III head and neck cancer. On *Int J Otolaryngol* 2:FA 1–8, 1997.
16. Benninger MS: Presentation and evaluation of patients with epidermoid head and neck cancers. *Henry Ford Hospital Med J* 1992; 40:144–148.
17. Sisson GA, Toriumi DM, Atiyah RA: Paranasal sinus malignancy: A comprehensive update. *Laryngoscope* 1989; 99:143–50.
18. Bush SE, Bagshaw MA: Carcinoma of the paranasal sinuses. *Cancer* 1982; 50:154–158.
19. Lee KJ, ed.: *Essential otolaryngology.* Medical Examination Publishing Co., New York, 1987.
20. Logemann JA: Swallowing disorders after treatment for laryngeal cancer. In Logemann JA: *Evaluation and treatment of swallowing disorders,* pp 187–209. Pro-ed, Austin, TX, 1983.
21. Hirano M, Hirade Y, Kawasaki H: Vocal function following carbon dioxide laser surgery for glottic carcinoma. *Ann Oto Rhino Laryng* 1985; 94:232–235.
22. Bastian RW, Collins SL, Kaanifl T, et al: Indirect video laryngoscopy versus direct endoscopy for larynx and pharynx cancer staging: Toward the elimination of preliminary direct laryngoscopy. *Ann Oto Rhino Laryng* 1988; 88:693–698.
23. Benninger MS, Enrique RR, Nichols RD: Symptom-directed selective endoscopy for evaluation of head and neck cancer. *Head Neck* 1993; 15:532–536.
24. Robins KT, ed.: *Pocket guide to neck dissection classification and TNM staging of head and neck cancer.* American Academy of Otolaryngology-Head and Neck Surgery, Washington, 1991.
25. Spector G: Cancer of the larynx, ear, and paranasal sinuses. In Lee KJ, ed., *Essential otolaryngology,* pp 493–514. Medical Examination Publishing Co., New York, 1987.
26. Amrein, P: Current chemotherapy of head and neck cancer. *J Oral Maxillofac Surg* 1991; 49:864–870.
27. Alessi DM, Hutcherson RW, Mickel RA: Production of lymphokine-activated lymphocytes: Lysis of human head and neck squamous cell carcinoma cell lines. *Arch Otolaryngol* 1989; 115:725–730.
28. Jones KR, Weissler MC: Blood transfusion and other risk factors for recurrence of cancer of the head and neck. *Arch Otolaryngol* 1990; 116:304–309.
29. Pellitteri PK, Kennedy TL, Vrobec DP, et al: Radiotherapy. The main-stay in the treatment of early glottic carcinomas. *Arch Otolaryngol Head Neck Surg* 1991; 117:297–301.
30. Stoicheff ML: Voice following radiotherapy. *Laryngoscope* 1975; 85:608–618.

31. Stoicheff ML, Ciampi A, Rassi JE, et al: The irradiated larynx and voice: A perceptual study. *J Speech Hear Res* 1983; 26:428–485.

32. Llewellyn-Thomas HA, Sutherland HJ, Hogg SA, et al: Linear analogue self-assessment of voice quality in laryngeal cancer. *J Chronic Dis* 1984; 37:917–924.

33. Lehman JJ, Bless DM, Brandenburg JH: An objective assessment of voice production after radiation therapy for stage I squamous cell carcinoma of the glottis. *Otolaryngol Head Neck Surg* 1988; 98:121–129.

34. Morgan DAL, Robinson HF, Marsh L, et al: Vocal quality 10 years after radiotherapy for early glottic cancer. *Clin Rad* 1988; 39:295–296.

35. McGuist FW, Koufman JA, Balock D: Voice analysis of patients with endoscopically treated early laryngeal carcinoma. *Ann Otol Rhinol Laryngol* 1996; 101:142–146.

36. Benninger M, Gillen J, Thieme P, et al: Factors associated with recurrence and voice quality following radiation therapy for T_1 and T_2 glottic carcinomas. *Laryngoscope* 1994; 104:294–298.

37. Nichols RD, Mickelson SA: Partial laryngectomy after irradiation failure. *Ann Otol Rhinol Laryngol* 1991; 100:176–180.

38. Pfister DG, Harrison LB, Strong EW, et al: Current status of larynx preservation with multimodality therapy. *Oncology* 1992; 6:33–38.

39. Benninger MS. Medical liasons for continuity of head and neck cancer care. *Head Neck* 1992; 14:28–32.

40. Casper JK, Colton RH: *Clinical manual for laryngectomy and head and neck cancer rehabilitation.* Singular, San Diego, 1993.

41. Groher ME, Gonzalez EE. Mechanical disorders of swallowing. In Groher ME, ed., *Dysphagia diagnosis and management,* 2nd ed., pp 53–84. Butterworth-Heinemann, Stoneham, MA, 1992.

42. Weber RS, Ohlms L, Bowman J, Jacob R, Goepfert H. Functional results after total or near total glossectomy with laryngeal preservation. *Arch Otolaryngol Head Neck Surg* 1991; 117:512–515.

43. Hamlet SL, Patterson RL, Fleming SM. A longitudinal study of vowel production in partial glossectomy patients. *J Phonetics* 1992; 20:209–224.

44. Schaff NG: Maxillofacial prosthetics and the head and neck cancer patient. *CA* 1984; 54:2682–2690.

45. Keith RL, Thomas JE: *A handbook for the laryngectomee,* 4th ed. Pro-ed, Austin, TX, 1996.

46. Salmon SJ: Artificial larynxes: Types and modifications. In Keith RL, Darley FL, eds., *Laryngectomy rehabilitation,* 3rd ed., pp 155–178. Pro-ed, Austin, TX, 1994.

47. Robbins J: Acoustic differentiation of laryngeal, esophageal, and tracheoesophageal speech. *J Speech Hear Res* 1984; 27:577–585.

48. Robbins J, Fisher HB, Blom ED, Singer ML: A comparative acoustic study of normal, esophageal, and tracheoesophageal speech production. *J Speech Hear Dis* 1984; 49:202–210.

49. Singer ML, Blom ED: An endoscopic technique for restoration of voice after laryngectomy. *Ann Oto Rhino Laryng* 1980; 89:529–533.

50. Blom ED, Singer MIm Hamaker RC: Tracheostoma valve for postlaryngectomy voice rehabilitation. *Ann Otol Rhinol Laryngol* 1982; 91:576–578.

51. Andrews JC, Mickel MD, Monahan GP, Hanson, DG, Ward PH: Major complications following tracheoesophageal puncture for voice rehabilitation. *Laryngoscope* 1987; 97:562–567.

52. Logemann JA: Effects of aging on the swallowing mechanism. *Otolaryngol Clin North Amer* 1990; 23:1045–1056.

53. Kronenberger MB, Meyers AD: Dysphagia following head and neck cancer surgery. *Dysphagia* 1994; 9:236–244.

Appendix A
Information Resources for Head and Neck Cancer Patients

American Cancer Society, Inc.
National Home Office
1599 Clifton Road NE
Atlanta, GA 30329–4251
1–800–ACS–2345

Bivona Medical Technologies (voice restoration products and laryngectomy supplies)
5700 West 23rd Avenue
Gary, IN 46406
1–800–348–6064

Blom-Singer (voice restoration products and laryngectomy supplies)
1110 Mark Avenue
Carpinteria, CA 93013–2918
1–800–477–5969

Bruce Medical Supplier (laryngectomy supplies)
411 Waverly Oaks Road
P.O. Box 9166
Waltham, MA 02254

Cancer Information Service (Canada)
755 Concession Street
Hamilton, Ontario L8V 1C4
1–800 939–3333

Let's Face It (support for people with facial
   difference)
Box 29972
Bellingha, WA 98228–1972
(360) 676–7325

Luminaud (laryngectomy supplies)
8688 Tyler Blvd.
Mentor, OH 44060–4348
(216) 255–9082

Siemens Hearing Instruments, Inc. (Servox
   electrolarynx)
16 E. Piper Lane, Suite 128
Prospect Heights, IL 60070
1–800–333–9083

Words+, Inc. (assistive communication
   devices)
40015 Sierra Highway
Building B-145
Palmdale, CA 93550
1–800–869–8521

Appendix B
Suppliers of Tracheoesophageal Voice Restoration Products

Bivona Medical Technologies
5700 West 23rd Avenue
Gary, IN 46406
(800) 348–6064

Blom-Singer
1110 Mark Avenue
Carpinteria, CA 93013–2918
(800) 477–5969
(805) 684–9337

Appendix C
Competencies for Speech–Language Pathologists Working with Head and Neck Cancer Patients

1. Thorough knowledge of normal head and neck anatomy and physiology.
2. Thorough knowledge of changes in head and neck anatomy and physiology as a result of cancer treatment.
3. Ability to predict likely changes in speech and swallowing following head and neck cancer treatment.
4. Provide parsimonious explanation of anatomical and physiological alterations that result from head and neck cancer surgeries to patients.
5. Participate in a multidisciplinary tumor board meeting.
6. Counsel the patient with regard to changes in speech and swallowing.
7. Provide explanation and demonstration of alaryngeal voice restoration methods.
8. Assess patient for use of oral prosthesis.
9. Assess candidacy of patient for tracheoesophageal speech.
10. Perform esophageal insufflation and interpret results.
11. Fit a tracheoesophageal voice prosthesis.
12. Explain and demonstrate procedures for tracheoesophageal voice prosthesis care and use.
13. Explain and demonstrate procedures for use of tracheostoma valve.
13. Provide patients and medical personnel with updated information on speech, swallowing, and voice restoration products.
14. Assist patient in establishing most efficient communication method based on each patient's individual communication needs.
15. Apply appropriate swallowing strategies based on clinical and radiologic findings.

Appendix D
Form for Laryngectomy Counseling Session

Laryngectomy Counseling Check List

Name _____

Address _____

Telephone _____

Sex _____ Date of Birth _____ Age _____

Medical Record Number _____

Contact Person _____

Surgeon _____ Surgery Date _____

Surgical Procedure(s) _____

Type of Insurance _____

Discuss structural changes in respiration, speech, and swallowing.

Discuss the following:

taste	cough	dentures	water sports
smell	sneezing	hygiene	tissue vs. handerchief
sniff	throat clearing	sex	bathing
sleeping	smoking	laughing	crying
showering	lifting	drinking	shampooing
blowing	emergency help	yelling	shaving
nose blowing	first aid	radiation	defecation
humidity	atomizer	numbness	cold air
work	body odors	neck size	jewelry
whistle	sun bathing	vocal intensity	musical instruments
cooling food	stoma covers	swallowing	

Discuss stoma and oral hygiene.

Discuss laryngeal speech methods.

Discuss laryngectomy visitor and information resources.

Appendix E
Letter of Necessity for Ordering an Electrolarynx

Date _____

RE: Order for an artificial larynx/electrolarynx

Patient _____

Medical Record Number _____

Address _____

Telephone _____

Date of Birth _____

SS No. _____

Surgeon _____

To Whom This Concerns:

This letter of necessity requesting an artificial larynx/electrolarynx is for the person named above. This person had a total laryngectomy on (date) _____ and is unable to speak. This person has/has not had radiation treatment to the neck. This person has been assessed by me and has shown:

____ *Good general physical ability*   ____ *Good manual dexterity*

____ *Alertness and attentiveness*   ____ *Physical ability to use an electrolarynx*

____ *Potentially frequent use of the*   ____ *Ability to follow multistep directions*
electrolarynx for communication   ____ *Production of comprehensible speech with*

____ *Correct use of the electrolarynx*   *the electrolarynx*

I am requesting a (type of device)_____, a battery, and a battery recharger. DO/DO NOT include an oral adapter with tubes. Enclosed is the physician's prescription and a photocopy of the patient's medical insurance information. Please send the device to me at the address listed below, and call me if you need additional information. Thank you for your assistance with this matter.

Sincerely,

Name of speech pathologist
Address of speech pathologist
Telephone number of speech pathologist

24

Pediatric Voice and Resonance Disorders

ANN W. KUMMER AND JANET H. MARSH

CHAPTER OUTLINE

Normal Phonation and Resonance

Early Development of Vocal Function

Voice Disorders: Characteristics and Causes

Evaluation

Treatment

Resonance Disorders: Characteristics and Causes

Evaluation

Treatment

Voice and resonance disorders are commonly seen in a pediatric speech pathology practice. In various surveys, the incidence of voice and resonance problems in children has been estimated to be between 6 and 9% of the general population.[1] In one survey of the caseloads of school speech–language pathologists, 6.7% of children were being treated for voice or resonance problems.[2] In this population of children, the three most common problems noted were vocal nodules (23%), hoarseness without obvious pathology (18%), and resonance problems, usually hypernasality (12%). Given this incidence, the pediatric speech–language pathologist needs to be knowledgeable about the different types of voice and resonance disorders commonly seen in children, and be competent in basic evaluation and treatment protocols.

This chapter begins with information regarding the normal production of voice and resonance, and the development of vocal function in children. This is followed by a discussion of the common types of voice and resonance disorders found in the pediatric population as well as the causes of these disorders. Basic information is then given regarding evaluation and treatment protocols.

This chapter is not meant to be all inclusive. Instead, it is intended to be a guide for basic information regarding pediatric voice and resonance disorders and a source of where to go for additional information when needed.

NORMAL PHONATION AND RESONANCE

With every instrument that is capable of producing sound, there must be at least three components: (1) a vibrating mechanism that can be set in motion to produce sound, (2) a stimulating mechanism that can set the vibration in motion, and (3) a resonating mechanism to reinforce or amplify the sound. In human speech, the vocal folds are the vibrating bodies, the force of breath pressure is the stimulating force, and the cavities of the vocal tract provide the mechanism for resonating the sound energy.[3] The acoustic product is then altered for different speech sounds by varying the size and shape of the oral cavity through placement and movement of the articulators and by raising and lowering the velum to change the focus of resonance.

Phonation is initiated when subglottal air pressure from the lungs forces the gently approximated vocal folds apart, causing them to vibrate. The theory of vocal fold vibration is based on three mechanical divisions of the vocal folds. These divisions are the cover (epithelium and superficial layer of the lamina propria), the transition layer (the deep layer of the lamina propria), and the body (the vocalis muscle). During phonation, the mass and stability is provided by the body while the cover level oscillates.[4–7]. This oscillation creates a wave motion in three vibratory phases: horizontal (medial to lateral movement), longitudinal (anterior to posterior movement), and vertical (inferior to superior movement). During speech, there is continuous adduction of the vocal folds as they vibrate for voiced phonemes, and periodic abduction of the folds with pauses and the production of voiceless sounds (Figure 24–1). Subtle changes in vocal fold length and mass also occur, which affect pitch and intonation.

Normal resonance depends on the size and shape of the resonating cavities and the activity of the velopharyngeal structures. During the production of oral phonemes, the velum moves in a superior and posterior direction with a type of "knee action" to achieve closure against the posterior pharyngeal wall (Figure 24–2). The posterior pharyngeal wall often moves anteriorly to assist in achieving contact. The lateral pharyngeal walls move medially to close against the velum, or in some cases, to meet in midline behind the velum.

There are three basic patterns of normal velopharyngeal closure. Some normal speakers demonstrate closure primarily through the action of the velum and posterior pharyngeal wall (coronal pattern), while with other normal speakers, closure is achieved primarily from the medial movement of the lateral pharyngeal walls, which meet in midline (sagittal pattern). In some speakers, all structures move equally to achieve closure (circular pattern). Regardless of the basic closure pattern, velopharyngeal closure occurs as a valve or sphincter through the coordinated action of these structures.[8,9] The velopharyngeal valve closes for the production of oral sounds and opens with the production of nasal sounds.

EARLY DEVELOPMENT OF VOCAL FUNCTION

Phonation begins with the birth cry. This is the first time that the infant is able to coordinate respiration, phonation, and velopharyngeal movement to produce sounds. Although the neonate is able to vocalize at birth, control over vocal productions has not yet been achieved. In addition, the neonate's voice quality is very different from the voice quality of an older child or adult due to the differences in the anatomy of the larynx and vocal tract.

At birth, the neonate's larynx is very high in the neck relative to its position in an adult. Soon after birth, the larynx begins to descend and continues to descend throughout childhood. As the larynx descends, there is a correlated decrease in

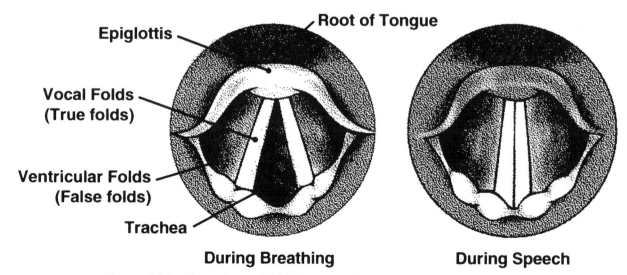

During Breathing   **During Speech**

Figure 24–1. Normal vocal fold function during breathing and speech.

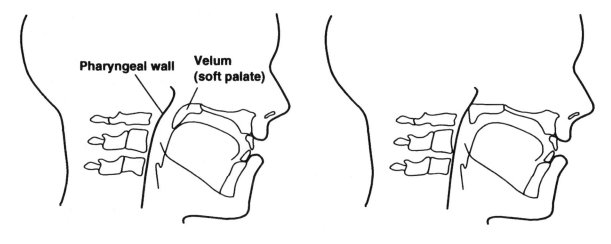

Velum at rest during nasal breathing.

Velum during speech.

Figure 24–2. Normal velopharyngeal function during breathing and speech.

the average pitch of the voice.[10,11] This occurs as the pharyngeal tube elongates, which enhances the resonance of lower fundamental frequencies. While the adult larynx has a cylinder shape, the infant's larynx is hourglass shaped, with the narrowest portion being the subglottic area. The shape of the larynx, the vocal fold length, glottal width, and infraglottal dimensions all change as the infant grows and develops, and these changes result in a change in the acoustic product of the voice.[5, 10–13]

As the anatomic changes in the vocal tract begin to occur, the infant also learns to manipulate the vocal mechanism. Within the first few months of age, the baby learns to alter phonation and develops different cries for pleasure, hunger, and pain. The baby begins to coo using vowel sounds between two to four months of age, and babble with consonant sounds around six months. Along with the development of cooing and babbling, the baby learns to use different intonational patterns with variations in pitch, intensity, and stress. In addition, the baby learns to produce both nasal and oral phonemes by opening and closing the velopharyngeal valve during articulation. By the child's first birthday, he or she has developed sufficient control over the vocal tract to be able to make fluctuations in phonation and resonance as appropriate for communication.

VOICE DISORDERS: CHARACTERISTICS AND CAUSES

Perceptual Characteristics

When the laryngeal mechanism does not function normally, abnormal voice quality may result. Re-

gardless of etiology, voice disorders tend to have certain perceptual characteristics in common. These characteristics may include the following:

Hoarseness: The perception of hoarseness is appreciated when there is aperiodic vibration of the vocal folds as they vibrate. The voice may also be described as having a "raspy" or "rough" quality.

Breathiness: Breathiness is the result of incomplete adduction of the vocal folds during phonation; this allows excess air to pass through the glottis during speech.

Glottal fry: Glottal fry occurs when the voice is produced at the very bottom of the normal pitch range. The vibratory pattern of the folds is so slow that individual vibrations are heard. This is perceived as a low pitched, staccato production.

Hard glottal attack: A hard glottal attack is characterized by rapid and complete vocal fold adduction prior to the initiation of phonation. This results in a sudden and explosive burst of phonation.

Abnormal pitch: Pitch is the perceptual counterpart of the fundamental frequency of vocal fold vibration. Pitch is considered abnormal if the habitual pitch is unusually high or low for the child's age or gender.

Diplophonia: Diplophonia is the perception of two different pitches at the same time. This can occur when the vocal folds are vibrating at different frequencies.

Inappropriate loudness: Loudness is the perceptual counterpart of vocal intensity, which is driven by subglottal air pressure.

Increased loudness is achieved by an increase in subglottal air pressure that drives the vocal folds, increasing the amplitude of the vibration. By contrast, the voice which is too soft is often the result of inadequate subglottal air pressure to drive the vocal fold vibration. When there is poor approximation of the vocal folds, resulting in breathiness, there is also a decrease in intensity secondary to a loss of subglottal air pressure.

Aphonia: Aphonia is the lack of vocal fold vibration, causing speech to be whispered. This can occur when breath support is severely compromised, resulting in inadequate subglottal air pressure to support continuous phonation.

Dysphonia: Dysphonia is a general term used to describe abnormal voice quality due to any of the above characteristics.

Common Causes

Voice disorders have a variety of causes. Some have an organic etiology, which may be either congenital or acquired. A pattern of vocal misuse or abuse can also cause a voice disorder. Some voice disorders have a psychogenic etiology.

The more common causes of voice disorders in children are noted below. Other laryngeal pathologies that are less often associated with voice disorders include congenital cysts, granuloma, polyps, and laryngeal malacia.[14]

Vocal Fold Nodules

A common cause of voice disorders in children is vocal fold nodules. Vocal nodules result from misuse (i.e., inappropriate pitch or loudness) or abuse (i.e., screaming, throat clearing, and vocal noises) of the vocal folds. Vocal misuse or abuse can cause hyperadduction and increase the friction between the vocal folds as they vibrate.[15] This can result in possible submucosal hemorrhage, followed by redness and edema of the vocal fold edges. This is later followed by a growth of hyperkeratotic epithelium with underlying fibrosis.[11] As the nodules develop, they present as white or gray protuberances on the edges of the vocal folds.

Vocal nodules are usually bilateral and located at the junction of the anterior and middle third of the vocal folds (Figure 24–3). This is the point of maximum vocal fold approximation. Vocal nodules alter the vocal fold edges and prevent the folds from complete adduction, resulting in a breathy voice quality. The extra mass on the vocal folds alters their vibratory behavior and increases the stiffness of the vocal folds,[16] resulting in a tendency for hoarseness and low pitch.

Vocal Fold Paralysis

Vocal fold paralysis comprises about 10% of all congenital anomalies of the larynx.[17] In children, laryngeal paralysis is often associated with other neurologic conditions.[18,19] Unilateral paralysis can also be associated with trauma or cardiac conditions.[20]

Lesions of the vagus nerve (CN X) and its branches at any point along the pathway from the brainstem to the laryngeal muscles can cause paresis (weakness) or total paralysis of the laryngeal muscles. The paresis or paralysis can present as either unilateral or bilateral. The folds may be paralyzed in the adducted or paramedian position

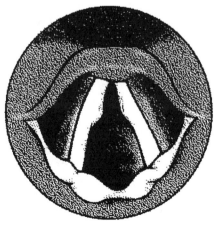
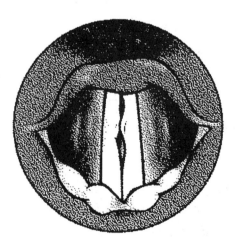

During Breathing   **During Speech**

Figure 24–3. Vocal folds with vocal nodules.

(abductor paralysis) or abducted position (adductor paralysis).[1,7,11] Bilateral abductor paralysis can be a life-threatening situation and may be treated with tracheostomy to provide the child with an adequate airway. Bilateral adductor paralysis can cause swallowing problems and a significant risk for aspiration.

The effect of paresis or paralysis on voice production depends on the location of the lesion, whether the damage involves one or both of the paired nerves, and the position of the vocal fold fixation. The voice of the child with bilateral abductor paralysis can appear normal because the vocal folds are in the median or paramedian position, allowing the subglottic air pressure to set the folds into vibration. However, inspiratory stridor may be noted. Bilateral adductor vocal fold paralysis frequently results in aphonia because the folds are unable to approximate for vibration. At times, supraglottic movement is noted during phonation attempts as a means of compensation for the paralysis.[21] Children who exhibit unilateral adductor vocal fold paralysis usually present with at breathy, hoarse voice quality with a limited pitch range or diplophonia.[1,22] Overall, the quality of phonation depends on how close the folds are able to approximate midline.

Subglottic Stenosis

Subglottic stenosis is a narrowing of the airway from the vocal folds down to the cricoid area below the glottis. Congenital subglottic stenosis is due to arrested embryonic development of the cricoid cartilage. If treatment is necessary, a tracheostomy is performed with anticipated decannulation by age two following growth of the larynx. Acquired subglottic stenosis can occur as a result of damage to the laryngeal mechanism secondary to prolonged endotracheal intubation. This is particularly common in patients with a history of prematurity. It can also occur following traumatic intubation. The degree of obstruction in acquired subglottic stenosis is usually greater than in congenital subglottic stenosis; therefore, this condition often requires long-term tracheostomy. Laryngotracheal reconstruction has proven successful in allowing earlier and successful decannulation for many of these patients.[23,24]

The effect of subglottic stenosis on phonation depends on the location and severity of the tracheal narrowing. Vocal fold damage is also common in these patients, and this can further affect phonation. Therefore, patients with subglottic stenosis often demonstrate breathiness, hoarseness, restricted pitch range, and reduced intensity.[21] Even when the patient is decannulated following laryngotracheal reconstruction, dysphonia may persist.

Papilloma

A papilloma is a neoplastic growth thought to be caused by a virus. Papillomas are the most common laryngeal tumors in children and usually occur between the ages of 2 and 4. Papillomas can present as a single growth or can occur in clusters. They can be found in various areas of the larynx, including the subglottal area, the level of the vocal folds, or the supraglottal area. They range in size from small to large enough to occlude the airway, making this a potentially life-threatening problem in children. Treatment may include medication, laser removal, surgical excision, and immunotherapy.[25,26] In children, the disease process usually resolves in adolescence, although it can persist into adulthood.

Papillomas can cause hoarseness, low pitch, and breathiness. In more severe cases, aphonia may result.[16,25] Once the papilloma has resolved, the voice quality may be affected by the residual damage to the folds.

Laryngeal Web

A laryngeal web is a congenital abnormality often detected soon after birth. It results from the lack of total separation of the connective tissue of the vocal folds during embryonic development of the larynx. When present, the web usually involves the anterior portion of the glottis at the level of the vocal folds.[1,16] Webs can also be located in the supraglottic and infraglottic areas as well. The size of a web can vary from small to very large. If the web is large enough to close a significant area of the glottis, the resulting obstruction of the airway is potentially life threatening.[27]

A laryngeal web can affect voice quality in several ways, depending on the web's location and extent. If the web shortens the available portion of the vocal folds for vibration, a high-pitched voice is the result.[1] Hoarseness, aphonia, and inspiratory stridor can also be noted. Thin laryngeal webs can usually be treated with endoscopic lysis, using either a laser or scalpel. This may need to be repeated several times with dilatation to prevent reformation of the web. Thicker webs usually required tracheostomy in addition to a reconstructive procedure with placement of a keel.[27,28]

Subglottic Hemangioma

A subglottic hemangioma is a congenital mass consisting of dilated blood vessels. Hemangiomas may cause dyspnea (labored breathing) and feeding problems, and can be large enough to interfere with the airway. Treatment may include laser surgery, steroids, or even tracheostomy.[27,28] Hemangiomas may gradually regress in size and usually disappear by age 2.

Although subglottic hemangiomas can potentially affect phonation by causing hoarseness and breathiness, they usually resolve before the child has fully developed speech.

Dysphonia Due to Tracheostomy

Indications for tracheostomy vary and include airway obstruction, persistent aspiration, and the need for prolonged mechanical ventilation.[29] When the problem is airway obstruction, there may also be secondary anomalies of the larynx, such as a laryngeal web, hemangioma, subglottic stenosis, or bilateral vocal fold paralysis.

A tracheostomy can cause changes in voice production, even when the laryngeal mechanism is normal. Phonation may be totally precluded if the tracheostomy tube is tight fitting in the trachea, as is needed for adequate mechanical ventilation[30] or in cases of subglottic stenosis. When a tight fitting tracheostomy tube limits the amount of air leak around that tube, airflow cannot be adequately maintained for vocal fold vibration. Manual closure of the tracheostomy tube during speech or the use of a one-way trach valve, such as the Passy-Muir trach valve,[31] can facilitate voicing by forcing the airflow around the trach tube and up to the larynx. If the tracheostomy tube is narrow compared to the size of the trachea, this may allow sufficient airflow between the tracheostomy tube and the trachea for phonation.

Conversion Aphonia/Dysphonia

A conversion aphonia/dysphonia is characterized by the inability to produce a normal voice, often resulting in whispering, in the absence of vocal fold pathology.[32,33] The onset is usually sudden and frequently follows complaints of a cold, sore throat or respiratory infection.[7] On recovery from this acute condition, the dysphonia remains or develops into aphonia. This condition tends to be associated with emotional stress or psychosocial problems. However, a thorough examination of the laryngeal mechanism is needed to rule out any organic pathology.

Puberphonia (Mutational Falsetto)

Puberphonia, also referred to as mutational falsetto, is a type of voice disorder in which the voice remains high-pitched and immature sounding, despite the completion of puberty. This problem is primarily noted in males, although women may demonstrate a high-pitched, childlike voice in the adult years.[16] In addition to the high pitch, the voice may sound thin, breathy, hoarse, mono-pitched, and weak. An organic etiology should be ruled out in patients who demonstrate these symptoms, although the cause is typically related to psychosocial factors.

EVALUATION

The evaluation of pediatric voice disorders is done through a combination of medical, perceptual, and instrumental procedures.

Medical Assessment and Endoscopy

While the majority of referrals for voice evaluations come from otolaryngologists, some patients are referred to speech–language pathologists by either the classroom teacher or directly by the parents. While the speech–language pathologist can proceed with the voice assessment in these circumstances, treatment should not be initiated until a medical examination has been completed. This is necessary to rule out an organic pathology for which medical treatment is indicated. The following case study illustrates this point.

CASE ONE

B.W. was a 7-year-old female who presented for a voice evaluation due to severe hoarseness. Of interest was the fact that the child was being treated for "asthma" with inhalers. The speech–language pathologist was concerned about the severity of the child's voice, and arranged for an immediate examination by an otolaryngologist, at which time multiple papillomas were diagnosed. B.W. was immediately admitted to the hospital for laser surgery. Lack of medical referral and treatment for this child could have meant severe airway compromise with serious consequences.

The medical examination by the laryngologist commonly includes an endoscopic examination of the larynx and vocal folds. This can be done through nasal or oral endoscopy. For an excellent guide to videoendoscopy of the larynx, please refer to Karnell[34] or Chapter 22.

When a strobe light is added to the endoscopy examination, the procedure is called stroboscopy, or videostroboscopy if the procedure is videotaped. The stroboscopic assessment is often done by the speech–language pathologist since it allows assessment of not only the anatomy, but also of the vibratory pattern of the vocal folds.[35–40] Stroboscopy simulates a slow-motion view of vocal fold vibration so that the mucosal wave can be assessed. The information that can be obtained from a laryngeal stroboscopic assessment includes:

- The extent and configuration of glottic closure
- The condition of the vocal fold edge
- The amplitude or excursion of the vocal folds during vibration
- The symmetry of the folds during the vibratory cycle
- The integrity of the mucosal wave
- The amount of supraglottic activity
- The integrity of the nonvibrating portion of the vocal folds.

Interview

The perceptual assessment of voice should be preceded by an interview to determine the history of the disorder, possible causes, and contributing factors.[7,41] The use of a questionnaire may be helpful in eliciting this information. The examiner should try to determine information such as the following: when the problem was first noticed; whether the onset was sudden or gradual; whether the onset was associated with any emotional or physical problems; if the patient has any chronic medical problems; if the patient is taking any medications on a regular basis; if there has been any variability in the perceptual features of the disorder; and finally, if any vocally abusive behaviors have been noted. Taking a thorough history can help the examiner to determine possible causes of the disorder and to develop an appropriate treatment plan.

Perceptual Assessment

The examiner should assess voice quality, pitch, and intensity by evaluating the voice in connected speech and with vowel prolongation. The examiner should determine if any abnormalities are present, such as: hoarseness, breathiness, glottal fry, hard glottal attack, inappropriate pitch level, restricted pitch range, diplophonia, or inappropriate volume. When present, these abnormalities can be rated on a scale of severity from mild to severe.[1,7] The quality of breath support and the type of breathing pattern should also be noted.

Instrumental Assessment

The Visi-Pitch-II (Kay Elemetrics Corp.) and Computerized Speech Lab (Kay Elemetrics Corp.) are two instruments available for objective analysis of the acoustic parameters of voice. Measures commonly used include fundamental frequency, frequency range, jitter (cycle to cycle variability in frequency), habitual intensity and intensity range, shimmer (cycle to cycle variation in amplitude), and signal to noise ratio.[3,42–44]

Various instruments, such as the Aerophone (Kay Elemetrics Corp.) or the Nagashima Phonatory Function Analyzer, can provide information regarding the aerodynamic parameters of voice production. These parameters may include airflow rate and volume, maximum phonation time, subglottal air pressure, and glottal resistance.[3,40,45,46] While normative data for aerodynamic evaluations in the pediatric population are limited, having objective data at the onset of treatment can allow the clinician to compare measures pre- and post-treatment, which may be very useful.

TREATMENT

The goal of voice therapy is to return the voice to its optimum state. If the patient demonstrates permanent alterations in anatomy or physiology, the goal of voice therapy should be optimal voice function considering these abnormalities, since a normal voice may not be possible.

The first phase of treatment is development of an understanding of the problem. The child and parent need to have a basic understanding of normal voice function, and then be knowledgeable about the cause of the child's voice disorder. If the cause of the vocal dysfunction is still present, as in vocal misuse, abuse, or emotional problems, this cause must be addressed early in the treatment process.

Some examples will now be given of basic management approaches for common voice problems in children. For more detailed information regarding treatment procedures, please refer to the texts listed in the references.

Voice Disorders of Hyperfunction

The most common result of hyperfunction in children is the development of vocal fold nodules. Nodules can be removed surgically, but this is rarely done because the nodules usually reappear if the original cause continues.[47,48] Therefore, voice therapy is most appropriate with this problem.

When vocal nodules have been identified, the first step of treatment is to identify all vocally abusive behaviors and note their frequency of occurrence. Charting the occurrence of vocally abusive behaviors over a brief period can be helpful in developing the child's awareness of these behaviors when they occur.

Reduction and eventual elimination of vocal abuses is critical to the resolution of the voice disorder. In the young child, it may mean offering a substitute for vocal noises. For example, the "raspberries" sound can be used as a substitution for a "motor" sound. For the child who is always yelling to other children on the playground, a whistle may be a viable substitute.

Hydration is an area that also needs to be addressed in the voice therapy program.[42] Drinking caffeinated soft drinks or the frequent use of drying medications, such as antihistamines, tends to dry out the superficial layer of the vocal folds. This can increase friction and irritation of the folds during phonation. Eliminating caffeinated soft drinks and increasing water intake can increase hydration and restore the folds to a healthier state. This can ultimately reduce the friction with phonation.

Another integral part of treatment is the restoration of laryngeal muscular strength and balance during phonation. This can be done through vocal function exercises. These exercises usually involve a warm-up phase, vocal fold stretching and contracting through pitch changes, and adduction power exercises.[7,42,49,50]

Some children with vocal fold nodules demonstrate a back-focused type of phonation. With these children, placing the voice is an important component to the treatment program. Instructing the child to actually "place" the voice on an object, such as a straw, is suggested. This is slowly transferred to placing the voice in the oral cavity. This technique is similar to a technique suggested by Laukkanen et al.[51] They found that using a voiced bilabial fricative may help to change the focus of the voice and this approach yielded improved vocal economy.

Voice Disorders of Hypofunction

Adductor vocal fold paralysis or paresis, whether unilateral or bilateral, results in incomplete closure of the glottis during phonation. This can cause breathiness, decreased intensity, diplophonia, and even aphonia.[11] The focus of voice therapy, therefore, is on encouraging vocal fold adduction for phonation.

Vocal fold adduction can often be improved through the use of effort closure techniques. These techniques are based on the fact that during exertion, as in pushing and pulling, the vocal folds close the glottis to prevent air from escaping from the lungs. During this closure, the true vocal folds adduct and there is general adduction of the laryngeal walls, including the false folds.[11] In treatment, vocal fold adduction can be stimulated by using pushing and pulling exercises with phonation attempts. When a vocal fold is affected by paresis, these activities can stimulate increased movement of the affected fold. When the effort closure techniques are used along with endoscopy, the patient can be provided with the additional benefit of biofeedback. Success of therapy often depends on the location of the paralyzed fold and whether touch closure can be achieved.

When therapy alone is not successful in improving vocal quality with adductor paralysis or paresis, a surgical approach can be considered. This could include vocal fold medialization (thyroplasty) or augmentation of the affected fold.[47,48,52,53] These procedures must be carefully considered because over time the paralyzed fold may become more flaccid and may migrate toward midline without intervention. In addition, airway compromise can occur following either procedure.[53]

Children who present with a history of bilateral abductor vocal fold paralysis may be treated initially with a tracheostomy, since airway concerns are paramount. For those children who are trached, many are able to achieve adequate voicing from air pressure around the trach, especially if the trach is plugged. The use of a one-way trach valve can also help the patient to achieve adequate phonation. If the patient continues to have significant difficulty phonating with the trach, augmentative measures should be considered to improve the child's ability to communicate. These might include an amplification system for the voice, an artificial larynx, sign language, a communication board, or a computerized communication system.

Surgical techniques for bilateral abductor paralysis, such as arytenoidectomy, can allow lateralization of one paralyzed vocal fold that could permit ultimate decannulation.[47,48,54] However, this may result in a breathy voice quality resulting from a now incomplete glottal closing with phonation.

Voice Disorders Secondary to Laryngeal Pathology

Children who exhibit laryngeal pathology, such as subglottic hemangioma or papillomas, are usually not candidates for voice therapy until the disease process has resolved. In some cases, however, therapy may be helpful in maintaining an acceptable voice between occurrences of the active disease process.[16] For those patients who have undergone surgical treatment, voice therapy may result in some improvement.

In patients with subglottic stenosis, surgical treatment, such as a laryngeotracheoplasty, is usually done with the primary purpose of improving the airway. When the airway has been improved and the child is decannulated, then the focus should be on improving the child's voice.

When the voice has been affected by a laryngeal pathology, a combination of symptomatic therapy and vocal function exercises may be appropriate for achieving an improvement in the voice. However, the parents and patient need to be made aware of the fact that any residual damage to the laryngeal mechanism may continue to affect the quality of the voice.[21]

Voice Disorders Secondary to Psychosocial Factors

When treating a patient with conversion aphonia/dysphonia, the examiner should attempt to establish a normal voice in the first session. Eliciting nonspeech sounds, such as coughing and throat clearing,[16,55] and then shaping them into vowels and speech is a starting point in establishing phonation. Using visual feedback, as can be done with the Visi-Pitch-II, the Computerized Speech Lab, the Video Voice or Speech Viewer, may also prove beneficial. If muscle tension is associated with a strained voice, then relaxation exercises would also be appropriate. Once a voice is established, the next goal is to stabilize the voice during subsequent sessions. In many cases, the impaired coordination of breath and voice has become habitually fixed,[32] so carryover can take time. A psychological evaluation may also be needed, since the child with a functional voice disorder may have deeper problems that need attention.[16]

The following case is an example of a conversion aphonia.

CASE TWO

J.G. was a 14-year-old female who had a history of acute laryngitis, but remained aphonic 9 months later. She had been seen by an otolaryngologist who diagnosed a functional voice disorder and recommended voice therapy. J.G. was then seen briefly by a speech–language pathologist in her school, who recommended treatment by a voice specialist. Unfortunately, the family did not pursue treatment until the new school year was to begin and the patient realized she would not be able to participate in choir.

When J.G. was finally seen by the voice specialist, voice was established during the first visit, although it was strained. By the next visit, a normal voice was produced, although she expressed some fear about using her voice with her family. At this time, counseling by a psychologist was recommended and accepted. Within a few weeks, normal voice production had returned to all situations. One year after treatment, she was still maintaining a normal voice.

When the patient demonstrates puberphonia (mutational falsetto), the therapy begins with an explanation for the voice problem. It can be helpful to associate this problem with difficulty coordinating the muscles of the larynx as they grow. The next step is helping the patient to achieve an appropriate pitch level and then recognize this level as the target. This can be done by using various techniques, including coughing, humming at a lower pitch, saying "uh hum" and progressively lowering the pitch, producing a hard glottal attack, and even having the patient imitate another person's lowered pitch. At times, digital manipulation of the larynx is helpful in getting the patient to lower the pitch.[11,41,56] This can be done by holding the larynx with the thumb and index finger and gently guiding it to a lower position in neck during phonation. Once an appropriate pitch level is established, carryover to connected speech is the goal. The patient's concept of a normal voice usually will change with reinforcement and practice.

RESONANCE DISORDERS: CHARACTERISTICS AND CAUSES

Abnormal resonance may be noted when the velopharyngeal mechanism does not function adequately, or when there is a blockage in the resonating cavities. Anything that disrupts the transmission of sound or the normal balance of oral and nasal resonance can cause a resonance disorder.

Hypernasality

Hypernasality is the result of too much resonance in the nasal cavity during speech. Hypernasality usually occurs as a result of velopharyngeal inadequacy (VPI), although a large fistula can also result in inappropriate or excessive nasal resonance with speech. Hypernasality is particularly perceptible on vowel sounds since these sounds are voiced and relatively long in duration. Hypernasality may be noted to increase with an increase in connected speech due to the additional demands on the velopharyngeal mechanism.

When hypernasal resonance is noted, there is often audible nasal air emission during consonant production. As the patient attempts to build up air pressure in the oral cavity for pressure sensitive sounds (plosives, fricatives, and affricates), air pressure leaks through the valve and is emitted nasally. Turbulent airflow, often called a nasal rustle, is a very loud and distracting form of nasal air emission. It is felt to be the result of a large amount of air being forced through a small velopharyngeal opening, causing a sound due to friction and the bubbling of secretions.[57,58]

When air leaks through the velopharyngeal valve, this may also reduce the amount of air pressure available for consonant production. As a result, consonants may be weak in pressure and intensity, or may be omitted completely.[3,59] With hypernasality and weak consonants, the speech often sounds muffled. The loss of air pressure can also affect utterance length because frequent breaths are required to replace air pressure. When intraoral air pressure is inadequate for normal speech, compensatory articulation productions are often acquired. Patients with VPI often demonstrate compensatory articulation productions by making use of the air stream in the pharynx before it is lost through the velopharyngeal port. These sounds can be articulated with what appears to be normal placement, but actually is not. For example, the patient may appear to be producing a normal /p/ phoneme with bilabial closure, while

coarticulating the plosive portion with a glottal stop. Common compensatory productions include glottal stops, pharyngeal stops, and pharyngeal fricatives. Other compensatory articulation productions have also been described.[60]

Velopharyngeal inadequacy (VPI) is a generic term that may be used to describe abnormal velopharyngeal function due either an anatomical deficiency or a physiological deficiency. Velopharyngeal dysfunction (VPD) is another generic term commonly used in the literature.

Velopharyngeal insufficiency refers to an anatomical deficit that would cause the velum to be short relative to the posterior pharyngeal wall (Figure 24–4). This often occurs due to a history of cleft palate or a submucous cleft palate. Congenital palatal insufficiency (CPI) can also occur for a variety of reasons, including a deep pharynx or cranial base abnormalities.[59,61] Velopharyngeal insufficiency may occur after an adenoidectomy,[62–64] especially if closure was achieved against the adenoid pad or was tenuous from the start. A Le Fort I maxillary advancement procedure can potentially result in velopharyngeal insufficiency, since the velum can move anteriorly with the maxilla.[65,66] Finally, large tonsils can restrict lateral pharyngeal wall motion, or can intrude into the nasopharynx and thus interfere with velopharyngeal closure.[67–69]

Velopharyngeal incompetence refers to a physiological deficiency that results in poor movement of the velum and pharyngeal structures (Figure 24–5). This can occur following a cleft palate repair due to poor muscle function, or in patients with submucous cleft palate and abnormal muscle insertion in the velum. Velopharyngeal incompetence can be noted in patients with oral-motor dysfunction, as in a dysarthria, due to poor movement

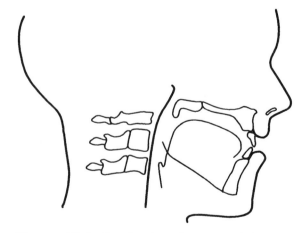

Figure 24–4. A short velum resulting in velopharyngeal insufficiency.

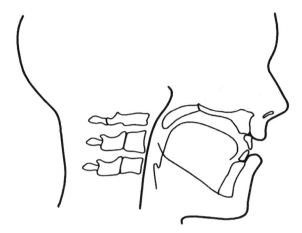

Figure 24–5. Poor velar movement resulting in velopharyngeal incompetence.

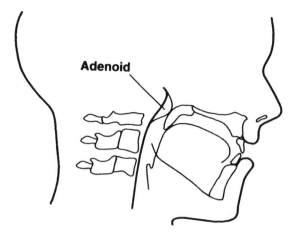

Figure 24–6. Upper airway obstruction causing hyponasality due to a large adenoid pad.

of the velopharyngeal structures.[70] In patients with either congenital or acquired cranial nerve damage, specific velopharyngeal paralysis or paresis (usually unilateral) can occur in the absence of other oral-motor deficits.

Velocardiofacial syndrome is commonly found in patients who present with velopharyngeal dysfunction as a result of congenital palatal insufficiency or submucous cleft palate.[71–73] Other characteristics of this syndrome include language deficits, learning disabilities, facial anomalies, and minor cardiac anomalies. Patients with any of these characteristics should be referred for a genetics assessment.

Hyponasality and Denasality

Hyponasality occurs when there is a reduction in nasal resonance during speech as a result of blockage in the nasopharynx or the entrance to the nasal cavity. If the nasal cavity is completely occluded, resonance would be denasal. Hyponasality and denasality affect the quality of vowels, but particularly affect the production of the nasal consonants (m, n, and ng). When nasal resonance is eliminated for the nasal consonants, these consonants sound similar to their oral phoneme cognates (b, d, and g).

The cause of hyponasality or denasality is always obstruction somewhere in the nasopharynx or nasal cavity. This obstruction may be due to adenoid hypertrophy (Figure 24–6), swelling of the nasal passages secondary to allergic rhinitis or the common cold, a deviated septum, choanal atresia (which is a congenital blockage of the opening into the nasopharynx from the nasal fossa), a stenotic naris, midface deficiency, and others. Since the cause of reduced nasal resonance is strictly obstruction, further evaluation and treatment should be done by a physician.

Cul-de-Sac Resonance

Cul-de-sac resonance occurs when the transmission of acoustic energy is trapped in a blind pouch with only one outlet. The speech is perceived as muffled and has been described as "potato-in-the-mouth" speech.[69] This can occur, for example, in patients with very large tonsils and adenoid hypertrophy.[67,68] As the sound energy travels superiorly, the sound may be blocked from the nasal cavity by the adenoid pad. The tonsils can also restrict sound transmission into the oral cavity. As a result, the sound energy is trapped and vibration occurs primarily in the pharynx. Resonance can also be perceived as cul-de-sac when there is VPI and anterior blockage of the nasal cavity. This blockage could be due to a deviated septum, nasal polyps, or stenotic nares. This type of resonance disorder requires medical intervention to eliminate the source of blockage.

Mixed Resonance

Some patients demonstrate characteristics of both hypernasality and hyponasality. Mixed hyper- and hyponasality can occur when there is VPI in addition to significant nasal airway blockage. In this case, hypernasality may be the predominate characteristic of connected speech, but hyponasality is noted on the nasal consonants. Mixed resonance can also occur in patients with oral-motor disorders, due to inappropriate timing of the upward or downward movement of the velum for speech.[74]

EVALUATION

Perceptual Evaluation

Resonance

Resonance should always be evaluated by judging connected speech, preferably spontaneous connected speech. Connected speech increases the demands on the velopharyngeal valving system to achieve and maintain closure. Therefore, hypernasality is often more apparent in connected speech than in single words or short utterances. In evaluating connected speech, the examiner should determine whether the quality or the intelligibility of speech is affected by abnormal transmission of acoustic energy in the vocal tract. Resonance can be rated on a simple scale as either denasal, hyponasal, normal, or hypernasal to a mild, moderate, or severe degree. The clinician should be sure to make a judgment as to whether there is any evidence of cul-de-sac nasality or mixed resonance.

Nasal Air Emission

When resonance is abnormal due to VPI, nasal air emission may also occur with consonant production. This can be evaluated by noting the occurrence and consistency of nasal air emission in connected speech. A single word articulation test can also be used to determine if the nasal air emission occurs primarily on certain types of phonemes, such as sibilants, or on all types of pressure sensitive sounds.

Articulation

Since compensatory articulation errors are common in patients with hypernasality, it is important to carefully evaluate articulation.[75] The examiner should determine which articulation errors are compensatory due to velopharyngeal valving problems versus those that are merely placement errors. The occurrence of compensatory articulation errors can be determined by using any single word articulation test.

In addition to articulation errors, the examiner should evaluate the adequacy of oral air pressure. If consonants are weak in intensity, it can be assumed that oral air pressure is compromised because of VPI. As previously mentioned, the examiner should note the occurrence of audible nasal air emission (including nasal rustle) during the production of pressure sensitive phonemes.

Assessing stimulability is an important component of the evaluation. The patient may be stimulable for a reduction or elimination of nasal air emission with a change in articulatory placement. This may be a good prognostic indicator for improvement or correction with therapy. It may also suggest that the patient demonstrates "functional" hypernasality or phoneme-specific nasal air emission. This may be caused by articulation errors or the faulty learning of movement patterns, rather than a primary velopharyngeal valving disorder.

Phonation

When problems in resonance are noted, the quality of phonation should also be assessed. Breathiness or hoarseness may indicate the presence of vocal nodules, which are commonly found in patients with mild VPI. These children may demonstrate laryngeal hyperfunction in an attempt to compensate for the effects of VPI. In addition, compensatory valving activities and the use of glottal stops may also contribute to the development of nodules.[76,77]

Additional Informal Tests

Additional informal tests are often needed to more clearly identify the abnormality of resonance. Using these informal tests, the examiner should listen for the type of resonance and the presence of nasal air emission, including nasal rustle (turbulence). The following informal speech tests may be helpful in that they are sensitive to velopharyngeal valving problems:

Nasal Sentences: To rule out hyponasality or denasality, the examiner can have the child produce nasal sounds repetitively or sentences loaded with nasal consonants. If the nasal phonemes are distorted or sound closer to their oral cognates, hypo- or denasality due to upper airway obstruction is suggested. Mouth breathing is also indicative of airway obstruction.

Cul-de-Sac Test: If the examiner is unsure of the type of abnormal resonance being presented, the cul-de-sac test can be used. With this informal test, the child is asked to produce a vowel or repeat a sentence completely devoid of nasal consonants. The child should then repeat the same utterance with the nares occluded. In normal speech, there should be no perceptible difference in the quality of the production since the nasal cavity is already closed by the velopharyngeal valve. If there is a difference in quality with closure of the nasal cavity at the nares, this suggests that resonance is hypernasal because sound is resonating in the nasal cavity. If resonance is perceived as abnormal, but closure of the nares results in no change in quality, this can suggest either cul-de-sac resonance or hyponasality.

Phoneme Repetition: To determine the presence of nasal air emission and compensatory articulation productions, have the child produce pressure sensitive phonemes (plosives, fricatives, affricates) in a repetitive manner (pa, pa, pa, pa, etc.).

Sentence Repetition: Another way to test for nasal air emission and compensatory articulation productions is to have the child repeat sentences that are loaded with pressure sensitive phonemes. It can be particularly helpful if these sentences contain similar phonemes in terms of articulatory placement. Sample sentences might include:

p	Popeye plays baseball.	v	Drive the van.
b	Buy baby a bib.	s	Sissy sees the sun in the sky.
t	Take Teddy to town.	z	I saw a zebra at the zoo.
d	Do it for Daddy.	sh	She went shopping.
k	I like cake and ice cream.	ch	I eat cherries and cheese.
g	Go get the wagon.	j	John told a joke to Jim.
f	Fred has five fish.		

Counting: Have the child count from 60 to 70. The sixties can be particularly diagnostic since these numbers contain a combination of sibilants, velar plosives, and alveolar plosives. These sounds require a build-up and continuation of intraoral air pressure, which can particularly tax the velopharyngeal mechanism and result in nasal air emission if there is VPI.

Tactile Feedback Test: The examiner should feel the sides of the nares as the child repeats pressure sensitive sounds repetitively. (It is important to eliminate nasal phonemes from the speech sample for obvious reasons.) If vibration is felt, this could indicate nasal air emission or hypernasality.

Visual Feedback Tests: In addition to listening and feeling for nasal air emission, the examiner can actually see nasal air emission by using an "air paddle."[78] A small paddle can be cut from a piece of paper and placed underneath the nares during speech. If the paddle moves during the production of pressure sensitive sounds, this indicates that there is nasal air emission. The See Scape (Speech Bin) is a simple tool that consists of a nasal olive, a tube, and a small styrofoam stopper in a cylinder. If there is nasal air emission with phoneme production while using this tool, the styrofoam stopper rises in the cylinder.

Fistula Test: To determine if a fistula is the cause of hypernasality or nasal air emission, the examiner can attempt to occlude the fistula with chewing gum or a tissue, and then evaluate whether there is a change in resonance and nasal emission. Even without occluding the fistula, the examiner can determine if there is a difference in the degree of nasal air emission for anterior sounds (p, b, t, d) and posterior sounds (k, g). More nasal air emission on anterior than posterior sounds is often suggestive of a symptomatic anterior fistula.

Instrumental Assessment

The nasometer (Kay Elemetrics Corp.) is a computer-based instrument designed to measure acoustic energy from the nasal cavity and oral cavity during speech. The nasometer computes the ratio of nasal acoustic energy to total (nasal plus oral) acoustic energy and displays this in real time. An average "nasalance" score can be computed for a given speech segment. When one of the standardized passages is used, the nasalance score can be compared to normative data. This instrument can be very useful in a clinical examination because it provides objective information regarding resonance and nasality.[79] However, the examiner must interpret the scores based on knowledge regarding resonance and articulation. A combination of hyponasality and nasal air emission can affect the nasalance score to a significant degree.[80] The use of nasal phonemes and compensatory articulation productions can also affect the score.

Using aerodynamic principles, instrumentation is now available to assess air pressure and airflow to evaluate velopharyngeal function. With the pressure-flow technique, simultaneous measurements are made of airflow through the velopharyngeal port and the pressure drop across the port. With this data, a formula can be used to calculate an estimate of velopharyngeal orifice size.[81–84]

Intraoral Examination

An intraoral examination should always be done as part of the resonance evaluation. However, the examiner should be aware that an intraoral view is not adequate for a judgment regarding velopharyngeal function. Closure occurs behind the velum and is above the level of the oral cavity, usually on the plane of the hard palate. In addition, the examiner cannot see the point of maximum lateral pharyngeal wall movement from an intraoral perspective.

In an intraoral examination, the clinician can determine palatal and velar integrity. The presence and location of a palatal fistula should always be noted since a large fistula, especially one in a posterior position, can cause hypernasality and nasal air emission. The examiner should judge the relative length of the velum because a very short velum may suggest velopharyngeal insufficiency. Velar mobility during phonation should be observed. The velum should raise and the velar "dimple" should be back approximately 80% of the length of the soft palate.[85] Poor velar mobility or asymmetrical movement may suggest VPI.

If there is no history of cleft palate, the examiner should look for signs of a submucous cleft. These signs may include a bifid or hypoplastic uvula, a bluish or transparent appearing velum, or a V shape in the hard palate. In palpating the posterior nasal spine, the examiner may feel a notch in the bony structure that would suggest a submucous cleft. During phonation, the velum often appears to "tent up" into an inverted V shape when there is a submucous cleft that extends through the velum.

Videofluoroscopic Speech Study

A videofluoroscopic speech study is a radiographic evaluation that allows the direct visualization of all aspects of the velopharyngeal sphincter during speech.[86] It is important to assess both the anatomical and physiological abnormalities causing VPI to determine the optimal surgical or prosthetic treatment for the patient. During the speech study, the patient is asked to repeat standard sentences so that the velopharyngeal structures can be observed during connected speech. Since multiple views are used, the examiner can evaluate the motion of the velum and posterior pharyngeal walls and then assess the movement of the lateral pharyngeal walls.

With multiview videofluoroscopy, the examiner can confirm the presence of the velopharyngeal opening and determine the relative size of the opening. The cause of VPI can also be differentiated between a short velum, poor velar movement, and/or poor lateral pharyngeal wall motion. For more indepth information regarding the videofluoroscopy technique for speech studies, please refer to Skolnick and Cohn.[87]

Nasopharyngoscopy (Endoscopy)

Nasopharyngoscopy is an endoscopic technique that can be a useful tool in evaluating velopharyngeal function.[88,89] This technique allows direct observation of the velopharyngeal portal during speech and can be performed by a physician or a well-trained speech–language pathologist.

The nasopharyngoscopy procedure requires the introduction of a topical anesthetic (i.e., xylocaine, lidocaine, or pontocaine) into the nasal cavity. Once numbing has occurred, the nasopharyngoscope is passed through the middle meatus and back to the area of velopharyngeal closure. The patient is asked to repeat sentences so that velopharyngeal function can be directly observed. The entire procedure is usually videotaped to allow for an in-depth analysis at a later time.

Through the nasopharyngoscopy procedure, the examiner can view the nasal aspect of the velum, the posterior pharyngeal wall, and lateral pharyngeal walls. The adenoid pad can be easily seen through this technique. Nasopharyngoscopy is a particularly good technique for evaluating the effectiveness of a retropharyngeal implant, sphincteroplasty, or pharyngeal flap, since the results of these procedures can be easily viewed. Please refer to Karnell[34] or Chapter 23 for more detailed information regarding the nasopharyngoscopy procedure.

TREATMENT

Surgical Intervention

Surgical intervention is indicated whenever there is hypernasality caused by a structural or physiological abnormality that renders the patient unable to achieve normal velopharyngeal closure. If the patient was born with a cleft palate, obviously this needs to be repaired before normal velopharyngeal function can be expected. Most surgeons repair the palate around the age of 12 months.[90,91] If the patient was born with a submucous cleft palate and has characteristics of VPI, the speech pathologist and surgeon may opt to try a primary palate repair first before considering secondary surgical procedures designed to correct VPI.

An oronasal fistula is an opening in the hard palate or velum that occurs occasionally after a cleft palate repair, particularly following maxillary expansion. When hypernasality is noted, the examiner should carefully evaluate whether the hypernasality is due to the fistula or if it results from VPI so that the appropriate surgical procedure is done. Closure of the fistula may be required to correct the hypernasality.

If VPI is the cause of hypernasality or nasal air emission, surgical intervention is typically the preferred course of treatment. One common procedure is the superiorly based pharyngeal flap (Figure 24–7). This procedure involves the creation of a soft tissue flap from the posterior pharyngeal wall, which is then sutured into the velum. This results in partial occlusion of the velopharyngeal space. Lateral ports on either side of the flap remain open for normal nasal breathing, but during speech the lateral walls move in to close around the flap.[59,90,91]

Another surgical procedure for correction of VPI is the sphincter pharyngoplasty. This surgery attempts to create a dynamic sphincter in the pharynx by repositioning the posterior tonsillar pillars, including the palatopharyngeous muscles, and suturing these lateral flaps on the posterior pharyngeal wall.[92–94] Some surgeons also elevate a posterior pharyngeal flap and attach it to the lateral flaps.

In cases of very mild VPI, pharyngeal augmentation is sometimes done. Various materials, such as a Teflon, Silastic, and cartilage, have been used for this purpose.[95,96] With this procedure, the material is injected into the pharyngeal wall in the area of the velopharyngeal opening to push that area forward. As the velum closes against the pharyngeal wall, this material serves to fill in the opening.

When the abnormal resonance is caused by a blockage somewhere in the resonating chambers, as in hyponasality, denasality, or cul-de-sac resonance, medical intervention is required. This could simply involve antihistamine/decongestant therapy. In many cases, surgical intervention is indicated, such as an adenoidectomy, a tonsillectomy, a septoplasty, or even midface advancement. Speech therapy is not appropriate in these cases.

Prosthetic Management

Prosthetic management should be considered for correction of VPI when surgery is not an option for medical or psychological reasons.[97] Prosthetic devices are typically made of acrylic and attach to the teeth with wires.

A palatal obturator is a prosthetic device that is used to cover an open defect, such as an unrepaired cleft or a fistula. A palatal lift can be used in cases where the velum is long enough to achieve closure, but does not move well. A palatal lift can be particularly effective for dysarthric patients, when hypernasality is a primary contributor to intelligibility deficits, and articulation, phonation, and respiration are not severely compromised (see References for further guidelines[70,98–101]). Finally, a speech bulb obturator can be considered when the velum is too short to close completely against the posterior pharyngeal wall. The bulb serves to fill in the pharyngeal space for speech.

Although a prosthesis is appropriate for some patients, it has some distinct disadvantages, particularly for children. Unlike surgery, a prosthesis is not a permanent correction. It usually needs to be removed at night and during eating. It can cause ulceration of the mucosa, making it uncomfortable to wear. Compliance can be a problem as a result. In young children, it needs to be remade periodically due to growth.

Speech Therapy

Speech therapy is appropriate for treatment of hypernasality and nasal air emission *only* under the following conditions:

- The characteristic is mild.
- The characteristic is inconsistent.
- The child is stimulable for a reduction or elimination of the characteristic.
- The characteristic results from faulty articulation (i.e., nasal air emission with pharyngeal fricatives, or nasality due to an associated /ng/ tongue position with an anterior phoneme, such as /l/).
- The characteristic is associated with oral-motor dysfunction or dysarthria.
- The characteristic occurs primarily when the patient is tired.
- The velopharyngeal opening is slight or inconsistent, as demonstrated by videofluoroscopy or nasopharyngoscopy.

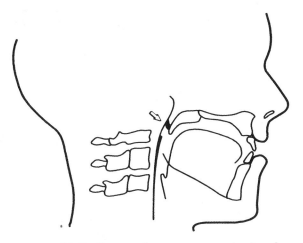

Figure 24–7. Surgical management of velopharyngeal insufficiency through a pharyngeal flap.

- Surgical correction of VPI has been done, and the patient needs therapy to increase velar or lateral pharyngeal wall motion to improve the function of the revised structures.

It is important to note that speech therapy cannot change structure, and therefore, surgical intervention is needed to correct VPI. On the other hand, surgery cannot change function. Even when VPI is corrected surgically, the child may need to be taught appropriate articulatory placement and oral airflow before normal speech can be achieved. This principle is nicely demonstrated by the following case report.

CASE THREE

L.W. presented at the age of 3 years, 4 months with a history of bilateral complete cleft lip and palate. The lip and velum were repaired at another center, but the hard palate was left unrepaired since the cleft was so wide. Speech was severely hypernasal due to the open palate and a very short, essentially nonfunctional velum. Articulation was characterized by the use of nasal phonemes and glottal stops for all oral sounds. Nasometric testing showed a significant degree of nasalance. On the Zoo passage, the nasalance score was 49.11 (mean = 15.53, s.d. = 4.86). A palate repair and pharyngeal flap were recommended and finally done at the age of 3 years, 8 months.

Three months after surgery, there was little change in speech. L.W.'s postoperative nasalance score was 51.07, which is actually a little higher than the preoperative score. She continued to use nasal phonemes and glottal stops for all oral sounds. Therefore, speech therapy was recommended.

L.W. was seen for speech therapy near her home for 10 months and then returned for a follow-up evaluation. On this evaluation, dramatic improvement in speech was noted. With the exception of a few developmental errors, L.W. was producing all oral phonemes normally with good oral pressure and no evidence of nasal air emission. Resonance was judged to be normal, and this was confirmed by the nasometric score of 10.41.

This case illustrates the point that when there is VPI, surgical intervention is needed to correct the structure and improve the potential for normal speech. However, if the child continues to produce nasal phonemes and glottal stops for all oral sounds, speech will remain defective and sound hypernasal. At this point, speech therapy is indicated to change the function of the velopharyngeal mechanism by helping the child learn to use this mechanism appropriately for speech.

If speech therapy is indicated, the techniques are similar to articulation therapy. The goal of therapy should be to eliminate compensatory articulation productions, eliminate inconsistent nasal air emission, and improve oral resonance by changing the focus of articulation. Specific techniques have been published,[102,103] but should be customized for the patient's needs.

Therapy should incorporate the use of visual or auditory biofeedback whenever possible. This can greatly facilitate progress.[104] The nasometer is an excellent tool for providing visual feedback regarding oral-nasal resonance and nasal air emission. Therefore, it can be very useful in the treatment process.

In addition to the use of the nasometer, other therapy techniques can be effective in treating the various characteristics of VPI. Kuehn[105] reported case studies where continuous positive airway pressure (CPAP) was used as a treatment for VPI. The CPAP instrument delivers a continuous flow of air into the nasal airway via a mask and hose, which is connected to a flow generator. In therapy, the patient attempts to block the flow of air through resistance of the velopharyngeal muscles during speech tasks.

In all cases, speech therapy should continue as long as the child is making progress. However, if the child demonstrates persistent hypernasality, nasal air emission, or weak consonants, speech therapy alone may not be appropriate. Instead, further evaluation of velopharyngeal function should be done through videofluoroscopy or nasopharyngoscopy for consideration of surgical intervention.

SUMMARY

In summary, voice and resonance disorders are commonly seen in the pediatric population. These disorders may be congenital, or due to disease or trauma, vocal abuse or misuse, or even psychosocial factors. The pediatric speech–language pathologist should be knowledgeable of the characteristics of these disorders and basic evaluation and treatment protocols. If the problem is complex, referral to a voice specialist or a center that specializes in this type of disorder is highly recommended.

If a referral to a voice specialist is indicated, this specialist can usually be found by checking with area hospitals, particularly pediatric or teaching hospitals. Voice specialists are often associated with the otolaryngology department of a university, hospital, or private practice.

If additional evaluations are needed for disorders of resonance, a referral should be made to a craniofacial anomaly team whenever possible. This ensures that the patient will receive appropriate services by a speech–language pathologist and other professionals who are knowledgeable and experienced in dealing with a variety of resonance disorders. If there is no team in the area, the Cleft Palate Foundation of the American Cleft Palate-Craniofacial Association can assist in finding appropriate professionals.

STUDY QUESTIONS

1. What are the various perceptual characteristics of a voice disorder and possible causes of each?

2. What is the potential impact of the following on voice production: vocal fold nodules, laryngeal web, tracheostomy?

3. What is the reason for a medical examination of the vocal folds prior to the initiation of voice therapy?

4. What kind of information regarding phonation can be obtained through various instrumental techniques? What information is obtained through videostroboscopy?

5. When vocal fold nodules are identified, how is this disorder typically treated?

6. What are the different types of resonance disorders and possible causes for each?

7. In addition to hypernasality, what are some other effects of velopharyngeal insufficiency on speech production?

8. In evaluating a patient with a resonance disorder, what information can be obtained from an intraoral assessment? Why is this information limited?

9. What information regarding velopharyngeal function can be obtained from videofluoroscopy and nasopharyngoscopy?

10. Under what circumstances is speech therapy appropriate for patients who demonstrate hypernasality?

REFERENCES

1. Wilson DK: *Voice problems of children,* 3rd ed. Williams & Wilkins, Baltimore, 1987.

2. Shearer W: The diagnosis and treatment of voice disorders in children. *J Speech Hear Dis* 1972; 37: 215–221.

3. Baken RJ: *Clinical measurement of speech and voice.* College-Hill Press, Boston, 1987.

4. Hirano M: Strucure and behavior of the vibratory vocal folds. In Sawashima T, Cooper D, eds., *Dynamic aspects of speech production,* pp 13–27. University of Tokyo Press, Tokyo, 1977.

5. Hirano M, Kurita S, Nakashima T: Growth, development and aging of human vocal folds. In Bless DM, Abbs JH, eds., *Vocal fold physiology,* pp 24–43. College-Hill Press, San Diego, 1983.

6. Hirano M, Yoshida T, Tanaka S: Vibratory behavior of human vocal folds viewed from below. In Gauffin F, Hammarberg B, eds., *Vocal fold physiology,* pp 1–6. Singular Publishing, San Diego, 1991.

7. Stemple JC, Glaze LE, Gerdeman BK: *Clinical voice pathology theory and management.* Singular Publishing Group, San Diego, 1995.

8. Skolnick ML, McCall GN, Barnes M: The sphincteric mechanism of velopharyngeal closure. *Cleft Palate J* 1973; 10:286–305.

9. Moon J, Kuehn D: Anatomy and physiology of normal and disordered velopharyngeal function for speech. *National Center for Voice and Speech* 1996; 9 April 143–158.

10. Kent R: Anatomic and neuromuscular maturation of the speech mechanism: Evidence for acoustic studies. *J Speech Hear Res* 1976; 19:421–446.

11. Aronson AE: *Clinical voice disorders,* 3rd ed. Thieme, New York, 1990.

12. Kahane JC: Growth of the human prepubertal and pubertal larynx. *J Speech Hear Res* 1982; 25:446–455.

13. Netsell R, Lotz WK, Peters JE, Schulte L: Developmental patterns of laryngeal and respiratory function for speech production. *J Voice* 1994; 8(2):123–131.

14. Dobres R, Lee L, Stemple JC, et al: Description of laryngeal pathologies in children evaluated by otolaryngologists. *J Speech Hear Dis* 1990; 55:526–532.

15. Hillman RE, Homberg EB, Perkell JS, et al: Objective assessment of vocal hyperfunction: An experimental framework and initial results. *J Speech Hear Res* 1989; 32:373–392.

16. Colton RH, Casper JK: *Understanding voice problems,* 2nd ed. Williams & Wilkins, Baltimore, 1996.

17. Holinger LD, Holinger PC, Holinger PH: Etiology of bilateral abductor vocal cord paralysis: A review of 389 cases. *Ann Otol Rhinol Laryngol* 1976; 85: 428–436.

18. Cohen S, Geller Ka, Birns JW: Laryngeal paralysis in children: A long term retrospective study. *Ann Otol Rhinol Laryngol* 1982; Jul-Aug 91:417–424.

19. Dedo DD: Pediatric vocal cord paralysis. *Laryngoscope* 1979; Sep. 89:1378–1384.

20. Rosin DF, Handler SD, Potsic WP, et al: Vocal cord paralysis in children. *Laryngoscope* 1990; 100(11): 1174–1179.

21. Smith ME, Marsh JH, Cotton RT et al: Voice problems after pediatric laryngotracheal reconstruction: Videolaryngostroboscopic, acoustic and perceptual assessment. *Int J Pediatr Otorhinolaryngol* 1993; 25: 173–181.

22. Tucker HM: Vocal cord paralysis in small children: Principles in management. *Ann Otol Rhinol Laryngol* 1986; 95:618–621.

23. Cotton RT: Pediatric laryngotracheal stenosis. *J Pediatr Surg* 1984; 19(6):699–704.

24. Cotton RT, Myer CM, O'Connor DM, et al: Pediatric laryngotracheal reconstruction with cartilage grafts and endotracheal tube stenting: The single-stage approach. *Laryngoscope* 1995; 105:818–821.

25. Borkowsky W. Martin D, Lawrence HS: Juvenile laryngeal papillomatosis with pulmonary spread. *Am J Dis in Child* 1984; 138:667–669.

26. Robbins KT, Woodson GE: Current concepts in the management of laryngeal papillomatosis. *Head and Neck Surg* 1984; Mar/April:861–866.

27. Richardson MA, Cotton RT: Anatomic abnormalities of the pediatric airway. *Pediatr Clin North Am* 1984; 31(4):821–834.

28. Cotton RT, Richardson MA: Congenital laryngeal anomalies. *Otolaryngol Clin North Am* 1981; 14(1): 203–218.

29. Motoyama EK: Physiologic alterations in tracheostomy. In Myers EN, Stool SE, Johnson JT, eds., *Tracheotomy.* 177–197. Churchill Livingstone, New York, 1985.

30. Fowler SM, Simon BM, Handler SD: Communication development in children. In Myers EN, Stool SE, Johnson JT, eds., *Tracheotomy,* 271–284. Churchill Livingstone, New York, 1985.

31. Mason MF, Meehan K, Holinger LD: Tracheostomy and tracheostomy tubes. In Mason MF, ed., *Speech pathology for tracheotomized and ventilator dependent patients.* Voicing, Newport Beach, 1993.

32. Kinzl J, Biebl W, Rauchegger H: Functional aphonia: Psychosomatic aspects of diagnosis and therapy. *Folia Phoniatr* 1988, 40(3):131–137.

33. Harris C, Richards C: Functional aphonia in young people. *J Laryngol Otol* July 1992; 106:610–612.

34. Karnell MP: *Videoendoscopy: From velopharynx to larynx.* Singular Publishing, Inc., San Diego, 1994.

35. D'Antonio LL, Chait DH, Lotz WK et al: Pediatric videonasoendoscopy for speech and voice evaluation. *Otolaryngol Head Neck Surg* 1986; 94:578–583.

36. Bless DM, Hirano M, Feder RJ: Videostrobic evaluation of the larynx. *Ear Nose Throat J* 1987; July 66(7): 289–296.

37. Woo P, Colton R, Casper J, et al: Diagnostic value of stroboscopic examination on hoarse patients. *J Voice* 1991; 5:231–238.

38. Casiano R, Zaveri V, Lundy D: Efficacy of videostroboscopy in the diagnosis of voice disorders. *Otolaryngol Head Neck Surg* July 1992; 107(1):95–100.

39. Hirano M, Bless DM: *Videostroboscopic examination of the larynx.* Singular Publishing, San Diego, 1993.

40. Lotz WK, Antonio L, Chait D, et al: Successful nasoendoscopic and aerodynamic examinations of children with speech/voice disorders. *Int J Pediatr Otorhinolaryngol* 1993; 26(25):165–172.

41. Boone DR: *The voice and voice therapy,* 4th ed. Prentice-Hall, Englewood Cliffs, 1988.

42. Stemple JC: *Voice therapy: Clinical studies.* Mosby Year-Book, St. Louis, 1993.

43. Bless DM: Measurement of vocal function. *Otolaryngol Clin North Am* 1991; 24:1023–1033.

44. Sataloff RT, Spiegel RJ, Carroll LM et al: Objective measures of voice function. *Ear Nose Throat J* 1987; Aug. 66(8):307–312.

45. Tanaka S, Gould WJ: Vocal efficiency and aerodynamic aspects in voice disorders. *Ann Otol Rhinol Laryngol* Jan–Feb 1985; 94:29–33.

46. Zajac D, Farkas Z, Dindzans L, Stool S: Aerodynamic and laryngographic assessment of pediatric vocal function. *Pediatr Pulmonol* 1993; 15:44–51.

47. Snow, JB: Surgery therapy for vocal dysfunction. *Otolaryngol Clin North Am* 1984; 12:91–100.

48. Choi SS, Cotton RT: Surgical management of voice disorders. *Pediatr Clin North Am* 1989; 46(6):1535–1549.

49. Stemple JC, Lee L, D'Amico B, et al: Efficiency of vocal function exercises as a method of improving voice production. *J Voice* 1994; 8(3):271–278.

50. Andrews M: *Management of voice treatment: Pediatrics through geriatrics.* Singular Publishers, San Diego, 1995.

51. Laukkanen A, Lindholm P, Vilkman E et al: A physiological and acoustical study on voiced bilabial fricative as a vocal exercise. *J Voice* 1996; 10(1):67–77.

52. Rontal E, Rontal M, Morse G: Vocal cord injection in the treatment of acute and chronic aspiration. *Laryngoscope* 1976; 86(5):625–634.

53. Levine B, Jacobs I, Wetmore R et al: Vocal cord injection in children with unilateral vocal cord paralysis. *Arch Otolaryngol Head Neck Surg* 1995; 121(1): 116–119.

54. Rosin E, Handler SD, Potsic WP, et al: Vocal cord paralysis in children. *Laryngoscope* 1990; 100(11): 1174–1179.

55. Prater RJ, Swift RW: *Manual of voice therapy.* Little, Brown, Boston, 1984.

56. Prater RJ: Voice therapy: Techniques and applications. *Otolaryngol Clin North Am* 1991; 24:1075–1091.

57. Kummer AW, Neale HW: Changes in articulation and resonance after tongue flap closure of palatal fistulas: Case reports. *Cleft Palate J* 1989; 26:51–55.

58. Kummer AW, Curtis C, Wiggs M, et al: Comparison of velopharyngeal gap size in patients with hypernasality, hypernasality and nasal emission, or nasal turbulence (rustle) as the primary speech characteristic. *Cleft Palate-Craniofac J* 1992; 29:152–156.

59. McWilliams BJ, Morris HL, Shelton RL: *Cleft palate speech.* B.C. Decker, Boston, 1990.

60. Trost JE: Articulatory additions to the classical descriptions of the speech of person with cleft palate. *Cleft Palate J* 1981; 18:193–203.

61. Peterson-Falzone SJ: Velopharyngeal inadequacy in the absence of overt cleft palate. *J Craniofac Genet Dev Biol* 1985; Suppl 1, 97–124.

62. Andreassen ML, Leeper HA, MacRae DL: Changes in vocal resonance and nasalization following adenoidectomy in normal children: Preliminary findings. *J Otolaryngol* 1991; 20:237–242.

63. Kummer AW, Myer CM, Smith ME, Shott SR: Changes in nasal resonance secondary to adenotonsillectomy. *Amer J Otolaryngol* 1993; 14:285–290.

64. Van Gelder L: Open nasal speech following adenoidectomy and tonsillectomy. *J Commun Dis* 1974; 7:263–267.

65. Kummer AW, Strife JL, Grau WH, et al: The effects of LeFort I osteotomy with maxillary movement on articulation, resonance, and velopharyngeal function. *Cleft Palate J* 1989; 26:193–199.

66. Witzel MA, Munro IR: Velopharyngeal insufficiency after maxillary advancement. *Cleft Palate J* 1977; 14: 176–180.

67. Shprintzen RJ, Sher AE, Croft CB: Hypernasal speech caused by tonsillar hypertrophy. *Int J Pediat Otorhinolaryngol* 1986; 14:45–56.

68. Kummer AW, Billmire DA, Myer CM: Hypertrophic tonsils: The effect on resonance and velopharyngeal closure. *Plastic Reconstr Surg* 1993; 91:608–611.

69. Finkelstein Y, Bar-Ziv J, Nachmani A, et al: Peritonsillar abscess as a cause of transient velopharyngeal insufficiency. *Cleft Palate-Craniofac J* 1993; 30: 421–428.

70. Yorkston KM, Beukelman DR, Bell KR: *Clinical management of dysarthric speakers.* College-Hill Press, Boston, 1988.

71. Shprintzen RJ, Goldberg RB, Lewin ML, et al: A new syndrome involving cleft palate, cardiac anomalies, typical facies, and learning disabilities: Velo-cardio-facial syndrome. *Cleft Palate J* 1978, 15:56–62.

72. Shprintzen RJ, Goldberg RB, Young D, et al: The velo-cardio-facial syndrome: A clinical and genetic analysis. *Pediatrics* 1981, 67(2):167–172.

73. Finkelstein Y, Zohar Y, Nachmani A, et al: The otolaryngologist and the patient with velocardiofacial syndrome. *Arch Otolaryngol Head Neck Surg* 1993; 119:563–569.

74. Netsell R: Evaluation of velopharyngeal function in dysarthria. *J Speech Hear Dis* 1969; 34:113–122.

75. Trost-Cardamone JE, Bernthal JE: Articulation assessment procedures and treatment decisions. In Moller KT, Starr CD, eds., *Cleft palate: Inter-disciplinary issues and treatment,* pp 307–336. PRO-ED. Austin, TX, 1993.

76. McWilliams BJ, Bluestone CD, Musgrave RH: Diagnostic implications of vocal cord nodules in children with cleft palate. *Laryngoscope* 1969; 79:2072–2080.

77. McWilliams BJ, Lavorato AS, Bluestone CD: Vocal cord abnormalities in children with velopharyngeal valving problems. *Laryngoscope* 1973; 83:1745–1753.

78. Bzoch KR: *Communicative disorders related to cleft lip and palate,* 3rd ed. College-Hill Press, Boston, 1989.

79. Dalston RM, Warren DW, Dalston ET: A preliminary investigation concerning the use of nasometry in identifying patients with hyponasality and/or nasal airway impairment. *J Speech Hear Res* 1991b; 34:11–18.

80. Dalston RM, Warren DW, Dalston ET: Use of nasometry as a diagnostic tool for identifying patients with velopharyngeal impairment. *Cleft Palate-Craniofac J* 1991a; 28:184–189.

81. Warren DW; DuBois A: A pressure-flow technique for measuring velopharyngeal orifice area during continuous speech. *Cleft Palate J* 1964; 1:52–71.

82. Warren DW: Perci: A method for rating palatal efficiency. *Cleft Palate J* 1979; 16:279–285.

83. Smith B, Weinberg B: Prediction of velopharyngeal orifice area: A re-examination of model experimentation. *Cleft Palate J* 1980; 17:277–282.

84. Warren DW: Aerodynamics of Speech. In Lass NJ, McReynolds LV, Northern JL, Yoder DE, eds., *Handbook of Speech–Language Pathology and Audiology,* pp 191–214. B.C. Decker, Philadelphia, 1988.

85. Mason RM, Simon C: Orofacial examination checklist. *Lang Speech Hear Services Schools* 1977; 8:161–163.

86. Skolnick ML: Videofluoroscopic examination of the velopharyngeal portal during phonation in lateral and base projections—A new technique for studying the mechanics of closure. *Cleft Palate J* 1970; 7: 803–816.

87. Skolnick ML, Cohn ER: *Videofluoroscopic studies of speech in patients with cleft palate.* Springer-Verlag, New York, 1989.

88. D'Antonio LL, Muntz HR, Marsh JL, et al: Practical application of flexible fiberoptic nasopharyngoscopy for evaluating velopharyngeal function. *Plastic Reconstr Surg* 1988; 82:611–618.

89. Watterson TL, McFarlane SC: Transnasal videoendoscopy of the velopharyngeal port mechanism. *Sem Speech Lang* 1990; 11:27–37.

90. Cooper HK, Harding RL, Krogman WM, et al., eds., *Cleft palate and cleft lip: A team approach to clinical management and rehabilitation of the patient.* W. B. Saunders, Philadelphia, 1979.

91. Grabb WC, Rosenstein SW, Bzoch K: *Cleft lip and palate.* Little, Brown, Boston, 1971.

92. Orticochea M: Construction of a dynamic muscle sphincter in cleft palates. *Plastic Reconstr Surg* 1968; 41:323–327.

93. Jackson IT, Silverton JS: The sphincter pharyngoplasty as a secondary procedure in cleft palates. *Plastic Reconstr Surg* 1977; 59:518–524.

94. Riski JE, Serafin D, Riefkohl R, et al: A rationale for modifying the site of insertion of the orticochea pharyngoplasty. *Plastic Reconstr Surg* 1984; 73:882–894.

95. Sturim HS, Jacob CT: Use of Teflon in hypernasal speech. *Rhode Island Med J* 1972; 55:317–320.

96. Smith JK, McCabe BF: Teflon injection in the nasopharynx to improve velopharyngeal closure. *Ann Otol Rhinol Laryngol* 1977; 86:559–563.

97. Posnick WR: Prosthetic management of palatopharyngeal incompetency for the pediatric patient. *J Dent Child* 1977; 44:117–121.

98. Schweiger J, Netsell R, Sommerfield R: Prosthetic management and speech improvements in

individuals with dysarthria of the palate. *J Am Dent Assoc* 1970; 80:1340.

99. Riski JE, Gordon D: Prosthetic management of neurogenic velopharyngeal incompetency. *N C Dent J* 1979; 62:24–26.

100. Dworkin JP, Johns DF: Management of velopharyngeal incompetence in dysarthria: A historical review. *Clin Otolaryngol* 1980; 5:61–74.

101. Johns DF, ed., *Clinical management of neurogenic communicative disorders.* Little, Brown, Boston, 1990.

102. Kummer AW, Lee L: Evaluation and treatment of resonance disorders. *Lang Speech Hear Serv Schools* 1996; 27:271–281.

103. Tomes L, Kuehn D, Peterson-Falzone S: *Behavioral therapy for speakers with velopharyngeal impairment.* Status and Progress Report, National Center for Voice and Speech 1996; 9 April:159–180.

104. Moller KT, Starr CD, eds.: *Cleft palate: Interdisciplinary issues and treatment.* Pro-Ed, Austin, TX, 1993.

105. Kuehn DP: New therapy for treating hypernasal speech using continuous positive airway pressure (CPAP). *Plastic Reconstr Surg* 1991; 88:959–966.

Appendix A
Professional Resources

Computerized Speech Lab (CSL),
Nasometer, Visi-Pitch-II, Aerophone
Kay Elemetrics Corp.
2 Bridgewater Lane
Lincoln Park, NJ 07035-1488
(800) 289–5296

Nagashima Phonatory Function Analyzer
Kelleher Medical Inc.
9710 Farrar Court Suite N
Richmond Virginia 23236–3666
(804) 323–4040

See Scape
Speech Bin
1965 25th Ave
Vero Beach, FL 32960

Speech Viewer and Speech Viewer-II
P.O. Box 1328
Boca Raton, FL 33429–1328
(800) 426–3333

Video Voice
Micro Video
210 Collingwood, Suite 100
P.O. Box 7357
Ann Arbor, MI 48107
(800) 537–2181

Passy-Muir Trach Valve
Passy-Muir, Inc.
4521 Campus Drive, Suite 273
Irvine, CA 92715
(714) 833–8255

American Cleft Palate-Craniofacial Association
1218 Grandview Ave.
Pittsburgh, PA 15211
(412) 481–1376

The Voice Foundation
1721 Pine Street
Philadelphia, PA 19103
(215) 735–7999

Appendix B
Pediatric Voice and Resonance Disorders
Basic Competencies

The clinician should have basic knowledge of the anatomy and physiology of the vocal tract, and understand how abnormalities in the tract can affect the acoustic product during voice production.

The clinician should be aware of the common causes of voice and resonance disorders in the pediatric population.

The clinician should be able to identify various characteristics of voice and resonance disorders through a perceptual assessment.

The clinician should be knowledgeable about the various instruments and techniques available for the visualization of structures and function, and also for the acoustic and aerodynamic measurement of the parameters related to voice and resonance.

The clinician should have basic knowledge of treatment protocols for patients with voice and resonance disorders, and know how to refer to a specialist if the problem is complex.

SECTION V

Psychiatry and the Speech–Language Pathologist

25

Overview of Psychiatric Disease for the Speech–Language Practitioner

CATHY FRANK

CHAPTER OUTLINE

Prevalence of Psychiatric Disorders

Classification of Mental Disorders

The Psychiatric Assessment

Common Psychiatric Disorders

When to Refer to a Psychiatric Specialist

Psychiatry plays an important role in the diagnosis and treatment of speech and language disorders for three reasons. First, mental illness may manifest itself as a speech or language problem (e.g., elective mutism). Second, disorders of speech may point to a psychiatric etiology of a disease (e.g., pressured speech as a manifestation of mania or neologism in schizophrenia). Last, patients plagued with speech and language problems may develop co-morbid psychiatric disorders such as depression and anxiety disorders. In an effort to help speech–language pathologists utilize psychiatric knowledge in their work, this chapter presents a summary of psychiatric assessment, psychopathology, and treatment. The review will include the prevalence of psychiatric disorders; the classification of mental disorders; a general approach to psychiatric symptoms as well as how to perform a mental status examination; common psychiatric illnesses and their treatment; and guidelines as to when to refer patients to a psychiatric specialist.

PREVALENCE OF PSYCHIATRIC DISORDERS

The most comprehensive epidemiologic study examining the prevalence of mental illness in the United States is the National Institute of Mental Health (NIMH) Epidemiology Catchment Area Program, in which researchers canvassed populations in five representative cities in the United States to ask questions about mental illness.[1] The study estimated that approximately 32% of individuals in the United States have a lifetime prevalence of a mental disorder. Anxiety disorders are the most common group of illnesses, with a lifetime prevalence of 14.6%. Mood disorders are second with the prevalence rate of 9% of the population with a lifetime prevalence of major depression, and 1% to 2% afflicted with bipolar disorder. Schizophrenia affects 1% of the population. The National Co-Morbidity Study[2] suggests even higher rates of psychiatric illness, with nearly 50% of respondents having at least one lifetime disorder. One-sixth of the population studied had a history of three or more co-morbid disorders. Surprisingly, the majority of mental health care is provided by primary care physicians, with only 15% treated by a mental health professional. Thus, it is imperative for nonpsychiatric practitioners to recognize mental illness and appropriately refer for treatment.

CLASSIFICATION OF MENTAL DISORDERS

The *Diagnostic and Statistical Manual of Mental Disorders-IV* (DSM-IV),[3] psychiatry's diagnostic standard published by the American Psychiatric Association, groups an array of psychiatric signs and symptoms into recognizable diseases and syndromes. DSM-IV utilizes a descriptive approach, without regard to etiology, that allows clinicians to speak a common language and gather data to study these illnesses. This classification utilizes the biopsychosocial model of disease, proposed by Engel,[4] that stresses a systematic, integrated approach to understanding disease and human behavior. This systems theory approach argues that to understand any disease one must understand its *biology*, which emphasizes structural, anatomical, and molecular aspects of the disease and its impact on the biological functioning of the patient; the *psychology*, which emphasizes behavioral, dynamic, and personality factors, and its impact on the patient—the patient's reaction to, and experience of, the disease; and its *sociology*, which emphasizes the family, culture, and environment and their impact on the patient's experience of the disease. DSM-IV integrates this model into its nomenclature by proposing a multiaxial evaluation of each patient along five dimensions or axes.

Axis I

The first Axis encompasses clinical syndromes, which include all the major mental disorders that affect mood (e.g., major depression, bipolar disorder, dysthymia), anxiety (e.g., panic disorder, post-traumatic stress disorder, generalized anxiety disorder), psychosis (e.g., schizophrenia, delusional disorder), dementia (e.g., Alzheimer's disease), and somatoform disorders (e.g., conversion reaction). Axis I also includes other conditions that may be a focus of clinical attention, such as marital problems, bereavement, or parent–child conflict. Table 25–1 provides a complete list of psychiatric disorders as categorized by the DSM-IV.

Axis II

The second Axis lists personality disorders, which consists of clusters of character traits that become maladaptive, causing impairment in social or occupational functioning and/or subjective distress. All human beings have character traits (e.g., the spouse who remains passive when angry, the shy partygoer), which usually do not cause problems in daily life. It is only when these traits create interpersonal or occupational havoc that they become pathological.

Axis III

The third Axis lists any physical illnesses that may be causative of the mental disorder (e.g., post-stroke depression); those related to a mental disorder (e.g., cirrhosis of the liver secondary to alcohol

Table 25–1. Classification of Adult DSM-IV Disorders

Delirium, dementia, amnestic, and other cognitive disorders

Mental disorders due to a general medical condition, not elsewhere classified

Substance-related disorders

Schizophrenia and other psychotic disorders

Mood disorders

Anxiety disorders

Somatoform disorders

Factitious disorders

Dissociative disorders

Sexual and gender identity disorders

Eating disorders

Sleep disorders

Impulse control disorders

Adjustment disorders

Personality disorders

Source: From DSM-IV, *Diagnostic and Statistical Manual of Mental Disorders,* 4th ed. American Psychiatric Association, Washington, DC, 1994.

dependence); or those that are potentially relevant to the understanding of the mental disorder.

Axis IV

The fourth Axis indicates the psychosocial stressors that may be contributing to the development or perpetuation of the mental disorder. Stressors may include problems in the family, problems related to the social environment, educational problems, occupational problems, financial problems, and the like.

Axis V

The fifth Axis provides a 100-point scale, called the global assessment of functioning (GAF), which enables the clinician to rate the patient's level of functioning. The scale takes into account markers of social, psychological, and occupational functioning. The scale ranges from a score of 100 for superior mental functioning to 1, indicating inability to function. Clinicians typically rate the current functioning, and the highest level of functioning within the last year. The GAF is presented in Table 25–2.

Purpose of the Axes

The Axes attempt to give the clinician a global description of the patient's biopsychosocial functioning. For example, a 55-year-old Caucasian widow, who lost her husband two weeks ago and now presents with mutism would be described, using the DSM-IV Axis evaluation as:

Axis I	Bereavement, Conversion Disorder
Axis II	Deferred
Axis III	General good health
Axis IV	Death of spouse two weeks ago
Axis V	Current 35; highest in last year 95

DSM-IV describes psychiatric disorders that occur in childhood, adolescence, adulthood, and old age. These disorders may be due to a known organic etiology (e.g., mood disorder caused by hypothyroidism), due to primary psychiatric pathology (e.g., mood disorders have a genetic loading and tend to run in families), or of unknown causation (e.g., generalized anxiety disorder). Whenever a psychiatric diagnosis is considered, it is imperative that the clinician evaluate the causative factors or co-morbid illnesses that may aggravate the psychiatric disorder. It is particularly important to inquire about substance use and abuse, because the use of these agents may mimic depression, mania, psychosis, and cognitive complaints.

THE PSYCHIATRIC ASSESSMENT

As in most areas of medicine, the key to psychiatric diagnosis is the history. Usually the diagnosis is clinical, with laboratory, radiographic, and psychological tests used to exclude other diagnoses. As part of the assessment, a variety of screening questions may be asked. Tables 25–3 and 25–4[5] highlight key areas that must be emphasized in the psychiatric history. To refine the psychiatric diagnosis, all patients should be asked the following:

History of presenting illness: Includes onset of symptoms, course of illness, duration, precipitating and palliating factors.

Past psychiatric history: Includes inpatient and outpatient treatment, with presenting symptoms for each, diagnoses, and which therapies were successful or unsuccessful.

Past medical history: Includes a thorough review of systems; past illnesses and surgeries; allergies; current medications; current alcohol intake, and history of abuse and dependence (any history of driving under the influence, withdrawal, seizures, blackouts); current illicit drug use, and history of abuse and dependence. The clinician should rule out any organic cause for the disorder, as many illnesses may mimic psychiatric disorders.

Psychosocial history: Includes a family history of psychiatric illness (many disorders are familial including major depression, bipolar disorder, panic disorder, obsessive-compulsive disorder, schizophrenia, alcoholism, attention deficit hyperactivity disorder); the current level of social support (e.g., lives alone, married, children); interpersonal relationships; education level; and employment status. Historic data such as prenatal/birth, childhood, adolescence history are important in understanding the patient's experiences. The adult history should include interpersonal strengths and weaknesses.

Mental status examination: This is the second key tool in the psychiatric assessment. The mental status examination is the psychiatric review of systems and ensures that the

Table 25–2. Global Assessment of Functioning (GAF) Scale

Consider psychological, social, and occupational functioning on a hypothetical continuum of mental health–illness. Do not include impairment in functioning due to physical (or environmental) limitations.

Code   *Note:* Use intermediate codes when appropriate (e.g., 45, 68, 72).

100   Superior functioning in a wide range of activities, life's problems never seem to get
 | out of hand, is sought out by others because of his or her many positive qualities.
91   No symptoms.

90   Absent or minimal symptoms (e.g., mild anxiety before an exam), good functioning
 | in all areas, interested and involved in a wide range of activities, socially effective,
 | generally satisfied with life, no more than everyday problems or concerns (e.g., an
81   occasional argument with family members).

80   If symptoms are present, they are transient and expectable reactions to psycho-
 | social stressors (e.g., difficulty concentrating after family argument); no more than
 | slight impairment in social, occupational, or school functioning (e.g., temporarily
71   falling behind in schoolwork).

70   Some mild symptoms (e.g., depressed mood and mild insomnia) OR some diffi-
 | culty in social, occupational, or school functioning (e.g., occasional truancy, or
 | theft within the household), but generally functioning pretty well, has some mean-
61   ingful interpersonal relationships.

60   Moderate symptoms (e.g., flat affect and circumstantial speech, occasional panic
 | attacks) OR moderate difficulty in social, occupational, or school functioning (e.g.,
51   few friends, conflicts with peers or co-workers).

50   Serious symptoms (e.g., suicidal ideation, severe obsessional rituals, frequent
 | shoplifting) OR any serious impairment in social, occupational, or school function-
41   ing (e.g., no friends, unable to keep a job).

40   Some impairment in reality testing or communication (e.g., speech is at times
 | illogical, obscure, or irrelevant) OR major impairment in several areas, such as
 | work or school, family relations, judgment, thinking, or mood (e.g., depressed man
 | avoids friends, neglects family, and is unable to work; child frequently beats up
31   younger children, is defiant at home, and is failing in school).

30   Behavior is considerably influenced by delusions or hallucinations OR serious im-
 | pairment in communication or judgment (e.g., sometimes incoherent, acts grossly
 | inappropriately, suicidal preoccupation) OR inability to function in almost all
21   areas (e.g., stays in bed all day; no job, home, or friends).

20   Some danger of hurting self or others (e.g., suicide attempts without clear expecta-
 | tion of death; frequently violent; manic excitement) OR occasionally fails to main-
 | tain minimal personal hygiene (e.g., smears feces) OR gross impairment in
11   communication (e.g., largely incoherent or mute).

10   Persistent danger of severely hurting self or others (e.g., recurrent violence) OR
 | persistent inability to maintain minimal personal hygiene OR serious suicidal act
1   with clear expectation of death.

0   Inadequate information.

Source: From DSM-1V, Diagnostic and Statistical Manual of Mental Disorders, 4th ed. American Psychiatric Association, Washington, DC, 1994.

clinician has asked questions that examine the major areas of pathology discussed earlier: symptoms of a mood disturbance, anxiety, psychosis, and cognitive impairment. The mental status examination summarizes the clinician's observation of the patient at the time of the interview. The mental status examination always reviews the following areas (see Table 25–5):

1. *Appearance:* This should convey the overall physical impression the clinician has of the patient, including posture, clothing, and grooming. Is the appearance consistent with the patient's education, occupation, and social strata? Poor eye contact, psychomotor retardation, and tearfulness, for example, are more likely to be seen in patients with depression.

Table 25–3. The Psychiatric History

Identifying information

Chief complaint

History of present illness

    Extended information about chief complaint

    Onset

    Duration/course

    Precipitants

    Exaggerating and alleviating factors

Psychiatric history

Medical history (drugs, alcohol)

Family history of psychiatric disorders and
    treatment

Personal history

    Prenatal/birth history

    Childhood

    Adolescence

    Adulthood

        Educational

        Occupational

        Interpersonal/social

        Sexual

Mental status examination

Table 25–4. Psychiatric Screening Questions for Patients

Depression
"Have you been feeling sad or depressed? Is this accompanied by trouble with sleep or appetite, low energy, or decreased interest in doing things? Do you have feelings of guilt or thoughts of harming yourself?"

Mania
"Do you feel on top of the world? Is this out of proportion to your usual self such that you talk more, don't need as much sleep, your thoughts race, or your enthusiasm gets you into trouble?"

Psychosis
"Have you heard or seen things that others didn't? Do you feel that you have special powers? Have you felt that others were watching or following you? Have you received peculiar or special messages or felt that others knew or controlled your thoughts?"

Alcoholism
"Have others thought you had a drinking problem? Has drinking alcohol caused problems with friends or relatives, caused you to miss work or lose a job, resulted in arrest, or caused health problems? Do you use recreational drugs?"

Anxiety disorder
"Have you had trouble with nervousness, anxiety, or feeling like you are going to panic?"

Anorexia nervosa
"Do you take special measures to keep your weight at its current level?"

Source: Stoudemire A: *Clinical psychiatry for medical students,* 2nd ed. J. B. Lippincott, Philadelphia, 1994. Reprinted with permission.

2. *Attitude:* Attitude can be described as cooperative, friendly, seductive, defensive, apathetic, hostile, guarded and so on. This presentation aids in the differential diagnosis, as for example, a paranoid patient may be guarded or suspicious.

3. *Motor activity:* Included in this category are mannerisms, gestures, stereotyped behavior, hyperactivity, agitation, rigidity, gait, restlessness, and retardation. Tardive dyskinesia or other extrapyramidal movements should be noted.

4. *Speech:* Speech can be described in terms of rate of production, quality, and quantity. Impairments (e.g., stuttering), spontaneity, and rhythm (e.g., dysprosody) are included. Speech may be described as slow, pressured, slurred, dysarthric, and so on. For example, a depressed patient may speak slowly and quietly, whereas an anxious patient may have rapid, nonpressured speech that is expressive.

5. *Mood/Affect:* Mood is defined as the patient's pervasive and sustained emotional state. Common descriptors include depressed, irritable, anxious, angry, expansive, euphoric, and frightened. Affect is defined as the patient's current emotional responsiveness and is what the clinician infers and observes during the interview. Affect may be described as congruent or incongruent to mood, constricted, blunt, or flat. The patient's ability to initiate, sustain, or end an emotional response should be noted, as well as the appropriateness of the response. A patient with schizophrenia, for example, may have inappropriate affect, such as laughing when describing a tragic event.

6. *Thought* is divided into two parts: process and content. Process is defined

Table 25–5. Mental Status Examination

Appearance, attitude, psychomotor activity, and behavior
Speech
Mood and affect
Thought and language
 Form
 Content
Suicidal and homicidal ideation
Perceptions
 Hallucinations/illusions
 Depersonalization
 Derealization
Cognitive function
 Level of consciousness
 Orientation
 Concentration
 Memory
 Intelligence
Insight and judgment

as the way a patient puts together ideas and associations, and is the form of thinking. Process may be logical and coherent or illogical. Thoughts may be vague or empty, with a poverty of ideas. Thought process can be described as a flight of ideas, loose associations, blocking, circumstantial, tangential, word salad, or neologisms. Poverty of thought, for example, is commonly seen in schizophrenia, although it can also be observed in profoundly depressed patients. Content of thought refers to the focus of the patient's conversation, his or her ideas, preoccupations, and any disturbances in content. Disturbances include obsessions, compulsions, phobias, and ideas of reference. Manic patients may have delusions of grandeur, believing they are God, with the delusions congruent to the euphoric mood. Schizophrenic patients, on the other hand, often have mood incongruent delusions, believing for example, that others can read or control their thoughts.

7. *Suicidal ideation:* All patients, and in particular those with depression, panic disorder, psychosis, chronic pain, or substance abuse, should explicitly be asked about current suicidal thoughts. If suicidal thoughts are present, the clini-

cian must ask if there is a plan, availability of weapons, and intent to act on the plan. A history of a previous attempt, and family history of suicide, are added risk factors. There is a myth that asking about suicide may "put the thought in the person's head." On the contrary, asking will help assess risk and potentially save a life.

8. *Homicidal ideation:* Psychotic patients, substance abusers, impulsive, and sociopathic patients, in particular, should be asked about current thoughts of violence to others. If homicidal thoughts are present, the clinician must ask regarding current plan, availability of weapons, and intent. A history of violence is a significant risk factor. All health professionals are required, by virtue of legal precedent (*Tarasoff v. Regents of University of California*), to protect an intended victim if a risk exists. A failure to protect places the clinician legally at risk. A mental health professional and/or legal consultant should be consulted if a potential risk of violence exists.

9. *Perceptual disturbances:* Hallucinations can involve a host of sensory apparatus, including visual, auditory, olfactory, gustatory, and tactile hallucinations. It is imperative to ask if the auditory hallucinations are command in nature, because this may put the patient at risk for acting out suicide or homicide intent.

10. *Orientation:* Orientation to time (i.e., today's date, day of the week, year, season), place (i.e., what place is this, what city, what state), and person (i.e., name, age) should be asked. Impairment to person is exceedingly rare. Impairment usually occurs in the following order: time, place, person, and reverses in that order.

11. *Attention/concentration:* Patients with impaired attention may require repetition of questions and are easily distracted. Formal tests of concentration may include digit span (ask the patient to repeat a sequence of numbers: average response is six digits forward and five backward), or ask the patient to spell the word "WORLD" backward, making sure he or she can spell it forward.

12. *Memory:* The clinician should be able to test anterograde memory (ability to

form new memories) and retrograde memory (ability to retrieve and recite information previously stored). Immediate memory can be tested by asking the patient to repeat three words (also tests attention); recent or short-term memory by asking the patient to repeat the words in five minutes; and remote memory by asking the patient to recite verifiable historical data. If a patient cannot attend or concentrate on the task, then the test of memory may not be reliable. Memory can be impaired in a wide range of disorders including dementia, depression (so-called pseudodementia), substances-related disorders, and chronic schizophrenia. Cognitive impairment requires further evaluation by a psychiatrist or psychologist.

13. *Judgment:* This can often be inferred from an understanding of how the patient leads his/her life, and handles the current medical complaints. Other forms of assessing judgment include asking what a person would do if he or she found a stamped, addressed, sealed envelope on the sidewalk, or what the person would do if he or she smelled smoke in a movie theater. An assessment of judgment helps the clinician gauge the patient's safety and ability to handle day-to-day activities, as well as how the person may accept treatment for the illness.

14. *Insight:* This can usually be inferred by the patient's presentation and interest in receiving help. Insight is the patient's degree of awareness and understanding that he or she is ill.

COMMON PSYCHIATRIC DISORDERS

It would be impossible to chronicle and detail all the DSM-IV disorders in this limited space. This overview will describe the more common disorders afflicting the general population, and particularly those patients with speech and language disorders.

Mood Disorders

Major depression is the most common mood disorder, in a class that includes bipolar disorder, dysthymia, cyclothymia, and mood disorder due to a general medical condition or substance use. Table 25–6 presents a classification of mood disorders. It

Table 25–6. Classification of Mood Disorders

Mood disorders
  Bipolar disorders
    Bipolar disorder
    Cyclothymia
  Depressive disorders
    Major depression
    Dysthymia (depressive neurosis)
Mental disorders due to . . .
  General medical condition
  Substance induced
Adjustment disorders
  Adjustment disorder with depressed mood
Conditions not attributable to a mental disorder
  Uncomplicated bereavement

has been estimated that 13 to 20% of the population has some symptoms of depression at any given time[6]; in medical settings, the rate may be as high as 15%. Depression is a symptom, not a disorder, and, as stated above, has a wide differential diagnosis. When depression is elicited, it is important to determine if it is a normal response to a stressor (e.g., bereavement), or if it is due to a primary psychiatric illness (e.g., major depression) or an identifiable organic disorder (e.g., hypothyroidism).

Major Depression

Major depression, the most common mood disorder, affects women twice as commonly as men. There are a number of risk factors for major depression including history of early loss, poor social support, gender, psychosocial stressors, and a family history of depression. The last factor is an important genetic indicator because the risk of major depression is two to five times greater in relatives of depressed patients than in relatives of controls. In addition to this biological abnormality, there are other markers including REM and non-REM sleep abnormalities, neuroendocrine abnormalities, and abnormalities at the neurotransmitter level. Major depression is clearly a biological disorder, with psychosocial precipitants and consequences. It is also a chronic disorder in that more than half of those with one episode will have a second. DSM-IV criteria for major depression, as listed in Table 25–7, mandate that the individual has at least a two-week period of depressed mood or loss of interest or pleasure in activities accompanied by a number of psychological and somatic symptoms. A helpful mnemonic, developed for remembering the key symptoms of major depression, developed

Table 25–7. Criteria for Major Depressive Episode

Five (or more) of the following symptoms have been present during the same 2-week period and represent a change from previous functioning; at least one of the symptoms is either (1) depressed mood or (2) loss of interest or pleasure.

1. Depressed mood most of the day, nearly every day, as indicated by either subjective report (e.g., feels sad or empty) or observation made by others (e.g., appears tearful). *Note:* In children and adolescents, can be an irritable mood.

2. Markedly diminished interest or pleasure in all, or almost all, activities most of the day, nearly every day (as indicated by either subjective account or observation made by others).

3. Significant weight loss when not dieting or weight gain (e.g., a change of more than 5% of body weight in a month), or decrease or increase in appetite nearly every day. *Note:* In children, consider failure to make expected weight gains.

4. Insomnia or hypersomnia nearly every day.

5. Psychomotor agitation or retardation nearly every day (observable by others, not merely subjective feelings of restlessness or being slowed down).

6. Fatigue or loss of energy nearly every day.

7. Feelings of worthlessness or excessive or inappropriate guilt (which may be delusional) nearly every day (not merely self-reproach or guilt about being sick).

8. Diminished ability to think or concentrate, or indecisiveness, nearly every day (either by subjective account or as observed by others).

9. Recurrent thoughts of death (not just fear of dying), recurrent suicidal ideation without a specific plan, or a suicide attempt or a specific plan for committing suicide.

The symptoms caused clinically significant distress or impairment in social, occupational, or other areas of functioning.

The symptoms are not due to the direct physiological effects of a substance (e.g., a drug of abuse, a medication) or a general medical condition (e.g., hypothyroidism).

The symptoms are not better accounted for by bereavement, i.e., after the loss of a loved one; the symptoms persist for longer than 2 months or are characterized by marked functional impairment, morbid preoccupation with worthlessness, suicidal ideation, psychotic symptoms, or psychomotor retardation.

Source: From DSM-IV, *Diagnostic and Statistical Manual of Mental Disorders*, 4th ed. American Psychiatric Association, Washington, DC, 1994.

by Dr. Carey Gross at Massachusetts General Hospital is SIG: E CAPS, as if you were writing a prescription for E capsules. The letters stand for:

S Sleep disturbance, usually insomnia with early morning awakening, but hypersomnia may also exist.

I Interest in activity is diminished, anhedonia.

G Guilt for real or imagined transgressions.

E Energy is diminished; the patient complains of fatigue.

C Concentration is impaired (e.g., patient cannot follow a story line on TV).

A Appetite is usually diminished, with anorexia. Hyperphagia may also exist.

P Psychomotor activity is usually retarded, but may be agitated.

S Suicidal ideation, plan, and/or intent or thought of death are prominent. To ask regarding suicidal ideation is therapeutic and helps assess the patient's safety. Detail specifically the plan and intent, and if weapons are available.

In a very "cookbook" fashion, if five of eight of these symptoms are present, major depression is likely. Major depression's symptoms must cause marked distress or social or occupational impairment. The symptoms may not be due to an identifiable medical disorder. These symptoms may be accompanied by psychotic symptomatology such as delusions or hallucinations. Somatic symptoms and preoccupation may be a prominent focus, especially in the elderly.

Major depression, when recognized, is a very treatable disorder. It is estimated that 65 to 70% of depressed patients respond to treatment. Treatment for moderate to severe depression is usually psychopharmacology and psychotherapy, although mild depression may respond solely to the latter. There are two types of psychotherapy that are well researched and effective in the treatment of major depression: cognitive therapy and interpersonal therapy. Cognitive therapy is based on the premise that people who are depressed focus on the negative, rather than the positive. Beck, Rush, Shaw, et al.[7] described a triad of three conditions as the basis for depression: negative view of self, negative interpretation of experiences, and negative expectations of the future. This brief psychotherapy, which can be in the form of individual or group therapy, focuses on these negative misinterpretations and helps the patient change these thought distortions. The basis for interpersonal psychotherapy is that depression occurs in the context of a relationship, and understanding that context, and the impact of depression on the relationship, will alter the depression.

The mainstay of the treatment of major depression, however, is psychopharmacology. All the antidepressants currently on the market are equally effective, although one patient may differentially respond to one rather than another. The agents differ in their side effect profile, pharmacokinetics, and pharmacodynamics. Newer agents, such as the selective serotonin reuptake inhibitors (e.g., Prozac, Zoloft) are better tolerated than the older agents, which are more sedating. Unfortunately, the antidepressants may take up to three to four weeks to work, so patients must be encouraged to continue a medication trial until its completion. The first episode of depression is usually treated for six to nine months after remission. Those patients with three or more episodes of depression may need to be on long-term antidepressants.

Dysthymia

Dysthymia, formally depressive neurosis, is a *chronic* form of depression, in which patients are depressed, more days than not, for at least two years. Instead of meeting criteria for 5 out of 8 "SIG E CAPS," as discussed earlier, the patient must meet criteria for 2 out of 8. These patients are treated similarly to those with major depression.

Bipolar disorders

Bipolar disorder, popularly known as manic depression, has mania as its cardinal feature, although bipolar patients may have prominent episodes of depression too. Mania, as described in

Table 25–8, is a distinct period in which the patient's mood is either elevated, expansive, or irritable with several associated symptoms including pressured speech, racing thoughts, grandiosity or inflated self-esteem, hyperactivity, and involvement in activities that may be potentially dangerous, even though seemingly pleasurable (e.g., spending sprees). Psychotic symptoms, such as delusions, hallucinations, thought broadcasting (the belief that others can read your thoughts) or thought insertion (the belief that others can put thoughts into your head) may accompany the mood disturbance. The mood disturbance in mania is severe enough to cause marked impairment in social or occupational functioning or require hospitalization. In contract, the term hypomania is used when the symptoms do not cause *marked* impairment, nor require hospitalization, or have accompanying psychotic symptoms. Patients may have episodes of mania, hypomania, or depression, or a mixture of all three. The distinction between major depression and bipolar disorder is an important one, as the treatment, risks, and prognosis differ. The mainstay of treatment for bipolar disorder is psychopharmacology, with the treatment strategy depending on whether the presentation is manic, depressed, or mixed.

Substance Abuse/Dependence

Surveys suggest that approximately 90% of the U.S. population uses at least some alcohol, and that 72.4 million Americans, age 12 or older, or 37% have used illicit drugs at least once in their life (1988 National Household Survey of Drug Abuse). Abuse is defined as a maladaptive pattern of use that causes significant impairment in social, occupational, or health functioning. Dependence incorporates abuse, but adds the needed factors of either tolerance (the need for increased amounts of the substance to achieve the desired effect); withdrawal; unsuccessful attempts to cut down or control the use; great deal of time spent in activities necessary to get the substance, take the substance, or recover from its effect; or important social or occupational activities are given up or reduced because of the substance. There are many psychoactive agents, as listed in Table 25–9, that may cause a variety of psychiatric disorders such as abuse, dependence, intoxication, withdrawal, delirium, a mood disturbance, psychosis, or dementia.

Alcoholism

Alcoholism is the most common form of substance dependence, affecting 5 to 7% of U.S. citizens in a

Table 25–8. Criteria for Manic Episode

A distinct period of abnormally and persistently elevated, expansive, or irritable mood, lasting at least 1 week (or any duration if hospitalization is necessary).

During the period of mood disturbance, three (or more) of the following symptoms have persisted (four if the mood is only irritable) and have been present to a significant degree:

1. Inflated self-esteem or grandiosity
2. Decreased need for sleep (e.g., feels rested after only 3 hours of sleep)
3. More talkative than usual or pressure to keep talking
4. Flight of ideas or subjective experience that thoughts are racing
5. Distractibility (i.e., attention too easily drawn to unimportant or irrelevant external stimuli)
6. Increase in goal-directed activity (either socially, at work or school, or sexually) or psychomotor agitation
7. Excessive involvement in pleasurable activities that have a high potential for painful consequences (e.g., engaging in unrestrained buying sprees, sexual indiscretions, or foolish business investments)

The mood disturbance is sufficiently severe to cause marked impairment in occupational functioning or in usual social activities or relationships with others, or to necessitate hospitalization to prevent harm to self or others, or there are psychotic features.

The symptoms are not due to the direct physiological effects of a substance (e.g., a drug of abuse, a medication, or other treatment) or a general medical condition (e.g., hyperthyroidism).

Source: From DSM-IV, *Diagnostic and Statistical Manual of Mental Disorders,* 4th ed. American Psychiatric Association, 1994.

Table 25–9. Classes of Psychoactive Substances in DSM-IV

Alcohol

Amphetamine

Caffeine

Cannabis

Cocaine

Hallucinogen

Inhalants

Nicotine

Opioid

Phencyclidine

Sedative, hypnotic, or anxiolytic

Others (e.g., anabolic steroids)

Source: From DSM-IV, *Diagnostic and Statistical Manual of Mental Disorders,* 4th ed. American Psychiatric Association, Washington, DC, 1994.

given year. It affects men three times more frequently than women. Alcoholism is a familial disorder, with clear genetic loading. Alcoholism has far-reaching biopsychosocial implications. Biologi-cal complications range from cirrhosis of the liver, to alcoholic dementia, to cerebellar dysfunction and subdural hematoma, to name a few. Psychological impact is significant with a high co-morbidity of other disorders including depression, anxiety disorders, schizophrenia, and other substance abuse and dependence disorders. The social implications include a higher rate of homicide, accidents, fetal alcohol syndrome, and divorce.

The key to diagnosis of alcoholism, or any other substance-related disorder, is to consider it in the differential diagnosis. A well-accepted screening tool is the CAGE questionnaire,[8] which takes only minutes to administer. This highly sensitive test uses the word CAGE as a mnemonic:

Have you ever felt the need to Cut down on drinking?

Have you ever felt Annoyed by criticisms of drinking?

Have you ever had Guilty feelings about drinking?

Have you ever taken a morning Eye opener?

A "yes" to one question is suggestive of alcohol abuse, and to two or more indicates alcoholism. In addition, the physical examination of alcoholics may show signs of liver disease, telangiectasis of the face, parotid gland enlargement, facial edema, and peripheral neuropathy. Intoxicated patients may appear drowsy, with incoordination, slurred speech, and irritability. Laboratory tests may support the diagnosis with macrocytic anemia and increased liver isoenzymes.

The major focus in the treatment of this chronic disorder is abstinence and relapse prevention, although there are some groups that support the idea of controlled drinking. The mainstay of treatment remains the self-help groups Alcoholics Anonymous (AA) and Recovery. Psychotherapy is usually supportive, exploring the toll on families, or behavioral, helping with stress reduction, self-control strategies, and relaxation. Treatment of any co-morbid disorders such as depression and anxiety is essential. There are also pharmacologic agents that have some success in either preventing alcohol consumption or limiting its use. Disulfiram (Antabuse) is an adjunctive treatment that prophylaxes against alcohol consumption by making the individual seriously ill (nausea, vomiting, shortness of breath, flushing) if he or she consumes alcohol. Naltrexone (Trexan), which is also used to treat opioid dependence, appears in early studies to allow more days of abstinence, lower rates of relapse, and fewer drinks per day.

Other Abused Substances

In addition to alcohol, there are a host of other psychoactive agents including amphetamines, cannabis, cocaine, hallucinogens, inhalants, opiates, phencychdine, sedatives, hypnotics, and steroids, which are implicated in abuse and dependence. Patients may not readily admit to substance abuse, but certain patterns of behavior such as impulsivity, unexplained job changes, violence, family instability, "lost weekends," and the like may suggest substance abuse. The focus in the treatment of all substance abuse is the medical, behavioral, and social sequela of the use.

Anxiety Disorders

Anxiety disorders are the most prevalent group of disorders afflicting Americans. This diagnostic category encompasses a number of disorders: panic disorder, agoraphobia, social phobia, generalized anxiety disorder, specific phobias, obsessive-compulsive disorder, acute stress disorder, and post-traumatic stress disorder, all of which have anxiety as a cardinal feature. As with depression, it is important to remember that anxiety is not a syndrome, but a symptom. It may be a very normative response to a situation (e.g., walking down a dark street you hear footsteps behind you), a key symptom in a primary anxiety disorder (e.g., panic attack in panic disorder), or represent an underlying organic illness (e.g., pheochromocytoma, mitral valve prolapse).

Panic Disorder

Panic disorder, which affects women twice as commonly as men, has as its hallmark spontaneous, episodic periods of acute anxiety that last from minutes to hours (see Table 25–10). The anxiety is accompanied by a host of somatic symptoms, which may include shortness of breath, sweating, trembling, nausea, chest pain, dizziness, paresthesia, or heart palpitations. The onset of this disorder is usually in the middle to late twenties and becomes disabling, as patients restrict their activity, becoming fearful of situations in which they had attacks. Patients develop secondary phobia avoidance and anticipatory anxiety. As noted by the diagnostic criteria in Table 25–11, panic attacks may be isolated events that never evolve into panic disorder, or they may be part of other disorders, such as post-traumatic stress disorder. Panic disorder is treatable with a combination of antidepressants and/or benzodiazepines and cognitive/behavioral psychotherapy.

Table 25–10. Criteria for Panic Attack

A discrete period of intense fear or discomfort, in which four (or more) of the following symptoms developed abruptly and reached a peak within 10 minutes:

1. Palpitations, pounding heart, or accelerated heart rate
2. Sweating
3. Trembling or shaking
4. Sensations of shortness of breath or smothering
5. Feeling of choking
6. Chest pain or discomfort
7. Nausea or abdominal distress
8. Feeling dizzy, unsteady, lightheaded, or faint
9. Derealization (feelings of unreality) or depersonalization (being detached from oneself)
10. Fear of losing control or going crazy
11. Fear of dying
12. Paresthesia (numbness or tingling sensations)
13. Chills or hot flushes

Source: From DSM IV, *Diagnostic and Statistical Manual of Mental Disorders,* 4th ed. American Psychiatric Association, Washington, DC, 1994.

Table 25–11. Diagnostic Criteria for Panic Disorder

Both 1 and 2:

1. Recurrent unexpected panic attacks

2. At least one of the attacks has been followed by 1 month (or more) of one (or more) of the following:

   (a) Persistent concern about having additional attacks

   (b) Worry about the implications of the attack or its consequences (e.g., losing control, having a heart attack, "going crazy")

   (c) A significant change in behavior related to the attacks

The panic attacks are not due to the direct physiological effects of a substance (e.g., a drug of abuse, a medication) or a general medical condition (e.g., hyperthyroidism).

The panic attacks are not better accounted for by another mental disorder, such as a social phobia (e.g., occurring on exposure to feared social situations), specific phobia (e.g., on exposure to a specific phobic situation), obsessive-compulsive disorder (e.g., on exposure to dirt in someone with an obsession about contamination), post-traumatic stress disorder (e.g., in response to stimuli associated with a severe stressor), or separation anxiety disorder (e.g., in response to being away from home or close relatives).

Source: From DSM-IV, *Diagnostic and Statistical Manual of Mental Disorders,* 4th ed. American Psychiatric Association, Washington, DC, 1994.

Generalized Anxiety Disorder

This disorder is characterized by excessive, uncontrollable, pervasive worry about multiple life circumstances. In addition to the anxiety and worry, the patient is plagued by physical correlates such as muscle tension, restlessness, fatiguability, impaired concentration, insomnia, and irritability. These patients find it impossible to put aside their fears, and may enjoy little of their successes. There is less research on treatment strategies in this disorder that affects men and women equally. Supportive or cognitive/behavioral psychotherapy are the mainstay of treatment. Trials of antidepressants or benzodiazepines may also be warranted.

Schizophrenia

Schizophrenia is an illness that affects approximately 1% of the population, often affecting teenagers and young adults in their key developmental period. Schizophrenia is an organic brain disorder, with a sweeping effect on thinking, affect, and behavior. The key features of this illness, as described in Table 25–12, include the so-called positive symptoms (i.e., hallucinations, delusions, disorganized or catatonic behavior, disorganized speech) and the negative symptoms (i.e., alogia, anhedonia, flat affect, apathy, and lack of motivation). This is a heterogeneous group of disorders, which are secondarily identified by their key feature: paranoid type, disorganized type, catatonic type, undifferentiated type, and residual type.

A key in the diagnosis is the presence of a formal thought disorder, which is an abnormality in the form of thought. Examples of a formal thought disorder include loose associations (the sequential connection between thoughts is difficult to follow because the patients talks in a totally unrelated sequence of subjects), tangentiality (thoughts wander in loosely connected fashion, unable to return to the original point), and incoherence (impossible to follow the line of thought). Speech may be incomprehensible due to clanging, word salad, and neologisms.

Schizophrenia is a chronic disorder, and one that has a poorer treatment response, particularly in regards to the negative symptoms. Treatment involves pharmacotherapy and psychosocial therapy. Antipsychotic medications are effective against the positive symptoms such as hallucinations and delusions, but usually less effective against the negative symptoms. Psychosocial treatment changes over the course of the illness and may involve hospitalization, day hospital, family therapy, behavioral therapy, supportive therapy, and crisis intervention.

Dementia

Dementia is an etiologically heterogeneous group of disorders, which have in common the development of memory impairment in addition to the deterioration of at least one other cognitive domain (e.g., language, executive functioning). The deficits must cause impairment in social or occupational functioning. The prevalence of severe dementia is

Table 25–12. Diagnostic Criteria for Schizophrenia

Characteristic symptoms: Two (or more) of the following, each present for a
significant portion of time during a 1-month period (or less if successfully treated):
1. Delusions
2. Hallucinations
3. Disorganized speech (e.g., frequent derailment of incoherence)
4. Grossly disorganized or catatonic behavior
5. Negative symptoms (i.e., affective flattening, alogia, or avolition)

Note: Only one symptom is required if delusions are bizarre or hallucinations consist
of a voice keeping up a running commentary on the person's behavior or thoughts, or
two or more voices conversing with each other.

Social/occupational dysfunction: For a significant portion of the time since the onset
of the disturbance, one or more major areas of functioning such as work,
interpersonal relations, or self-care are markedly below the level achieved prior to
the onset (or when the onset is in childhood or adolescence, failure to achieve
expected level of interpersonal, academic, or occupational achievement).

Duration: Continuous signs of the disturbance persist for at least 6 months.

Source: From DSM-IV, *Diagnostic and Statistical Manual of Mental Disorders,* 4th ed. American
Psychiatric Association, Washington, DC, 1994.

estimated at 1.3 million cases in the United States, with 50 to 60% of these the Alzheimer's type. The majority of nursing home residents suffer from dementia. Dementia usually develops insidiously and progresses gradually. The initial evaluation must rule out reversible causes (e.g., hypothyroidism).

The most common form of dementia is Alzheimer's disease, which presents a major public health problem as our population ages (see Table 25–13). The dementia is defined by preeminent memory deficits, which begin as short-term memory deficits and progress to more global deficits, including aphasia, apraxia, and agnosia. Alzheimer's disease is a terminal illness, progressing to death on an average of seven years after its onset. Multiinfarct dementia is the second leading cause of dementia. The cognitive deficits are similar to those of Alzheimer's disease, but differ in that they are accompanied by focal neurologic signs and symptoms (e.g., extensor plantor response, gait disturbance) and laboratory evidence of cerebral vascular disease that is judged etiologic of the disorder. The disease often progresses in a stepwise fashion with advancing vascular disease. There are other types of dementia including AIDS dementia complex, Pick's disease, Parkinson's dementia, and that associated with multiple sclerosis, to name a few.

Demented patients often suffer from co-morbid psychiatric illness, including depression, paranoia, and delirium, which are treatable. Treatment of this group of disorders focuses on providing supportive medical care to the patient, emotional support to the patient and family, and treatment of co-morbid conditions and troublesome behaviors

(e.g., wandering). Most communities have a chapter of the Alzheimer's Disease and Related Disorders Association (ADRDA), an organization that offers education and support to families.

In addition to the aggressive psychopharmacology of co-morbid disease (e.g., antidepressants for depression; antipsychotics for paranoia), there are agents such as tacrine HCl (Cognex) and Donepezil (Aricept), which are FDA approved for the treatment of cognitive deterioration of Alzheimer's disease. Although the response rate is relatively low, patients with mild to moderate disease deserve a treatment trial.

Somatoform Disorders

Somatoform disorders have in common the expression of unconscious conflict or gain through somatization. This abnormal behavior can be expressed through physical complaints or symptoms, inappropriate use of medical services, and/or maintenance of the sick role. It has been estimated that this pathology may account for between 5 to 40% of patient visits in clinical settings.[9] This group of disorders includes somatization disorder, conversion disorder, hypochondriasis, body dysmorphic disorder, and pain disorder. See Table 25–14 for critical features of each disorder.[10]

Somatization Disorder

Somatization disorder, once known as Briquet's syndrome, affects mostly women, with onset before the age of 30. These patients have multiple recurrent somatic complaints for which they repeatedly

Table 25–13. Diagnostic Criteria for Dementia of the Alzheimer's Type

The development of multiple cognitive deficits manifested by both

1. Memory impairment (impaired ability to learn new information or recall previously learned information)
2. One (or more) of the following cognitive disturbances:
   (a) aphasia (language disturbance)
   (b) apraxia (impaired ability to carry out motor activities despite intact motor function)
   (c) agnosia (failure to recognize or identify objects despite intact sensory function)
   (d) disturbance in executive functioning (i.e., planning, organizing, sequencing, abstracting)

The cognitive deficits in Criteria 1 and 2 each cause significant impairment in social or occupational functioning and represent a significant decline from a previous level of functioning.

The course is characterized by gradual onset and continuing cognitive decline.

The cognitive deficits in Criteria 1 and 2 are not due to any of the following:

1. Other central nervous system conditions that cause progressive deficits in memory and cognition (e.g., cerebrovascular disease, Parkinson's disease, Huntington's disease, subdural hematoma, normal-pressure hydrocephalus, brain tumor)
2. Systemic conditions that are known to cause dementia (e.g., hypothyroidism, vitamin B_{12} or folic acid deficiency, niacin deficiency, hypercalcemia, neurosyphilis, HIV infection)

Source: From DSM-IV, *Diagnostic and Statistical Manual of Mental Disorders,* 4th ed. American Psychiatric Association, Washington, DC, 1994.

seek medical attention. The complaints fall into four broad categories: pain, gastrointestinal, sexual/reproductive, or pseudoneurologic. The goal of treatment is management, rather than cure, for this disorder responds poorly to treatment. These patients are often resistant to psychiatric referral and are best managed by the primary care physician. Regularly scheduled appointments, irrespective of the clinical course, support, and judicious use of medical interventions are important.

Conversion Disorder

Conversion disorder is diagnosed when motor, sensory, or convulsive neurologic symptoms are the predominant complaint, yet cannot be explained on the basis of a known pathophysiologic etiology. The onset of the symptoms is usually preceded by a stressor and occurs predominantly in women. This disorder, with a prevalence of 20 to 25% in a general medical setting,[9] is usually brief in duration. The conversion, which is unconsciously motivated, may remit spontaneously, with encouragement or brief psychotherapy.

Hypochondriasis

Hypochondriasis, by contrast, is characterized by preoccupation with a specific disease. Despite medical assurance to the contrary, these patients are convinced that the disease exists and often misinterpret bodily symptoms. The triad of disease fear, disease conviction, and bodily preoccupation are the key elements of this disorder, which often becomes the bane of primary care physicians and specialists. Although the onset can be at any age, it typically begins in middle age, affecting men and women equally. These patients are often resistant to psychiatric referral and are often treated in a "holding environment" by the family physician.

Factitious Disorder and Malingering

These patients, like patients with somatoform disorder, express emotional conflict via physical complaints. In factitious disorder, however, somatizing patients *voluntarily* produce the physical signs and symptoms, with the goal of achieving the role of patient. In other words, they knowingly fake the symptoms, but do so for psychological reasons that are unconscious. Munchausen's syndrome, an extreme form of this disorder, is characterized by feigned illness, pathological lying, and wandering around the country in search of multiple medical opinions. Treatment may include gentle confrontation and a psychiatric referral. Setting limits on medical interventions is imperative be-

Table 25–14. Somatoform Disorders: A Comparison

Somatoform Disorder	General Description	Temporal and Other Requirements
Somatization disorder	History of many physical complaints: pain in at least four different sites or functions, two non-pain gastro-intestinal, one sexual or reproductive, one pseudoneurological (conversion or dissociative).	Onset before age 30. Occurs over a period of several years. Treatment sought for significant impairment in social, occupational, or other important areas of functioning.
Conversion disorder	Symptoms of deficits affecting voluntary motor or sensory function suggesting a neurological or other general medical condition. Not limited to pain or sexual dysfunction.	Psychological factors associated. Clinically significant distress or impairment in social, occupational, or other important areas of functioning; or warrants medical evaluation.
Pain disorder	Pain as predominant focus of clinical presentation. Of sufficient severity to warrant clinical attention.	Clinically significant distress or impairment in social, occupational, or other important areas of functioning. Psychological factors have an important role.
Hypochondriasis	Preoccupation with fears of having, or the idea that one has, a serious disease based on the misinterpretation of bodily symptoms. Persists despite appropriate medical evaluation and reassurance.	Duration of at least 6 months. Clinically significant distress or impairment in social, occupational, or other important area of functioning.
Body dysmorphic disorder	Preoccupation (may be of delusional intensity) with imagined defect in appearance or markedly excessive concern with slight physical anomaly.	Clinically significant distress or impairment in social, occupational, or other important areas of functioning.

Source: From Hales RE, et al. eds: *The American Psychiatric Textbook of Psychiatry.* American Psychiatric Press, Washington, DC, 1994.

cause these patients often may have had multiple surgeries, for example, by well-meaning surgeons, looking for an occult etiology of symptoms.

Malingering also involves intentional simulation of illness, but is motivated by conscious *external* incentives, such as financial compensation, avoiding legal procedures, obtaining drugs and so on. Usually these patients will not cooperate with the clinical evaluation and are noncompliant. The presence of sociopathic tendencies or a clear medical/legal context should make one consider this disorder in the differential diagnosis. Firm but empathetic confrontation is essential.

WHEN TO REFER TO A PSYCHIATRIC SPECIALIST

As noted earlier, primary care physicians are the principle providers of psychiatric care in the United States. Most feel competent to treat the common disorders, such as major depression, dysthymia, panic disorder, generalized anxiety disorder, and insomnia. There are some disorders, particularly in the acute phase, that are best managed by a psychiatric specialist. These may include psychotic disorders (i.e., schizophrenia, psychotic major depression), bipolar disorder, and acutely suicidal or homicidal patients. Those patients with any psychiatric disorder refractory to conventional treatment may also benefit from seeing a specialist as well as those with multiple co-morbid psychiatric disorders.

The majority of psychiatric specialists are psychiatrists, psychologists, social workers, and nurse clinicians. Psychiatrists specialize in the diagnosis and treatment of mental disorders and are the only psychiatric professionals who are physicians with training in the medical management of these disorders. Psychologists have traditionally had expertise in psychological and neurological testing.

Table 25–15. Examples of the Clinical Uses of Common Psychological Tests

Clinical Questions	Test(s) Indicated[a]	Information Derived
Intellectual functioning	WAIS-R, Stanford-Binet	IQ estimate, cognitive strengths/ weaknesses
Academic achievement	WRAT-R, K-TEA, Woodcock-Johnson	Academic skills and strengths and weaknesses
Adaptive behavior	Vineland	Capacity to effectively meet environmental demands
Vocational skills	SVIB, MBTI	Job and career suitability and interests according to interests/personality preferences
Brain impairment	Halstead-Reitan, Luria-Nebraska	Presence and effects of brain lesions
Psychiatric diagnosis	SCID	DSM diagnostic considerations
Psychosis	Rorschach, MMPI-2	Disordered thinking, impaired reality testing
Mood disorder	Rorschach, MMPI-2, BDI, SCL-90	Depression, mania, affect, regulation
Global personality functioning	Rorschach, MMPI-2, TAT, MCMI	Self-esteem, interpersonal style, dynamic conflicts

[a] Key: WAIS-R = Weschler Adult Intelligence Scale-Revised; WRAT-R = Wide Range Achievement Test-Revised; K-TEA = Kaufman Test of Educational Achievement; SVIB = Strong Vocational Interest Blank; MBTI = Myers-Briggs Type Indicator; SCID = Structured Clinical Interview for DSM-IIIR; MMPI-2 = Minnesota Multiphasic Personality Inventory; BDI = Beck Depression Inventory; SCL-90 = Symptom Checklist-90; TAT = Thematic Apperception Test; MCMI = Millon Clinical Mutiaxial Inventory
Source: Adapted with permission from Stoudemire A: *Clinical psychiatry for medical students,* 2nd ed. J. B. Lippincott. Philadelphia, 1994.

(See Table 25–15 for an overview of commonly administered tests and the clinical questions they attempt to answer.) They, as well as psychiatrists, are adept at an array of psychotherapies. Social workers, although historically trained in family theory and dynamics, are also experts in psychotherapy, and are the major providers of this service in the United States. All these clinicians work as a multidisciplinary team and offer consultation as well as treatment.

A case example follows to highlight issues related to psychiatric assessment and treatment.

CASE ONE

A 65-year-old Caucasian married male is referred to the speech pathology department for evaluation two months after a stroke. He had been hospitalized after suffering right arm and right lower face weakness and aphasia. On examination, the patient has weakness of the right arm. He has a paucity of speech, which consists almost exclusively of short phrases. Articulation is impaired and cadence is irregular. He appears to have normal comprehension, and can follow most commands. However, the patient could not blow out an imaginary match or protrude his tongue in different directions although he could use the same muscles automatically. The diagnosis is left frontal lobe stroke, with damage to Broca's area. The patient has residual right arm and face paresis, nonfluent aphasia, and buccofacial apraxia.

In evaluating this patient, you learn that he had no previous psychiatric history or medical history, or a history of substance abuse. He is an executive at a major firm and has always been somewhat of a workaholic, although he is currently on a medical leave. He had no hobbies other than work, according to his wife. He has had a happy marriage, but now notes marital discord because he and his wife argue because she wants him to start socializing whereas he does not. The couple have two grown children and five grandchildren. There is no family history of psychiatric illness. You note that he is depressed, and he admits to crying spells daily. He is unable to sleep with middle and late insomnia, anorexia, anhedonia, fatigue, and inability to concentrate. When questioned, he reveals that he has thoughts of ending his life, but has no plan, and would never do so as it would hurt his family. He has no prior history of depression or suicide attempts. On mental status examination, he is alert and tearful, and cooperative with the interviewer. He does not think that speech therapy will be helpful, and despairs that he will ever get better. He is neatly dressed and groomed, with notable right arm and hand weakness. His speech is consistent with the nonfluent aphasia. His mood is depressed, and affect is congruent with decreased range. His thoughts appear to be goal directed. No delusions, obsessions, or compulsions are noted. No phobias are elicited, but he appears embarrassed at leaving his home, feeling that others will notice his disability. He has no current homicidal ideation or history of violence. There are no signs of inappropriate laughing or crying, or signs of mania or hypomania. He denies perceptual disturbances. On cognitive testing he is oriented to time, place, and person. His concentration is mildly impaired. He spelled WORLD backwards as DLORW. Digit span was 5 numbers forward and 3 backward. His immediate memory was 3/3; recent 2/3; and remote fair.

From the mental status examination, you determine that in addition to the neurological deficits, he has signs and symptoms of depression, such as dysphoria, anhedonia, insomnia, impaired concentration, anorexia, and hopelessness. He has cognitive deficits in terms of concentration and memory, but it is unclear if this is due to his depression, or signs of an underlying organic illness, such as a dementia. From a biopsychosocial perspective, you surmise that the cerebrovascular insult to his left frontal lobe makes him at risk for developing a mood disturbance. Psychologically, you are aware that for this independent harddriving executive, neurological impairment will be a severe narcissistic injury, and one that will be difficult to grieve. The loss of his job, which is how he defined himself, is traumatic. The stroke and its sequelae have affected him and his wife, as they struggle to come to terms with their grief and a dramatic change in their lifestyle, both socially and financially. Your DSM-IV diagnoses are:

Axis I   Mood disorder due to left hemispheric stroke
Adjustment disorder with depressed mood

Axis II   Deferred
Axis III   Left hemispheric stroke with nonfluent aphasia, left paresis, and buccofacial apraxia
Axis IV   Problems with primary support group, conflict with wife
Axis V   Current 65; Highest in last year 95

Your treatment plan is to discuss your concerns about his depression with his neurologist. You feel that depression is a treatable illness, and worry that his dysphoria and hopelessness may impair his ability to work in speech–language therapy. You discuss this with the couple, and they both agree that medication and family therapy may help them grieve this sudden trauma. The neurologist will retest cognition once the patient's depression has improved.

CONCLUSION

Knowledge of psychiatric illness may aid speech–language pathologists in their daily work. Patients afflicted with speech and language disorders may develop secondary grief, depression, or anxiety in response to their illness. In addition, because of the speech symptoms, the psychiatric patient may present first to the speech–language pathologist or the primary care provider. It is imperative that the speech–language therapist has a working knowledge of psychopathology and psychiatric diagnosis and how to facilitate treatment of these disorders.

STUDY QUESTIONS

1. What is the biopsychosocial model of disease?

2. What do the five axes of the *Diagnostic and Statistical Manual of Mental Disorders* (DSM-IV) represent?

3. What are the key elements of a mental status examination?

4. What are the key signs and symptoms of major depression?

5. What is bipolar disorder?

6. What is the CAGE questionnaire and how can it be used to diagnose alcohol abuse or dependence?

7. What are the signs and symptoms of panic disorder?

8. What are the so called positive and negative symptoms of schizophrenia?

9. What is the most common form of dementia?

10. How does conversion disorder differ from hypochondriasis?

11. How does one differentiate facticious disorder from malingering?

12. What factors determine when a patient should be referred to a psychiatric specialist?

REFERENCES

1. Regier DA, Farmer ME, Race DS, et al: One month prevalence of mental disorders in the US and sociodemographic characteristics: The Epidemiologic Catchment Area Study. *Acta Psychiatr Scand* 1993; 88:35–47.

2. Kessler R, McGonagle KA, Zhao S, et al: Lifetime and 12 month prevalence of DSM-IIIR psychiatric disorders in the United States. *Arch Gen Psych* 1994; 51:8–19.

3. American Psychiatric Association: DSM-IV, *Diagnostic and Statistical Manual of Mental Disorders,* 4th ed. Washington, DC, 1994.

4. Engel GL: The need for a new medical model: A challenge for biomedicine. *Science* 1977; 196: 129–136.

5. Stoudemire A, ed: *Clinical psychiatry for the medical student.* J.B. Lippincott, Philadelphia, 1994.

6. Weisman MM, Boyd JH: The epidemiology of affective disorders. In Post, RM, Ballenger, JC, eds., *Neurobiology of mood disorders.* Williams and Wilkins, Baltimore, 1984.

7. Beck A, Rush AJ, Shaw B, et al: *Cognitive theory of depression.* Guilford Press, New York, 1979.

8. Ewing JA: Detecting alcoholism: The CAGE questionnaire. *JAMA* 1984; 252:1905–1907.

9. Ford CV: *The somatizing disorders: Illness as a way of life.* Elsevier, New York, 1983.

10. Hales RE, Yudofsky SC, Talbott JA, eds: *The American psychiatric press textbook of psychiatry,* 2nd ed. American Psychiatric Press, Washington, DC, 1994.

26

Psychogenic Communication Disorders

GREG MAHR

CHAPTER OUTLINE

Terminology

Classification

Epidemiology

Psychiatric Comorbidity

Assessment

Treatment

After a violent assault, a young man suddenly develops dysfluent speech. His speech superficially resembles stuttering, but he blocks on every word, has no struggle behaviors, and no history of speech disturbance. A woman newly diagnosed with leukemia suddenly stops talking, despite the abscence of any neurological pathology. In such cases, although the presenting symptom is a disturbance in communication, the underlying pathology involves emotional and psychological issues. These disorders are psychogenic: They superficially resemble physical illnesses but are in fact caused or exacerbated by emotional or mental factors.

Psychogenic communication disorders are very important in the practice of speech–language pathology in the medical setting. Psychogenic speech and voice disorders accounted for 4.5% of all acquired communication disorders evaluated at the Mayo Clinic between 1987 and 1990.[1] As in most psychogenic disorders, an appropriate diagnosis is often established only after multiple costly medical evaluations. Patients with psychogenic problems tend to see many doctors and seek aggressive medical

work-ups. Almost half of speech–language pathologists do not feel comfortable treating patients with psychogenic speech and voice disorders.[2] Effective and efficient diagnosis and treatment of these disorders requires a team approach and multidisciplinary collaboration. Speech–language pathology, mental health, and medical and surgical disciplines working as a team can minimize unneccessary and repetitive evaluations and provide effective coordinated care.

In this chapter we will describe the various psychogenic speech and voice disorders, explore issues of psychiatric co-morbidity, and then discuss assessment and treatment.

TERMINOLOGY

Psychogenic symptoms have been called "functional," "histrionic" or "hysterical," "nonorganic," and "psychosomatic." None of these terms is satisfactory, including the term "psychogenic." The term "functional" implies a spurious dichotomy between structure and function. The terms "hysterical" and "histrionic" carry historical connotations that are sexist and pejorative. The term hysteria originally referred to the alleged wandering of the uterus in the female body. Historically, women's symptoms have been dismissed as "hysterical" by male physicians. The term nonorganic is clumsy and suggests a radical dichotomy between organic pathology and "other" pathology. The term psychosomatic refers specifically to illnesses such as duodenal ulcer, ulcerative colitis, and asthma, where some have suggested that chronic stress and autonomic overactivity lead to organic pathology.

"Psychogenic" is the least objectionable term available, and the term that will be used in this chapter. Although the term psychogenic still implies a dualistic view of mind and body, it is at least nonpejorative. This term also reminds the user that mental pathology is more than just the absence of organic pathology.

CLASSIFICATION

While the psychogenic communication disorders in general have yet to be clearly described or categorized, several classification schemes have been devised for the psychogenic voice disorders.

Aronson identified five groups of psychogenic voice disorders: (1) the musculoskeletal tension disorders involving excess muscle tension and vocal abuse with resultant inflammation, nodules, and ulcers; (2) the conversion voice disorders, including conversion muteness, aphonia, dysphonia, and adductor spastic dysphonia; (3) mutational falsetto; (4) transsexualism; and (5) childlike speech in adults.[3] Koufman and Blalock developed a similar classification scheme, but included a separate category for habitual hoarseness and postoperative dysphonia.[4] Based on a retrospective review of 1000 patients, Morrison et al. described three types of psychogenic dysphonia: (1) muscle tension dysphonia, (2) functional or psychological dysphonia, and (3) spasmodic dysphonia. He and his associates detailed the anatomic and laryngoscopic findings in the various psychogenic voice disorders.[5]

According to these schemes the muscle misuse or tension disorders are distinct from the conversion or psychological dysphonias. The misuse disorders are bad habits that may relate in a general way to personality style; the conversion voice disorders are specific symptoms of psychopathology and symbolically depict emotional conflicts.

Morrison and Rammage, in fact, argues that the term psychogenic should be restricted to the conversion voice disorders.[6]

In practice, conversion and muscle misuse disorders are difficult to distinguish. In dysphonia, for instance, conversion symptoms necessarily involve changes in muscle tension. The diagnosis of conversion is based on theoretical constructs that must be inferred from observed data. Such inferences are often difficult to make. Distinctions between the two groups of disorders cannot be made on laryngoscopic or clinical grounds, but only on the basis of an interpretation of the nature and meaning of psychopathology. Such distinctions are inherently unreliable.

The three classification schemes described above are restricted to voice disorders and do not include closely related disorders of speech, such as psychogenic stuttering. Table 26–1 compares the classification schemes developed by Aronson, Koufman, and Morrison. In Table 26–2, a comprehensive classification scheme, detailed below, that encompasses the full range of the major psychogenic communication disorders is suggested.

Muscle Tension Disorders

Abnormal muscle tension is present in all the psychogenic communication disorders, but is particularly important in muscle tension disorders. The laryngeal musculature responds to emotional stress with hypercontraction. As shown in Figure 26–1, such tension can be observed and palpated by encircling the larynx with the thumb and middle finger in the region of the thyrohyoid space. In the relaxed state the larynx is mobile and the thyrohyoid space distinct and palpable; when the laryngeal musculature is tense the larynx rises and the thryohyoid space narrows.[7] Tension can also be palpated in the submandibular region.

Muscle tension or muscle misuse disorders develop when the laryngeal muscles are chronically and habitually misused or hypercontracted. Polyps, nodules, and scarring can develop as a result of chronic muscle misuse. While patients with muscle tension disorders are sometimes anxious, they do not display the more specific forms of mental illness seen in conversion disorders. Patients with muscle tension voice disorders misuse their voices in one or more of the following ways: (1) overuse, (2) speaking with abnormal muscle tension in the larynx and neck muscles, or (3) using an abnormally low pitch.[4]

Anatomical subtypes of muscle tension disorders have been described in detail by Morrison

Table 26–1. Classification Schemes for Psychogenic Speech and Voice disorders

Aronson	Koufman	Morrison
Muscle tension	Voice abuse	Muscle tension
Conversion	Hysterical	Functional
Muteness	aphonia	
Aphonia	dysphonia	
Dysphonia		
Spastic dysphonia		Spasmodic
Mutational falsetto	Falsetto	
Transexualism		
Child-like speech		
	Habitual hoarseness	
	Post-op dysphonia	

and Rammage.[6] Anatomical patterns seen in conversion and muscle misuse disorders may overlap, adding to the complexity of differential diagnosis.

Types of Muscle Tension Disorders

The most common type of muscle tension disorder is the laryngeal isometric, usually seen in untrained individuals who use their larynx excessively, such as cheerleaders or amateur singers. This pattern of misuse has also been called habitual hyperkinetic dysphonia and is one of the most common vocal complaints in adults. Sustained hypertonicity of the posterior cricoarytenoid muscle deflects the arytenoid cartilage and produces a posterior glottal chink. Phonation has a characteristic "whispery/breathy" quality and secondary mucosal injury can occur.

Lateral contraction and/or hyperadduction, where the larynx is squeezed in a side-to-side direction, is also common. When this occurs at a glottic level, it is usually as a result of poor vocal technique. Glottic contraction can be triggered by an upper respiratory infection that causes hoarseness, which then is maintained by poor vocal technique after the viral irritation has resolved.

Supraglottic contraction is also known as ventricular dysphonia or plica ventricularis. This vocal pattern involves the abnormal participation of the false vocal cords in phonation. Supraglottic contraction is commonly noted in the conversion dysphonias, but can occur in injury to the true vocal cords.

An anteroposterior contraction of the supraglottic larynx has also been described. Koufman and Blalock[4] labeled this disorder the "Bogart–Bacall" syndrome. Such patients display a tension dysphonia and effortful voice at the bottom of their vocal ranges but can talk freely at a higher pitch.

Hypokinetic dysphonia results from the inadequate movements of laryngeal muscles during phonation. Such patients have bowed vocal cords on indirect laryngoscopic examination and weak, husky breathy voices. These patients typically suffer from conversion disorders, but hypokinetic dysphonia may result from habitual hoarseness following an upper respiratory tract infection.

Table 26–2. The Psychogenic Communication Disorders

Muscle tension disorders

Conversion communication disorders

   Aphonia

   Dysphonia

   Psychogenic stuttering

Mutational falsetto

Spasmodic dysphonia

   Neurogenic type

   Conversion type

Conversion Communication Disorders

The term "conversion disorder" describes a broad range of pseudoneurological symptoms that develop as a result of emotional stress and conflict. In conversion psychic conflict is "converted" into a physical symptom. Conversion symptoms can be distinguished from true neurological symptoms

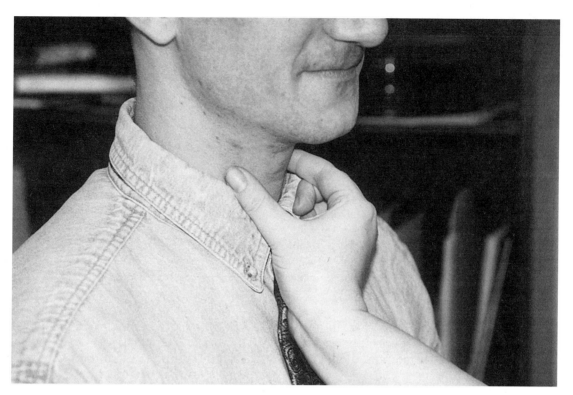

Figure 26–1. Assessing tension in the laryngeal musculature.

because conversion symptoms are *ideogenic*. They correspond not to the actual anatomy and physiology of a neurological disorder, but to a person's idea of what such a disorder might be like. For instance, in a conversion paralysis of the arm a patient might be unable to move his or her arm from the elbow down. He or she does not understand the innervation of the arm, and does not realize that such a pattern of paralysis is implausible, but develops a symptom pattern that corresponds to his or her mental idea of a paralysis. Similarly, in conversion aphonia a patient might still be able to cough or sing even though he or she attests that he or she cannot phonate.

Conversion cannot be diagnosed by exclusion. Just because a symptom has no known anatomical or physiological explanation does not mean that it is a conversion. To diagnose conversion, a clear temporal relationship between a symptom and a psychological stressor must be present. In chronic conversion reactions such temporal relationships can be difficult to elucidate. The criteria for conversion disorder are shown in Table 26–3.

Initially, a conversion reaction provides *primary gain*. The conversion symptom helps keep a painful emotional conflict out of conscious awareness. *Secondary gain* refers to those benefits that indirectly accrue from the conversion symptom; these include time off work, disability payments,

extra nurturance from one's spouse, and relief from family responsibilities and chores. Secondary gain helps maintain conversion symptoms and make them less responsive to treatment. A common conversion symptom in past decades was "Saturday night amnesia." A young woman involved in a weekend sexual indiscretion that she found morally and socially unacceptable would present to the emergency room as amnestic for the prior night. The amnesia would serve the primary gain of protecting the patient from the guilt and shame of her sexual encounter and the secondary gain of giving the support and protection from her family that the sick role offers.

Conversion symptoms are often accompanied by "la belle indifference"; the sufferer is relatively unconcerned about a neurological symptom that one would expect to be very troubling and frightening. True neurologically based amnestic episodes

Table 26–3. Criteria for Conversion Disorder

Symptoms affecting voluntary motor or sensory function suggesting a neurological condition.

Psychological factors are temporally associated with the onset or exacerbation of the symptom.

Symptom is not intentionally produced or feigned.

Symptom cannot be explained by a medical condition.

are frightening and troubling, but the victim of "Saturday night amnesia" might seem untroubled by her symptoms.

Patients with psychogenic disorders also tend to be *alexithymic*. Alexithymia literally means "no words for feelings." Patients with alexithymia are concrete, show little insight into emotional issues, and lack fantasy and imaginative life. Patients with alexithymia are less likely to benefit from psychotherapy. The process of "talking through" problems and talking about feelings has no meaning for alexithymic patients.

Conversion symptoms start early in life and are more common in women. Cultural factors may explain the gender differential in conversion disorders. The example of "Saturday night amnesia" cited previously illustrates this point. Such conversion reactions never occurred in males because sexual indiscretion was more acceptable for men, and they did not face the guilt and social stigma that women faced. Somatic symptoms may empower women in cultural and social contexts where other avenues for empowerment are denied.

Malingering and Factitious Disorders

Malingering and factitious disorders can resemble conversion disorder. Unlike conversion, where the patient is not aware that he or she is producing the symptoms, the malingering patient deliberately and consciously feigns symptoms for secondary gain. In factitious disorder, also known as Münchhausen's syndrome, the patient deliberately and knowingly produces medical symptoms not for secondary gain, but for the purpose of assuming the sick role. In factitious disorder, patients are aware that they are feigning symptoms, but not aware of their own motivations.

In practice, conversion, factitious, and malingering disorders are difficult to distinguish. For instance, a patient with a conversion symptom may consciously feign or magnify his or her illness when undergoing a disability evaluation. Jonas and Pope felt that these disorders were indistinguishable and should be called "the dissembling disorders."[8] In their view, all these patients dissembled or lied. Pure classical conversion patients lie to themselves and successfully fool even themselves. The relationship between conversion, factitious, and malingering disorders is depicted in Table 26–4.

Types of Conversion Disorders

Conversion speech symptoms are protean; their variety is limited only by the imagination of the sufferer. Conversion speech disorders are classified on

Table 26–4. The Dissembling Disorders

Disorder	Symptom Production	Motivation
Conversion	Unconscious	Unconscious
Malingering	Conscious	Conscious
Factitious	Conscious	Unconscious

the basis of the observed speech pattern. In conversion muteness the patient neither whispers nor articulates despite normal laryngeal and oral motor function. In conversion aphonia the patient whispers involuntarily despite normal vocal cord function on laryngoscopic examination and in cough. Conversion dysphonia is psychogenic hoarseness and can resemble laryngitis. The ideogenic nature of conversion symptoms is confirmed by the incongruities in the clinical presentation, like an inability to adduct the vocal cords during phonation in the presence of normal cough or laugh.

Psychogenic stuttering is also a form of conversion speech disorder. Like other conversion disorders, psychogenic stuttering shows ideogenic and atypical features. In contrast to typical developmental stuttering, psychogenic stutterers show stereotyped repetitions, lack of improvement with choral reading, and the absence of islands of fluency, secondary symptoms, or avoidance behaviors.[9,10] Developmental stuttering shows an insidious onset in early childhood, while psychogenic stuttering begins acutely and can occur at any age after an emotional trauma. Psychogenic stuttering must be carefully distinguished from fluency disturbances that can occur in brain diseases such as Parkinson's or after traumatic brain injury. The differences between developmental stuttering, psychogenic stuttering, and neurogenic fluency disorders are summarized in Table 26–5.

Mutational falsetto, or adolescent transitional dysphonia, can be a habitual pattern or a form of conversion disorder. The adolescent male with mutational falsetto appears to resist the development of the normal lower pitch by adopting a falsetto voice. The larynx is raised and the glottis is tense and hyperadducted to maintain elevated pitch in the face of masculinized laryngeal anatomy. Mutational falsetto is relatively uncommon and represents only 2 or 3% of patients presenting for the treatment of voice disorders.[11] Most cases present in adolescence. Occasionally, adults will present because of pitch breaks, which actually are intervals of normal pitch in a mutational falsetto that has been habitually maintained for years or decades.[3]

Table 26–5. Fluency Disorders

	Developmental Stuttering	Neurogenic Fluency Disorders	Psychogenic Stuttering
Age	Early childhood	Age of onset of neurologic illness	After trauma
Onset	Gradual	Same as neurologic illness	Sudden
Secondary mannerisms, struggle behaviors	Common	Rare	Rare
Improves with repetition, choral reading, delayed auditory feedback	Yes	No	No
Related psychiatric history	No	No	Other psychiatric illness or conversion symptoms

Aronson has described a pattern of childlike speech in adults.[3] Such individuals show pitch and vocal qualities suggesting the speech of a child, as well as childlike facial expressions and mannerisms. Childlike speech in adults is probably best considered a rare form of conversion disorder.

Individuals undergoing sex change surgery may seek voice therapy. Such patients, called transsexuals, are usually male and have a persistent discomfort about their assigned gender and a persistent preoccupation with losing their primary and secondary sexual characteristics and acquiring those of the opposite gender.[12] Transsexual patients are typically required to live for a year as a member of the opposite gender before undergoing definitive surgical procedures. Before or after surgery they may wish to modify their voices with respect to gender-specific traits. The goal of such therapy is not the treatment of vocal pathology or conversion symptoms, but voice modification for the purposes of gender change. Transsexual patients should be considered to have psychopathology, but not voice pathology.

Spasmodic Dysphonia

Spasmodic dysphonia, also known as spastic dysphonia, is a rare and disabling disorder of unknown etiology. Patients with spasmodic dysphonia have characteristic episodes of jerky and effortful vocalization with laryngoscopic evidence of involuntary vocal fold spasm. Spasmodic dysphonia has been described as a "stuttering" of the vocal folds. Spasms can involve true vocal folds, false vocal folds, or both. Severe tension in the entire phonatory system is evident, with grimacing, facial flushing, eye blinks, and tics that are reminiscent of stuttering. At times speech is quite normal, especially when the patient is taken off guard and using nonprepositional speech. Laughing, singing, whispering, and speaking in a falsetto are also often normal.[13]

Two variants of spasmodic dysphonia have been described.[14] Most common is adductor spastic dysphonia with intermittent hyperadduction of the vocal folds. Much more rare is the abductor variant with weak or breathy phonation.

Traditionally spasmodic dysphonia has been considered a psychogenic disorder.[15] Investigators have pointed to the episodic nature of the disorder and the clear evidence of normal vocal fold function in singing or whispering to suggest that spasmodic dysphonia is a conversion disorder.

On the other hand, clear correlations between emotional stressors and the onset of spasmodic dysphonia often cannot be made. Izdebski et al. studied comprehensive case history profiles of 200 spasmodic dysphonia patients and 200 controls.[16] Only 20% of patients associated stress or emotional trauma with the onset of their spasmodic dysphonia.

In the last decade, investigators have focused on potential organic causes for spasmodic dysphonia. Auditory brainstem responses and visceral efferent brainstem pathways, such as the cardia reflex and cephalic-vagal reflex, show abnormalities in spasmodic dysphonia patients. MRI, SPECT and BEAM studies have been inconclusive, showing a range of lesions that do not correlate well with brainstem findings.[17] Spasmodic dysphonia resembles other focal dystonias, such as blepharospasm and torticollis. Blitzer and others have suggested that spasmodic dysphonia be

Cognitive Techniques

Cognitive techniques are a natural and vital component of a therapy regimen for psychogenic voice disorders. Education about vocal functioning and proper vocal techniques aids patients to gain a sense of mastery and control, and helps them be partners in their own care. Education helps negate the attitudes of passivity, helplessness, and self-blame that complicate the treatment of psychogenic speech and voice disorders.

Response to Treatment

As might be expected in such a heterogenous group of disorders, response to treatment is variable. In practice most patients are treated for 6 to 10 sessions.[2] Outcomes have not been systematically studied, but the best evidence suggests that about half of patients recover completely over 3 to 6 months, and another quarter are at least significantly improved by speech therapy. A significant minority of patients do not appear to do well.[23] Butcher et al. studied 19 nonresponders. They were found to be anxious and to have significant problems with interpersonal relationships.[27]

Referral to a mental health professional may be of benefit, especially in treating nonresponders or those in whom emotional issues are clearly evident. Referral is also useful for the treatment of co-morbid problems like anxiety, depression, or somatization. In Butcher's study of patients with psychogenic voice disorders who did not respond to standard speech therapy, nearly half improved in a conjoint therapy program with a psychologist and a speech pathologist.

Somatizing patients may reject mental health referrals. They may be very strongly invested in having their problem be "medical"; and a referral to a mental health provider may be seen as trivializing their voice problems. A referral to mental health treatment is best presented as an adjunct to speech therapy, not as a substititute for it.

A referral to a mental health professional might be worded as follows: "I have noticed that anxiety may be contributing to your voice problem. I work with Dr. X., who is an expert in anxiety problems, and can help us with that aspect of your speech problem."

Unfortunately, the results of mental health referrals can be disappointing. Psychiatrists, psychologists, and therapists often lack knowledge or experience in speech and voice problems. Few clinical settings allow for clinical interactions between speech–language pathologists and mental health professionals, and most speech–language pathologists feel uncertain when and to whom to refer patients. Treatment failures, who are less likely to benefit from any intervention, are usually the ones referred.

A multidisciplinary team approach can obviate some of these difficulties. A patient is more likely to accept a referral to a practitioner who is part of the "team." Each team member brings his or her unique expertise to the program and the team as a whole develops a comprehensive approach to patient care. Communication between disciplines is facilitated, allowing the patient's needs to be efficiently and effectively addressed.

SUMMARY

In this chapter we have described the various psychogenic speech and voice disorders and presented methods for diagnosis and treatment. Figure 26–3 graphically depicts a model for the treament of the psychogenic speech and voice disorders, including the role of psychiatric and psychological assessment.

STUDY QUESTIONS

1. What are the different types of psychogenic speech and voice disorders?

2. What is meant by co-morbid pathology?

3. How are conversion speech and voice disorders treated?

REFERENCES

1. Duffy JR: *Motor speech disorders.* Mosby, New York, 1995.
2. Elias A, Raven R, Butcher P, Littlejohns DW: Speech therapy for psychogenic voice disorder: A survey of current practice and training. *Br J Dis Comm* 1989; 24:61–76.
3. Aronson AE: *Clinical voice disorders.* Thieme, New York, 1990.
4. Koufman JA, Blalock PD: Classification and approach to patients with functional voice disorders. *Ann Otol Rhinol Laryngol* 1982; 91:372–377.
5. Morrison MD, Nichol H, Rammage LA: Diagnostic criteria in functional dysphonia. *Laryngoscope* 1986; 94:1–8.
6. Morrison MD, Rammage LA: Muscle misuse voice disorders: Description and classification. *Acta Otolaryngol (Stockh)* 1993; 113:428–434.

7. Case JL: *Clinical management of voice disorders.* Pro-ed, Austin, TX, 1996.

8. Jonas JM, Pope HG: The dissimulating disorders: A single diagnostic entity? *Comp Psych* 1985; 26:58–62.

9. Roth CR, Aronson AE, Davis LJ: Clinical studies in psychogenic stuttering of adult onset. *J Speech Hear Dis* 1989; 54:634–636.

10. Mahr G, Leith W: Psychogenic stuttering of adult onset. *J Speech Hear Res* 1992; 35:283–286.

11. Hammarberg B: Pitch and quality characteristics of mutational voice disorders before and after therapy. *Folia Phoniat* 1987; 39:204–216.

12. American Psychiatric Association: *Diagnostic and statistical manual of mental disorders.* APA Press, Washington, DC, 1994.

13. Stoicheff ML: The present status of adductor spastic dysphonia. *J Otolaryngol* 1983; 311–314.

14. Aronson AE, Brown JR, Litin EM, Pearson JS: Spastic dysphonia. Comparison with essential tremor and other neurological and psychogenic dysphonias. *J Speech Hear Dis* 1968; 33:219–231.

15. Cannito MP: Emotional considerations in spasmodic dysphonia: Psychometric quantification. *J Commun Disord* 1991; 24:313–329.

16. Izdebski K, Dedo HH, Boles L: Spastic dysphonia: A patient profile of 200 cases. *Am J Otolaryngol* 1984; 5:7–14.

17. Finitzo T, Freeman F: Spasmodic dysphonia, whether and where: Results of seven years of research. *J Speech Hear Res* 1989; 32:541–555.

18. Blitzer A, Brin MF et al: Clinical and laboratory characteristics of focal laryngeal dystonia: Study of 110 cases. *Laryngoscope* 1988; 98:636–640.

19. Blitzer A, Brin MF et al: Localized injections of botulism toxin for the treatment of focal laryngeal dystonia (spastic dysphonia). *Laryngoscope* 1988; 98:193–197.

20. Blitzer A, Brin MF: Spastic dysphonia (laryngeal dystonia). Current therapy in otolaryngology. *Head Neck Surg* 1990; 4:346–349.

21. Aronson AE, De Santo LW: Adductor spastic dysphonia: Three years after recurrent laryngeal nerve resection. *Laryngoscope* 1983; 93:1–8.

22. Ludlow CL, Naunton RF et al: Effects of botulinum toxin injections of speech in adductor spasmodic dysphonia. *Neurology* 1988; 38:1220–1225.

23. Bridger MWM, Epstein R: Functional voice disorders: A review of 109 patients. *J Laryngol Otol* 1983; 97:1145–1148.

24. Butcher P, Elias A, Raven R: *Psychogenic voice disorders and cognitive behavioral therapy.* Singular Publishing, San Diego, 1993.

25. Beck, AT: *Cognitive therapy and emotional disorders.* International Universities Press, New York, 1976.

26. Seligman MEP: *Helplessness.* Freeman, San Francisco, 1975.

27. Butcher P, Elias A, Raven R, Yeatman J, Littlejohns D: Psychogenic voice disorder unresponsive to speech therapy: Psychological characteristics and cognitive-behavioral therapy. *Brit J Dis Comm* 1987; 22:81–92.

Current Issues in Health Care Delivery and the Speech–Language Pathologist

27

Clinical Service Delivery Reform

ARLENE PIETRANTON

CHAPTER OUTLINE

The Changing World of Clinical Service Delivery

Managed Care Dominance

Treatment Outcomes

Clinical Protocols

Alternative Personnel Options

Innovative Service Delivery Models

This chapter discusses: (1) the financial, political, and market-based factors that are rapidly reshaping clinical service delivery in the United States today including the rising costs of health care, the shift of political power from the federal to the state level, and the rapid growth of managed care; and (2) four trends that speech–language pathologists must master to survive and thrive in this era of reform: treatment outcomes, clinical protocols, alternative personnel options, and innovative service delivery models.

THE CHANGING WORLD OF CLINICAL SERVICE DELIVERY

It has been said that the rate of sociopolitical change accelerates in the final decade of a century. This certainly appears to be the case for clinical service delivery in the United States. The magnitude of change in that arena alone makes it tempting to contemplate whether the acceleration accelerates as one approaches the turn of a millennium. Stark realities such as funding cutbacks,

cost containment strategies, legislative changes, organizational redesign initiatives, and heightened demands for accountability are essentially reshaping the delivery of clinical services in the United States. Simply put, it is no longer "business as usual." This chapter reviews the changing world of clinical service delivery and its impact on medical speech–language pathology services and practitioners.

The Driving Force Behind the Changes

The primary driving force behind the changes has been concern over the dramatic and steady upward spiral of health care costs that occurred in the United States between the late 1960s and the mid 1990s. In 1960, health care expenditures accounted for approximately 5.3% ($27 billion) of the U.S. gross national product (GNP). By 1994, they consumed nearly 16% ($903 billion) of the GNP. This rate of growth, if left unchecked, would have resulted in health care costs consuming 100% of the GNP by the year 2050.[1] Public concern over these escalating costs reached a crescendo in 1994, the year of the "National Health Care Reform that wasn't." That year witnessed a myriad of reform bills and debates at the federal level that eventually capitulated to partisan politics and failed to produce any federally mandated system-wide reform. Congress subsequently attempted various "incremental reforms" in 1995 and early 1996, most of which also fell prey to political tactics. By the mid-1990s, federal legislators were deeply entrenched along party lines. Their primary concern appeared to be the potential impact their voting actions could have on election outcomes. It seems reasonable to posit that, for the remainder of this century, the greatest variable in the success of future federal health care reform efforts will be party alignment (or lack thereof) between the majority party in Congress and the presidency.

The New Locus of Power

Although health care reform may have stalled at the federal level in the mid-1990s, the outcome of the 1994 elections dramatically altered the political climate in the United States. There was a clear shift of power from the federal level to the state and local levels, along with overt promotion of business-sector opportunities and influence. The previous decades' dominant strategies of federal regulation and funded mandates drew to an end. Funds that traditionally were earmarked for education and/or health services were threatened by the mixing bowl of block grants. Legislative mandates specifying services and provider qualifications were targeted for eradication. Speech–language pathology services, like many other clinical services, had prospered under federally legislated mandates and entitlement programs that were increasingly in danger of being dismantled as power shifted to the state and private sector.

MANAGED CARE DOMINANCE

Against this backdrop, managed care thrived in the early 1990s and has quickly grown to dominate clinical service delivery. Contrary to what many may believe, however, managed care is not a "90s" phenomenon. Managed care, primarily in the form of Health Maintenance Organizations (HMOs), has been an viable health care option in the United States since the early 1960s. Over the ensuing decades, managed care demonstrated moderate growth as a choice of health care coverage until the early 1990s, when it began growing at a staggering

rate (see Table 27–1). By 1996, it was estimated that more than 70% of all health insurance in the United States was under the umbrella of managed care.

The percentage of persons covered by Medicare and Medicaid under managed care also grew rapidly. According to the Health Care Financing Administration, the branch of the U.S. Department of Health and Human Services responsible for administering Medicare, the relative growth (i.e., the percentage of increase each year over the previous year's enrollment) in Medicare HMO enrollment steadily increased from a rate of 6% in 1988 to 25% in 1994.

Managed care is not simply a different health care funding strategy. It is an entirely different framework of service delivery with an altogether different set of ground rules (see Table 27–2). Speech–language pathologists have become well acclimated to the fee-for-service reimbursement ground rules with their associated opportunities and pitfalls. Under fee-for-service, the fundamental steps typically involve verifying that the health plan covers the services needed, securing appropriate authorization as necessary, providing the services, submitting interim progress reports as required, billing for services provided, and receiving reimbursement (or a retroactive denial) some 30,

Table 27–1. Under the Managed Care Umbrella

The number of individuals enrolled in HMOs grew from 10.8 million in 1982 to 46 million in 1993.

In December 1987, approximately 12 million individuals were enrolled in Preferred Provider Organizations (PPOs). Over 60 million were enrolled by December 1993.

The number of HMOs increased from 566 in October 1993 to 628 one year later.

The number of PPOs grew from 895 in October 1993 to 1107 one year later.

In 1985, 84.7% of Blue Cross/Blue Shield's (BC/BS) customer base was enrolled in traditional indemnity plans. By the second quarter of 1994, 83% were in managed care programs

In 1991, among firms of 200 or more employees, 53% offered their employees conventional insurance coverage; 47% offered managed care coverage (i.e., Health Maintenance Organizations [HMOs], Preferred Provider Organizations [PPOs], or Point of Service [POS]. By 1994, that balance had more than reversed itself: 35% offered conventional insurance coverage; 65% offered managed care coverage.

Source: American Managed Care and Review Association: *Managed care—Quality, Choice, Satisfaction.* AMCRA, Washington, DC, 1995.

Table 27-2. Fee for Service Versus Managed Care

Fee for Service	Managed Care
Retrospective reimbursement	Prospective reimbursement
Financial risk on payor	Financial risk on provider
Per visit/procedure payment	Capitated rate for covered population
Authorization needed	Clinical autonomy
Provider driven system	Payor-driven system
More visits/procedures generate more charges (i.e., more potential revenue)	Fewer visits/procedures reduce costs (i.e., more potential profit)
Payor wants provider to do as little as possible (control costs)	Payor wants provider to do everything possible
Provider wants to do as much as clinically justified	Provider wants to provide minimum services necessary (control costs)

60, or 90 days later—less and less of which holds true under managed care.

The New Financial Ground Rules

The ultimate goal of managed care is to shift the financial risk from the payor to the provider through capitated contractual arrangements. Under capitation, a predetermined fee (usually on a per-member per-month basis) is negotiated for each individual who is covered as a potential recipient of the specified services (regardless of how much or how little) from the provider. That fee is multiplied by the number of covered lives (eligible individuals within the plan) and paid to the provider at the agreed-on interval (typically monthly). The provider does not have to seek authorization, submit charges, or hope for retroactive reimbursement. In that sense, the provider is empowered to exercise his or her clinical judgment autonomously. However, the provider must now shoulder the financial risk associated with the cost of the services and the resources expended in the course of the patients' treatment. If the cost of the care exceeds the capitated amount of the reimbursement received, the provider must absorb the excess cost as a loss. If the cost of services rendered is less than the capitated amount of reimbursement, the provider keeps the excess payment and realizes a profit. Clinical productivity monitors that measure charges generated as a means to judge efficiency are not meaningful under capitation. The crucial variables to be monitored are the actual cost of providing each unit of service and population-based utilization rates. From the perspective of the program's financial well-being, under capitation less (services provided or charges generated) is now more (profit).

Cost Effectiveness

Under a service delivery system dominated by managed care, efficiency and effectiveness are paramount considerations. Clinicians can no longer assume that one-on-one treatment for as long as progress can be demonstrated is a viable option. Many of today's health care practitioners entered their chosen discipline with a strong commitment to helping others and a firm belief that continued treatment is warranted until a patient plateaus. Today we must demonstrate that our services make a functional difference—and that they do so with optimum efficiency.

Collectively as a profession, and individually as service providers, speech–language pathologists must explore, embrace, and master four major trends to help assure that individuals in need of speech–language pathology services continue to have access and funding. These four major trends are: treatment outcomes, clinical protocols, alternative personnel options, and innovative service delivery models.

TREATMENT OUTCOMES

Treatment outcome is the natural starting point in considering these trends because it provides the objective framework and tools for assessing the effectiveness of the care provided and the variables involved.

"Satisfaction guaranteed," "money back warranty," "the best value for your dollar"—these time-honored concepts from the American marketplace have entered the realm of clinical service delivery. It is no longer enough to show that what you do is effective—you must demonstrate the relationship between the costs involved and the benefits derived. Simply put, payors are no longer interested in paying for clinical services. Today they want to buy measurable outcomes. Clinical providers are being asked to furnish proof of the measurable value of their services. They are being confronted with such questions as "Why does it matter?" "What functional difference will it mean for this individual?" "How will it measurably improve this individual's social, educational, and/or vocational performance?" Decisions regarding benefits packages, what they cover, by whom they're provided, for how long, and at what cost, are increasingly outcomes driven.

Accountability is not a new concept to the profession of speech–language pathology. The profession has a long-standing and well-documented commitment to judging its effectiveness via clinical research, peer review, quality assurance, and quality improvement activities. However, treatment outcomes are not the same as efficacy, nor are they retrospective, and they do not focus on process. Rather, outcomes measures are intended to relate observed clinical changes (e.g., survival, recovery, restoration of function) directly to specific variables (e.g., patient characteristics, frequency, duration, cost, provider characteristics) of the intervention provided—in real world circumstances.

Outcomes Measures

Treatment outcomes measures focus on patients' initial status, their demographics and habits, the process of treatment (what was done, who did it, how long it took, etc.), in relationship to their status at discharge (or exit from treatment). Harry Wetzler, director of technology and research at the Health Outcomes Institute in Bloomington, MN, advises that outcomes measures are multidimensional and that one must include measures in at least the following five areas:

1. Clinical status (traditional anatomical and physiological findings)
2. Functional status (skills related to social, academic, or vocational activities)
3. Well-being (mental and emotional health, amount of pain, energy, vitality, etc.)
4. Satisfaction with care
5. Cost—to the patient and the system[2]

Wetzler also points out that the different dimensions are of different levels of interest depending on one's vantage point. For example, the successful outcome of fitting a tracheoesophageal voice prothesis could be measured as: increased ease and confidence in speaking by the **patient**; improved scores on an assessment battery administered by the **clinician**; or return to gainful employment by the **payor**. A measurement tool must balance the perspectives of all the stakeholders if it is to be a valid indicator of outcomes. Many existing databases were designed to answer questions from a different era and as such do not offer this balance.

There is a rapidly growing cadre of outcomes resources available (see Chapter 28). Selecting the "best fit" for your program and needs requires careful scrutiny of a number of salient features (see Table 27–3). Whether choosing to subscribe to a nationally aggregated database, purchasing an off-the-shelf software shell that can be customized, constructing a sophisticated in-house system, or designing a paper and pencil tool—today's clinical practitioners must collect outcome data. The profession of speech–language pathology faces a challenge in selecting outcomes measurement tools that can credibly answer the questions being asked today. Many of the well-established tools are outgrowths of a physical or medical systems orientation to status assessment and treat the complicated act of communication simply, measuring only broadly diverse aspects of communication such as "expressive" (a.k.a. speaking) and "receptive" (a.k.a. listening) skills. Such global measures cannot adequately differentiate the discrete components of communication, and the resulting measurements are likely to overlook meaningful functional gains in communication.

ASHA's Task Force on Treatment Outcome and Cost Effectiveness

In its efforts to construct treatment outcomes data collection instruments sufficiently sensitive to measure changes in communication, ASHA's Task Force on Treatment Outcomes and Cost Effectiveness reviewed and expanded the Functional Communication Measures (FCMs; see Table 27–4) that had been developed as part of ASHA's Program Evaluation System in the late 1980's. In the Task Force's Data Collection Instruments, only those FCMs related to areas that are addressed in treatment are scored (see Table 27–5 for an example of the scoring guidelines—"Comprehension of Spoken Language"). Recognizing that one set of measures may not be appropriate for all individuals who demonstrate a communication disorder, the Task Force chose to develop and refine instruments that are customized for the adult health, au-

Table 27–3. Features to Consider in Selecting Treatment Outcomes Tools

Nationally Aggregated Service vs. In-House System

Nationally aggregated systems have the advantage of name recognition, assumed neutrality (therefore, perceived enhanced credibility), and the ability to benchmark against large databases, but usually offer little by way of customization. There are subscription fees and extra charges for additional reports. In-house systems allow you to select those measures and scales that are meaningful to your practice and provide greater flexibility in analyzing and cross-tabulating the data to answer the question of the moment—as long as you have access to the needed expertise.

Method of Data Collection

The array of data collection options is limited only by the user's creativity. Popular options include: paper and pencil tools with hand tallies and calculations; scannable forms completed by hand, then electronically read into a database; computer keyboard data entry into a database; and wandpen data entry from a screen. Deciding which option is for you usually involves a trade-off between the ease of ongoing use by clinical and support staff and the financial resources available.

Compatibility with the Program's Mission

If your goal is to measure overall rehab gains to market your rehabilitation program, global measures (i.e., "receptive" and "expressive") may meet your needs. However, if you need to document the additional benefits of eight versus two sessions of voice treatment, you will need a more precisely delineated instrument.

Dedicated Raters

Some outcomes systems allow raters to score any of the items, including those that would not be considered within their scope of practice (i.e., a speech–language pathologist could score mobility and transfer items, etc.). Others specify which disciplines can rate which items. An analysis of LORS-III items by Formations in Health Care, Inc., revealed that communication and cognition ratings at admission by speech–language pathologists were statistically significantly lower than those by other raters, underscoring the importance of having discipline-designated raters coding admission and discharge scores on specified items in order to minimize the effect of inter-rater reliability[a]

Scoring Every Item

Some insurance requires that all patients be scored on all items (i.e., total hip replacement patients would be scored on communication items, regardless of whether or not they present with a communication deficit). Such a requirement also means that all items are scored regardless of whether or not the deficit area is being addressed in treatment. The resulting data obviously is not related to intervention by clinical practitioners. When aggregated with measurements of patients who did demonstrate the presence of, and receive treatment for, a deficit in a given area, such data can alter the amount of measured change attributed to the intervention. Other instruments code these situations with a "N/A" or a "0" to assure that data was not omitted. In those cases, the resulting measurements have not been contaminated by a pool of data from patients who are not in need of, or who did not receive, treatment.

Recording the Amount of Treatment

Most instruments record the date of admission and discharge, but many do not capture other variables such as the amount of treatment provided (i.e., frequency and duration; interruptions to the course of treatment; whether discharge occurred before the patient completed the course of treatment; if the amount of treatment received was consistent with the amount recommended/needed); the level of practitioner (i.e., professional, assistant, aide) who provided the care, etc., which may affect the outcome.

[a]Pietranton A: A primer in outcomes measurements: What are they and where did they come from? TEJAS 1994/1995; 20(2):3–5.

Table 27–4. Functional Communication Measures (FCMs)

Speech production disorder

Voice disorder

Disorder of rate, rhythm, or fluency

Ability to swallow function

Comprehension of spoken language

Production of spoken language

Recognition of nonspoken language

Production of nonspoken language

Comprehension of written language

Production of written language

Cognitive communication

Hearing sensitivity

Central auditory processing

No FCM (i.e., "Other")

diology, pediatric, and birth to kindergarten populations. The validity of the instruments is being assessed through a series of Treatment Outcomes Grants awarded through the American Speech–Language-Hearing Foundation. A variety of distribution options for these instruments (i.e., making them available as stand-alone products, partnering with outcomes systems and consultants to have the scales from the instruments incorporated into other outcomes systems, etc.) are being explored.

CLINICAL PROTOCOLS

Outcomes data are more than just a negotiating tool; they are also an internal feedback loop about what works and what does not. To use outcomes data this way, we must be able to relate the measured outcome to the specifics of the clinical intervention in a predictable fashion—in other words, what clinical approach, or protocol, produced the observed results?

Traditionally, a high degree of variation has been tolerated in the delivery of health care services under the heading of "clinical judgment." John E. Wennberg is one of the pioneering researchers of variation in clinical practice. Some of his early studies in the 1960s focused on variations within individual states in the utilization rate for specific surgical procedures. Among his reported findings was a 250% variation in hysterectomy rate before age 70 between two locations less than 100 miles apart in the same state.[3] Innumerable other examples of variation across the spectrum of clinical practice have been cited, including the number of caesarean sections, the number of tonsillectomies, the rate of radical versus modified mastectomies, and on and on.

Research in clinical practice variation studies the relationship between the appropriateness of care and overutilization as well as underutilization. Although those relationships are not yet completely understood, it is now clear that a substantial portion of medical and surgical care does not benefit the patient who receives that care.

Table 27–5. Sample Scoring Guidelines for FCMs (Comprehension of Spoken Language)

Level 0   Unable to test

Level 1   No comprehension of spoken language

Level 2   Comprehension of spoken language is limited to familiar words and/or phrases related to personal needs; most responses are inaccurate or inappropriate

Level 3   Comprehension of spoken language consists primarily of simple statements about personal topics; repetition and/or rephrasing required. Accuracy of comprehension is erratic.

Level 4   Comprehension of spoken language is limited to the primary activities of daily living needs and simple ideas and frequently requires repetition and/or rephrasing.

Level 5   Comprehension of spoken language is normal for activities of daily living, but limited in complexity of form, content or use; self-monitoring is inconsistent.

Level 6   Comprehension of spoken language is normal in most situations, although minimal difficulty may occur; self-monitoring/self-correcting are present.

Level 7   Comprehension of spoken language is normal in all situations.

According to Donald Berwick, president and CEO of the Institute for Healthcare Improvement in Boston, MA, the proportion of inappropriate care varies with the procedure, test, drug, or surgery, but is rarely less than 10% and in some cases exceeds 50%.[3] Just as it is not unreasonable to ask questions such as: "Is MRI [magnetic resonance imaging], at a considerably greater cost, a substantially more effective diagnostic procedure than CT [computerized tomography] scan for a particular set of clinical symptoms?" or "Does surgical intervention, with a potential price tag in excess of $50,000 in combined hospital and professional fees, yield a better survival rate for a given cardiac condition than long-term pharmacological management?," it is not unreasonable to ask, "How do the measurable results differ from one speech–language pathology intervention to another?"

To study these differences, we must assure that the specifics of the interventions measured are the same from time to time, patient to patient, and practitioner to practitioner—in other words, that a clinical protocol was followed (or that the variation was purposeful and documented). The Joint Commission on Accreditation of Healthcare Organizations defines a clinical protocol as:

> A description of steps to be taken in patient care in specified circumstances, such as a description of the steps to be taken in the care of adult patients presenting with nontraumatic chest pain. This approach makes use of branching logic and of all pertinent data, both about the patient and from epidemiologic and other sources, to arrive at decisions that yield maximum benefit and minimum risk.[4]

A clinical protocol is comparable to what the profession of speech–language pathology defines as a "practice guideline"—a recommended set of procedures for a specific area of practice, based on research findings and current practice, that details the procedures involved and the knowledge and skills needed to perform the procedures competently.[5] It is an explicit commitment on the part of a provider or program to do things a certain way, unless documented otherwise. For that reason, clinical protocols are typically diagnosis-driven and customized to the patient population and setting. They usually vary from one program to another, unless each program has specifically chosen to adopt and follow the same clinical protocol(s). At a minimum, clinical protocols need to specify certain kinds of information (see Table 27–6).

With a large enough database, providers who deliver care according to established clinical protocols and collect outcomes data can easily assess the

Table 27–6. Clinical Protocols

Clinical Protocols Need to Specify:

Population—who should receive these services (i.e., age, primary and secondary diagnosis, setting, etc.)?

Provider—which discipline(s) and what level of practitioner (i.e., professional, assistant, aide) provide the service?

Clinical indications—what are the risk factors, symptoms, referral conditions, etc., that must be present to warrant the services?

Clinical process—what are the components of the services (i.e., the assessment tools, intervention methods, etc.)?

Setting/equipment specifications—what instrumentation and/or environmental resources are required to provide the services?

Documentation requirements—what information must be recorded and where is it filed (i.e., background, procedures, results and interpretation, prognosis, recommendations, etc.)?

Expected outcomes—what should be accomplished as a result of the services (i.e., information acquired, functional gains, etc.)?

Source: From American Speech–Language-Hearing Association: Preferred practice patterns. *Asha* 1993; 35(3).

effectiveness of their clinical protocol(s) and identify opportunities for improvement. Aggregating such information on a regional or national basis allows clinical providers to compare outcomes across protocols, thus objectively determining the most effective way of managing different patient populations and diagnoses. Clinical protocols are also another tool in one's negotiating armamentarium. They are an indication to the purchaser that you, the provider, have determined what means will be used to achieve the desired ends or outcomes.

Clinical Pathways

In those environments where speech–language pathologists are one of several disciplines working with a patient, their discipline-specific clinical protocols should in turn tie into clinical pathways (also known as critical paths, care maps, etc.). Clinical pathways are a multidisciplinary framework for coordinating the health care team's work in order to streamline and conform the delivery process (i.e., reduce the variation—see Table 27–7). They are a clinical management tool used to organize, sequence, and time the major interventions of the health care providers involved.[6] Like protocols, pathways stipulate the preferred pattern

Table 27-7. Goals and Quality Benchmarks for Stroke Clinical Pathway (Initial Stroke—First Admission)

PARTICIPANT NEEDS	WEEK #1	WEEK #2	WEEK #3	WEEK #4
1. <u>Medical Management</u>: (MD, RN, ARNP, OT, PT) Medical Problems Stroke Risk Factors Potential altered skin integrity Medication Administration	Medical problems, stroke risk factors, and appropriate treatment for these are identified; participant is able to verbalize these. Participant & family initiate preventive skin program. Participant participates in self-medication program.	Participant & family are unable to verbalize medical problems and stroke risk factors. Able to provide assistance with skin care strategies, participates in self-medication program.	Participant completes self-medication program. Participant & family able to inspect & perform skin care independently.	Participant & family verbalize understanding of discharge instructions and medical follow-up.
2. <u>Communication</u>: (ST, OT, RN) Comprehension: Expression:	Participant is able to follow simple directions and simple conversation. Needs cueing 75% of the time. FIM-2 Participant is able to respond to yes/no personal information questions. Needs cueing 75% of the time. FIM-2	Participant is able to follow simple directions & simple conversation. Needs cueing 50% of the time. FIM-3 Participant is able to communicate basic needs. Needs cueing less than 50% of the time. FIM-3	Participant is able to follow simple directions & simple conversation. Needs cueing 25% of the time. FIM-4 Participant is able to communicate basic needs. Needs cueing less than 25% of the time. FIM-4	Participant is able to follow simple directions & simple conversation. Needs cueing less than 10% of the time. FIM-5 Participant is able to communicate basic needs. Needs cueing less than 10% of the time. FIM-5
3. <u>Cognitive</u>: Memory: (ST, OT, RN, PT) Problem Solving/Safety Fall Risk: (ST, OT, RN, PT)	Participant recognizes and remembers 25%–50% of the time; needs prompting more than 50% of the time. FIM-2 Participant identifies that a routine problem exists and is able to initiate sequence to correct/scan environment less than 50% of the time. FIM-2	Participant refers to environmental cues without verbal cue 50% of the time. FIM-3 Participant initiates sequence to self-correct problems/scan environment 50–75% of the time. FIM-3	Participant refers to environmental cues 75% of the time. FIM-4 Participant is able to self-correct problems/scan environment 75–90% of the time. FIM-4	Participant refers to environmental cues 90% of the time. FIM-5
4. <u>Activities of Daily Living</u>: Self-Care Deficits (OT, RN, KT)	Participant performs self-care activities of feeding, bathing, personal grooming, and dressing/undressing 50% of the time. FIM-3	Participant performs self-care activities with adaptive equipment 50–75% of the time. FIM-3	Participant performs self-care activities with adaptive equipment more than 75% of the time. FIM-4	Participant is able to perform self-care activities with set-up and supervision, using adaptive equipment. FIM-5

Table 27-7. (continued)

PARTICIPANT NEEDS	WEEK #1	WEEK #2	WEEK #3	WEEK #4
5. Dysphagia: Dietary (ST, OT, RN)	Participant is able to indicate awareness of swallowing difficulty & possible aspiration. Participant receives adequate nutrition via appropriate mode (TF, 6T, altered food/liquid consistency, PO)	Participant is able to demonstrate safe compensatory safe swallowing techniques with maximum to moderate supervision.	Participant is able to perform compensatory techniques with moderate to minimum supervision.	Patient is able to perform compensatory techniques in safe swallowing techniques.
6. Continence: Bowel Management Neurogenic Bowel (RN)	Bowel accidents less often than daily. FIM-3	Participant is continent of bowel with bowel care Q.O.D. with suppository. FIM-4	Participant is continent of bowel with diet supplement and/or stool softener. FIM-6	
Bladder Management Neurogenic Bladder (RN)	Bladder accidents less often than daily. FIM-3	Participant uses urinal for voiding with setup; uses external urinary device at night. Accidents occur less often than weekly. FIM-4	Participant is continent, using toilet during waking hours; uses urinal for night voiding only. FIM-5	Participant is continent of bladder with no accidents. Independent with urinal. FIM-6
7. Mobility & Fall Prevention: (PT, KT, OT, RN) Balance Transfers	Participant is able to perform transfers with 50–25% assistance. FIM-3	Participant is able to perform transfers with 25% assistance. FIM-4	Participant performs transfers with supervision/stand-by assistance. FIM-5	
Wheelchair Mobility	Requires assistance with wheelchair mobility 50–25% of the time. FIM-3	Participant is independent in wheelchair mobility for short distances on the ward and in P.T. clinic. FIM-5	Participant is independent in wheelchair mobility on the ward and to/from therapies for short distances. FIM-5	Independent in wheelchair mobility on all terrain, inclines, curbs, and carpeting. FIM-6
Gait/Ambulation	Participant is able to initiate pre-gait/balance activities in the parallel bars with 75% assistance. FIM-2	Requires 25% assistance with long-distance wheelchair mobility. FIM-4 Participant is able to initiate gait activities with assistive device with 50% assistance. FIM-3	Participant ambulates with assistive device and with 50% assistance. FIM-3	Participant ambulates independently a minimum of 150 feet with assistive device and/or orthosis with contact guard/25% assistance. FIM-4
8. Sexuality: (MD, RN, ARNP)	Participant & spouse will identify sexuality issues.	The participant & spouse will understand common problems of stroke participants with sexuality issues.	Participant & spouse can identify supportive resources.	

677

Table 27-7. (continued)

PARTICIPANT NEEDS	WEEK #1	WEEK #2	WEEK #3	WEEK #4
9. Discharge Planning: (SWS, PT, OT, ST, RN)	Participant & family identify current social service needs. Participant & family identify tentative discharge needs. Participant & family present model of home environment.	Participants & family are aware of discharge options. Participant & family follow-up on social service referrals (i.e., food stamps, public assistance, etc.).	Participant & family finalize discharge plans (i.e., home, NHCU, HBHC, Home Health Care Agency, OP, other VA).	Participant & family acknowledge discharge plans completed. Successful discharge accomplished and appropriate follow-up established.
10. Equipment:	Participant receives initial assessment of ADL and functional status to determine basic equipment needs.	Participant begins training in use of assistive devices/adaptive equipment. Participant & family receive necessary equipment for use on therapeutic weekend pass; receive appropriate training in use of equipment.	Participant equipment needs are adjusted according to changing status. Participant & family demonstrate safe use of equipment 80% of the time.	Participant receives all necessary equipment for post-discharge use. Participant & caregiver understand safe effective use of all equipment.
11. Psychosocial Needs: (SWS) Spiritual (RT) Leisure (VRT) Vocation	Participant & family participate in interview with SWS to assess psychosocial needs. Primary caregiver is identified. Leisure & vocational needs identified.	Participant & family receive ongoing supportive therapeutic contact, leisure alternatives, and participate in vocational evaluation.	Participant & family aware of community resources for spiritual, leisure, and vocational needs.	Participant & family demonstrate improved coping/adjustment to lifestyle change.
12. Education: (MD, RN, PT, OT, KT, ST, RT, VRT, SWS, ARNP)	Participant & family are aware of learning needs.	Participant & family demonstrate readiness to learn/begin participation in program.	Participant & family able to perform home exercise programs, safe use of equipment, and safety techniques with supervision.	Participant & family able to demonstrate knowledge of meds, diet, home care, exercises, equipment use, and follow-up care.
Concur with rehab goals:				
Barriers to goal attainment:				
Tentative discharge date:				
Next review date:				

Source: From the James A. Haley Veterans' Hospital, Tampa, FL, Physical Medicine and Rehabilitation Service. Reprinted with permission.

of service delivery, while recognizing that variation will undoubtedly occur. Monitoring and tracking variances from the established pathway are an integral part of using clinical pathways. Variances are typically coded into different categories (i.e., patient/family, provider, setting, community, or event not applicable). This way the causes of the variation can be identified and tracked. All the providers involved are on the "same sheet of music" in terms of the what, when, and how of delivering care, but always have the option—and the responsibility—of altering the plan when the patient or circumstances warrant.

ALTERNATIVE PERSONNEL OPTIONS

There are over 200 different recognized clinical disciplines in the health arena alone. Concern over the continued expansion and specialization of clinical disciplines throughout this century, coupled with a desire to decrease costs by increasing efficiencies, has led some to question the composition of, and boundaries within, the current clinical workforce. An adjunct to identifying the best approach(es) to and amount(s) of service is determining the most appropriate level(s) of provider(s) for the service. Two categories of alternative clinical personnel are receiving heightened consideration: support personnel and multiskilled personnel.

Speech–Language Pathology Assistants

Clinical support personnel, or assistants, have been used by some speech–language pathologists for decades as a cost-effective way of extending speech–language pathology professionals. Assistants provide those clinical services that are more repetitive or routine. The American Speech–Language-Hearing Association (ASHA) Position Statement for the Training, Credentialing, Use, and Supervision of Support Personnel in Speech–Language Pathology was approved in 1994,[7] followed by the Guidelines for the Training, Credentialing, Use, and Supervision of Speech–Language Pathology Assistants in 1995.[8] The Guidelines state that "support personnel are people who, following academic and/or on-the-job training, perform tasks as prescribed, directed, and supervised by certified speech–language pathologists."[8] According to the ASHA guidelines, support personnel can be used to increase the frequency, efficiency, and availability of services; they can assist the supervising speech–language pathologist with generalization of learned skills to mul-

tiple settings; they can assist with habilitation and restorative programs; and they can perform nonclinical duties, freeing up more of the speech–language pathologists' time for clinical services.

The appropriate use of support personnel can increase access to care for diverse and underserved patient/client populations, and enhance diversity in the work force by having different levels of entry into the profession. The use of well-trained and well-supervised support personnel is one way of increasing the frequency of services while maintaining their quality. Certain tasks, procedures, or activities used with individuals with communication disorders can be performed successfully by persons other than certified speech–language pathologists (see Table 27–8) if those conducting the activity are properly trained and supervised by ASHA-certified speech–language pathologists. The decision to shift responsibility for implementation of the more repetitive, mechanical, or routine clinical activities to assistants should be made only by qualified professionals and only when the quality of care and the level of professionalism will not be compromised (see Table 27–9). Professional judgment should always be at the heart of the selection, management, supervision, and use of support personnel.[8]

Multiskilled Personnel

Like support personnel, the concept of multiskilled personnel is not new. Multiskilled personnel, or multiskilling, has been discussed for decades by the American Hospital Association, W. K. Kellogg Foundation, the Pew Health Professions Commission, and some health professions. To date, there is no universally accepted or officially approved definition of the term. However, a national Multiskilled Health Practitioner Clearinghouse was established in 1987 at the University of Alabama at Birmingham's School of Health Related Professions that defines multiskilled health practitioners as:

> Persons cross-trained to provide more than one function, often in more than one discipline. These combined functions can be found in a broad spectrum of health-related jobs ranging in complexity from the nonprofessional to the professional level, including both clinical and management functions. The additional functions (skills) added to the original health care worker's job may be of a higher, lower, or parallel level.[9]

The intent of multicompetency is the more efficient and effective use of human resources. A 3-year study by Booz, Allen, and Hamilton found

Table 27–8. Scope of Responsibilities for a Speech–Language Pathology Assistant

Provided that the training, supervision, documentation, and planning are appropriate, the following tasks may be designated to a speech–language pathology assistant:

Conduct speech–language screenings (without interpretation) following specified screening protocols developed by the supervising speech–language pathologist.

Provide direct treatment assistance to patients/clients identified by the supervising speech–language pathologist.

Follow documented treatment plans or protocols developed by the supervising speech–language pathologist.

Document patient/client progress toward meeting established objectives as stated in the treatment plan, and report this information to the supervising speech–language pathologist.

Assist the speech–language pathologist during assessment of patient/clients, such as those who are difficult to test.

Assist with informal documentation (e.g., tallying notes for the speech–language pathologist to use), prepare materials, and assist with other clerical duties as directed by the speech–language pathologist.

Schedule activities, prepare charts, records, graphs, or otherwise display data.

Perform checks and maintenance of equipment.

Participate with the speech–language pathologist in research projects, in-service training, and public relations program.

Source: American Speech–Language-Hearing Association: *Guidelines for the training, credentialing, use, and supervision of speech–language pathology assistants. Asha* 1996; 38(2):21–34.

that, of every dollar a hospital spends on wages, 20 cents goes to structural idle time (in Brider[10]). Current viewpoints about multiskilling run the gamut from acquiring additional basic patient care skills, to taking lead responsibility for administrative functions, to developing new professions such as a "rehab specialist" who could practice across multiple scopes of practice.

ASHA's Ad Hoc Committee on Multiskilling developed a technical report on Multiskilling.[11] It discusses the dimensions of multiskilling (see Table 27–10) and issues related to the heterogeneity of the health care workforce with regard to preparation, autonomy, and level of patient contact. An ASHA Position Statement on Multiskilled Personnel was approved in 1996 and states:

> It is the position of the American Speech–Language-Hearing Association that multiskilling is not a unidimensional concept and that it cannot be evenly applied across the diverse clinical workforce. Specifically, cross-training of clinical skills is not appropriate at the professional level of practice (i.e., audiologists or speech–language pathologists). Cross-training of basic patient care skills, professional nonclinical skills, and/or administrative skills is a reasonable option that clinical practitioners at all levels of practice may need to consider depending on the service delivery setting, geographic location, patient/client population, and clinical workforce resources.[12]

As evidenced by input from speech–language pathologists attending ASHA Town Meetings in 1996, there is mixed opinion regarding the appropriateness of the use of alternative personnel to deliver speech–language pathology services. Those in favor of speech–language pathology assistants cite the need of lowering the costs of delivering services to assure continued access and funding for patients and the opportunity for professional level practitioners to focus more of their time on those services that require ongoing clinical judgment and decision making. Opponents believe that the use of speech–language pathology assistants will lower professional standards and result in fewer jobs for certified speech–language pathologists. Advocates for multiskilling identify its potential benefits as enhanced opportunities for professional growth and development, expanded scopes of practice, increased employability and job security, improved efficiency and coordination of clinical services, and the opportunity for professional-level practitioners to focus on the more clinically challenging services. Adversaries believe that the risks associated with multiskilling include potential decreases in the quality and outcome of clinical services, loss of specialized clinical services, loss of autonomy, erosion of scopes of practice, loss of revenue, and reduced numbers of positions for some clinical service providers.

Table 27–9. Activities Outside the Scope of Responsibilities of a Speech–Language Pathology Assistant

The speech–language pathology assistant may not

Perform standardized or nonstandardized diagnostic tests, formal or informal evaluations, or interpret test results.

Participate in parent conferences, case conferences, or any interdisciplinary team without the presence of the supervising speech–language pathologist or other ASHA-certified speech–language pathologist designated by the supervising speech–language pathologist.

Provide patient/client or family counseling.

Write, develop, or modify a patient/client's individualized treatment plan in any way.

Assist with patients/clients without following the individualized treatment plan prepared by the speech–language pathologist or without access to supervision.

Sign any formal documents (e.g., treatment plans, reimbursement forms, or reports; the assistant should sign or initial informal treatment notes for review and co-signature by the supervising professional).

Select patients/clients for services.

Discharge a patient/client from services.

Disclose clinical or confidential information either orally or in writing to anyone not designated by the supervising specch–language pathologist.

Make referrals for additional service.

Communicate with the patient/client, family, or others regarding any aspect of the patient/client status or service without the specific consent of the supervising speech–language pathologist.

Represent himself or herself as a speech–language pathologist.

Source: American Speech–Language-Hearing Association: *Guidelines for the training, credentialing, use, and supervision of speech–language pathology assistants. Asha* 1996; 38(2):21–34.

Various health care decision makers, including some state legislatures, are making decisions and implementing changes related to the clinical workforce. The time has come for speech–language pathologists to move beyond discussion and debate regarding the use of alternative personnel. While the existing resource documents concerning speech–language pathology assistants and multiskilled personnel provide a framework for their role, each speech–language pathology program must determine the best use of such personnel based on the nature of the population served, type of setting, other provider resources available, and the mission of the organization.

INNOVATIVE SERVICE DELIVERY MODELS

As caseloads change and clinicians are faced with mounting budgetary restrictions, the demand for innovative service delivery models has increased. While there is a wide array of possibilities, four in particular demand exploration: prevention-focused services, new treatment models, contin-

uum shifts and employment opportunities, and responding to market needs.

Prevention

Historically, prevention of communication disorders has not been a focus of service delivery for speech–language pathologists, who have tended to focus on the identification, assessment, and treatment of communication disorders. Given that communication is the most fundamental and essential of all human skills and that reliable communication skills are a requisite for individuals to achieve their social, educational, and vocational potentials, such services will continue to be critical in our culture. However, in a increasingly capitated reimbursement environment, prevention is not only of intrinsic value, it is of financial value as well since the up-front expenditure of human and financial resources to prevent a disorder from occurring are usually more then offset by the savings from decreased utilization of evaluation and treatment services further down the road. An additional benefit is that public health and prevention-oriented initiatives are viewed as a commitment to the larger

Table 27–10. Dimensions of Multiskilling

Cross-Training of Basic Patient Care Skills that includes routine, frequently provided, easily trainable, low-risk procedures such as suctioning patients, monitoring vital signs, and transferring and positioning patients. Identifying a facility/agency/ program-specific set of patient care skills that can be performed by various practitioners in that particular setting may lead to less fragmented and less costly patient care (e.g., bedside treatment sessions do not have to be delayed waiting for another practitioner to suction the patient; home care patients' compliance with prescribed medications can be verified by clinicians already coming to the home on a regular basis; diabetic preschoolers' blood sugar levels can be monitored by on-site clinicians).

Cross-Training of Clinical Disciplines that involves training practitioners in one discipline to perform services traditionally regarded as within the purview or scope of practice of another discipline in an attempt to more efficiently deploy the clinical workforce to meet the needs of the patient caseload as it fluctuates at any particular time. Examples include training respiratory therapists to perform EEGs (electroencephalograms), or medical technologists to perform certain radiological procedures.

Cross-Training of Professional, Nonclinical Skills that includes skills and services such as patient education, technical writing, and team dynamics/communication/ leadership. Establishing competency standards for such skills across the workforce may enhance the overall quality, efficiency, and coordination of service delivery.

Cross-Training of Administrative Skills that includes programmatic activities such as quality improvement, case management, systems design, and the management of clinical services. As organizations downsize, increasingly, such responsibilities are no longer centralized into one or more "administrative positions," but often distributed among clinical practitioners. Doing so may result in more efficient use of staff and better integration of these functions with clinical service delivery.

Clinical Skills That Span a Discipline need to be recognized and acknowledged. Some clinical practitioners already possess knowledge and skills that span a complex and essential domain of human function and already are able to provide a variety of services to an array of patients as a result of their broad and complex scopes of practice. Speech–language pathologists and audiologists are such practitioners as evidenced by the range of services they provide (i.e., audiologists diagnose hearing loss and related disorders, fit hearing aids, provide aural rehabilitation, perform and interpret site-of-lesion testing, etc.; speech–language pathologists evaluate and treat cognitive-communication, language, memory, swallowing, fluency, and/or voice disorders, etc.).

Source: American Speech–Language-Hearing Association: *Technical report of the Ad Hoc Committee on Multiskilling. Asha* 1996; 38(2): 53–61.

community and well received from a community relations perspective. Speech–language pathology prevention services require increased efforts to eliminate the onset of communication disorders and their causes and promote the development and maintenance of optimal communication. ASHA's Committee on Prevention of Speech, Language, and Hearing Disorders described three levels of prevention activity related to communication disorders[13] (see Table 27–11).

New Treatment Models

Determining the most appropriate and effective use of group, consultative, collaborative, technology-assisted, and family/volunteer-assisted approaches to treatment is no longer desirable—it is mandatory. Likewise, the most effective combination of frequency, length, and duration of treatment services must be ascertained. Clinical protocols that systematically control for these variables, coupled with careful analysis of the resulting treatment outcomes, are needed to determine the optimum combinations for different patient population and circumstances.

Continuum and Employment Opportunities

As hospital lengths of stay decrease, an increasing percentage of speech–language pathology services are being provided in subacute, rehabilitation,

Table 27–11. Prevention of Communication Disorders

Primary prevention

The elimination or inhibition of the onset and development of a communication disorder by altering susceptibility or reducing exposure for susceptible persons.

Secondary prevention

The early detection and treatment of communication disorders. Early detection and treatment may lead to the elimination of the disorder or the retardation of the disorder's progress, thereby preventing further complications.

Tertiary prevention

The reduction of a disability by attempting to restore effective functioning. The major approach is rehabilitation of the disabled individual who has realized some residual problem as a result of the disorder.

Source: American Speech–Language-Hearing Association: *Position statement on prevention of communicable disorders.* Washington, DC, 1988.

skilled nursing, home health, hospice, and outpatient settings. Concomitantly, there is widespread consolidation of departments, elimination of middle managers, and implementation of patient-focused care in many clinical settings, leading to the decline of the traditional departmental structure. It is very likely that the number of full-time employee positions that are compensated via an annual salary and benefits package will decline as more organizations seek to limit their costs through the use of contract and/or per diem providers. More than ever, speech–language pathologists must be innovative in seeking and identifying professional opportunities. Today's practitioners need to be entrepreneurs who are skilled at marketing their skills, promoting their cost-effectiveness, and creating a demand for their services so that they maximize their career opportunities, strengthen their financial security, and ensure their clinical autonomy.

Market Needs

The clinical characteristics, distinguishing features, and social demographics of speech–language pathology caseloads are changing. Currently, approximately 12% (28 million) Americans are over the age of 65. By the year 2040, that number is projected to increase to 68 million. The fastest growing segment of our population is the "old-old," those over 80, which is projected to increase more than 400% over the next 25 years. By the turn of

this century, it is anticipated that one-third of the U.S. population will be members of racial and linguistic minorities. There is substantial regional variation in the distribution of such demographic variables throughout the United States, which in turn produces differences in the incidence and prevalence of various communication needs. When coupled with such factors as access to, and community saturation of professional resources, the result is tremendous variability in "market-needs" from one community to another. Another rapidly growing factor is the demand for "corporate-communication" skills such as vocal use, accent reduction and the like. Today's speech–language pathologists need to assess the needs and opportunities of their local market.

SUMMARY

Clinical service delivery is changing at a sometimes dizzying pace in the final decade of the twentieth century. Change is all around us as we head toward the year 2000. The World Wide Web, little more than a nebulous curiosity to most just a few years ago, is now a daily reality for many—including preschoolers and elementary school children. Cellular phones, compact discs, and minivans, now taken for granted as ordinary resources, were rare as recently as 5 years ago. So it is also true for the clinical arena where speech–language pathologists now routinely assess and treat communicative-cognitive disorders, conduct videoflouroscopic examinations, fit and dispense tracheoesophageal voice protheses—aspects of clinical practice that not so long ago were considered "cutting edge."

Much has been written about change—how to cope with it, how to facilitate it—how to accept it for the reality that it is.[14] The legacy of W. Edwards Deming, the founding father of quality improvement,[15] is that change is required. To paraphrase the writings of Charles Darwin offers an even more compelling perspective on change—adapt or die. Perhaps the best way to align the mix of emotions change generates is to keep in mind the Chinese word for crises, which is represented by a combination of the symbols for danger and opportunity. So it is with change—a combination of challenges and opportunities. During this era of clinical service delivery reform, medical speech–language pathologists must accept and address the challenges so that they may help shape the solutions—and seize the opportunities that emerge for new and innovative ways of serving individuals with communication and related disorders.

STUDY QUESTIONS

1. Why are the escalating costs of health care and the shift of political power and decision making from the federal to the state level of concern regarding access to and funding of speech–language pathology services?

2. How does a capitation payment system differ from fee-for-service coverage of clinical services?

3. Why is clinical efficiency a paramount issue in a managed care dominated system of clinical service delivery?

4. What kind of questions do treatment outcomes measures intend to answer? How are they different from treatment efficacy questions?

5. Identify and describe the pros and cons of at least four features that should be considered in selecting a treatment outcomes tool.

6. What is a clinical protocol and how does it help reduce clinical variation?

7. What are the pros and cons associated with the use of alternative personnel in the delivery of speech–language pathology services?

8. Describe at least two examples (including the circumstances under which they might be considered) for each of the following: cross-training of basic patient care skills; cross-training of clinical disciplines; and, cross-training of administrative skills.

9. Why is prevention an increasing important service delivery option? What are some examples of prevention services in speech–language pathology?

10. How do demographics influence the need for speech–language pathology services?

REFERENCES

1. Banja JD: Ethics, outcomes, and reimbursement. *REHAB Manag* 1994; 7(1): 61–65, 136.

2. Hengst WG: The cutting edge for improving care. *Adv Dir Rehab* 1994; 3(7): 29–33.

3. Berwick D: Improving the appropriateness of care. *Qual Connect* 1994; 3(1): 4–6.

4. Joint Commission on Accreditation of Healthcare Organizations: *Lexikon: Dictionary of health care terms, organizations, and acronyms for the era of reform.* JCAHO, Oakbrook Terrace, IL, 1994.

5. American Speech–Language-Hearing Association: *Preferred practice patterns. Asha* 1993; 35(3).

6. Shekim L: Critical pathways. *Quality improvement digest.* American Speech–Language-Hearing Association, Rockville, MD, 1994.

7. American Speech–Language-Hearing Association: *Position statement for the training, credentialing, use and supervision of support personnel in speech–language pathology. Asha* 1995; 37 (Suppl. 14): 21.

8. American Speech–Language-Hearing Association: *Guidelines for the training, credentialing, use, and supervision of speech–language pathology assistants. Asha* 1996; 38(2): 21–34.

9. Bamberg R, Blayney KD, Vaughn DG, Wilson, BR: *Multiskilled health practitioner education: A national perspective.* University of Alabama at Birmingham, School of Health Related Professions, National Multiskilled Health Practitioner Clearinghouse, 1989.

10. Brider P: The move to patient-focused care. *Amer J Nurs* 1992; 9: 26–33.

11. American Speech–Language-Hearing Association: *Technical report of the Ad Hoc Committee on Multiskilling. Asha* 1996; 38(2), 53–61.

12. American Speech–Language-Hearing Association: *Position statement on multiskilled personnel. Asha* 1996; 39(2), 13.

13. American Speech–Language-Hearing Association: *Position statement on prevention of communication disorders.* Washington, DC, Author, 1988.

14. Pietranton A: Health care reform: What does it mean for speech–language pathologists and audiologists? *Hearsay* 1995; 10(1), 13–18.

15. Walton M: *The Deming management method.* Perigee, New York, 1986.

28

Outcomes Assessment in Speech–Language Pathology

CAROL M. FRATTALI

CHAPTER OUTLINE

Current Requirements

Outcomes Assessment: Definitions, Measures, and Methods

Using Outcomes Data for Decision Making

The U.S. health care system, particularly in its hybrid forms of managed care, has become a business not unlike the manufacturing business. While the analogy is a poor one given that the health care product to which is referred is the clinical management of the complexities of human disease or injury processes and its outcomes, a buyer's expectation is that the value of health care services, like other products or services, can be determined on the basis of objective and meaningful performance data.

Consider, for example, the process of buying a car. Before purchasing, consumers expect to see specifications of the car's physical features, comfort, gas efficiency, and ergonomics; how it handles on city roads and interstates; its maintenance record and availability of parts; its safety record. Consumers also want to know the cost so that they can estimate its value. They seldom will buy the least expensive, but rather, the best for the money. Without both performance and cost data, consumers would not consider buying; with this information against which to compare the features of other cars, consumers will shop around.

Suppliers of manufactured goods have learned that they cannot engage in successful business practices without objective performance data, nor can they generate meaningful data without seeking and factoring in the opinions of the buyers themselves. Suppliers do this to continually improve their products and offer buyers precisely what they want to meet their expectations (sometimes even more than they want in an effort to exceed their expectations), if only to survive in a competitive marketplace. Progress and innovation become by-products of the process.

When health care is purchased, its buyers (either consumers themselves or the agents working in their behalf) expect objective information similar to that for manufactured goods. They want data about the performance of providers, their qualifications, and their competence and track record in conducting specific clinical procedures; the amenities of care (convenient parking, comfort, privacy and confidentiality, access to the most advanced technologies); the relative risks of morbidity and mortality; rates of cure; and rates of functional improvement. Also, as with cars, consumers want

685

to know what health care costs so they may estimate its value. These calculations require access to outcomes data, as well as data from the perspectives of health care consumers themselves. If the perceived benefits are not considered to be worth the cost, consumers (including large employers and public payers) most certainly will seek provision of health care from other providers.

This chapter details the current accreditation and payer requirements that are driving the need for collecting and managing outcomes data; offer definitions and a conceptual model of patient outcomes and their measurement; describe various measures and methods in use in the field of speech–language pathology; and suggest ways in which outcomes data can be used for decision making.

CURRENT REQUIREMENTS

The business of health care today, given the choices of health plans and the active participation of consumers in making these choices, begs the question, "Whom do health care providers need to satisfy?" There would be little argument that, foremost, providers need to satisfy their patients by meeting their individual needs. Second, providers need to satisfy payors and regulators who have the tough job of managing limited resources. These parties, particularly in managed care environments, are largely responsible for the decisions surrounding provision of both effective and efficient care. In large measure, they determine what services will be provided to whom, by whom, in what setting, for how long, and at what cost. Their interest is in getting the "best" for the dollars spent. Thus, the primary measure of health care is in determining its *value* (good care at a low cost).

Particularly noteworthy, in terms consistent with a common mindset among payers, is a quote from a payor who addressed an audience of rehabilitation professionals at a national meeting:[1]

> If I (the buyer of care) give you (the provider of care) X dollars, I get one point on a functional status measure. If other providers can give me two points after the same treatment time, I'll buy from them. I'm a buyer. I want to get more for my money. I am paying you to maximize the level of independence.

What this buyer was seeking was, in his words, a "quantitative measure of a qualitative product" (i.e., rehabilitative services). Thus, functional status measures have become the measure of choice among many payors because they speak in meaningful terms (e.g., levels of independence in daily

life activities) and translate into dollars saved by suggesting the need for fewer health care resources as the patient's independence is attained. This cost perspective, which favors functional status as a desired or expected outcome of medical rehabilitation, is reflected in several important accreditation agency standards and payer guidelines (Table 28–1).

Accreditation agencies and payors are emphasizing the use of outcome measures, particularly for assessing functional status and patient satisfaction, to document the benefits of treatment. The requirements specify that these outcome measures should be used for comparative purposes (i.e., for comparing patient progress to baseline performance or one program's performance to another's). They do not, however, dictate which specific measures or methods should be used. These decisions are left to the provider who must identify, from the wide array of measures and methods available, the most appropriate for their particular patient populations and in their particular health care settings.

OUTCOMES ASSESSMENT: DEFINITIONS, MEASURES, AND METHODS

Measuring outcomes is a complex activity because of the scope of their defining characteristics, growing number of measures currently available with their varying purposes and psychometric properties, and various methods of assessment. A simple comparison of the results yielded from pre- and post-treatment measures for individual patients can be considered outcomes assessment; so can statistical analysis of aggregate data generated from automated outcomes management systems that capture multiple outcomes of treatment while adjusting for various risks for large patient groups. Outcomes assessment can involve a case report or randomized controlled clinical trials. Outcome measures can be simple rating scales developed by group consensus, or highly standardized tests supported by rigorous psychometric research. Given the range of measures and methods that constitute "outcomes assessment," it is important to clarify what is meant by the term using currently accepted definitions and a conceptual model of patient outcomes.

Definitions of Terms

Simply defined, an *outcome* is the result of an intervention. In the context of health care, Donabedian[7] describes the multifactorial nature of the term *outcome,* defining it as:

Table 28–1. Examples of Accreditation Agency and Payor Requirements

Source	Excerpts from Requirements/Guidelines
Joint Commission on Accreditation of Healthcare Organizations[2]	**Assessment of Patient Function (PE):** The goal of the patient assessment function is to determine what kind of care is required to meet a patient's initial needs as well as his or her needs as they change in response to care. PE 1.3 Functional status is assessed when warranted by the patient's needs or condition. PE1.3.1 All patients referred to rehabilitation services receive a functional assessment.
CARF . . . The Rehabilitation Accreditation Commission[3]	**Principle #4:** Based on the informed choices of the persons served, the organization, using a team approach, provides coordinated, individualized, goal-oriented services leading to desired outcomes. **Accreditation Criteria #3: The Organization Meets the Policy on Outcomes** The organization should demonstrate that systems are in place to measure outcomes including effectiveness, efficiency, satisfaction of persons served, and status of the persons served after discharge (follow-up). These outcome measures should be in place for all programs for which the organization is seeking accreditation. The organization should demonstrate the utilization of outcome information throughout its planning activities. This information should be provided to the persons served, personnel, payers, and if requested, CARF.
American Speech–Language-Hearing Association's Professional Services Board[4]	**Standard 3.0 Quality Improvement and Program Evaluation Implementation** The plan for ongoing quality improvement periodically addresses all standards, with particular attention to services that are of high volume or that carry added risk, emphasizing client evaluation and/or treatment outcomes; these may include, but are not limited to, identification of disorder, acceptance of recommendations, functional change in status, client/family satisfaction, and others appropriate to the population.
Medicare: Intermediary Manual Part 3—Claims Process[5]	Progress reports. Obtain: The initial functional communication level of the patient. The present functional level of the patient and progress. The medical reviewer may approve the claim if there is still a reasonable expectation that significant improvement in the patient's overall functional ability will occur . . . The speech–language pathologist may choose how to demonstrate progress. However, the method chosen and the measures used generally remain the same for the duration of treatment. The provider must interpret reports of test scores or comparable measures and their relationship to functional goals.
Medicare: Outpatient Rehabilitation Services Forms 700 (Plan of Care and Assessment) and 701 (Updated Plan of Care and Patient Progress)[6]	Form 700 requires an initial assessment detailing the level of function at the start of care, and documentation of functional goals. Also requires documentation of the patient's functional level at the end of the billing Form 701 requires an update of functional goals and a statement of functional level at the end of each billing period as compared to the previous month or initial assessment.

A change in a patient's current and future health status that can be attributed to antecedent health care. Change includes improvement of social and psychological function in addition to the more usual emphasis on the physical and physiological aspects of performance. By still another extension, [change includes] patient attitudes (including satisfaction), health-related knowledge acquired by the patient, and health-related behavioral change. All of these can be seen either as components of current health or as contributions to future health (pp. 82–83).

A clinical intervention, therefore, does not result in a single outcome; it results in several and reflects the varying perspectives of the patients and their agents, including families, physicians, payers, employers, and administrators. Thus, outcomes can be:

- *Clinically derived* (e.g., ability to sustain phonation, accuracy in naming, type and frequency of disfluencies in a speech sample, integrity of the swallowing mechanism)
- *Functional* (e.g., ability to communicate basic needs, use the telephone, read the newspaper)
- *Social* (e.g., employability, ability to learn, community reintegration)
- *Patient-defined* (e.g., satisfaction with treatment; quality of life)

Outcomes may also define programmatic characteristics and desired operational changes. They, therefore, can also be:

- *Administrative* (e.g., patient referral patterns, average lengths of stay, rates of missed sessions, productivity levels in direct patient care)
- *Financial* (e.g., cost-effective care, cost/benefit of care, rate of rehospitalizations, levels of independence as an economic factor)

Outcomes as a Factor of Time

Outcomes can occur at any point during or after the course of clinical interventions, with their temporal order giving rise to the terms *intermediate, instrumental,* and *ultimate outcomes.*[8] *Intermediate outcomes* determine, from session to session, whether treatment is benefiting the patient. These outcomes allow investigation of the treatment process and can, for example, determine whether certain treatment methods (e.g., oral/facial exercises, head positioning) are necessary for adequate chewing and swallowing. *Instrumental outcomes* activate the learning process. These are outcomes that, when reached, trigger the ultimate outcome. Theoretically, once an instrumental outcome is reached, treatment is no longer necessary, for the patient will continue to improve on his or her own. It raises the "how long to treat" question, a question of particular interest to payers. Finally, *ultimate outcomes* are those that demonstrate the social or ecological validity of interventions, such as functional communication, reemployability, and social integration. Ultimate outcomes are most meaningful to patients and their families: "How will this treatment make me a more effective communicator?" "How will it enhance my ability to learn in school?" "To get a job?"

Considering outcomes as a factor of time, both short- and long-term effects of interventions can be measured. While most would agree that long-term outcomes are of greater significance as indicators of treatment benefit, they are the most difficult to measure for several reasons. First, patients can be lost to follow-up: patients die, develop secondary morbidities, relocate, or lose interest in participating in research activities. Second, it becomes more difficult to link treatment and outcome when other intervening variables outside the control of investigators fill the time gap. Finally, it requires considerable human and financial resources to conduct longitudinal studies, often an activity unsupported by payors of care who are focused on quick results and initial expenses of rehabilitation, rather than long-term savings to the health care system.

Measurable Aspects of Outcomes

In the field of speech–language pathology, a goal or desired outcome of treatment might be to improve the patient's functional communication. Thus, if a clinician wants to capture functional communication, it must be measured in some manner. The focus on assessment, particularly if the clinician wants it to be objective and measurable, requires operational definition. Thus, the clinician must determine what exactly is meant by "functional." In the hospital setting, it may mean communicating basic needs to hospital staff. If focused at the outset of treatment on discharge, functional communication may be regarded as communication that allows the individual to function independently (e.g., telephone interactions, responding in an emergency, social communication, understanding TV/radio). As time passes, our focus on functional communication may involve the ability to become reemployed or return to school. Thus, functional communication becomes more individually defined and may involve higher level skills (e.g., writing business letters, completing forms, reading and comprehending books, following complex instructions, preparing and delivering oral presentations). The term "communication" must also be defined. For example, does the term mean auditory comprehension and verbal expression only? Does it include nonverbal skills? With a partner? In a group? Does it include reading and writing skills? Does it include speech intelligibility or does it mean only that a message was conveyed regardless of articulatory precision? The questions lead to answers that form the content of operational definitions and, consequently, selection of appropriate instruments that are believed to accurately and sensitively capture the targeted behavior.

Deming[9] devotes an entire chapter of his book, *Out of the Crisis,* to formulation of operational definitions as requisite to measurement:

> Adjectives like good, reliable, uniform, round, tired, safe, unsafe . . . have no communicable meaning until they are expressed in operational terms of sampling, test, and criterion. . . . We have seen in many places how important it is that buyer and seller understand each other. They must both use the same kind of centimetre. . . . This requirement has meaning only if instruments are in statistical control. Without operational definition, a specification is meaningless (p. 277).

Indeed, providers are best advised to measure "changes," whether clinically derived, functional, social, administrative, or financial, by means of instruments that stem from operational definitions. Further, these instruments must be reliable and valid if the derived data are to be meaningful. In addition, the perspectives of payors would add to the desired features of outcome measures in that they are quantitative (results expressed in scores or ratings) and comprehensible (written in language understandable or meaningful to the layperson).

A Conceptual Framework of Patient Outcomes

The range and interrelationships among patient outcomes, as well as their defining characteristics, have been expressed in several conceptual frameworks found in the professional literature. These models have been described and applied directly to the care of individuals in diagnosis and treatment, evaluation of treatment results, assessment for work and school, and facilitation of communication between various categories of health care workers and coordination between different levels of care. While the international classification scheme of the World Health Organization (WHO)[10] is perhaps the most widely known, other models have been proposed (e.g., References 11, 12), with classifications distinguishing functional limitations and disabilities and (instead of handicaps), and social science and biomedical paradigms becoming more accepted.

Even though the World Health Organization[10] International Classification of Impairments, Disabilities and Handicaps (ICIDH) has been the subject of criticism (e.g., its use of the politically incorrect term "handicap"; its perceived lack of designation of the interrelationships among its classifications; its biomedical versus social science

orientation), it still remains a useful and widely used model, particularly for identifying the consequential phenomena of disease or injury. (Currently, an ICIDH-2 is in Beta testing, with classifications including impairments, activities, and participation. This new model is expected to be finalized by 1999.)

The ICIDH[10] links a chain of principal events that occur in the development of illnesses or injuries:

1. Something abnormal happens (a pathology occurs).
2. Someone becomes aware of such an occurrence (recognition of *impairment*).
3. The individual's performance or behavior may be altered and common activities may be restricted (giving rise to a *disability*).
4. The individual is placed at a disadvantage relative to others, thus socializing the experience (creating a *handicap*).

The WHO, then, defines the consequences of disease as follows:

Impairment: Any loss or abnormality of psychological, physiological, or anatomical structure or function. It represents deviation from a norm.

Disability: Any restriction of lack of ability to perform an activity in a manner or within a range considered normal for a human being. A disability is the functional consequence of an impairment manifested in integrated activities represented by tasks and skills.

Handicap: A disadvantage resulting from an impairment or disability that limits or prevents the fulfillment of a role that is normal (depending on age, sex, and social and cultural factors) for that individual. A handicap is the social consequence of an impairment or disability, defined by the attitudes and responses of others. Thus, the state of being handicapped is relative to other people.

If the WHO framework is applied to the field of speech–language pathology, one can use the example of the person with cerebral vascular disease who sustains a left-hemisphere stroke. The resultant impairment is aphasia (characterized by dysnomia, agrammatism, dysgraphia, and reduced auditory and visual comprehension), which can lead to a communication disability manifested in the performance of daily life activities such as communicating with family members or friends, using the telephone, making grocery lists, and reading the newspaper. The disability can, in turn, lead to handicaps of social isolation and loss of job.

Each consequential phenomenon along the WHO continuum defines a class of patient outcomes, and thus a class of measures to capture these outcomes: (1) traditional diagnostic, instrumental, and behavioral measures to determine differential diagnosis and identify specific strengths and weaknesses; (2) functional communication measures to identify the effects of these deficits on communication in everyday life activities; and (3) quality-of-life or wellness measures that assess the social, environmental, and economic effects of impairments and/or disabilities from the perspectives of patients and/or their caregivers.

Although health-related consequences do not necessarily occur in a linear direction, the WHO model adequately portrays a problem-solving sequence in the context of clinical intervention. That is, intervention at the level of one element has the potential to modify or prevent succeeding elements. Batavia[13] states, "With appropriate rehabilitative intervention, an impairment does not necessarily result in a disability. Similarly, with appropriate social and environmental interventions, a disability does not necessarily results in a handicap" (p. 3). The focus on problem-solving, then, is largely considered to define the ultimate outcomes of medical rehabilitation, which are to optimize independence and quality of life.

Outcome Measures

Once the concept of outcomes assessment is described by way of definitions and accepted conceptual models, one can select appropriate measures from the array of available instruments. This, however, is not an easy task. Clinicians will find it difficult to select the most appropriate or best measures: ones that are sufficiently sensitive, reliable, and valid; relatively quick and easy to administer; quantitative in their results; comprehensible and meaningful to key decision makers in patient care; and useful across the continuum of health care settings for defined patient populations.

At a minimum, clinicians must consider at least three classes of measurement to capture the impairments, disabilities and handicaps associated with disease, disorder, or injury. Also, clinicians need to select instruments with strong psychometric properties so that they can have confidence in the quality of derived test data.

Clinicians are advised to avoid the practice of *measurement generalization;* that is, use of a measure beyond its intended purposes. For example, a functional communication measure will never yield the sensitive information necessary for differential diagnosis and thus appropriate treatment planning. Consider the patient with hoarseness who is found to have independent communication in daily activities as evidenced by scores on a functional status measure, but who has a malignant growth on the left vocal cord, only detectable by instrumental procedures such as laryngoscopy, that is causing the hoarseness. Consider also the patient with dementia who "looks good" on standardized tests of language processes but whose communication in everyday life situations, assessed by measures of functional communication, is markedly reduced. Such standardized tests typically are not designed to capture the integrative aspects or contextually based domains of functional communication.

Instrument sensitivity must also be addressed. Once cannot, for example, expect to capture small increments of change using a measure designed as a minimum data set or screening tool, or using a general- rather than condition-specific measure for particular patient populations.

Test Selection Considerations

Outcome measures should possess certain characteristics that can be used as a checklist against which to judge their appropriateness and ability to capture targeted behaviors. An outcome measure should be:

- **Valid**: Measures what it claims to measure. A measure can be reliable but not valid. For example, the *Functional Independence Measure,*[14] may be reliable but not valid as a measure of functional communication. The question of validity is raised by a school of thought in the discipline of communication sciences and disorders that upholds the concept of functional communication assessment as an integrated and contextually based (e.g., assessment domains of social communication, communication of basic needs) rather than modality-specific (e.g., assessment domains of verbal expression, auditory comprehension, reading and writing) construct.
- **Reliable**: Consistent in results yielded across time and by different examiners. The chance of error can never completely be eliminated from a measure (e.g., due to the patient's anxiety level, quality and quantity of observations, time of day and fatigue factors), but to the extent that error is slight, scores derived from that measure are reliable.
- **Sensitive**: Able to detect small but meaningful increments of change. An instrument is

only sufficiently sensitive *for its intended purposes.* Thus, if it is a screening measure, it should be sensitive enough to identify problems vs. no problems. If it is a diagnostic measure, it should be sufficiently sensitive to differentially diagnose among the patient populations for which it was validated. If it is a general measure it will seldom yield the depth of information sought by specialists for condition-specific populations. Therefore, tools should not be used beyond the limits of their intended purposes. If a measure is sensitive, it must be able to detect targeted change if change occurs.

- **Practical:** Should be feasible for use by both examiners and examinees. The utility of an instrument typically is determined by the mode of administration required, the time it takes to administer, requirements in use of stimulus materials and other needed equipment, need for special training of examiners, burden to the respondent, and complexity of scoring.

- **Comprehensible:** Should be understandable to end users of the information. Often, treatment decisions are made on the basis of test results. These decisions can include eligibility for services, payment for services, continuation of services, and judgments about the quality of services. Often, decision makers are not clinicians. The information yielded from tests, therefore, should be understandable to other professionals as well as the layperson.

These considerations should be incorporated into any evaluation of "best measures." Otherwise, measurement can become encumbered in conceptual, psychometric, and practical problems that can lead to misuse of time, effort, and resources.

Measures of Impairment

If the consequences of disease or injury are considered along a continuum, outcomes assessment usually begins with identification of modality-specific behaviors, and identification of changes in these behaviors over time. The WHO[10] describes *impairment* as an exteriorization of a pathological state. Thus, aphasia and dysphagia resulting from stroke, cognitive disturbances resulting from head injury or dementia, aphonia resulting from laryngectomy, delayed speech and language resulting from mental retardation are all examples of impairments.

The assessment of impairment historically has been the focus of the speech–language pathologist's evaluations. Included in this category are the instrumental and behavioral diagnostic procedures that assess specific anatomical structures, physiological function, and behavioral processes of speech, language, voice, fluency, cognition, and swallowing.

Test Design Features

Impairment-level measures are typically designed to test separate behavioral processes (e.g., speech, language, voice) that, considered collectively, constitute human communication. A range of behaviors within each modality (e.g., aspects of auditory comprehension and verbal expression for the modality of language) usually is measured by each instrument. Tests of acquired language dysfunction in adults, for example, could measure confrontation naming, word fluency, verbal repetition, grammatical structure, proverb interpretation, spontaneous speech, auditory comprehension of one-, two-, and three- step commands, auditory retention, and so on.

According to Sarno,[15] traditional clinical tests are designed to discover whatever residuals a patient may have in each modality. In this respect, these tests are more often a measure of communication potential than actual use. Examples include instrumental procedures, such as vocal tract visualization and imaging (e.g., flexible fiberoptic nasendoscopy, stroboscopy), instrumental diagnostic procedures for swallowing (e.g., fiberoptic endoscopic examination of swallowing [FEES], electromyography, ultrasonography), and evaluation for tracheoesophageal fistulization/puncture. Examples also include the standardized tests of acquired language disorders in adults, such as the *Boston Diagnostic Aphasia Examination,*[16] *Minnesota Test for Differential Diagnosis of Aphasia,*[17] *Porch Index of Communicative Ability,*[18] and *Western Aphasia Battery.*[19]

Separate behaviors within a particular modality can also be assessed by a single test. Examples are found in the area of childhood language assessment, with tests designed to assess specific behaviors involving syntax, semantics, morphology, phonology, and pragmatics. They include the *Peabody Picture Vocabulary Test,*[20] *Expressive One-Word Picture Vocabulary Test—Revised,*[21] mean length of utterance, *Developmental Sentence Scoring,*[22] and *Northwestern Syntax Screening Test.*[23]

Because of their clinical objectivity and psychometric strengths, standardized tests of impairment have been typically used for purposes of controlled clinical studies. Thus, the field of speech–language pathology currently knows more about the effects of interventions on impairment-level phenomena than on resultant functional abilities or quality of life.

Measures of Disability

Disability, according to the WHO,[10] is the functional consequence of an impairment, manifested in the performance of daily life activities. In this context, specific speech, language, voice, fluency, and cognitive impairments can lead to communication disabilities (e.g., problems in social communication, communication of basic needs, daily planning). Similarly, impairments in swallowing can lead to an eating disability that can interfere with adequate intake and nutrition.

Test Design Features

Unlike impairment-level measures, disability measures typically are not designed to assess separate modalities. Rather, their designs coincide with the concept of communication as an integration of specific speech, language, and cognitive behaviors that allow the ability to perform everyday life activities. For example, the ability to use the telephone requires a range of specific skills (e.g., auditory comprehension, verbal expression, speech intelligibility, voice intensity and quality) that, considered together, allow the ability to perform the activity. Further, because disability often is measured by what patients do rather than can do (i.e., performance vs. potential), many are designed to rate abilities on the basis of direct observations.

A review of available measures, however, blur the lines between impairment and disability measurement. Tables 28–2 and 28–3 summarize the features of a sample of functional status measures, with inconsistencies in design noted particularly when comparing general rehabilitation and global measures to discipline-specific measures.

Among available rehabilitation and global measures, functional communication measures typically are embedded as separate sections. Rehabilitation-oriented instruments of this nature include, for example, the *Patient Evaluation and Conference System* (*PECS*),[24] the *Level of Rehabilitation Scale—III* (LORS),[25] and the *Functional Independence Measure, Version 4.0* (*FIM*).[14] The *Assessment of Needs for Continuing Care*[30] and the

Minimum Data Set for Nursing Facility Assessment and Care Screening[31] are among the global measures that incorporate sections on communication. These measures, all of which use rating scales (ranging from 4 to 7 points) along a continuum of independence, were developed to yield a relatively quick estimate of functional communication. The extent to which communication functions are considered, however, varies considerably across measures. For example, PECS addresses 12 areas of communication and related abilities; while the FIM, designed as a minimum data set, addresses 5 areas. Of note, however, are their assessment domains (e.g., auditory comprehension, verbal expression, speech production, impairment in thought processing), which depart from the concept of disability measurement as reflected in functional communication measures designed within the field of speech–language pathology.

Table 28–3 describes the features of a sample of measures developed exclusively for assessing functional communication. These include the *Communicative Abilities in Daily Living* (*CADL*),[33,34] the *Communicative Effectiveness Index* (*CETI*),[35] and the *ASHA Functional Assessment of Communication Skills for Adults* (*ASHA FACS*).[41] In contrast to the designs of communication sections of general rehabilitation or global measures, these measures are based on an integrative construct that addresses communication in various everyday contexts. Common assessment domains, for example, include communication of basic needs, social need, life skills, social communication, and daily planning.

Holland[42] tells clinicians to add three words to their usual treatment goals to reach what is functional: "*In order to. . . .*" Thus, a goal might be to improve auditory comprehension *in order to* engage in telephone conversations or understand what is heard on television, or to improve reading comprehension *in order to* understand environmental signs and follow prescriptions. The bridge is helpful in understanding the concept of functional communication, and in developing conceptual frameworks for its measurement.

Measuring Handicap

If handicap pertains to the social, environmental and economic effects of impairments or disabilities, then outcomes assessment pertains largely to measuring health-related quality of life. By its very nature, quality of life is an inherently subjective concept, best judged not by clinicians but by the patients themselves. Thus, quality of life measurement reflects personal values, beliefs, and

Table 28-2. Characteristics of Selected Functional Status Measures

Instrument (Reference)	Instrument Type	Assessment Domains	Aspects of Communication and Related Areas Addressed	Assessment Method	Reliability/ Validity
Patient Evaluation and Conference System (PECS)[24]	General rehabilitation for adults	Functions related to rehabilitation medicine, rehabilitation nursing, physical mobility, ADL, communication, medications, nutrition, assistive devices, psychology, neuropsychology, social issues, vocational educational activity, therapeutic recreation, pain, pulmonary rehabilitation pastoral care	Hearing, comprehension of spoken language, production of verbal language, comprehension of written language, production of written language, production of speech, swallowing, knowledge of assistive devices, skill in speaking with assistive communication devices, utilization of assistive communication devices, impairment in thought processing, comprehension and use of gestures	7-point ordinal scale from dependent to independent function combined into 6 interval Life Scales	Studies are ongoing. Preliminary studies found range of interrater reliability from .68 to .80. Content and construct validity are reported.
Level of Rehabilitation Scale-III (LORS III)[25]	General rehabilitation for adults	ADL, mobility, communication, cognitive ability	Auditory comprehension, oral expression, reading comprehension, written expression	5-point interval scale	Interrater reliability of item ratings ranges from .53 to .70 at admission and from .64 to .76 at discharge. Face validity based on agreement by experts in the field of rehabilitation is reported

693

Table 28–2. (continued)

Instrument (Reference)	Instrument Type	Assessment Domains	Aspects of Communication and Related Areas Addressed	Assessment Method	Reliability/ Validity
Rehabilitation Institute of Chicago Functional Assessment Scale '95 (RIC-FAS)[26]	General rehabilitation for adults	Functions related to the following services: physical medicine, nursing, physical therapy, occupational therapy, communication disorders, psychology, social work, vocational rehabilitation, therapeutic recreation	Hearing, auditory comprehension, oral expression, reading comprehension, written expression, speech production, chewing/swallowing, alternative/augmentative communication, money management	7-point ordinal scale ranging from normal to severe ability	Interrater reliability for RIC-FAS ranges from .66 to 1 across item scores, with 75% to 100% agreement on most items. Interrater reliability for communication items ranges from .90 to 1 (<.0001); 100% on all except written and pragmatic (97% agreement) and speech production (93% agreement)
Neurological Outcome Scale, an Evaluation System for Out-patient Rehabilitation Programs[27]	General rehabilitation for adults	Physical restoration, cognitive retraining, communication skills development, community re-entry, social involvement	Expressive skills (written, verbal), comprehension (auditory, reading)	5-point ordinal scale from 0 to 100% function	Based on pilot data from 36 clients, interitem reliability of the scale item ratings range from .81 to .93 (admission) and .47 (for communication skills) to .94 (discharge). Face validity is being tested.
Functional Independence Measure (FIM) Version 4.0[14]	General rehabilitation for adults	Self-care, sphincter control, transfers, locomotion, communication, social cognition	Comprehension (auditory), expression (vocal), comprehension (visual), expression (nonvocal), eating, problem solving, memory, social interaction	7-point scale from complete independence to total assistance	Intraclass correlation coefficients (ICC) range from .89 to .96 for FIM domain scores. FIM item Kappa range: .53 (memory) to .66 (stair climbing). Interrater reliability ranges from .97 to .98 for FIM domain scores; FIM item Kappa range: .69

694

Table 28–2. (continued)

Instrument (Reference)	Instrument Type	Assessment Domains	Aspects of Communication and Related Areas Addressed	Assessment Method	Reliability/Validity
					(memory) to .84 (bladder management). Reported face-, construct-, and criterion-related (predictive and concurrent) validity (for minutes of help per day for stroke, multiple sclerosis, and traumatic brain injury)
WeeFIM[28]	General rehabilitation for children (6 mos. to 7 years and older)	Self-care, transfers, locomotion, sphincter control, communication, and social cognition	Comprehension (auditory or visual), expression (verbal, nonverbal)	7-point scale from complete independence to total assistance	Reliability and validity studies underway. Statistical comparisons will examine the relationship of ratings on the WeeFIM with scores on the *Battelle Developmental Screening Inventory Test* and the *Vineland Adaptive Behavior Scales*
Pediatric Evaluation of Disability Inventory[29]	General rehabilitation for children (6 mos. to 7.5 years)	Self-care, mobility, social function	Comprehension of word meanings, comprehension of sentence complexity, functional use of expressive communication, complexity of expressive communication, problem-resolution, social interactive play, peer interactions, self-information, time orientation, community function	Part 1: Functional skills (0 = unable; 1 = capable of performing item in most situations) Part 2: Caregiver assistance (5-point scale of independence) Part 3: Modifications (N = no modifications; C = Child-oriented modifications; R = Rehabilitation equipment; E = Extensive modifications)	Content validity reported rehab. professionals; standardized on a normative sample (N = 412); PEDI highly correlated with *WeeFIM* and *Battelle;* PEDI selectively responsive to change in certain clinical samples; reliability data unavailable.

695

Table 28-2. (continued)

Instrument (Reference)	Instrument Type	Assessment Domains	Aspects of Communication and Related Areas Addressed	Assessment Method	Reliability/ Validity
Assessment of Needs for Continuing Care (ANCC)[30]	Global for adults	Health status, functional status (ADLs, IADLs), communication, environmental factors in post-discharge care, nursing and other care requirements, family and community support, patient/family goals and preferences, options for continuing care	Comprehension, expression, usual mode(s) of communication	4-point ordinal scale from independent to dependent function	Information is currently unavailable.
Minimum Data Set for Nursing Home Resident Assessment and Care Screening (MDS)[31]	Global for adults	Cognitive patterns, communication/hearing patterns, vision patterns, physical functioning and structural problems (including ADLs), continence, psychosocial well-being, mood and behavior patterns, activity pursuit patterns, disease diagnoses, health conditions, oral/nutritional status, oral/dental status, skin condition, medication use, special treatment and procedures	Hearing, communication devices/techniques, models of expression, making self understood, ability to understand others, change in communication/hearing	4-point ordinal scale	Based on published field test results, select interrater reliability values for key functional indicators are: making self understood, .92; hearing: .78; locomotion, .92; eating, .94; bladder continence, .93; cognitive skills, .93; vision, .85; wandering, .83; weight loss, .85; pressure ulcers, .92.

Source: From Frattali C: Measuring modality-specific behaviors, functional status, and quality of life. In C Frattali, ed., *Measuring outcomes in speech–language pathology.* Thieme Medical Publishers, Inc., New York, 1998. Reprinted with permission.

Table 28–3. Characteristics of Selected Functional Communication Measures

Instrument (Reference)	Communication Components	Assessment Method	Applicable Populations	Reliability/Validity
Functional Communication Profile (FCP)[32]	45 communication behaviors in: movement (e.g., gestures), speaking, understanding, reading, miscellaneous (e.g., writing, calculation)	9-point scale	Adults with aphasia	Concurrent and predictive validity (correlates with measures of auditory memory span and CADL); high inter-examiner reliability; test-retest reliability described as significant
Communicative Abilities in Daily Living (CADL)[33,34]	68 items incorporating everyday language activities in: content/form (production, comprehension), use (role-playing, speech acts)	3-point scoring system (0 = wrong, 1 = adequate, 2 = correct)	Adults with aphasia, mental retardation or Alzheimer's disease; experienced hearing aid users	Concurrent validity (correlates with Boston Diagnostic Aphasia Examination,[16] Porch Index of Communicative Ability,[18] FCP, and direct observations of communication behavior); high inter-examiner and test-retest reliability
Communicative Effectiveness Index (CETI)[35]	16 communication items categorized by social need, life skill, basic need, health threat	10-cm visual analogue scale from "not at all able" to "as able as before the stroke"	Adults with aphasia secondary to stroke	Based on evaluation of 22 patients with aphasia (11 recovering, 11 stable); has good test-retest and interrater reliability; face and construct validity (correlates with global ratings of language & communication by spouses)
Revised Edinburgh Functional Communication Profile (EFCP)[36]	Communication functions and modalities used: greetings, acknowledging, responding, requesting, initiating	5-point effectiveness scale, and modality used is noted	Adults with aphasia, developmental disorders, mental retardation, cerebral palsy who use AAC systems	Concurrent validity; content validity evaluated by scoring 16-minute language samples and comparing with 10 exchanges; interrater reliability based on 14 patients

Table 28-3. (continued)

Instrument (Reference)	Communication Components	Assessment Method	Applicable Populations	Reliability/ Validity
A Performance Status Scale for Head and Neck Cancer Patients[37]	Eating in public, understandability of speech, normalcy of diet	Total of 3 ratings (one on each subscale). In each subscale, items are arranged hierarchically to describe a continuum, with total incapacitation at one end to full, normal functioning at the other end	Adults with head and neck cancer	Based on 181 patients, interrater reliability between research team members was .88 for normalcy of diet; .64 for understandability of speech; and .78 for eating in public. Interrater reliability for untrained professionals was .84 (normalcy of diet), .43 (understandability of speech), and .81 (eating in public); moderate correlations were found when compared with Karnofsky Performance Status Rating Scale [Karnofsky & Burchenal, 1949].[63]
Amsterdam Nijmegan Everyday Language Test (ANELT)[38]	Two parallel versions, each consisting of 10 items constructed as scenarios of familiar daily life activities	Two 5-point scales: A-scale (understandability of the message) and B-scale (intelligibility of the utterance). Points on rating scale: not at all, a little, medium, reasonable, and good	Adults with aphasia	Psychometric analysis showed perfect parallelism for both test versions. Based on 60 adult subjects with no history of neurological impairment and 60 subjects with aphasia, interrater reliability ranged from .70 to .92. Concurrent validity (correlates with Aachen Aphasia Test-Communicative Behavior Scale) is reported.
Communication Profile: A Functional Skills Survey[39]	26 daily communication skills involving speaking, reading comprehension, verbal comprehension, writing, and math comprehension	5-point scale (face-to-face interview) that allows clients or family members to rate communication skills from "very important" to "not important at all"	Adults with language impairments from diffuse neurological disorders, hearing impairments, mental retardation, stroke, and traumatic brain injury	On the basis of 65 subjects, internal consistency of items was .95. Internal consistency of subscales was reportedly high. Test-retest reliability was .92. Validity between total score and client self-assessment of severity was .63.

Table 28–3. (*continued*)

Instrument (Reference)	Communication Components	Assessment Method	Applicable Populations	Reliability/ Validity
Functional Linguistic Communication Inventory[40]	Assessment areas include greeting/naming, answering questions, writing, comprehension of signs/ pictures, following commands, conversation, reminiscing, gesture, pantomine, and word reading/comprehension	32 items that require the examiner to judge whether a correct response was provided. The number of correct responses are totaled, and subtest scores can be compared to performance on standardization study subjects by severity level.	Adults with moderate and severe dementia	Test-retest reliability for 20 patients with dementia, using the coefficient of determination and the probability of concordance, were high and significant for all subtests except gesture. Criterion validity using the Arizona Battery for Communication Disorders of Dementia[40] (Bayles & Tomoeda, 1993) was strong, $r = .78$ ($p < .002$).
ASHA Functional Assessment of Communication Skills for Adults (ASHA FACS)[41]	43 items within 4 assessment domains: social communication; communication of basic needs; reading, writing, and number concepts; daily planning	7-point scale of independence; 5-point scale of qualitative dimensions of communication (i.e., adequacy, appropriateness, promptness, and communication sharing)	Adults with aphasia secondary to left-hemisphere stroke; adults with cognitive-communication disorders secondary to traumatic brain injury	Inter-rater reliability ranged from .72 to .95. Intra-rater reliability ranged from .94 to .99. Moderate correlations with Western Aphasia Battery and Scale of Cognitive Abilities for Traumatic Brain Injury. High internal consistency, measure sensitivity, and social validity reported.

Source: From Frattali C: Measuring modality-specific behaviors, functional status, and quality of life. In C Frattali, ed., *Measuring outcomes in speech–language pathology.* Thieme Medical Publishers, Inc., New York, 1998. Reprinted with permission.

preferences. Environmental factors, such as societal attitudes and social/psychological supports also directly influence perceptions about quality of life.

Health-related quality of life (HQL) typically refers to the individual's ability to function in a variety of roles and derive satisfaction from them, despite the presence of an impairment and/or disability. These measures often assess multiple dimensions of life (the objective component) and attach values to each dimension (the subjective component). This area of outcomes measurement is perhaps the most important contribution made during the last 10 years, consistent with the growing consensus that the patient's point of view is central to measuring clinical outcomes. It is also an area in great need of research and development.

Design Features

Assessment domains of HQL measures can be all encompassing and include performance of activities of daily living, social roles (e.g., return to work, school), social interaction, emotional state, intellectual functioning, and general satisfaction and perceived well-being. The concept, therefore, subsumes the narrower concepts of functional limitations or disabilities, but the dimensions of health-related quality of life are broader than those found in disability measures. Emotional well-being, overall life satisfaction, energy, and vitality are all legitimate components of quality of life.

The major distinguishing feature of HQL measures is that their dimensions are on the personal/social level; therefore, values are typically assigned by patients (or their family members) and reflect their personal values and beliefs. These measures often take the form of self-administered surveys, interviewer-administered questionnaires, and open-ended interviews.

A sample of HQL measures is described in Table 28–4. These are primarily general measures—measures that are relevant to individuals generally rather than specific to one condition or diagnostic group. In addition, these measures were developed to measure outcomes of primary medical care, although they are being used increasingly to measure the outcomes of medical rehabilitation. Two exceptions included in Table 28–4, specific to the discipline of communication sciences and disorders, are the *Hearing Handicap Inventory for the Elderly* (HHIE)[53] and the *Voice Handicap Index* (VHI).[54] Both measures assess the quality of life for patients with hearing disorders or voice disorders, respectively. The HHIE assesses the situational effects

and the emotional and social adjustment of elderly people to hearing impairment. Two subscales make up the measure: emotional consequences, and social and situational effects. The VHI measures physical symptoms, functional factors, and emotional factors.

Cost Measures

An outcome of primary interest to payors relates, not surprisingly, to cost. In the minds of payors, positive clinical outcomes must viewed in terms of their relationship to total costs. This relationship often is expressed by dollars spent or length of stay. Two types of cost analyses can be conducted to determine how certain outcomes compare to their costs: *cost-benefit* and *cost-effectiveness* analyses. Both are conducted for comparative purposes in determining which provider can achieve the same or better outcomes at a lower cost. This type of analysis requires that cost and outcomes be linked.

A cost-benefit analysis determines the economic efficiency of a program expressed as the relationship between dollars spent to dollars saved. In contrast, a cost-effectiveness analysis explores the effectiveness of a program in achieving targeted intervention outcomes in relation to program costs (e.g., dollars spent or length of stay per points on a functional outcome measure).

The Uniform Data System for Medical Rehabilitation, which incorporates use of the *Functional Independence Measure*,[14] calculates what it calls a *length of stay efficiency* by dividing the FIM change by the length of stay to determine the mean change in FIM score per day. A higher length of stay efficiency denotes a more efficient program.

Satisfaction Measures

As health care becomes more patient centered, health care practitioners as well as administrators are turning their attention to patients' judgments about the quality of care. These measures, commonly designed as self-assessment questionnaires, solicit the judgments of patients about several dimensions of care and determine the extent to which a program fulfils patients' expectations. Dimensions of assessment address three basic areas:

1. Access to care (e.g., signs and directions to treatment facility, waiting room time, clinic hours)
2. Physical environment (e.g., cleanliness of reception area, noise level, condition of treatment space)

Table 28–4. Characteristics of Selected Quality of Life Measures

Measure (Reference)	Assessment Domains	Assessment Method	Length	Time Requirements	Reliability/Validity
Medical Outcome Study (MOS) Health Status Questionnaire (SF-36)[43]	Physical; role limitations due to physical and emotional problems; social functioning; general mental health; pain; energy/fatigue; general health perceptions	Self-report	360 items	10 minutes	Reliability estimates for all SF-36 scales were .78 or higher. Multitrait scaling analyses support item convergence for hypothesized scales and item discrimination across scales.
COOP Charts[44]	Physical: mental; role; social; pain; overall health change; social resources; life quality	Self-report or clinical rating	9 items	<10 minutes	Charts correlate with validity indicator variables, indicating convergent and discriminant validity. Reliability data unavailable.
Duke-UNC Health Profile[45]	Symptom status; physical function; emotional function; social function	Self-report	64 items	15–20 minutes	Based on 395 ambulatory patients in a family medicine center, temporal stability ranged from .52 to .82. Cronbach's alpha for internal consistency was .85 for emotional function. Convergent and discriminant validity supported by strong associations with the Sickness Impact Profile, and other measures.
Sickness Impact Profile (SIP)[46]	Physical: ambulation, mobility, body care; psychosocial: social interaction, communication, alertness, emotional behavior; other: sleep/rest, eating, work, home management, recreational pastimes	Self-report	136 items	30 minutes	Based on large field trial on a random sample of prepaid group practice enrollees and smaller trials on samples of patients with hyperthyroidism, rheumatoid arthritis, and hip replacements, test-retest reliability ($r = .92$) and internal consistency ($r = .94$). Clinical validity (with clinical measures of disease) was moderate to high.

Table 28-4. (continued)

Measure (Reference)	Assessment Domains	Assessment Method	Length	Time Requirements	Reliability/ Validity
McMaster Health Index Questionnaire (MHIQ)[47]	Physical: mobility, self-care, communication, global physical function; Social: general well-being, work/social role, performance, social support and participation, global self-function; Emotional: self-esteem, personal relationships, critical life events, global emotional function	Self-report	59 items	20 minutes	Retest reliability coefficients of .53, .70, and .48 for physical, emotional, and social function scores, respectively, were observed in physiotherapy patients. In psychiatry patients, coefficients were .95, .77, and .66 respectively. Scores correlate with global assessment made by health professionals. Physical function scores were responsive to change.
Nottingham Health Profile (NHP)[48]	Six domains of experience: pain, physical mobility, sleep, emotional reactions, energy, social isolation	Self-report	45 items	10 minutes	High face, content and criterion validity. NHP scores effectively differentiated between well and ill groups. Intra-rater reliability ranged from .44–.89 in groups with chronic illness. Norms for general population and employed population established.
Quality of Well-being Scale (QWB)[49]	Functional performance: self-care, mobility, institutionalization, social activities; symptoms and problems	Self-report	50 items	12 minutes	Sensitivity to changes over time in patients with AIDS demonstrated in a 52-week multi-center trial.
Craig Handicap Assessment and Reporting Technique (CHART)[50]	Physical independence, mobility, occupation, social integration, economic self-sufficiency	Self-report	327 questions	20 minutes	Based on data from 135 individuals with spinal cord injury, test-retest reliability for overall CHART score was .93. Rasch analysis verified CHART scaling and scoring procedures. Validity supported by overall differences in total and subscale scores between high-handicap and low-handicap

702

Table 28–4. (continued)

Measure (Reference)	Assessment Domains	Assessment Method	Length	Time Requirements	Reliability/ Validity
Community Integration Questionnaire (CIQ)[57]	Home integration, social integration, integration into productive activities	Interview	15 questions	10 minutes	Based on data from 16 individuals with moderate to severe traumatic brain injury and a family member for each, test-retest reliability for the overall CIQ was .91 for individuals and .97 for family members' assessment of individuals. Good internal consistency reported.
Functional Status Questionnaire (FSQ)[52]	Physical: basic and intermediate activities of daily living; emotional function: anxiety and depression, quality of social interaction; social performance: occupational function, social activities; other: sexual, global disability, global health satisfaction, social contacts	Self-report	34 items	10 minutes	Intra-reliability for the 6 scale scores ranged from .64 to .82. Scale scores correlated with scores on 7 health measures. Inverse relationship found between age and performance on intermediate activities of daily living, and age and social activity. Satisfaction with health is positively correlated with each scale score.
Hearing Handicap Inventory for the Elderly[53]	Perceived problems caused by hearing loss (i.e., emotional consequences and social and situational effects)	Self-report	25-items	10 minutes	Reported reliability (by assessing internal consistency) as well as construct and content validity
Voice Handicap Index[54]	Physical symptamotology, functional factors, emotional factors	Self-report	30 items	15 minutes	Based on 65 subjects, internal consistency of items was .95. Internal consistency of subscales was high. Test-retest reliability was .92. Validity between total score and patient self-assessment of severity was .63.

Source: From Frattali C: Measuring modality-specific behaviors, functional status, and quality of life. In C Frattali, ed., *Measuring outcomes in speech–language pathology.* Thieme Medical Publishers, Inc., New York, 1998. Reprinted with permission.

3. Care received (i.e., both interpersonal and technical aspects)

The adage, "keep the customer happy" carries new significance in the current health care marketplace as managed care organizations compete for market share. Today's patients typically have a choice of provider, and they exercise this choice if dissatisfied.

Outcomes Assessment Methods

Any approach to outcomes assessment can be considered research if one attempts to systematically answer a question or test a hypothesis. A common question is, "Does clinical intervention make a difference? Attempts to answer this inquiry lead to investigation. While research usually carries a definition of scientific or scholarly investigation that implies explicit protocols and well-controlled conditions aimed at proving cause and effect, not all research proves causation. Thus, important differences have evolved between efficacy research and outcomes research.

Efficacy Research vs. Outcomes Research

Treatment efficacy is the ability of an applied treatment to produce a predicted result. It measures the results of treatment as it is applied under *ideal* circumstances. Conceptually, it is distinguished from outcomes research that measures the results of treatment as it is applied to a *typical* circumstance. Outcomes studies seldom incorporate experimental research designs because their focus is on the influence of the applied treatment over numerous facets in the patient's life that typically cannot be experimentally controlled. In general, efficacy research is designed to prove; outcomes research can only identify trends, describe, or make associations or estimates.

It is commonly held that efficacy research is reserved for the controlled conditions of a laboratory, and outcomes research for the variable conditions of the real-world including the health care setting. Interpretations of research findings, therefore, must be approached with caution. For example, statements of cause and effect (e.g., speech–language pathology treatment can shorten the length of stay for inpatients with dysphagia resulting from stroke) cannot be made when one has not adequately controlled for the possible intervening variables that could influence the outcome or outcomes under study (e.g., spontaneous recovery, severity of the clinical condition, age,

type of clinical procedures, comorbidities, adherence to a treatment regimen).

Classifying Outcomes Assessment Methods

Outcomes assessment methodologies can be classified into three categories:

1. **Experimental:** Studies that involve random or fully specifiable assignment to intervention and control groups or phases. Examples include randomized controlled clinical trials and time series research using single subject designs.
2. **Quasi-experimental:** Studies that involve nonrandom and not fully specifiable assignment to intervention and control groups or phases. Examples include program evaluation studies and quality improvement studies. Epidemiologic studies also are often categorized as quasi-experimental.
3. **Non-experimental:** Studies that involve no clear comparison groups or phases. Case reports and data registries are examples.

Two approaches of particular interest to individuals who work in health care settings are program evaluation and quality improvement processes. Over time, these two methods are losing their distinguishing features. Major components of both approaches are: (1) measurement of patient outcomes, and (2) management of those outcomes to continually improve the quality of care.

Program Evaluation

Program evaluation methods were designed primarily to determine whether a program is meeting its goals. Both clinical and administrative goals are monitored. The term "program evaluation" is defined by CARF, The Rehabilitation Accreditation Commission, as a system that enables the organization to identify the outcomes of its programs, the satisfaction of the persons served, and follow-up on outcomes achieved by the persons served.[55] Patton[56] describes program evaluation as the systematic collection of information about the characteristics (structure), activities (process), and outcomes of programs and services that help administrators reduce uncertainty in the decisions they make regarding those same program and services they administer. Program evaluation, therefore, is a planned process of gathering and analyzing data to help reduce the risk of decisions. Wilkerson[57] refers to program evaluation as an enterprise that depends on aggregations of data collected about individuals receiving services. She details its key steps:

- Establish program goals, clarifying what outcomes are really important
- Specify quanitifiable objectives to meet those goals
- Select measures that indicate progress toward objectives
- Measure program performance on those measures
- Compare performance to desired objective
- Identify potential changes in the program likely to enhance performance toward desired objectives
- Implement program changes
- Measure program performance once again, comparing to the objective
- Re-enter the cycle

Thus, both measurement and management components constitute the approach to program evaluation.

Quality Improvement

Both measurement and management are also the primary aspects of quality improvement methods. However, a greater emphasis is placed on measurement of work processes (which are directly attributable to desired or expected outcomes). Quality improvement methods were designed initially to determine whether actual care complies with preestablished gold standards (e.g., standards of practice, preferred practice patterns, practice guidelines, practice parameters, or critical/clinical paths). However, with recognition that methods can also be designed to acquire new knowledge, quality improvement activities can result in establishing or modifying gold standards.

Quality assessment and improvement are defined broadly by the Joint Commission on Accreditation of Healthcare Organizations[58] as follows:

PI.3.1 The hospital collects data on important processes or outcomes related to patient care and organization functions.

PI.4.2 The hospital makes internal comparisons of its performance of processes and outcomes over time (pp. 134–135).

The methods typically involve a Plan-Do-Study-Act (PDSA) cycle:

Plan: A work process for study is selected and an improvement trial is developed.

Baseline data are collected.

Do: The trial is performed, and data are collected.

Study: The data are studied and compared to previous knowledge (i.e., baseline data).

Act: Changes are made based on the new knowledge, or a new plan is developed and the cycle starts again.

The PDSA cycle, in fact, mirrors the clinical process. A clinician collects baseline data to document a patient's current condition and develops a plan of treatment to improve the condition (Plan). The clinician then carries out the plan (Do), observes and records the effects using objective outcome measures to determine if treatment results in improved abilities (Study). Finally, the clinician applies what is learned to either continue, discontinue, or modify the plan of treatment (Act), thereby starting the cycle of learning and improvement over again.

The Emergence of Automated Systems

Historically, rehabilitation professionals had no universally accepted terminology with which to communicate about disability. They also did not have uniform measures for capturing disability. These needs gave rise to the development of the Uniform Data Set for Medical Rehabilitation (UDS MR),[14] which is a system that incorporates the *Functional Independence Measure* (*FIM*) and documents, in a uniform way, severity of patient disability and the outcomes of medical rehabilitation. While criticized for its lack of sufficient sensitivity or design flaws in capturing communication disabilities, it is widely known as the industry standard. Currently, inpatient medical rehabilitation facilities in 49 states enrolled as UDS participants, and over 300,000 patient records are entered into the data base in the United States. Thus, patients can be tracked from hospital admission through discharge and follow-up, with periodic reassessment measuring changes in patient performance over time to determine rehabilitative outcomes. Included in the data set are patient demographic characteristics, diagnoses, impairment groups, lengths of rehabilitation inpatient stay, and rehabilitation changes as measured by the *FIM*. Primary data can be adjusted for certain risk factors (e.g., age, diagnosis) and aggregated to show trends pertaining to the benefits of rehabilitation.

In the field of speech–language pathology, a few automated systems have recently become available. Two commercially available systems are the Beaumont Outcome Software System (BOSS)[59] and OUTCOME.[60] Their features and hardware requirements are summarized in Table 28–5. Keatley and Miller[59] are credited with introducing the concept of automated outcomes management specific to speech–language pathology; Merson, Rolnick, and Wiener[60] are credited with introducing a user-friendly system with development of the BOSS. As in any new area of development, however, flaws are found. The BOSS, in its simplicity, can only incorporate outcome measures using 7-point scales. Its suggestion that any standardized test or other measure can be converted into 7-point scales seriously threatens reliability and validity. Also, the BOSS can only adjust for two risk factors at any one time to account for variance in outcome; therefore, treatment outcome data are open to incomplete interpretations. The OUTCOME software offers more in the number of risk factors that can be controlled at any one time and in its sophisticated data analysis capabilities. However, the system is considered complex to learn and use, and its applications not transparent to the user.

These two software programs will likely be refined with use and with access to better outcome measures once they are developed. The area of automation will continue to advance, with other automated systems in the field already in formative stages of development.

USING OUTCOMES DATA FOR DECISION MAKING

Once outcomes are measured, they must be managed if they are to have a purpose. This belief forms the basis of Ellwood's[61] approach to *outcomes management,* which involves the use of outcomes data for decision making. Providers may find, for example, that the costs of certain clinical procedures do not justify the minimal progress made with certain patient populations, especially when less costly alternatives to treatment (e.g., family instruction or group treatment) have a similar result. Thus, a decision can be made to allocate more resources to underserved patient populations in which significant improvements can be documented.

The management of outcomes leads to the development of data-based standards of care and clinical management tools such as critical paths (i.e., treatment regimes, supported ideally by patient outcomes research, that include only those vital elements that have been proved to affect pa-

tient outcomes) to improve the effectiveness and efficiency of care.

The methods of program evaluation and quality improvement, described above, are examples of managing outcomes once they are measured. Both suggest a continuous cycle of investigation and change. Ellwood[61] describes the field of outcomes management as:

A technology of patient experience designed to help patients, payers, providers make rational [health care]-related choices based on better insight into the impact of these choices on the patient's life. Outcomes Management consists of:

- Common patient-understood language of health outcomes;
- A national data base containing clinical, financial and health outcome information and analysis that estimates as best we can the relationship between [health care] interventions and health outcomes, as well as the relationship between health outcomes and money;
- An opportunity for each decision-maker to have access to those analyses that are relevant to the choices they must make (p. 4).

Dissemination of outcomes data for the purposes of decision making not only by practitioners on a local level but by payors, legislators, and regulators on state, regional, and national levels becomes necessary. The ambitious work of the ASHA Task Force on Treatment Outcomes and Cost Effectiveness[62] is a prime example of systematic collection and planned dissemination of outcomes data on a national level to improve access to and the quality of speech–language pathology services.

Good outcomes data can exist without the knowledge of professional groups. For outcomes to be managed, outcomes data must be translated into practice guidelines and protocols, which in turn should be distributed and applied widely in efforts to change ineffective or inefficient ways of rendering services.

SUMMARY

This chapter has addressed outcomes assessment requirements, measures, and methods. It has included definitions of terms in current use and also addressed some ways in which to proceed from measurement to management so that we may effectively improve care and, by extension, enhance patients' lives. Given the time demands of clinicians, the application of outcomes assessment is still largely perceived as a burden or add-on to busy clinical schedules. However, the demands for

Table 28–5. Features of Two Automated Outcomes Management Systems in Speech–Language Pathology

Software	Developer	Features	Applicable Patient Populations	Hardware Requirements
Beaumont Outcome Software System (BOSS)[59]	Parrot Software P.O. Box 250755 West Bloomfield, MI 48325 1-800-Parrot-1	Reports clinical and financial outcomes. Uses 7-point clinical scales only. Data elements include clinical site, communication diagnosis, diagnosis code, evaluation and treatment procedures, fees charged, clinicians providing the service. Variables that account for variance in outcomes are clinical site, age, gender, severity, diagnosis, clinician, or patient. Outcome variables include admission status, discharge status, treatment outcome, total procedures, length of stay, and cost per case (in total charges). Outcome data can be reported in tables and bar graphs. Demo disk available.	Adult and pediatric populations. Multiple speech/language swallowing diagnoses.	386 (or higher) PC compatible system. Microsoft WINDOWS 3.x or WINDOWS 95, VGA graphics, 4 megabytes of RAM, 3 megabytes of memory.
OUTCOME[60]	Evaluation Systems International, Inc.	Accepts any outcome scales and independent variables. Programmed for ASHA's Functional Communication Measures. Analyzes functional outcome data for patient improvement, financial variables, critical pathways, length of stay/number of sessions, effectiveness of treatment techniques and patient demographics. Adjusts for severity and predicts outcomes for defined patient populations. Exports data for other applications. Produces multiple reports, color graphics. Demo disk available.	Adult and pediatric populations. Multiple diagnosis can be evaluated.	386 or higher IBM PC compatible. Microsoft WINDOWS, 8 megabytes of RAM, 2.5 megabytes of memory, VGA color monitor, mouse driver (optional).

data should support and sustain these types of activities, if only to maintain patients' access to care and preserve its quality.

Established methodologies, the growing number of outcome measures in the field, and advancing technologies allow the systematic and accurate assessment of outcomes data for answering some of the pressing questions being asked by both consumer representatives and payors. In this era of managed care, in which cost and clinical outcome predictions form the basis of financial and clinical viability, the data are critically necessary to maintain a position as a qualified provider of health care to those in current and future need.

STUDY QUESTIONS

1. Cite various payor and accreditation agency requirements for outcomes assessment.

2. Give three examples of outcomes that can be measured and identify the key stakeholders who would be most interested in each outcome.

3. Identify a measure of impairment, disability, and handicap in the profession of speech–language pathology. How are they similar? How are they different?

4. Why is test reliability and validity important when measuring patient outcomes?

5. What is the difference between efficacy research and outcomes research?

6. How are quality improvement and program evaluation activities similar? How are these activities different?

7. How can outcomes data be *managed*?

8. Design an outcomes study. Which approach/method will you use? For which patient populations? Using which outcome measures? What systematic steps will you follow in conducting the study? What interpretations can you make based on the results of the study?

9. What is the danger in looking at outcomes without regard for the antecedent process of care?

10. What might be your predictions for the future of outcomes assessment in health care?

REFERENCES

1. Adamzyk J: Relevance of CIQI measures of quality and outcome to the payer/insurer—How to "buy smart." Presentation at Rehabilitation Medicine: Continuous Interdisciplinary Quality Improvement (CIQI). Conference sponsored by the Buffalo General Hospital and State University of New York at Buffalo, Buffalo, NY, 1991.

2. Joint Commission on Accreditation of Healthcare Organizations: Hospital Accreditation Standards. Oakbrook Terrace, IL, 1997.

3. CARF . . . The Rehabilitation Accreditation Commission: Accreditation standards for inpatient rehabilitation programs. Tucson, AZ, 1997.

4. American Speech–Language Hearing Association. Professional Services Board: PSB standards. Rockville, MD, 1994.

5. Health Care Financing Administration: Medicare intermediary manual, Part 3: Claims process. Baltimore, MD, 1991.

6. Health Care Financing Administration: Outpatient rehabilitation services forms 700 and 701. Baltimore, MD, 1993.

7. Donabedian A: *Explorations in quality assessment and monitoring. Volume I: The definition of quality and approaches to its assessment.* Health Administration Press, Ann Arbor, MI, 1980.

8. Rosen A, Procter E: Distinctions between treatment outcome and their implications for treatment evaluation. *J Consult Clin Psych* 1981; 49:418–425.

9. Deming WE: *Out of the crisis.* Cambridge, Massachusetts Institute of Technology, Center for Advanced Engineering Study, 1982.

10. World Health Organization: *International classification of impairments, disabilities, and handicaps: A manual for classification relating to the consequences of disease.* Geneva, Switzerland, 1980.

11. Pope AM, Tarlov AL, eds: *Disability in America: Toward a national agenda for prevention.* National Academy Press, Washington, DC, 1991.

12. Wilson IB, Cleary PD: Linking clinical variables with health-related quality of life: A conceptual model of patient outcomes. *JAMA* 1995; 273(1):59–65.

13. Batavia AI: Assessing the function of functional assessment: A consumer perspective. *Disab Rehab* 1992; 14:156–160.

14. State University of New York at Buffalo, Research Foundation: *Guide for use of the Uniform Data Set for Medical Rehabilitation: Functional Independence Measure.* Buffalo, NY, 1993.

15. Sarno MT: A measurement of functional communication in aphasia. *Arch Phys Med Rehab* 1965; 46:101–107.

16. Goodglass, Kaplan: *Assessment of aphasia and related disorders, 2nd ed.* Lea & Febiger, Philadelphia, 1972.

17. Schuell H: *The Minnesota Test for Differential Diagnosis of Aphasia.* University of Minnesota Press, Minneapolis, 1965.

18. Porch BE: *Porch Index of Communicative Ability.* Consulting Psychologists Press, Palo Alto, CA, 1971.

19. Kertesz, A: *Western Aphasia Battery.* Grune & Stratton, New York, 1982.

20. Dunn LM, Dunn LM: *Peabody Picture Vocabulary Test—Revised.* American Guidance Service, Circle Pines, MN, 1981.

21. Gardner MF: *Expressive One-word Picture Vocabulary Test—Revised.* Academic Therapy Publications, Novato, CH, 1990.

22. Lee LL: *Developmental Sentence Scoring.* Northwestern University Press, Evanston, IL, 1974.

23. Lee LL: *Northwestern Syntax Screening Test.* Northwestern University Press, Evanston, IL, 1971.

24. Harvey RF, Jellinek HM: *Patient evaluation and conference system: PECS.* Marianjoy Rehabilitation Center, Wheaton, IL, 1979.

25. Formations in Health Care: *Level of Rehabilitation Scale—III.* Chicago, 1995.

26. Cichowski K: *Rehabilitation Institute of Chicago Functional Assessment Scale—Revised.* Rehabilitation Institute of Chicago, Chicago, 1995.

27. Santopoalo RD, Carey D: *Neurological Outcome Scale: An Evaluation System for Outpatient Rehabilitation Programs.* Parkside Associates, Park Ridge, IL, 1991. (Now available from Formations in Health Care, Chicago).

28. State University of New York at Buffalo, Research Foundation: *Functional Independence for Children (WeeFIM),* Version 1.5. Buffalo, NY, 1991.

29. Haley SM, Coster WJ, Ludlow LH, Haltiwanger JT, Andrellos PJ: *Pediatric Evaluation of Disability Inventory, Version 1.0.* New England Medical Center Hospitals, Inc., Boston, 1992.

30. Health Care Financing Administration: *Assessment of Needs for Continuing Care.* (Form HCFA-32; 10-89). Baltimore, MD, 1989.

31. Hawes C, Morris JN, Phillips CD, Mor V, Fries BE, Nonemaker S: Reliability estimates for the minimum data set for nursing facility resident assessment and care screening (MDS). *Gerontologist* 1995; 35(2):172–178.

32. Sarno MT: *Functional communication profile.* Institute of Rehabilitation Medicine, New York University Medical Center, New York, 1969.

33. Holland AL: *Communicative abilities in daily living.* University Park Press, Baltimore, MD, 1980.

34. Holland AL, Frattali CM, Fromm D: *Communicative abilities in daily living—Revised.* ProEd, Austin, TX, in press.

35. Lomas J, Pickard L, Bester S, Elbard H, Finlayson A, Zoghaib C: The Communicative Effectiveness Index: Development and psychometric evaluation of a functional communication measure for adults. *J Speech Hear Dis* 1989; 54:113–124.

36. Wirz S, Skinner C, Dean E: *Revised Edinburgh Functional Communication Profile.* Communication Skill Builders, Tucson, AZ, 1990.

37. List MA, Ritter-Sterr C, Lansky SB: A performance status scale for head and neck cancer patients. *Cancer,* 1990; 66:564–569.

38. Blomert L, Kean ML, Koster C, Schokker J: Amsterdam-Nijmegen Everyday Language Test: Construction, reliability, and validity. *Aphasiology* 1994; 8(4):381–407.

39. Payne J: Communication Profile: A Functional Skills Survey. Communication Skill Builders, San Antonio, TX, 1994.

40. Bayles K, Tomoeda C: Functional Linguistic Communication Inventory. Canyonlands Publishing, Inc., Phoenix, AZ, 1994.

41. Frattali CM, Thompson CK, Holland AL, Wohl CB, Ferketic MM: *Functional Assessment of Communication Skills for Adults.* ASHA, Rockville, MD, 1995.

42. Holland AL: Presentation during ASHA teleconference: Developing a functional communication measure. ASHA, Rockville, MD, 1995.

43. Ware J, Sherbourne C: The MOS 36-item Short Form Health Survey (SF-36). *Medical Care* 1992; 30:473–483.

44. Nelson E, Wasson J, Kirk J, et al: Assessment of function in routine clinical practice: Description of the COOP Chart Method and preliminary findings. *J Chronic Disab* 1987; 40 (suppl) 1:55S–69S.

45. Parkerson GR, Gehlbach SH, Wagner EH, et al: The Duke-UNC Health Profile: An adult health status measure. *Medical Care* 1981; 19:787–805.

46. Bergner MB, Kaplan RM, Ware JE: Evaluation health measures: Commentary: Measuring overall health: An evaluation of three important approaches. *J Chronic Dis* 1987; 40 (Suppl. 1):23S–26S.

47. Chambers LW, MacDonald LA, Tugwell P, et al: The McMaster health index questionnaire as a measure of quality of life for patients with rheumatoid disease. *J Rheumatol* 1982; 9:780–784.

48. McEwen J: The Nottingham Health Profile. In S Walker, R Rosser, eds., *Quality of life: Assessment and application,* p. 95. MTP Press, Lancaster, England, 1988.

49. Fanshel S, Bush JW: A health-status index and its application to health-services outcomes. *Operations Research* 1970; 18:1021–1066.

50. Whiteneck GG, Charlifue SW, Gerhart KA, Overholser JD, Richardson GN: Quantifying handicap: A new measure of long-term rehabilitation outcomes. *Arch Phys Med Rehab* 1992; 73:519–526.

51. Willer B, Rosenthal M, Kreutzer JS, Gordon WA, Rermpel R: Assessment of community integration following rehabilitation for traumatic brain injury. *J Head Trauma Rehab* 1993; 8(2):75–87.

52. Jette AM, Davies AR, Cleary PD, et al: The Functional Status Questionnaire: Reliability and validity when used in primary care. *J Gen Int Med* 1986; 1(3): 143–149.

53. Ventry I, Weinstein BE: The Hearing Handicap Inventory for the Elderly: A new tool. *Ear and Hearing,* 1982; 3:128–134.

54. Jacobson B, Johnson A, Silbergleit A, Benninger M: *Voice Handicap Index.* Henry Ford Hospital, Detroit, MI, in progress.

55. CARF . . . The Rehabilitation Accreditation Commission: *Accreditation standards for inpatient rehabilitation programs.* Tucson, AZ.

56. Patton MQ: *Practical evaluation.* SAGE Publications, Beverly Hills, CA, 1982.

57. Wilkerson D: Program evaluation. In CM Frattali, ed., *Measuring outcomes in speech–language pathology.* Thieme, New York, in press.

58. Joint Commission on Accreditation of Health Care Organizations: *Accreditation manual for hospitals.* Oakbrook Terrace, IL, 1997.

59. Merson R, Rolnick MI, Weiner F: Beaumont Outcome Sofware System. Parrot Software, W. Bloomfield, MI, 1995.

60. Keatley MA, Miller T: OUTCOME. Evaluation Systems International, Denver, CO, 1994.

61. Ellwood P: Shattuck lecture—Outcome management: A technology of patient experience. *N Eng J Med* 1988; 318(23):1549–1556.

62. American Speech–Language-Hearing Association: Task force on clinical outcome and cost effectiveness. Report update. Rockville, MD, 1995.

63. Karnofsky DA, Burchenal JH: The clinical evaluation of chemotherapeutics in cancer. In C.M. McCloud, ed., *Evaluation of Chemotherapeutic Agents.* New York: Columbia Press, 1949.

Index